RUSH UNIVERSITY MEDICAL CENTER

Review of Surgery

Steven D. Bines, M.D.
Associate Professor of Surgery; Associate Attending Surgeon, Department of General Surgery, RUSH University Medical Center, Chicago, Illinois

José M. Velasco, M.D.
Professor of Surgery, Senior Attending Surgeon, Department of General Surgery, RUSH University Medical Center, Chicago, Illinois; Chairman, Department of Surgery, RUSH North Shore Medical Center, Skokie, Illinois

Keith W. Millikan, M.D.
Professor of Surgery; Senior Attending Surgeon, Department of General Surgery; Associate Dean and Vice President of Surgical Sciences and Services, RUSH University Medical Center, Chicago, Illinois

Theodore J. Saclarides, M.D.
Professor of Surgery; Head, Section of Colon and Rectal Surgery; Senior Attending Surgeon, Department of General Surgery, RUSH University Medical Center, Chicago, Illinois

Richard A. Prinz, M.D.
Helen Shedd Keith Professor of Surgery; Chairman, Department of General Surgery, RUSH University Medical Center, Chicago, Illinois

Walter J. McCarthy, III, M.D.
Associate Professor of Cardiovascular-Thoracic Surgery; Chief, Section of Vascular Surgery, Department of Cardiovascular-Thoracic Surgery, RUSH University Medical Center, Chicago, Illinois

Linnea S. Hauge, Ph.D.
Associate Professor, Educational Specialist, Department of General Surgery, RUSH University Medical Center, Chicago, Illinois

Daniel J. Deziel, M.D.
Professor of Surgery; Senior Attending Surgeon, Department of General Surgery, RUSH University Medical Center, Chicago, Illinois

RUSH UNIVERSITY MEDICAL CENTER

Review of Surgery

Fourth Edition

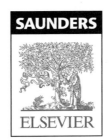

SAUNDERS

ELSEVIER

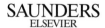

SAUNDERS
ELSEVIER

1600 John F. Kennedy Blvd.
Suite 1800
Philadelphia, PA 19103-2899

RUSH University Medical Center Review of Surgery, Fourth Edition

ISBN-13: 978-0-7216-0304-9
ISBN-10: 0-7216-0304-1

Notice

Knowledge and best practice in this field are constantly changing. As new research and experience broaden our knowledge, changes in practice, treatment, and drug therapy may become necessary or appropriate. Readers are advised to check the most current information provided (i) on procedures featured or (ii) by the manufacturer of each product to be administered, to verify the recommended dose or formula, the method and duration of administration, and contraindications. It is the responsibility of the practitioner, relying on their own experience and knowledge of the patient, to make diagnoses, to determine dosages and the best treatment for each individual patient, and to take all appropriate safety precautions. To the fullest extent of the law, neither the Publisher nor the Editors assume any liability for any injury and/or damage to persons or property arising out of or related to any use of the material contained in this book.

The Publisher

Library of Congress Cataloging-in-Publication Data

RUSH University medical center review of surgery / [edited by] Steven D. Bines ... [et al.] -- 4th ed.
 p. ; cm.
 Includes bibliographical references.
 ISBN 0-7216-0304-1
 1.   Surgery--Examinations, questions, etc. 2. Surgery, Operative--Examinations,
questions, etc. I. Bines, Steven D. II. Rush University. III. Title: Review of surgery.
 [DNLM: 1.   Surgery--Examination Questions. 2.   Surgical Procedures, Operative--
Examination Questions.   WO   18.2 R953   2007]
 RD31.R85 2007
 617.0076--dc22   2006044889

Acquisitions Editor: Judith Fletcher
Developmental Editor: Ryan Creed
Publishing Services Manager: Tina Rebane
Project Manager: Mary Anne Folcher
Design Direction: Lou Forgione
Marketing Manager: Emily Christie

Printed in the United States of America

Last digit is the print number: 9   8   7   6   5   4   3   2   1

All of us are keenly aware of the many persons in our lives—parents, wives, and children, teachers and mentors, residents and students, and surely others—who, at different times and in varying ways, have so critically molded our lives and influenced our careers. We are honored to dedicate this book to them.

Contributing Editors

Alberto Aviles, M.D.
Plastic Surgery Fellow, Medical College of Wisconsin and Sroedtert Hospital, Milwaukee, Wisconsin
Chapter 54, Plastic and Reconstructive Surgery

Katherine F. Baker, M.D.
Assistant Professor, RUSH University Medical Center, Chicago; Attending Physician, RUSH North Shore Medical Center, Skokie, Illinois
Chapter 23, Oncology: C, Radiation Therapy

Robert L. Barkin, Pharm. D., F.A.C., M.B.A.
Associate Professor, Anesthesiology, Family Medicine, and Pharmacology; Clinical Pharmacologist, Anesthesiology, Pain Center, RUSH University Medical Center, Chicago, Illinois; Clinical Pharmacologist, RUSH North Shore Medical Center, Skokie, Illinois
Chapter 11, Pharmacology

Eric Berkson, M.D.
Clinical and Research Fellow, Massachusetts General Hospital, Boston, Massachusetts
Chapter 51, Orthopedics

Steven D. Bines, M.D.
Associate Professor of Surgery; Associate Attending Surgeon, Department of General Surgery, RUSH University Medical Center, Chicago, Illinois
Chapter 2, Fluids and Electrolytes; Chapter 10, Wound Healing; Chapter 17, Burns; Chapter 20, Surgical Technology; Chapter 24, Skin; Chapter 25, Breast; Chapter 50, Neurosurgery; Chapter 53, Hand Surgery; Chapter 54, Plastic and Reconstructive Surgery; Chapter 55, Genetics; Chapter 56, Biostatistics and Data Management

Marc I. Brand, M.D.
Assistant Professor of Surgery, Department of General Surgery, Colon and Rectal Surgery Section, RUSH University Medical Center, Chicago, Illinois
Chapter 33, Small Intestine

Wahab Brobbey, M.D.
Attending Physician, Metro Infectious Disease Consultants, LLC., Hinsdale; Chairman, Infection Control Committee, Trinity Medical Center, Rock Island; Section of Infectious Diseases, RUSH University Medical Center, Chicago, Illinois
Chapter 18, Surgical Infections

Eric R. Brown, M.D., Ph.D.
Assistant Professor, Departments of Obstetrics/Gynecology and Biochemistry; Director, Section of Gynecology; Director, Medical Student Programs; Director, Continuing Medical Education Programs, RUSH University Medical Center, Chicago, Illinois
Chapter 49, Gynecology

Christopher M. Bulger, M.D.
Vascular Fellow, Department of Vascular Surgery, Manchester Memorial Hospital, Manchester, Connecticut
Chapter 44, Vascular Surgery: A, Principles; B, Cerebrovascular Disease

Richard W. Byrne, M.D.
Associate Professor of Neurosurgery, RUSH University Medical Center, Chicago, Illinois
Chapter 50, Neurosurgery

Edie Y. Chan, M.D.
Transplant Fellow, Department of Transplantation, University of Washington, Seattle, Washington
Chapter 28, Parathyroid; Chapter 41, Spleen

John D. Christein, M.D.
Assistant Professor, Department of Surgery, University of Alabama at Birmingham, Birmingham, Alabama
Chapter 31, Esophagus

Mitchell Jay Cohen, M.D.
Assistant Professor in Residence, Department of Surgery, University of California, San Francisco, San Francisco, California
Chapter 6, Complications; Chapter 16, Trauma

James A. Colombo, M.D.
Attending Anesthesiologist/Intensivist, Advocate Lutheran General Hospital, Park Ridge, Illinois
Chapter 12, Anesthesia

Christopher L. Coogan, M.D.
Associate Professor of Urology, RUSH University Medical Center, Chicago, Illinois
Chapter 48, Urology

Gordon H. Derman, M.D.
Assistant Professor of Plastic Surgery; Director of Hand Surgery, Department of Plastic and Reconstructive Surgery, RUSH University Medical Center, Chicago, Illinois
Chapter 10, Wound Healing; Chapter 53, Hand Surgery

Daniel J. Deziel, M.D.
Professor of Surgery; Senior Attending Surgeon, Department
of General Surgery, RUSH University Medical Center,
Chicago, Illinois
*Chapter 19, Transmissible Diseases and the Surgeon: Prevention
and Management; Chapter 21, Principles of Laparoscopy;
Chapter 22, Principles of Ultrasound; Chapter 32, Stomach and
Duodenum; Chapter 38, Portal Venous System; Chapter 39,
Biliary System; Chapter 40, Pancreas; Chapter 43, Pediatric
Surgery*

S. Forrest Dodson, M.D.
Assistant Professor of Surgery; Director of Abdominal
Transplantation, Department of Surgery, RUSH University
Medical Center, Chicago, Illinois
Chapter 14, Transplantation

Alain Domkam, M.D.
Adjunct Instructor, Department of Vascular Surgery,
RUSH University Medical Center, Chicago, Illinois
Chapter 44, Vascular Surgery: A, Principles

Mark R. Edwards, M.D.
General Surgery Resident,
Department of General Surgery, RUSH University Medical
Center, Chicago, Illinois
*Chapter 22, Principles of Ultrasound; Chapter 43, Pediatric
Surgery*

Nadine Duhan Floyd, M.D.
Colon-Rectal Surgeons of Fort Wayne Lutheran Hospital,
Fort Wayne, Indiana
Chapter 5, Acute Abdomen

Michael J. Gaffud, M.D.
Resident Physician, Department of General Surgery,
RUSH University Medical Center, Chicago, Illinois
Chapter 55, Genetics

Mehra Golshan, M.D.
Instructor in Surgery, Harvard Medical School;
Associate Surgeon, Department of Surgery, Brigham and
Women's Hospital; Surgical Oncologist, Dana-Farber Cancer
Institute, Boston, Massachusetts
Chapter 25, Breast

Irina Goncharova, M.D.
Adjunct Instructor, Department of Cardiovascular-Thoracic
Surgery, RUSH University Medical Center, Chicago, Illinois
Chapter 45, Peripheral Venous and Lymphatic Disease

Linnea S. Hauge, Ph.D.
Associate Professor, Education Specialist, Department of
General Surgery, RUSH University Medical Center,
Chicago, Illinois
Chapter 56, Biostatistics and Data Management

Tina J. Hieken, M.D.
Associate Professor of Surgery, Attending Surgeon, Department
of General Surgery, RUSH University Medical Center; Chicago,
Illinois; Attending Surgeon, Department of Surgery, North Shore
Medical Center, Skokie, Illinois
*Chapter 23, Oncology: A, Principles; Chapter 26, Head
and Neck*

Robert S.D. Higgins, M.D., M.S.H.A.
Chairman, Professor of Cardiovascular-Thoracic Surgery,
Director of Thoracic Residency Program, RUSH University
Medical Center, Chicago, Illinois
Chapter 47, Cardiac Surgery

Edward F. Hollinger, M.D., Ph.D.
Transplant Surgery Fellow, Indiana
University School of Medicine, Indianapolis, Indiana
Chapter 20, Surgical Technology

Chad E. Jacobs, M.D.
Assistant Professor, Cardiovascular-Thoracic Surgery, RUSH
University Medical Center, Chicago, Illinois
*Chapter 44, Vascular Surgery: E, Peripheral: Lower Extremity;
Chapter 52, Amputations*

Edward Kaplan, M.D.
Assistant Professor of Medicine, RUSH University Medical
Center, Chicago, Illinois
Chapter 23, Oncology: D, Systemic Therapy

Richard Keen, M.D.
Chair, Vascular Surgery, Stroger Cook County Hospital,
Chicago, Illinois
Chapter 45, Peripheral Venous and Lymphatic Disease

Anthony W. Kim, M.D.
Fellow, Department of Cardiovascular-Thoracic Surgery,
RUSH University Medical Center, Chicago, Illinois
*Chapter 1, Cell Biology; Chapter 2, Fluids and
Electrolytes*

Edward H. Kolb, M.D.
Surgeon, Orthopedic and Sports Medicine Center, Normal, Illinois
Chapter 51, Orthopedics

George J. Kouris, M.D.
Assistant Professor of Plastic Surgery, Plastic and
Reconstructive Surgery, RUSH University Medical
Center, Chicago, Illinois
Chapter 10, Wound Healing

Miguel Mandariaga, M.D.
Assistant Professor of Medicine, University of Nebraska Medical
Center, Omaha, Nebraska
Chapter 18, Surgical Infections

Walter J. McCarthy, III, M.D.
Associate Professor of Cardiovascular-Thoracic Surgery;
Chief, Section of Vascular Surgery, Department of
Cardiovascular-Thoracic Surgery, RUSH University Medical
Center, Chicago, Illinois
*Chapter 44, Vascular Surgery; Chapter 45, Peripheral Venous
and Lymphatic Disease; Chapter 47, Cardiac Surgery; Chapter 52,
Amputations; Chapter 56, Biostatistics and Data Management*

Bruce C. McLeod, M.D.
Professor of Medicine and Pathology; Director, Blood Center,
RUSH University Medical Center, Chicago, Illinois
Chapter 7, Hemostasis and Transfusion

Janet Millikan, M.S., R.D., L.D.
Registered Dietician
Bloomingdale, Illinois
Chapter 8, Nutrition

Keith W. Millikan, M.D.
Professor of Surgery, Senior Attending Surgeon, Department of
General Surgery, Associate Dean and Vice President of Surgical
Sciences and Services, RUSH University Medical Center,
Chicago, Illinois
*Chapter 8, Nutrition; Chapter 9, Morbid Obesity; Chapter 18,
Surgical Infections; Chapter 31, Esophagus; Chapter 37, Liver;
Chapter 42, Hernia, Abdominal Wall, and Retroperitoneum;
Chapter 48, Urology; Chapter 51, Orthopedics*

Laura J. Moore, M.D.
Fellow, Trauma and Critical Care Department, University of
Texas Health Science Center, Houston, Texas
Chapter 17, Burns

Jonathan A. Myers, M.D.
Assistant Professor of General Surgery; Assistant Attending
Surgeon, General Surgery, RUSH University Medical Center,
Chicago, Illinois
Chapter 37, Liver

Douglas R. Norman, M.D.
Assistant Professor of Cardiovascular-Thoracic Surgery, RUSH
University Medical Center, Chicago, Illinois; Attending Surgeon,
Cardiovascular-Thoracic Surgery, Department of Surgery, RUSH
North Shore Medical Center, Skokie, Illinois
Chapter 46, Chest

Eric J. Okum, M.D.
Assistant Professor of Cardiovascular Surgery,
Department of Cardiovascular-Thoracic Surgery, RUSH
University Medical Center, Chicago, Illinois
Chapter 47, Cardiac Surgery

Srdjan Andrei Ostric, M.D.
Assistant Professor, Plastic Surgery, RUSH University Medical
Center, Chicago, Illinois
Chapter 53, Hand Surgery

Samuel M. Parnass, M.D.
Associate Professor of Anesthesiology, RUSH University
Medical Center, Chicago, Illinois; Chairman, Department of
Anesthesiology, RUSH North Shore Medical Center,
Skokie, Illinois
Chapter 4, Perioperative Care

R. Anthony Perez-Tamayo, M.D., Ph.D.
Assistant Professor, Department of Cardiovascular-Thoracic
Surgery, RUSH University Medical Center; Chairman, Division
of Cardiothoracic Surgery, John H. Stroger Jr., Hospital of Cook
County, Chicago, Illinois
Chapter 47, Cardiac Surgery

Richard A. Prinz, M.D.
Helen Shedd Keith Professor of Surgery; Chairman, Department
of General Surgery, RUSH University Medical Center, Chicago,
Illinois
*Chapter 3, Endocrine and Metabolic Response to Injury; Chapter
6, Complications; Chapter 13, Immunology; Chapter 14,
Transplantation; Chapter 16, Trauma; Chapter 27, Thyroid;
Chapter 28, Parathyroid; Chapter 29, Pituitary; Chapter 30,
Adrenal*

Roderick Michael Quiros, M.D.
Fellow in Surgical Oncology, Department of Surgery, Fox Chase
Cancer Center, Philadelphia, Pennsylvania
*Chapter 3, Endocrine and Metabolic Response to Injury;
Chapter 27, Thyroid*

Heather Rossi, M.D.
Adjunct Instructor of Surgery, Division of Colon and Rectal
Surgery, Colon and Rectal Surgery Associates, Ltd., University
of Minnesota, Minneapolis, Minnesota
Chapter 34, Appendix

Theresa W. Ruddy, M.D.
Resident Physician, RUSH University Medical Center, Chicago,
Illinois
Chapter 13, Immunology; Chapter 30, Adrenal

Theodore J. Saclarides, M.D.
Professor of Surgery; Head, Section of Colon and Rectal Surgery;
Senior Attending Surgeon, Department of General Surgery;
RUSH University Medical Center, Chicago, Illinois
*Chapter 5, Acute Abdomen; Chapter 7, Hemostasis and
Transfusion; Chapter 11, Pharmacology; Chapter 12, Anesthesia;
Chapter 33, Small Intestine; Chapter 35, Colon and Rectum;
Chapter 36, Anus and Perianal Disease; Chapter 49, Gynecology*

Edward B. Savage, M.D.
Medical Director, Heart and Vascular Services, St. John's Mercy
Medical Center, St. Louis, Missouri
Chapter 47, Cardiac Surgery: B, Acquired Diseases

David M. Simon, M.D., Ph.D.
Assistant Professor of Medicine, Section of Infectious Diseases,
RUSH University Medical Center, Chicago, Illinois
Chapter 18, Surgical Infections

Carmen C. Solorzano, M.D.
Assistant Professor of Surgery, RUSH University Medical Center,
Chicago, Illinois
Chapter 30, Adrenal

Apostolos K. Tassiopoulos, M.D.
Assistant Professor of Thoracic and Cardiovascular Surgery,
RUSH University Medical Center; Senior Attending Vascular
Surgeon, The John H. Stroger, Jr., Hospital of Cook County,
Chicago, Illinois
*Chapter 44, Vascular Surgery: C, Thoracic Aorta; D, Abdominal
Aorta; F, Renal Disease; G, Mesenteric Disease*

Kenneth J. Tuman, M.D.
Professor of Anesthesiology and Chairman,
Department of Anesthesiology, RUSH University Medical Center
Chicago, Illinois
Chapter 12, Anesthesia

Leonard A. Valentino, M.D.
Associate Professor, RUSH University Medical Center, Chicago,
Illinois
Chapter 7, Hemostasis and Transfusion

José M. Velasco, M.D.
Professor of Surgery, Senior Attending Surgeon, Department of
General Surgery, RUSH University Medical Center, Chicago,
Illinois; Chairman, Department of Surgery, RUSH North Shore
Medical Center, Skokie, Illinois
*Chapter 1, Cell Biology; Chapter 4, Perioperative Care;
Chapter 15, Critical Care; Chapter 23, Oncology; Chapter 26,
Head and Neck; Chapter 34, Appendix; Chapter 41, Spleen;
Chapter 46, Chest*

Scott M. Wilhelm, M.D.
Assistant Professor, Department of Surgery, University
Hospitals of Cleveland, Case Western Reserve University,
Cleveland, Ohio
Chapter 29, Pituitary

Thomas R. Witt, M.D.
Associate Professor, Department of General Surgery,
RUSH University Medical Center, Chicago, Illinois
Chapter 25, Breast

Edward Yastrow, M.D.
Associate Professor of Anesthesia, RUSH North Shore
Medical Center, Skokie, Illinois
Chapter 4, Perioperative Care

Preface

The first three editions of *RUSH University Review of Surgery* were favorably received. They provided their targeted audiences—residents in training, young surgeons preparing for General Surgery Boards, those already certified or preparing for recertification, and those simply wishing to remain abreast of current surgical knowledge—an encompassing yet concise and self-contained review of surgery and its subspecialties in a format that stimulated self-examination. At the same time they encouraged further reading of more comprehensive texts and current periodical literature.

Since publication of the Third Edition, surgical information has increased appreciably, and new subjects about which surgeons should be knowledgeable have expanded dramatically. This has led to heightened expectations for the *RUSH University Medical Center,* Fourth Edition, to which we have responded appropriately. The entire book was examined minutely to ensure that it continues to contain the fullest information in the field of general surgery. With respect to the subspecialties, we have focused on fundamental information that a general surgeon might wish to know or be required to know by accreditation boards. Thus, this edition can serve residents in general surgery and in most of the subspecialties. Subspecialty residents reading *RUSH Review* before sitting for their board examination can expect an exposition of subjects in general surgery that should satisfy many of their needs. In similar fashion, a general surgeon can feel confident of a rich storehouse of information on general surgery and exposure to the fundamentals of the surgical subspecialties.

This comprehensive offering was developed by extensively rewriting many chapters and bringing the remaining ones to a current state. In addition, *seven new chapters* were added. Those include: Chapter 4—Perioperative Care; Chapter 5—Acute Abdomen; Chapter 6—Complications; Chapter 9—Morbid Obesity; Chapter 19—Transmissible Diseases and the Surgeon: Prevention and Management; Chapter 21—Principles of Laparoscopy; and Chapter 22—Principles of Ultrasound. We believe that these numerous additions and revisions were necessary, not only because of the dictates of newer and more precise information but also because of the practical expectation that those who already have access to previous editions can combine them with the Fourth Edition for an even fuller compendium of ready surgical information.

We have continued our emphasis on basic science in keeping with the increased sophistication of care of patients and with the need for surgeons to be well versed in the fundamental scientific components of clinical practice. From a practical standpoint, it is logical to expect that accrediting bodies will rightfully have higher expectations in this respect as well.

As a consequence of these changes, we expect that *RUSH University Medical Center Review of Surgery,* Fourth Edition, will enable the reader to gain a breadth of knowledge in general surgery and closely associated subspecialty subjects in a manner that can be readily translated to clinical use as well as provide a deeper understanding of the fundamentals of surgical diseases and practices.

Acknowledgments

The *RUSH University Medical Center Review of Surgery,* Fourth Edition, was written in a whirlwind of separate and then converging activity by the editors, augmented by a sizeable supportive team of talented contributors. An integral part of all this was a huge flow of manuscripts, revised drafts, and new writings, resulting in penultimate copies that were then refined and assembled into the final chapters. Thanks to Drs. Carl Tommaso and Christopher Najafi for lending their expertise to the chapter, *Critical Care.*

This daunting project was made logistically possible and infinitely easier for us by the unmatched skill and dedication of our secretaries, Kathy Martin, Gabriela Gonzalez, and Eileen Pehanich. We express our sincere gratitude to them for this marvelous effort. A special thanks to Eileen Pehanich, who was the captain of this endeavor. Again, many thanks, Eileen. We wish to also thank Ryan Creed for his editorial contributions.

Finally, we are especially indebted to our editor, Judith Fletcher, whose steady and unerring guidance was critical to the completion of this Fourth Edition of *RUSH University Medical Center Review of Surgery.*

How to Use this Text

A reader's approach to any book may vary from rapid scanning for basic concepts to meticulous outlining, note-taking, and underlining for detail. In an effort to satisfy these needs, this book includes an appropriate mixture of detail (found primarily in the Questions) and conceptual information (found primarily in the Comments).

The questions are organized principally in an organ-system manner. None of the questions is intentionally "tricky"; many, however, require the careful attention to detail that should characterize all students of surgery. To allow readers the opportunity to answer the question on their own and yet enable them to check their response without the ponderous flipping back and forth of pages, the correct answer is spatially separated from the question by the interposed Comment. For readers who wish to go to the basic source material before answering the question, such material is referenced immediately after the question. Although a number of popular textbooks serve as sources for further reading, many additional references (e.g., more specialized monographs and review articles) are cited in this Fourth Edition as supplemental sources of information. All of the sources used in a given chapter are listed at the end of the chapter and are referred to by number, as appropriate, after each question. Because sufficient factual information is provided in the Comments section to answer each question, the referenced materials do not include specific page numbers but are offered as sources of general reading on the topic at hand, so overall conceptual knowledge can be enhanced.

The Comments are offered to provide amplification and elucidation of the facts brought out in the Question and to provide a conceptual framework within which to view the factual data. Of necessity, several Comments have the latitude of editorial license and reflect individual and pooled clinical experience that amplify the cited references. As there are many areas of controversy in surgery, the reader may disagree with some of the more judgmental statements made in the Comments. We trust, however, that our editorial and consultant review of the Comments has successfully resulted in the avoidance of factual errors.

We hope that readers will find *RUSH University Medical Center Review of Surgery* an enjoyable means by which not only to test their knowledge of the art and science of surgery but to expand it as well.

Contents

C H A P T E R   1

Cell Biology

Anthony W. Kim, M.D., and José M. Velasco, M.D.

1. Which of the following statements regarding lipids in the cell membrane is/are not true?

A. Membrane lipids provide a permeable barrier for the cell.

B. Arachidonic acid is a constituent of membrane phospholipids.

C. Phophatidylinositols serve as protein anchors.

D. Cell membrane lipids are inert.

E. All of the above

Ref.: 2, 3

COMMENTS: Phospholipids, cholesterol, and glycolipids constitute the three main lipid classes found in cell membranes. • They are not necessarily inert, since they may function as mediators or protein anchors. • The basic function of membrane lipids is to provide a permeable barrier for the cell.

Phospholipids play a primary role in membrane fluidity, which accounts for the lateral and rotational movement. • Arachidonic acid is a common constituent of membrane phospholipids and is released in response to the local action of activated phopholipases. • Upon their release, they can be oxidized via the cyclooxygenase or lipoxygenase pathways, and the products of these pathways play important roles as mediators of several biologic disorders.

Cholesterol lies between the phospholipids and decreases the fluidity of the plasma membrane.

Glycolipids are structurally similar to the glycerol-based phospholipids. • Their function is unclear, although roles in intercellular interactions and transmembrane signaling have been supported by evidence. • Phosphatidylinositols constitute another class of membrane lipids. • They serve as the anchoring mechanism for a diverse group of external cell-surface proteins, including alkaline phosphatase, carcinoembryonic antigen, and acetylcholinesterase. • Their mobile configuration allows for their quick release in both normal and abnormal biochemical pathways.

A N S W E R :
D

2. What is the term for proteins that firmly are anchored to the cell membrane?

A. Peripheral proteins

B. Integral proteins

C. Primary structure proteins

D. Tertiary structure proteins

E. Quaternary structure proteins

Ref.: 3

COMMENTS: **Peripheral proteins** are bound loosely to the plasma membrane. • Their superficial attachment allows for their easy removal. • **Integral proteins** are anchored to the plasma membrane by either covalent bonding with surface lipids or incorporation into the hydrophobic ions. • **Primary structure proteins** are the most basic units of proteins and are genetically determined by a specific set of amino acids. • **Secondary structure proteins** are three-dimensional arrangements of amino acids in a specific segment of a protein molecule. • **Tertiary structure proteins** are protein configurations resulting from the complex patterns of folding by protein polypeptides. • **Quaternary structure proteins** result from the spatial relationships that develop between multiple polypeptide chains of proteins.

A N S W E R :
B

3. Which of the following statements regarding plasma membranes is/are not true?

A. Approximately 60% of the plasma membrane is composed of carbohydrate.

B. The major lipids in the membrane are phospholipids, glycolipids, and cholesterol.

C. The ability of proteins to move around in the plasma membrane depends primarily on the amount of cholesterol in the membrane.

D. Plasma membrane lipids have a high degree of polarity.

E. Approximately 40% of the plasma membrane is composed of lipid.

Ref.: 6–8

COMMENTS: Plasma membranes are a common feature of all cells. • They are composed of a lipid bilayer in which proteins are essentially floating. • Carbohydrate is a minor component (approximately 1–10%), whereas approximately 60% is protein and 40% is lipid. • The major lipids in the plasma membrane are the phospholipids, glycolipids, and cholesterol. • Examples of the commonest phospholipids include phosphatidylcholine and phosphatidylethanolamine. • The more cholesterol in the membrane, the greater the membrane fluidity and therefore the easier it is for intramembrane proteins to move and interact. • Plasma membrane lipids are quite polar, containing both hydrophilic and hydrophobic components. • The hydrophilic portions of the lipid generally orient in a direction perpendicular to the membrane plane and point toward either the cytoplasm or the extracellular space. • The hydrophobic lipid chains are sandwiched between the hydrophilic portions.

ANSWER:
A

4. Which of the following statements regarding plasma membrane proteins is/are not true?

   A. Transmembrane proteins traverse the entire lipid bilayer.

   B. Membrane proteins are always attached by a covalent bond to a membrane lipid.

   C. Transmembrane proteins within the membrane plane possess an α-helical configuration.

   D. Membrane proteins within the membrane plane are free to move in a fluid mosaic.

   E. Sialic acid residues help maintain a negative charge on the outer cell surface.

   Ref.: 5

COMMENTS: Membrane proteins can be divided into a few basic types. • **Transmembrane** proteins extend across the lipid bilayer one or more times. • This group includes receptor molecules linked to intracellular enzymes, transport molecules, and ion-conductance channels. • Although some proteins are **covalently** attached to the lipid bilayer by a direct covalent link to a lipid or, less commonly, indirectly through an oligosaccharide link to a lipid, other proteins are associated with the plasma membrane by **noncovalent** interactions with transmembrane proteins such as those linking the cytoskeleton to membrane junctions.

Proteins that pass through the membrane are generally in an α-helical configuration. • Proteins and lipids within the plane of the membrane are not covalently bound but are free to move in a fluid mosaic. • Some complex polysaccharides are not covalently associated with the membrane. • However, glycolipids and glycoproteins generally have covalently linked carbohydrate chains that are oriented toward the extracellular space. • On glycoproteins, sialic acid residues comprise the terminal residue on the oligosaccharide chain. • Sialic acid residues help maintain a negative charge on the outer cell surface and may be involved in maintaining cell independence by inhibiting cell contact.

ANSWER:
B

5. Which of the following statements regarding the electrical properties of cell membranes is/are not true?

   A. Ions flow through hydrophilic channels formed by specific transmembrane proteins.

   B. Lipids provide the ability to store electrical charge (capacitance).

   C. Active ionic pumps maintain the ionic gradients necessary for a resting membrane potential.

   D. Large numbers of sodium ions *rush in* during the initial phase of a nerve action potential.

   E. Capacitance is required for maintenance of a resting membrane potential.

   Ref.: 4, 5

COMMENTS: The lipid component of the plasma membrane provides the capability of storing electrical charge (**capacitance**), and the protein component provides the capability of resisting electrical charge (**resistance**). • Specific transmembrane proteins provide hydrophilic paths for the ions (primarily Na^+, K^+, Ca^{2+}, and Cl^-) involved in electrical signaling. • The amino acid sequence in specific regions of these proteins determines the selectivity for specific ions.

The establishment and maintenance of a resting cell membrane potential require the separation of charge maintained by membrane capacitance, selective permeability of the plasma membrane, concentration gradients (intracellular versus extracellular) of the permeant ions, and impermeant intracellular anions. • Active pumping by the sodium (Na^+/K^+-ATPase) or calcium pumps generally maintains the ionic concentration gradients.

Action potentials are regenerative (self-sustaining) transient depolarizations caused by activation of voltage-sensitive sodium and potassium channels. • Only a small volume of sodium ions is necessary to initiate an action potential. • In fact, the amount of sodium ions that flow into a typical nerve cell during an action potential would change the intracellular Na^+ concentration by only a few parts per million.

ANSWER:
D

6. Which of the following statements regarding cell-surface antigens is/are true?

   A. Cell-surface antigens are generally glycoproteins or glycolipids.

   B. Histocompatibility antigens are not cell-surface antigens.

   C. ABO antigens are glycoproteins.

   D. HLA antigens have an extracellular hydrophobic region and an intracellular hydrophilic region.

   E. All of the above.

   Ref.: 6–8

COMMENTS: Cell-surface antigens are generally glycoproteins or glycolipids that are anchored to either a protein or a lipid. • Common examples include the ABO blood group antigens and the histocompatibility antigens. • **Antigens of the ABO** system are glycolipids whose oligosaccharide portions are responsible for the antigenic properties. • The structures of the blood group oligosaccharides occur commonly in nature and lead to the stimulation needed to produce anti-A or anti-B antibodies after a few months of life.

HLA antigens are two-chain glycoproteins that are anchored in the cell membrane at the carboxyl terminal. • These antigens contain an extracellular hydrophilic region, a transmembrane hydrophobic region, and an intracellular hydrophilic region. • It is thought that this transmembrane structure may allow extracellular signals to be transmitted to the interior of the cell.

ANSWER:
A

7. Which of the following statements regarding "second-messenger" systems is/are true?

   A. Inositol triphosphate (IP_3) inhibits intracellular calcium release.

   B. Adenylate cyclase stimulates conversion of cyclic adenosine monophosphate (cAMP) to adenosine triphosphate (ATP).

C. Diacylglycerol (DAG) and calcium lead to the activation of protein kinase C.

D. Thyroid-stimulating hormone (TSH) release is mediated by conversion of IP$_3$ to membrane phospholipid.

E. All of the above.

Ref.: 4, 6–8

COMMENTS: The interaction of ligands with cell-surface receptors results in activation of the second-messenger systems. • Well-described examples of second messengers include IP$_3$, DAG, calcium, and cAMP. • Stimulation of the cell-surface receptor leads to increased calcium concentration in the cytoplasm by either causing a membrane permeability change that increases calcium influx from outside the cell or allowing intracellular calcium release. • In the latter system, receptor stimulation activates the enzyme phospholipase C, which converts membrane phospholipids (phosphoinositols) to IP$_3$ and DAG. • IP$_3$ mediates release of calcium from intracellular reservoirs, such as the endoplasmic reticulum, sarcoplasmic reticulum in muscle, and mitochondria. • DAG works in concert with calcium to activate protein kinase.

Cell-surface receptor activation stimulates the enzyme adenylate cyclase, which breaks down ATP to cAMP, with release of pyrophosphate. • cAMP regulates the activation of protein kinases, which in turn stimulate a variety of metabolic pathways by activation of many other enzymes via phosphorylation. • Examples of cAMP-dependent hormones include adrenocorticotrophic hormone (ACTH) and TSH. • Receptors that increase cAMP are coupled to adenylate cyclase through intermediary guanosine triphosphate (GTP)-binding proteins (G proteins). • The interaction with G proteins may result in normal regulation (permissive actions of hormones) or toxin action (e.g., pertussis toxin).

ANSWER:
C

8. Match the receptors in the left-hand column with one or more of the items in the right-hand column.

A. Tyrosine kinase receptors	a. Guanosine-5′-triphosphate
B. G-protein receptor	b. Gated ionic channel
C. Nicotinic acetylcholine receptor	c. Epidermal growth factor
D. Integrin receptor	d. von Willebrand factor

Ref.: 3

COMMENTS: The **G-protein–linked receptor** family is a member of the guanosine triphosphatase (GTPase) superfamily. • These receptors are associated with a ubiquitous molecular switch with on and off positions triggered by the binding and hydrolysis of guanine nucleotide. • They all have a seven-membrane spanning domain, which distinguishes them from other receptors. • When catecholamines, most peptide hormones, several pharmacologic agents, and proto-oncogenes bind to these receptors, they are coupled to heterotrimeric G proteins, causing them to interact with guanosine-5′-triphosphate (GTP). • This activates a second-messenger system or opening of ion channels. • In a common second-messenger system, membrane-bound adenyl cyclase is stimulated, leading to the generation of cAMP, which, together with calcium, controls the activity of various protein kinases. • These enzymes, in turn, catalyze the phosphorylation of specific cytoplasmic proteins, thereby inducing changes in their behavior. • G4 protein binding may also cause the degradation of phosphatidylinositol, a membrane phospholipid, to inositol-1,4,5,- triphosphate (IP$_3$) and DAG. • Cytosolic IP$_3$ promotes calcium release from intracellular stores, allowing for the formation of calcium-calmodulin complexes, which stimulate further protein phosphorylation. • Similarly, increases in DAG stimulate protein kinase C activation, which acts to modulate membrane function and activate gene transcription. • When coupled to ion channels, once there is receptor activation, these channels open to allow entry of various cations.

The protein **tyrosine kinase receptor** family controls cellular events by phosphorylation of tyrosine residues located in certain intracellular proteins. • The covalent binding of phosphate groups to proteins at specific sites is catalyzed by protein kinase and induces a conformation change sufficient to initiate a specific intracellular response. • This receptor family is composed of single-membrane–spanning polypeptides and includes growth factors, such as epidermal growth factor, platelet-derived growth factor, and transforming growth factor α.

The **nicotinic acetylcholine receptor** is the historically typical neurotransmitter gated ionic channel. • These receptors are composed of four different polypeptide chains located around a single ion channel. • Acetylcholine binds to the receptor, thus mediating transmission of nerve impulses to muscle at the motor endplate. • This receptor also included the γ-aminobutyric acid and glycine-receptor–gated channels, which share considerable structural homology. • It is structurally unrelated to the muscarinic acetylcholine receptors that belong to the G-protein family.

The **integrin receptor** is composed of receptors that are essential for adhesion of cells to the extracellular matrix proteins. • They are active in cell-to-cell adhesions. • They provide anchorage, cues for migration, and signals for growth and migration. • Structurally, they are composed of two disulfide links, membrane-spanning glycoprotein subunits. • The external ligand-binding site is formed by sequences from both units, whereas the internal domain forms links with the cystoskeleton. • Known ligands include the extracellular matrix proteins; the intercellular adhesion proteins of other cells; intracellular adhesion molecule (ICAM)-1, ICAM-2, and vascular cell adhesion molecule-1; and some components of the coagulation system, including platelets, fibrinogen, and von Willebrand factor.

ANSWER:
A-c; B-a; C- b; D-d

9. Which of the following statements regarding mechanisms of cell transport is/are true?

A. Hydrophilic substances facilitate simple diffusion.

B. Facilitated diffusion requires a carrier for transport and does not require ATP.

C. Facilitated diffusion requires ATP.

D. The sodium-potassium pump is an example of active transport not requiring ATP hydrolysis.

E. The sodium-potassium pump is an example of facilitated transport requiring ATP hydrolysis.

Ref.: 6

COMMENTS: There are two basic types of cell transport: diffusion and active transport. • The driving force of **diffusion** is simply a concentration gradient; therefore, it does not require energy in the form of ATP. • *Simple* diffusion is generally greater with more hydrophobic substances, whereas hydrophilic substances penetrate less easily. • Pores of specific size limit simple diffusion of larger molecules. • Oxygen, carbon dioxide, and urea pass easily through the membrane by diffusion. • *Facilitated* (carrier-mediated) diffusion requires a carrier for transport. • In addition, unlike simple diffusion, which is not saturable, the number of carrier proteins limits facilitated diffusion.

Active transport requires ATP for energy. • The sodium-potassium pump—in which a higher potassium concentration and lower sodium concentration are maintained inside the cell relative to the concentrations in the extracellular space—is an example of active transport. • In this case, both sodium and potassium are pumped against concentration gradients, an effect resulting from energy released by ATP hydrolysis.

ANSWER:
B

10. Which cell junction acts as a transmembrane linkage without intracellular communication function?

　　A. Tight junction

　　B. Gap junction

　　C. Desmosome

　　D. Connexon

　　E. All of the above

Ref.: 3, 6–8

COMMENTS: There are three major types of cell junction: gap junctions, desmosomes, and tight junctions. • **Gap junctions** are the commonest type and function primarily for intercellular communication but also for cellular adhesion. • The connection between cells maintained by the gap junction is not particularly stable; it depends on a variety of complexes on each cell but not on connecting proteins (hence the term *gap*). • Gap junctions serve as a pathway of permeability between cells for many different molecules up to weights of 1000 daltons. • **Connexons** are protein assemblies formed by six identical protein subunits. • They span the intercellular gap of the lipid bilayer to form an aqueous channel connecting the bilayers. • **Desmosomes** function as cellular adhesion points but do not provide a pathway of communication. • They are linked by filaments that function as transmembrane linkers, but desmosomes are not points of true cell fusion. • **Tight junctions**, in contrast, are true points of cell fusion and are impermeable barriers. • They prevent leakage of molecules across the epithelium in either direction. • They also limit the movement of membrane proteins within the lipid bilayer of the plasma membrane and therefore maintain cells in a differentiated polar state.

ANSWER:
C

11. Which of the following statements regarding the endoplasmic reticulum is/are not true?

　　A. Rough endoplasmic reticulum is the site of lipid synthesis.

　　B. Smooth endoplasmic reticulum mediates synthetic reactions and chemical modifications of protein synthesis.

　　C. Endoplasmic reticulum may be differentiated from plasma membrane by its higher protein/lipid ratio and lower cholesterol content.

　　D. There are three general shapes of endoplasmic reticulum: lamellar, vesicular, and tubular.

　　E. Rough endoplasmic reticulum is the site of synthesis of membrane and secreted proteins.

Ref.: 6–8

COMMENTS: Endoplasmic reticulum is part of a network that includes mitochondria, lysosomes, microbodies, the Golgi complex, and the nuclear envelope. • This network forms an intracellular circulatory system that allows vital substrates to reach the cell interior for transportation and assembly. • There are **two types** of endoplasmic reticulum: *rough* endoplasmic reticulum, which is coated with ribosomes and functions as the site of synthesis of membrane and secreted proteins, and *smooth* endoplasmic reticulum, which is the site of synthetic reactions and chemical modifications of protein synthesis. • Thus, cells that synthesize a large amount of protein have abundant rough endoplasmic reticulum, whereas cells that make a large amount steroids (e.g., those in the adrenal cortex) generally have more smooth endoplasmic reticulum.

Endoplasmic reticulum is found in **three general forms**: *lamellar*, which is made up of collections of flattened membrane sacs and is the commonest; *vesicular*, which is particularly common with smooth endoplasmic reticulum; and *tubular*, which mainly is a form of smooth endoplasmic reticulum. • Endoplasmic reticulum may be differentiated from plasma membrane in that it has a higher protein/lipid ratio and a lower concentration of cholesterol. • Both of these properties give it more structural stability. • The endoplasmic reticulum, however, is thinner than the plasma membrane.

ANSWER:
A

12. Which of the following statements regarding microbodies is/are not true?

　　A. Peroxisomes contain catalases and oxidases.

　　B. The microbody membrane is essentially impermeable.

　　C. Microbodies use molecular oxygen to oxidize substrate, with generation of hydrogen peroxide.

　　D. Microbodies degrade hydrogen peroxide to water and oxygen.

　　E. Glyoxisomes are found primarily in plants.

Ref.: 6–8

COMMENTS: Microbodies may be distinguished from other cell organelles by the fact that they contain catalase. • There are two microbody classes: the **peroxisome**, which is found in both plants and animals and contains catalases and oxidase, and the **glyoxisome**, which is found mainly in plants and contains part or all of the enzymes of the glyoxylate cycle. • Like the endoplasmic reticulum, the microbody membrane is thinner than the plasma membrane.

The microbody membrane is freely permeable to a number of natural substrates of the enzymes within. • These substrates include amino acids, hydroxy acids, and uric acid. • In general, microbody enzymes are a specialized group of oxidation enzymes that degrade a fairly limited number of substrates.

Microbodies protect cells from high oxygen toxicity and compartmentalize purine-pyrimidine catabolism and amino acid destruction. • They use molecular oxygen to oxidize a given substrate, with the generation of hydrogen peroxide. • They then degrade the hydrogen peroxide to water and oxygen to protect the cell from the toxic effect of hydrogen peroxide.

ANSWER:
B

13. Which of the following statements regarding phagocytosis is/are not true?

    A. Phagocytosis refers to engulfment of particulate matter.

    B. Opsonins increase phagocytosis by exposing the hydrophilic tail portion of the antibody–foreign particle complex.

    C. Opsonins increase phagocytosis by exposing the hydrophobic tail portion of the antibody–foreign particle complex.

    D. Phagocytosis is not temperature dependent.

    E. Pinocytosis refers to the engulfment of soluble materials.

Ref.: 6–8

COMMENTS: Phagocytosis is accomplished by several cells in the body, including macrophages and polymorphonuclear leukocytes. • **Endocytosis** is, generally, cellular engulfment of *foreign* particles. • **Phagocytosis** specifically refers to the engulfment of *particulate* material. • **Pinocytosis** is the engulfment of *soluble* materials. • Increased hydrophobicity of a foreign particle or increased hydrophilicity of the phagocyte increases phagocytosis. • **Opsonins** are antibody molecules that increase phagocytosis as a result of combining the hydrophilic antigen-binding portion of the antibody with a foreign particle, thereby exposing the hydrophobic tail of the antibody. • Once a particle is engulfed by a phagocyte, it forms a **phagosome**, which combines with a **lysosome** to form a **phagolysosome**. • Phagocytosis is temperature-dependent in that it does not occur below a critical temperature threshold. • Because pinocytosis involves the uptake of already soluble molecules, it is not affected by this critical temperature threshold.

ANSWER:
B, D

14. Which of the following statements regarding lysosomes is/are true?

    A. Cathepsins are a form of oxidative enzyme found in lysosomes.

    B. Heterolysosomes are not involved in the endocytosis of extracellular material.

    C. Primary lysosomes are formed by fusion with a phagosome and are referred to as phagolysosomes.

    D. Acid phosphatase is a marker enzyme for lysosomes.

    E. Lysosomal membranes have a high proportion of proteins in a micellular configuration.

Ref.: 6–8

COMMENTS: Lysosomes are membrane-bound cellular structures that contain two or more acid hydrolases. • Heterolysosomes are involved in the endocytosis and digestion of extracellular material, whereas autolysosomes are involved in digestion of the cell's own intracellular material. • Lysosomes are formed in the Golgi complex by the packaging of enzymes formed in the rough endoplasmic reticulum. • A primary lysosome is formed by the cell before digestive activity. • Combining a primary lysosome with a phagosome creates a **secondary lysosome**, or **phagolysosome**. • Lysosomal enzymes are hydrolases that are resistant to autolysis. • Acid phosphatase is the principal marker enzyme for lysosomes. • Cathepsins are a type of acid hydrolase found in lysosomes.
One of the distinguishing characteristics of lysosomal membranes is their ability to fuse with other cell membranes. • Lysosomal membranes have a high proportion of lipids in a micellular configuration, primarily because of the presence of the phospholipid lysolecithin. • This increased micellular configuration in the membrane facilitates membrane fusion of lysosomes with phagosomes for digestion and with the plasma membrane for secretion. • Steroids are thought to work partially by stabilizing lysosomal membranes, thereby inhibiting membrane fusion and enzyme release. • Lysosomes may engage in some autophagocytosis, which is thought to be responsible for cell turnover, cell remodeling, and tissue changes.

ANSWER:
D

15. Which of the following statements regarding the Golgi complex is/are true?

    A. The Golgi complex is a system of round membrane sacs scattered throughout the cytoplasm.

    B. The Golgi complex is oriented so that a maturing face is close to the endoplasmic reticulum and a forming face points toward the cell surface.

    C. The Golgi complex is responsible for the breakdown of carbohydrate-rich macromolecules.

    D. The Golgi complex is involved in the breakdown of integral membrane proteins and lysosomes.

    E. Glycosyltransferase is a marker enzyme for the Golgi complex.

Ref.: 6–8

COMMENTS: The Golgi complex is a highly pleomorphic system of membrane sacs arranged in a stacked form. • It is surrounded by vesicles and tubules, with an orientation such that the forming face is close to the endoplasmic reticulum and the mature face points toward the cell surface, where secretory materials may be exported. • The Golgi complex contains a variety of enzymes, including glycosyltransferase, which is its best marking enzyme. • The Golgi complex is responsible for the assembly of carbohydrate-rich macromolecules. • It is partially responsible for the synthesis of integral membrane glycoproteins and the synthesis of lysosomes.

ANSWER:
E

16. Which of the following statements regarding mitochondria is/are true?

    A. There is an inverse relationship between the number of mitochondria and the metabolic demands on a cell.

    B. Ribosomes are rarely found in association with the mitochondrial matrix.

    C. The lamellar form of cristae is common in steroid-producing cells.

    D. The matrix contains soluble enzymes of the tricarboxylic acid cycle.

    E. All of the above.

Ref.: 6–8

COMMENTS: Mitochondria are organelles bounded by two membranes separated by a space called the **intermembrane space**. • Although the membranes appear separate, they are in fact continuous. • The highly invaginated inner membrane, or **crista,**

projects into the innermost space of the organelle, referred to as the **matrix**. • The matrix contains soluble enzymes of the tricarboxylic acid cycle. • Although the matrix appears smooth, it may also contain ribosomes and filaments of DNA. • There are two forms of mitochondrial cristae: the lamellar form, which is relatively stacked and the commonest, and the tubular form, which is common in steroid-producing cells. • The inner membranes contain all the enzymes necessary for electron transport, from reduced coenzymes to molecular oxygen, as well as the coupled process of phosphorylation. • There appears to be a direct relationship between the number of mitochondria per cell and the metabolic demands on the cell.

ANSWER:
D

17. Which of the following statements regarding oxidative phosphorylation and mitochondria is/are true?

   A. Metabolic products from glycolytic reactions outside mitochondria enter the mitochondria and are acted on by nuclear enzymes of the tricarboxylic acid cycle.

   B. Oxyreductase enzymes sequester electrons and then load reduced nicotinamide adenine dinucleotide phosphate and flavine adenine dinucleotide phosphate onto electron carriers.

   C. Electrons flow through a system of membranes, thereby releasing energy, which is captured by phosphorylation of ADP to ATP.

   D. Twelve ATP molecules are generated per mole of oxygen consumed.

Ref.: 6–8

COMMENTS: Metabolic products of glycolysis outside the mitochondria enter the mitochondria and are acted on by enzymes of the tricarboxylic acid cycle located in the matrix, not in the nucleus. • Oxyreductase enzymes sequester electrons from these substrates and then load onto electron carriers. • The electrons flow through three membrane systems, the energy being released and stored by the phosphorylation of ADP to ATP. • This electron flow is coupled to phosphorylation in such a way that three ATP molecules are generated for each mole of oxygen consumed. • In the mitochondria of muscle cells, the process of aerobic glycolysis breaks down glycogen to carbon dioxide and water, releasing the energy necessary for conversion of ADP to ATP.

ANSWER:
C

18. Which of the following statements regarding cellular motility and contractility is/are not true?

   A. The interactions between actin and myosin that underlie the contraction of skeletal muscle require Ca^{2+} but not ATP.

   B. The proteins kinesin and dynein are required for directional transport of cellular components along the microtubules.

   C. Microtubules are involved in the movement of cilia and flagella.

   D. The spindle apparatus is formed by cytoskeletal microtubules.

   E. Actin forms the stress fibers of fibroblasts.

Ref.: 6–8

COMMENTS: Actin is found in muscle cells and many other cell types. • Actin microfilaments form a cortical layer beneath the plasma membrane of most cells, the stress fibers of fibroblasts, and the cytoskeleton of microvilli of intestinal epithelial cells. • The cycle of interaction between the heads of **myosin** ("thick filaments") and actin ("thin filaments") in skeletal muscle requires hydrolysis of ATP to separate the myosin from the actin filament at the end of the power stroke. • **Calcium and troponin C** (an actin-associated protein) are required to expose the binding site for myosin on the actin filament.

   Cilia and flagella contain a column of doublet microtubules in a "9 + 2" arrangement (nine doublets in a circle surrounding two central doublets). • Movement is accomplished by the doublets' sliding along each other, mediated by *dynein,* an associated protein, and requiring the hydrolysis of ATP. • Microtubules form part of the cytoskeletal network and arise from the microtubule-organizing center (sometimes called the *centrosome*). • The microtubule-organizing center is found near the nucleus and contains a pair of *centrioles*. • Movement of cellular components, such as vacuoles, along the microtubules requires ATP and the involvement of either of two associated proteins: *kinesin* for movement away from the microtubule-organizing center and *dynein* for movement toward it.

   Microtubules are in a constant dynamic equilibrium between assembly from subunits and disassembly. • Assembly of the mitotic spindle involves (1) replication and splitting of the microtubule-organizing center into the two spindle poles and (2) reorganization of the cytoskeletal microtubules to form the spindle apparatus.

ANSWER:
A

19. Which intermediate filament is characteristic of cells of mesenchymal origin?

   A. Desmin

   B. Vimentin

   C. Keratin

   D. Glial protein

   E. Neurofilaments

Ref.: 4, 5

COMMENTS: Intermediate filaments are a group of related molecules that form stable mechanical components of the cytoskeleton. • Nuclear lamins are intermediate filaments that form the nuclear lamina on the inner surface of the nuclear envelope. • One or more specific intermediate filaments are characteristic of certain cell types. • Immunocytochemical identification of intermediate filament proteins is used to determine the cell-type origin of some tumors. • **Desmin** is an important intermediate filament protein found in smooth muscle cells and in the mechanical junctions (**desmosomes**) that link epithelial cells. • **Vimentin** is an intermediate filament characteristic of fibroblasts and other mesenchymal cells. • **Keratin** is characteristic of epithelial cells and epidermal derivatives such as hair and nails. • **Glial protein**, or glial fibrillary acidic protein, is found in all glial cells (e.g., astrocytes). • **Neurofilaments** are characteristic of neuronal tissue (e.g., neurons).

ANSWER:
B

20. Which one of the following constitutes the major element of the extracellular matrix?

   A. Collagen

   B. Noncollagenous glycoproteins

   C. Laminins

   D. Proteoglycans

   E. Glycosaminoglycans

Ref.: 3–5

COMMENTS: The **extracellular matrix**, a meshwork of various macromolecules, is particularly prominent in connective tissue, where it is secreted by fibroblasts. • **Collagens**, the major constituents of the extracellular matrix, are glycoproteins characterized by their tertiary structure. • **Noncollagenous glycoproteins** are adhesive macromolecules that interact with cells and other extracellular matrix components. • They promote adhesion, migration, and proliferation to influence gene expression. • **Laminins** are multidomain glycoproteins located primarily in the basement membrane, where they can interact with many cells and other extracellular-matrix components. • **Proteoglycans**, such as hyaluronate, chondroitin, dermatan, keratin, and heparin, are large molecules composed of protein cores to which are attached side chains of glycosaminoglycans. • They form bulky, hydrated gels that fill most of the extracellular space, providing an environment in which water-soluble molecules can readily diffuse and easily migrate.

ANSWER:
A

21. Which of the following statements regarding the nuclear envelope is/are true?

   A. The nuclear envelope is a double-membrane sheath that joins at several areas called tight junctions.

   B. Pore complexes are made up of a cylindrical structure called the annulus and a central granule.

   C. The nuclear envelope is impermeable to inorganic ions and small organic molecules.

   D. The nucleus moves throughout the cell because of its free-floating nature.

Ref.: 6–8

COMMENTS: The **nuclear envelope,** which surrounds the nucleus, is made up of two membranes that are essentially parallel except in areas where they join as a pore complex. • The space between the membranes is referred to as the **perinuclear space**. • The outer membrane of the nuclear envelope occasionally has attached ribosomes and may be continuous with the endoplasmic reticulum. • The nuclear side of the inner membrane, referred to as the **nuclear lamina**, is a fibrous layer of electron-dense material. • The nuclear lamina is thought to function as an organizing frame for the nuclear envelope and as a site of attachment for chromosomes. • The **pore complexes** are composed of a cylindrical structure called the **annulus**, which forms the rim of the pore, and an inner **central granule**. • A large number of pore complexes is associated with heavy traffic between the nucleus and the cytoplasm. • There are fewer pore complexes in slowly metabolizing or nonproliferating cells than in highly proliferating cells. • The nuclear envelope is highly permeable to inorganic ions and small organic molecules and may permit passage of materials up to the molecular weight of proteins needed inside the nucleus for nucleic

acid replication and transcription. • The nucleus does not appear to be free-floating in the cell. • It may be held in position by a web of filaments extending from the surface throughout the cell interior.

ANSWER:
B

22. Which of the following statements regarding the nucleus is/are true?

   A. The nucleus is made up of a nuclear envelope, a nucleolus, chromatin, and a structural network called the matrix.

   B. The matrix is thought to be involved in replication and transcription only.

   C. The matrix functions as a depot for RNA and protein being assembled into preribosomal subunits.

   D. The nucleolus contains a fibrillar zone in which ribosomes are condensed with RNA.

Ref.: 6–8

COMMENTS: The nuclear region is divided into a **nuclear envelope**, a **nucleolus**, **chromatin**, and a structural network called the **matrix**. • The **matrix** is proposed to be involved in replication, transcription, and post-transcriptional processing and transport. • The **nucleolus** functions as a depot for RNA and protein being assembled into preribosomal subunits. • The nucleolus is divided into a fibrillar zone and a granular zone. • The fibrillar zone has sites where ribosomal RNA is transcribed, and the granular zone has sites where ribosomes and proteins are condensed with the ribosomal RNA.

ANSWER:
A

23. Which of the following statements regarding chromosomes is/are not true?

   A. The nucleus contains the entire cellular DNA.

   B. Interactions between DNA and proteins stabilize chromosome structure.

   C. Interactions between DNA and proteins expose specific genes and control their expression.

   D. During mitosis, the spindle apparatus attaches to the chromosome at the centromere.

   E. Telomeres maintain the chromosomal length through replication cycles.

Ref.: 4, 5

COMMENTS: Chromosomes are formed by the combination of double-stranded helical **DNA** with histones and other proteins. • The interactions between DNA and proteins stabilize the chromosomal structure. • Most cellular DNA is located in the **nucleus**, although a small portion is found in the mitochondria. • Each chromosomal double helix contains approximately 10^8 base pairs. • There are several levels of organizational restructuring: progression from the DNA and histones forming chromatin to the complex folded structure of the chromosome. • To express a gene, that portion of the chromosome must be unfolded and unwrapped, exposing the DNA double helix. • Gene expression is regulated by the binding of nonchromosomal proteins (*transcription factors*) to specific regions of the DNA (*enhancer elements* and *promoter elements*). • Several distinct regions of chromosomes are identifiable: *origins of replication* (sites of initiation of DNA synthesis), the *centromere* (site of spindle attachment during mitosis), and *telomeres* (specialized end structures that maintain the length of the chromosome through replication cycles).

ANSWER:
A

---

24. Which of the following statements regarding the nucleolus is/are true?

    A. The nucleolus is the functional site for the generation of DNA.

    B. The nucleolus has a limiting double-membrane sheath.

    C. The fibrillar component of the nucleolus is involved in associating genes for ribosomal RNA.

    D. The nucleolus is characterized by a granular component, which is a site for RNA transcription and protein synthesis.

    E. The primary function of the nucleolus is generation of ribosomes.

Ref.: 6–8

COMMENTS: The primary function of the nucleolus is generation of ribosomes. • It is functionally and structurally associated with the nuclear envelope and the lamina. • The nucleolus has no limiting membrane and is made up of a fibrillar component and a granular component. • The fibrillar center of the nucleolus functions to associate nucleolar-organizing regions, which are genes for ribosomal RNA. • The dense fibrillar component is involved in the transcription of ribosomal RNA genes and the assembly of pre-ribosomal subunits. • The granular component is involved in the processing and maturation of preribosomes.

ANSWER:
C, E

---

25. Which phase of mitosis is associated with re-formation of the nucleolus and nuclear envelope?

    A. Prophase

    B. Anaphase

    C. Metaphase

    D. Telophase

    E. None of the above

Ref.: 6–8

COMMENTS: Mitosis is a progressive cell change, characterized by several phases, that leads to two identical daughter cells. • **Prophase**, the first phase, includes shortening of the chromosomes, followed by disappearance of both the nucleolus and the nuclear envelope and formation of the spindle apparatus. • Centrioles replicate, and the two centrioles move to opposite ends. • At this stage, the identical shortened chromosomes, referred to as chromatids, are temporarily held together by a centromere. • **Metaphase** occurs with movement of the chromosomes toward the center so that the centromeres align on a plane called the *equatorial plate*. • The centromeres then attach to spindle fibers from the spindle apparatus. • At the same time, the centromeres of each chromatid duplicate. • **Anaphase**, the next portion of mitosis, is marked by migration of the chromatids to

opposite poles. • When separated, the chromatids are referred to as chromosomes. • **Telophase** occurs shortly thereafter and involves decondensation of the chromosomes, with simultaneous nucleolar and nuclear envelope re-formation.

ANSWER:
D

---

26. Which phase of the cell cycle is associated with DNA synthesis?

    A. S

    B. G_1

    C. G_2

    D. M

Ref.: 6–8

COMMENTS: The cell cycle is composed of a long **interphase** and a comparatively short **mitosis** phase. • Interphase is initiated by a G_1 phase, followed by an *S* phase (during which DNA synthesis occurs and two sister chromosomes are generated) and then by a G_2 quiescent phase. • RNA and protein synthesis occurs during both the G_1 and G_2 phases. • Mitosis (characterized by a prophase, a metaphase, an anaphase, and a telophase, during which two identical daughter cells are generated) then occurs, and the cycle is repeated.

ANSWER:
A

---

27. Which of the following statements regarding protein synthesis is/are not true?

    A. Transcription of messenger RNA takes place in the nucleus.

    B. Messenger RNA moves from the nucleus to the cytoplasm and attaches to free ribosomes in the cytoplasm.

    C. The enzyme RNA polymerase catalyzes the transcription of messenger RNA from DNA.

    D. Free ribosomes are involved in the synthesis of proteins that are inserted in the endoplasmic reticulum.

    E. Ribosomal RNA is transcribed in the nucleolus.

Ref.: 4, 6–8

COMMENTS: The sequence of nucleotides in DNA determines the amino acid sequence of the protein. • Protein synthesis involves (1) *transcription* of messenger RNA from the gene that codes for the protein, (2) *translation* of the messenger RNA into a protein, and (3) *post-translational processing* of the protein, in which there may be enzymatic cleavage or glycosylation of the protein.

Transcription takes place in the nucleus, whereas translation and post-translational processing occur in the rough endoplasmic reticulum, Golgi complex, or free ribosomes in the cytoplasm. • Transcription of messenger RNA from DNA occurs by assembly of complementary base pairs on the DNA template one nucleotide at a time. • This step is catalyzed by the enzyme RNA polymerase. • Eukaryotic genes are interrupted by noncoding regions called *introns*. • Introns are removed from the RNA transcript by *splicing*.

The resulting messenger RNA is moved to the cytoplasm, in which it binds to ribosomes to begin *translation*. • Ribosomes are composed of proteins and ribosomal RNA. • Ribosomal RNA is transcribed in the *nucleolus,* where it is combined with ribosomal proteins to form ribosomal subunits. • The ribosomal subunits are transported to the cytoplasm, where they are assembled into two populations of ribosomes: *free ribosomes*, which are engaged in the synthesis of proteins that remain in the cytoplasm, and *membrane-bound ribosomes*, which become attached to the *rough endoplasmic reticulum* and are involved in the synthesis of proteins that are inserted in the endoplasmic reticulum.

The initial step of protein synthesis is attachment of the messenger RNA to a ribosome that is preloaded with *transfer RNA* that recognizes the start codon (three bases) AUG and thus sets the reading frame for the translation. • Subsequent binding of aminoacyl-transfer RNA to the ribosomes that match the three nucleotide codons that specify each amino acid results in peptide synthesis as the ribosome moves along the messenger RNA molecule. • The first portion of the protein that is synthesized is an amino terminal leader called the *signal peptide*. • At this stage, the ribosome becomes attached to the rough endoplasmic reticulum through interactions between the signal peptide, a cytoplasmic signal recognition peptide, and a signal recognition peptide receptor protein in the rough endoplasmic reticulum. • As translation continues, the signal peptide is inserted in the rough endoplasmic reticulum membrane by another transmembrane protein and later cleaved as the peptide elongates.

ANSWER:
D

28. Which of the following is not an RNA transcription factor?

    A. Zinc finger

    B. Helix turn helix

    C. Leucine zipper

    D. TATA box

Ref.: 3

COMMENTS: Transcription factors are proteins that play key roles in regulating the initiation of transcription by associating either directly with the DNA or indirectly via other mediators. • They can be categorized into three major families, depending on their amino acid homologies and protein structures. • Receptors in the **zinc finger** family have a domain in the protein structure that contains zinc atoms that bind to multiple amino acid with looped zinc-finger regions. • Steroid and glucocorticoid receptors, including thyroid hormone, retinoic acid, and vitamin D_3 receptors, are included in this family. • Zinc fingers bind to hormone-responsive elements in the DNA. • When a hormone binds to this receptor, the zinc finger–ligand complex is transported to the nucleus and binds to DNA, activating transcription. • **Helix-turn-helix** structures play a critical role in development and are expressed characteristically and temporally in subsets of embryonic cells. • The best known example in eukaryotes is the homeo domain protein, which is encoded by the homeobox regions of DNA. • **Leucine zippers** are short coils of two parallel α helices with approximately eight turns per helix. • The zipper motif of the protein characteristically occurs as a Y-shaped scissors-grip structure within the molecule. • These motifs are found in some eukaryotic transcription factors and some nuclear oncogenes. • The **TATA box**, a promoter element, is a thymine-adenine–rich region upstream from the start region along the DNA in RNA synthesis.

ANSWER:
D

29. Where do steroid hormones initiate their regulatory mechanism on the DNA?

    A. Cell membrane

    B. Nucleus

    C. Cytoplasm

    D. Endoplasmic reticulum

    E. Nucleolus

Ref.: 3

COMMENTS: Steroid hormones are synthesized from cholesterol and are lipophilic. • They can cross cell membranes easily. • Along with other molecular signals, such as thyroid hormone, vitamin D_3, and retinoic acid, steroids form complexes with **cytoplasmic receptors**. • These receptors become activated and rapidly move into the nucleus to bind to regulatory units on the DNA.

ANSWER:
C

30. Which one of the following is not associated with matrix metalloproteinases (MMPs)?

    A. Neurologic diseases

    B. Arthritis

    C. Emphysema

    D. Inhibition of tumor invasion

    E. Cardiovascular diseases

Ref.: 3

COMMENTS: MMPs are a family of extracellular zinc-dependent proteinases. • In addition to cardiovascular disease, neurologic disease, arthritis, and emphysema, MMPs have been implicated in mechanisms of tumor invasion and metastases generation. • Controlled degradation of the basement membrane and other extracellular membrane components is the mechanism through which these are achieved. • The expression of MMP genes has been influenced by several oncologic factors, including up regulation by growth factors, cytokines, stress, and medications. • Down regulation has been mediated by retinoic acid, glucocorticoids, transforming growth factor β, and tissue inhibitors of metalloproteinases.

ANSWER:
D

31. Which of the following methods relies on the transfer and binding of proteins to study macromolecules separated by gel electrophoresis?

    A. Southern blotting

    B. Northern blotting

    C. Western blotting

    D. Polymerase chain reaction

    E. Eastern blotting

Ref.: 3

COMMENTS: Blotting is a method used to study macromolecules separated by gel electrophoresis and transferred onto membrane filters. • The macromolecules can be visualized by specific probes and/or staining methods. • **Southern** blotting relies on the transfer and binding of DNAs and allows probing for expression of specific genes. • **Northern** blotting relies on the transfer and binding of RNAs and allows probing for DNA expression of specific genes. • **Western** blotting relies on the transfer and binding of proteins and allows for comparative protein analysis. • It is augmented by the use of protein-specific antibodies to establish the identity of macromolecules. • Eastern blotting remains to be developed.

A N S W E R :
C

32. Which DNA recombinant technology specifically relies directly on the selective cleavage of bacterial DNA over native DNA?

    A. Polymerase chain reaction

    B. DNA sequencing

    C. Restriction nucleases

    D. DNA cloning

    E. None of the above

Ref.: 3

COMMENTS: Polymerase chain reaction is a technique by which DNA may be amplified a billion-fold. • Primers or oligonucleotides are synthesized to complement one strand of the DNA double helix to be amplified. • Also added to the polymerase chain reaction mixture are the DNA sequence or template, two primers, heat-stable DNA polymerase, and the four types of deoxynucleotide triphosphate. • Amplification involves three temperature-cycled steps: (1) heating for separation of the double-helix structure into two single strands, (2) cooling for hybridization of each single strand with its primer, and (3) heating for DNA synthesis. • When RNA is used, reverse transcriptase is employed to transcribe it to DNA initially. • **DNA sequencing** is based on an enzymatic method requiring in vitro DNA synthesis. • It is a rapid technique that allows the determination of the boundaries of a gene and the amino acid sequence of the protein that is encoded. • **Restriction nucleases** are bacterial enzymes that splice the DNA double helix at specific sequences of four to eight nucleotides. • These enzymes are derived from various species of bacteria and can recognize several sequences. • They protect the bacterial cell from foreign DNA, whereas native DNA is protected from cleavage by methylation at vulnerable nucleotides. • Commonly used restriction enzymes often recognize palindromic sequences. • Each restriction enzyme cuts a DNA molecule into a series of specific fragments. • When utilized appropriately, **DNA cloning** allows identification of a gene of interest from the human genome. • It relies on the joining of DNA fragments to self-replicating genetic elements, such as viruses or plasmids, via transfection. • The transected cells are able to produce large copies of these genetic elements with the incorporated DNA fragments.

A N S W E R :
C

33. Which of the following does not distinguish cellular apoptosis from necrosis?

    A. It begins under the precise control of diverse intracellular and extracellular signals.

    B. It acts mainly through its effect on the mitochondria.

    C. It represents the cellular response to injuries such as ischemia or irradiation.

    D. Its progression is regulated by a variety of genes.

    E. It follows a fixed sequence of events.

Ref.: 2, 3

COMMENTS: Necrosis represents the cellular response to injury, such as ischemia, irradiation, or the effects of toxins. • Apoptosis is a natural cellular process that begins under the precise control of a variety of intracellular and extracellular signals and follows a fixed sequence of events. • These signals are variable and include oxidant stress, radiation, viral infection, trauma, and the action of cytokines.

Apoptosis involves the initiation of a cellular suicide program that may be either receptor independent or receptor dependent. • Sphingomyelin breakdown and DNA damage from radiation or oxygen free radicals are examples of receptor-independent initiation of apoptosis. • Receptor-dependent induction of apoptosis occurs through the activation of a tumor necrosis factor (TNF) receptor superfamily also known as the death receptor. • The Fas antigen and TNFRI are the primary receptors that have been described. • They are activated by the FasL and TNF ligands, respectively. • Regardless of the initiation pathway, the induction of the genes to promote pro-apoptotic proteins is the first point in the common pathway.

Normally, there is an intercellular balance between pro-apoptotic and anti-apoptotic genes and their proteins. • The Bcl-2 and Bax (including Bax, Bad, Bid, and Bim) families of genes are the best-characterized examples of anti-apoptotic and pro-apoptotic genes, respectively. • Once the apoptosis is signaled, there is a down regulation of the Bcl-2 gene and therefore a relative up regulation of the Bax gene.

The proteins ultimately produced from these genes converge on the mitochondrial membrane, where apoptosis begins with a battle for the regulation of cytochrome c migration out of the cell. • With apoptosis, the permeability of the outer mitochondrial membrane rapidly increases, thus allowing the release of factors that activate caspases (catabolic hydrolases) and nucleases. • These activated enzymes then degrade proteins in the cellular skeleton, cytoplasm, and nucleus. • Cellular budding and fragmentation ensue. • The resultant apoptotic bodies are then phagocytosed rapidly by macrophages and neighboring cells.

A N S W E R :
C

34. Select the basic units of DNA packaging.

    A. Centrioles

    B. Nucleosomes

    C. Histones

    D. Solenoids

    E. All of the above

Ref.: 3

COMMENTS: A hierarchy of DNA organization exists to allow for tight packaging of 46 chromosomes into the nucleus. • **Nucleosomes** are the basic units of DNA packaging and are coils of DNA. • **Histones** are small basic proteins that bind tightly but nonspecifically with the more acidic DNA segments. • Each nucleosome is formed by the wrapping of nearly 200 base pairs of DNA twice around an octameric composed of two copies each of four histones (H2A, H2B, H3, and H4). • **Solenoids** develop when an additional histone, H1, promotes the coiling of six or more nucleosomes to form larger complexes. • **Centrioles** are cytoplasmic microtubules containing structures that migrate to opposite sides of the nucleus during mitosis.

ANSWER:
B

35. What enzyme is responsible for the catalyzation of deoxynucleoside triphosphates into DNA?

    A. DNA helicase

    B. DNA ligase

    C. DNA polymerase

    D. DNA primase

    E. All of the above

Ref.: 6

COMMENTS: DNA polymerases are enzymes that catalyze the polymerization of deoxynucleoside triphosphates into DNA. • There are several types of DNA polymerases. • For example, DNA polymerase III promotes DNA elongation by nucleotide linkage, whereas DNA polymerase I functions to fill gaps and repair DNA. • **DNA helicase** is the enzyme involved in the unwinding step of DNA replication. • **DNA primase** catalyzes the formation of RNA primers used to initiate DNA synthesis. • **DNA ligase** joins DNA fragments generated by the degradation of RNA primers.

ANSWER:
C

36. In DNA replication, what type of mutation specifically is associated with the generation of a stop codon?

    A. Point mutation

    B. Missense mutation

    C. Nonsense mutation

    D. Frame-shift mutation

Ref.: 1

COMMENTS: A change in a single base pair is known as a **point mutation**. • A single amino acid change resulting from a point mutation is known as a **missense mutation,** which may cause changes in the structure of the protein, leading to altered biologic activity. • **Nonsense mutations** occur if a point mutation results in the replacement of an amino acid codon with a stop codon. • Nonsense mutations lead to premature termination of translation and often result in the loss of encoded protein. • **Frame-shift mutations** occur when there are additions or deletions of a few base pairs, leading to the introduction of unrelated amino acids or stop codons.

ANSWER:
C

REFERENCES

1. Townsend CM, Beauchamp RD, Evers BM, et al (eds): *Sabiston Textbook of Surgery: The Biological Basis of Modern Surgical Practice,* 16th ed. Saunders, Philadelphia, 2001.
2. Greenfield LJ, Mulholland MW, Oldham KT, et al (eds): *Surgery: Scientific Principles and Practice*, 3rd ed. Lippincott, Williams & Wilkins, Philadelphia, 2001.
3. O'Leary JP (ed): *Physiologic Basis of Surgery,* 3th ed. Lippincott, Williams & Wilkins, Philadelphia, 2002.
4. Darnell J, Lodish H, Baltimore D: *Molecular Cell Biology.* Scientific American Books, New York, 1990.
5. Alberts B, Bray D, Lewis J, et al: *Molecular Biology of the Cell.* Garland Publishing, New York, 1989.
6. Thorpe NO: *Cell Biology.* John Wiley & Sons, New York, 1984.
7. Carroll M: *Organelles.* Guilford Press, New York, 1989.
8. Karp G: *Cell Biology.* McGraw-Hill, New York, 1984.

C H A P T E R **2**

Fluids and Electrolytes

Anthony W. Kim, M.D., and Steven D. Bines, M.D.

1. Which of the following statements regarding total body water is/are true?

A. In males, approximately 60% of total body weight is water.

B. In general, the percentage of total body weight that is water is higher in males than in females.

C. Lean individuals have a greater proportion of water (relative to body weight) than do obese individuals.

D. The percentage of total body water increases with age.

E. The majority of our body water is intestinal.

Ref.: 1

COMMENTS: Approximately 50–75% of body weight is water. • In males, 60% (±15%) of body weight is water, and, in females, 50% (±15%) of body weight is water. • Age and lean body mass also contribute to differences in the percentage of total body weight that is water. • Since fat contains little water, lean individuals have a greater proportion of body water than do fat individuals of the same weight. • Because females have more subcutaneous fat in relationship to lean mass than do males, they have less body water. • Total body water decreases with age as a result of decreasing lean muscle mass. Infants have an unusually high ratio of total body water to body weight: up to 75–80%. • By 1 year of age, however, the percentage of body water approaches that of adults.

Body water is divided into three functional compartments: the *intracellular* fluid compartment (40% of body weight), the *interstitial* (extravascular) fluid compartment (15% of body weight), and the *intravascular* (plasma) fluid compartment (5% of body weight). • Together, the interstitial and intravascular compartments constitute the *extracellular* fluid compartment.

A N S W E R :
A, B, C

2. Which of the following statements regarding the distribution and composition of the body fluid compartments is/are not true?

A. Most intracellular water is in skeletal muscle.

B. The major intracellular cation is sodium.

C. The major extracellular cation is sodium.

D. The major extracellular anions are chloride and bicarbonate.

Ref.: 1

COMMENTS: The intracellular fluid compartment (accounting for 40% of total body weight) is contained mostly within skeletal muscle. • The principal intracellular cations are potassium and magnesium, whereas the principal anions are proteins and phosphates. • In the extracellular fluid compartment (20% of total body weight), subdivided into the interstitial compartment (extravascular) and the intravascular compartment (plasma), the principal cation is sodium, and the principal anions are chloride and bicarbonate. • The interstitial compartment has a rapidly equilibrating functional component and a slowly equilibrating, relatively nonfunctional component consisting of fluid within connective tissue and cerebrospinal and joint fluids. • The water in the cerebrospinal fluid and joint spaces is called transcellular water. • The nonfunctional component represents only one half of body weight. Intravascular fluid (plasma) has a higher concentration of nondiffusible organic proteins than do interstitial fluids. • These plasma proteins act as multivalent anions. • As a result, the concentration of *inorganic* anions is lower, but the total concentration of cations is higher, in intravascular fluid than in interstitial fluid. • This relationship is explained by the **Gibbs-Donnan** equilibrium equation: the product of the concentrations of any pair of diffusible cations and anions on one side of a semipermeable membrane equals the product of the same pair on the other side.

In each body compartment, the concentration of osmotically active particles is 290–310 mOsm. • Although total osmotic pressure represents the sum of osmotically active particles in a fluid compartment, the effective osmotic pressure depends on osmotically active particles that do not freely pass through the semipermeable membranes of the body. • Nonpermeable proteins in plasma are responsible for the effective osmotic pressure between the plasma and the interstitial fluid compartment (the colloid osmotic pressure). • The effective osmotic pressure between the extracellular fluid and intracellular fluid compartments is due mainly to sodium, the major extracellular cation, which does not freely cross the cell membrane. • Because water moves freely between compartments, the effective oncotic pressures within the various body fluid compartments are considered equal. • An increase in the effective oncotic pressure of the extracellular fluid compartment, such as results from an increase in sodium concentration, causes movement of water from the intracellular space to the extracellular space until the osmotic pressures equalize. • Conversely, loss of sodium (hyponatremia) from the extracellular space results in movement of water into the intracellular space. • Thus, the intracellular fluid contributes to correcting the concentration and composition changes in the extracellular fluid. • Isotonic extracellular volume losses (volume losses without change in concentration) generally do not cause transfer of water from the intracellular space as long as the osmolarity remains unchanged. • Isotonic volume losses result in extracellular fluid volume changes.

A N S W E R :
B

3. Which of the following statements regarding the chemical composition and osmolarity of the body fluids is/are true?

   A. From a physiologic standpoint, the numbers of millimoles, milliequivalents, and milliosmoles are interchangeable.

   B. The osmolality of body fluids is between 290 and 310 mOsm.

   C. The effective osmotic pressure of a body compartment is determined by the presence of nondiffusible proteins.

   D. Because water diffuses freely between compartments, the effective osmotic pressures within the various fluid compartments are considered equal.

Ref.: 1, 2

COMMENTS: From a physiologic and chemical standpoint, the terms *millimoles, milliequivalents*, and *milliosmoles* are not interchangeable. • *Millimole* refers to the number of particles per unit volume, *millequivalent* to the number of electrical charges per unit volume, and *milliosmole* to the number of osmotically active particles per unit volume. • In solution, the number of milliequivalents of cations present is balanced by the number of milliequivalents of anions (a balance that the body maintains in a steady state). • In each body compartment, the concentration of osmotically active particles is 290–310 mOsm. • Although total osmotic pressure represents the sum of osmotically active particles in a fluid compartment, the effective osmotic pressure depends on osmotically active particles that do not freely pass through the semipermeable membranes of the body. • Nonpermeable proteins in plasma are responsible for the effective osmotic pressure between the plasma and the interstitial fluid compartment (the colloid osmotic pressure). • The effective osmotic pressure between the extracellular fluid and intracellular fluid compartments is mainly due to sodium, the major extracellular cation, which does not freely cross the cell membrane. • Because water moves freely between compartments, the effective oncotic pressures within the various body fluid compartments are considered equal. • An increase in the effective oncotic pressure of the extracellular fluid compartment, such as results from an increase in sodium concentration, causes movement of water from the intracellular space to the extracellular space until the osmotic pressures equalize. • Conversely, loss of sodium (hyponatremia) from the extracellular space results in movement of water into the intracellular space. • Thus, the intracellular fluid contributes to correcting the concentration and composition changes in the extracellular fluid. • Isotonic extracellular volume losses (i.e., volume losses without change in concentration) generally do not cause transfer of water from the intracellular space as long as the osmolarity remains unchanged. • Isotonic volume losses result in extracellular fluid volume changes.

A N S W E R :
B, C, D

4. Which of the following statements regarding volume status changes of the extracellular fluid compartment is/are true?

   A. Hyponatremia is diagnostic of extracellular fluid volume excess.

   B. Hypernatremia is diagnostic of extracellular fluid volume depletion.

   C. Tissue signs of acute volume loss appear early after acute volume loss.

   D. Extracellular volume excess is usually iatrogenic.

Ref.: 1, 2

COMMENTS: The concentration of serum sodium is not necessarily related to the volume status of the extracellular fluid compartment. • Volume deficit or excess can exist with high, low, or normal serum sodium concentrations. • **Volume deficit** is the commonest volume disorder encountered during surgery. • Its commonest cause is loss of isotonic fluid (i.e., fluid having the same composition as extracellular fluid), for example, through hemorrhage, vomiting, diarrhea, fistulas, or third spacing. • With acute volume loss, central nervous system symptoms (e.g., sleepiness and apathy progressing to coma) and cardiovascular signs (e.g., orthostasis, hypotension, tachycardia, and coolness in the extremities) appear first, along with decreasing urine output. • Tissue signs (e.g., decreased turgor, softness of the tongue with longitudinal wrinkling, and atonicity of muscles) usually do not appear during the first 24 hr. • In response to hypovolemia, the body temperature may be decreased slightly (varying with the environmental temperature). • It is therefore important to monitor the body temperature of hypovolemic patients. • Signs and symptoms of sepsis may be depressed in volume-depleted patients. • The abdominal pain, fever, and leukocytosis associated with peritonitis may be absent until the extracellular fluid volume is restored. • **Volume overload** generally is either iatrogenic or the result of renal insufficiency or heart failure. • Both plasma and interstitial fluid spaces are involved. • The signs are those of circulatory overload and include distended veins, bounding pulse, functional murmurs, edema, and basilar rales. • These signs may be present in young, healthy patients, but these patients can compensate for moderate-to-severe volume excess without developing overt failure or pulmonary edema. • In elderly patients, however, congestive heart failure with pulmonary edema may develop quite rapidly.

A N S W E R :
D

5. When calculating the amount of solutes per unit of water, the concentrations of which of the following serum values is not required?

   A. Sodium

   B. Glucose

   C. Urea

   D. Chloride

Ref.: 1, 3

COMMENTS: Serum osmolality is described as the amount of solutes per unit of water. • It can be measured with an osmometer or it can be calculated. • It is reported as milliosmoles per liter. • Calculating serum osmolality is performed using the following equation:

$$\text{Calculated serum osmolality} = [2 \times Na^+ + urea/2.8 + glucose/18]$$

The concentrations of serum sodium, urea, and glucose are required, whereas that of serum chloride is not required for the calculation. • Simply doubling the serum sodium concentration provides an adequate estimate of serum osmolality.

A N S W E R :
D

6. Within the vascular compartment, what percentage of fluid resides in the arterial system?

   A. 85%

   B. 50%

   C. 30%

   D. 15%

Ref.: 3

COMMENTS: Approximately 85% of the extracellular fluid that is within the vascular compartment resides in the venous circulation. • Therefore, the remaining 15% resides within the arterial system. • The vascular compartment, otherwise known as the plasma fluid, constitutes approximately one third of the extracellular fluid. • The interstitial fluid (i.e., the fluid between the cells) makes up approximately two thirds of the extracellular fluid. • The extracellular fluid constitutes one third of the total body water, whereas the intracellular fluid constitutes two thirds.

ANSWER:
D

7. Which one of the following is not a stimulus for extracellular fluid expansion?

   A. Hemorrhage leading to reduction of blood volume

   B. Increased capillary permeability after major surgery

   C. Peripheral arterial vasoconstriction

   D. Negative interstitial fluid hydrostatic pressure

Ref.: 3

COMMENTS: The expansion of extracellular fluid is primarily driven by three mechanisms, all of which have the final common stimuli of reduction of intravascular volume. • The first mechanism, hemorrhage, is directly responsible for the reduction of blood volume. • Through various pathways, this drop in volume signals the retention and sequestration of fluid in the intravascular space. • Increased capillary permeability, the second mechanism, occurs following major surgery and is due to the loss of endothelial integrity. • This loss of integrity is mediated by several humoral factors that act on the endothelium. • The end result of the loss of endothelial integrity is the extravasation of protein-rich fluid into the interstitium, with a consequent increase in the interstitial fluid space. • This constitutes the third mechanism of extracellular fluid expansion.

ANSWER:
C

8. Which of the following humoral factors increases arterial vasodilatation while not decreasing protein permeability in the capillary membranes?

   A. Bradykinin

   B. Nitric oxide

   C. Atrial natriuretic factor

   D. Histamine

   E. Platelet-activating factor

Ref.: 1

COMMENTS: The protein permeability characteristics of capillary membranes are quantified by a numeric value termed the reflection coefficient. • This value ranges from 0 to 1 and is conceptualized as the fraction of plasma protein that "reflects" back from the capillary wall when water crosses. • The higher the coefficient, the more impermeable the capillary is to protein. • Therefore, the oncotic pressure of the plasma volume declines as the reflection coefficient decreases. • Certain intravascular factors can reduce the reflection coefficient and increase arterial vasodilation. • Bradykinin, atrial natriuretic factor, histamine, and platelet-activating factor increase the microvascular membrane permeability while causing arterial vasodilation. • Nitric oxide, while it causes arterial vasodilation, does not increase the microvascular membrane permeability. • Membrane permeability causes a shift of fluid and plasma proteins into the interstitium and thereby decreases the intravascular compartment. • The protein-rich edema in the interstitium can adversely affect the ability to combat infection.

ANSWER:
B

9. Which of the following statements regarding volume excess in postoperative patients is/are not true?

   A. This situation can be produced by the administration of isotonic salt solutions in amounts that exceed volume loss.

   B. Acute overexpansion of the extracellular fluid space is usually well tolerated in healthy individuals.

   C. Avoidance of volume excess requires daily monitoring of intake and output and determinations of serum sodium concentrations to guide accurate fluid administration.

   D. The earliest sign of volume excess is peripheral edema.

Ref.: 1, 2

COMMENTS: The earliest sign of volume excess during the postoperative period is **weight gain**. • Normally, during this period the patient is in a catabolic state and is expected to *lose weight* (¼–½ pound per day). • Circulatory and pulmonary signs of overload appear late and usually represent a massive overload. • Peripheral edema does not necessarily indicate volume excess. • In a patient with edema but without additional evidence of volume overload, other causes of peripheral edema should be considered. • The commonest cause of volume excess in a surgical patient is administration of isotonic salt solutions in amounts that exceed volume loss. • In a healthy individual, such overload is usually well tolerated, but, if excess administration of fluid continues for several days, the ability of the kidneys to secrete sodium may be exceeded and hypernatremia may result.

ANSWER:
D

10. When loop diuretics are used in pulmonary edema, which of the following mechanisms of action come into play?

   A. Inhibition of active sodium absorption

   B. Increased blood flow to the kidney

   C. Increased venous capacitance

   D. Augmented catecholamine sensitivity to α-adrenergic receptors

Ref.: 3

COMMENTS: Loop diuretics are typically used in pulmonary edema because they are the most potent drugs for this condition. • Loop diuretics decrease pulmonary edema through several mechanisms. • First, they inhibit active sodium absorption in the thick ascending loop of Henle. • Second, they increase blood flow to the kidneys by stimulating vasodilatory prostaglandins. • Third, they increase venous capacitance.

ANSWER:
A, B, C

11. When patients are resistant to boluses of loop diuretics, by what percentage will starting a continuous intravenous dose augment urine output?

   A. 5%

   B. 30%

   C. 66%

   D. 90%

Ref.: 3

COMMENTS: When patients are resistant to boluses of loop diuretics, the initiation of continuous intravenous infusion of loop diuretics can be employed to substantially increase diuresis. • Continuous administration of loop diuretics may augment urine output by approximately 30% volume.

ANSWER:
B

12. Which of the following pairings is/are correct?

   A. Daily insensible loss, 2000–2500 ml

   B. Average stool loss, 250 ml

   C. Average insensible loss, 600 ml

   D. Average urine volume, 800–1500 ml

   E. Daily water consumption, 3500 ml

Ref.: 2

COMMENTS: The average individual has an intake of 2000–2500 ml of water per day: 1500 ml is ingested orally and the remainder through solid food. • Daily losses include 250 ml in the stool, 800–1500 ml in urine, and approximately 600 ml as insensible loss. • To excrete the products of normal daily catabolism, an individual must produce at least 500–800 ml of urine. • In normal individuals, 75% of insensible loss is through the skin and 25% through the lungs. • Insensible loss from the skin occurs through loss of water vapor through the skin and not the evaporation of water secreted by sweat glands. • In febrile patients, insensible skin loss may increase to 250 ml/day for each degree of fever. • Losses from sweating can be as high as 4 L/hr. • In a patient with a tracheostomy who is ventilated with unhumidified air, insensible loss from the lungs may increase to 1500 ml/day.

ANSWER:
B, C, D

13. Which of the following secretions and sodium concentrations is/are incorrectly paired?

   A. Pancreatic secretions, 140 mEq/L

   B. Sweat, 40 mEq/L

   C. Gastric secretions, 50 mEq/L

   D. Saliva, 100 mEq/L

   E. Ileostomy output, 125 mEq/L

Ref.: 3

COMMENTS: Normal daily salt intake varies from 50–90 mEq sodium chloride. • Normal kidneys maintain balance and excrete excess salt as it is encountered. • Under conditions of reduced intake or increased extrarenal loss, the kidneys can reduce sodium excretion to less than 1 mEq/day. • Conversely, in patients with nonfunctioning kidneys, sodium loss may be as high as 200 mEq/L of urine.

   The electrolyte composition of sweat and gastrointestinal secretions vary (Table 2-1). • Sweat represents a hypotonic loss of fluids. • The average sodium concentration in sweat is 15–60 mEq/L. • Insensible loss from skin and lungs is pure water. • Note that *insensible* skin loss is not the same as water lost from sweat glands. • Although the various gastrointestinal secretions vary in composition, gastrointestinal losses are usually isotonic or slightly hypotonic. • Pancreatic fluids and bile have high bicarbonate concentrations. • Stomach, small intestine, and biliary fluids have relatively high chloride concentrations. • Duodenal, ileal, pancreatic, and biliary fluids contain levels of sodium that approximate those seen in the plasma. • Saliva is relatively high in potassium, a fact that is important to remember when managing a patient with a salivary fistula.

Table 2-1 Electrolyte Composition

Fluid	Na⁺	K⁺	H⁺	Cl⁻	HCO₃
Sweat	30–50	5	45–55	—	—
Gastric	40–65	0	90	100–140	—
Biliary	135–155	5	—	80–110	70–90
Pancreatic	135–155	5	—	55–75	70–90
Ileostomy	120–130	10	—	50–60	50–70
Diarrhea	25–50	35–60	—	20–40	30–45

ANSWER:
D

14. How many milliequivalents of chloride are in a liter of lactated Ringer's solution?

   A. 77 mEq

   B. 154 mEq

   C. 513 mEq

   D. 109 mEq

Ref.: 3

COMMENTS: Lactated Ringer's solution contains 130 mEq/L of sodium and 109 mEq/L of chloride. • It also contains 4 mEq/L of potassium, 3 mEq/L of calcium, and 28 mEq/L of lactate. • This is in contrast to 0.9% normal saline solution, which contains 154 mEq/L of both sodium and chloride. • Each fraction of 0.9% normal saline solution contains that fraction of sodium and chloride. • For example, half or 0.45% normal saline solution contains one half the 0.9% normal saline concentrations. • On the other hand, hypertonic 3% saline solution contains 513 mEq/L of both sodium and chloride, which is essentially a multiple of 3 times the normal saline concentration. • Five percent dextrose in water contains 50 g/L of glucose.

• Increasing percentages of dextrose in water contain concentrations of glucose that are multiples of 5% dextrose in water.

ANSWER:
D

15. With regard to distributional shifts during an operation, which of the following statements is/are true?

   A. The surface area of the peritoneum is not great enough to account for significant third-space loss.

   B. Sequestered extracellular fluid is predominantly isotonic.

   C. The formula for replacing intraoperative fluid loss follows strict guidelines based on body weight and serum sodium concentration.

   D. Third-space volume losses include evaporative loss from the open wound.

Ref.: 1, 2

COMMENTS: The functional extracellular fluid volume decreases during major abdominal operations largely as the result of sequestration of fluid in the operative site as a consequence of (1) extensive dissection, (2) fluid collection within the lumen and wall of the small bowel, and (3) accumulations of fluid in the peritoneal cavity. • The surface area of the peritoneum is 1.8 m². • When irritated, it can account for a functional loss of several liters of fluid that is not readily apparent. • It is generally agreed that this lost volume should be replaced during the course of an operation with isotonic saline solution as a "mimic" of sequestered extracellular fluid. • Although there is no set formula for intraoperative fluid therapy, useful guidelines for replacement include the following. • (1) Blood is replaced as it is lost, regardless of additional fluid therapy. • (2) Lost extracellular fluid should be replaced during the operative procedure; delay of replacement until after the operation is complicated by adrenal and hypophyseal compensatory mechanisms that respond to operative trauma during the immediate postoperative period. • (3) Approximately 0.5–1.0 L/hr of fluid is needed during the course of an operation, to a *maximum* of 2–3 L during a 4-hr procedure unless there are measurable losses.

ANSWER:
B

16. With regard to intraoperative management of fluids, which of the following statements is/are true?

   A. In a healthy person, up to 500 ml of blood loss may be well tolerated without the need for blood replacement.

   B. During an operation, the functional extracellular fluid volume is directly related to the volume lost to suction.

   C. Functional extracellular fluid losses should be replaced with plasma.

   D. Administration of albumin plays an important role in the replacement of functional extracellular fluid volume loss.

Ref.: 1, 2

COMMENTS: It is now believed that the addition of albumin to blood and extracellular fluid replacement intraoperatively is not indicated and may be potentially harmful. • Maintenance of cardiac and pulmonary function by replacing blood with blood products and extracellular fluid with "mimic" solutions can be obtained without the addition of albumin. • In general, it is believed that blood should be replaced as it is lost. • However, it is usually unnecessary to replace blood loss of less than 500 ml. • Operative blood loss is usually underestimated by the surgeon by 15–40% compared to the isotopically measured loss, a factor that may contribute to the detection of anemia during the immediate postoperative period. • There is an understandable hesitancy to perform transfusions unless absolutely necessary. • In cases involving rapid loss of large volumes of blood, there is not much room for debate. • In more controlled situations, careful clinical judgment is needed.

ANSWER:
A

17. With regard to postoperative fluid management, which of the following statements is/are not true?

   A. Insensible loss is approximately 600 ml/day.

   B. Insensible loss may increase to 1500 ml/day.

   C. About 800–1000 ml of fluid is needed to excrete the catabolic end products of metabolism.

   D. Lost urine should be replaced milliliter for milliliter.

   E. Lost gastrointestinal fluids should be replaced milliliter for milliliter.

Ref.: 1, 2

COMMENTS: Administration of fluids to the postoperative patient begins with an assessment of the patient's volume status and a check for concentration or compositional disorders. • Familiarity with the usual routes of fluid loss is of central importance. • All measured and insensible losses should be treated by replacement with appropriate fluids. • In patients with normal renal function, the amount of potassium given is 40 mEq/day for replacement of renal excretion. • An additional 20 mEq should be given for each liter of gastrointestinal loss. • Insensible water loss is usually constant in the range of 600 ml/day. • It can be increased to 1500 ml/day by hypermetabolism, hyperventilation, or fever. • Insensible loss is replaced with 5% dextrose in water. • Insensible loss may be offset by an insensible gain of water from excessive catabolism in postoperative patients who require prolonged intravenous fluid therapy. • Approximately 800–1000 ml/day of fluid is needed to excrete the catabolic end products of metabolism. • Because the kidneys are able to conserve sodium in a healthy individual, this amount can be replaced with 5% dextrose in water. • A small amount of salt is usually added, however, to relieve the kidneys of the stress of sodium resorption. • If there is a question regarding urinary sodium loss, measurement of urinary sodium levels helps determine the type of fluid that can best be used. • Urine volume should not be replaced milliliter for milliliter, because a high output may represent diuresis of fluids given during operation or the diuresis that takes place to eliminate excessive fluid administration. • Sensible or measurable losses such as those from the gastrointestinal tract are usually isotonic and therefore should be treated by replacement in equal volumes with isotonic salt solutions. • The type of salt solution selected depends on the determination of serum sodium, potassium, and chloride levels. • In general, replacement fluids are administered at a steady rate over 18–24 hr as losses are incurred.

ANSWER:
D

18. With regard to derangement of the serum sodium concentration, which of the following statements is/are true?

   A. Changes in serum sodium concentration usually produce changes in the status of the extracellular fluid volume.

B. The chloride ion is the main determinant of the osmolarity of the extracellular fluid space.

C. Extracellular hyponatremia leads to depletion of intracellular water.

D. Dry, sticky mucous membranes are characteristic of hyponatremia.

Ref.: 1, 2

COMMENTS: Whereas extracellular volume may change without a change in serum sodium concentration (as occurs after isotonic volume losses), changes in serum sodium concentration usually produce changes in extracellular fluid volume because the serum sodium concentration is the main determinant of the **osmolarity** of the extracellular fluid space. • Alterations in its concentration produce concomitant shifts in water volume. • Signs and symptoms of hyper- and hyponatremia generally are not present unless the changes are severe or the change in sodium concentration occurs rapidly.

Hyponatremia is caused by excessive intake of hypotonic fluids or salt losses that exceed water loss. • With hyponatremia, decreased extracellular osmolarity causes a shift of water *into* the intracellular compartment. • When this occurs, central nervous system symptoms caused by increased intracranial pressure develop, and tissue signs of excess water are noted. • The central nervous system symptoms include muscle twitching, hyperactive tendon reflexes, and, when the hyponatremia is severe, convulsions and hypertension. • Tissue signs include salivation, lacrimation, watery diarrhea, and "fingerprinting" of the skin. • When hyponatremia develops rapidly, signs and symptoms may appear at sodium concentrations of less than 130 mEq/L. • Chronic hyponatremia develops slowly, and patients may develop sodium levels as low as 120 mEq/L before becoming symptomatic. • Severe hyponatremia may be associated with the onset of irreversible oliguric renal failure. • Patients with a closed head injury are sensitive to even mild hyponatremia owing to increased intracellular water, which exacerbates the increased intracranial pressure associated with the head injury. • In symptomatic patients, the administration of hypertonic (3%) solutions of sodium salt may be indicated to correct the acute problem. • In less severe cases, free water restriction and judicious infusion of normal saline solution usually are sufficient.

Hypernatremia is the result of excessive free water loss or salt intake. • The central nervous system signs and symptoms associated with hypernatremia include restlessness, weakness, delirium, and maniacal behavior. • The tissue signs are characteristic and include dryness and stickiness of mucous membranes, decreased salivation and tear production, and redness and swelling of the tongue. • The body temperature is usually elevated, occasionally to a lethal level. • The treatment consists of water replacement.

ANSWER:
A

19. Which of the following does not contribute to the development of hypernatremia?

A. Excessive sweating

B. Hyperlipidemia

C. Lactulose

D. Glycosuria

E. Inadequate maintenance fluids

Ref.: 3

COMMENTS: Hypernatremia is less common than hyponatremia in postoperative patients and is a reflection of elevated serum osmolality and hypertonicity. • It is indicative of a deficiency of free water relative to the sodium concentration. • Decreased intake of water, increased losses of water, or increased intake of sodium are the main mechanisms responsible for the development of hypernatremia. • Loss of the thirst mechanism and the inability to access free water are mechanisms by which hypernatremia due to decreased intake of water can develop. • Excessive sweating and large evaporative losses are mechanisms of loss of free water. • Agents such as lactulose, sorbitol, and carbohydrate malabsorption can cause osmotic diarrhea, resulting in relative losses of hypotonic fluid. • Similarly, hyperglycemia causing glycosuria or diuresis in a catabolic patient excreting excess urea can also cause an osmotic diuresis. • Both hyperlipidemia and hyperproteinemia are responsible for an entity known as **pseudohyponatremia**, which occurs when excess lipids or proteins displace water and create a falsely measured hyponatremia.

ANSWER:
B

20. Which of the following conditions is not associated with hypernatremia?

A. Diabetes insipidus

B. Primary polydipsia *[hypo handwritten above "poly"]*

C. Stevens-Johnson syndrome

D. Chemotherapy for abdominal tumors

E. Enterocutaneous fistula

Ref.: 1

COMMENTS: Diabetes insipidus is characterized by the excretion of large volumes of dilute urine, which can lead to hypernatremia. • Patients with primary hypodipsia, a rare neurologic deficit of the thirst center, have an impaired or absent thirst response to an increase in extracellular tonicity. • Tumor or infection may be responsible for this defect. • Dermatologic conditions such as second-degree burns and exfoliative dermatitis can substantially increase transcutaneous water loss, resulting in the rapid onset of dehydration and hypernatremia. • Dehydration from vomiting, diarrhea, or uncompensated losses of hypotonic gastrointestinal fluid, such as occurs with fistulas or endoluminal tubes, may cause hypernatremia. • Patients treated with chemotherapy using vinca alkaloids typically develop tumor lysis syndrome, which is not associated with hypernatremia.

ANSWER:
D

21. In hospitalized patients, what is the commonest cause of hypovolemic hyponatremia?

A. Intravenous fluids

B. Head trauma

C. Diuretic administration

D. Decreased renal function

Ref.: 3

COMMENTS: Diuretic administration in hospitalized patients is the commonest cause of hypovolemic hyponatremia. • Thiazide diuretics are more frequently responsible for the development of this type of hyponatremia than are loop diuretics. • The reason for this is that the site of action of thiazide diuretics is the distal convoluting tubule, where the dilutional urinary capacity is blunted. • This hyponatremia is typically mild and asymptomatic, but occasionally it can be acute and severe, lasting more than 48 hr.

ANSWER:
C

22. Which of the following statements is/are true in the correction of euvolemic hypernatremia?

    A. Treatment of modest SIADH should include fluid restriction of 7–10 mL/kg/day.

    B. Lithium may be used to correct SIADH.

    C. Three percent or 5% hypertonic saline solution may be used in the correction of SIADH.

    D. Correction of chronic hypernatremia should be less than 10–15 mEq/L of sodium over 24 hr.

    Ref.: 1

COMMENTS: The rapid correction of symptomatic hypernatremia associated with volume deficit can be achieved by slow, cautious infusion of 5% dextrose in water. • However, this treatment can cause a rapid reduction in extracellular osmolarity. • If this reduction is too rapid, it may cause convulsions and coma. • It may therefore be safer to correct the hypernatremia and the volume deficit with half-strength sodium chloride or half-strength lactated Ringer's solution. • In the absence of significant volume deficit, hypervolemia may result with the judicious infusion of water. • When treating symptomatic hypernatremia, frequent clinical observation and determination of serum sodium concentrations are mandatory.

ANSWER:
D

23. Which of the following conditions does not predispose patients to hypervolemic hyponatremia?

    A. Congestive heart failure

    B. Nephrotic syndrome

    C. Cirrhosis

    D. Gastrointestinal fistula

    Ref.: 1

COMMENTS: Patients with edema and ascites secondary to congestive heart failure, nephrotic syndrome, or cirrhosis can develop hyponatremia despite having an expanded overall volume of extracellular water. • They develop an excess of sodium but an even greater proportional increase in water volume. • Their pathophysiologic condition entails an overall contracted intravascular volume, which stimulates the release of vasopressin from the hypothalamus centrally. • Peripherally, renal hypoperfusion contributes to water retention. • Fluid restriction is crucial to the treatment of this type of hyponatremia. • In severe hyponatremia, small volumes of hypertonic saline solution may be given. • Diuresis may be used but is usually unsuccessful. • Hemodialysis may be used in extreme circumstances of fluid excess.

ANSWER:
D

24. With regard to postoperative hypernatremia, which of the following statements is/are not true?

    A. Hypernatremia may indicate a deficit of total body water.

    B. It may be caused by a high protein intake.

    C. Replacement of lost water with isotonic salt solutions can produce hypernatremia.

    D. A common cause is excessive extrarenal water loss.

    Ref.: 1, 2

COMMENTS: Hypernatremia can easily be produced when renal function is normal. • In surgical patients, hypernatremia most commonly arises from excessive or unexpected water loss, although it may result from the replacement of lost water with salt-containing solutions. • Excessive extrarenal water loss is most often associated with loss of water from excessive sweating and failure to humidify the air used to ventilate patients with a tracheostomy. • Another cause of water loss is the presence of granulating surfaces, and this loss may be significant in burn patients. • Increased renal water loss results from hypoxic damage to the distal tubules and collecting ducts or from central nervous system injury, causing diabetes insipidus (loss of antidiuretic hormone). • High protein intake produces an osmotic load of urea, which necessitates secretion of large volumes of water. • This can be avoided by allowing an intake of 7 ml of water per gram of dietary protein. • Finally, isotonic salt solutions can produce hypernatremia if they are used to replace pure water loss.

ANSWER:
C   ?

25. A 30-year-old 70-kg woman has symptomatic hyponatremia. Her serum sodium level is 120 mEq/L (normal level, 140 mEq/L). What is her sodium deficit calculated to be?

    A. 500 mEq/L

    B. 600 mEq/L

    C. 700 mEq/L

    D. 800 mEq/L

    Ref.: 1

COMMENTS: Correction of concentration changes depends in part on whether the patient is symptomatic. • If symptomatic hypernatremia or hyponatremia is present, attention is focused on prompt correction of the concentration abnormality to the point that symptoms are relieved. • Then attention is shifted to correction of the associated volume abnormality. • The sodium deficiency in this patient is estimated by multiplying the sodium deficit (normal sodium concentration minus observed sodium concentration) by total body water in liters (60% of body weight in males and 50% of body weight in females). • For the patient in question, the calculation is as follows: total body water = 70 kg × 0.5 = 35 L. • Sodium deficit = (140 − 120 mEq/L) × 35 L = 700 mEq sodium chloride.

Initially, half the calculated amount of sodium is infused as 3% sodium chloride. • The infusion is given slowly. • Rapid infusion can be associated with symptomatic hypovolemia. • Rapid correction of hyponatremia can be associated with irreversible central nervous system injury (central pontine and extrapontine myelinolysis). • Once symptoms are alleviated, the patient should be reassessed before additional infusion of sodium salt is begun. • In cases of profound hyponatremia, a correction of no more than 12 mEq/L/24 hr should be achieved. • If the original problem was associated with a volume deficit, the remainder of the resuscitation can be accomplished with isotonic fluids (sodium chloride in the presence of alkalosis, and M/6 sodium lactate (6 molar) in the presence of acidosis). • Care must be taken in treating hyponatremia associated with volume excess. • In this setting, after symptoms are alleviated with a small volume of hypertonic saline solution, water restriction is the treatment of choice. • Infusion of hypertonic saline solution in this setting has the potential to further expand extracellular intravascular volume and is contraindicated for patients with severely compromised cardiac reserve. • In such a case, peritoneal dialysis or hemodialysis may be preferred for removing excess water.

ANSWER:
C

---

26. A postoperative patient has a serum sodium concentration of 125 mEq/L and a blood glucose level of 500 mg/dl (normal level, 100 mg/dl). What would the patient's serum sodium concentration be (assuming normal renal function and appropriate intraoperative fluid therapy) if the blood glucose level were normal?

    A. 120 mEq/L

    B. 122 mEq/L

    C. 137 mEq/L

    D. 142 mEq/L

Ref.: 1, 2

COMMENTS: As a general rule, each 100-mg/dl rise in the blood glucose level above normal is equivalent to a 1.6–3.0-mEq/L fall in the apparent serum sodium concentration. • For example, a patient has a blood glucose level of 500 mg/dl, or 400 mg/dl above normal. • This is equivalent to a 12-mEq/L change in the serum sodium level. • If this patient has a measured sodium concentration of 125 mEq/L, he actually has a sodium concentration of 137 mEq/L once the excess extracellular water has been eliminated.

ANSWER:
C

---

27. With regard to postoperative hyponatremia, which of the following statements is/are not true?

    A. It may easily occur when water is used to replace sodium-containing fluids or when the water given exceeds the water lost.

    B. In patients with head injury, hyponatremia despite adequate salt administration is usually caused by occult renal dysfunction.

    C. In oliguric patients, cellular catabolism with resultant metabolic acidosis increases cellular release of water and can contribute to hyponatremia.

    D. Hyperglycemia may be a cause of hyponatremia.

Ref.: 1, 2

COMMENTS: Abnormalities of sodium concentration usually do not occur during the postoperative period if the functional extracellular fluid volume has been adequately replaced during the operation. • The sodium concentration usually remains normal because the kidneys retain the ability to excrete moderate excesses of water and solute administered during the early postoperative period. • Hyponatremia does occur when water is given to replace lost sodium-containing fluids or when the amount of water given consistently exceeds the amount of water lost.

In patients with head injury, hyponatremia may develop despite adequate salt administration because of excessive secretion of antidiuretic hormone, with resultant increased water retention. *SIADH*

Patients with preexisting renal disease and loss of concentrating ability may elaborate urine with a high salt concentration. • This salt-wasting phenomenon is commonly encountered in elderly patients and often is not anticipated because the blood urea nitrogen and creatinine levels are within normal limits. • When there is doubt, determination of urine sodium concentration can help clarify the diagnosis.

Oliguria reduces the daily water requirement and can lead to hyponatremia if not anticipated.

Cellular catabolism in patients without adequate caloric intake can lead to the gain of significant quantities of water released from the tissues.

Hyperglycemia may produce a depressed serum sodium level by exerting an osmotic force in the extracellular compartment, thus diluting serum sodium levels.

ANSWER:
B

---

28. The onset of sepsis predisposes an elderly patient with adult-onset diabetes mellitus to all but which one of the following conditions?

    A. Hypokalemia

    B. Hyperkalemia

    C. Nonketotic hyperosmolar coma

    D. Hypophosphatemia

    E. Hyponatremia

Ref.: 1

COMMENTS: Elderly patients with adult-onset diabetes mellitus are at risk of developing nonketotic hyperosmolar coma during sepsis. • As a result of the development of a nonketotic hyperglycemic hyperosmolar state, hypokalemia and hyperglycemia also may occur. • The treatment of these patients should include a reduction in the glucose load provided and the administration of isotonic fluid. • Patients may also benefit from the administration of insulin. • Systemic bacterial sepsis also is often accompanied by a drop in serum sodium concentration, possibly due to interstitial or intracellular sequestration. • It is treated by withholding free water, restoring extracellular fluid volume, and treating the source of sepsis.

ANSWER:
B

---

29. Which one of the following medications is not capable of causing diabetes insipidus (DI)?

    A. Desmopressin

    B. Lithium

    C. Demeclocycline

    D. Amphotericin B

    E. Glyburide

Ref.: 1

COMMENTS: Diabetes insipidus is characterized by the production of large volumes of dilute urine and the risk of developing hypernatremia. • There are two types of DI, distinguished by pathophysiologic characteristics. • Central DI is an endocrine disorder related to attenuated or absent synthesis of vasopressin in the hypothalamus or release from the pituitary. • Nephrogenic DI is a defect of the nephron that impairs or prevents the activity of vasopressin. • Clinically, patients complain of polyuria and polydipsia. • Patients with central DI have decreased levels of vasopressin, whereas those with nephrogenic DI have increased levels of vasopressin.

Central DI typically is caused by neurosurgery of the brain or head trauma, although there are other causes. • Nephrogenic DI can be caused by an intrinsic renal pathologic condition, such as chronic ureteral obstruction, sickle cell nephropathy, or medullary cystic disease. • Medications, including lithium, glyburide, foscarnet, demeclocycline, methoxyflurane, and amphotericin B, can cause an acquired form of nephrogenic DI.

Patients with a sustained urine output of greater than 100 mL/hr who develop hypernatremia should be evaluated for DI with tests of urine and serum osmolality. • Dilute urine with an osmolality of less than 300 mOsm/L in a patient whose serum sodium concentration is greater than 150 mEq/L suggests a diagnosis of DI. • The diagnostic test to differentiate central DI from nephrogenic DI is the administration of antidiuretic hormone, which will slow urine output in patients with central DI. • The vasopressin analogue desmopressin, also known as DDAVP (1-desamino-8-D-arginine-vasopressin) is the preferred drug for central DI because it activates water absorption in the nephron without acting as a vasopressor. • Failure to produce urine flow after administration of DDAVP indicates nephrogenic DI.

ANSWER:
A

30. Which one of the following clinical signs or symptoms is not associated with serum sodium concentrations below 125 mEq/L?

   A. Headache

   B. Hallucinations

   C. Bradycardia

   D. Hypoventilation

   E. Hyperthermia

Ref.: 2, 3

COMMENTS: In most cases of symptomatic hyponatremia, the serum sodium concentration decreases below 125 mEq/L. • When the concentration falls below 125 mEq/L, clinical signs and symptoms may occur. • These include headache, nausea, lethargy, hallucinations, seizure, bradycardia, hypoventilation, and occasionally coma. • Hypothermia, not hyperthermia, occurs.

ANSWER:
E

31. With regard to potassium, which of the following statements is/are not true?

   A. Normal dietary intake of potassium is 50–100 mEq/day.

   B. In patients with normal renal function, most ingested potassium is excreted in the urine.

   C. More than 90% of potassium in the body is located in the extracellular compartment.

   D. Dangerous hyperkalemia (>6 mEq/L) is rarely encountered if renal function is normal.

Ref.: 1, 2

COMMENTS: The average daily dietary intake of potassium is 50–100 mEq. • In patients with normal renal function and normal serum potassium levels, most ingested potassium is excreted in the urine. • More than 90% of the body's potassium is within the intracellular compartment at a concentration of 150 mEq/L. • Although the total extracellular potassium concentration is only 50–70 mEq (4.5 mEq/L), this concentration is critical for cardiac and neuromuscular function. • Significant quantities of intracellular potassium are released in response to severe injury, surgical stress, acidosis, and a catabolic state. • However, dangerous hyperkalemia (>6 mEq/L) is rarely encountered if renal function is normal.

ANSWER:
C

32. Which of the following electrocardiographic findings is not associated with hyperkalemia?

   A. Peaked T waves

   B. Prolonged PR interval

   C. Loss of P wave

   D. Narrowing of QRS complex

Ref.: 1, 3

COMMENTS: The signs of hyperkalemia are generally limited to cardiovascular and gastrointestinal symptoms. • Gastrointestinal symptoms include nausea, vomiting, intermittent intestinal colic, and diarrhea. • Cardiovascular symptoms are electrocardiographic. • Peaked T waves and prolonged PR interval are characteristic early findings. • These electrocardiographic changes may be seen with potassium concentrations greater than 6 mEq/L. • At higher potassium concentrations, loss of P waves, slurring or widening of QRS complexes, and terminal broad ventricular tachycardia indicate impending arrhythmia or asystole.

ANSWER:
D

33. Which one of the following need not be administered or performed within 1 hr to prevent the complications of hyperkalemia?

   A. Calcium salts

   B. Sodium bicarbonate

   C. K$^+$-binding resins

   D. Glucose and insulin

   E. Hemodialysis

Ref.: 1–3

COMMENTS: Hyperkalemia becomes an emergency with the occurrence of lethal arrhythmias or asystole, its most feared complications. • It is crucial that administration of both intravenous and oral potassium-containing supplements be stopped immediately. • It is imperative that calcium salts be administered within minutes. • This measure stabilizes the cell membrane through antagonizing the adverse membrane potential effects of hyperkalemia. • Calcium gluconate and calcium chloride are effective calcium salts. • In addition, sodium bicarbonate is administered intravenously, since this action drives K^+ into the cells. • The administration of glucose followed by intravenous insulin also drives K^+ into the cells. • In cases of rapid and severe hyperkalemia, hemodialysis is the definitive and most rapid method of decreasing K^+ in the extracellular fluid. • The administration of K^+-binding resins, such as sodium polystyrene sulfonate (Kayexalate), within hours of the onset of acute hyperkalemia is effective. • Rectal administration of these binding resins is more effective than oral administration. • Kaliuresis through the administration of diuretics, such as acetazolamide, within hours of the onset of acute hyperkalemia is also effective.

ANSWER:
C

34. With regard to hypokalemia, which of the following statements is/are not true?

    A. Potassium is in competition with hydrogen ion for renal tubular excretion in exchange for sodium resorption.

    B. Tubular excretion of potassium may be increased when large quantities of sodium are available for resorption.

    C. Flattening of the T waves and suppression of the ST segments are characteristic electrocardiographic changes associated with hypokalemia.

    D. Intravenous administration of potassium may exceed 100 mEq/hr.

Ref.: 1, 2

COMMENTS: Surgical patients exhibit hypokalemia more frequently than hyperkalemia. • This hypokalemia is the result of excessive renal excretion, prolonged administration of potassium-free parenteral fluids, parenteral hyperalimentation with inadequate potassium replacement, and loss of gastrointestinal secretions. • Some acid-base disturbances, including respiratory and metabolic alkaloses, result in excess potassium excretion. • Potassium is in competition with hydrogen ion for renal tubular excretion in exchange for sodium. • With alkalosis, the potassium ion is preferentially excreted in an attempt to preserve the hydrogen ion. • Another setting leading to increased tubular excretion of potassium exists when there is a large quantity of sodium available for resorption from the renal tubule. • Potassium is exchanged for sodium, and the serum potassium levels fall. • The loss of gastrointestinal fluids can be a significant cause of potassium depletion. • This problem is compounded if potassium-free fluids are used for replacement.

Signs of potassium deficit are related to failure of contractility of skeletal, smooth, and cardiac muscle. • Such signs include paralytic ileus and diminishing or absent tendon reflexes or weakness that may progress to flaccid paralysis. • Sensitivity to digitalis and electrocardiographic signs of low voltage, such as flattening of the T waves and suppression of ST segments, are characteristic.

The best treatment for hypokalemia is prevention. • Gastrointestinal losses should be treated by replacement with fluids containing potassium in quantities sufficient to replace the daily obligatory loss (20 mEq/day) as well as the additional loss related to the volume of gastrointestinal drainage. • As general guidelines, no more than 40–60 mEq of potassium should be added to each liter of intravenous fluid; the rate of administration should never exceed 40–60 mEq/hr; the electrocardiogram should be monitored during infusion; and potassium administration to oliguric patients should be withheld during the first 24 hr after severe surgical stress or trauma.

ANSWER:
D

35. Approximately what percentage of calcium exists in the ionized form?

    A. 10%

    B. 25%

    C. 50%

    D. 75%

Ref.: 1–3

COMMENTS: The body contains approximately 1000–1200 g of calcium. • Most of it is in the bone in the form of calcium carbonate and calcium phosphate. • Normal daily intake of calcium is 1–3 g, most of which is excreted via the gastrointestinal tract, with 200 mg or less excreted in the urine. • Approximately half of the normal serum calcium level (9–11 mg/ml) is nonionized and bound to plasma protein. • An additional 5% of nonionized calcium is bound to other substances in the plasma. • The remaining 45% is ionized and is the portion responsible for neuromuscular stability. • It is therefore important to determine the plasma protein level when assessing serum calcium levels. • A drop of 1 g of protein results in a 0.8-mg/dl decrease in measured total serum calcium. • Conversely, the total serum calcium level *increases* by 0.8 mg/dl for every 1-g/dl increment of the serum albumin level above a normal value of 4 g/dl. • The ratio of ionized to nonionized calcium is affected by the pH. • Acidosis increases and alkalosis decreases the ionized fraction. • Routine administration of calcium to surgical patients is not required unless there is a specific indication to do so, such as skeletal loss of calcium, which results in hypocalcemia in patients subjected to prolonged immobilization.

ANSWER:
B

36. Which one of the following is not a complication of hypocalcemia?

    A. Seizures in children

    B. Painful muscle spasms

    C. Perioral or fingertip tingling

    D. Cardiac dysfunction with shortening of the ST segments

Ref.: 1–3

COMMENTS: The signs and symptoms of hypocalcemia generally are seen at serum levels of less than 8 mg/dl. • The symptoms include numbness and tingling of the circumoral area and in the tips of the fingers and toes. • The signs include hyperactive deep tendon reflexes, positive Chvostek's sign, Trousseau's sign, muscle and abdominal cramps, tetany with carpal pedal spasm, convulsions, and prolongation of the QT interval on the electrocardiogram. • Symptoms may appear with a normal serum calcium level in patients with severe alkalosis as the result of a decrease in the ionized fraction of the total serum calcium. • Conversely, hypocalcemia without signs or symptoms may be present in patients with hypoproteinemia and a normal ionized fraction. • Acute symptoms can be relieved by intravenous administration of calcium gluconate or calcium chloride. • Patients requiring prolonged replacement can be treated with oral calcium given with or without vitamin D.

ANSWER:
D

37. Which one of the following clinical scenarios is not associated with acute hypocalcemia?

    A. Fluid resuscitation from shock

    B. Rapid infusion of blood products

    C. Improper administration of phosphates

    D. Vitamin D–deficient diets

    E. Acute pancreatitis

Ref.: 1

COMMENTS: The infusion of large volumes of isotonic fluid during the resuscitation of shock is associated with a modest reduction in calcium to a range of 0.8–1.0 mmol/L. • There is also a concomitant decrease in magnesium, which can impair the actions of vitamin D and contribute to difficulty in correcting the hypocalcemia from resuscitation.

The administration of a citrate load during the rapid transfusion of blood products can lead to severe hypocalcemia, hypotension, and myocardial failure. • In this setting, calcium should be replaced at a dose of 0.2 g/500 ml of blood transfused. • It is believed that most patients receiving slow, elective blood transfusions do not require calcium supplementation.

Rapid increases in serum phosphate levels can develop after the improper administration or excessive dosing of phosphate-containing fluids or cathartics. • In general, the total calcium dose should not exceed 3 g unless obvious signs and symptoms of hypocalcemia are present.

The saponification of fat to free calcium with acute pancreatitis is also implicated as a cause of severe hypocalcemia. • Other common causes of hypocalcemia include, necrotizing fasciitis, renal failure, gastrointestinal fistula, and hypoparathyroidism. • (Because of atrophy of the remaining glands, hypocalcemia can also develop transiently in patients who have a parathyroid adenoma removed.) Under ideal circumstances, calcium replacement should be monitored by measuring the concentration of ionized calcium.

ANSWER:
D

38. Which one of the following disturbances is not associated with tumor lysis syndrome?

    A. Hypocalcemia

    B. Hyperphosphatemia

    C. Hypermagnesemia

    D. Hyperkalemia

    E. Hyperuricemia

Ref.: 1

COMMENTS: Tumor lysis syndrome is a condition of electrolyte abnormalities that occurs rapidly after antineoplastic therapy. • It is due to massive tumor cell death. • Hypocalcemia, hyperphosphatemia, hyperuricemia, and hyperkalemia occur. • The occurrence of hypermagnesemia has not been described in the literature. • Chemotherapy directed against solid tumors and lymphomas has been associated with tumor lysis syndrome. • Acute renal failure can occur in patients with this syndrome, and this occurrence prevents the spontaneous correction of the electrolyte abnormalities. • Emergency dialysis may be the only therapy that provides adequate correction.

ANSWER:
C

39. An asymptomatic patient who is evaluated in the physician's office is found to have a serum calcium level of 13.5 mg/dL. Which of the following medications should either be discontinued or not recommended?

    A. Bisphosphonates

    B. Thiazide diuretics

    C. Mithramycin

    D. Calcitonin

    E. Corticosteroids

Ref.: 1

COMMENTS: The symptoms of hypercalcemia arise from the gastrointestinal, renal, musculoskeletal, and central nervous systems. • Early symptoms include fatigability, lassitude, weakness, anorexia, nausea, and vomiting. • Central nervous system symptoms can progress to stupor and coma. • Other symptoms may include headaches and the three P's: **pain**, **polydipsia**, and **polyuria**. • The critical serum calcium level for hypercalcemia is 16–20 mg/ml. • Prompt treatment must be instituted at this level, or the symptoms may progress to death.

The two major causes of hypercalcemia are hyperparathyroidism and metastatic disease. • Metastatic breast cancer in patients receiving estrogen therapy is the commonest cause of hypercalcemia associated with metastases. • In many patients, there is an associated volume deficit due to vomiting and polyuria. • Rapid volume replacement with saline solution quickly lowers the calcium level by dilution and by increasing renal excretion of calcium (saline diuresis). • Renal clearance of calcium can be increased by giving furosemide.

Oral or intravenous phosphates are useful for reducing hypercalcemia by inhibiting bone resorption and forming calcium phosphate complexes that are deposited in the soft tissues. • Intravenous phosphorus, however, has been associated with acute development of hypocalcemia, hypotension, and renal failure. • For this reason, it should be given slowly over 8–12 hr once daily for no more than 2–3 days. • Intravenous sodium sulfate is effective, but no more so than saline diuresis. • Bisphosphonates reduce serum calcium levels by suppressing the function of osteoclasts and thus reducing the bone resorption of calcium. • With some malignant conditions such as breast cancer, bisphosphonates may be administered prophylactically to prevent hypercalcemia.

Mithramycin lowers serum calcium levels in 24–48 hr also by inhibiting bone resorption. • A single dose may maintain a normal serum calcium level for up to several weeks.

Calcitonin is a hormone produced by parafollicular cells of the thyroid gland and functions by inducing renal excretion of calcium and suppressing osteoclast bone resorption. • Calcitonin can produce a moderate decrease in serum sodium levels, but the effect is lost with repeated administration as long-term tachyphylaxis, possibly due to the development of antibodies.

Because corticosteroids decrease resorption of calcium from bone and reduce intestinal absorption, they are useful for treating patients with sarcoidosis, myeloma, lymphoma, or leukemia who have hypercalcemia. • Their effects, however, may not be apparent for 1–2 weeks.

Chelating agents, such as ethylenediaminetetraacetic acid (EDTA) are not indicated, since they are associated with complication of metastatic calcification, acute renal failure, and excessive hypocalcemia. • Thiazide diuretics are contraindicated because they are calcium-sparing diuretics and are often implicated as a cause of iatrogenic hypercalcemia. • Acute hypercalcemic crisis in hyperparathyroidism is treated by immediate corrective operation after the patient is stabilized to the point at which anesthesia can be safely administered.

A N S W E R :
B

40. With regard to magnesium, which of the following statements is/are true?

    A. The distribution of nonosseous magnesium is similar to that of sodium.

    B. Obligate renal loss is 15–20 mEq/day.

    C. Magnesium depletion is characterized by depression of the neuromuscular and central nervous systems.

    D. The treatment of choice for magnesium deficiency is the oral administration of magnesium phosphate.

Ref.: 1, 2

COMMENTS: The total body content of magnesium is 2000 mEq, half of which is in bone. • Of the remaining magnesium, most is intracellular (a distribution similar to that of potassium). • Plasma levels range between 1.5 and 2.5 mEq/L. • Normal dietary intake is 240 mg/day, most of which is excreted in the feces. • The kidneys excrete some magnesium and effectively conserve magnesium in the presence of deficiency, excreting less than 1 mEq/day if necessary.

Hypomagnesemia is characterized by neuromuscular and central nervous system hyperactivity, signs and symptoms similar to those of calcium deficiency. • Deficiency is known to occur with starvation, malabsorption, protracted loss of gastrointestinal fluid, and prolonged parenteral therapy without proper magnesium supplementation. • When there is an accompanying calcium deficiency, the latter cannot be successfully treated until the hypomagnesemia is corrected.

Magnesium deficiency is treated by parenteral administration of magnesium sulfate or magnesium chloride. • In a patient with normal renal function, up to 2 mEq of magnesium per kilogram of body weight can be given on a daily basis. • When large doses of magnesium are given, vital signs and the electrocardiogram should be monitored for signs of magnesium toxicity, which can lead to cardiac arrest (increased PR interval, widening QRS, and elevated T waves).

Magnesium toxicity is treated by infusion of calcium chloride or calcium gluconate. • In fact, these substances should be on hand when magnesium is administered intravenously to severely depleted patients. • In depleted states, the extracellular concentration can be rapidly restored, but therapy must be continued for 1–2 weeks to replenish the intracellular component.

To avoid the development of magnesium deficiency, patients on hyperalimentation should receive 12–24 mEq of magnesium daily. • Magnesium should not be given to oliguric patients unless magnesium depletion has been demonstrated. • Oral supplementation (800 mg/day of magnesium oxide) or intramuscular injection (of magnesium sulfate, which is very painful) are alternative routes for replacement but are not preferred.

A N S W E R :
B

41. An elderly alcoholic man who has seen a physician in the past only for renewal of his loop diuretic medications comes to the clinic with signs and symptoms of hypocalcemia. Measures are taken to correct the hypocalcemia without success. What electrolyte abnormality must be corrected in order to correct his hypocalcemia?

    A. Calcium

    B. Potassium

    C. Magnesium

    D. Sodium

Ref.: 1, 3

COMMENTS: Magnesium stores in the intracellular fluid become substantially depleted in patients with chronic diarrhea or prolonged aggressive diuretic therapy. • Magnesium deficiency is common in patients who have a heavy intake of ethanol. • Diabetic patients with a persistent osmotic diuresis from glucosuria commonly have hypomagnesemia.

Correction is accomplished by intravenous administration of magnesium sulfate. • Correction of severe hypomagnesemia requires sustained therapy because equilibration of extracellular magnesium with intracellular stores is slow. • Commonly, the magnitude of magnesium deficiency parallels the magnitude of hypocalcemia. • Hypocalcemia in patients with magnesium deficiency is resistant to calcium replacement alone, and these patients should concurrently receive magnesium.

A N S W E R :
C

42. With regard to hypermagnesemia, which of the following statements is/are not true?

    A. It is most commonly seen in patients with severe renal insufficiency.

    B. It occasionally occurs in patients with severe alkalosis.

    C. The acute symptoms can be controlled by intravenous administration of calcium chloride or calcium gluconate.

    D. Persistent symptoms may be an indication for dialysis.

Ref.: 1, 2

COMMENTS: Symptomatic hypermagnesemia is most commonly seen in patients with severe renal insufficiency. • The serum magnesium levels tend to *parallel* changes in *potassium* concentration in such cases. • Because the use of magnesium-containing antacids and laxatives can produce symptomatic hypermagnesemia in patients with impaired renal function, these drugs should be avoided. • Other causes of symptomatic hypermagnesemia include burns, massive trauma, surgical stress, severe extracellular volume deficit, and severe acidosis.

The signs and symptoms include lethargy, weakness, and progressive loss of deep tendon reflexes. • The electrocardiographic changes resemble those seen with hyperkalemia. • In extreme cases, somnolence leading to coma and muscular paralysis may occur.

Treatment is aimed at correcting any existing acidosis, restoring depleted extracellular volume deficit, and withholding exogenous magnesium. • Acute symptoms can be controlled temporarily by the infusion of 5–10 mEq of calcium chloride or calcium gluconate. • If elevated levels of magnesium or the symptoms persist, peritoneal dialysis or hemodialysis may be required.

A N S W E R :
B

43. With regard to the acid-base buffering system of the extracellular fluid, which of the following statements is/are not true?

   A. The bicarbonate-carbonic acid system is the primary intracellular buffering system.

   B. The base bicarbonate/carbonic acid ratio determines the extracellular fluid pH.

   C. The functions of the extracellular buffering system are expressed in the Henderson-Hasselbalch equation.

   D. A bicarbonate/carbonic acid ratio of 20:1 is associated with a normal pH (7.4).

   Ref.: 1, 2

COMMENTS: Assessment of complex acid-base disorders requires an understanding of the given clinical situation and of acid-base physiology. • Important intracellular buffers include proteins and phosphates. • The bicarbonate-carbonic acid system is the primary extracellular buffering system. • In extracellular fluids, acids (inorganic acids, such as hydrochloric, sulfuric, or phosphoric acids, and organic acids, such as lactic, pyruvic, and keto acids) combine with sodium bicarbonate to form the sodium salt of the acid and carbonic acid. • Carbonic acid then dissociates into water and carbon dioxide. • In equation form, this interaction is as follows:

$$HCl + NaHCO_3 \leftrightarrows NaCl + H_2CO_3 \leftrightarrows H_2O + CO_2$$

ANSWER:
A

44. Intracellular buffering is dependent on which system?

   A. Ammonia buffer system

   B. Bicarbonate buffer system

   C. Citrate buffer system

   D. Phosphate buffer system

   Ref.: 1

COMMENTS: Buffering of intracellular fluid, in which the concentration of protons is 80–100 nmol/L, depends primarily on the phosphate buffer system. • The dibasic phosphate converts to a monobasic phosphate with the addition of a proton, and 33% of intracellular phosphate is in the monovalent form of $H_2PO_4^-$. • This buffer system enables the stabilization of cytosolic pH when there are sudden alterations in metabolism, such as occur during a hypoxic insult and rapid H^+ ion increase. • In addition to the phosphate buffer system, there are buffers within cells in the form of proton-binding sites on constitutive molecules such as proteins. • As the number of H^+ ions bound to proteins increases, the function of the proteins is altered.

The bicarbonate buffer system functions primarily in the extracellular fluid environment. Carbonic acid is a prime physiologic buffer because it has the capacity to convert to either a water-soluble buffer (bicarbonate) or a volatile gas (carbon dioxide). The kidneys function to adjust bicarbonate concentrations in blood by determining the proton concentration in excreted urine. The lungs function to extract and exhale CO_2 from the blood in the pulmonary capillaries during respiration.

ANSWER:
D

45. Which of the following is not one of the direct major stimuli for bicarbonate reabsorption in patients with normal renal function?

   A. Lactic acidosis

   B. Arterial volume depletion

   C. Mineralocorticoid excess

   D. Hypokalemia

   Ref.: 3

COMMENTS: Volume loss from within the arterial component increases proximal tubular reabsorption of bicarbonate. • Mineralocorticoids increase distal tubular acid excretion. • However, this contributes to the development of hypokalemia. • Hypokalemia, in turn, stimulates the increased reabsorption of bicarbonate while also increasing distal acid secretion. • Lactic acidosis does not directly enhance bicarbonate reabsorption but, on the contrary, may function to consume bicarbonate as a result of the bicarbonate buffering effect (i.e., titration of lactic acid).

ANSWER:
A

46. With regard to metabolic alkalosis, which of the following statements is/are not true?

   A. Metabolic alkalosis results from the loss of fixed acids or the gain of bicarbonate.

   B. Compensation is mainly renal.

   C. A common cause is prolonged nasogastric suctioning.

   D. Hydrochloric acid infusion to correct this disturbance is no longer used because of the high incidence of arrhythmias.

   Ref.: 1, 2

COMMENTS: Metabolic alkalosis results from the loss of fixed acids (as with prolonged nasogastric suction of an obstructed stomach) or the gain of bicarbonate (as occurs when renal tubular damage prevents its normal excretion). • Loss of acid or gain of bicarbonate leads to a relative increase in the numerator of the Henderson-Hasselbalch equation, an increase in the 20:1 ratio, and a rise in pH. • Compensation is mainly renal and occurs through the same mechanisms discussed for respiratory alkalosis. • With alkalosis, avoidance of hypokalemia is important. • Occasionally, a component of respiratory compensation leads to hypercarbia.

ANSWER:
D

47. With regard to metabolic acidosis, which of the following statements is/are true?

   A. The acute compensation for metabolic acidosis is primarily renal.

   B. Metabolic acidosis results from the loss of bicarbonate or the gain of fixed acids.

   C. The commonest cause of acid excess is prolonged nasogastric suction.

   D. Restoration of blood pressure with vasopressors corrects the metabolic acidosis associated with circulatory failure.

   Ref.: 1, 2

COMMENTS: Metabolic acidosis has several causes. • It results from retention or gain of fixed acids (e.g., through diabetic acidosis or lactic acidosis) or the loss of bicarbonate (e.g., through diarrhea, small bowel fistula, or renal tubular dysfunction). • Increased acid consumes bicarbonate, thereby lowering the numerator of the Henderson-Hasselbalch ratio and lowering the pH. • Bicarbonate loss causes the same change. • Initial compensation is respiratory (hyperventilation), which lowers carbonic acid concentration, decreasing the denominator and restoring the 20:1 ratio. • Renal compensation is slower and occurs through the same means as the renal compensation for respiratory acidosis: excretion of acid salts and retention of bicarbonate. • This compensation depends on normal renal function. • When kidney damage interferes with the ability to excrete acid and resorb bicarbonate, metabolic acidosis may rapidly progress to profound levels. • The commonest cause of metabolic acidosis in surgical patients is circulatory failure, with accumulation of lactic acid, resulting from tissue hypoxia and anaerobic metabolism.

Resuscitation with vasopressors or infusion of bicarbonate does not correct the underlying problem. • Volume replacement with a balanced electrolyte solution, blood, or both results in restoration of the circulation, hepatic clearance of lactate, consumption of the formed bicarbonate, and clearance of carbonic acid by the lung. • The excessive use of bicarbonate for resuscitation of patients can lead to severe metabolic alkalosis, which, in association with other possible sequelae, such as hypothermia and low levels of 2,3-diphosphoglycerate in banked blood, shifts the oxygen-hemoglobin distribution curve to the left, compromising oxygen delivery.

Acidosis resulting from circulatory arrest is well tolerated if the patient is well ventilated and has not previously been acidotic. • The use of excessive bicarbonate in such situations may induce a hypernatremic, hyperosmotic state. • It is therefore recommended that the initial dose of bicarbonate not exceed 50 ml of a 7.5% solution and that administration of additional doses be based on results of serial blood gas analysis.

ANSWER:
B

48. A 70-kg man with pyloric obstruction resulting from ulcer disease is admitted to the hospital for resuscitation after 1 week of prolonged vomiting. What metabolic disturbance is expected to occur?

A. Hypokalemic hyperchloremic metabolic acidosis

B. Hyperkalemic hypochloremic metabolic alkalosis

C. Hyperkalemic hyperchloremic metabolic acidosis

D. Hypokalemic hypochloremic metabolic alkalosis

Ref.: 1, 2

COMMENTS: A common problem seen in patients with persistent emesis in the presence of an obstructive pylorus is hypokalemic, hypochloremic metabolic alkalosis. • To compensate for the alkalosis associated with the loss of chloride and hydrogen ion–rich fluid from the stomach, there is increased bicarbonate excretion in the urine. • The bicarbonate usually is excreted as the sodium salt, but, in an attempt to conserve intravascular volume, aldosterone-mediated sodium absorption occurs, accompanied by potassium and hydrogen excretion, compounding the alkalosis and leading to a paradoxical aciduria. • The management of this derangement includes resuscitation with isotonic saline solutions and aggressive replacement of lost potassium.

ANSWER:
D

49. The same patient referred to in Question 48 is found to have a serum chloride level of 80 mEq/L (normal level, 103 mEq/L). What is his chloride deficit?

A. 23 mEq/L

B. 183 mEq/L

C. 640 mEq/L

D. 322 mEq/L

Ref.: 1, 2

COMMENTS: Severe metabolic alkalosis (such as that caused by renal or liver failure) may respond to infusions of dilute hydrochloride formulated by the addition of 150 ml of a 0.1 N hydrochloride solution in 1 L of normal saline solution or 5% dextrose in water. • When formulated with the use of normal saline solution, the additional chloride in the saline solution must be taken into account. • Such a solution (with 5% dextrose in water) yields 300 mEq of hydrogen and chloride ions and is infused over a 6- to 24-hr period, with measurement of the pH, PCO_2, and electrolytes every 4-6 hr. • To determine the volume of solution that should be infused, the **chloride deficit** can be calculated using the plasma chloride concentration and the presumed volume in which the chloride is dispersed (a volume equal to 20% of body weight). • For a 70-kg man with a serum chloride level of 80 mEq/L (normal level, 103 mEq), the deficit would be 20% of body weight $\times$ (normal chloride level − observed plasma chloride level), which equals $(0.2 \times 70) \times (103 - 80) = 322$ mEq.

ANSWER:
D

50. With regard to respiratory acidosis and alkalosis, which of the following statements is/are not true?

A. Respiratory acidosis is associated with an increased denominator in the Henderson-Hasselbalch ratio due to CO_2 retention, resulting in a ratio of less than 20:1.

B. Respiratory alkalosis is associated with a decreased denominator in the Henderson-Hasselbalch ratio due to loss of CO_2, resulting in a ratio of more than 20:1.

C. Compensation for respiratory acidosis is primarily renal.

D. Compensation for respiratory alkalosis is primarily pulmonary.

Ref.: 1, 2

COMMENTS: The four types of acid-base disturbances are respiratory acidosis, respiratory alkalosis, metabolic acidosis, and metabolic alkalosis. • **Respiratory acidosis** is a result of CO_2 retention secondary to decreased alveolar ventilation. • It leads to increased carbonic acid production, which in turn increases the denominator of the Henderson-Hasselbalch ratio. • This lowers the 20:1 ratio, and the pH falls.

Acute forms of this problem in previously healthy individuals can be corrected by restoring alveolar ventilation to normal values, such as by reversing central nervous system depression, removing mechanical airway obstruction, or increasing the rate of mechanical ventilation. • Compensation for chronic forms of decreased alveolar ventilation occurs in the kidney, in which increased resorption of bicarbonate occurs. • The reabsorbed bicarbonate raises the numerator, thus restoring the 20:1 ratio and raising the pH to a normal value. • In this compensated form, the plasma bicarbonate level is *higher* than in the normal, noncompensated state.

Respiratory alkalosis is caused by excessive loss of CO_2 secondary to increased alveolar ventilation. • It is characterized by a fall in arterial CO_2 pressure (PCO_2) and a rise in pH. • Carbonic acid production falls, lowering the denominator of the Henderson-Hasselbalch ratio, and the 20:1 ratio increases, leading to increased pH. • Renal compensation occurs when acid is *reabsorbed* in exchange for increased bicarbonate excretion. • The renal excretion of bicarbonate lowers the numerator, restores the 20:1 ratio, and brings the pH back down to 7.4. • In the acute phase of respiratory alkalosis, pH is elevated, PCO_2 falls, and the bicarbonate level may be normal. • In the compensated phase, pH normalizes, and the bicarbonate concentration falls and is *lower* than normal.

Of central importance when dealing with alkalosis is the avoidance of hypokalemia. • Potassium is in competition with hydrogen ions for resorption of sodium bicarbonate at the level of the renal tubule. • With alkalosis (where there is a relative lack of hydrogen ions), preferential excretion of potassium in exchange for sodium occurs at the level of the distal convoluted tubule. • Also, hypokalemia itself may contribute to alkalosis, because in hypokalemic states hydrogen ion rather than potassium is, by necessity, excreted for sodium resorption. • An additional factor in the development of hypokalemia in alkalotic states is the exchange of extracellular potassium for intracellular hydrogen ions (these changes are more pronounced for metabolic alkalosis than they are for respiratory alkalosis).

Part of the treatment for alkalosis—whether it be respiratory, metabolic, or a combination of the two—is adequate potassium replacement. • Adjusting the ventilatory rate and volume and adding dead space to the ventilation circuit are methods used to avoid respiratory alkalosis. • Adding 5% CO_2 to inspired air is poorly tolerated and not used.

ANSWER:
D

51. With regard to metabolic acidosis and alkalosis, which of the following statements is/are not true?

   A. Metabolic acidosis results from retention of fixed acid or a loss of bicarbonate, which causes a fall in the numerator of the Henderson-Hasselbalch ratio, leading to a ratio less than 20:1.

   B. Metabolic alkalosis results from loss of fixed acid or gain of bicarbonate, causing an increase in the numerator of the Henderson-Hasselbalch ratio and leading to a ratio greater than 20:1.

   C. With metabolic acidosis or alkalosis, rapid compensation is brought about by pulmonary mechanisms.

   D. With metabolic acidosis or alkalosis, slow compensation occurs via pulmonary mechanisms.

Ref.: 1, 2

COMMENTS: The major effects of metabolic acid-base derangements are exerted on the numerator of the Henderson-Hasselbalch ratio. • **Metabolic acidosis** due to retention of fixed acid or loss of bicarbonate causes a fall in the numerator relative to the denominator, a ratio less than 20:1, and a fall in pH. • **Metabolic alkalosis** results from a loss of fixed acid or a gain of bicarbonate, which causes a relative increase in the numerator of the Henderson-Hasselbalch ratio and produces a ratio greater than 20:1, with an associated rise in pH. • Rapid compensation for metabolic acid-base disturbances is provided via pulmonary mechanisms. • Increased ventilation compensates for metabolic acidosis, and decreased ventilation compensates for metabolic alkalosis. • In both instances, slow compensation occurs via renal mechanisms, as for respiratory acidosis and respiratory alkalosis.

ANSWER:
D

REFERENCES

1. Townsend CM, Beauchamp RD, Evers BM, et al (eds): Sabiston Textbook of Surgery, The Biological Basis of Modern Surgical Practice, 17th ed. Saunders, Philadelphia, 2004.
2. Brunicardi FC, Andersen DK, Billiar TR, et al (eds): Schwartz's Principles of Surgery, 8th ed. McGraw-Hill, New York, 2004.
3. O'Leary JP: *Physiologic Basis of Surgery*, 4th ed. Lippincott, Williams & Wilkins, Philadelphia, 2003.

CHAPTER 3

Endocrine and Metabolic Response to Injury

Roderick M. Quiros, M.D., and Richard A. Prinz, M.D.

1. The metabolic rate increases by what percentage for each 1°C elevation in body temperature?

   A. 1%

   B. 5%

   C. 10%

   D. 15%

   E. 20%

Ref.: 1–3

COMMENTS: In septic patients, O_2 consumption is typically elevated. • The presence of infection causes a rise in the metabolic rate, due in part to fever, which is often present. • The Q10 effect states that the metabolic rate increases by 10% for each elevation of 1°C in central temperature.

ANSWER:
C

2. Which of the following is the most important stimulus for triggering the endocrine response after injury?

   A. Afferent nerve stimuli from the injured area

   B. Hypovolemia

   C. Tissue acidosis

   D. Local wound factors

   E. Temperature changes

Ref.: 1–3

COMMENTS: The response to injury involves an integrated series of endocrine and metabolic changes designed to maintain homeostasis. • A variety of stimuli are involved in triggering these responses. • Of these, one of the earliest and most important stimuli is the signal carried by the afferent sensory nerves from the injured area. • This signal directly stimulates release of adrenocorticotropic hormone (ACTH), which begins the adrenocortical response to injury, and elaboration of arginine vasopressin (AVP), formerly called antidiuretic hormone (ADH). • ACTH is synthesized and stored in the chromophobe cells of the anterior pituitary. • Its release is stimulated by corticotropin-releasing factor (CRF) from the paraventricular nucleus of the hypothalamus. • CRF release

is induced by the neurogenic inputs (afferent nerve stimuli) generated by injury. • This hormonal response can be ablated experimentally by division of the peripheral nerves to the injured area, and it may be diminished clinically in patients with spinal anesthesia. • It is for this reason that paraplegic patients show a diminished corticosteroid response to injuries below the level of cord transection. • Perception of injury need not be conscious. • Individuals under general anesthesia are able to respond to stimuli present during injury.

ANSWER:
A

3. In addition to decreased effective circulatory volume, which of the following can stimulate the reflexes associated with injury?

   A. Oxygen, carbon dioxide, and hydrogen ion concentration

   B. Emotional arousal

   C. Hypoglycemia

   D. Alteration in body temperature

   E. Local response to wounds

Ref.: 1, 2, 3

COMMENTS: Although nearly all injuries are associated with loss of effective circulatory volume, which initiates the events previously discussed, stimuli other than hypovolemia and pain are capable of initiating many of the reflexes associated with injury. • Hypoxemia, hypercarbia, and acidosis are events sensed by chemoreceptors located in the carotid and aortic bodies. • Activation of these receptors stimulates the hypothalamus and sympathetic nervous system and inhibits the parasympathetic nervous system, resulting in tachycardia and increased cardiac contractility. • The respiratory rate increases, and ACTH and AVP release is stimulated. • Hypoxemia potentiates the response to hypovolemia, and hyperventilation often accompanies these events. • The perception or threat of possible injury, acting via the limbic system, affects the hypothalamus and stimulates secretion of injury-related hormones such as AVP, ACTH, cortisol, catecholamines, and aldosterone. • Hypoglycemia acting via central and autonomic pathways stimulates the release of these same injury-related hormones. • The inflammatory cells that accumulate and become activated in the environment around wounds can exert systemic effects that can stimulate neurohormonal responses such as those described above. • Exotoxin (from gram-positive bacteria) and endotoxin (from gram-negative bacteria) can activate such substances as interleukin-1 (IL-1) and tissue necrosis factor (TNF) and can stimulate the release of ACTH.

A N S W E R :

A, B, C, D, E

---

4. Match the items in the left-hand column with the appropriate items in the right-hand column.

Area	**Activity**
A. Posterior hypothalamic area	a. Controls ACTH and sympathetic activity
B. Paraventricular nucleus	b. Controls AVP, oxytocin, and ACTH
C. Ventromedial nucleus	c. Controls growth hormone and ACTH
D. Arcuate nucleus	d. Controls gonadotropin-releasing hormones
E. Supraoptic nucleus	e. Controls AVP and oxytocin
F. Superchiasmic nucleus	f. Controls circadian rhythms of ACTH and gonadotropins

Ref.: 1–3

COMMENTS: The afferent impulses stimulated by injury act via input into various hypothalamic nuclei (refer to Question 2). • The response to injury is variable and depends on the type of injury, its duration, and its severity. • It is not an all-or-none phenomenon, and physiologic potentiation is common. • An example of this potentiation is baroreceptor responsiveness to hypovolemia. • Hypovolemia increases baroreceptor responsiveness, which initiates catecholamine release. • Catecholamines, in turn, increase baroreceptor responsiveness.

A N S W E R :

A-a; B-b; C-c; D-d; E-e; F-f

---

5. True or false: The "fight or flight" response described by W. B. Cannon is a sympathetic event mediated by catecholamines.

Ref.: 1–3

COMMENTS: The "fight or flight" response to danger or pain is an event mediated primarily by the sympathetic nervous system and catecholamines. • It includes sweating, tremor, tachycardia, dry mouth, and pallor. • This response contrasts with the vasovagal response, mediated by the parasympathetic nervous system, which includes bradycardia and increased salivation.

A N S W E R :

True

---

6. Which of the following statements regarding the mediators of the response to injury is/are true?

A. Steroid hormones interact only with cell-surface receptors.

B. Peptide and amine hormones originally bind to cytosolic receptors in target cells.

C. The action of steroid hormones is faster and of shorter duration than the action of peptide hormones.

D. Peptide hormones act primarily via the second messenger system.

E. Cyclic adenosine monophosphate (cAMP) and calcium are the second messengers.

Ref.: 1, 2, 3

COMMENTS: See Question 7.

---

7. True or false: G proteins bind steroid hormones to the nuclear envelope.

Ref.: 1, 2, 3

COMMENTS: Steroid hormones bind to cytosolic receptors. • The receptor-steroid complex passes to the nucleus, where it binds to the nonhistone protein of nuclear chromatin, whereby it modulates the transcription of specific messenger RNA and ultimately the synthesis of effector proteins. • This process accounts for the 1- to 2-hr delay in the onset of action for most steroid hormones. • Peptide hormones, in contrast, bind to cell-surface receptors coupled to guanine nucleotide-binding proteins (G proteins), causing alteration in the intracellular concentration of either cAMP or calcium, the so-called second messengers. • Their onset of action is faster and of shorter duration than that of steroid hormones. • The second messengers activate or inactivate existing regulatory proteins and enzymes rather than initiate the synthesis of new proteins. • G proteins coupled to adenylate cyclase increase cAMP. • G proteins coupled to phospholipase C produce either diacylglycerol (DAG) or inositol triphosphate (IP_3). • DAG activates protein kinase C, which in turn opens membrane calcium channels. • IP_3 acts on the endoplasmic reticulum to release intracellular calcium. • The free calcium binds to calmodulin, a calcium-binding protein that activates phosphorylase kinase, the final step in activating the target enzyme. • The actions of cAMP and Ca^{2+} in the coupling of receptor activation with hormonal action is known as stimulus-response coupling.

A N S W E R S :

Question 6: D, E
Question 7: False

---

8. Which of the following statements regarding catecholamines is/are true?

A. Catecholamine levels increase immediately after injury.

B. Catecholamine levels peak 24–48 hr after injury.

C. Epinephrine generally reflects the activity of the sympathetic nervous system.

D. Norepinephrine generally reflects the activity of the adrenal medulla.

Ref.: 1–3

COMMENTS: Catecholamines include norepinephrine and epinephrine. • Norepinephrine is released from sympathetic postganglionic neurons. • Epinephrine is secreted by the adrenal medulla as a hormone acting at local and distant sites. • The effects of catecholamines differ according to target-cell receptor types. • Plasma catecholamine levels after injury are correlated most closely with the volume of blood lost. • A considerable psychological component affects these levels, depending on the mechanisms of injury. • Levels rise immediately and peak within 24–48 hr. • In general, changes in norepinephrine reflect changes in the activity of the sympathetic nervous system, whereas changes in epinephrine reflect the activity of the adrenal medulla. • The actions of these substances, mediated by α- and β-adrenergic receptors, are primarily metabolic and hemodynamic. • Epinephrine plays a major role in stress-induced hyperglycemia by increasing glucose production in the liver and decreasing glucose uptake in the periphery. • Epinephrine and norepinephrine cause increased secretion of glucagon (from pancreatic alpha islet cells) and decreased secretion of insulin (from pancreatic beta islet cells). • Hemodynamic effects include α_1-mediated vasoconstriction, β_2-mediated arterial vasodilatation, and β_1 receptor-mediated increases in heart rate, conductivity, and contractility. • The effects are dose dependent. • Those of low-dose epinephrine are primarily β_1 and β_2 mediated, whereas those of high-dose epinephrine are primarily α_1-mediated.

ANSWER:
A, B

9. Which of the following statements regarding the ebb phase after injury is/are true?

   A. It usually lasts 12–24 hr.

   B. Blood pressure, body temperature, and O_2 consumption are reduced.

   C. Hypermetabolism occurs.

   D. Cardiac output is increased as a compensatory mechanism.

   Ref.: 1–3

COMMENTS: The ebb phase, as described by D.P. Cuthbertson in the 1930s, occurs immediately after injury and is typically brief, lasting no more than 12–24 hours. • Blood pressure, cardiac output, body temperature, enzymatic activity, and oxygen consumption are reduced. • Cardiac output and core temperature are reduced, and lactic acidosis may be present. • The ebb phase is often associated with hemorrhage and resultant hypoperfusion and is thought to be a mechanism for preserving blood volume.

The flow phase is broken down into two phases: catabolic and anabolic. • During the catabolic phase, which occurs 3–10 days after injury, body temperature increases and a negative nitrogen balance ensues. • These effects are thought to occur as the body attempts to maintain energy. • During the anabolic phase, which occurs 10–60 days after injury, a positive nitrogen balance reflects the organism's replacement of lost tissue. • The flow phase is characterized by hypermetabolism, increased cardiac output and oxygen consumption, normalization of acidosis, and increased glucose production.

ANSWER:
A, B

10. Changes in glucose metabolism in the flow phase after stress or injury include which of the following?

    A. Hyperglycemia

    B. Hypoglycemia

    C. Increased insulin activity

    D. Increased insulin concentration

    E. Increased glucose uptake by the liver in response to insulin

    Ref.: 1–3

COMMENTS: In the ebb phase, elevation in blood glucose levels may parallel the degree of stress or injury. • Insulin levels are low, with normal to slightly elevated glucose production. • During the flow phase, insulin levels are often elevated, although hyperglycemia may persist or worsen despite the elevation. • This effect is thought to result from alterations in tissue sensitivity to insulin,

effectively leading to insulin resistance. • The elevation in blood glucose level is also maintained by glucagon, cortisol, and catecholamines because of their effects on hepatocytes and skeletal muscle cells, increasing glycogen breakdown and gluconeogenesis in these cells.

ANSWER:
A, D

11. Which of the following statements regarding the flow phase after injury is/are true?

    A. Hypoglycemia results as tissues deplete blood glucose stores.

    B. Glucagon breaks down glycogen stores.

    C. Hepatocytes produce glucose (gluconeogenesis).

    D. Fat breakdown occurs as a result of catecholamine stimulation.

    E. Growth hormone levels are elevated.

    F. Thyroid hormone levels are elevated.

    Ref.: 1–3

COMMENTS: With the onset of the flow phase, a hypermetabolic state ensues. • Glucagon levels are increased, with glycogenolytic and gluconeogenic effects on the liver. • Hepatocytes are thus stimulated to produce glucose. • Cortisol mobilizes amino acids from skeletal muscle to serve as gluconeogenic precursors for liver glucose production. • Catecholamines stimulate hepatic glycolysis and gluconeogenesis, increase lactate formation in skeletal muscle, increase the metabolic rate, and increase lipolysis. • Growth hormone levels are elevated despite the hyperglycemic state, and thyroid hormone levels are reduced to low or normal concentrations.

ANSWER:
B, C, D, E

12. Levels of which of the following substances is/are elevated during the acute response to injury?

    A. Glucagon

    B. Glucocorticoids

    C. Catecholamines

    D. Insulin

    E. Thyroid-stimulating hormone (TSH)

    Ref.: 1–3

COMMENTS: After injury, pain and hypovolemia are the primary stimuli that produce the subsequent neurohormonal events aimed at restoring hemodynamic stability and providing readily available energy substrates. • Direct stimulation of the hypothalamic-pituitary axis results in prompt increases in circulating ACTH, cortisol, AVP, and growth hormone. • Hypothalamic signals also result in sympathetic autonomic nerve stimulation that leads to the release of epinephrine and norepinephrine from the adrenal medulla and the sympathetic nerve endings themselves.

The catecholamines modulate the secretion of glucagon (from pancreatic alpha islet cells) and insulin (from pancreatic beta islet cells) via α- and β-adrenergic receptor stimulation (not related to the "alpha" and "beta" designation for islet cells). • α-Adrenergic receptors mediate inhibition, whereas β-adrenergic receptors mediate stimulation of glucagon and insulin secretion. • The alpha islet cell (the source of glucagon) is relatively rich in β-adrenergic (stimulatory) receptors. • Therefore, the predominant response to adrenergic stimulation is glucagon secretion. • The beta islet cell (the source of insulin) is relatively rich in α-adrenergic (inhibitory) receptors, and its response to adrenergic stimulation is inhibition of insulin secretion. • This inhibition is one reason why the hyperglycemia observed with acute injury does not elicit a reflex insulin response. • Elevated TSH levels are not thought to play an important role in the acute response to injury.

A N S W E R :
A, B, C

13. True or false: The neuroendocrine changes initiated by a loss of blood volume are proportional to the magnitude of the volume loss.

Ref.: 1–3

COMMENTS: The neuroendocrine and cardiovascular changes in response to volume loss are proportional to the magnitude of the loss. • Maximal response, however, is achieved when the volume is decreased by 30–40%.

A N S W E R :
True

14. True or false: The rate of change in volume loss is not an important parameter determining the neuroendocrine response to hypovolemia.

Ref.: 1–3

COMMENTS: For small hemorrhages (10–20%) of blood volume, the neuroendocrine response is independent of the rate of hemorrhage. • However, for larger-volume losses (>20%), the rate of hemorrhage does affect response. • Rapid losses are not as well tolerated as are slow losses.

A N S W E R :
False

15. Hypothalamically mediated responses to hemorrhagic shock include production of which of the following substances?

A. ACTH

B. AVP

C. Somatostatin

D. Growth hormone

E. Aldosterone

Ref.: 1–3

COMMENTS: When acute blood loss occurs, the decrease in the effective circulating volume activates high-pressure baroreceptors (in the aorta, carotid arteries, and renal arteries) and low-pressure stretch receptors (in the left atrium), which set into motion a series of compensatory responses. • The pressure and stretch receptors exert a tonic inhibitory effect on the neuroendocrine system. • Volume loss causes release or inactivation of this effect, initiating the compensatory cascade. • Receptor activity exerts its effect via direct hypothalamic stimulation, resulting in increases in ACTH,

AVP, and growth hormone levels. • AVP is synthesized in the hypothalamus and stored in the neurohypophysis. • In addition to changes in the effective circulating volume, an increase in plasma osmolality is a major stimulus for its release. • Other stimulators of ACTH activity are pain, catecholamines, angiotensin II, and cortisol. • The actions of ACTH are *osmoregulatory* (via resorption of solute-free water from the distal convoluted tubules and collecting ducts), *vasoactive* (via peripheral vasoconstriction, especially in the splanchnic bed), and *metabolic* (stimulating hepatic glycogenolysis and gluconeogenesis). • Growth hormone is synthesized and released from acidophilic cells of the adenohypophysis. • Decreased effective circulating volume causes its release after injury. • Growth hormone has many metabolic effects that lead to an increase in plasma glucose levels.

One of the most important responses to hypovolemia is the release of aldosterone, which is synthesized in the adrenal zona glomerulosa. • Aldosterone is released in response to a number of stimuli. • The two important stimuli for its release after injury are ACTH and angiotensin II. • ACTH stimulation is a calcium- and cAMP-dependent event that is short-lived. • Angiotensin II stimulation is a calcium-dependent, cAMP-independent event and is most important during injury. • Generation of angiotensin II is the result of activation of the renin-angiotensin system by stimulation of the juxtaglomerular cells in response to decreased renal arterial perfusion. • ACTH levels are elevated as a result of hypothalamic stimulation in hypovolemic shock. • Aldosterone increases Na+ and Cl− resorption in the early distal convoluted tubule and promotes Na+ resorption and K+ excretion in the late distal convoluted tubule and collecting ducts. • Water follows the sodium, and the net effect is an increase in intravascular volume.

A N S W E R :
A, B, D, E

16. True or false: There are many stimuli associated with injury and many areas where input can be registered, but the afferent (output) arm of the injury response is under local tissue control.

Ref.: 1–3

COMMENTS: There are several arms of the efferent limb of the neuroendocrine response to injury. • The endocrine response includes hormones under hypothalamic-pituitary control (cortisol, thyroxine, growth hormone, and AVP) and hormones under autonomic control (catecholamines, insulin, and glucagon). • Local tissue response includes release of cytokines such as the interleukins, TNF, and eicosanoids. • Vascular endothelium can respond by releasing endothelial cell mediators, including nitric oxide, endothelins, and prostaglandins.

A N S W E R :
False

17. Which of the following factors determine the host response to surgical stress?

A. Body composition

B. Nutritional status

C. Race

D. Type of stress

E. Age

F. Gender

Ref.: 1–3

COMMENTS: Several factors determine a patient's response to stress. • Body composition is a major determinant of the metabolic response, since post-traumatic nitrogen excretion correlates with the mass of total body protein. • Likewise, nutritional status can influence a patient's postoperative course. • Studies have shown a causal relationship between preoperative protein depletion and postoperative complications in elective major general surgical procedures. • Patients with protein depletion have a higher risk of respiratory complications, including postoperative pneumonia and decreased respiratory muscle strength, necessitating prolonged intubation. • Problems with wound healing and hepatic and muscle function may occur in malnourished patients. • The type, intensity, and duration of stress influence the activation of host mediators and the resulting physiologic changes in a patient. • An increase in fat mass and a decrease in muscle mass occur with aging even though body weight may remain constant. • The loss of strength that accompanies decreased muscle mass can have detrimental functional consequences, such as impaired respiratory function. • Moreover, cardiovascular and pulmonary diseases are more common with advancing age, and both affect a patient's ability to successfully tolerate surgical stress. • Lean body mass as a proportion of body weight is lower in women than in men, resulting in a decreased net nitrogen loss in women than in men after major general surgical operations. • Race per se is not a prime determinant of a patient's response to surgical stress.

ANSWER:
A, B, D, E, F

---

18. Match the hormones in the left-hand column with their site of production in the right-hand column.

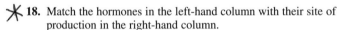

A. Growth hormone	a. Chromophobe cells of the anterior pituitary
B. Cortisol	b. Adrenal zona fasciculata
C. ACTH	c. Acidophilic cells of the anterior pituitary
D. Follicle-stimulating hormone and luteinizing hormone	d. Supraoptic and paraventricular nuclei
E. AVP	e. Basophilic cells of the anterior pituitary

Ref.: 1–3

COMMENTS: See Question 19.

19. Which of the following statements is/are true?

A. The cumulative effect of cortisol is "insulin like."

B. Peripheral conversion of thyroxine (T$_4$) to triiodothyronine (T$_3$) increases with injury.

C. Somatostatin potentiates growth hormone release.

D. The primary function of growth hormone is to promote protein synthesis.

Ref.: 1–3

COMMENTS: The chromophobe cells of the anterior pituitary synthesize ACTH and store it as a large molecule, propiomelanocortin. • This large molecule also contains ∃- and β-lipotropin, γ-melanocyte–stimulating hormone (γMSH), and β-endorphins. • ACTH is responsible for stimulating the release of cortisol from the adrenal zona fasciculata.

The primary role of cortisol is to maintain euglycemia during stress and injury. • It has widespread effects on metabolism and the utilization of glucose, amino acids, and fatty acids. • In the liver, cortisol stimulates gluconeogenic activity. • In skeletal muscle, it inhibits insulin-mediated glucose uptake. • Cortisol inhibits amino acid uptake and stimulates amino acid release. • In adipose tissue, cortisol stimulates lypolysis and decreases glucose uptake. • Cortisol also exerts immunologic and inflammatory effects. • It causes demargination of white blood cells and suppresses leukocyte synthesis of the cytokines associated with inflammation. • Cortisol inhibits phospholipase A$_2$, limiting the production of prostaglandins and leukotrienes.

Peripheral conversion of T$_4$ to T$_3$ is impaired following injury, burns, and surgery, leading to reduced circulating concentrations of both free and total T$_3$. • This cortisol-mediated event decreases the metabolic impact of thyroid hormone during injury.

Growth hormone is synthesized, stored, and released from acidophylic cells of the anterior pituitary. • It exerts a direct action as growth hormone and secondarily owing to release of insulin-like growth factors 1 and 2 (IGF-1 and IGF-2), formerly called somatomedins. • Secretion of growth hormone is stimulated by a variety of factors, including α-adrenergic stimulation, thyroxine, AVP, ACTH, αMSH, glucagon, and testosterone. • Its release is suppressed by somatostatin, β-adrenergic stimulation, cortisol, hyperglycemia, and increased plasma fatty acid concentration. • The primary action of growth hormone during stress is to promote protein synthesis (IGF-1–mediated) and enhance breakdown of lipids and carbohydrates. • Plasma concentrations of growth hormone increase following injury, hemorrhage, and operative stress.

ANSWERS:
Question 18: A-c; B-b; C-a; D-e; E-d
Question 19: D

---

20. Which of the following statements is/are true?

A. Suppression of gonadotropic hormones is the cause of post-traumatic amenorrhea.

B. Prolactin inhibits T-cell function.

C. Exogenous opioids act via a single receptor.

D. Head injury can cause both diabetes insipidus and syndrome of inappropriate secretion of ADH (SIADH).

Ref.: 1–3

COMMENTS: Follicle-stimulating hormone and luteinizing hormone are synthesized and stored by the basophilic cells of the anterior pituitary. • Their secretion is suppressed after injury, which is responsible for the menstrual dysfunction and decreased libido observed after injury.

Prolactin is synthesized and released by acidophilic cells of the anterior pituitary. • It acts metabolically to produce increased nitrogen retention and increased lipid mobilization. • It also has been shown to stimulate T-cell function. • The importance of prolactin action following injury is not well understood.

Endogenous opioids arise from precursors whose secretion increases during the response to injury. • ACTH is secreted as a large protein complex that exhibits β-endorphin activity. • Endogenous opioids act on several receptors and exert multiple effects, since none shows complete specificity for a single receptor type. • The endogenous opioids exert an analgesic effect and have cardiovascular, metabolic, and immunologic actions. • β-Endorphin is associated with hyperglycemia and is hypotensive. • The enkephalins are associated with hypertension. • Some opioid peptides have the ability to suppress immunologic function. • Their precise actions in response to hemorrhage and sepsis are still under investigation. • Arginine vasopressin (AVP, formerly called antidiuretic hormone, or ADH) arises from the supraoptic and paraventricular nuclei of the anterior hypothalamus and is stored in the posterior pituitary. • The primary stimulus for its secretion is increased plasma osmolality. • Its release is enhanced by β-adrenergic and angiotensin II stimulation. • Its actions are classified as osmoregulatory, vasoactive, and metabolic. • It mediates resorption of solute-free water in the distal tubules and collecting ducts as well as peripheral vasoconstriction, particularly in the splanchnic bed. • It stimulates hepatic glycogenolysis and gluconeogenesis. • Head injury can be associated with inappropriately high secretion of AVP (known as SIADH) and can, conversely, cause lack of AVP secretion, leading to diabetes insipidus (resulting from damage to the supraoptic hypophyseal system).

ANSWER:
A, D

---

21. Metabolic effects of the neuroendocrine response to injury include which of the following events?

   A. Gluconeogenesis

   B. Glycogen synthesis

   C. Lipolysis

   D. Proteolysis

   E. Hypoglycemia

   Ref.: 1–3

COMMENTS: Glucose is the primary fuel for vital organs, such as the heart, peripheral nerves, and renal medulla, as well as for the red blood cells and leukocytes. • For the human organism to survive serious injury, a ready supply of glucose must be made available. • This condition constitutes a critical effect of the many neurohormonal changes observed after injury. • Since the supply of hepatic glucose stored as glycogen is rapidly depleted, glucose must be obtained from other sources. • Gluconeogenesis occurs through the use of alanine and other amino acids generated from breakdown of skeletal muscle (proteolysis), glycerol derived from the breakdown of triglycerides in body fat (lipolysis), or lactate and pyruvate formed as a result of anaerobic glycolysis of glucose. • In addition, glucose entry into cells is impaired by the action of catecholamines and cortisol and by the decrease in serum insulin. • This impairment produces hyperglycemia rather than hypoglycemia.

ANSWER:
A, C, D

---

22. In septic patients, cytokine-mediated effects on trace element metabolism include which of the following?

   A. Increased serum iron levels

   B. Decreased serum iron levels

   C. Increased serum zinc levels

   D. Decreased serum zinc levels

   E. Increased serum copper levels

   F. Decreased serum copper levels

   Ref.: 1–3

COMMENTS: Cytokines alter trace element levels in stressed or septic patients. • TNF-α and IL-1 have been shown to cause decreased circulating levels of iron and zinc. • Decreases in serum iron levels are thought to benefit patients by inhibiting the growth rate of microbes that use iron as a growth factor. • Administration of iron to infected patients is contraindicated, since increased serum iron concentrations can impair resistance. • Copper levels usually rise as a result of increased ceruloplasmin, made by the liver as part of the acute-phase protein response.

ANSWER:
B, D, E

---

23. Which of the following statements is/are true?

   A. Insulin levels are elevated during the early phase of injury.

   B. The postinjury elevation of insulin is mediated by epinephrine.

   C. Serum glucose levels in injured patients are directly related to insulin levels.

   D. Serum insulin levels correlate well with the degree of injury.

   E. The insulin/glucose ratio is a better predictor of survival than is either level alone.

   Ref.: 1–3

COMMENTS: After injury, there is initial suppression of insulin secretion, mediated by catecholamines and sympathetic nervous system activity, followed by a period of normal or slightly increased secretion. • Injury produces peripheral block of insulin action. • Therefore, hyperglycemia can occur in the presence of a normal insulin level. • The insulin/glucose ratio is a better predictor of survival than is the insulin or glucose level alone.

ANSWER:
E

---

24. Which of the following statements is/are true?

   A. Insulin is the body's primary anabolic hormone.

   B. Cortisol exerts its effect on insulin by direct action on the beta islet cells of the pancreas.

   C. β-Endorphins contribute to stress-induced hyperglycemia by interfering with the peripheral action of insulin.

   D. Insulin exerts its metabolic effects via carbohydrate, fatty acid, and amino acid metabolism.

   Ref.: 1–3

COMMENTS: Insulin is secreted by beta islet cells of the pancreas. • Substrates that increase its secretion include glucose, amino acids, free fatty acids, and ketone bodies. • Normally, glucose is the most important stimulant. • Sympathetic nervous cell stimulation and epinephrine secretion inhibit insulin secretion in the presence of hyperglycemia. • Glucagon, somatostatin, β-endorphin, and IL-1 also inhibit insulin secretion via their effects on beta islet cells. • Cortisol, estrogen, and progesterone enhance injury-related hyperglycemia by interfering with the peripheral action of insulin. • Insulin is an anabolic hormone promoting storage of carbohydrates, proteins, and lipids. • The effects of insulin on carbohydrate include stimulation of glucose transfer into cells, stimulation of glycogenesis and glycolysis, and inhibition of hepatic gluconeogenesis. • Insulin stimulates lipid synthesis and inhibits lipid degradation. • Insulin promotes protein synthesis by increasing amino acid transfer into the liver and peripheral tissues and by inhibiting gluconeogenesis and amino acid oxidation.

ANSWER:
A, D

25. Which of the following statements is/are true?

 A. Major stimulants for secretion of glucagon include glucose, amino acids, and exercise.

 B. The effects of glucagon are inhibited by cortisol.

 C. Glucagon plays a major role in the development of postinjury hyperglycemia.

 D. Somatostatin potentiates glucagon effects.

Ref.: 1–3

COMMENTS: Glucagon originates from the alpha islet cells of the pancreas. • Its normal stimuli are glucose, amino acids, and exercise. • Hypoglycemia causes the release of glucagon, as does sympathetic nervous system α-adrenergic stimulation. • Parasympathetic and β-adrenergic input inhibits its glucagon secretion. • Glucagon stimulates glucogenolysis, gluconeogenesis, and ketogenesis in the liver. • Its effects on hepatic carbohydrate metabolism are potentiated by cortisol. • Although glucagon levels increase after injury, glucagon does not play an important part in postinjury hyperglycemia. • Somatostatin is synthesized in delta islet cells and in central and peripheral neurons. • It is an inhibitor of growth hormone, TSH, renin, insulin, and glucagon release.

ANSWER:
A

26. Match the items in the left-hand column with the appropriate choice in the right-hand column. Items in the right-hand column may be used more than once.

 A. C-reactive protein   a. With copper, helps clear oxygen-free radicals

 B. Ceruloplasmin   b. Protease inhibitor

 C. α₁-Antitrypsin   c. Functions as an opsonin and complement activator

 D. α₂-Macroglobulin

Ref.: 1–3

COMMENTS: See Question 27.

27. Which of the following statements is/are true?

 A. Both IL-1 and IL-2 act primarily as immunostimulants.

 B. IL-2 is used to generate lymphokine-activated killer cells.

 C. IL-6 is released from the anterior hypothalamus.

 D. IL-6 is responsible primarily for splanchnic vasoconstriction.

Ref.: 1–3

COMMENTS: Cells are capable of releasing a number of factors that participate in the response to injury, including cytokines, eicosanoids, and endothelial cell factors. • Cytokines are primarily involved in cell-to-cell (paracrine) functions, but some exert distant (hormonal) effects. • Those that affect immune function are termed lymphokines and include primarily the interleukins, TNF, and the interferons. • IL-1 activity is mediated by IL-1α and IL-1β and has a broad range of activities. • IL-1 augments T-cell proliferation. • It induces fever by stimulating local release of prostaglandins in the anterior hypothalamus. • Other centrally mediated effects include inducing anorexia, lessening pain perception (by increasing β-endorphin release), and increasing the basal metabolic rate and oxygen consumption. • Together with IL-6,

TNF, and interferon, IL-1 promotes synthesis of hepatic acute-phase proteins (ceruloplasmin, fibrinogen, haptoglobin, C-reactive protein, complement factors, α₁-antitrypsin, and α₂-macroglobulin). • IL-1 also promotes the breakdown of skeletal muscle into amino acids, some of which are oxidized and others used by the liver for protein synthesis. • The IL-1 effect on carbohydrate metabolism is a mild hyperglycemic response. • IL-2 is the true lymphokine, acting mainly as an immunostimulant. • Antigen stimulation of lymphocytes triggers the release of IL-2, which is used to generate lymphokine-activated killer cells. • IL-6 is a family of glycoproteins whose role is to enhance immune function and (with IL-1) to promote hepatic protein synthesis. • Surgical stress, viruses, bacterial products, and cytokines IL-1 and TNF cause its release by monocytes, fibroblasts, and endothelial cells.

ANSWERS:
Question 26: A-c; B-a; C-b; D-b
Question 27: B

28. Which of the following statements is/are true?

 A. TNF is also known as anabolin.

 B. Interferon is released by macrophages.

 C. TNF and interferon have similar effects.

 D. TNF is active in dimer, trimer, and pentamer forms.

Ref.: 1–3

COMMENTS: TNF, or cachectin, is produced as a pro-TNF molecule and undergoes proteolysis into dimer, trimer, and pentamer forms. • Its production is stimulated by complement activation. • Many cells can produce TNF, including monocytes, macrophages, Kupffer cells, mast cells, and endothelial cells. • TNF acts with IL-1 to produce hypotension, tissue necrosis, and death. • It causes prostaglandin E₂ (PGE₂) release and is cytotoxic for beta islet cells. • TNF and IL-2 induce eicosanoids and platelet-activating factor. • TNF may mediate the early phase and IL-2 the late phase of hypotension associated with sepsis. • Interferon γ is a glycoprotein released by T lymphocytes. • It activates macrophages to release IL-1 and TNF, increases monocyte IL-2 expression, and inhibits viral replication. • It inhibits PGE₂ release, thereby reducing the immunosuppressive effects of PGE₂ secretion.

ANSWER:
D

29. Which of the following cytokines is/are pyrogenic (fever producing)?

 A. IL-1

 B. IL-2

 C. IL-6

 D. IL-12

 E. TNF

Ref.: 1–3

COMMENTS: In response to stress, the host resets various set points in an attempt to maintain homeostasis. • Neuroendocrine changes in this process may be manifested by fever. • IL-1, IL-6, and TNF all stimulate PGE₂ synthesis. • PGE₂ directly affects the hypothalamus and increases the hypothalamic temperature set point, resulting in fever. • In addition, PGE₂ stimulates vasoconstriction and shivering, both of which increase body core temperature and contribute to the fever.

ANSWER:
A, C, E

30. Conflicting effects of which cytokine include both proinflammatory and apoptosis-inducing properties; procoagulant effects on endothelial cells via induction of platelet-activating factor, von Willebrand factor, thromboplastin, and tissue-type plasminogen activator inhibitor; and antithrombotic effects via induction of prostacyclin and urokinase-type plasminogen activator?

A. IL-6

B. IL-10

C. IL-13

D. TNF-α

E. IFN-γ

Ref.: 1–3

COMMENTS: IL-6, IL-10, and IL-13 are known as counter-regulatory cytokines. • IL-6 regulates the hepatic acute-phase response to injury or infection. • The proteins produced are involved in the homeostatic response to injury. • IL-6 expression is up-regulated by cytokines, bacterial endotoxins, platelet-derived growth factor, and fibroblast growth factor, among other substances. • IL-10 and IL-13 inhibit certain processes leading to signal transduction and gene activation in inflammatory pathways, but the precise mechanisms have yet to be characterized. • IL-10 is the strongest anti-inflammatory cytokine listed. • TNF-α has both procoagulant and antithrombotic effects via the mechanisms discussed above. • The net effect on vascular endothelium depends on the amount of each mediator produced and the vascular bed it affects. • IFN-γ is a pro-inflammatory cytokine that regulates cellular differentiation, cytotoxicity, cytokine production, and cellular adhesion. • It influences macrophage activity, including tumor-cell cytotoxicity, killing of intracellular pathogens, and antigen processing and presentation to lymphocytes.

ANSWER:
D

31. Which of the following statements regarding NFκB is/are true?

A. It is a cytokine.

B. It is anti-inflammatory.

C. It inhibits TNF and IL-1.

D. Its activation increases iNOS expression.

E. Its primary site of action is the cytoplasm.

Ref.: 1–3

COMMENTS: The inflammatory response depends on transcription of genes that encode effector proteins. • Gene expression is regulated by DNA-binding proteins called transcription factors. • NFκB is an important transcription factor in inflammation. • Its activation is crucial for maximal expression of TNF, IL-1, IL-6, and IL-8. • NFκB activation also leads to upregulation of COX-2 and iNOS, which then produce more inflammatory mediators. • NFκB is sequestered in the cytoplasm of inflammatory cells. • In response to stress, it enters the cell nucleus, where it binds

target gene promoters and induces gene expression and protein synthesis.

ANSWER:
D

32. Which of the following statements is/are true?

A. Eicosanoids are known as the glycoprotein mediators of shock.

B. Eicosanoids are derived from arachidonic acid.

C. Eicosanoids are stored in hepatic Kupffer cells.

D. Eicosanoids include thromboxane and prostaglandins.

Ref.: 1–3

COMMENTS: Eicosanoids, the lipid mediators of shock, are derived from arachidonic acid and are secreted by all enucleated cells except lymphocytes. • Stimuli for their secretion include hypoxia, ischemia, injury, fibrinogens, endotoxin, norepinephrine, AVP, angiotensin II, bradykinin, serotonin, and histamine. • The creation of eicosanoids begins with the action of the enzyme phosphorylase A on precursor fatty acids to form arachidonic acid. • This enzyme is activated by epinephrine, angiotensin II, bradykinin, histamine, and thrombin and is inhibited by lipocortin. • Eicosanoids, which include prostaglandins, thromboxane, and leukotrienes, are created from arachidonic acid by the activity of cyclooxygenase, thromboxane synthetase, and lipoxygenase, respectively.

The eicosanoids are not stored but are released de novo after injury, and their effects depend on what stimulates their production and which cells produce them. • For example, vascular endothelial cells produce prostacyclin (PGI_2) by the action of prostacycline synthetase on arachidonic acid, the cyclooxygenase pathway. • PGI_2 produces vasodilatation. • Platelets use thromboxane synthetase to convert prostaglandin to thromboxane (TxA_2), a vasoconstrictor and platelet-aggregating stimulator. • Leukotrienes include the slow-releasing substance of anaphylaxis. • They produce capillary leakage, bronchospasm, and vasoconstriction. • Prostaglandins are the major component of the inflammatory response. • Eicosanoids have been proposed as the cause of adult respiratory distress syndrome, pancreatitis, and some forms of renal failure. • β-Kinin release is stimulated by hypoxia and ischemia. • The kinins are vasodilators and produce capillary leakage, edema, pain, and bronchospasm.

ANSWER:
B, D

33. True or false: Although the endothelium can elaborate a number of active substances, the endothelial mass is small, limiting its effect on the response of the body to injury.

Ref.: 1–3

COMMENTS: The endothelial cell mass is large, approximately 1.5 kg in weight and 400 m² in surface area. • The endothelium secretes substances whose primary actions are vasomotor regulation and regulation of coagulation. • Endothelium-derived relaxing factor (EDRF) acts through the release of nitrous oxide (NO). • NO production is dependent on *l*-arginine. • The compound EDRF-NO is a potent vasodilator. • Endothelins, which are produced in response to injury, counteract this vasodilatory effect. • They are 21–amino-acid peptides and are 10 times more potent than angiotensin II. • Endothelial cells also produce prostacyclin and PGE_2. • These products promote vasodilatation and reduce platelet aggregation. • Release of platelet-activating factor (PAF) from endothelial cells is stimulated by TNF, IL-1, AVP, and angiotensin II. • PAF causes platelets to produce TxA_2 and increases endothelial cell permeability to albumin. • PAF may mediate the hemodynamic and metabolic effects of endotoxin. • Atrial natriuretic peptides (ANPs) are released by atrial tissue in response to volume change. • ANP is a potent inhibitor of aldosterone.

A N S W E R :
False

34. Which of the following is/are part of the vascular response to injury?

    A. Mast cell and macrophage activation of vascular endothelium

    B. Vasodilation of local arterioles

    C. Leukocyte margination

    D. Down regulation of leukocyte integrin

    E. Leukocyte inhibition

Ref.: 1–3

COMMENTS: In the vascular response to injury, vascular endothelial cells are activated by both the injury and local leukocytes, including mast cells and macrophages. • Endothelial cells are then able to release various factors, including histamine, serotonin, complement, prostaglandins, leukotrienes, PAF, and NO. • Release of these substances leads to vasodilation of local arterioles, resulting in tissue congestion, or reactive hyperemia, at the site of injury. • On a cellular level, leukocytes migrate to sites of injury through a response coordinated with endothelial cells. • Circulating leukocytes migrate to the vessel periphery, a process known as margination. • They then roll along the endothelium and form loose attachments to the endothelium mediated by E-selectin and P-selectin on the endothelium and L-selectin on the rolling leukocyte. • Leukocytes then become bound to the endothelial surface, in part due to integrins that are up-regulated as part of the activation response. • Integrins mediate both rolling and adhesion of leukocytes, with concomitant ICAM and VCAM expression by endothelial cells for adhesion. • Adherent leukocytes are then able to migrate between endothelial cells, in a process known as diapedesis, and enter the extracellular matrix en route to the site of injury, during the process of transmigration.

A N S W E R :
A, B, C

35. Which of the following statements regarding PAF is/are true?

    A. It is stored in white blood cells and released in response to injury.

    B. Its biologic effects are mediated through a G-protein–coupled PAF receptor.

    C. It may induce vasodilation and increased vascular permeability.

    D. It is a potent vasoconstrictor.

    E. It is synthesized by vascular endothelial cells.

Ref.: 1–3

COMMENTS: PAF is a lipid mediator of inflammation that is rapidly produced by activated inflammatory cells. • It has multiple biologic effects, including inducing of platelet aggregation and degranulation, increasing vasodilation and vascular permeability,

increasing bronchoconstriction, promoting adherence of activated inflammatory cells to endothelium, augmenting endotoxin-induced hypotension, and causing neutrophil and platelet accumulation in the lungs. • It is synthesized by neutrophils, platelets, basophils, monocytes, eosinophils, mast cells, and vascular endothelial cells. • The biologic effects of PAF are mediated through a G-protein–coupled PAF receptor.

A N S W E R :
B, C, E

36. In which of the following situations is ACTH release not inhibited by high plasma cortisol levels?

    A. Somatic pain

    B. Severe hypovolemia

    C. Sequential injury or operations

    D. Cushing's disease

    E. Endotoxic shock

Ref.: 1–3

COMMENTS: The pituitary-adrenal axis is normally under the control of a negative feedback mechanism wherein increased cortisol levels inhibit further release of ACTH. • This mechanism is operable in most situations of simple trauma, in which various stimuli lead to ACTH release. • Important exceptions are severe hypovolemia and scenarios involving sequential traumatic events or sequential operations. • In such settings, ACTH release is not suppressed by cortisol. • The mechanism of this physiologic facilitation, termed feed forward, is not known. • The secondary cortisol responses are often greater than is the initial response, a phenomenon known as potentiation. • Stimulation of ACTH persists until the intravascular volume has been replenished. • Lack of ACTH suppression by cortisol is also seen in the nontraumatic condition of Cushing's disease as the result of ACTH production by a pituitary adenoma.

A N S W E R :
B, C, D

37. Chronic adrenal insufficiency is characterized by which of the following?

    A. Hypothermia

    B. Hypertension

    C. Hyperkalemia

    D. Hyponatremia

    E. Hyperglycemia

Ref.: 1–3

COMMENTS: The adrenocortical response is a critical mechanism of survival in situations of shock, trauma, or sepsis. • When endogenous corticosteroid production is impaired and exogenous replacement insufficient, profound cardiovascular collapse occurs. • **Acute adrenal insufficiency** may result from bilateral adrenal hemorrhage (caused by severe sepsis or anticoagulation or occurring spontaneously), adrenalectomy, or, in particular, withdrawal of exogenous steroids that have been administered for a long time. • **Chronic adrenal insufficiency** may result from autoimmune destruction of the adrenal glands or, less commonly, from tuberculous or fungal disease. • The clinical manifestations of chronic adrenal insufficiency are those of combined mineralocorticoid and gluco-corticoid deficiency. • Characteristically, patients with chronic adrenal insufficiency have hyperpigmentation, weakness, weight loss, gastrointestinal symptoms, hyperkalemia, hyponatremia, and hypoglycemia. • In injured patients with adrenal insufficiency, hyperkalemia, hyponatremia, and hypoglycemia predominate. • Hyponatremia and hyperkalemia are a result of the loss of the sodium-retaining and kaliuretic properties of aldosterone. • Hypoglycemia results from the loss of the effect of cortisol on hepatic glucose production. • Fever and hypotension are the most prominent features of acute adrenal insufficiency. • If adrenal insufficiency is not recognized and promptly treated with exogenous supplementation, affected patients may die as a result of any medically stressful situation, such as an operation, an injury, or an infection.

A N S W E R :
C, D

38. Death after severe injury often is the result of which of the following events?

A. Adrenal failure

B. Respiratory failure

C. Renal failure

D. All of the above

Ref.: 1–3

COMMENTS: Death after injury does not result from adrenal exhaustion, except in patients with underlying insufficiency or those in whom acute adrenal failure develops during the course of their illness. • Severe illness or injury is characterized by marked adrenocortical stimulation and release of cortisol under the control of ACTH, which acts on the cells of the zona fasciculata via cAMP. • Plasma levels of corticosteroids and their metabolites are elevated in these patients, and the normal circadian rhythm is lost. • Levels remain elevated for up to 4 weeks after burns, 1 week after soft-tissue injury, and a few days after hemorrhage. • With pure hypovolemia, cortisol levels quickly return to normal when the patient becomes euvolemic. • During recovery, plasma corticosteroid levels decline. • Persistent elevation suggests ongoing injury or sepsis and is a bad prognostic sign. • Death after critical illness often involves multisystem organ failure, particularly pulmonary and renal decompensation.

A N S W E R :
B, C

39. Which of the following processes is/are important in the restoration of blood volume after hypovolemia?

A. Transcapillary refill

B. Increased interstitial osmolality

C. Decreased interstitial osmolality

D. Hepatic albumin synthesis

Ref.: 1–3

COMMENTS: Reduction of blood volume by 15–20% decreases capillary pressure and results in an initial shift of protein-free fluid from the interstitium back into the vascular compartments. • This mechanism only partially compensates for the volume loss, however, and is limited by the equilibrium established between intravascular oncotic pressure and interstitial fluid pressure.

• Further restoration of the intravascular volume depends on increases in the levels of plasma proteins, primarily albumin. • The albumin comes from the interstitium itself but can be moved across capillary membranes into the vascular system if the interstitial pressure (relative to the intravascular pressure) is adequate. • Critical to increasing interstitial pressure to accomplish this movement is an increase in the extracellular interstitial osmolality that occurs after injury. • This metabolic effect is the result of numerous hormonal influences, especially that of cortisol.

A N S W E R :
A, B

40. With regard to the renin-angiotensin system, which of the following statements is/are true?

A. Renin is an enzyme originating from the juxtaglomerular apparatus of the kidney.

B. Angiotensinogen is a potent vasoconstrictor synthesized in the liver.

C. Angiotensin I is converted to angiotensin II primarily in the kidney.

D. Angiotensin II stimulates aldosterone release from the adrenal cortex.

E. Aldosterone increases sodium resorption in the distal renal tubule.

Ref.: 1–3

COMMENTS: See Question 41.

41. Match each relationship described in the left-hand column with the appropriate physiologic effect in the right-hand column.

A. Effect of decreased renal artery perfusion on renin release	a. Stimulates
B. Effect of vasopressin on renin release	b. Inhibits
C. Effect of angiotensin II on renin release	c. Neither
D. Effect of angiotensin II on ADH release	

Ref.: 1–3

COMMENTS: The renin-angiotensin pathway is a physiologic mechanism critical for maintaining perfusion after hypovolemia. • Renin is elaborated in an inactive form, prorenin, in the myoepithelial cells (juxtaglomerular cells) of afferent renal arterioles. • It is converted to its active form in response to decreased perfusion pressure or to β-adrenergic stimulation of the juxtaglomerular body. • Its activation is also stimulated by decreased delivery of sodium chloride to the distal renal tubules, as sensed by the macula densa. • Renin converts angiotensinogen (renin substrate), produced in the liver, to the inactive intermediary peptide angiotensin I. • In the lung, angiotensin-converting enzyme converts angiotensin I to the active angiotensin II.

Angiotensin II is a potent vasoconstrictor, stimulates heart rate and myocardial contractility, and increases vascular permeability. • It stimulates the secretion and release of aldosterone from the adrenal cortex, which in turn increases sodium and water resorption from the renal tubules. • Angiotensin II has other physiologic effects, including stimulating the release of vasopressin and ACTH from the pituitary. • Metabolic activity includes stimulation of hepatic glycogenolysis and gluconeogenesis. • By a negative feedback mechanism, angiotensin II inhibits the release of renin. • Renin release is also inhibited by vasopressin and potassium.

• The normal circadian rhythm of renin release is lost after injury, when it can be suppressed by salt and water loading.

ANSWERS:
Question 40: A, D, E
Question 41: A-a; B-b; C-b; D-a

---

42. Which of the following statements regarding AVP is/are true?

A. The baroreceptor response to hypotension leads to increased AVP release from the anterior pituitary.

B. The counterregulatory effects of AVP on hypotension include diffuse arteriolar vasoconstriction and increased water resorption in the kidney.

C. AVP release is enhanced by high angiotensin II levels.

D. AVP may be secreted in nephrogenic diabetes insipidus (DI).

Ref.: 1–3

COMMENTS: Baroreceptor responses to hypotension augment the release of AVP from the supraoptic and paraventricular nuclei of the hypothalamus. • AVP induces arteriolar constriction and increased water resorption in the kidney. • In patients in shock, the renin-angiotensin-aldosterone system is also activated, leading to a decrease in renal sodium levels and to water loss. • High levels of angiotensin II can actually stimulate AVP release, linking the two endocrine compensatory responses. • AVP levels in nephrogenic DI are normal or elevated. • The defect lies in the inability of the renal tubule cells to respond to AVP, leading to excess water loss and resulting in increased excretion of very dilute urine.

ANSWER:
B, C, D

---

43. With regard to protein loss after injury, which of the following statements is/are true?

A. It results from impaired protein synthesis.

B. It occurs primarily from skeletal muscle.

C. It occurs primarily from the site of injury.

D. It can be prevented by total parenteral nutrition.

Ref.: 1–3

COMMENTS: Acute injury is associated with an obligatory nitrogen loss occurring primarily in the form of urinary nitrogen. • Generalized catabolism of skeletal muscle is the primary cause of this protein loss. • There is also impaired entry of amino acids into muscle cells as an effect of cortisol and other hormones. • Protein may also be lost when there are large, open wounds; extensive areas of necrotic tissue; peritonitis; or ascites. • Protein synthesis is not impaired after injury. • In fact, it may be accelerated, but, because of the marked increase in catabolism, the net protein balance is negative.

ANSWER:
B

---

44. Match the metabolic response in the left-hand column with the appropriate clinical situation in the right-hand column.

A. Hepatic glycogenolysis   a. Trauma
B. Hyperglycemia   b. Fasting

C. Protein catabolism that   c. Both
   exceeds energy needs
D. Gluconeogenesis from glycerol   d. Neither
E. Utilization of fat as the main
   energy source

Ref.: 1–3

COMMENTS: Response to injury or fasting requires energy substrates. • Normal circulating fuel sources in the form of glucose and plasma fats and triglycerides make up a small part of a person's total fuel composition and are not capable of providing the required calories. • Stored sources of fuel include hepatic and muscle glycogen, protein, and fat. • Hepatic glycogen stores are readily available but are limited and depleted within 24 hr. • The largest potential calorie source is body fat.

Following starvation or injury, body fat becomes a main provider of energy through oxidation of fatty acids and generation of glycerol to be used in gluconeogenesis. • A number of vital areas of the body, including the brain, renal medulla, red blood cells, leukocytes, and peripheral nerves, are glycolytic tissues, meaning that they require a glucose source of energy for metabolism and are unable to utilize fatty acids. • For this reason, a continuous supply of glucose must be available. • When the limited glycogen stores are depleted, this availability is accomplished by gluconeogenesis and by recycling incompletely metabolized glucose. • Primary sources of gluconeogenesis are (1) amino acids, derived from breakdown of muscle proteins, and (2) glycerol, derived from breakdown of triglycerides in adipose stores. • These processes are fueled by the oxidation of fatty acids.

With trauma, the hormonal milieu results in catabolism of protein stores beyond that necessary for energy needs alone. • With starvation, the body attempts to conserve proteins by adaptations that permit the use of fatty acids and ketones for fuel by nonglycolytic tissues and that promote gluconeogenesis. • With prolonged fasting, ketone bodies such as acetoacetate and β-hydroxybutyrate can be used in place of glucose for brain metabolism. • Lactate and pyruvate derived from incomplete utilization of glucose by glycolytic tissues can be regenerated into glucose through the use of energy provided by fatty acid oxidation, a process known as the Cori cycle. • The recycled glucose becomes the main source of available glucose during late starvation. • Another change observed during late starvation is a shift from the liver to the kidney as the primary source of gluconeogenesis. • This change occurs as alanine, the main source of gluconeogenesis from amino acids, is depleted in the liver. • The human organism does not have the enzymes necessary to utilize free fatty acids directly for gluconeogenesis. • The protein-conserving adaptations seen during late starvation do not occur with injury because of the hypermetabolic effects of cortisol, catecholamines, and other circulating hormones.

ANSWER:
A-c; B-a; C-a; D-c; E-c

---

45. Match the characteristic in the left-hand column with the appropriate response in the right-hand column.

A. High urine output   a. Inappropriate AVP secretion
B. High urinary osmolarity   b. DI
C. Hypernatremia   c. Both
D. Head trauma   d. Neither

Ref.: 1–3

COMMENTS: Afferent neural stimulation of the hypothalamus in response to injury or hypovolemia leads to release of AVP from the posterior pituitary gland. • The physiologic action of AVP (formerly known as ADH) is to increase water resorption from the distal renal tubule and collecting ducts. • A disturbance causing persistent release of AVP may produce a syndrome known as inappropriate release of ADH (SIADH). • The converse is DI, or absence of AVP secretion. • Either of these conditions may be associated with head injury.

With SIADH, secretion of AVP exceeds that required for normal homeostasis, resulting in *oliguria, urinary hyperosmolality,* and *dilutional hyponatremia.* • Hyponatremia may occur in patients with normal AVP response if they are given excess hypotonic fluids. • In DI, the failure of AVP secretion results in the production of large volumes of *dilute urine*, with the urine osmolality lower than the plasma osmolality, which is abnormally high. • If not recognized and treated appropriately, it leads to dehydration, hypernatremia, and hypotension. • DI is corrected by administering free water and exogenous AVP.

ANSWER:
A-b; B-a; C-b; D-c

---

46. Which of the following statements regarding DI is/are true?

    A. In central DI, severity is independent of the deficit in circulating AVP.

    B. Unlike patients with central DI, those with nephrogenic DI produce dilute urine and are hypernatremic.

    C. Lithium may cause nephrogenic DI.

    D. Dilute urine with an osmolatiy less than 300 mOsm/L in a hypernatremic patient suggests a diagnosis of DI.

    E. 1-Deamino-8-D-arginine-vasopressin (DDAVP) is the preferred therapy for patients with central DI.

    Ref.: 1–3

COMMENTS: DI is characterized by production of large amounts of dilute urine, often coupled with elevations in serum sodium levels. • These findings are seen in both central and nephrogenic DI and are accompanied by polydipsia.

Central DI is an endocrine disorder in which a patient has blunted or nonexistent synthesis and release of AVP from the posterior pituitary. • The severity of central DI is directly proportional to the deficit in circulating AVP. • Central DI may follow neurosurgery or brain injury or trauma, subarachnoid hemorrhage, or tumors involving the posterior pituitary.

Nephrogenic DI has the same symptoms as central DI, but AVP levels are typically normal or elevated. • The pathophysiologic defect in nephrogenic DI is poor response to AVP by the renal tubular cell. • Causes of nephrogenic DI include renal conditions (e.g., chronic ureteral obstruction or sickle cell nephropathy), drugs (e.g., lithium glyburide, foscarnet, demeclocycline, or amphotericin B), and electrolyte abnormalities (e.g., hypercalcemia or severe hypokalemia).

Differentiating between central and nephrogenic DI involves administration of AVP, which slows urine production in patients with central DI. • Desmopressin, an AVP analogue, is the drug of choice for patients with central DI. • Failure to reduce urine flow after DDAVP administration is suggestive of nephrogenic DI.

ANSWER:
C, D, E

---

47. With regard to renal conservation of salt and water after injury, which of the following statements is/are true?

    A. Normally, 25% of the cardiac output is directed to the kidneys.

    B. Normally, 180 L of plasma water are filtered per day.

    C. Glomerular filtration can be increased by changes in pressure at the renal afferent arteriole.

    D. Increased filtration fraction can maintain the glomerular filtration rate with renal perfusion pressure as low as 80 mmHg.

    E. Increased filtration fraction causes increased oncotic pressure of the blood perfusing the proximal tubule.

    Ref.: 1–3

COMMENTS: Volume loss causes a reflex increase in renal efferent arteriolar pressure, which allows maintenance of the glomerular filtration rate by increasing the filtration fraction. • When the amount of plasma water removed at the glomerulus is increased, the oncotic pressure of the remaining blood passing out of the glomerulus to the proximal tubule is increased. • This increased oncotic pressure of the capillary blood surrounding the proximal tubule causes a net transfer of water, sodium, chloride, and bicarbonate from the renal tubule into the blood. • As a result, sodium, chloride, and fluid volume delivery to the loop of Henle are decreased. • This, in turn, affects the normal osmotic gradient maintained in the renal medulla (this gradient depends on adequate delivery of Na^+ and Cl^- to the loop of Henle). • This fall in the medullary oncotic gradient decreases the ability of the kidney to concentrate urine and can lead to polyuric prerenal failure.

Volume loss also leads to a shift of glomerular blood flow to the juxtamedullary nephrons, which possess much longer loops of Henle, thereby allowing increased resorption of sodium. • This Na^+ resorption is dependent on the active resorption of chloride. • If chloride delivery is increased (as would occur with increased chloride resorption in the proximal tubule in response to an increased filtration fraction), there is increased delivery of sodium to the distal tubules, which produces hypokalemia and alkalosis as sodium is resorbed and K^+ and H^+ are secreted. • This process is augmented by the aldosterone secretion that accompanies injury. • In summary, sodium retention, a hallmark of injury, results from increased secretion of corticosteroids and aldosterone, an increased glomerular filtration fraction with an attendant increase in proximal tubule resorption of sodium, and increased flow of blood to the juxtamedullary nephrons.

ANSWER:
A, B, E

---

48. True or false: Injury and hypotension are characterized by an increase in water resorption.

    Ref.: 1–3

COMMENTS: Increased water resorption occurs after injury and is caused by several factors. • One factor is sodium retention (discussed in Question 47), which is associated with the passive resorption of water. • Another factor is the increased AVP secretion associated with injury. • The increased levels last 3–5 days. • The return of AVP levels to normal is associated with a brisk diuresis of free water and resolution of edema, as is seen in surgical patients on the third to fifth postoperative day.

ANSWER:
True

49. With regard to protein digestion and utilization, which of the following statements is/are true?

  A. Approximately 40% of ingested protein is stored in non-functional energy reserves.

  B. The stomach is unnecessary for protein digestion.

  C. Amino acid absorption occurs primarily in the proximal ileum.

  D. At least 10% of ingested protein is lost in the feces.

Ref.: 1–3

COMMENTS: Nearly all protein in the body is functional. • Although protein represents a large potential source of energy, there is no nonfunctional storage analogous to the storage of triglycerides in fat globules. • Protein digestion begins in the stomach, in which polypeptides are denatured and partially digested by the action of gastric acid and pepsin. • However, the stomach is not essential for protein digestion. • Most enzymatic digestion of protein occurs in the duodenum as the result of pancreatic enzyme activity. • More than 80% of protein absorption occurs in the first 100 cm of the jejunum. • Absorption of ingested protein is nearly 100% complete. • Almost all of the protein excreted in the feces is derived from bacteria, desquamated cells, and mucoproteins. • Ultimately, all protein is absorbed as amino acids by an active carrier-mediated transport mechanism. • Absorbed amino acids are necessary for daily protein synthesis to occur in a state of positive nitrogen balance.

Normal nonstressed adults require 0.8–1.0 g/kg/day of protein to maintain this balance (the average diet provides 70–80 g/day). • Daily synthesis is utilized to maintain skin and muscle mass, the structural proteins of the gut, plasma proteins, and enzymes and to provide a circulating pool of amino acids. • As Figure 3-1 indicates, little if any protein is used for daily energy requirements in normal nonstressed adults, and nearly every molecule of protein has a specific function. • An example of the disruption of this balance occurs during starvation, in which amino acids are shunted from muscle to liver to provide substrate for gluconeogenesis. • When this occurs, urinary excretion of nitrogen (not protein) increases dramatically.

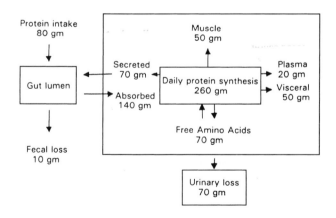

ANSWER:
B

50. In the acute-phase response to injury or trauma, levels of which of the following substances are increased?

  A. C-reactive protein

  B. Serum amyloid A

  C. Fibrinogen

  D. Ceruloplasmin

  E. Albumin

Ref.: 1–3

COMMENTS: Acute-phase proteins are those whose concentrations increase by at least 25% during inflammation. • After an initial delay of about 6 hr, the levels of acute-phase proteins increase in order to maintain homeostasis by a number of mechanisms. • C-reactive protein, whose levels increase by a thousand-fold, serves as an opsonin. • Levels of serum amyloid A, an apolipoprotein, also increase by a thousand-fold. • Levels of fibrinogen, which functions as an antiproteinase, increase by two- to five-fold. • Ceruloplasmin, whose levels increase 0.5-fold, serves as an antioxidant and in transport processes. • Albumin is actually an acute-phase reactant. • Levels of albumin decrease by 30–50% of the original baseline values in response to inflammatory stimulation, but the reasons for the decrease remain to be elucidated.

ANSWER:
A, B, C, D

51. Match the following major acute-phase reactants with their respective functions.

Acute-Phase Reactant	Function
A. C-reactive protein	a. Antiproteinase
B. Serum amyloid A	b. Oxygen scavenger, transport
C. α_2-macroglobulin	c. Apolipoprotein
D. Haptoglobin	d. Opsonin
E. Ceruloplasmin	e. Binds or removes hemoglobin

Ref.: 1–3

COMMENTS: Acute-phase proteins are produced by hepatocytes in response to stress and are regulated by IL-1 and/or IL-6. • They are primarily glycoproteins and have varying functions that enable the host to recover from injury or infection.

ANSWER:
A-d; B-c; C-a; D-e; E-b

52. Which of the following statements regarding heat-shock proteins (HSPs) is/are true?

  A. They are expressed under conditions of compromised O_2 delivery.

  B. They are constituitively or inducibly expressed.

  C. They are proinflammatory.

  D. They play little to no role in apoptosis.

Ref.: 1–3

COMMENTS: HSPs are expressed when O_2 delivery is compromised, as in conditions causing hemorrhage or ischemia. • They are either constituitive or are induced with heat shock or other stresses, including burns, radiation, trauma, toxins, heavy metals, bacteria, viruses, and allergens. • Constituitive HSPs are called molecular chaperones because of the role they play in protein processing. • While some HSPs may facilitate intercellular signals leading to NO formation by eNOS (and thus promoting inflammation), HSPs are primarily involved in down regulation of the inflammatory response. • HSPs are thus both pro- and anti-inflammatory. • HSPs also enhance the immune response, regulate apoptosis, promote hemostasis, and help protect against reactive oxygen species or oxygen free radicals.

ANSWER:
A, B, C

REFERENCES

1. Mulholland MW, Lillemoe KD, Doherty GM, et al: *Greenfield's Surgery: Scientific Principles and Practice,* 4th ed. Lippincott, Williams & Wilkins, Philadelphia, 2006.

2. Townsend CM, Beauchamp RD, Evers BM, et al (eds): *Sabiston Textbook of Surgery: The Biological Basis of Modern Surgical Practice,* 17th ed. Saunders, Philadelphia, 2004.
3. Brunicardi FC, Andersen DK, Billiar TR, et al (eds): *Schwartz's Principles of Surgery,* 8th ed, McGraw-Hill, New York, 2004.

CHAPTER 4

Perioperative Care

José M. Velasco, M.D., Samuel Parnass, M.D., and Edward Yastrow, M.D.

1. Regarding tight control of serum glucose levels in diabetic patients undergoing cardiac surgery, which of the following statements is/are true?

   A. It has no effect on postoperative complications.

   B. It significantly reduces the incidence of deep sternal wound infections.

   C. It enhances phagocytosis.

   D. It increases urine production.

   E. None of the above

   Ref.: 1–5

COMMENTS: Diabetes mellitus impairs wound healing. In addition, tissue perfusion is decreased due to both macrovascular and microvascular disease. • Hyperglycemia also may result in osmotic diuresis, which may lead to a decrease in effective hypovolemia. • Hyperglycemia is a known risk factor for postoperative deep sternal wound infection because it alters the normal physiologic response to infection. • It is associated with impaired phagocytosis, lymphocyte dysfunction, immunoglobulin inactivation, activation of C3 complement factor, and impaired wound collagen deposition. • Tight control of blood glucose levels in diabetic patients during the postoperative period via a continuous insulin infusion pump improves wound healing and reduces the incidence of postoperative sternal wound infections. • When blood glucose levels are maintained between 80 and 120 mg, the postoperative sternal wound infection rate approaches that found in nondiabetic patients. • Correction of the blood glucose level to normal limits restores both neutrophil chemotaxis and phagocytosis. • Moreover, it reverses the reduced CD4 cell counts found in patients with poorly controlled diabetes.

ANSWER:
B

2. The perioperative management of a patient whose diabetes has been controlled by diet alone consists of blood glucose level determinations and which of the following?

   A. Continuation of diet and determination of serum glucose level before surgery

   B. Subcutaneous administration of regular insulin

   C. Oral hypoglycemic agents initiated 3 days before surgery

   D. Insulin infusion beginning 1 hr before surgery

   E. Increased oral carbohydrate intake to prevent ketosis

   Ref.: 6

COMMENTS: Patients whose diabetes is controlled by diet alone do not require any special preoperative measures other than serum glucose monitoring. • Insulin and oral hypoglycemic agents are not necessary and may cause hypoglycemia. • Oral hypoglycemic agents stimulate insulin secretion (sulfonylurea) or decrease intestinal absorption (metformin). • Patients on oral hypoglycemic agents should stop taking them before any major operation, and their blood glucose level should be controlled with insulin as needed. • Increasing carbohydrate consumption will cause hyperglycemia, putting the patient at risk for infection.

ANSWER:
A

3. Regarding diabetic patients, which of the following statements is false?

   A. Glycosylated hemoglobin (HbA_{1c}) accounts for 4–7% of total hemoglobin.

   B. High levels of HbA_{1c} result in a higher complication rate.

   C. Long-acting insulin should be replaced with intermediate-acting insulin preoperatively.

   D. Operations commonly result in an elevation of blood glucose level and higher ketone body levels.

   E. Short-acting insulin and 5–10% glucose should be administered in separate bags to optimize the blood glucose control.

   Ref.: 5

COMMENTS: Management of diabetic patients is complex owing to the metabolic effects of the disease and the possible presence of complications such as cardiovascular, renal, and neurological diseases. • Tight control of the blood glucose level is imperative. • Ideally, blood glucose levels should be 80–110 mg/dl during fasting and below 180 mg/dl postprandially. • Normally, HbA_{1c} accounts for 4–7% of total hemoglobin. • Poor control of glycemia will result in higher HbA_{1c} levels. • However, there is no evidence that high levels of HbA_{1c} are associated with a higher risk of complications, provided that the blood glucose level is carefully monitored and controlled. • Diabetic and nondiabetic

[handwritten at top: ACTH 250mg IV X 1 / Cortisol: Baseline, 30min, 60min]

patients experience higher blood glucose levels due to suppression of endogenous insulin secretion, the action of counterregulatory hormones, and infusion of glucose solutions. • In preparing diabetic patients for major operations, all use of long-acting insulins and oral hypoglycemic agents should be suspended. • When renal function is impaired, metformin may lead to lactic acidosis.

ANSWER:
B

4. When evaluating a patient with known or suspected adrenal insufficiency, which of the following statements is/are false.

   A. When indicated, the dose of glucocorticoid (generally hydrocortisone) should be adjusted in response to the anticipated surgical stress.

   B. Signs and symptoms of acute adrenal insufficiency may mimic those of septic shock.

   C. Hyponatremia, hyperkalemia, and hypoglycemia are frequently present.

   D. Development of sudden hypotension in these patients should be immediately treated with 200 mg of hydrocortisone (intravenously).

   E. Appropriate laboratory studies, including determinations of serum cortisol and electrolyte levels, should be conducted and interpreted before initiation of therapy.

Ref.: 1–3

COMMENTS: Adrenal insufficiency can be classified as primary or secondary. • Three main causes of secondary insufficiency include exogenous glucocorticoids, operative correction of endogenous hypercortisolism, and abnormalities of the hypothalamus or pituitary gland. • The hypothalamus secretes corticotropin-releasing factor, which stimulates the anterior pituitary to release adrenocorticotropic hormone (ACTH). • ACTH stimulates adrenal production of cortisol. • Cortisol activates a negative feedback mechanism that affects both the hypothalamus and the anterior pituitary. • Acute, or relative, adrenal insufficiency is a rare condition that may present clinically as would septic shock. • It is associated with electrolyte abnormalities (hyponatremia and hyperkalemia), hypotension, nausea, vomiting, abdominal pain, weakness, and dizziness. • The diagnosis should be considered in any patient with a history of tuberculosis or any patient on long-term glucocorticoid therapy. • While laboratory studies are being conducted, suspected adrenal insufficiency should be treated with a 200-mg loading dose of hydrocortisone or its equivalent. • The laboratory studies should include determinations of cortisol, electrolyte, blood urea nitrogen, and creatinine levels as well as a complete blood count. • If the blood pressure fails to return to normal within 1–2 hr following administration of the hydrocortisone bolus, an adrenal crisis is unlikely. • If adrenal insufficiency is supported by the patient's response to hydrocortisone and a serum cortisol level less than 20 mg/dl, an ACTH stimulation test can be used to confirm the diagnosis.

ANSWER:
E

5. Regarding the ACTH stimulation test in patients with suspected adrenal insufficiency, which of the following statements is/are true?

   A. The ACTH stimulation test is useful in determining the functional status of the hypothalamic-pituitary-adrenal (HPA) axis.

   B. This test is based on the blood glucose response to a standard dose of ACTH.

   C. If the ACTH test result is abnormal, a 6-week perioperative steroid coverage is indicated.

   D. This test is not indicated for a patient on chronic topical steroid preparations.

   E. All of the above

Ref.: 1, 2, 3, 5

COMMENTS: In conditions of adrenal gland suppression or adrenal insufficiency, it is important to determine whether the HPA axis is intact. • Basically, the ACTH test determines the response of a patient's adrenal gland (cortisol) after ACTH stimulation. • A normal response includes a baseline cortisol level greater than 20 μg/dl and an elevation of the cortisol level of at least 7 μg/dl following an ACTH bolus. • A patient who demonstrates a normal response to ACTH stimulation (i.e., a cortisol level >600 mg/L *[handwritten: ?]* at 30 min) does not need additional glucocorticoid therapy. • An abnormal response to ACTH stimulation indicates that either the HPA axis is not intact, the adrenal gland is insufficient, or both. • In patients for whom surgical intervention results in the need for perioperative glucocorticoid therapy, the ACTH stimulation test can be used to determine when the function of the HPA axis normalizes. • In addition, this test should be used to assess the integrity of the HPA axis in patients on chronic inhaled or topical steroid preparations.

ANSWER:
A

6. A patient with a long-term history of rheumatoid arthritis is scheduled for an emergency colon resection. Which of the following statements is/are true?

   A. Sudden hypotension and tachycardia should be treated with a 200-mg hydrocortisone bolus and perioperative glucocorticoid treatment.

   B. The patient is at increased risk for infection.

   C. The patient might benefit from an epidural catheter.

   D. Before elective reversal of the colostomy, the patient needs an ACTH stimulation test.

   E. All of the above

Ref.: 3, 5

COMMENTS: The patient suffers from a medical condition often treated with long-term steroid therapy that may lead to acute adrenal insufficiency, particularly during periods of stress. • Acute adrenal crisis can present as a shocklike syndrome. • Treatment should be instituted while investigating possible causes. • If acute adrenal insufficiency is present, the patient will improve following the hydrocortisone injection, and administration of perioperative glucocorticoid should be continued. • Patients on long-term steroid therapy are at increased risk for postoperative infection, impaired wound healing, increased skin friability, and increased risk of gastrointestinal bleeding. • Epidural anesthesia reduces the perioperative stress response in patients at risk for adrenal insufficiency. • The ACTH stimulation test assesses the integrity of the HPA axis. • While a negative test result indicates that perioperative glucocorticoids are not necessary, a positive result indicates that steroid replacement therapy may be helpful but does not predict the clinical response to surgical stress. • There is considerable variation in cortisol secretion among individuals undergoing operations. • However, cortisol secretion rates greater than 200 mg/day in the first postoperative day are rare. • Patients who have received more than 80 mg/day of hydrocortisone or its equivalent for longer than 3 weeks can be considered to have suppression of the HPA axis. • They require perioperative stress therapy with 100 mg of hydrocortisone, followed by 100–150 mg in three divided doses. • Tapering to preoperative maintenance doses can be accomplished in 2–3 days. • In general, patients who have taken any dose of corticosteroid for less than 3 weeks or who are on chronic alternative therapy should take the same dose perioperatively.

ANSWER:
E

7. Which of the following statements concerning preoperative management of patients with pheochromocytoma is/are true?

   A. α-Adrenergic blockade with phenoxybenzamine requires a minimum of 4–6 weeks of therapy.

   B. A β-blocker is indicated in patients with persistent tachycardia despite adequate α-adrenergic blockade.

   C. Determination of 24-hr urine metanephrine levels confirms adequate α-adrenergic blockade.

   D. Intraoperative hypotension following resection of the tumor is best treated with vasopressors and glucocorticoids.

   E. Morphine and phenothiazines should be avoided preoperatively.

Ref.: 1, 7

COMMENTS: Preoperative management of patients with pheochromocytoma requires control of hypertension, α-adrenergic blockade to prevent intraoperative hypertensive crisis, and fluid resuscitation to prevent hypovolemia following successful removal of the tumor. • Several classes of medication have been investigated, including α-adrenergic and β-adrenergic blockers, calcium channel blockers, and alpha-methyl *para*-tyrosine. • Phenoxybenzamine is the drug of choice for α-adrenergic blockade. • Initial doses begin around 10 mg/day in two divided doses with ranges from 10–240 mg/day being required. • The average dose is about 45 mg/day, and therapy may require 2–3 weeks to become effective. • Therapy is considered effective when a patient's symptoms have disappeared and there is adequate blood pressure control (blood pressure ≤160/90) and in the presence of orthostatic hypotension (blood pressure <85/50). • The absence of ST-segment depression on the electrocardiogram and the presence of no more than one premature ventricular contraction per 5-min period are indicators of adequate treatment and predictors of relatively few perioperative complications. • If a patient's symptoms have not resolved or if the pulse is higher than 100 beats per minute, β-adrenergic blockade therapy is added. • To avoid hypertensive crisis, β-adrenergic blockers should not be utilized until α-blockade has been established.

The half-life of phenoxybenzamine and the long duration of therapy may result in certain side effects, including reflex tachycardia, nasal congestion, and an inability to ejaculate. • Once the catecholamine-secreting tumor is removed, persistent vasodilation may result in hypovolemia, increasing the need for intravenous fluids. • Therefore, a central-venous pressure monitor or a pulmonary catheter may prove to be useful in the perioperative management. • Also, patients may seem somnolent or sedated as a result of α-adrenergic blockade therapy that may last as long as 24-hr postoperatively. • Morphine and phenothiazines may precipitate hypertensive crisis and should be avoided preoperatively. • Anesthetic agents may trigger catecholamine secretion. • Enflurane and isoflurane have been used successfully.

• Intraoperative hypertension is treated with sodium nitroprusside, and cardiac arrhythmias are best treated with short-acting β-blockers.

ANSWER:
B, E

8. A 33-year-old woman is scheduled for elective cholecystectomy. Preoperative evaluation shows the presence of mild-to-moderate hypothyroidism. Select the next most appropriate action.

   A. Proceed with surgery with the knowledge that minor perioperative complications could develop.

   B. Postpone surgery until a euthyroid state is achieved.

   C. Proceed with surgery while beginning treatment with L-thyroxin.

   D. Proceed with surgery while beginning treatment with thionamides.

   E. Proceed with surgery if severe clinical symptoms are not present.

Ref.: 8–16

COMMENTS: Mild-to-moderate hypothyroidism is a diagnosis that applies to patients who are not in myxedema coma and do not exhibit severe clinical symptoms. • Hypothyroidism causes a decrease in cardiac output by reducing heart rate and contractility. • Hypoventilation may be present because of respiratory muscle weakness and impaired pulmonary response to hypoxia and hypercapnia. • These patients have decreased gut motility, constipation, and hyponatremia due to reduction in free-water clearance. • Hypothyroidism is also associated with a decrease in red blood cell mass, causing normochromic normocytic anemia. • Although elective procedures may be performed on these patients safely, the patients are at risk for increased incidence of hypotension and congestive heart failure, along with postoperative gastrointestinal and neuropsychiatric complications. • In these patients, elective operations should be postponed while urgent and/or emergent ones can proceed, provided that thyroid replacement is begun with L-thyroxine. • Thionamides are used for the treatment of hyperthyroidism.   ↳ propylthiouracil, methimazole

ANSWER:
B

9. Regarding thyroid dysfunction in surgical patients, which of the following statements is/are true?

   A. An operation can precipitate myxedema coma in patients with severe hypothyroidism.

   B. Iodine administration is more likely to trigger an exacerbation of hyperthyroidism in patients with Graves' disease than in those with toxic multinodular goiter.

   C. Both

   D. Neither

Ref.: 12–15, 17–20

COMMENTS: Severe hypothyroidism is a medical emergency with a high mortality rate (50%). • Symptoms and signs include decreased mental status, hypoventilation, and hypothermia. • In both Graves' disease and toxic multinodular goiter, iodine may worsen hyperthyroidism. • Antithyroid medication (thionamide) should be administered at least 1 hr before administration of iodine.

• Postoperative hypothyroidism can occur in any patient with chronic hypothyroidism when replacement therapy is not resumed within 10 days. • Treatment of severe hypothyroidism consists of administration of hydrocortisone followed by thyroxine. • Fluid restriction may be necessary if hyponatremia exists.

ANSWER:
A

10. Which of the following agents is not a recommended treatment for the management of thyroid storm crisis?

A. β-Blockers

B. Thionamide

C. Iodine solution

D. Aspirin

E. Acetaminophen

Ref.: 21

COMMENTS: Patients with hyperthyroidism should not undergo a surgical procedure until clinical euthyroidism has been achieved. • **β-Blockers** will control symptoms of increased adrenergic tone, whereas **thionamides** will block new hormone synthesis. • **Iodine solution** has been used both to decrease vascularity of the gland and to block the release of thyroid hormone. • **Acetaminophen** is preferred over aspirin to treat hyperpyrexia because aspirin can cause increases in serum free-T4 and -T3 concentrations by interfering with protein binding. • In emergency situations, hydration, cooling blankets, and a combination of glucocorticosteroids, β-blockers, and iopanoic acid therapy can restore patients with thyrotoxicosis to an acceptable state of clinical euthyroidism within 5 days, even if this treatment does not normalize the thyroid-stimulating hormone levels.

ANSWER:
D

11. Regarding the use of epidural anesthesia in patients with severe chronic obstructive pulmonary disease (COPD) undergoing upper abdominal operations, which of the following statements is/are true?

A. Epidural anesthesia is preferred to avoid the respiratory depressant effects of general anesthetics.

B. The use of epidural anesthesia has consistently led to a decreased incidence of postoperative pulmonary complications.

C. Postoperative epidural analgesia leads to a higher incidence of postoperative respiratory depression than does patient-controlled analgesia with morphine.

D. None of the above

E. All of the above

Ref.: 22, 23

COMMENTS: In general, epidural or spinal anesthesia is preferred for patients with severe COPD scheduled to undergo operations outside the abdominal cavity, particularly lower-extremity operations. • Although procedures involving the lower abdomen frequently can be performed with epidural or spinal anesthesia, upper abdominal operations usually require supraumbilical incisions that would necessitate higher levels of epidural anesthesia. • Patients with

severe COPD may not tolerate such high levels, which may result in decreased expiratory reserve volume, ineffective cough, and inability to clear secretions. • General anesthesia allows for better control of ventilation in these patients, thus optimizing ventilation and oxygenation. • Studies have been inconclusive as to whether epidural anesthesia results in a decreased incidence of postoperative pulmonary complications. • Generally, it is believed that the risk of postoperative pulmonary complications is independent of the choice of **intraoperative** anesthesia. • However, **postoperative** epidural analgesia may decrease the risk of complications after upper abdominal and thoracic surgery. • Ideal anesthesia for patients with severe COPD would include an epidural catheter for postoperative pain control and general anesthesia for intraoperative management. • Intravenous narcotics are associated with higher postoperative respiratory depression, and they may not be as effective in treating pain in these patients.

ANSWER:
D

12. Regarding preoperative pulmonary function tests (PFTs), which of the following statements is/are false?

A. PFTs help predict postoperative pulmonary complications in patients undergoing abdominal operations.

B. PFTs conducted before and after bronchodilator therapy are useful in determining optimal management.

C. History and physical examination are more useful tools than are PFTs in predicting postoperative pulmonary complications.

D. Patients with a functional residual capacity less than 50% of forced vital capacity should undergo ventilation-perfusion testing before undergoing a pneumonectomy.

E. All of the above

Ref.: 22, 23

COMMENTS: Routine use of preoperative PFTs for all patients with preexisting pulmonary disease is controversial. • PFTs have a positive predictive value for postoperative pulmonary complications in patients undergoing lung resection. • However, the routine use of PFTs for abdominal operations often does not predict postoperative pulmonary complications. • Instead, PFTs can be used as tools to provide optimal preoperative management and assist in postoperative care of patients (i.e., patients with bronchospastic disease whose PFT results improve after bronchodilator therapy). • Clinical findings such as smoking, wheezing, and increased sputum production on preoperative workup are more predictive of potential postoperative complications. • Patients with a functional residual capacity less than 50% of forced vital capacity who are scheduled for lung resection should undergo ventilation-perfusion studies to determine predicted postoperative pulmonary function.

ANSWER:
A

13. A 25-year-old asthmatic is scheduled for elective inguinal hernia repair. In the holding area, he has severe wheezing bilaterally. Which of the following would be the best initial approach?

A. Administer local anesthesia with sedation, and avoid unnecessary airway manipulation.

B. Administer albuterol nebulizer treatment in the holding area, and proceed with the operation if the patient is not wheezing.

C. Postpone surgery until the patient's asthma is under control.

D. Administer spinal anesthesia and intravenous corticosteroids.

E. Provide supplemental steroids intraoperatively if the patient states that he uses steroid inhalers.

Ref.: 22, 23

COMMENTS: This patient may have uncontrolled or poorly controlled asthma. • Although inguinal hernia repairs are considered low-stress operations, unexpected complications can occur with both the surgical procedure and anesthesia. • Since this is an elective procedure, the patient's asthmatic attack should be managed preoperatively. • A single treatment may not be sufficient for adequate therapy. • The use of spinal or local anesthesia with sedation does not ensure that the patient will not require a general anesthetic, particularly if the spinal block or sedation is inadequate. • Patients using inhaled steroids as part of their asthma management do not require supplemental steroids.

ANSWER:
C

14. An 85-year-old with severe COPD is scheduled for an elective cholecystectomy. Preoperatively, which one of the following steps will not help reduce the risk of postoperative pulmonary complications?

A. Cessation of smoking for 2 weeks

B. Prophylactic antibiotics for patients with productive yellowish sputum

C. Preoperative incentive spirometry

D. Laparoscopic cholecystectomy

E. None of the above

Ref.: 22, 23

COMMENTS: Patients with COPD are at increased risk for postoperative pulmonary complications. • The risk can be reduced if effective measures are taken in the perioperative period. • Patients should be instructed to stop smoking. • Often, however, there is insufficient time to allow for the beneficial effects of this maneuver. • It takes at least 8 weeks of cessation before any decrease in postoperative pulmonary complications can be realized. • Cessation for 2 weeks will improve carbon monoxide levels, but secretions still can be a problem, and ciliary function may take longer to return. • Patients with COPD should be free of any acute exacerbations of bronchospasm or infection. • Increased sputum production, or change in color of sputum, is an indication that an underlying infection could exist. • If pulmonary infection exists, antibiotic therapy should be instituted and the patient treated for the appropriate amount of time before undergoing surgery. • Incentive spirometry may help prevent postoperative pulmonary complications, along with deep breathing, coughing, and chest physical therapy. • In patients with COPD, if at all possible, the cholecystectomy should be done via laparoscopy to avoid a painful upper abdominal incision and to preserve better diaphragmatic function.

ANSWER:
A, B

15. In morbidly obese patients, obstructive sleep apnea often results in all but which one of the following conditions?

A. Right ventricular failure

B. Hypoxemia

C. Hypercapnia

D. Polycythemia

E. Left ventricular failure

Ref.: 22

COMMENTS: Morbidly obese patients (body mass index >40) have an increased incidence of obstructive sleep apnea (25%). • Right ventricular failure can occur secondary to the effects of obstructive sleep apnea. • Chronic arterial hypoxemia and hypercarbia often lead to polycythemia, pulmonary hypertension, and right heart failure. • These patients are at an increased risk of developing left ventricular failure but not as a direct result of sleep apnea. • Increased stroke volume may lead to left ventricle enlargement. • In addition, systemic hypertension causes left ventricular hypertrophy, which, added to the effects of an increased stroke volume, ultimately results in systolic and diastolic dysfunction. • The higher incidence of ischemic heart disease found in these patients also increases the risk of left ventricular failure.

ANSWER:
E

16. Obese patients have an increased risk for deep vein thrombosis for all but which one of the following reasons?

A. Increased abdominal weight and venous stasis

B. Polycythemia

C. Infrequent ambulation

D. Increased incidence of ischemic heart disease

E. Lengthy operations because of difficult exposure

Ref.: 22

COMMENTS: Obese patients are at a much higher risk for deep vein thrombosis than are nonobese patients. • **Venous stasis** increases the risk of deep vein thrombosis. • Increased abdominal weight leads to decreased venous return secondary to compression of the inferior vena cava. • **Polycythemia** leads to decreased vascular flow. • If an obese patient has difficulty walking preoperatively, it is likely that postoperative mobilization will be unsatisfactory, leading to an increased risk. • **Prolonged operations** result in longer periods of venous stasis during the intraoperative course, increasing the risk. • Preventive therapy should be instituted before induction of anesthesia by administering regular heparin or low–molecular-weight heparin along with intermittent sequential venous compression boots. • It is important to encourage **early ambulation** in this patient population.

ANSWER:
D

17. Regarding tracheal intubation in morbidly obese patients, which of the following statements is/are true?

A. The body habitus of these patients (i.e., short, thick necks) makes intubation difficult. However, it does not compromise ventilation.

B. The diagnosis of obstructive sleep apnea should not alter management of the airway.

C. Hypoxemia following induction of anesthesia and during intubation is the result of a diminished functional residual capacity.

D. Awake intubation is contraindicated.

E. All of the above.

Ref.: 22

COMMENTS: Management of the morbidly obese patient's airway can be difficult. • The approach to intubation must take into consideration a number of factors. • Such patients often have short, thick necks; large tongues; limited mouth and neck mobility; and increased thoracic and abdominal pressure. • For these reasons, both ventilation and intubation can be difficult. • Patients with obstructive sleep apnea often have redundant soft tissue in the airway, making it extremely difficult to visualize the vocal cords. • In fact, obese patients with sleep apnea and abnormalities on airway examination should be considered for an awake intubation. • In experienced hands, an awake fiberoptic intubation with prior topical application of local anesthetic and small amounts of sedation is ideal. • If general anesthesia is induced and difficulty with intubation and ventilation ensues, obese patients can become rapidly desaturated and hypoxemic. • This is due both to an increased rate of oxygen consumption and a decreased functional residual capacity. • Oxygenation with 100% oxygen before induction of anesthesia helps decrease the rate of desaturation but does not eliminate this risk.

ANSWER:
C

18. A 65-year-old patient with no significant past medical history and normal laboratory test values is scheduled for a laparoscopic inguinal hernia repair. While waiting in the preoperative holding area, his electrocardiographic monitor demonstrates an irregularly irregular rhythm without P waves. His heart rate varies between 70 and 85 beats per minute. Which of the following constitutes appropriate management of this patient?

A. Cancel the operation, and order a stress test.

B. Cancel the operation, and immediately start the patient on digoxin.

C. Perform a transthoracic echocardiogram, and proceed with the operation if the result is normal and the heart rate is controlled.

D. Proceed with the operation, and place the patient on aspirin postoperatively.

E. Administer cardioversion.

Ref.: 24

COMMENTS: This patient has atrial fibrillation. • Arrythmias in this setting typically appear in elderly patients and are frequently associated with pain or with severe anxiety. • The possibility of a new arrhythmia in association with these diseases is less than 1% in the absence of signs suggesting cardiac disease or thyrotoxicosis. • Therefore, immediate stress testing is unnecessary. • This patient's heart rate is within normal limits, making digoxin unwarranted. • Proceeding with surgery is an acceptable course of management, provided the ventricular rate is controlled and there are no signs of acute illness. • A transthoracic echocardiogram should rule out structural heart disease and atrial clot. • Anticoagulation is recommended only if the risk of thromboembolism is high compared to the risk of postoperative bleeding. • Intravenous heparin and initiation of oral warfarin, not aspirin, is the anticoagulation therapy of choice.

Cardioversion is not indicated as the initial management step on this patient since there is no hemodynamic instability. • Moreover, 85% of the patients who develop atrial fibrillation revert to sinus rhythm with medication. • Of those who are discharged from the hospital with atrial fibrillation, 98% revert to sinus rhythm within 2 months of the operation. • Perioperative atrial fibrillation may be related to autonomic nervous system changes associated with an inflammatory response. • While it may seem logical that rhythm conversion would be more advantageous than rate control, this is not true. • Controlling the ventricular response rate either pharmacologically or through a-v nodal ablation and pacemaker implantation allows for the use of less toxic medications, resulting in fewer adverse drug reactions and hospitalizations.

ANSWER:
C

19. A patient in the post-anesthesia care unit is in no apparent distress. The vital signs are stable except for a heart rate of 128 beats per minute that is irregularly irregular with no P waves. Which of the following treatment options would not be an appropriate initial therapy?

A. Metoprolol

B. Diltiazem

C. Digoxin

D. Adenosine

E. Direct-current cardioversion

Ref.: 25

COMMENTS: This patient has atrial fibrillation with a rapid ventricular response. • Treating this patient with β-blockers such as metoprolol or calcium channel blockers such as diltiazem would be appropriate. • **Calcium-channel blockers** are especially advantageous in those patients who cannot tolerate β-blockade, such as those with bronchospastic disease or congestive heart failure. • **Digoxin** may also be used, although recent studies suggest that it may be ineffective in high adrenergic states such as those that are present postoperatively. • Supraventricular tachycardia, not atrial fibrillation, responds to **adenosine**. • Direct-current **cardioversion** is not an appropriate first-line therapy in a hemodynamically stable patient. • Had the aforementioned patient been hypotensive, complaining of angina, or in pulmonary edema, cardioversion would have been appropriate.

ANSWER:
D, E

20. A 65-year-old patient develops atrial fibrillation 4 days after a coronary arterial bypass graft. The vital signs are stable, and the laboratory test values are normal. Which of the following statements pertains to this patient?

A. The patient is at increased risk for stroke.

B. The duration and cost of the patient's hospital stay will be increased.

C. The duration of atrial fibrillation is inconsequential.

D. Anticoagulation therapy with heparin should be started immediately.

E. All of the above

Ref.: 25, 26

COMMENTS: The risk of stroke in postoperative cardiac patients who develop atrial fibrillation doubles compared to those without atrial fibrillation. • The duration of the hospital stay will increase by an average of 1 to 2 days, and the median cost of will increase by $1,600. • The duration of atrial fibrillation is crucial to determining therapy. • The risk for thromboembolism in patients without a sinus rhythm is markedly increased after 48 hr. • Therefore, anticoagulation should be strongly considered in patients with an indeterminate duration of atrial fibrillation, even in the immediate postoperative period. • A reasonable treatment plan consists of intravenous heparin, titrated to maintain a partial thromboplastin time 2 to 3 times normal, and subsequent warfarin administration to maintain an international normalized ratio between 2.0 and 3.0.

ANSWER:
A, B

21. Indicate which of the following statements in regard to delaying elective noncardiac surgery is/are not true.

A. Elective noncardiac surgery should be delayed for at least 2 weeks, and optimally 4–6 weeks, after coronary artery stenting.

B. Elective noncardiac surgery should be delayed at least 3 months after myocardial infarction (MI).

C. Elective noncardiac surgery should be delayed at least 1 week after coronary artery angioplasty without stent placement.

D. Elective noncardiac surgery should be delayed in patients with stage 3 hypertension.

Ref.: 23, 27

COMMENTS: The "6-month rule" formerly observed for delaying elective noncardiac surgery after acute MI was based on the results of perioperative management of patients with recent MI reported nearly three decades ago. • Current management and risk stratification does not use the 3- and 6-month intervals traditionally discussed in the past. • Rather, current management of MI provides for risk stratification during convalescence, and the risk of adverse perioperative complications depends more on the amount of residual myocardium at risk of severe ischemia and infarction than the age of the previous MI. • Although no specific current studies have evaluated timing of elective noncardiac surgery after MI, it appears reasonable to delay elective surgery 4–6 weeks after uncomplicated MI, assuming noninvasive testing does not indicate residual myocardium at risk.

Timing of elective surgery after percutaneous coronary intervention (PCI) involving angioplasty with or without stenting depends on the temporally related risks of vessel thrombosis, restenosis, and bleeding related to the antiplatelet therapy used in the acute phase after PCI. • Delaying surgery for at least 1 week after balloon angioplasty has the theoretical benefits of allowing healing of the vessel injury and reducing the risk of vessel thrombosis. • Delaying elective surgery for 2 weeks, and ideally for 4–6 weeks will allow for partial endothelialization of a coronary stent as well as decrease the risk of bleeding related to antiplatelet therapy (typically used for 4–6 weeks after stenting). • Stage 3 hypertension (systolic blood pressure 180 mmHg and diastolic blood pressure 110 mmHg) should be controlled before elective surgery. • Effective control of blood pressure can often be achieved with oral antihypertensive medication over several days to weeks. • If an operation is urgent, more aggressive therapy can reduce blood pressure preoperatively, but there is a significantly greater risk of intraoperative blood pressure lability, with potential development of hypotension and severe hypertension.

ANSWER:
B

22. A 65-year-old man with a long-standing history of hypertension and a 25-pack-per-year history of smoking is scheduled for elective laparoscopic hernia repair. On examination, his blood pressure is 150/90. The electrocardiogram (ECG) shows nonspecific ST-segment changes. Appropriate interventions would include which of the following?

A. Obtaining old medical records and any previous ECGs

B. Obtaining a more detailed history regarding level of exercise and daily activity

C. Requesting a cardiac consultation

D. Perioperative administration of a β-blocker and changing the operation to an open hernia repair with local anesthesia

E. None of the above

Ref.: 23, 27

COMMENTS: Current recommendations regarding preoperative cardiac evaluation for noncardiac surgery are based on the theory that random testing and screening for cardiac disease in the absence of clinical findings or changes in a patient's history are not cost-effective, nor do they appear to reduce perioperative cardiovascular morbidity and mortality. • The approach to the patient needs to consider both the surgical risk factors for a cardiac complication and the patient's cardiac risk factors.

High-risk predictors of cardiac complications include known coronary artery disease, unstable angina, severe stenotic valvular disease, essential hypertension, and recent documented myocardial infarction. • Intermediate predictors of coronary disease include advanced age, poor exercise tolerance, congestive heart failure, rhythm other than sinus rhythm, and insulin-dependent diabetes. • High-risk surgical procedures include any emergency procedure, procedures involving the aorta or other major vasculature, and long procedures entailing large blood loss and fluid shifts. • Intermediate procedures involve major orthopedic procedures and prostate, carotid artery, and head and/or neck operations.

For a patient undergoing a low-to-intermediate risk procedure who has more than two intermediate-to-high predictors of cardiac risk, the history and physical findings will guide the necessity for further workup. • If the history and exercise tolerance have been stable and routine laboratory studies such as ECGs are unchanged, then elective procedures of low-to-intermediate risk can proceed without additional intervention. • When additional history or records cannot be obtained, the urgency of surgery must be considered in situations where history and physical findings suggest a progression of coronary artery disease.

Cardiac consultation should be utilized to answer specific questions regarding disease status and not simply to request "clearance." Appropriate use of consultation services may include further testing when indicated by changes in a patient's history or findings on examination. • As a general rule, if nothing in the history or examination findings indicates a need for intervention, then an intervention is not required simply because the patient is undergoing an operation.

While available data indicate that appropriate β-blockade therapy may reduce the incidence of preoperative morbidity and mortality, there is no evidence that one type of anesthetic technique is superior to another. • The approach should involve optimizing the patient's condition and making reasonable predictions of risk rather than attempting alternative measures in the hope of reducing the likelihood of complications.

ANSWER:
A, B

23. A patient is scheduled for colon resection secondary to diverticulitis. The patient's history is significant for coronary artery disease, hypertension, and insulin-dependent diabetes. The patient had a two-vessel angioplasty 6 months ago and is symptom free, exercising three times per week. Appropriate preoperative testing would include which of the following?

A. ECG

B. Treadmill stress test

C. Dobutamine echocardiographic stress test

D. Angiogram

E. None of the above

Ref.: 23, 27

COMMENTS: In the absence of a change in a patient's clinical history or physical findings, only routine testing appropriate for age and gender needs to be conducted. • In a patient who has had coronary artery bypass grafting within 5 years or normal findings during an interventional cardiac workup within 2 years, no further testing is warranted unless dictated by changes in history and/or findings on physical examination. • When indicated, exercise stress testing is the preferred test. • Routine **treadmill testing** provides much useful information, including the patient's functional capacity, areas of myocardium where ischemia may occur, and a heart rate at which ischemia may occur. • For patients who cannot exercise on a treadmill, **chemical stress testing** is the next preferred method of assessing ventricular function. • An **angiogram** is generally reserved for patients with known cardiac disease, recent MI or unstable angina, or severe stenotic valvular disease. • In such patients, an acute intervention such as angioplasty (stenting) or balloon valvuloplasty may be indicated before noncardiac surgery. • In addition, while coronary artery bypass grafting is generally not indicated to improve the outcome of noncardiac surgery, angioplasty may identify patients who do require coronary artery bypass grafting and/or valve replacement before elective noncardiac surgery. • When surgery is urgent or emergent, the patient's condition should be medically optimized and interventional studies reserved for the postoperative period.

ANSWER:
A

24. In patients with intermediate predictors of cardiac risk who are scheduled for intermediate or high-risk surgical procedures, which of the following interventions can reduce perioperative morbidity and mortality?

A. Continuous intraoperative ST-segment monitoring

B. Regional anesthesia when indicated

C. Transesophageal echocardiography

D. Routine use of intravenous nitroglycerin

E. β-Blockade therapy

Ref.: 23, 27

COMMENTS: It is unclear whether certain anesthetic techniques or intraoperative monitors can reliably reduce perioperative morbidity and mortality. • **Continuous ST-segment monitoring** is a noninvasive, safe, readily available, inexpensive component of routine intraoperative monitoring. • While it has proven useful in early detection of myocardial ischemia, it has not been shown to favorably affect the overall incidence of perioperative MI or death. • Although **regional anesthesia** seems safer than general anesthesia, there are no studies corroborating such a claim. • **Transesophageal echocardiography** is very safe and provides pertinent information regarding volume status, contractility, and regional wall-motion abnormalities. • However, it requires an experienced operator, since adequate views may not always be obtainable, particularly during procedures involving the thorax and upper abdomen.

Perioperative **nitroglycerin administration** has been used to optimize cardiac perfusion in high-risk patients, since it causes dilatation of epicardial vessels and is an effective therapy for angina. • Topical nitrates are not recommended in the operating room, since absorption may be adversely affected by changes in body temperature and cutaneous blood flow. • While intravenous nitroglycerin is commonly employed, no studies have clearly demonstrated its efficacy in reducing perioperative cardiac morbidity and mortality. • **β-Blockade therapy** reduces perioperative and long-term complications related to myocardial morbidity and death from MI. • It is thought to reduce the incidence of myocardial complications via several mechanisms, including reduction of myocardial oxygen demand and stabilization of intravascular plaques and thrombi. • Even when therapy is instituted 3–4 hours preoperatively, cardiac complications are reduced in patients followed 2 years postoperatively. • Other drugs, such as calcium-channel blockers and α_2-agonists, have not been shown to have the same effect as does β-blockade.

ANSWER:
E

25. Which of the following statements regarding perioperative β-blocker use is/are true?

A. Perioperative β-blockade can reduce intraoperative myocardial ischemia in at-risk patients.

B. Perioperative β-blockade can reduce postoperative myocardial ischemia in at-risk patients.

C. Perioperative β-blockade can reduce postoperative cardiac death and nonfatal MI after major vascular surgery.

D. Perioperative β-blockade should be initiated preoperatively and continued for several days postoperatively in patients at risk of cardiac events.

E. All of the above

Ref.: 23, 24, 28

COMMENTS: In 2001, the Agency for Healthcare Research and Quality found sufficient clinical evidence to justify widespread implementation of perioperative β-blockade. • Patients with known coronary disease, positive preoperative stress evaluation results, or known risk factors for cardiac complications and those undergoing intermediate- to high-risk procedures will likely benefit from perioperative β-blockade. • This observation has been best documented in vascular surgery patients, in whom reductions in intraoperative and postoperative ischemia, perioperative MI, and cardiac mortality have been demonstrated. • The greatest benefit appears to accrue in patients with more than one of the following risk factors: high-risk surgery, known coronary artery disease, cerebrovascular disease, diabetes mellitus, or chronic renal insufficiency. • Although specific guidelines have not yet been developed, continuing β-blockade for up to a month postoperatively appears logical. • The risk of perioperative MI is greatest in the first 24–96 hr after surgery, but it persists up to 1 week postoperatively.

ANSWER:
E

26. Regarding the several scenarios listed below, which one of the operations should proceed as scheduled?

A. An 80-year-old scheduled for cataract surgery who has a pulse of 60 and blood pressure of 180/110 and is completely asymptomatic

B. A 67-year-old scheduled for left total hip arthroplasty who has a pulse of 80 and blood pressure of 180/110, is asymptomatic, and takes β-blockers

C. A 65-year-old hypertensive scheduled for bilateral total knee arthroplasty who has a pulse of 90 and blood pressure of 130/70 and who takes angiotensin-converting enzyme (ACE) inhibitors

D. An 80-year-old scheduled for bilateral laparoscopic hernia repair who has a pulse of 42 and blood pressure of 100/60 and who has a pacemaker and takes β-blockers

Ref.: 22, 27

COMMENTS: The management of hypertension in the perioperative period remains controversial. • However, several studies consistently have shown that a preoperative diastolic blood pressure higher than 110 confers increased risk of major morbidity. • Aggressive perioperative normalization may not reduce the risk. • However, the patient in scenario A is scheduled for a low-risk operation, unlike the patient in scenario B. • Therefore, the operation in scenario A can be performed safely as long as the patient has adequate follow-up. • ACE inhibitors have been associated with severe perioperative hypotension during major surgery, especially in patients who receive an epidural catheter as part of their management. • The patient in scenario D may have a pacemaker malfunction that needs to be evaluated. • β-Blockers have been shown to decrease intraoperative ischemia and should be continued. • Calcium-channel blockers and diuretics may be continued.

ANSWER:
A

27. Which of the following strategies is not important for obtaining positive outcomes in geriatric surgical patients?

A. Preoperative evaluation of medical physiologic status

B. Optimization of physical and cognitive function

C. Minimization of perioperative nutritional deficiency

D. Postoperative patient assessment for rehabilitation options

E. Surgical risk assessment based on a specific diagnosis

Ref.: 26

COMMENTS: There are several important factors in obtaining positive surgical outcomes in geriatric patients. • Assessment of a patient's preoperative physical and cognitive function, along with optimization of these variables, is critical in elderly patients. • Ignorance of these variables may result in more aggressive surgical procedures and poor outcomes. • As risks of surgical therapy increase, elderly patients may opt for palliative procedures, which allow for resumption of preoperative independence and activities of daily life, as opposed to more radical procedures, which entail a prolonged convalescence and a questionable quality of life. • Elderly patients may be at risk for malnutrition due to physical and cognitive disabilities, poverty, and lack of awareness of the importance of a balanced diet. • Proper preoperative rehabilitation planning results in quicker resumption of independent living, as shown in studies of patients with hip fractures. • Surgical risk assessment is multifactorial and not based on a specific diagnosis.

• Physical fitness, cognitive fitness, and social factors (e.g., family and financial support), in addition to a specific diagnosis and surgical plan, are part of a thorough preoperative risk assessment.

ANSWER:
E

28. Following small bowel resection, a 75-year-old patient is agitated, calling out for his deceased wife. He requires restraints. Which of the following statements is incorrect regarding his condition?

A. Postoperative delirium may occur in up to 15% of patients 70 years of age or older.

B. Postoperative delirium increases the risk of other complications.

C. A preoperative assessment of cognitive function should be routine in patients older than 75 years of age for major elective surgery.

D. Postoperative delirium may indicate the onset of another disease process.

E. In geriatric patients, regional anesthesia is associated with a lower incidence of postoperative delirium than is general anesthesia.

Ref.: 26, 29

COMMENTS: Postoperative delirium is a common and serious problem in the geriatric population. • Delirium occurs in 15% of patients 70 years of age and older. • The risk is greater following orthopedic procedures, with rates as high as 60%. • A baseline assessment of cognitive function is a valuable tool in assessing risk and implementing preventive strategies. • A mini-mental status examination is a useful tool for cognitive assessment. • New-onset postoperative delirium may be caused by multiple factors, including drugs, disease, and depression. • Controversy exists as to whether the anesthetic technique has an effect on postoperative delirium. • However, recent studies indicate no relationship between severity of postoperative delirium and anesthetic technique.

ANSWER:
E

29. With regard to the physiologic changes associated with aging, which of the following is/are true?

A. Tachypnea is a less reliable sign of respiratory failure

B. The cough mechanism is less effective

C. Normal creatinine values decrease

D. Hypothermia becomes more prevalent

E. Fever is a reliable sign of infection

Ref.: 26, 29

COMMENTS: Pulmonary complications are among the commonest complications in elderly surgical patients. • Decreased strength and endurance of respiratory muscles, decreased lung volumes, and decreased compensatory responses to hypoxia or hypercarbia make tachypnea a less reliable sign of impending respiratory failure. • Decreased airway sensitivity, mucociliary clearance dysfunction, and decreased muscle strength all contribute to a decreased cough mechanism. • Because decreased muscle mass occurs with aging, normal creatinine levels are lower in the elderly. • Geriatric patients are at increased risk of hypothermia due to impaired mechanisms of heat conservation. • Decreased muscle mass and metabolic heat production, malnutrition, and increased heat loss due to thinning skin all contribute to this phenomenon. • Fever is not a reliable indicator of infection in elderly patients. • Malnourished geriatric patients or the extremely old may be unable to mount a febrile response to infection.

ANSWER:
A, B, C, D

30. Following a cholecystectomy, an 82-year-old patient has an oxygen saturation of 88% on 2 L of oxygen by nasal cannula. Which of the following is not a likely explanation for this phenomenon?

A. A decrease in glomerular filtration rate

B. Postoperative shivering

C. A spurious pulse oximetry reading

D. Repositioning of the patient from a supine to a sitting position

E. Conversion of a laparoscopic cholecystectomy to an open cholecystectomy

Ref.: 26, 30

COMMENTS: One of the numerous effects of aging on the renal system is a decrease in glomerular filtration rate, particularly after the fifth and sixth decade of life. • The resultant decreased ability to excrete an acute salt load or water load places the patient at risk of pulmonary edema from overzealous hydration. • Shivering, a common postoperative phenomenon, dramatically increases oxygen consumption, which could cause hypoxia. • In addition, the patient's movement could result in a spurious pulse oximetry reading. • The patient's positioning has a direct effect on ventilation-perfusion mismatch and the alveolar-arterial oxygen gradient. • The supine, as opposed to the sitting, position results in closure of small airways in the dependent lung, resulting in ventilation-perfusion mismatch and subsequent hypoxemia. • Therefore, placing a patient in the sitting position should result in improved oxygenation. • Unlike a laparoscopic cholecystectomy, an open cholecystectomy entails an upper abdominal incision, resulting in a decreased tidal volume, impaired diaphragmatic excursion with resultant hypoxemia, and an increased risk of atelectasis and pneumonia.

ANSWER:
D

31. Evidence-based strategies for perioperative renal protection include which of the following?

A. Fenoldopam: 0.01 µg/kg/min IV

B. Mannitol: 0.5–1 g/kg IV

C. Lasix: 20–40 mg IV

D. None of the above

Ref.: 22, 27, 31

COMMENTS: None of the above has been approved as a renoprotective agent by the U.S. • Food and Drug Administration, and none has consistently shown clear benefit, although all have theoretical benefits. • **Fenoldopam** preserves medullary blood flow without significant systemic effects. • **Mannitol** promotes diuresis,

which should minimize sludging of tubular fluid, and seems to be a free-radical scavenger. • However, it increases osmolarity and may lead to hypovolemia. • Loop diuretics, such as **Lasix**, reduce the metabolism of tubular cells and should enable patients to better tolerate ischemia.

ANSWER:
D

32. Regarding urinary retention after ambulatory surgery, which of the following statements is/are true?

A. Urinary retention is most frequently associated with herniorrhaphy and anorectal procedures.

B. Spinal anesthesia, but not general anesthesia, is a predisposing factor for postoperative urinary retention.

C. Postoperative urinary retention frequently can be asymptomatic.

D. Ambulatory surgery patients must void as a criterion for discharge.

E. Overzealous administration of intravenous fluids (>1,200 ml) can cause urinary retention.

Ref.: 1–3, 22

COMMENTS: Patients at risk for postoperative urinary retention include those with a previous history of retention and those undergoing procedures such as herniorrhaphy and anorectal operations. • Both spinal anesthesia and general anesthesia are predisposing factors, especially when the latter is associated with use of anticholinergic drugs. • Although bladder overdistention is a significant contributing factor in postoperative urinary retention, many patients are asymptomatic with bladder volumes exceeding 600 ml. • While low-risk patients may be safely discharged without the requirement to void, consideration should be given to catheterization of high-risk patients before discharge. • Patients at high risk of postoperative urinary retention should have ready access to a medical facility and be instructed to return to a medical facility if still unable to void 8–12 hr after discharge from an ambulatory surgical facility. • Judicious use of intravenous fluids may reduce the incidence of postoperative urinary retention in patients at high risk.

ANSWER:
A, C, E

33. Initial treatment of a postoperative headache 24 hr after spinal anesthesia for outpatient knee arthroplasty includes all but which of the following?

A. Oral fluids

B. Bed rest

C. Oral analgesics

D. Caffeine

E. Epidural blood patch

Ref.: 23

COMMENTS: Postdural puncture headache (PDPH) results from decreased intracranial pressure caused by leakage of cerebrospinal fluid from the dural defect caused by the spinal needle. • The incidence of PDPH can be decreased primarily by reducing the needle size and, to a lesser extent, by using needles of improved design. • Increased oral fluid intake, remaining recumbent, and use of oral analgesics can reduce cephalgia as well as other symptoms, such as visual disturbances, auditory disturbances, and nausea. • Caffeine may also be helpful in reducing symptoms. • An epidural blood patch is a more aggressive approach typically reserved for severe, persistent symptoms. • Epidural injection of 10–20 ml of autologous blood collected from a fresh venipuncture is associated with successful relief of severe, persistent PDPH symptoms in 90% of cases.

ANSWER:
E

---

34. Indicate whether each statement about postoperative nausea and vomiting (PONV) after ambulatory surgery is true or false.

A. PONV is associated with opioid use.

B. PONV occurs less frequently following anesthetic induction with propofol than with thiopental.

C. PONV prophylaxis should be administered to all patients before ambulatory surgery.

D. PONV is decreased in adults who are not required to ingest oral fluids before discharge.

Ref.: 22

COMMENTS: PONV is one of the most prevalent factors leading to delay in discharge from ambulatory surgical centers or unanticipated hospitalization after outpatient procedures. • Both pain and the treatment of pain with opioids are associated with increased risk of PONV. • "Balanced analgesia," with use of nonopioids, such as ketorolac (a nonsteroidal anti-inflammatory drug), and adjuvant methods of analgesia, such as wound infiltration with local anesthetic, and local or regional nerve blocks can substantially reduce the use of opioids and associated PONV. • Use of propofol as an induction drug is known to reduce the incidence of PONV, although the effect is lessened after long surgical procedures unless an infusion of propofol is used during the procedure or another dose of propofol is administered toward the conclusion of a long procedure. • Because of the cost and side effects of antiemetic drugs, prophylaxis for all patients undergoing ambulatory surgery is not recommended. • However, prophylaxis for patients at high risk for PONV can be cost effective by reducing the length of the postoperative stay and improving patients' satisfaction.

Risk factors for PONV include ophthalmic, middle ear, breast, and laparoscopic procedures; previous history of PONV; and history of motion sickness. • Although oral fluid intake before discharge does not increase the risk of PONV in adult patients, eliminating oral fluid intake as a discharge criterion does not reduce the risk of PONV. • Therefore, patients should be allowed to decide to accept or decline oral fluids as they desire before discharge.

ANSWER:
A-True; B-True; C-False; D-False

---

35. Regarding skin preparation in a 35-year-old man scheduled for an inguinal hernia repair, which of the following is/are effective measures?

A. Clip the hair from the operative site.

B. Paint the operative site with chlorhexidine gluconate.

C. Give a preoperative antiseptic bath.

D. All of the above

E. None of the above

Ref.: 1, 3

COMMENTS: The sole reason for preparing the patient's skin before an operation is to reduce the risk of wound infection. • A preoperative antiseptic bath is not necessary for most surgical patients. • Hair should not be removed from the operative site unless it physically interferes with accurate anatomic approximation of the wound edges. • If hair must be removed, it should be clipped in the operating room. • Shaving hair from the operative site, particularly on the evening before operation or immediately before wound incision, increases the risk of wound infection. • The necessary reduction in microorganisms can be achieved by using povidone-iodine or chlorhexidine gluconate both for mechanical cleansing of the intertriginous folds and the umbilicus and for painting the operative site. • Simply applying the agents (painting or spraying) is an effective means of disinfection of the skin. • Povidone-iodine should be allowed to dry.

ANSWER:
A, B

---

36. Regarding the risk of surgery in patients with liver disease, which one of the following is not true?

A. Halothane and enflurane reduce hepatic arterial blood flow.

B. Hypercarbia increases portal blood flow.

C. Fentanyl, not morphine or meperidine, is the preferred narcotic agent.

D. Child's class B cirrhosis patients undergoing cardiac operations have a high mortality rate.

E. Laparoscopic cholecystectomy can be performed safely in patients with compensated cirrhosis, even in the presence of portal hypertension.

Ref.: 32

COMMENTS: Routine laboratory screening of otherwise healthy surgical candidates for unsuspected liver disease is controversial. • However, a carefully taken history to identify risk factors for liver disease permits adequate initial evaluation. • Isoflurane is preferred over halothane because it increases hepatic arterial blood flow. • Hypercarbia should be avoided, since it triggers a sympathetic splanchnic stimulation, leading to decreased portal flow. • Fentanyl or sufentanyl are the narcotic agents of choice. • The metabolism of morphine and diazepam can be prolonged in patients with liver disease. • Lorazepam is preferred, since it is eliminated by glucoronidation. • Cardiac operations are associated with a high mortality rate in patients with cirrhosis Child's class B because of the higher risk of infection and bleeding. • Celiotomy leads to a greater reduction in hepatic arterial blood flow than do extra-abdominal or laparoscopic operations. • In patients with cirrhosis, the Child-Pugh classification is the most useful predictor of mortality and morbidity. • Postoperatively, bilirubin levels and prothrombin time should be closely monitored. • Preoperative correction of coagulopathic states is mandatory.

ANSWER:
B

REFERENCES

1. Townsend CM, Beauchamp RD, Evers BM, et al (eds): *Sabiston Textbook of Surgery: The Biological Basis of Modern Surgical Practice*, 16th ed. Saunders, Philadelphia, 2001.
2. Schwartz SI, Shires GT, Spencer FC (eds): *Principles of Surgery*, 7th ed. McGraw-Hill, New York, 1999.

3. Greenfield LJ, Mulholland MW, Oldham KT, et al (eds): *Surgery: Scientific Principles and Practice*, 3rd ed. Lippincott, Williams & Wilkins, Philadelphia, 2001.

4. Fumary AP, Zerr KJ, Grunkemier GL, et al. Continuous intravenous insulin infusion reduces the incidence of deep sternal wound infection in diabetic patients after cardiac surgical procedures. *Ann Thorac Surg* 67:352–362, 1999.

5. Bartlett RH, Rich PB. Endocrine problems. American College of Surgeons ACS Surgery Principles and Practice. Retrieved May 2003 from www.acssurgery.com.

6. Ansara MF, Gryer PE, Scharp DN. Diabetes mellitus. American College of Surgeons ACS Surgery Principles and Practice. Retrieved May 2003 from <www.acssurgery.com>.

7. Kinney MAO, Narr BJ, Warner MA. Perioperative management of pheochromocytoma. *J Cardiothorac Vasc Anesth* 6:359–369, 2002.

8. Abbott TR. Anaesthesia in untreated myxoedema. Report of two cases. *Br J Anaesth* 39:510–514 1967.

9. Kim JM, Hackman L. Anesthesia for untreated hypothyroidism: report of three cases. *Anesth Analg* 56:299–302, 1977.

10. Weinberg AD, Brennan MD, Gorman CA, et al. Outcome of anesthesia and surgery in hypothyroid patients. *Arch Intern Med* 143:893–897, 1983.

11. Ladenson PW, Levin AA, Ridgway EC, et al. Complications of surgery in hypothyroid patients. *Am J Med* 77:261–266, 1984.

12. Appoo JJ, Morin JF. Severe cerebral and cardiac dysfunction associated with thyroid decompensation after cardiac operations. *J Thorac Cardiovasc Surg* 114:496, 1997.

13. Catz B, Russell S. Myxedema, shock and coma. *Arch Intern Med* 108:407–417, 1961.

14. Holvey DN, Goodner CJ, Nicoloff JT, et al. Treatment of myxedema coma with intravenous thyroxine. *Arch Intern Med* 113:89–96, 1964.

15. Ragaller M, Quintel M, Bender HJ, Albrecht DM. Myxedema coma as a rare postoperative complication. *Anaesthesist* 42:179–183, 1993.

16. Bennett-Guerrero E, Kramer DC, Schwinn DA. Effect of chronic and acute thyroid hormone reduction on perioperative outcome. *Anesth Analg* 85:30–36, 1997.

17. Roti E, Robuschi G, Gardini E, et al. Comparison of methimazole and saturated solution of potassium iodide in the early treatment of hyperthyroidism Graves' disease. *Clin Endocrinol* 28:305–314, 1988.

18. Baeza A, Aguayo J, Barria M, et al. Rapid preoperative preparation in hyperthyroidism. *Clin Endocrinol* 35:439–442, 1991.

19. Nabil N, Miner DJ, Amatruda JM. Methimazole: an alternative route of administration. *J Clin Endocrinol Metab* 54:180–181, 1982.

20. Walter RM, Bartle WR. Rectal administration of propylthiouracil in the treatment of Graves' disease. *Am J Med* 88:69–70, 1990.

21. Burch HB, Wartofsky L: Hyperthyroidism. *Curr Ther Endocrinol Metab* 5:64–70, 1994.

22. Stoelting RK, Dierdorf SF: *Anesthesia and Co-Existing Disease*, 4th ed. Churchill Livingstone, Philadelphia, 2000.

23. Barash PG, Cullen BF, Stoelting RK: *Clinical Anesthesia*, 4th ed. Lippincott Williams & Wilkins, Philadelphia, 2001.

24. Eagle KA, Berger PB, Calkin H, et al. ACC/AHA guideline update for perioperative cardiovascular evaluation of non-cardiac surgery: a report of the American College of Cardiology/American Heart Association Task Force on Practice Guidelines 2002. Retrieved June 2003 from <www.acc.org/clinical/guidelines/perio/update/periupdate_index.htm>.

25. Amar D, Zhang H, Leung DH, et al. Older age is the strongest predictor of postoperative atrial fibrillation. *Anesthesiology* 96:352–356, 2002.

26. Bharucha D, Marinchak R, Kowey P. Arrhythmias after cardiac surgery: atrial fibrillation and atrial flutter. Up to Date 2003.

27. Miller RS. *Anesthesia*, vol. 2, 5th ed. Churchill Livingstone, Philadelphia, 2000.

28. Mangano DT, Layug EI, Wallace A, et al. Multicenter study of perioperative ischemia research group: effect of atenolol on mortality and cardiovascular morbidity after noncardiac surgery. *N Engl J Med* 335:1713–1720, 1996.

29. Pavlin DJ, Pavlin EG, Fitzgibbon DR, et al. Management of bladder function after outpatient surgery. *Anesthesiology* 91:42–50, 1999.

30. Leung JM, Liu LL. Current controversies in the perioperative management of geriatric patients. ASA refresher course in anesthesiology. 29:175–187, 2001.

31. Newman MF (ed). *Perioperative Organ Protection*. Lippincott, Williams & Wilkins, Philadelphia, 2003.

32. Friedman LS. The risk of surgery in patients with liver disease. *Hepatology* 29:1617–1623, 1999.

CHAPTER 5

Acute Abdomen

Nadine L. Duhan Floyd, M.D.

1. With regard to C fibers and peritoneal innervation, which of the following statements is/are true?

   A. They are myelinated, polymodal nociceptors.

   B. They travel bilaterally with the sympathetic chains.

   C. Their stimulation is interpreted as localized, sharp pain.

   D. They conduct rapidly (<0.5 m/s).

   E. They refer pain to dermatomes.

Ref.: 1–4

COMMENTS: See Question 3.

2. Which one of the following is not a trigger of visceral pain?

   A. Ischemia

   B. Traction

   C. Distention

   D. Heat

   E. Inflammation

Ref.: 1–4

COMMENTS: See Question 3.

3. Match the organs in the left-hand column with the location of their referred pain in the right-hand column. Items in the right-hand column may be used more than once.

   A. Gallbladder   a. Epigastrium

   B. Jejunum   b. Periumbilical

   C. Rectum   c. Hypogastrium

   D. Pancreas   d. Shoulder

   E. Appendix

Ref.: 3, 4

COMMENTS: The visceral peritoneum is innervated by C fibers coursing with the autonomic ganglia. • C fibers are unmyelinated, slow-conducting (0.5–5.0 m/s), polymodal nociceptors that travel bilaterally with the sympathetic and parasympathetic fibers.

• Visceral pain is a response to injury of the visceral peritoneum. • Distention, stretch, traction, compression, torsion, ischemia, and inflammation trigger visceral pain fibers. • Abdominal organs are insensate to heat, cutting, and electrical stimulation.

Visceral pain is typically vague and crampy and is perceived in the region of origin of the embryologically derived autonomic ganglia. • **Foregut** organs (proximal to the ligament of Treitz) refer pain to the celiac chain, and the pain is felt in the epigastrium. • The organs of the **midgut** (small intestine and ascending colon) refer pain to the superior mesenteric chain (periumbilical pain) and those of the **hindgut** (transverse and descending colon, sigmoid colon, and rectum) to the inferior mesenteric ganglia and hypogastrium.

ANSWERS:
Question 1: B
Question 2: D
Question 3: A- a,d; B- b; C- c; D- a; E- b

4. An 18-year-old male has a 12-hr history of vague abdominal pain, anorexia, and nonbilious vomiting. The pain has now localized to the right lower quadrant. On examination, he is found to have tenderness over McBurney's point, with involuntary muscle rigidity. Which of the following best explains the localization of pain?

   A. Inflammation of the visceral peritoneum produces localizing pain.

   B. Pain over McBurney's point is caused by distention of the appendiceal lumen.

   C. Unmyelinated fibers carry pain signals with thoracic and lumbar spinal nerves.

   D. Movement of the inflamed parietal peritoneum induces rebound tenderness.

Ref.: 1–4

COMMENTS: Typically, early in the course of appendicitis, **distention** of the appendiceal lumen triggers visceral nerves that course with the superior mesenteric artery ganglia, producing vague pain that is perceived in the periumbilical region. • As appendiceal **inflammation** progresses and involves the parietal peritoneum, somatic pain fibers are triggered. • Somatic pain travels via thinly myelinated fibers. • These fibers are fast conducting and course with spinal nerve roots T7–L2. • Movement of the inflamed parietal peritoneum will trigger the fibers and is the cause of "rebound tenderness." Muscle rigidity is involuntary spasm of the abdominal muscles in response to peritoneal inflammation.

ANSWER:
D

5. Which of the following is not an ominous sign in a patient with abdominal pain?

A. Diaphoresis

B. Pallor

C. Hypotension

D. Patient lying still

E. Jaundice

Ref.: 1–4

COMMENTS: Initial evaluation of patients with acute abdominal pain should include assessment for signs of shock. • Shock may be secondary to hypovolemia or a systemic inflammatory response. • **Signs include tachycardia, hypotension, pallor, dry mucous membranes, poor skin turgor, and slow capillary refill.** • Immediate intravenous access and resuscitation should be initiated. • A patient writhing with colicky pain may have distention or obstruction of a hollow viscus (e.g., ureter or intestine), whereas a patient lying very still probably has diffuse peritoneal inflammation and a perforated viscus. • A patient with right upper quadrant pain, fever, jaundice, and signs of septic shock may have ascending cholangitis, requiring emergent decompression of the biliary tree. • However, jaundice itself is not necessarily an ominous sign.

ANSWER:
E

6. Regarding peritoneal fluids, which of the following statements is/are true?

A. The abdominal cavity normally contains 150–200 ml (3 g/dl of isotonic fluid).

B. The protein content of peritoneal fluid is 3 g/dl.

C. Mesothelial cells absorb solutes via endocytosis.

D. Inflammation of the peritoneum decreases its permeability.

E. Bacteria contaminating the peritoneum enter the systemic circulation through subdiaphragmatic lymphatics.

Ref.: 1

COMMENTS: Normally, the peritoneum contains 50 to 100 ml of fluid, with solute concentrations equal to those found in plasma. • The protein content is less than that of plasma (3 g/dl). • Fluid is absorbed by the mesothelial cells lining the peritoneum through endocytosis. • Solutes with molecular weight less than 30 kD are easily absorbed. • Inflammation of the peritoneum increases its permeability. • Gravity and the negative pressure created by exhalation under the diaphragm effect movement of the peritoneal fluid. • The right paracolic gutter allows unhindered movement of fluid from the pelvis to the right subdiaphragmatic area, whereas the phrenicocolic ligaments obstruct flow through the left paracolic gutter. • Subdiaphragmatic lymphatics play a major role in the absorption of peritoneal fluid and the clearance of solutes and bacteria into the thoracic duct.

ANSWER:
C, E

7. Which of the following will not alter the natural flow of peritoneal fluid?

A. Fibrin

B. Bowel obstruction

C. Cirrhosis

D. Positive-pressure ventilation

E. Previous appendectomy

Ref.: 1

COMMENTS: Adhesions, fibrin, paralytic ileus, and positive-pressure mechanical ventilation all obstruct the normal flux of peritoneal fluid. • Adhesions from prior surgery may create compartments within the abdominal cavity that are sequestered from the natural flow of peritoneal fluid. • Fluid loss may occur in long-standing bowel obstruction that alters the dynamics of fluid secretion and absorption.

ANSWER:
C

8. Regarding bacterial contamination of the peritoneal cavity, which of the following statements is not true?

A. Bacterial contamination of the peritoneum triggers degranulation of mesothelial cells, which initiates the systemic inflammatory response.

B. Once the systemic response is initiated, the endothelial cells increase their permeability to complement, opsonins, and fibrin.

C. Serum levels of catecholamines decrease in feedback to mast cell degranulation.

D. Ninety percent of the bacteria are cleared by phagocytosis and the reticular endothelial system.

Ref.: 1

COMMENTS: Bacterial contamination triggers mast cells to degranulate, initiating a local and systemic cascade of events. • Locally, the mesothelial and endothelial cells increase their permeability, allowing products of complement, opsonins, and fibrin to enter the peritoneal cavity freely. • This increased permeability depletes intravascular volume as fluid shifts into the peritoneal cavity. • The systemic inflammatory response syndrome (SIRS) is initiated and consists of an increase in serum levels of catecholamines, glucocorticoids, aldosterone, and vasopressin. • The combination of hypovolemia and SIRS causes hyperdynamic hemodynamics. • Once bacteria enter the abdomen, they circulate via the subdiaphragmatic lymphatics and enter the systemic circulation through the thoracic duct. • Once circulating, more than 90% will be cleared by Kupffer cells and the reticuloendothelial system.

ANSWER:
C

9. Regarding the initial assessment of a patient who comes to the emergency department with acute abdominal pain, which of the following statements is/are not true?

A. Conducting thin-cut computerized tomographic (CT) scanning with contrast is the first step in evaluating the acute abdomen.

B. Absence of bowel sounds rules out the presence of a mechanical obstruction.

C. Hypoactive bowel sounds may suggest an intra-abdominal infection.

D. Plain radiographic studies can demonstrate abdominal free air, pelvic fluid, intra-abdominal abscess, and intestinal pneumatosis.

Ref.: 1, 2

COMMENTS: In a stable patient, a good history and physical examination are paramount to determining the potential cause of the acute abdomen and directing the initial work-up. • Distention and high-pitched bowel sounds may represent an **early** mechanical bowel obstruction. • Decreased or absent bowel sounds are suggestive of an ileus secondary to an infectious process but may also be found in cases of **long-standing** obstruction. • For a patient with a diffusely rigid abdomen, plain radiographs (upright chest x-ray or lateral decubitus films) may identify free air, suggestive of perforated viscus. • Plain radiographs can also demonstrate loculated extraluminal air-fluid levels, suggestive of abscess, pneumatosis intestinalis, or loss of psoas shadow and fat lines, suggesting edema or fluid in the pelvis. • Computed tomographic and ultrasound imaging can also demonstrate these abnormalities and more accurately characterize intra-abdominal fluid or abscess. • These modalities may also permit therapeutic percutaneous treatment of fluid collections.

ANSWER:
A, B

10. A 55-year-old man comes to the emergency department with a history of 6 hr of acute, diffuse abdominal pain. On examination, his heart rate is found to be 115 beats per minute, his blood pressure 95/60, his respiratory rate 22 breaths per minute, and his pulse oximetric results 93% on a 4-L nasal cannula. He has diffuse abdominal rigidity. Plain radiographic studies demonstrate extraluminal free air. Regarding resuscitation of the patient in the emergency department before transfer to the operating room, which of the following statements is/are true?

A. Intravenous administration of antibiotics is the first priority.

B. The intravenous access of choice is a Swan-Ganz catheter.

C. Two to 3 L of crystalloid should be administered intravenously.

D. Endotracheal intubation should be established immediately.

Ref.: 1, 3

COMMENTS: The initial evaluation of a patient with abdominal pain should include evaluation for signs of hemodynamic instability, including tachycardia, hypotension, pallor, decreased skin turgor, and decreased urine output. • **Establishing intravenous access and starting intravenous hydration should be undertaken immediately,** and, for a patient with hypotension, boluses of crystalloid (lactated Ringer's or normal saline solution) should be given. • Routine pulmonary artery catheterization is not required unless there is a known history of serious cardiac disease or renal failure. • However, if there is no evidence of active bleeding and the blood pressure does not improve after a minimum of 3 L of crystalloid have been infused, cardiac status should be reassessed and pulmonary artery catheterization considered. • Not all patients require mechanical ventilation, but if there is evidence of rapid shallow breathing, impending ventilatory failure (hypercapnea, $PaCO_2 > 50$; pH <7.35), or a shunt refractory to oxygen failure (hypoxia, $PaO_2 < 60$ on FIO_2 100%), endotracheal intubation and mechanical ventilation should be established.

ANSWER:
C

11. Regarding the patient with a rigid abdomen and free air on plain film, which of the following statements is/are true?

A. No further radiologic work-up is required.

B. CT scanning with contrast medium is required to confirm the diagnosis.

C. Bedside sonographic imaging is preferred to CT imaging to confirm the diagnosis of free air.

D. Narcotics are contraindicated in patients with an acute abdomen.

E. Preoperative prophylactic steroids are indicated in patients with free air.

Ref.: 1, 2

COMMENTS: For a patient with a rigid abdomen and free air revealed by plain film imaging, no further radiographic work-up is required. • **Time would be unnecessarily wasted pursuing CT or sonographic imaging for a patient who needs prompt surgical exploration.** • Narcotics may be given after a patient has been adequately examined, a differential diagnosis established, and a treatment plan instituted. • However, caution should be taken in administering narcotics to a hypotensive, incompletely resuscitated patient. • There is no role for prophylactic steroid administration except for patients who use steroids chronically and are experiencing abdominal pain or an addisonian crisis.

ANSWER:
A

12. A 35-year-old woman experiences acute onset of epigastric and right upper quadrant pain several hours after a large dinner. She has had similar episodes in the past that resolved after a few hours. This episode persists, and she has fever and nonbilious vomiting. What is the most likely source of abdominal pain?

A. Perforated ulcer

B. Acute appendicitis

C. Perforation following bowel obstruction

D. Cholecystitis

E. Diverticulitis

Ref.: 2–4

COMMENTS: See Question 17.

13. A 60-year-old man with chronic alcoholism awakens at 3 AM with severe, sharp epigastric pain that 3 hr later becomes diffuse abdominal pain. What is the most likely source of abdominal pain?

A. Perforated ulcer

B. Acute appendicitis

C. Perforation following bowel obstruction

D. Cholecystitis

E. Diverticulitis

Ref.: 2–4

COMMENTS: See Question 17.

14. A 55-year-old man with a 2-day history of abdominal distention, vomiting, crampy abdominal pain, and obstipation is experiencing severe, diffuse abdominal pain. What is the most likely source of abdominal pain?

   A. Perforated ulcer

   B. Acute appendicitis

   C. Perforation following bowel obstruction

   D. Cholecystitis

   E. Diverticulitis

Ref.: 2–4

COMMENTS: See Question 17.

15. A 22-year-old man awakens with periumbilical abdominal pain followed by nonbilious vomiting. What is the most likely source of abdominal pain?

   A. Perforated ulcer

   B. Acute appendicitis

   C. Perforation following bowel obstruction

   D. Cholecystitis

   E. Diverticulitis

Ref.: 2–4

COMMENTS: See Question 17.

16. A 65-year-old man with a history of chronic constipation has had loose bowel movements, fever, and lower left quadrant pain for 2 days. What is the most likely source of the abdominal pain?

   A. Perforated ulcer

   B. Acute appendicitis

   C. Perforation following bowel obstruction

   D. Cholecystitis

   E. Diverticulitis

Ref.: 2–4

COMMENTS: See Question 17.

17. A 65-year-old man with a history of chronic constipation has a 3-day history of abdominal distention without a bowel movement. He has fever and abdominal rigidity. What is the most likely source of abdominal pain?

   A. Perforated ulcer

   B. Acute appendicitis

   C. Perforation following bowel obstruction

   D. Cholecystitis

   E. Diverticulitis

Ref.: 2–4

COMMENTS: The examples in Questions 12–17 demonstrate the importance of an adequate history in determining a patient's diagnosis and tailoring a patient's initial work-up. • Differentiating between patients who require immediate intervention and those who require a more gradual work-up is also essential in order to avoid unnecessary delays in treatment. • Biliary pain is typically mid-epigastric, with radiation to the right upper quadrant and right subscapular area. • It often occurs after fatty food intake. • It may be intermittent, crampy pain or constant, severe pain associated with nausea and vomiting.

Patients with perforated ulcer will classically remember the exact moment in time when perforation occurred. • There may be an initial period of diminished pain followed by severe pain when diffuse chemical peritonitis sets in. • Risk factors include a prior history of peptic ulcer disease and untreated *Helicobacter pylori* infection, use of medications such as steroids and nonsteroidal anti-inflammatory drugs, and alcohol abuse.

When vomiting is part of the history, it is important to differentiate between patients with a mechanical obstruction of the bowel, bile duct, or pancreatic duct and patients who have an ileus in response to pain from a nonintestinal source. • A patient with acute appendicitis and periumbilical pain may have one or two episodes of nonbilious emesis before localization of pain in the lower right quadrant. • The early abdominal pain and vomiting of appendicitis may resemble gastroenteritis. • However, in gastroenteritis the vomiting is typically more profuse and frequent and may be associated with profuse diarrhea as well.

Complications of bowel obstruction, a history of weight loss or new-onset obstipation, and changes in stool patterns may suggest a colorectal malignancy. • Although such a diagnosis is possible, it is critical to determine whether urgent surgery is required. • A patient with a 3-day history of obstructive symptoms (i.e., distention, crampy pain, and vomiting) who has peritonitis and fever is likely to have a complicated obstruction (e.g., ischemic, gangrenous, or perforated bowel) requiring immediate intervention. • If the pain is diffuse, it may be due to a free perforation, causing diffuse contamination of the peritoneal cavity. • If the pain is localized, it may represent a contained perforation, as can occur with diverticulitis. • This type of pain is typically in the lower left quadrant.

A N S W E R S :
Question 12: D
Question 13: A
Question 14: C
Question 15: B
Question 16: E
Question 17: C

18. A 65-year-old man with a history of chronic alcohol abuse has been experiencing epigastric and periumbilical pain associated with nonbilious vomiting for 1 day. He denies any melena or hematemesis. In the past, he has had several episodes of similar pain, which sometimes radiated to the back, and he was hospitalized for several days 2 months ago. He denies any prior surgery or medical problems. His vital signs are stable. His abdomen is not distended and does not exhibit surgical scars. Bowel sounds are present but diminished. His abdomen is soft, and he exhibits voluntary guarding of the epigastrium. His serum amylase level is 550 units per 100 ml. Regarding management of this patient, which of the following is the most reasonable next step?

   A. Establish intravenous access.

   B. Conduct sonographic studies to demonstrate cholelithiasis.

   C. Conduct CT scanning to diagnose a pancreatic pseudocyst.

D. Perform an esophagogastroduodenoscopy (EGD) to evaluate for varices and complications of cirrhosis.

E. Initiate a low-fat diet and antilipid medication.

Ref.: 1, 2

COMMENTS: A patient with pancreatitis can have severe abdominal pain and rigidity. • Surgery should be avoided except for complications (e.g., necrotizing pancreatitis or symptomatic pseudocyst). • Management of a patient with acute pancreatitis should include bowel rest, intravenous resuscitation, parenteral nutrition, and monitoring in the intensive care unit when appropriate. • Sources of pancreatitis should be investigated, including gallstones, hyperlipidemia, and drugs (i.e., thiazides). • Alcohol abuse is a common cause of pancreatitis, but the fact that a patient abuses alcohol should not dismiss the necessity for a thorough work-up. • After stabilization and resuscitation, diagnostic studies to define the pancreas and biliary tree are conducted. • Sonographic studies can screen for stones but cannot provide a good evaluation of the retroperitoneum. • CT scanning with a contrast medium reveals good pancreatic and retroperitoneal detail in most patients.

For patients with recurrent or chronic pancreatitis, a CT scan should be performed to look for complications of pancreatitis, including a pancreatic pseudocyst, fistula, or mass. • EGD is not usually used to make the diagnosis of pancreatitis. • It may be a useful adjunctive diagnostic tool during the course of the disease. • Patients should receive nothing by mouth initially and are not fed.

ANSWER:
A, B, C

19. Five days later, the patient described in Question 18 returns with worsening pain. He states that he stopped the prescribed treatment 3 days ago because he felt better. He now has fever and had diarrhea this morning. On examination, he is found to have fullness in the lower left quadrant with guarding. What would the best management now include?

A. Hospitalization

B. Immediate operative exploration

C. Air-contrast enema

D. Colonoscopy

E. CT scan of the abdomen and pelvis

Ref.: 1, 2

COMMENTS: In complicated cases, such as those involving fever, a mass, and localized peritonitis, hospitalization with bowel rest, broad-spectrum intravenous antibiotics, and serial examinations should be initiated. • CT scanning should be performed to differentiate between phlegmon and abscess. • The latter can be drained percutaneously. • Elective resection should be undertaken after successful nonoperative treatment of an abscess. • The patient who becomes hemodynamically unstable during a period of conservative management or does not improve with nonoperative measures will require urgent surgical exploration with drainage and bowel diversion. • In this setting, resection of the diseased segment is generally possible, but the surgeon may elect to perform fecal diversion alone if the phlegmon is adherent and resection is too dangerous.

ANSWER:
A, E

20. A 55-year-old man comes to the physician's office with complaints of lower left quadrant abdominal pain. He reports chronic constipation but denies any nausea or vomiting. He denies melena or bright-red blood, fever, or anorexia. On examination, his abdomen is not found to be distended and exhibits no surgical scars. He has mild tenderness in the lower left quadrant without guarding. Of the following, which is the best, most likely next step?

A. Administer oral antibiotics and clear diet.

B. Immediately conduct operative exploration.

C. Begin bowel preparation for a colonoscopy.

D. Administer an air-contrast barium enema.

Ref.: 1, 2

COMMENTS: Diverticulitis is a common source of abdominal pain that often does not require immediate intervention. • Mild cases without evidence of peritonitis or mass, suggesting a phlegmon, can be treated on an outpatient basis with oral antibiotics. • However, it is important to have a reliable and compliant patient who will return if worsening pain or fever develops. • Once the episode subsides, a work-up including a colonoscopy and/or a barium enema should be performed to confirm evidence of diverticulosis and to rule out malignancy. • However, these tests should not be performed during an acute exacerbation, since the instrumentation and distention of the inflamed bowel entail a higher risk of perforation. • In a patient with multiple episodes of diverticulitis, it is best to "cool" the inflammation down and perform a planned resection on cleansed bowel.

ANSWER:
A

21. Regarding peritonitis, which of the following statements is/are not true?

A. Primary peritonitis is commoner in children with nephrosis and adults with cirrhosis than in patients without such conditions.

B. Primary peritonitis is usually monomicrobial.

C. Chemical peritonitis often precedes bacterial contamination.

D. Multiple organisms are commonly cultured from peritoneal dialysis catheters.

E. Tuberculosis peritonitis has an insidious onset.

Ref.: 1, 2

COMMENTS: Primary, or spontaneous, peritonitis occurs in the absence of a known intra-abdominal source. • More often occurring in children, single microbes are isolated. • The most commonly cultured organisms include pnemococcus and hemolytic *Streptococcus*. • Among adults, patients with cirrhosis with ascites and patients on peritoneal dialysis are at higher risk, and *Escherichia coli* and *Klebsiella* are more commonly cultured. • Secondary peritonitis is more commonly encountered by the surgeon and implies inflammation secondary to a known intra-abdominal source (e.g., perforated viscus). • Chemical peritonitis is most commonly caused by sterile body fluids, including gastric contents, bile, urine, pancreatic fluid, and blood. • Chemical peritonitis is often followed by bacterial contamination, as in the case of perforated peptic ulcer. *peritoneal dialysis*

Patients with ~~chronic obstructive pulmonary disease~~ catheters are prone to peritonitis. • These infections are monomicrobial and may respond to intraperitoneal and systemic antibiotics. • If multiple organisms are grown from peritoneal fluid cultures, intestinal perforation should be suspected. • Tuberculous peritonitis usually occurs in chronically ill or malnourished patients and may accompany pulmonary reactivation. • Onset is usually insidious, with several weeks of fever, weight loss, anorexia, ascites, and dull, diffuse abdominal pain.

ANSWER:
D

REFERENCES

1. Brunicardi FC, Andersen DK, Billiar, TR, et al (eds): *Schwartz's Principles of Surgery,* 8th ed. McGraw-Hill, New York, 2004.
2. Townsend CM, Beauchamp RD, Evers BM (eds): *Sabiston Textbook of Surgery, The Biological Basis of Modern Surgical Practice,* 17th ed. Saunders, Philadelphia, 2004.
3. Silen W (ed): *Cope's Early Diagnosis of the Acute Abdomen,* 19th ed. Oxford University Press, New York, 1996.
4. Martin RF, Ricardo LR: The acute abdomen: an overview and algorithms. *Surg Clin North Am* 77(6):1227–1243, 1997.

CHAPTER 6

Complications

Mitchell Jay Cohen, M.D.

1. A 67-year-old woman undergoes a reversal of a Hartman's procedure. The procedure goes well, with no spillage of bowel contents. On postoperative day 5, the patient has a fever of 102°F (38.8°C), and erythema and drainage are noted around and from her wound. The wound is opened, revealing purulence and intact fascia. Which of the following should be considered risk factors for the development of wound infection?

   A. Her age

   B. The presence of foreign body in the wound

   C. The case classification as dirty

   D. A and B

   E. A, B, and C

   Ref.: 1–3

COMMENTS: See Question 2.

2. Which of the following perioperative interventions has been shown to affect the probability of wound infection?

   A. Hair removal the night before surgery

   B. Three days of perioperative antibiotics

   C. Strict maintenance of blood glucose level below 110 mg/dl

   D. Iodine-based, rather ~~of~~ than alcohol-based, scrub

   Ref.: 1–3

COMMENTS: Wound infection remains the most common nosocomial infection in surgical patients. • Surgical site infections account for 38% of all infections in surgical patients. • Contamination of the surgical site, most commonly from seeding from the patient's skin or gastrointestinal tract, allows a bacterial inoculum to begin multiplying. • An inoculum of 10^5 microorganisms is necessary for the formation of clinical infection. • Several factors, including the presence of a foreign body, devitalized tissue, hematoma, and altered patient immunologic function (e.g., due to diabetes or steroid use), reduce the number of bacteria necessary to cause clinical infection to as low as 10^3. • Other risk factors associated with infection include smoking, obesity, distant infection, and length of operative procedure. • The National Academy of Science classifies cases in four categories according to the likelihood of wound infection: clean (0–1%), clean contaminated (2–7%), contaminated (10–20%), and dirty (20–40%). • Hair removal, 3 days of

perioperative antibiotics, and iodine, as opposed to alcohol, scrubs have not been shown to affect the probability of a wound infection.

ANSWERS:
Question 1: E
Question 2: C

3. Approximately 30 min after the induction of general anesthesia for an exploratory laparotomy, the patient's end-tidal CO_2 begins to rise, and the anesthesiologist notes that the patient's core temperature is 105°F. What is the next appropriate step for the care of this patient?

   A. Continue the procedure, working quickly to finish, and place a cooling blanket on the patient.

   B. Quickly terminate the procedure and inhalation of any anesthetic agent, hyperventilate with 100% oxygen, administer dantrolene (2 mg/kg), and actively cool the patient with a saline bolus and cooling blanket.

   C. Continue the operation, switch to a different inhaled anesthetic agent, administer dantrolene, and actively cool the patient with a saline bolus and cooling blanket.

   D. Quickly terminate the procedure and inhalation of any anesthetic agent, and administer calcium-channel blockers.

   Ref.: 1–3

COMMENTS: See Question 4.

4. True or false: A prior history of malignant hyperthermia is a contraindication for future general anesthetics.

   Ref.: 1–3

COMMENTS: Malignant hyperthermia is a rare complication caused by uncontrolled calcium metabolism at the muscle level. • It results from a genetic defect in calcium metabolism at the sarcoplasmic reticulum. • It can be triggered by inhaled anesthetics, local amide anesthetics, or depolarizing muscle relaxants. • It has an incidence of 1 in 50,000 adults and a mortality rate of 30%. • Although muscle biopsy is necessary for pathologic confirmation, clinical symptoms of high end-tidal CO_2 and high core temperature are sufficient to make the diagnosis.

When the diagnosis is suspected in the operating room, rapid treatment is necessary to reverse progression and prevent death.

• The procedure should be immediately abandoned and any inhaled or local anesthetic discontinued. • The patient should be rapidly cooled by using cooling blankets and pads, administering cooled intravenous solutions, and, if the abdomen is open, lavage with cooled saline solution. • Dantrolene should be administered, since it blocks the release of calcium from the sarcoplasmic reticulum. • In addition, calcium may be administered, and any electrolyte abnormalities should be corrected. • Despite the risk, a prior episode of malignant hypothermia is not a contraindication to general anesthetic but should give rise to careful monitoring and choice of anesthetic.

A N S W E R S :
Question 3: B
Question 4: False

5. A 56-year-old man is recovering from a right hemicolectomy for tumor. On postoperative day 2, he becomes acutely short of breath. His pulse oximeter reads 85% on room air. His heart rate is 110. Because of difficulty with pain control, he has remained in bed since the operation. What is the next appropriate step in his management?

   A. Administration of 40 mg of Lasix and placement of a Foley catheter

   B. Sublingual nitroglycerin

   C. Initiation of anticoagulation with heparin, an electrocardiogram, arterial blood gas determinations, and a spiral chest computerized tomographic (CT) scan

   D. 5000 units of subcutaneous heparin and ventilation perfusion (VQ) scan

Ref.: 1–3

COMMENTS: Pulmonary embolism (PE) is a significant cause of morbidity and mortality in postoperative patients. • It is estimated to occur in about 100,000 patients per year. • PE may be characterized by symptoms ranging from minor tachypnea to sudden cardiac arrest and death. • It results from clots usually originating in the deep venous system in the legs. • Risk factors for deep vein thrombosis are any that predispose to stasis and hypercoagulability. • They include age over 40 years, chronic heart disease, coagulation deficiencies, malignancy, obesity, paralysis, prolonged surgical procedures, traumatic injuries, and orthopedic fractures. • A high index of suspicion is necessary when approaching a patient with respiratory difficulty. • Any suspicion of PE requires empiric treatment with heparin anticoagulation while the work-up is being completed. • The work-up should include arterial blood gas determinations, an electrocardiogram, and a spiral CT scan of the chest.

A N S W E R :
C

6. Which of the following statements regarding the perioperative management of a hypertensive patient is/are true?

   A. Moderate hypertension has little effect on surgical outcome and can be managed by having the patient take any antihypertensive medication the morning of surgery and restarting the medication as soon as the patient can tolerate intake by mouth.

   B. Hypertension can be managed with general anesthetic agents after induction.

   C. Good blood pressure control should be maintained in all patients undergoing elective or emergent surgery.

   D. Postoperative hypertension usually lasts 24 hr and should be controlled with a combination of analgesic and antihypertensive medication.

Ref.: 1–3

COMMENTS: Hypertension affects 50–60 million adults in the United States. • It contributes to surgical morbidity and mortality and is a primary risk factor for myocardial infarction (MI), cardiac arrest, stroke, renal failure, and bleeding. • Perioperatively, patients should be kept on any antihypertensive medications. • β-Blockade has the additional benefit of being cardiac protective. • Hypertension cannot and should not be assumed to be controlled by general anesthesia. • Surgical stimulation, hemodynamic changes, and depth of anesthesia all affect blood pressure and cannot reliably maintain blood pressure in the normal range. • Hence, careful maintenance of blood pressure is mechanically similar in surgical and nonsurgical patients. • While adequate analgesia is often necessary to prevent pain-induced hypertension and tachycardia, analgesia alone is not sufficient for maintenance of normotension. • Postoperative hypertension is not self-limiting and is independent of the time since operative intervention.

A N S W E R :
C

7. A 69-year-old patient who suffered an MI 2 months ago comes to the emergency department with biliary colic. With regard to his cardiac risk, which of the following statements is/are true?

   A. Since the patient has suffered no additional effects from his MI and has had no angina or cardiac symptoms, his risk of perioperative MI is 10%.

   B. Even though the patient has suffered no additional effects from his MI and has had no angina or cardiac symptoms, his risk of periopererative MI is 27%.

   C. The mortality rate associated with a perioperative MI is approximately equal to that associated with any MI in this patient.

   D. Since the risk of perioperative MI decreases 5% per month, the patient should postpone surgery until 9 months have passed since his MI if possible.

Ref.: 1–3

COMMENTS: Perioperative MI in patients undergoing noncardiac surgery remains a significant problem and risk. • In the elderly population, MI is the number-one cause of death in those undergoing noncardiac surgery. • In addition, the number of patients requiring both elective and emergent surgery who have suffered from a past MI or have significant heart disease is increasing in a rapidly aging population. • Because of this phenomenon, attempts have been made to stratify patients and assign risk in order to decide timing of surgery. • Patients who have had an MI in the past 3 months have a perioperative reinfarction rate of 27%. • Patients who are in the 3–6 month time frame have a 10% perioperative reinfarction rate. • After 6 months since an MI, patients have a 5–8% perioperative reinfarction rate, approximately equal to the reinfarction rate without surgery. • Because the mortality rate associated with perioperative MI is much higher than that associated with a nonperioperative MI (50–90% versus 12%), it is advisable to wait as long as possible, ideally at least 6 months, before performing elective or semi-elective surgery.

A N S W E R :
B

8. With regard to the patient in Question 7, which of the following perioperative interventions should be employed to minimize his cardiac risk from surgery?

A. Risk stratification using a scheme such as the Goldman classification

B. Perioperative β-blockade

C. Perioperative administration of lidocaine

D. Preoperative noninvasive cardiac testing

E. All of the above

Ref.: 1–3

COMMENTS: The aim of preoperative stratification and testing is to identify patients who are at increased cardiac risk. • Schemes such as the Goldman classification use various criteria with assigned points to predict surgical cardiac risk. • These risk criteria include age over 70 years, previous MI within 6 months, jugular venous distention (JVD) or S3 gallop on physical examination, electrocardiographic changes and premature ventricular contractions, and laboratory test result abnormalities. • In addition, points are assigned according to the type and acuity of surgery. • Based on this classification scheme, a patient's cardiac risk can be predicted. • If the patient's risk is sufficient, noninvasive cardiac testing can select patients who should undergo cardiac catheterization or revascularization procedures before noncardiac surgery. • Perioperatively, the goal is to maximize oxygen delivery and minimize cardiac work. • With this in mind, perioperative β-blockers are cardiac protective. • Hypotension or hypertension should be avoided, and euvolemia is the goal. • Patients who have normal noninvasive cardiac testing do not require any additional studies.

ANSWER:
E

9. A 32-year-old patient undergoes an appendectomy. During recovery, the patient has not voided for 4 hr. Her vital signs are normal. What is the next appropriate step in management?

A. Administer a 1-L bolus of 0.9 normal saline solution.

B. Continue the intravenous solution at the current rate for an additional 2 hr, and, if the patient still has not voided, insert a Foley catheter.

C. Insert a Foley catheter.

D. Straight-catheterize the patient.

E. Continue the intravenous solution at the current rate for an additional 2 hr, and, if the patient still has not voided, straight-catheterize the patient.

Ref.: 1–3

COMMENTS: Urinary retention occurs in approximately 5% of patients after general anesthesia. • It is caused by the prevention of α-adrenergic inhibition, which prevents relaxation at the bladder neck, which is necessary for urination. • It is more common in men than in women and is commonest after anorectal procedures and groin hernia repairs. • In these procedures, urinary retention can occur in approximately 40% of patients. • Additional contributing factors include postoperative pain, epidural anesthesia, and bladder expansion caused by overly aggressive fluid resuscitation. • The approach to a patient who experiences urinary retention must include elimination of causes for anuria. • However, once these causes are ruled out, a straight catheter

should be inserted after 6 hr of urinary retention. • If a second episode occurs and a second straight catheterization is necessary, a Foley catheter should be inserted and maintained for 2–5 days.

ANSWER:
E

10. With regard to acute renal failure (ARF), which of the following statements is/are true?

A. ARF occurs in 20% of surgical patients.

B. ARF is commonest in cardiopulmonary bypass and vascular procedures.

C. Damage to the tubular epithelia from toxins is the commonest reason for ARF.

D. Preexisting renal disease has little or no relationship to the risk of perioperative ARF.

E. B and D

Ref.: 1–3

COMMENTS: ARF occurs in 5–10% of patients after surgery. • Although toxin-induced injury is a common cause of ARF, most perioperative ARF is caused by decreased renal perfusion. • Despite mechanisms to maintain constant renal blood flow, even modest hypotension can lead to sequelae of vasoconstriction, tubular epithelial sloughing, and altered tubular permeability. • Additional damage is caused by exposure to toxins such as medications, anesthetics, and blood products. • Patients with preexisting renal disease are at greatest risk. • Patients with a serum creatine level of 2 mg/100 ml already have a 75% filtration deficit and are hence predisposed to renal failure with even small amounts of damage.

ANSWER:
B

11. A 55-year-old man is admitted to the hospital and treated with broad-spectrum antibiotics for uncomplicated diverticulitis. On day 5 of his hospital stay, increasing leukocytosis, abdominal pain, and constant, foul-smelling diarrhea develop. Which of the following diagnoses is most likely?

A. Pseudomembranous colitis

B. Progression of the diverticulitis

C. Infectious colitis

D. Retained colonic blood

Ref.: 1–3

COMMENTS: Pseudomembranous colitis is caused by overgrowth of *Clostridium difficile*. • While antibiotic-associated diarrhea can occur in up to 70% of patients treated with broad-spectrum antibiotics, infection with *C. difficile* accounts for 50% of antibiotic-associated colitis. • The usual symptoms include abdominal cramping; copious, foul-smelling diarrhea; and leukocytosis. • The white blood cell count can be as high as 60,000/mm³. • Pseudomembranes form primarily in the sigmoid colon and rectum. • Diagnosis is made by a high index of suspicion and an assay for the *C. difficile* toxin. • Equivocal cases can be diagnosed by the presence of pseudomembranes on sigmoidoscopy. • Even a single dose of antibiotic can cause colitis up to 6 weeks after administration. • The mortality rate is low but can reach 20% in comorbid patients and is usually a result of toxic megacolon and perforation, causing diffuse peritonitis. • Patients should be treated with oral antibiotics against *C. difficile*, including metronidazole (Flagyl) and vancomycin.

ANSWER:
A

12. A 35-year-old woman who underwent a laparoscopic chole-cystectomy 1 week ago comes to the emergency department with a history of 3 days of abdominal pain, nausea, vomiting, and jaundice. Which of the following diagnoses is most likely?

  A. Bile duct injury with intra-abdominal bile collection

  B. Normal postoperative nausea and discomfort

  C. Postoperative bowel obstruction or ileus

  D. Duodenal injury with leakage

Ref.: 1–3

COMMENTS: See Question 13.

13. For the patient described in Question 12, what is the next step in diagnosis and management?

  A. Abdominal sonographic studies

  B. Dimethyl iminodiacetic acid (HIDA) scan

  C. CT scan

  D. Endoscopic retrograde cholangiopancreatogram (ERCP)

  E. Percutaneous transhepatic cholangiogram (PTC)

Ref.: 1–3

COMMENTS: Although laparoscopic cholecystectomy has become commonplace, unrecognized bile duct injury remains a significant cause of morbidity. • Bile leakage after cholecystec-tomy occurs in 1% of patients, and 25% of the leaks occur from injuries to the major bile ducts. • It is estimated that the rate of subclinical or late-manifesting bile duct injuries is much higher. • Although some recent studies have shown no difference between open and laparoscopic cholecystectomy in terms of the incidence of bile duct injury, multiple studies have shown that there can be a fourfold increase in injuries during laparoscopic procedures. • Any patient who has sustained a bile duct injury during a laparo-scopic operation should immediately undergo open surgery to repair it. • Depending on the severity and location of the injury, the repair can range from primary repair over a T tube to a Roux-en-Y biliary enteric anastomosis.

Patients with delayed onset of abdominal pain, nausea, vomiting, and jaundice should be assumed to have a bile duct injury with a leak or biloma until proven otherwise. • Although sonographic studies can often identify a bile collection, bowel gas and postoperative changes often hinder the resolution of such imaging studies. • A CT scan can evaluate the entire abdomen and diagnose a bile collection. • A HIDA scan is a useful adjunct test to diagnose a bile leak or collection in cases with equivocal sonographic and CT findings. • Once a bile leak and bile collec-tion are diagnosed, the collection should be percutaneously drained. • After drainage, which will often improve the patient's symptoms, the injury should be defined with a combination of ERCP and PTC. • The timing of operative repair depends on the health of the patient and the amount of inflammation assumed to be present. • The time of greatest inflammation is between

7 and 21 days after initial injury, and the patient should be treated temporarily with drainage of the bile collection until that time has passed. • The repair to be performed depends on the severity and location of the injury. • Small leaks without transection (e.g., as seen in cystic duct stump leaks) can often be stented via ERCP. • Larger leaks or complete transactions usually require a Roux-en-Y biliary enteric anastomosis.

ANSWERS:
Question 12: A
Question 13: C

14. What is the commonest cause of low-grade fever (99–101°F, or 37.2–38.3°C) in the 48-hr period immediately following abdominal surgery?

  A. Atelectasis

  B. Urinary tract infection

  C. Pulmonary embolism

  D. Wound infection

  E. Pseudomembranous colitis

Ref.: 1–3

COMMENTS: See Question 15.

15. For intubated, severely injured patients, which is the best predictor for the likelihood of contracting pneumonia?

  A. Thoracic, as opposed to abdominal, surgery

  B. Pre-existing obstructive pulmonary disease

  C. Length of time on the ventilator

  D. Systemic antibiotic use

Ref.: 1–3

COMMENTS: Pneumonia remains the number-one cause of noso-comial infection in the hospital population. • The progression from minor atelectasis to full-blown pneumonia has been well documented and described. • The commonest causes of postoperative fever can easily be remembered using the mnemonic the *five W's*. • The first *W* stands for *wind*, which refers to atelectasis. • (See the Comments for Question 17 for discussion of the remaining four W's.) Atelectasis is the lack of expansion of the distal alveoli because of a nonexpan-sive pulmonary effort. • Perioperative patients often lack adequate respiratory effort because of surgical pain, oversedation, and their nonambulatory, bedridden state. • Collapse of distal alveoli causes type II pneumonocytes to release interleukin-6, which leads to low-grade fever. • Prevention includes adequate pain control, early ambulation, and deep breathing and coughing.

If unchecked, atelectasis can progress to pneumonia in the particularly susceptible collapsed distal lung segments. • The inci-dence of pneumonia is greatest in intensive care units, where pro-longed mechanical ventilation is the greatest risk factor. • The risk of acquiring pneumonia is directly proportional to the length of time a patient undergoes mechanical ventilation. • Ten to 20% of patients in intensive care units develop pneumonia, and the mortality rate is as high as 50%.

ANSWERS:
Question 14: A
Question 15: C

16. A 54-year-old patient undergoes a right hemicolectomy and on postoperative day 1 has a low-grade fever to 100.4°F (38°C). He complains of no additional symptoms. The patient's work-up should include which of the following?

    A. History, physical examination, chest x-ray, CT scan of the abdomen, blood cultures, and urinalysis

    B. History, physical examination, chest x-ray, CT scan of the abdomen, and blood cultures

    C. History, physical examination, chest x-ray, and blood cultures

    D. History, physical examination, chest x-ray, blood cultures, and urinalysis

    E. History and physical examination

    Ref.: 1–3

COMMENTS: See Question 17.

17. The patient described in Question 16 has a fever of 102.2°F (39°C) on postoperative day 3. The patient's work-up should include which of the following?

    A. History, physical examination, chest x-ray, CT scan of the abdomen, blood cultures, and urinalysis

    B. History, physical examination, chest x-ray, CT scan of the abdomen, and blood cultures

    C. History, physical examination, chest x-ray, and blood cultures

    D. History, physical examination, chest x-ray, blood cultures, and urinalysis

    E. History and physical examination

    Ref.: 1–3

COMMENTS: The common causes of postoperative fever can be remembered by using the mnemonic *5 W's: wind, water, wound, walking,* and *wonder drugs.* • In the absence of an obvious source of infection, such as a preexisting infection or contamination during the surgical procedure, the commonest cause of fever in the first 48–72 hr is atelectasis *(wind).* • As described in Question 15, lack of pulmonary expansion and proper pulmonary toilet cause distal alveoli to collapse, leading to the release of proinflammatory mediators by type II pneumonocytes, causing fever.

The work-up during early postoperative fever centers on ruling out known infectious causes. • Very high fevers can be caused by necrotizing infection with clostridial and streptococcal species. • Any high fever in the immediate postoperative period mandates *wound* inspection. • If a very high fever is seen with an erythematous wound with drainage, necrotizing infection should be suspected and the patient emergently returned to the operating room for dèbridement. • In a patient with low-grade fever, no additional cultures and/or imaging studies are warranted. • The commonest cause of fever after 72 hr is urinary tract infection *(water).* • The risk period for wound and intra-abdominal infection typically begins after the third postoperative day. • At this point, a complete work-up to determine the cause of fever includes a history, physical examination, chest x-ray, blood cultures, and urinalysis. • Wound infection is usually manifested 3–7 days after operation and is characterized by fever, erythema, and drainage. • Treatment involves opening the wound. • Simple drainage and packing are usually adequate, and antibiotics are not necessary.

The two remaining *W's* are *walking,* which refers to fever secondary to deep vein thrombosis (DVTs), and *wonder drugs,*

which refers to drug fever. • Both are exceedingly rare causes of fever and are not commonly seen in surgical patients. • These causes should be considered only after all others are ruled out.

ANSWERS:
Question 16: E
Question 17: D

18. A 74-year-old diabetic man undergoes an exploratory laparotomy for a small-bowel resection. On postoperative day 6, erythema is noted around the wound, and the wound is opened. A moderate amount of pus is evacuated from the wound, which is packed open. The next day, a 3-cm defect is noted in the fascia at the inferior aspect. What treatment should be performed?

    A. Return to the operating room, fascial dèbridement and closure, and closure of the skin

    B. Return to the operating room, fascial dèbridement and closure over absorbable mesh, and packing of the open wound

    C. Wet-to-dry packing of the abdominal wound

    D. Return to the operating room and closure of the skin with retention sutures

    Ref.: 1–3

COMMENTS: Fascial dehiscence is defined as a separation of the fascial layer. • Its severity ranges from minor openings of 1 cm or less to complete disruption of the wound with evisceration of the abdominal contents. • The rate of fascial disruption ranges from 0.2 to 5%. • The highest rates occur in the elderly population and in patients with poor wound healing from diabetes, steroid use, or other co-morbid factors. • The key to preventing dehiscence is meticulous technique coupled with minimization of co-morbid factors to help reduce the risk of disruption. • Wounds should be closed without tension and with evenly spaced sutures from fascia to fascia. • Diligence is also necessary in diagnosing and treating wound infections early before the fascial layer can become infected and weakened. • At the first sign of wound infection, the outer skin layer should be opened and the layer above the fascia drained and packed with moist gauze. • Wounds that are grossly infected should be left open to facilitate drainage and bacterial clearance. • When dehiscence is discovered, treatment should be individualized. • Most small-to-moderate disruptions may be packed, allowing granulation tissue to form, along with of a small hernia, which can be repaired later. • For larger disruptions with significant exposure of the bowel or evisceration, emergency surgery should be performed to attempt closure and coverage.

ANSWER:
C

19. A patient undergoes removal of an abdominal wall tumor with primary closure. Two weeks later, the patient experiences swelling and fullness at the wound site. There is a small amount of serous drainage at the inferior aspect of the wound. The patient has experienced no fever, and the wound is without pain or erythema. What is the next step in management?

    A. Sonographic studies of the wound

    B. Abdominal CT scan

    C. Return to the operating room for wound exploration and drainage

    D. Broad-spectrum antibiotics and observation

E. Aspiration with an 18-gauge needle, pressure dressing, or binder

Ref.: 1–3

COMMENTS: Seromas are sterile collections of lymph and serum in the potential space of a wound. • Disruption of lymph channels leads to leakage and collection in the wound space. • Meticulous ligation of any lymph channels encountered during surgery can decrease the likelihood of seroma formation. • The rate of seroma formation is highest in operations that disrupt lymph channels, such as groin hernia repairs or explorations. • The use of closed-suction drains and pressure dressings has been shown to decrease the leakage rate, and some reports indicate measured success with fibrin glue injection. • Seromas can be differentiated from wound infections by the lack of erythema, pain, and warmth at the site. • In addition, aspiration of seromas produces a thin, noninfected, clear or straw-colored fluid, as opposed to the purulent, foul-smelling fluid from an abscess. • Patients with a seroma should be initially treated with aspiration and pressure drainage. • Repeated aspirations are sometimes necessary. • Recurrent seromas can sometimes require wound exploration, fibrin glue injection, and closure over closed-suction drains.

ANSWER:
E

20. A debilitated cachectic nursing home patient undergoes small-bowel resection for bowel obstruction with a primary anastomosis. Which of the following are considered risk factors for anastomotic breakdown?

A. Stapled anastomosis

B. Hand-sewn anastomosis

C. Use of a systemic anticoagulant postoperatively

D. Chronic obstructive pulmonary disease requiring steroid treatment

Ref.: 1–3

COMMENTS: Reduction of the risk of anastomotic leakage requires optimization of wound healing, gastrointestinal mucosal health, and meticulous surgical technique. • Patients who are severely malnourished, with a serum albumin level below 3 g/ml, should receive nutritional supplementation if the surgery can be delayed. • Bowel preparation also decreases the rate of leakage. • Meticulous technique, with mucosal opposition, adequate blood supply, perfect hemostasis, and minimal tension, is mandatory. • No difference has been shown between stapled and hand-sewn anastomosis or between one-layer and two-layer anastomosis. • Systemic anticoagulation does not increase wound or anastomotic breakdown. • Chronic obstructive lung disease and steroid use both adversely affect wound healing and are associated with anastomotic breakdown.

ANSWER:
D

21. Which anastomosis location has the highest leakage rate?

A. Jejunojejunostomy after a Roux-en-Y reconstruction

B. Pancreaticojejunostomy

C. Esophagojejunostomy

D. Rectosigmoid anastomosis

Ref.: 1–3

COMMENTS: The leakage rate is highest in the pancreatic anastomosis, followed by esophagojejunostomy, rectosigmoid anastomosis, and jejunojejunostomy.

ANSWER:
B

22. Based on the x-ray shown, what should be the next step in management?

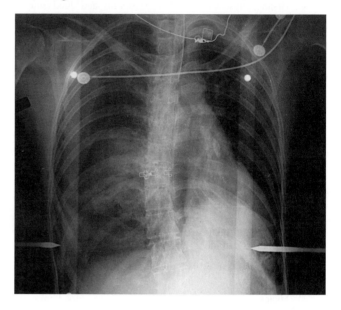

A. Complete abdominal series x-rays

B. Endotracheal intubation

C. Ventilation-perfusion scan

D. Right needle thoracostomy

E. Anteroposterior and lateral chest x-ray

Ref.: 1–3

COMMENTS: This patient's x-ray demonstrates the classic findings of a right tension pneumothorax. • With a tension pneumothorax, air continues to accumulate under increasing pressure as a result of each inspiration. • Increasing intrapleural pressure causes lung collapse and a mediastinal shift to the opposite side. • The pressure must be relieved immediately so that interference with ventilation in the opposite lung and impairment of cardiac function from decreased venous return can be avoided. • Appropriate treatment for a tension pneumothorax is the prompt insertion of a 14-gauge angiocath in the second intercostal space at the mid-clavicular line on the affected side. • This procedeure is followed by a rush of air and relief of the tension pneumothorax. • A chest tube is then immediately inserted. • Since there is no free or loculated fluid collection, there is no concern for hemothorax. • A ventilation scan may demonstrate the gradual accumulation of isotope in the pleural space and ultimately confirm the diagnosis of pneumothorax. • However, a ventilation scan is unnecessary and would cause considerable delay. • There is no evidence of pneumonia to suggest the need for antibiotic therapy. • Repeat films are unnecessary and would delay prompt life-saving treatment.

ANSWER:
D

23. With regard to afferent loop syndrome, which of the following statements is/are true?

A. It is most often the result of jejunogastric intussusception.

B. It usually becomes apparent several months following gastrectomy.

C. Its classical symptoms are abdominal pain and diarrhea.

D. It can usually be diagnosed by the appearance of the afferent loop on barium x-ray studies of the stomach.

E. It constitutes a surgical emergency if the obstruction is complete.

Ref.: 1–3

COMMENTS: The afferent loop syndrome is caused by acute or chronic obstruction of the duodenum and jejunum proximal to the site of a Billroth II gastroenterostomy. • Only rarely is it caused by jejunogastric intussusception. • In most cases, it occurs within the first postoperative week. • The classic symptoms of partial obstruction are postprandial epigastric fullness and pain, relieved by vomiting of bilious material. • X-ray studies with a barium swallow may demonstrate delayed gastric emptying but often fail to visualize the afferent loop. • The serum amylase level may be elevated because of stasis of pancreatic secretions in the obstructed loop. • Chronic bacterial overgrowth may produce vitamin B_{12} deficiency. • Complete obstruction requires prompt surgical treatment, since it may cause duodenal necrosis and perforation.

ANSWER:
E

24. Which of the following statements regarding pulmonary embolism is/are true?

A. Known risk factors include gastric cancer, the postpartum period in women, and AIDS.

B. Prompt heparin therapy will dissolve formed thrombi and prevent thrombus formation.

C. Most patients manifest dyspnea, pain, and hemoptysis.

D. Fifty percent of all pulmonary emboli originate in the lower extremities.

E. Free-floating ileofemoral thrombi are an indication for a caval filter.

Ref.: 1–3

COMMENTS: Known risk factors for pulmonary embolism include processes leading to vascular stasis, abnormalities in the vessel wall, or alterations in coagulation. • Risk factors include use of birth control pills, congestive heart failure, obesity, sickle cell anemia, fractures, pregnancy, the postoperative period, stasis, and carcinoma. • An increased risk of pulmonary embolism has not been identified in AIDS patients. • Heparin therapy is indicated to help prevent thrombus formation and propagation but will not dissolve thrombi. • The classic triad of dyspnea, pain, and hemoptysis is seen only in 30% of patients. • Approximately 85–90% of all pulmonary emboli originate in the lower extremities. • Free-floating thrombi in the iliac veins are an indication for caval interruption.

ANSWER:
E

25. Which of the following statements regarding central venous catheters is/are true?

A. Before catheter placement, platelet transfusions should be given routinely if the platelet count is less than 100,000/mm³.

B. Deadly arrhythmias frequently result from overinsertion of the guide wire or catheter.

C. The presence of fever with or without leukocytosis mandates removal of the central venous catheter.

D. Catheter tunnel infections rarely respond to antibiotic treatment alone.

E. Low-dose anticoagulants reduce the incidence of catheter-related thrombosis.

Ref.: 1–3

COMMENTS: The two most important predictors of complications associated with insertion of central venous catheters are the physician's experience and the accuracy in emergency placement. • Improperly positioned catheters may lead to arrhythmias, venous thrombosis, vascular perforation, and false readings. • A history of central venous thrombosis warrants preoperative imaging studies. • Successful placement of central venous catheters in thrombocytopenic patients (platelet count <50,000/mm³) can be achieved by cutdown on the cephalic vein and/or by preoperative transfusion of platelets for patients with severe thrombocytopenia. • Arrhythmias frequently result from overinsertion of the guide wire or catheter but reverse when the wire or catheter is withdrawn.

The incidence of catheter-related sepsis per 100 patient days varies from 0.08 to 0.14 episodes. • The clinical definition of catheter-related sepsis is fever with or without leukocytosis that resolves with removal of the catheter. • With the use of clinical criteria alone, as many as 85% of catheters would be removed unnecessarily. • Semiqualitative cultures of the catheter tip distinguish catheter colonization from catheter infection. • No episodes of bacteremia occur with fewer than 15 colony-forming units. • The commonest organisms involved are coagulase-negative *Staphylococcus aureus* and yeast organisms. • In patients with nontunneled central venous catheters, clinically suspected catheter-related sepsis warrants exchange of a catheter over a guide wire as a method of bacteriologic sampling. • Catheter tunnel infections respond to antibiotic treatment alone in only 25% of patients. • However, combined local treatment and systemic antibiotic therapy permit salvage of the catheter in about 70% of patients. • The use of low-dose heparin and warfarin has been shown to reduce the likelihood of development of catheter-related thrombosis in high-risk patients.

ANSWER:
E

REFERENCES

1. Townsend CM, Beauchamp RD, Evers BM, et al (eds): *Sabiston Textbook of Surgery, The Biological Basis of Modern Surgical Practice*, 17th ed. Saunders, Philadelphia, 2004.
2. Brunicardi FC, Andersen DK, Billiar TR, et al (eds): *Schwartz's Principles of Surgery*, 8th ed. McGraw-Hill, New York, 2004.
3. Mullholland MW, Lillemoe KD, Doherty GM, et al (eds): *Greenfield's Surgery: Scientific Principles and Practice*, 4th ed. Lippincott, Williams & Wilkins, Philadelphia, 2006.

CHAPTER 7

Hemostasis and Transfusion

Leonard A. Valentino, M.D., and Bruce C. McLeod, M.D.

1. With regard to normal hemostasis, which of the following statements is/are true?

   A. Vascular disruption is followed by vasoconstriction mediated by vasoactive substances released by activated platelets.

   B. Platelet adhesion is mediated by fibrin monomers.

   C. The endothelial surface supports platelet adhesion and thrombus formation.

   D. Heparin inhibits adenosine diphosphate (ADP)-stimulated platelet aggregation.

   E. A prolonged bleeding time may be due to thrombocytopenia, a qualitative platelet defect, or reduced amounts of von Willebrand factor.

   Ref.: 1–3

COMMENTS: Blood fluidity is maintained by the action of inhibitors of blood coagulation and by the nonthrombogenic vascular surface. • Three physiologic reactions mediate initial hemostasis following vascular injury: (1) vascular response (vasoconstriction) to injury; (2) platelet activation, adherence, and aggregation; and (3) generation of thrombin, with subsequent conversion of fibrinogen to fibrin. • Injury exposes subendothelial components and induces vasoconstriction independent of platelet participation, resulting in decreased blood flow but an increase in local shear force. • Within seconds, platelets are activated by the increase in shear force and adhere to exposed subendothelial collagen by a mechanism dependent on the participation of von Willebrand factor. • Adhesion stimulates release of platelet ADP, mediating recruitment of additional platelets. • Fibrinogen binds to activated platelet receptors, and platelet aggregation follows, creating a primary hemostatic plug. • Formation of the plug requires calcium and magnesium and is not affected by heparin. • Bleeding time measurements reflect the time it takes to form this platelet plug. • A reduction in platelet number or function, loss of vascular integrity, or a reduction in the amount or function of von Willebrand factor may prolong the bleeding time.

ANSWER:
E

2. With regard to drug effects and platelet function, which of the following statements is/are true?

   A. Vasoconstricting agents such as epinephrine, prostaglandins G_2 and H_2 (PGG_2 and PGH_2), and thromboxane A_2 reduce levels of cyclic adenosine monophosphate (cAMP) and induce platelet aggregation.

   B. Vasodilators such as prostaglandin E_1 (PGE_1), prostacyclin (PGI_2), theophylline, and dipyridamole elevate cAMP levels and block platelet aggregation.

   C. Aspirin and indomethacin interfere with platelet release of ADP and inhibit aggregation.

   D. Furosemide competitively inhibits PGG_2 and platelet aggregation.

   E. The effect of aspirin is reversible in 2–3 days.

   Ref.: 1–4

COMMENTS: Aspirin, indomethacin, and most other nonsteroidal anti-inflammatory drugs (NSAIDs) are inhibitors of prostaglandin synthesis. • They block the formation of PGG_2 and PGH_2 from platelet arachidonic acid and, as a result, inhibit platelet aggregation. • PGI_2, PGE_2, and thromboxane A_2 stimulate cAMP production, whereas dipyridamole and theophylline derivatives block its degradation. • Aspirin inhibits thromboxane production, acetylates fibrinogen, interferes with fibrin formation, and makes fibrin susceptible to accelerated fibrinolysis. • The effect of aspirin begins within 2 hr, is irreversible, and lasts the 7- to 9-day life span of affected platelets. • The clinical result is increased bruising and bleeding and increased risk of surgical bleeding. • Platelet counts are normal, but there is a prolonged bleeding time. • Furosemide competitively inhibits ADP-induced platelet aggregation and reduces the response of platelets to PGG_2. • Furosemide may also cause thrombocytopenia. • A wide variety of drugs inhibit platelet function.

ANSWER:
A, B

3. With regard to blood coagulation, which of the following statements is/are true?

   A. The principal complex initiating blood coagulation is tissue factor (TF)–factor VIIa complex.

   B. Coagulation is initiated in the fluid phase of blood.

   C. Many cells, including monocytes and fibroblasts, express TF.

   D. Factor Xa-Va complex converts prothrombin to thrombin in quantities sufficient to activate platelets.

   E. Antithrombin III is the main regulator of blood coagulation.

   Ref.: 1, 2

COMMENTS: Coagulation is initiated on a phospholipid surface, such as the monocyte or fibroblast membrane, following expression of TF. • TF binds factor VII, which is then activated by minor proteolysis through an autocatalytic mechanism or by the action of thrombin or other serine proteases. • The TF-factor VIIa complex is a potent serine protease that activates factors X and IX. • Factor Xa combines with factor Va on the phospholipid surface to convert prothrombin to thrombin. • The amount of thrombin generated by this reaction is insufficient for formation of a stable fibrin clot. • It is sufficient, however, to activate platelets, dissociate factor VIII from von Willebrand factor, and activate factors V, VIII, and XI. • Factor IXa, formed by the action of the TF-factor VIIa complex, binds to activated platelets and associates with factor VIIIa, which then recruits circulating factor X to the platelet surface, converting it to factor Xa. • Platelet-bound factor Xa and its cofactor, factor Va, generate sufficient quantities of thrombin to form a stable fibrin clot. • The catalytic activity of the TF–factor VIIa–factor Xa complex is regulated by tissue factor pathway inhibitor (TFPI). • TFPI binds to factor Xa, limiting the activity of the complex.

ANSWER:
A, C, D

4. With regard to fibrinolysis, which of the following statements is/are true?

   A. Plasmin is essential to fibrinolysis.

   B. Plasminogen deficiency results in a clinical bleeding disorder.

   C. Plasmin acts only on cross-linked fibrin polymers.

   D. Ischemia is a potent activator of the fibrinolytic system.

   E. There is no such thing as "physiologic" fibrinolysis.

Ref.: 1–3

COMMENTS: Plasminogen is converted to plasmin by a number of enzymes, including blood-borne activators and tissue activators such as thrombin, streptokinase, urokinase, and kallikrein. • Ischemia is also a potent stimulator of the activation of the fibrinolytic system. • Plasmin acts on fibrin, fibrinogen, factor V, and factor VIII. • Physiologic fibrinolysis is the result of the natural affinity of plasminogen for fibrin. • Plasminogen is incorporated into the clot, and fibrinolysis is locally controlled. • Pathologic fibrinolysis occurs when plasminogen that is free in plasma is activated, resulting in proteolysis of fibrinogen, fibrin, and other coagulation factors. • Unrestrained fibrinolysis can result in bleeding for several reasons: small fibrin fragments are capable of interfering with normal platelet aggregation; large fibrin fragments join the clot instead of the normal monomers, producing an unstable clot; fibrin fragments interfere with thrombin cleavage of fibrinogen; and destruction of clotting factors other than fibrin results in a consumptive coagulopathy. • Blood and platelets contain antifibrinolytic substances capable of plasminogen inhibition. • Physiologic fibrinolysis plays an important role in tissue repair, cancer metastasis, ovulation, and embryo implantation. • Disorders of fibrinolysis can result from excessive activity (bleeding) or insufficient activity (thrombosis).

ANSWER:
A, D

5. With regard to the measurement of bleeding times, which of the following statements is/are true?

   A. Spontaneous bleeding rarely occurs with platelet counts higher than 40,000/µl.

   B. Platelet counts higher than 150,000/µl exclude the possibility of a primary hemostatic disorder.

   C. Bleeding time is prolonged by a variety of drugs.

   D. Platelet counts higher than 50,000/µl are usually associated with a normal bleeding time and adequate surgical hemostasis.

   E. Normal bleeding time excludes von Willebrand's disease as a potential factor affecting surgical hemostasis.

Ref.: 1, 3

COMMENTS: The bleeding time is a crude measure of platelet function, the number of platelets, or both. • The normal value is 3–9 minutes and implies normal platelet function and counts of more than 50,000/µl. • Bleeding time is prolonged in patients with normal platelet counts in whom qualitative abnormalities are present as a primary platelet disorder or one secondary to drugs, uremia, or liver disease or in those who have thrombasthenia or a variety of other platelet function defects. • Patients with defective platelets or capillaries, those with von Willebrand's disease, and those with a history of recent ingestion of aspirin, NSAIDs, antibiotics (penicillins and cephalosporins), and a wide variety of miscellaneous drugs also have prolonged bleeding times. • False-negative (normal) bleeding times are frequently due to the technical difficulty of performing the test and its lack of sensitivity. • For example, only 60% of patients with von Willebrand's disease have a prolonged bleeding time. • Other tests of platelet function include assessment of platelet aggregation in response to a variety of agonists and serotonin release.

ANSWER:
A, C, D

6. Match each item in the left-hand column with the appropriate item in the right-hand column.

   A. Prolonged in hemophilia and von Willebrand's disease
   B. Prolonged owing to factor VIII deficiency
   C. Detects deficiencies of factors II, V, and X and fibrinogen
   D. Detects deficiencies of factors II, V, X, VIII, IX, XI, and XII and fibrinogen
   E. Preferred method of monitoring warfarin (Coumadin) anticoagulation
   F. Prolonged by use of heparin

   a. Prothrombin time (PT)
   b. Partial thromboplastin time (PTT)
   c. Both
   d. Neither

Ref.: 1, 2

COMMENTS: The one-stage PT is used to measure the function of fibrinogen and factors II, V, X, and VII. • The PTT reflects the function of fibrinogen and factors II, V, X, VIII, IX, XI, and XII. • Fibrinogen and factors II, V, and X are common to both tests. • Both tests require comparison with normal control values obtained daily in the laboratory. • Because of the antithrombin effect of heparin, even trace amounts prolong the PT, PTT, and thrombin time. • At least 5 hr must elapse after the last dose of intravenous heparin before the PT can be reliably interpreted. • The thrombin time is a measure of the ability to generate fibrin and is prolonged by deficiencies and abnormalities of fibrinogen or the presence of heparin or fibrinogen degradation products. • The thrombin time, together with the PT and PTT, can distinguish whether factor deficiencies exist in the first or second stage of coagulation. • A normal PT and thrombin time with an abnormal PTT in the absence of clinical bleeding suggests deficiencies of factor XII, high-molecular-weight kininogen, or prekallikrein or the presence of a lupus anticoagulant. • The same laboratory values obtained for a bleeding patient suggest deficiency of factor VIII, IX, or XI. • A normal PTT and thrombin time with an abnormal PT suggests factor VII deficiency. • A prolonged thrombin time with abnormal PTT and PT suggests the presence of hepatocellular liver disease or a consumptive coagulopathy if the platelet count is decreased or an abnormality of fibrinogen if the platelet count is normal. • Factor VIII is synthesized in endothelial cells of the liver and is therefore not affected by hepatocellular disease. • A decrease in factor VIII can be used to differentiate consumptive coagulopathy (reduced levels of all factors) from hepatocellular liver disease (reduced levels of all factors except factor VIII). • The PTT also is prolonged by heparin administration and can be used to monitor its efficacy. • Calculation of the international normalized ratio (INR) from the PT is the preferred method of controlling anticoagulation with warfarin (Coumadin). • Vitamin K is necessary for the full function of factors II, VII, IX, and X, and therefore its deficiency is reflected by prolongation of both the PT and PTT.

ANSWER:
A-b; B-a; C-c; D-b; E-a; F-c

7. True or false: The thrombin time aids in detecting qualitative abnormalities of fibrin, circulating anticoagulants, and inhibition of fibrin polymerization.

Ref.: 1, 2

COMMENTS: The thrombin time is a measurement of the clotting time of plasma. • In the absence of heparin or the by-products of fibrinolysis, fibrinogen abnormalities or deficiencies may be detected. • Pathologic fibrinolysis causes a prolonged thrombin time as well as rapid whole blood clot dissolution. • Whole blood clot lysis, which normally takes as long as 48 hr, may occur in as little as 2 hr in the presence of increased fibrinolysis. • The presence of a paraprotein may cause false-positive results for the thrombin time and other tests based on whole blood clotting measurements.

ANSWER:
True

8. With regard to evaluating bleeding in surgical patients, which of the following statements is/are true?

A. All surgical wounds, no matter how small, must be evaluated.

B. The commonest cause of surgical bleeding is incomplete mechanical hemostasis.

C. ε-Aminocaproic acid is an excellent topical hemostatic agent.

D. Isolated bleeding from a surgical wound implies poor local hemostasis.

Ref.: 1, 2, 4

COMMENTS: Bleeding from the surgical wound suggests ineffective local hemostasis, particularly if associated wounds (e.g., drain sites, tracheostomy wounds, or intravenous infusion sites) are not bleeding. • An exception is isolated bleeding from a resected prostatic bed, in which prostate-borne plasminogen activators can be activated by urokinase. • Activation is inhibited by ε-aminocaproic acid. • Blood transfusions can lead to bleeding via a number of mechanisms. • Transfusion of more than one blood volume produces thrombocytopenia by dilution. • Patients bleeding after a large number of blood transfusions should be considered thrombocytopenic and treated as such. • Nonetheless, additional

evaluation is indicated because an alternative explanation for transfusion-associated bleeding is a hemolytic transfusion reaction. • In such an instance, disseminated intravascular coagulopathy (DIC) is caused by thromboplastic activity of factors liberated from the stroma of lysed red blood cells. • Extracorporeal circulation may induce hemostatic failure owing to thrombocytopenia, inadequate reversal of heparinization, or overadministration of protamine. • Septic surgical patients may bleed because of endotoxin-induced thrombocytopenia. • Defibrination and bleeding may occur with meningococcemia, *Clostridium welchii* sepsis, or staphylococcal sepsis. • Uncommonly, an operation on tissues rich in fibrinolytic activity, such as those of the pancreas, liver, or lungs, may lead to pathologic fibrinolysis and bleeding.

Table 7-1. Examples of DIC Syndromes

"Fast" DIC	"Slow" DIC
Amniotic fluid embolus	Acute promyelocytic leukemia
Abruptio placentae	Dead fetus syndrome
Septic abortion	Transfusion of activated prothrombin complex concentrates
Septicemia	Carcinomas
Massive tissue injury	Kasabach-Merritt syndrome
Incompatible blood transfusion	Liver disease
Purpura fulminans	

ANSWER:
A, B, D

9. When evaluating a patient who bleeds unexpectedly, which of the following statements is/are true?

A. The most reliable way of detecting patients at risk for bleeding is with a platelet count.

B. Infants who do not bleed during circumcision have normal hemostatic function.

C. An isolated episode of gastrointestinal bleeding is often associated with generalized hemostatic disorders.

D. Menorrhagia is common in women with generalized hemostatic disorders.

E. The presence of healthy parents and siblings does not exclude the possibility of a primary hemostatic disorder.

Ref.: 2, 3

COMMENTS: No single test for detecting patients at risk for bleeding exists. • The best protocol is a complete history and physical examination. • Many normal individuals consider themselves to have a positive bleeding history. • Because aspirin is contained in a wide variety of over-the-counter medications, its use is easily overlooked in the patient's medical history. • Circumcision typically involves significant trauma to tissues and activation of the TF-factor VIIa pathway. • Only 30% of affected males bleed following circumcision. • Only rarely do patients with a bleeding disorder undergo tooth extraction or tonsillectomy without encountering a bleeding problem. • Some patients with a severe bleeding disorder experience bleeding with tooth eruption. • Isolated gastrointestinal bleeding is unusual in patients with congenital bleeding disorders. • Epistaxis is one of the commonest symptoms of von Willebrand's disease and platelet disorders. • Excessive menstrual flow (menorrhagia), but not intermenstrual bleeding, is common in patients with hemostatic disorders. • Because inherited bleeding defects may be autosomal dominant, autosomal recessive, or sex-linked recessive, an inquiry into the family history should account for grandparents, aunts, uncles, and cousins.

Because patients' assessment of severity is subjective, objective indicators should be sought, such as need for a prolonged hospital stay for minor surgery, transfusion, and anemia. • A search for ecchymosis or petechiae, particularly near pressure points, is essential. • The lesions of hereditary hemorrhagic telangiectasia are found on the lips, underneath the fingernails, and around the anus. • Signs of liver disease suggest the presence of acquired deficiency of the prothrombin complex, not a predisposition to primary hemostatic disorders.

ANSWER:
D, E

10. With regard to classic hemophilia, which of the following statements is/are true?

A. The incidence in the general population is 1:10,000.

B. A given patient's baseline factor VIII or IX level remains constant.

C. Muscle compartment bleeds are the commonest orthopedic problem.

D. Factor VIII replacement therapy is required before any elective surgery.

E. Therapy with cryoprecipitated plasma is free of risk for hepatitis.

Ref.: 1–3

COMMENTS: Bleeding in hemophiliacs usually appears during early childhood. • Hemarthrosis is the commonest orthopedic problem. • Epistaxis, hematuria, and intracranial bleeding may occur. • Equinus contracture, Volkmann's contracture of the forearm, and flexion contracture of elbows or knees are sequelae of these bleeding episodes. • Retroperitoneal or intramural intestinal bleeding may produce abdominal symptoms. • The level of factor VIII or IX in the plasma (which tends to remain stable throughout life) determines the tendency to bleed. • Spontaneous bleeding is frequent in patients with severe disease, defined as less than 1% factor VIII or IX activity. • Bleeding typically occurs with trauma in patients with moderately severe disease, defined as 1–5% factor activity. • In patients with mild hemophilia A or B, defined as 6–25% factor activity, bleeding typically only occurs with major trauma or surgery. • The factor VIII or IX level must be raised to at least 30% to achieve hemostasis and control minor hemorrhage. • A level of approximately 50% is required to control joint and muscle bleeding, while a level of 80–100% is necessary to treat life-threatening hemorrhage (central nervous system, retroperitoneal, or retropharyngeal bleeding) and to prepare patients for elective surgery. • After elective surgery, levels of 25% should be maintained for at least 2 weeks. • Transmission of hepatitis or human immunodeficiency virus (HIV), development of neutralizing antibodies, and qualitative platelet dysfunction are possible complications of factor replacement therapy.

ANSWER:
A, B, D

11. A 12-year-old boy with known factor VIII deficiency has a painful, swollen, immobile right knee. The clinician suspects a hemarthrosis. Therapeutic options include which of the following?

A. Immediate aspiration and compression dressings to prevent cartilage necrosis

B. Compression dressings and immobilization to prevent further bleeding

C. Immediate aspiration after appropriate factor VIII replacement therapy

D. Initial trial of factor VIII therapy, compression dressings, cold packs, and rest followed by active range-of-motion exercises

Ref.: 1, 2

COMMENTS: Treatment of joint bleeding is aimed at preventing chronic synovitis and degenerative arthritis. • Early, intensive factor VIII therapy is critical for limiting the extent of hemorrhage. • Factor VIII replacement therapy is most effective when initiated before swelling of the joint capsule. • Often, replacement therapy is initiated before the onset of any objective physical findings, when the patient perceives only subtle signs of joint hemorrhage. • Factor VIII therapy, joint rest, compression dressing (Ace wrap), and cold packs constitute the usual initial therapy. • Aspiration is to be avoided. • The goal of treatment of hemarthrosis is maintenance of range of motion. • Active range-of-motion exercises should begin 24 hr after factor VIII therapy. • Compression and cold packs should be continued for 3–5 days.

ANSWER:
D

12. With regard to von Willebrand's disease, which of the following statements is/are true?

A. It is more common than hemophilia.

B. It is best treated with cryoprecipitated plasma.

C. Factor VIII levels may vary over time in a given patient.

D. There is an associated platelet abnormality in 70% of patients.

E. Bleeding following elective surgery is rare.

Ref.: 1, 2

COMMENTS: Von Willebrand's disease is the commonest congenital bleeding disorder, affecting 1% of the population. • The prevalence of patients with symptomatic bleeding is approximately 1:1000. • Most patients have mild disease unless challenged by trauma or surgery. • Von Willebrand's disease is associated with a variable deficiency of both von Willebrand factor and factor VIII. • A platelet defect is also present in most patients. • The severity of coagulation abnormalities varies from patient to patient and from time to time for a given patient. • In all but 1–2% of patients, bleeding manifestations are milder than those of classic hemophilia. • In the same group of patients with type 3 von Willebrand's disease, bleeding is more severe than in hemophilia. • Bleeding is treated with desmopressin (DDAVP), which induces the release of von Willebrand factor from storage sites in endothelial cells and platelets. • The effect of desmopressin is rapid, reaching maximal procoagulant effects in 1–2 hr. • The effects dissipate quickly, necessitating repeated dosing. • When more than two or three doses of DDAVP are given, the effects may diminish or are absent. • Desmopressin is most effective for type 1 disease and is not effective for type 3 disease. • Because of a risk of thrombocytopenia, DDAVP is specifically contraindicated for type 2B disease but may be effective for other forms of type 2 disease.

ANSWER:
A, C, D

13. With regard to hereditary hemostatic disorders, which of the following statements is/are true?

A. Deficiencies of any of the four vitamin K-dependent factors (II, V, VII, and X) may be treated with stored plasma.

B. Factor VII has the shortest intravascular half-life of any clotting factor.

C. Factor IX deficiency is clinically indistinguishable from factor VIII deficiency.

D. Factor V is known as a labile factor.

E. Factor XI deficiency is treated with plasma.

Ref.: 2, 4

COMMENTS: Factor V is not vitamin K–dependent. • Factor VIII and IX deficiencies are clinically indistinguishable. • Bleeding with factor IX deficiency (Christmas disease) is treated with recombinant factor IX concentrate. • The use of prothrombin complex concentrate (PCC) may be complicated by thrombosis or DIC. • In older patients, administration of PCC should be accompanied by prophylactic administration of low-dose heparin. • Deficiency of factor XI (Rosenthal's syndrome) or factor V is treated with plasma. • Because factor V is labile and activity is lost with storage, fresh plasma is necessary. • Deficiencies of factors VII, X (Stuart-Prower deficiency), or II are also treated with plasma. • The duration and frequency of treatment with plasma-derived products is inversely proportional to the intravascular half-life.

ANSWER:
B, C, D, E

14. True statements regarding acquired hypofibrinogenemia include which of the following?

A. Introduction of thromboplastic materials into the circulation is the commonest cause of DIC.

B. Release of excessive plasminogen activators causes pathologic fibrinolysis.

C. Primary fibrinolysis can be differentiated from DIC on the basis of the PT, PTT, and thrombin time.

D. The most important aspect of the treatment of DIC is adequate heparinization.

Ref.: 1–3

COMMENTS: DIC results from the introduction of thromboplastic materials into the circulation, leading to activation of the coagulation system, with secondary "protective" fibrinolysis. • Transfusion reactions, crush injuries, hemorrhagic perinatal complications, disseminated cancer, and bacterial sepsis have been implicated as causes. • The release of excessive plasminogen-activating substances leads to primary pathologic fibrinolysis. • Shock, hypoxia, sepsis, disseminated prostate cancer, cirrhosis, portal hypertension, and peritoneovenous shunts are possible causes. • Differentiation between DIC and "protective" fibrinolysis on laboratory grounds alone is difficult, although thrombocytopenia is rarely seen with pure fibrinolysis. • For both entities, treating the underlying medical or surgical problem is the most important single step. • With DIC, maintenance of a patent microcirculation is important. • Adequate fluid volumes and heparinization may be necessary. • Active bleeding should be appropriately treated with factor replacement and does not accelerate DIC. • Clotting factors can be replenished with fresh-frozen plasma. • Heparin alone is rarely useful for treatment of acute DIC. • Antithrombin III concentrates may be beneficial. • Fibrinolytic inhibitors may be useful for DIC after appropriate heparinization. • Giving heparin to patients with primary pathologic fibrinolysis can be dangerous, as is giving ε-aminocaproic acid to patients with secondary fibrinolysis. • Correction of the underlying cause is the most important component in the treatment of DIC.

ANSWER:
A, B

15. With regard to polycythemia vera, which of the following statements is/are true?

A. Spontaneous thrombosis is a complication of polycythemia vera.

B. Spontaneous hemorrhage is a possible complication of polycythemia vera.

C. The reason for bleeding is a deficit of platelet function.

D. A hematocrit of less than 48% and a platelet count of less than 400,000/μl are desirable before an elective operation is performed on a patient with polycythemia vera.

Ref.: 2, 3

COMMENTS: Patients with untreated polycythemia vera are at high risk of postoperative bleeding or thrombosis. • The complication rate is highest with uncontrolled erythrocytosis. • Increased viscosity and platelet count, along with a tendency toward stasis, may explain the spontaneous thrombosis seen in patients with polycythemia vera. • Patients most likely to bleed are those with platelet counts greater than 1.5 million/μl. • Polycythemia vera may be caused by a qualitative defect in platelet function. • When possible, operation should be delayed until the hematocrit and platelet count can be medically reduced. • Phlebotomy may help in acute situations. • Complication rates as high as 46% have been reported among patients with polycythemia vera undergoing operation. • Spontaneous hemorrhage, thrombosis, a combination of hemorrhage and thrombosis, and infection are the major complications.

ANSWER:
A, B, C, D

16. With regard to anticoagulation, which of the following statements is/are true?

A. Warfarin (Coumadin) inhibits the activity of vitamin K-dependent factors (II, VII, IX, and X).

B. Heparin enhances the effect of antithrombin on thrombin-mediated conversion of fibrinogen to fibrin.

C. Theoretically, 1.28 mg of protamine neutralizes 1 mg of heparin.

D. The effects of vitamin K reversal take 48 hr.

E. An INR of more than 1.5 is considered safe for operation.

Ref.: 2, 5

COMMENTS: With meticulous hemostatic technique, many operations can be performed on patients with an INR greater than 1.5. • Exceptions include operations on the eye or the prostate, neurosurgical procedures, or a blind needle aspiration. • In these cases, an INR of less than 1.2 is required. • Patients who are receiving anticoagulant treatment with warfarin and who require emergency surgery may be given plasma to immediately reverse the warfarin effect. • Alternatively, vitamin K may be given orally or subcutaneously at least 6 hr preoperatively to reverse the effect of warfarin on vitamin K–dependent factors. • The INR should be obtained again before surgery and, if it is not below 1.5, plasma should be administered. • The efficacy of recombinant activated factor VII (rFVIIa) in reversing the INR has been demonstrated in several clinical scenarios. • This mediation has the advantage of directly activating the hemostatic mechanism and generating high concentrations of thrombin. • Use of rFVIIa should be reserved for patients with life-threatening hemorrhage and a significantly elevated INR (>6) in whom emergency surgery is anticipated. • An INR greater than 1.5 is a contraindication to intramuscular medications.

ANSWER:
A, B, C, E

17. With regard to the storage of banked blood, which of the following statements is/are true?

    A. Packed red blood cells stored in AS-3 and kept at 4°C are suitable for transfusion for 3 months.

    B. Platelets in banked blood retain their function for 3 days.

    C. Factors II, VII, IX, and XI are stable at 4°C.

    D. An increase in red blood cell oxygen affinity occurs during storage as a result of a decrease in 2,3-diphosphoglycerate (2,3-DPG) levels.

    E. There is a significant rate of hemolysis in stored blood.

Ref.: 4

COMMENTS: Packed red blood cells properly collected and stored at 4°C in AS-3 additive solution are "good" for 42 days. • The proportion of cells removed from the circulation within 24 hr of transfusion increases with the time the blood is in storage, reaching about 25% at 42 days. • This percentage defines satisfactory shelf life. • Any blood component that has been stored in an "open" system (e.g., frozen red blood cells after thawing and deglycerolization) has a useful life of only 24 hr owing to concerns about contamination. • Cells that survive the first 24 hr live out their remaining life span, and some transfused cells can be detected for up to 120 days—the life span of the normal red blood cell. • Platelets in packed red blood cells become nonfunctional during the first 6 hr of storage. • Red blood cell ATP and 2,3-DPG levels fall during storage. • Oxygen affinity is increased until 2,3-DPG levels rise again after transfusion. • Factors II, VII, IX, and XI are stable at 4°C, whereas factors V and VIII are not. • To maintain factor V and VIII activity, plasma must be frozen shortly after the blood is drawn (fresh-frozen plasma). • Lactic acid concentrations increase, and pH falls in packed red blood cells during storage, while potassium and ammonia concentrations rise steadily. • The citrate used for preservation may reduce plasma ionized calcium if large volumes are transfused. • These metabolites are especially significant in pediatric patients and in patients with impaired liver or renal function (or both).

ANSWER:
C, D

18. True or false: In a major crossmatch, donor cells are compared with recipient serum, whereas, in a minor crossmatch, donor serum is compared with recipient cells.

Ref.: 4

COMMENTS: Because of the high degree of sensitivity of the antibody screening performed on donor blood, virtually all unexpected antibodies are detected, and the minor crossmatch has been rendered unnecessary. • Recipient alloimmunization to "minor" antigens may occur after multiple transfusions, in which case red blood cells lacking the relevant antigen must be transfused. • To detect or exclude such alloimmunization, recipient serum samples should be screened for antibodies. • This screening should be repeated every 48–72 hr if multiple transfusions are given. • It can take several hours to identify the antibody specificity (e.g., anti-C and anti-K antibodies) and find donor red blood cells that lack the relevant antigen(s). • This unavoidable delay can be problematic for same-day surgery patients who have not had a blood bank sample drawn in advance.

ANSWER:
True

19. With regard to leukocytes in cellular blood components (red blood cells and platelets), which of the following statements is/are true?

    A. Leukocytes and their secretions cause some febrile transfusion reactions.

    B. Washing red blood cells with saline solution is the best way to remove leukocytes.

    C. Leukocyte reduction lowers the rate of febrile reactions to cellular components from 10 to 1%.

    D. Leukocyte reduction of cellular components lowers the risk of alloimmunization to HLA antigens in transfusion recipients.

    E. Leukocyte reduction of cellular components lowers the risk of wound infection in transfused surgical patients.

Ref.: 4

COMMENTS: Transfused leukocytes may interact with pre-existing recipient HLA antibodies. • In addition, leukocytes in platelets that are stored at room temperature may elaborate pyrogenic cytokines, such as IL-6, during storage. • Either mechanism may cause a febrile reaction in a susceptible recipient. • Leukocyte-reduction filters are 100–1000 times more effective than is washing for removing leukocytes from packed red blood cells. • Thus, filtration is the preferred method. • (Washed red blood cells are virtually free of plasma proteins and can be given safely to patients who have had severe allergic or anaphylactic reactions to plasma.) Less than 1% of transfusions cause a (usually mild) febrile reaction. • Fifty to 70% of these reactions may be prevented by leukocyte reduction. • Use of leukocyte-reduced components to avoid febrile reactions is only justified for patients who have repeated reactions despite premedication with antipyretics. • A more important indication for leukocyte-reduced components is to prevent formation of HLA antibodies in candidates for kidney, heart, and/or lung transplantation and in patients expected to need long-term platelet support. • Despite a long-standing suspicion that transfusions may be immunosuppressive, large prospective controlled studies have not shown lower mortality rates, shorter hospital stays, or lower rates of postoperative infection in transfused surgical patients who received only leukocyte reduced cellular components.

ANSWER:
A, D

20. With regard to hemolytic transfusion reactions, which of the following statements is/are true?

    A. They are generally caused by ABO incompatibility.

    B. Urticaria and pruritus are the commonest symptoms.

C. Acidification of the urine prevents precipitation of hemoglobin.

D. Intravenous diphenhydramine (Benadryl) should be given immediately.

E. The laboratory findings include a positive direct hemoglobin test result and a free hemoglobin concentration higher than 5 mg/dl in a post-transfusion blood sample.

Ref.: 4

COMMENTS: The commonest cause of fatal hemolytic transfusion reaction is a clerical error that results in transfusion of red blood cells of the wrong ABO type of blood. • Because the severity is proportional to the antigen dose, constant awareness, early recognition, and immediate intervention are important. • Hemolytic reactions lead to complement-mediated intravascular red blood cell destruction, hemoglobinemia, and hemoglobinuria. • They also lead to the release of vasoactive amines through the activation of complement. • This in turn leads to shock, renal ischemia, tubular necrosis, and renal failure proportional to the depth and duration of hypotension. • Red blood cell lipids initiate DIC in 8–30% of patients in whom a full unit of mismatched blood has been transfused. • However, as little as 10 ml can produce serious hypotension and DIC. • Typical signs and symptoms include chills, fever, lumbar and chest pain, pain at the infusion site, and hypotension. • In anesthetized patients, diffuse bleeding and continued hypotension suggest the diagnosis. • Laboratory criteria are positive direct antiglobulin test results; hemoglobinemia, with free hemoglobin concentrations higher than 5 mg/dl; and serologic confirmation of incompatibility. • Because hemoglobin is a highly chromogenic molecule, small amounts (as little as 30 mg/dl) can be detected visually. • The hemoglobin from as little as 5 ml of red blood cells makes the plasma pink and produces hemoglobinuria. • Treatment includes stopping the transfusion, inserting a bladder catheter, and administering mannitol and bicarbonate to encourage excretion of alkaline urine. • This helps prevent precipitation of hemoglobin in the renal tubules, which could contribute to tubular necrosis. • If oliguria develops, appropriate fluid management and possibly dialysis are begun. • The most important treatment is restoration of blood pressure and renal perfusion. • Vasopressors may be necessary. • A sample of the recipient's blood is compared to pretransfusion samples to confirm incompatibility. • The direct antiglobulin test result remains positive for as long as incompatible red blood cells continue to circulate. • The serum bilirubin level can be monitored to follow the increase in indirect bilirubin caused by hemolysis.

ANSWER:
A, E

21. With regard to complications of transfusion, which of the following statements is/are true?

A. Febrile reactions are rare.

B. Gram-positive organisms are the commonest contaminants of stored blood.

C. Even small amounts of intravenous air are poorly tolerated.

D. Transfusions lasting longer than 6 hr increase the risk of infection by contaminated blood.

E. Malaria, Chagas' disease, human T-cell leukemia virus I (HTLV-I), acquired immunodeficiency syndrome (AIDS), and hepatitis can be transmitted by blood transfusions.

Ref.: 1, 4

COMMENTS: Febrile reactions are the commonest reactions to red blood cell and platelet transfusions and occur once per 100 units given. • Fever and chills are the usual symptoms. • If they are mild, these symptoms respond to antipyretics. • In severe cases, they are treated with opiates. • Urticarial reactions are the commonest reaction to plasma transfusions. • They usually respond to antihistamines. • Anaphylactic reactions are rare and are treated with epinephrine and steroids. • Although unusual, gram-negative organisms capable of surviving at 4°C are the commonest cause of bacterial contamination of banked blood. • Platelets, which are optimally stored at room temperature and are being used increasingly, are a more frequent source of sepsis, usually with gram-positive organisms. • Air embolus has become rare since bottles have been replaced by collapsible plastic containers. • Even small volumes of air have the potential to cause fatal complications and should be avoided whenever possible. • Hepatitis viruses B and C (HBV and HCV), HIV, HTLV I and II, malaria, Chagas' disease, and other infections can be transmitted by transfusion. • Specific testing of donors is available for HBV, HCV, HIV, and HTLV. • Health, immigration, and travel histories are used to exclude donors who may harbor malaria or Chagas' disease and are being used to control a perceived "theoretical risk" of variant Creutzfeldt-Jakob disease.

ANSWER:
C, D, E

22. In cirrhotic patients who are actively bleeding, the coagulopathy of end-stage liver disease can be differentiated from DIC most readily by estimation of which of the following factors?

A. Factor II

B. Factor V

C. Factor VII

D. Factor VIII:C

E. Factor X

Ref.: 3

COMMENTS: Of all of the coagulation factors, only factor VIII:C is not produced by hepatocytes. • It is manufactured by reticuloendothelial cells, and levels are typically increased in the presence of cirrhosis. • Reductions in factor VIII:C are observed in patients with DIC because it is consumed along with the other coagulation factors.

ANSWER:
D

REFERENCES

1. Townsend CM, Beauchamp RD, Evers BM, et al (eds): *Sabiston Textbook of Surgery: The Biological Basis of Modern Surgical Practice*, 17th ed. WB Saunders, Philadelphia, 2004.
2. Brunicardi FC, Andersen DK, Billiar TR et al (eds): *Schwartz's Principles of Surgery*, 8th ed. McGraw-Hill, New York, 2004.
3. Colman RW, Hirsh J, Marder VJ, et al (eds): *Hemostasis and Thrombosis: Basic Principles and Practice*. JB Lippincott, Philadelphia, 1994.
4. Rossi EC, Simon TL, Moss GS (eds): *Principles of Transfusion Medicine*, 2nd ed. Williams & Wilkins, Baltimore, 1996.
5. Sorensen B, Johansen P, Nielsen GL, et al: Reversal of the international normalized ratio with recombinant activated factor VII in central nervous system bleeding during warfarin thromboprophylaxis: clinical and biochemical aspects. *Blood Coagul Fibrinol* 14(5):469–477, 2003.

CHAPTER 8

Nutrition

Janet Millikan, M.D.

1. For an adult patient consuming a normal diet, which of the following energy sources is most abundant?

A. Fat

B. Water

C. Protein

D. Carbohydrate

Ref.: 1

COMMENTS: Understanding body composition is important for understanding metabolic changes that occur in various clinical settings. • The science of nutrition is primarily the study of nutrient metabolism at the cellular level. The digestive tract allows nutrient utilization via various mechanisms of digestion, including ingestion of food, separation of nutrients from food (digestion), movement of nutrients into the body for use (absorption), and release of by-products. • Interruption of any of these stages of intake, digestion, and absorption creates a deviation from normal nutrition and can lead to unfavorable nutritional status.

A normal diet provides sufficient amounts of energy, protein, water, vitamins, minerals, and other nutrients to meet the needs of the individual. • Variations of the normal diet are designed to allow for restrictions or additions for individuals with specific dietary requirements due to their disease state (e.g., a lactose-restricted diet, a mechanical soft diet, or a low-sodium diet). • Understanding the pathologic features of various diseases and the body's response allows for proper dietary management of patients.

For a 70-kg adult male, body composition can be generalized as follows in terms of percentage of body weight: 40% intracellular fluid; 20% extracellular fluid, composed of 13% interstitial fluid, 2% transcellular fluid, and 5% plasma; 7% minerals; 18% protein; and 15% lipid. • Fat stores can equal 160,000 kcal, with higher (unlimited) stores in obese individuals. • Lean body mass proteins can supply 30,000 kcal of the body's energy stores. • While energy in the diet is provided entirely by carbohydrates (4 kcal/g), fats (9 kcal/g), proteins (4 kcal/g), alcohol (7 kcal/g), water, and maintenance of fluid status are essential for nutrient use and nutritional equilibrium. • The end products of protein, carbohydrate, and fat oxidation include water. • The water of metabolism is released in constant amounts. • One gram of carbohydrate yields 0.6 ml of water; 1 g of protein 0.42 ml, and 1 g of fat 1.07 ml. • Additional sources of fluid are ingested through fluid intake. • In addition, the gastrointestinal tract may secrete and reabsorb as much as 8–10 L/day of water as digestive juices in the following estimated amounts: saliva, 1500 ml; gastric juice, 2500 ml; bile,

500 ml; pancreatic juices, 700 ml; intestinal juices, 3000 ml; and water intake, 2000 ml. • Regulation of fluid via the thirst mechanism and antidiuretic hormone (ADH) allow for stable fluid status. • Excessive fluid losses require diligent replacement and monitoring.

The body's largest component, water, provides no energy. • Protein and fat supply much of the body's energy. • Protein is an inefficient calorie source, since it requires one quarter of the amount of the energy produced to synthesize protein. • Fat is stored in an anhydrous state, allowing for large storage amounts of this energy source. • Carbohydrates are the largest component of the oral diet besides water, and their major role is as an energy source.

Reserves of carbohydrate can be depleted within 24–48 hr, since the body's storage capacity is relatively low. • Energy supplied to the body via protein mobilization in the amount of 80–100 g/day leads to lean body mass loss. • Compromised body cell mass, with losses of 50–60%, likely lead to death. • Monitoring of a patient's nutritional status ensures appropriate nutritional interventions in various disease states and during medical and surgical therapies.

ANSWER:
D

2. Which of the following statement or statements most accurately describe muscle glycogen?

A. Muscle glycogen remains within the muscle because muscle tissues lack glucose-6-phosphatase.

B. Muscle glycogen is a significant contributor to plasma glucose level maintenance.

C. Muscle glycogen levels can exceed 120 g in a 70-kg adult male.

D. Glucagon mobilizes muscle glycogen to allow for use by the liver.

Ref.: 2

COMMENTS: See Question 5.

3. Which of the following statements regarding hormonal regulation of the blood glucose level is/are true?

A. An increased glucagon/insulin ratio allows mobilization of liver glycogen.

B. An increased circulating insulin level with glucose intake allows decreased glucagon secretion.

C. Insulin allows tissues, such as liver, muscle, and adipose tissue, to release glucose.

D. Glucagon stimulates the cyclic adenosine monophosphate (cAMP) cycle to store glucose as glycogen to meet the body's future needs.

E. All of the above

Ref.: 2

COMMENTS: See Question 5.

4. To prevent gluconeogenesis, glucose administration must be carefully monitored. The protein-sparing effect of glucose administration begins to be manifested after administration of how much glucose?

A. 100 g

B. 200 g

C. 75 g

D. 150 g

Ref.: 3

COMMENTS: See Question 5.

5. Which of the following statements regarding carbohydrate metabolism is/are true?

A. Like dietary fiber, starch is readily digested in the small intestine and used as a source of energy.

B. Digestion occurs primarily in the small intestine via pancreatic enzymes.

C. To prevent stimulation of protein for use in gluconeogenesis during times of stress, only 50 g/day of glucose may be supplied exogenously.

D. Glucagon secretion is increased with the intake of glucose, which allows uptake of glucose by the liver, muscle, and adipose tissue.

E. All of the above

Ref.: 3, 4

COMMENTS: Dietary carbohydrates provide 4 kcal/g and can be complex (polymeric) or simple (monomeric or dimeric). • The major role of carbohydrates in the body is to provide energy for body tissues to use for metabolic processes. • Approximately 30–60% of calories consumed are in the form of carbohydrates.

Digestion of starches begins orally via salivary amylase. • As the starches are passed from the stomach to the small intestine, pancreatic and intestinal enzymes (amylase and disaccharidases) reduce complex carbohydrates to disaccharides (maltose, sucrose, and lactose), which can then be hydrolyzed to primary derivatives of carbohydrates—the monosaccharides or hexoses (glucose, fructose, and galactose)—via specific disaccharidases. • Glucose is the preferred fuel in humans, with all metabolism beginning or ending with this hexose. • The monosaccharides are absorbed into the intestinal mucosa and transported to the liver via the portal circulation. • Their final fate is to be used to form pyruvate or glycogen or to be transported back to the blood for use by red blood cells or the brain or in the formation of fat in adipose tissue.

In a 70-kg man, the liver can store as much as 70 g of glycogen (10% of the liver's wet weight), allowing a 12- to 24-hr nutritional reservoir during fasting, and 120 g (1–2%) of the wet weight of the muscle mass can be attributed to glycogen. • Muscle glycogen has the role of maintaining fuel within muscle tissue. • Release of muscle glycogen to the bloodstream, as seen with liver glycogen, cannot occur because muscle tissue lacks the necessary enzyme for release: glucose-6-phosphatase. • Free glucose from muscle glycogen is not a significant contributor to plasma glucose. • Thus, liver glycogen is the glucose reserve used to maintain blood glucose levels as needed.

Blood glucose levels are regulated by hormones in response to carbohydrate intake. • Insulin secretion increases with intake of glucose, and glucagon secretion declines, allowing increased uptake of glucose by liver, muscle, and adipose tissue. • Conversely, glucagon mobilizes liver glycogen via the cAMP protein kinase system when blood glucose levels decrease owing to decreased intake. • Glucose tolerance is determined by the rate at which mechanisms of glucose removal can operate. • Administration of 100 g of glucose (or 1 mg/kg/min) has a protein-sparing effect, suppressing the use of nitrogen (from amino acids) for gluconeogenesis.

All major pathways of carbohydrate metabolism start or end with glucose. • The three major types of glucose metabolism are (1) glycolysis, a process by which all cells can oxidize glucose to pyruvate and lactate; (2) oxidation of acetyl coenzyme A (CoA) from carbohydrates, fat, or protein for use by the tricarboxylic acid cycle; and (3) the hexose monophosphate shunt (pentose phosphate shunt), which produces NADPH, a reducing agent, and enables the degradation of sugars other than hexoses. • In addition to glucose from outside sources, **gluconeogenesis** (formation of glucose from a large variety of noncarbohydrate substrates, including amino acids, lactate, pyruvate, propionate, and glycerol) and **glycogenolysis** (formation of glucose from glycogen) allow glucose production endogenously when exogenous sources are not available. • Endogenous glucose production allows maintenance of plasma glucose levels in the fasting state at a rate of approximately 2–3 mg/kg/min. • Given the availability of endogenous glucose, excess infusion of parenteral glucose can lead to unwanted side effects, including (1) elevated blood glucose levels; (2) increased rate of fat synthesis, leading to fatty liver; and (3) increased water and carbon dioxide production, which can lead to respiratory compromise and possible water overload. • Glucose administration should be kept below 5 mg/kg/min to prevent these complications.

Dietary fiber is a form of complex carbohydrate, classified based on its structure. • It is enzymatically digested and is not considered a source of nourishment. • Fiber includes cellulose (insoluble) and noncellulose (soluble) forms (including pectins, gums, mucilages, and hemicelluloses), which are broken down by bacterial flora of the gut and degraded primarily in the colon. • Soluble fiber is thought to have numerous benefits, including (1) hypocholesterolemic effects; (2) production of short-chain fatty acids, which have trophic effects throughout the intestinal tract; (3) improvement of blood glucose levels by decreasing the rate of glucose absorption; and (4) protection from bacterial translocation.

A N S W E R S :

Question 2: A

Question 3: A, B

Question 4: A

Question 5: B

6. Which of the following is considered a nonessential amino acid for an unstressed patient but has been shown to be conditionally essential for a stressed patient?

A. Lysine

B. Valine

C. Glutamine

D. Phenylalanine

Ref.: 5, 6

COMMENTS: See Question 9.

7. Which of the following statements regarding the metabolism of amino acids (proteins) is/are true?

A. Branched-chain amino acids (BCAAs) can be metabolized outside the liver by muscle.

B. The liver can biosynthesize nonessential amino acids important for maintaining the equilibrium of proteins in the body.

C. Amino acids cannot be oxidized for energy.

D. Amino acids regulate insulin production.

Ref.: 7

COMMENTS: See Question 9.

8. What is the dietary protein recommendation for a 70-kg man with intact protein stores?

A. 2–3 g/kg/day (140–210 g/day)

B. 4 g/kg/day (280 g/day)

C. 5–7 g/kg/day (340–410 g/day)

D. 0.8–1.0 g/kg/day (56–70 g/day)

Ref.: 8

COMMENTS: See Question 9

9. In which of the following amino acid categories would leucine, isoleucine, and valine be placed?

A. Branched-chain amino acids

B. Essential amino acids

C. Nonessential amino acids

D. A and B

E. A and C

F. None of the above

Ref.: 7

COMMENTS: Body proteins are made up of 20 different amino acids, each of which has a different metabolic fate and function in the body. • Amino acids commonly have a central α-carbon atom with a carboxylic acid group, an amino group, and a hydrogen atom covalently bonded. • The α-carbon atom is the site at which a side chain, different for each amino acid, is attached. • Unlike carbohydrates and fat, proteins (amino acids) contain nitrogen. • There are three categories of amino acids (Table 8-1): (1) essential amino acids, which cannot be synthesized by the body; (2) nonessential amino acids, which can be synthesized de novo in the body; and (3) conditionally essential amino acids, consisting of nonessential amino acids that are considered essential during stress or trauma if their use exceeds the body's capacity for synthesis and an outside source is required. • The dietary protein requirement for adults is 0.8 g/kg/day; that is, approximately 20% of calories consumed should be in the form of protein. • Overconsumption of protein is common in the typical Western diet, often exceeding the need for essential amino acids.

Protein consumed is used as a source of amino acids for (1) creating essential nitrogenous substances, (2) growth, and (3) maintenance. • Degradation and absorption of protein-derived amino acids is efficient, with protein being recycled continuously. • Protein digestion is a result of sequential hydrolysis of peptide bonds of the protein to form amino acids and peptides. • It begins in the stomach with the action of pepsin and proceeds to the small intestine, where pancreatic enzymes (trypsin, chymotrypsin, and carboxypolypeptidase) continue the process. • All protein metabolism depends on numerous endogenous mediators, including endocrine hormones (insulin and glucagon), prostaglandins, cytokines, and lymphokines, with health status and intake determining which substance takes precedence. • The free amino acids and small peptides resulting from protein digestion are absorbed into the brush border of intestinal epithelial cells. • Once in the portal system, free amino acids are distributed to the liver and muscles.

Endogenous protein production is estimated at 70 g/day, with approximately 250 g of protein mobilized daily within the body. • Protein breakdown is thought to match protein input, with 60% of protein intake converted to urea, 25% used to form new amino acids, and 15% used for new protein synthesis. • Urine contains 90% of all nitrogen lost, with small amounts lost via the skin and stool. • Cellular protein and amino acids are thought to be in constant equilibrium in terms of degradation and synthesis. • Continuous turnover of protein and amino acids (the amount of synthesis or degradation occurring over time) occurs at the following rates: 30% in muscle, 50% in the viscera, and 20% in plasma, without which daily protein requirements would be higher. • The liver is the site of urea production, biosynthesis of nonessential amino acids, and degradation of all amino acids. • Excess amino acids can be oxidized for energy, stored as fat or glycogen, or excreted. • Glutamate dehydrogenase, present in both the cytoplasm and mitochondria of the liver, is the primary enzyme

Table 8-1 Classification of Amino Acids

Nonessential Essential Amino Acids	Conditionally Essential Amino Acids	Amino Acids
Isoleucine	Alanine	Glutamine
Leucine	Arginine	Cysteine
Lysine	Asparagine	Histidine
Methionine	Glutamic acid	Tyrosine
Phenylalanine	Glutamine	
Threonine	Glycine	
Tryptophan	Proline	
Valine	Serine	

responsible for transamination of amino acids to the end products α-ketoglutarate and ammonia.

One special class of amino acids are the branched-chain amino acids, which include leucine, isoleucine, and valine. • The branched-chain amino acids are similar in terms of chemical structure and degradation steps, and they are the only amino acids metabolized outside the liver. • Branched-chain amino acids are extensively oxidized by muscle and adipose tissue and are a local source of energy for muscle, indicating their importance for patients with severe liver disease.

A N S W E R S :
Question 6: C
Question 7: A, B
Question 8: D
Question 9: D

---

10. Match the statements in the left-hand column with the substances in the right-hand column.

A. Cholesterol is primarily composed of this substance.   a. Glycerides

B. Fats are stored in the body in this form.   b. Phospholipids

C. These substances can be directly absorbed via portal blood, bypassing the lymphatic system.   c. Sterols

d. Medium-chain fatty acids

Ref.: 8

COMMENTS: See Question 11.

11. Lipolysis is the breakdown of fat. Which of the following statements regarding this process is/are true?

A. Insulin stimulates fat breakdown.

B. Lipolysis results in the formation of glycerol.

C. Glucagon is a hormone that can stimulate lipolysis.

D. With increased lipolysis, ketones are formed and released into the circulation.

Ref.: 9

COMMENTS: Fat is considered the most calorie-dense macronutrient in the diet, providing 9 kcal/g. • The structure of fat is characterized by its relative lack of oxygen, necessitating longer oxidative processes than do the less calorie–yielding carbohydrates. • Three main forms of fat are found in the body: glycerides, phospholipids, and sterols. • **Glycerides**, principally triglycerides or triglycerol (fatty acid and glycerol), are the storage forms of fat and are the most abundant forms in food, making up approximately 95–98% of ingested fat and in tissues. • Essential fatty acids are a form of triglyceride characterized by an unsaturated bond within the last seven carbons of the fatty acid chain at the methyl end. • The essential fatty acids (linoleic, linolenic, and arachidonic acids) cannot be synthesized by humans. • **Phospholipids** are ingested in small amounts and are mainly constituents of cell membranes and myelin sheaths. • **Sterols** consist primarily of cholesterol.

The functions of each type of fat are as follows. • Triglycerides are the most efficient form for storing calories. • In adipose tissue, they serve to protect organs, act as insulators, and contribute to body shape. • Cholesterol and phospholipids make up cell membranes and are substrates for other essential substances. • Cholesterol is the substrate for the formation of bile acids (primary bile acids are cholate and chenodeoxycholate) and steroid hormones (aldosterone, progesterone, estrogen, and androgens). • Phospholipids are substrates for prostaglandins, leukotrienes, and thromboxanes.

Dietary fat is digested in the small intestine, where emulsification by bile salts greatly increases the surface area of fat globules, allowing hydrolysis by lipases on the surface of fat. • The end products of triglyceride digestion are free fatty acid and two monoglycerides. • These end products combine with bile salts to form micelles, which are transported to brush borders of epithelial cells. • Bile salts are released back to chyme when monoglycerides and free fatty acids make their way to the brush border. • Cholesterol (esters) and phospholipids are hydrolyzed by pancreatic cholesterol ester hydrolase and phospholipase A_2, respectively. • Again, the bile salts form micelles, which are delivered to the brush border. • Once absorbed, the triglycerides, cholesterol esters, and phospholipids are formed and combined with small amounts of protein to form lipoproteins. • Lipoproteins (very low density, low density, and high density) act as transporters for various forms of fat to their ultimate destination (i.e., liver and adipose tissue). • It should be noted that only medium-chain fatty acids, which are made up of fewer than 12 carbons, can be directly absorbed via the portal circulation, bypassing the lymphatic system.

Various hormonal and substrate factors influence rates of adipose tissue lipolysis. • Utilization of fat energy relies on adipose cell lipase, which is regulated by epinephrine, norepinephrine, glucagon, and adrenocorticotrophic hormone. • Insulin inhibits the lipolysis. • Lipolysis results in the formation of glycerol and eventually glucose or pyruvate in the liver. • If fat breakdown exceeds carbohydrate degradation for energy, which is common in diabetic patients and in the fasting state, fatty acids are converted to ketones (acetoacetate and β-hydroxybutyrate), and oxidation by the tricarboxylic acid cycle is decreased. • The ketones are released into the circulation from the liver and converted back to acetyl CoA for use in the citric acid cycle in peripheral tissues. • In the heart, muscle, and renal cortex, ketone acetoacetate is the predominant fuel, whereas in the brain and red blood cells, glucose is the predominant fuel.

A N S W E R S :
Question 10: A-c; B-a; C-d
Question 11: B, C, D

---

12. Which of the following statements regarding vitamins is/are true?

A. They are produced in the body and do not require exogenous supplies.

B. They are a source of energy.

C. Some are necessary for the release of energy from carbohydrate, fat, and protein.

D. All are water soluble and can be eliminated easily from the body if excesses are consumed.

Ref.: 8, 10

COMMENTS: Vitamins and minerals are not a source of energy, but some are necessary for the release of energy from carbohydrate, fat, and protein; for oxygen transfer and delivery; and for tissue repair. • In addition, ongoing scientific research shows that vitamins and minerals have potentially important roles in controlling acute and chronic diseases and improving outcomes during recovery.

Vitamins are chemically unrelated organic substances required for specific metabolic reactions in the cell and must be supplied in the diet to prevent deficiency, since they cannot be synthesized in the body. • The biochemical roles of many vitamins are not precisely known. • However, it is known that some vitamins serve primarily as coenzymes to aid in the action of enzymes. • Vitamins can be either water soluble (e.g., vitamins C, B_1, B_3, B_6, and B_{12}) or fat soluble (i.e., soluble in organic solvents, e.g., vitamins A, D, E, and K). • Excess water-soluble vitamins can be excreted in the urine, but excess fat-soluble vitamins can be toxic.

Minerals exist as organic ions and include calcium, phosphorus, potassium, sodium, chloride, magnesium, iron, and sulfur. • To be considered essential, they must perform functions that are vital for life, growth, and maintenance.

The recommended daily intake for vitamins and minerals should be met in the clinical setting unless restrictions are necessary. • Early detection of deficiencies may be difficult, but ensuring adequate intake can be therapeutic in recovery. • Patients with malnutrition should be assumed to have inadequate vitamin and mineral intake. • Results of ongoing research will only improve the application of specialized vitamin and mineral use in stressed patient populations.

A N S W E R :
C

13. Laboratory tests to determine the status of which of the following visceral proteins yield results in 1–2 days?

    A. Albumin

    B. Transferrin

    C. Thyroxine-binding pre-albumin

    D. Retinol-binding protein

Ref.: 11, 12

COMMENTS: See Question 16.

14. When evaluating a patient's nutritional status, which of the following indicate(s) declining or poor nutritional status?

    A. The patient has a history of one and a half weeks of poor or negligible oral intake without supplemental feedings and has a serum albumin level of 2.1 g/dl.

    B. The nitrogen balance is −1.

    C. Indirect calorimetric studies indicate that the patient requires 1600 kcal/day, and the patient has been consuming 1600–1800 kcal/day.

    D. A patient receiving tube feedings has not met the goal tube feeding rate of 1500 ml/day for 2 weeks, and problems with nausea and vomiting prevent oral intake.

Ref.: 13, 14

COMMENTS: See Question 16.

15. A patient has gained 5 pounds in the 3 days since surgery. What is most likely the cause of the weight increase?

    A. Poor eating habits established before admission to the hospital

    B. Increase in dietary intake over the past 3 days that exceeds nutritional requirements

    C. Fluid retention

    D. Consumption of high-calorie beverages on a liquid diet

Ref.: 15, 16, 17

COMMENTS: See Question 16.

16. Which of the following would be a likely calorie recommendation for a postsurgical patient weighing 160 pounds who is neither obese nor a burn victim?

    A. 1250–1450 kcal

    B. 1375–2100 kcal

    C. 1500–2225 kcal

    D. 1820–2545 kcal

Ref.: 18

COMMENTS: Malnutrition is common in hospitalized patients, with significant increases in morbidity and mortality in surgical or highly stressed patients. • As many as 50% may have moderate malnutrition, causing a suboptimal response to surgery or medical therapies. • Diagnosis of malnutrition is important early in the patient's care, since rapid depletion of the body's energy and protein stores can occur. • Nutritional status can be determined through a review of the patient's medical history, physical examination, anthropometric characteristics, and laboratory data related to ingestion, digestion, absorption, and excretion. • There is no official formula for diagnosis of malnutrition, but surgical candidates and postoperative patients are highly susceptible to nutritional anomalies.

In reviewing the *medical history*, the surgeon should evaluate how past and present medical problems and therapies can affect current nutritional status and have knowledge of each disease state as it relates to nutrition (i.e., medical problems including recent surgery, sepsis, chronic illness, gastrointestinal disorders, psychosocial problems, or abnormal diets). • The *physical examination* can identify frank signs of malnutrition (i.e., marasmus or physical effects of specific vitamin or mineral deficiencies).

In terms of *anthropometric data*, height and weight help relate body size to nutritional needs. • Drastic changes in weight within a short time (days) is an indication of fluid shifts and should be evaluated appropriately. • Adjustments to weight expectations and macronutrient needs should be made for obese patients and those with amputations. • Estimates of fat and muscle mass using the midarm circumference and triceps skinfold thickness are not widely used for assessment of hospitalized patients, given issues with technique and time for data collection, but they have shown merit in patients followed long term.

Several *laboratory tests* may be used to evaluate nutritional status. • Visceral protein stores are commonly assessed, including albumin (half-life, 18–21 days), transferrin (half-life, 8–10 days), thyroxine-binding prealbumin (half-life, 1–2 days), and retinol-binding protein (half-life, 10 hr). • Albumin is the visceral protein universally used as an indicator of nutritional status and is typically the least expensive to assess. • Shorter–half-life proteins are most useful in acute-care settings. • All can be affected by other variables unrelated to nutrient intake (e.g., surgery or fluid status), and these variables must be considered when evaluating protein status. • The adequacy of protein supplied to maintain lean body mass is typically evaluated by assessing nitrogen balance, which is the state when protein intake (nitrogen input) and nitrogen output are equal. • Nitrogen output is monitored through 24-hr urine collection and determination of urinary urea nitrogen (UUN) levels. • One gram of protein equals 6.25 g of nitrogen.

• Therefore, the protein input (24-hr UUN + 4 for insensible losses) equals the nitrogen balance. • A positive nitrogen balance is an indication of anabolism (goal, +2–+4), and a negative nitrogen balance indicates a catabolic or starvation state. • The total lymphocyte count and the results of delayed hypersensitivity testing to measure compromised immune function resulting from malnutrition may be affected by many nonnutritional factors. • Therefore, the validity of these tests as a measure of malnutrition is debated.

The commonest type of malnutrition seen in hospitalized patients is protein-calorie malnutrition due to partial or total starvation. • Seven days is the absolute maximum period for which a patient should have severely limited nutritional intake. • Therefore, determination of the need for oral supplements or a more aggressive feeding regimen (i.e., enteral or parenteral nutrition) is important and requires knowledge of a patient's daily nutritional requirements. • The consequences of underfeeding (i.e., weight loss and nutrient deficiency) or overfeeding (i.e., hepatic lipogenesis and increased carbon dioxide production) are significant. • Therefore, specific, individualized estimates of each patient's nutritional requirements are important.

Many equations and formulas have been developed and studied to determine energy expenditure, including the most widely used **Harris-Benedict equation** for measuring basal energy expenditure (BEE). • The Harris-Benedict equation for males is 66 + 13.7(weight) + 5(height) − 6.8(age), and that for females is 65 + 9.6(wt) + 1.8(ht) − 4.7(age), where wt is weight given in kilograms (pounds ÷ 2.2), ht is height in centimeters, and age is given in years. • The BEE is typically adjusted for injury and activity factors, but overestimation of needs with these considerations do occur. • The most accurate means of measuring energy expenditure in the hospital setting is to use indirect calorimetric measurements (via a metabolic cart) to measure resting energy expenditure (REE). • Typically, calorie requirements of hospitalized adults range from 25 to 35 kcal/kg.

The recommended daily allowance for protein is 0.8 g/kg in healthy adults. • An increased need for protein is seen with the catabolic response to injury, with 1.2–1.5 g of protein per kilogram or higher necessary for protein synthesis in stressed patients (i.e., postsurgery or sepsis). • Calculating nitrogen balance is the commonest way to determine whether protein needs are being met. • Patients with severe injuries or burns typically require larger amounts of calories and protein. • Protein synthesis requires calories from sources other than protein to fuel production. • A nonprotein calorie/nitrogen ratio of 150:1 in a nonstressed individual or 80–100:1 in a stressed individual is typically recommended. • For patients with hepatic disease, protein requirements are based on stress level. • A patient with encephalopathic episodes requires use of branched-chain amino acids, since they do not require metabolism by the liver and can be converted to energy locally in the muscle. • Patients with renal disease and acute failure, without dialysis, are typically permitted only 0.4–0.6 g/kg of protein. • Protein needs increase with dialysis, and the needs should be determined on an individual basis.

ANSWERS:
Question 13: C
Question 14: A, B, D
Question 15: C
Question 16: D (25–35 kcal/kg)

17. Which of the following statements regarding simple starvation is/are true?

    A. It results in a respiratory quotient of 0.6–0.7, which is indicative of fat as a primary fuel source.

    B. The Cori and alanine cycles provide carbon for gluconeogenesis in the liver.

    C. Energy expenditure decreases in response to decreased intake.

    D. Lipogenesis ensures maintenance of fat reserves.

Ref.: 11, 18

COMMENTS: See Question 19.

18. Which of the following tissues are obligatory glucose users?

    A. Cardiac muscle

    B. Red blood cells

    C. Brain

    D. Skeletal muscle

Ref.: 11, 18

COMMENTS: See Question 19.

19. When calculating protein losses in nitrogen balance studies, how much protein is lost per gram of nitrogen?

    A. 1.00 g

    B. 2.50 g

    C. 3.40 g

    D. 6.25 g

Ref.: 19

COMMENTS: Surgical patients may be at risk for both simple starvation and stress hypermetabolism, depending on the severity of disease, length of recovery, and the surgical procedure performed and its consequences. • Simple starvation results when nutrient intake does not meet energy requirements. • Energy expenditure characteristically decreases to help match energy intake, and metabolic responses occur to preserve muscle mass. • Initially, during early fasting, glycogen from glycogenolysis supplies glucose for obligatory glucose-using tissues (i.e., red blood cells and brain). • Lipogenesis is curtailed, since lactate, pyruvate, and amino acids are not diverted to glucose production. • The Cori cycle is then activated, which allows the glucose produced by gluconeogenesis in the liver to be converted back to lactate through glycolysis in the peripheral tissues. • Skeletal muscle releases amino acids via the alanine cycle, which provides carbon for gluconeogenesis in the liver. • The Cori and alanine cycles are important because tissues that use only glucose (i.e., brain, blood, renal medulla, and bone marrow) depend on hepatic gluconeogenesis, primarily from lactate, glycerol, and alanine, during starvation. • The alanine and Cori cycles supply glucose but do not provide carbon for net synthesis of glucose. • They only replace the glucose that is used to produce lactate in peripheral tissues. • Even as fuel in the gut is diminished, glucose is still required. • Glycerol and protein are important substrates for net glucose synthesis.

Protein metabolism adapts to starvation, as follows: (1) synthesis of protein decreases because energy sources to generate production are not available; (2) protein catabolism is reduced as other fuels become primary sources of energy for many tissues; (3) decreased ureagenesis and urinary nitrogen loss reflect protein sparing (in the initial stages of starvation, the rate of urea nitrogen loss is more than 10 g/day, with a decline to less than 7 g/day after weeks of starvation). • In calculating protein losses, each gram of nitrogen lost in urine reflects 6.25 g of protein lost.

Alanine, glutamine, and glycine are released in large amounts to be used by the liver and kidney for net glucose formation. • Glucose synthesis in the liver during simple starvation is linked to synthesis of urea because of the increased transamination. • The adipose tissue during starvation is important because the insulin/glucagon ratio is decreased, which allows activation of lipolysis and suppression of lipogenesis. • Levels of fatty acids are increased during starvation and are used as alternative fuels by many tissues that prefer fat as a fuel source (i.e., kidney, cardiac muscle, and skeletal muscle). • The liver uses fatty acids to meet energy needs for gluconeogenesis. • The acetyl CoA generated by oxidation of fatty acids in the liver is converted to ketones. • As ketones (acetoacetate and β-hydroxybutyrate) rise, they can cross the blood-brain barrier to supply fuel, but some glucose is still required. • The use of fatty acids as a primary fuel source allows the sparing of body proteins for gluconeogenesis. • This sparing effect is important for maintenance of immune functions and liver and respiratory muscle function. • A respiratory quotient of 0.6–0.7 during simple starvation reflects the fact that fat is the body's primary fuel source during simple starvation.

ANSWERS:

Question 17: A, B, C

Question 18: B, C

Question 19: X D

20. Which phase of hypermetabolism can last for an extended period of time, leading to adverse effects on nutritional status?

A. Ebb phase

B. Flow phase

C. Cycling phase

D. Imbalance phase

Ref.: 11, 20

COMMENTS: See Question 21.

21. Which of the following occurs during stress hypermetabolism?

A. Decreased need for linoleic and arachidonic acids

B. Increased proteolysis

C. Elevated REE

D. Positive nitrogen balance

Ref.: 1, 20, 21

COMMENTS: In contrast simple starvation, activation of stress hypermetabolism occurs following surgery, trauma, or sepsis to provide energy and substrates for tissue repair and to activate immune function and the inflammatory response. • In the initial period, known as the ebb phase, a decline in oxygen consumption is seen, along with poor circulation, fluid imbalance, and cellular shock lasting 24–36 hr. • As the body adapts (flow phase), there are increased cellular activity and increased hormonal stimulation, leading to elevated metabolic rate, body temperature, and nitrogen loss. • This phase can last days, weeks, or months.

Nutrients are used during hypermetabolism in response to the stress hormonal and inflammatory mediator response to the injury. • The earliest stages of response are characterized by increases in gluconeogenesis, REE, proteolysis, ureagenesis, and urinary nitrogen loss. • Clinical signs include tachypnea, increased body temperature, and tachycardia, with laboratory results showing increased leukocytosis, hyperlactatemia, azotemia, and hyperglycemia. • Liver production of glucose during stress is increased through gluconeogenesis and glycogenolysis (Cori cycle), which are stimulated by endocrine (hormonal) changes: increased cortisol, increased glucagon,

increased catecholamines, and decreased insulin. • Overall use of protein as an oxidative fuel source by the liver is increased, and typically there is increased turnover of branched-chain amino acids.

Hyperglycemia is characteristic during stress, with (1) increased glycogenolysis occurring initially to elevate the blood glucose level followed by (2) increased glucose production and (3) reduced peripheral utilization later in response to the stress. • Gluconeogenesis in the liver continues despite hyperglycemia. • Typically, neither glucose nor insulin infusion can control blood glucose levels (or gluconeogenesis) during times of extreme stress. • As a result, protein stores are depleted and insulin resistance continues. • Unsuppressed glucose production leads to low rates of glycogen storage, lipolysis, and oxidation of fat. • Continuous circulation of insulin, resulting from high plasma glucose levels, prevents extended use of the body's vast fat stores for energy. • Increased fatty acid oxidation occurs with hypermetabolism, resulting in decreased plasma linoleic and arachidonic acid levels, which can lead to essential fatty acid deficiency in 10 days if exogenous sources are not supplied.

ANSWERS:

Question 20: B

Question 21: X, C
     B

22. What is the appropriate course of action for a patient with a respiratory quotient (RQ) of 1.01?

A. Increase supply of protein.

B. Increase supply of lipids.

C. Decrease total calorie load owing to overfeeding.

D. Maintain current feeding regimen.

Ref.: 22, 23

COMMENTS: See Question 23.

23. Indirect calorimetric data include which of the following in determining energy requirements?

A. Oxygen consumption

B. Carbon dioxide produced

C. REE obtained by applying the Weir equation

D. RQ

E. All of the above

F. None of the above

Ref.: 22

COMMENTS: Energy expenditures and the resulting caloric needs can be estimated for stressed patients through various developed equations. • Approximately 190 equations estimating energy expenditure exist, and controversy continues as to the optimal equation. • Energy expenditure is the ability to do external and internal work, and methods exist for performing accurate patient-specific measurements. • Energy exists in the body in many forms, including chemical energy, mechanical energy, thermal energy, and electrical energy. • Nutrients are chemical forms of energy converted to various other forms to be utilized by the body.

Indirect calorimetric studies measure a hospitalized patient's energy released and gas exchange via a portable metabolic cart at the patient's beside. • Both ventilator-dependent and non–ventilator-dependent patients can have accurately determined energy expenditure to allow for the provision of optimal macronutrient prescription. • The indirect calorimeter measures O_2 consumption (VO_2) and CO_2 production (VCO_2), enabling the calculation of

REE and RQ. • One liter of O_2 consumed indicates 3.9 kcal generated, and 1 L of CO_2 exhaled produces 1.1 kcal. • The abbreviated **Weir equation** is REE = 1.44 [3.9(VO_2) + 1.1(VCO_2)], where VO_2 is O_2 consumption in milliliters per minute, VCO_2 is CO_2 production on milliliters per minute, and REE is in kilocalories per day.

REE is typically 10% greater than BEE (measurement of kilocalorie expenditure in a thermally regulated environment 12–18 hr after dietary intake at rest, an expensive and impractical procedure in a hospital setting). • REE is typically obtained using the metabolic cart for an alert person in a postabsorptive state. • A steady state is achieved when three consecutive 1-min readings of REE are within 10% of each other and the correlating RQ values are within 5% of each other. • This value reflects 75–90% of total energy expenditure (TEE). • An additional factor of 1.1–1.3 is required to account for the thermodynamic effects of food, shivering, physical activity, illness, and injury in TEE estimations. • Therefore, the REE measurement obtained, multiplied by 1.1–1.3, equals the patient's daily energy requirements.

When the REE value obtained through indirect calorimetric studies is compared to predicted results using the Harris-Benedict equation, the following assessments can be made regarding a patient's metabolic state: (1) 110% greater than predicted REE = hypermetabolism, (2) 90–100% of predicted REE = normometabolism, and (3) REE measured at 90% less than predicted REE = hypometabolism. • Calculation of the RQ provides verification of the substrate utilization for energy at the time of testing. • This information allows the clinician to alter nutrient content of feedings to optimize macronutrient intake. • The RQ is the ratio of CO_2 expired (VCO_2) to the amount of O_2 inspired (VO_2): RQ = VCO_2/VO_2.

• The RQ value obtained indicates type of substrate utilization, as summarized in the following table:

Substrate	RQ
Ethanol	0.67
Fat oxidation	0.71
Protein oxidation	0.82
Mixed substrate oxidation	0.85–0.95 (ideal)
Carbohydrate oxidation	0.9–1.0
Lipogenesis	1.01
Hyperventilation	>1.1
Ketosis	<0.6

In general, the following nutritional changes can be suggested for the RQ values obtained. • RQ > 1 indicates excessive calorie load and necessitates decreased caloric intake. • RQ = 1.0 indicates a need to decrease carbohydrates and/or increase lipids. • RQ < 0.82 requires an increase in total energy intake. • Mixed substrate oxidation with an RQ of 0.85–0.95 is considered ideal. • Normal deviations in RQ can be seen after eating (RQ = 1.0), in diabetes (RQ = 0.71), and in starvation (RQ = 0.83). • Anything that can alter breathing must be considered when performing indirect calorimetric studies and interpreting the RQ value. • Ongoing comparisons between estimated energy expenditure (e.g., obtained using the Harris-Benedict equation) and actual results obtained using indirect calorimetric studies are helpful in monitoring feeding regimens and making nutritional recommendations.

A N S W E R S :

Question 22: C

Question 23: E

Chart 1:Algorithm to Determine Method of Nutritional Support		
Action	**Gut Functioning**	**Gut Not Functioning**
Proceed with oral feedings.	Determine best enteral route (e.g., nasogastric or jejunostomy gastric feedings).	Consider TPN if expected length of time without intake to exceed 5–7 days total.
Order patient-appropriate diet.	Assess fluid, calorie, and protein needs.	Place access device.
	Determine best formula, rate, and method of administration.	Assess fluid, calorie, protein, and electrolyte needs.
	Monitor laboratory study results, weight, and fluid status tolerance to feedings.	Formulate TPN to meet patient's requirements.
		Monitor appropriate laboratory study results, blood glucose levels, weight, fluid status, and tolerance to TPN.

---

24. Which of the following is a contraindication for enteral nutrition support?

    A. Recent surgery

    B. Poor oral intake

    C. Weight loss and functional gastrointestinal tract

    D. Bowel obstruction

    Ref.: 24–27

COMMENTS: See Question 26.

25. Which of the following is appropriate action when a patient experiences diarrhea during the course of a tube-feeding regimen?

    A. Stop the tube feedings immediately to ensure that the patient does not become dehydrated.

    B. Switch to a more concentrated formula to provide less free water to the patient.

    C. Evaluate the patient's medications, if any, and determine whether they contribute to the diarrhea.

    D. Rule out *Clostridium difficile* colitis.

    E. Slow the rate of feedings or consider antidiarrheal medications when *C. difficile* is ruled out as a cause of the diarrhea.

    Ref.: 24–27

COMMENTS: See Question 26.

26. Which condition contraindicates using enteral feedings?

    A. Recent surgery

    B. High-output enteric fistula

    C. Head trauma

    D. Cachexia

    Ref.: 28, 29

COMMENTS: Enteral nutrition is the provision of a liquid formula diet by mouth or tube into some area of the gastrointestinal tract to maintain or improve nutritional status. • Research indicates that enteral nutrition is generally well tolerated and cost effective and allows for gut mucosal growth, development, and integrity when prescribed appropriately. • The decision to use enteral nutrition is based on the premise that if the gut works, use it. • Patients receiving enteral feedings have been found to have fewer septic complications than those receiving total parenteral nutrition (TPN), probably because there is less bacterial translocation in the gut in the former. • The functional capacity of the gut must be considered before prescribing enteral nutrition therapy. • There must be (1) at least 100 cm of small intestine for nutrient absorption, (2) an intact ileocecal valve, and (3) adequate airway protection. • Conditions contraindicating use of the gastrointestinal tract include gastroparesis, intestinal obstruction, paralytic ileus, high-output enteric fistula, short bowel syndrome, and hemodynamic instability.

Once it has been established that the patient cannot consume adequate nutrition by mouth and that the enteral route can be used, the clinician determines where in the gastrointestinal tract to establish the feeding and which technique to use for tube placement. • Nasogastric tubes are preferred for short-term feedings (< 4 weeks) and can be inserted in the stomach, duodenum, or jejunum. • Poor results with beside nasogastric nasoenteric placement (80–85% success rate) have led to placement of feeding tubes using fluoroscopic or endoscopic guidance (85–95% success rate in postpyloric tube placement). • Long-term feedings (> 4–6 weeks) require placement of a more permanent gastrointestinal access device: (1) a percutaneous enteral device (gastric, gastric jejunal, or direct jejunal), (2) a laparoscopically placed tube (gastrostomy or jejunostomy), or (3) a surgically placed tube (gastrostomy or jejunostomy). • The gastrostomy tube tends to be the most popular for long-term patient feeding. • The patient's status, the ability to tolerate the procedure, cost, and techniques available to the institution all influence selection of the tube feeding technique.

Decisions regarding tube feeding rate, frequency, and amount depend on the patient's medical condition, the tube feeding type, and the enteral feeding site. • There are three methods for administering enteral feedings: (1) bolus or gravity, in which 250–500 ml of formula is administered quickly several times per day to patients with relatively normal digestion and absorption; (2) intermittent feeding, administered several times per day over at least a half-hour to allow gastric emptying similar to that seen with normal eating; and (3) continuous feeding, which requires a kangaroo-type pump to administer feedings over 10–24 hr for patients who require consistent delivery of nutrients to prevent dumping. • In continuous feeding, the formula is typically full strength, initiated at a slow rate (20–40 ml/hr) and advanced as tolerated until the goal rate is reached. • A patient's goal rate is based on nutritional requirements for fluid, calories, and protein. • A typical advancement schedule may include increasing the tube feeding rate by 20–30 ml every 6 hr, as tolerated, until the goal rate is reached, depending on the patient.

Most complications associated with tube feeding can be prevented with proper monitoring. • Complications can be metabolic (e.g, overhydration or underhydration), gastrointestinal (e.g., diarrhea, nausea, vomiting, delayed gastric emptying, constipation, or abdominal distention), or mechanical (e.g., the wrong tube size or a cracked tube). • To prevent complications for enterally fed patients, the clinician should ensure that the patient is in a semi-upright position for gastric feeding, confirm the tube position, and initiate feedings slowly, with gastric residuals checked frequently (i.e., every 4–6 hr, with residuals >150 ml rechecked and tube feedings or other contributing factors adjusted appropriately). • All patients should be instructed about flushing to keep lines clear and to provide adequate hydration upon discharge. • Note that the typical tube feeding regimen requires additional water to ensure adequate hydration.

Diarrhea has been estimated to occur in 2.3% of the enteral population and in 34–41% of critically ill patients. • Diarrhea may be related to (1) factors not associated with the feeding formula, including medications or antibiotics, fecal impaction, hypoalbuminemia, enteric pathogens, pre-existing medical conditions, inflammatory syndromes, or sepsis; or (2) factors related to the tube feeding formula, including a too rapid infusion rate, a too rapid initiation or progression, lactose intolerance, microbe contamination, lack of fiber, the osmolality of the formula, or a high fat content in the formula. • Diarrhea may be controlled by (1) medication, such as Lomotil, Imodium, or paregoric if not contraindicated; (2) changing to continuous feeding; or (3) slowing the rate of tube feeding until tolerance is established. • *C. difficile* must be ruled out as a cause of the diarrhea before initiation of medication to control the problem. • Careful monitoring of conditions surrounding the onset of diarrhea is important when evaluating the cause.

ANSWERS:
Question 24: D
Question 25: C, D, E
Question 26: B

27. Specialty enteral products are available for which of the following patient populations?

   A. Liver patients

   B. Renal patients

   C. Pulmonary patients

   D. All of the above

   E. None of the above

Ref.: 30

COMMENTS: See Question 28.

28. Match the descriptions in the left-hand column with the formulas in the right-hand column.

A. High-density formula with decreased water content	a. Elemental formula (e.g., Alitraq)
B. Contains hydrolyzed macronutrients and is low in fat	b. Blenderized formula (e.g., Compleat)
C. Formula may be used for patients with increased protein needs	c. Fiber-containing formula (e.g., Jevity)
D. Formula used to help eliminate diarrhea	d. Concentrated formula (e.g., Two-cal HN)
E. Contains regular food in liquid form	e. High-nitrogen formula (e.g., Osmolite HN)
F. Formula designed for patients with renal failure	f. Disease-specific formula (e.g., Nepro)

Ref.: 30

COMMENTS: Many formulas exist for use in tube-fed patients. • Whereas the hospital formulary dictates what is available for use in the hospital, any formula can be obtained for tube-fed outpatients or specially ordered for inpatients. • Carbohydrate is usually provided from intact macronutrient sources, including maltodextrin, hydrolyzed cornstarch, corn syrup solids, and sucrose. • Protein sources are casein, soy, whey, lactalbumin, or free amino acids. • Fat content may consist of long-chain triglycerides derived from vegetable oil or medium-chain triglycerides derived from coconut or palm kernel oil. • Appropriate selection is key to successful tube feeding.

Six product categories exist for enteral formulas. • *Standard* formula mimics the American diet, with 50–60% of calories from carbohydrates, 10–15% from protein, and 25–40% from fat (e.g., Isocal and Osmolite). • These formulas are isosmolar to blood (300 mOsmol/kg) and are used for patients with functioning gastrointestinal tracts who have been receiving nothing by mouth for less than 7 days. • *Concentrated* formula is similar to standard formula in terms of content to meet the patient's nutritional requirements, but the density per milliliter is greater than that of standard formulas because of the decreased water content (e.g., Ensure Plus and Impact 1.5). • It is typically used for patients with fluid restrictions. • *High nitrogen-protein* formulas contain more than 15% of calories supplied by nitrogen and protein (e.g., Isosource HN, Osmolite HN, and Replete). • These formulas are used for patients with higher than normal protein needs (e.g., malnourished, catabolic, or elderly patients with increased protein requirements). • *Elemental* formulas are advocated for patients who have been receiving nothing by mouth for more than 7 days and patients with partially functioning gastrointestinal tracts (e.g., Alitraq and Peptamen). • They contain hydrolyzed macronutrients, which require less digestion and are potentially better tolerated until the patient is able to transition back to intact nutrients. • Generally, the formulas are low in fat or contain fewer long-chain triglycerides and are hyperosmolar (>450 mOsm/kg). • *Fiber-containing or blenderized* formulas contain fiber supplied from added soy polysaccharides or natural food sources, respectively. • Fiber formulas are intended to regulate bowel function by eliminating diarrhea and constipation (e.g., Jevity and Enrich, which is Ensure with fiber). • Blenderized formulas differ from fiber formulas in that they are regular foods and therefore contain all components of nutrients naturally occurring in foods (e.g., Compleat). • *Specialty* products are available for patients with liver, renal, and pulmonary disease (e.g., for pulmonary disease, Pulmocare; for liver disease, Hepatic Aid II; and for renal failure, Nepro). • Their composition varies, depending on the disease state, but they generally have high osmolality and are nutritionally inadequate. • The benefit of such formulas remains controversial. • Some enteral products contain lactose, which causes bloating, cramping, and diarrhea in some patients. • Lactose-free products should be used if intolerance is expected or symptoms arise.

Because of electrolyte imbalances or the need for varied macronutrient content, some patients have needs that cannot be met by available commercial products. • Enteral feeding modules can be used to create a patient-specific formula (modular formula). • Carbohydrate modules include Sumacal and Polycose powder. • Protein modules available include ProMod and Propac. • Fat sources are MCT oil and Microlipid. • Vitamins and mineral products are available. • Modular formulas are made by adding water to specific amounts of these products to best suit a patient's needs. • Adding to the complexities of nutritional management of the tube-fed patient is the wide variety of enteral products available. • Dietitians and nutrition support teams are typically responsible for determining the best formulas for a hospital formulary to carry, based on current research and cost constraints.

ANSWERS:
Question 27: D
Question 28: A-d; B-a; C-e; D-c; E-b; F-f

29. How many calories per gram are contained in the anhydrous form of dextrose used in parenteral formulas?

   A. 3.4

   B. 4.0

   C. 7.0

   D. 9.0

Ref.: 6, 31

COMMENTS: See Question 31.

30. Which is true of perioperative nutritional support?

   A. A patient with mild malnutrition should postpone surgery to allow for 5 days of nutritional support.

   B. TPN should be used for moderately malnourished patients even if oral or enteral routes can be used.

   C. Seven to 10 days of optimal nutrition should be provided via TPN to severely malnourished patients if surgery can be postponed.

   D. Macronutrient dosages should exceed daily requirements to allow for "catch-up" before surgery in moderately malnourished patients.

Ref.: 32, 33

COMMENTS: See Question 31.

31. How many calories are provided in one 500-ml bottle of 10% intravenous fat solution?

   A. 150 kcal

   B. 550 kcal

   C. 800 kcal

   D. 1000 kcal

Ref.: 31

COMMENTS: Parenteral nutrition (including TPN and hyperalimentation) is the provision of nutrients (carbohydrates, protein, fat, vitamins and minerals, and sterile water) via a hyperosmolar solution delivered into a central vein, typically the superior vena cava. • All components must be individualized to the patient, based on diagnosis, the presence of a chronic disease state, fluid and electrolyte status, acid-base balance, and specific nutritional goals. • The patient whose nutritional needs cannot be met via the oral or enteral route requires TPN, the basic goal of which is to meet nutritional needs and maintain or improve metabolic balance.

Disease state indications for TPN include a nonfunctioning gastrointestinal tract (i.e., short-bowel syndrome, intractable vomiting, or diarrhea), the need for bowel rest (e.g., as in severe pancreatitis), and severe malnutrition, when the patient has been unable to eat for 5–7 days or more. • Two types of solution exist: (1) traditional dextrose and amino acid solutions in which lipids are piggybacked into the solution and (2) total nutrient admixture (TNA), which contains all three macronutrients dispensed from a single container. • An automated compounding device is needed for accurate mixing, and as with all TPN, mixing should be done under laminar airflow to control bacterial contamination.

Various concentrations of macronutrients are available to develop a patient-specific, nutritional regimen that helps prevent overfeeding or underfeeding. • The composition of TPN is limited by maximum concentrations of various amino acid and dextrose solutions that are physically achievable. • Crystalline protein and synthetic amino acids are the protein sources for TPN solutions, with standard base solutions ranging from 8.5 to 10.0% amino acids (0.5 L of 8.5% solution contains 42.5 g protein). • Hepatamine 8% is an amino acid solution sometimes used for patients with encephalopathy, since it contains an increased percentage of branched-chain amino acids. • Commercially available dextrose solutions contain 5–70% glucose (50–700 g/L). • The final solution (i.e., after all solutions are added) typically contains 15–35% dextrose. • The monohydrate form of dextrose is used for TPN, providing 3.4 kcal/g upon oxidation. • Dextrose can be provided peripherally, through the process of peripheral venous nutrition, at concentrations of less than 10% and should be administered only short term. • Higher concentrations may promote thrombosis due to low peripheral blood flow, thereby preventing the provision of adequate calories or protein (or both) via this method.

Fat solutions are considered isotonic and can be administered peripherally or centrally without concern about thrombosis. • Carbohydrates should be administered at a rate no greater than 5 mg/kg/min via TPN, which is the maximum oxidation rate of glucose. • Fat solutions are available in 10 and 20% solutions, which provide 1.1 and 2.0 kcal/ml, respectively. • Fats can be administered intermittently, continuously, or via TNA. • Monitoring clearance by checking triglyceride levels is key to ensuring tolerance to lipid infusions. • Patients should also be monitored for signs of chills, fevers, headaches, or back pain with initiation of fat to rule out intolerance. • Fat should be administered at no more than 2.5 g/kg/day. • Lipid solutions should be administered cautiously to patients with respiratory distress syndrome, severe liver disease, or increased metabolic stress, since fat may exacerbate these conditions. • Patients with hypertriglyceridemia (>250 mg/dl), lipid nephrosis, egg allergy, or acute pancreatitis associated with hyperlipidemia should not be given fat emulsions.

Vitamins and minerals should be supplied to meet the recommended daily allowance. • Vitamin K must be ordered separately based on coagulation status. • Electrolytes are added to TPN to maintain or achieve electrolyte homeostasis, with individual electrolyte needs depending on disease state, renal function, drug therapy, hepatic function, and nutritional status (Table 8-2). • A problem sometimes seen in malnourished patients with initiation of feedings is the refeeding syndrome, which is characterized by rapid depletion of potassium, phosphorus, and magnesium owing to lean tissue synthesis and the shift of metabolism intracellularly with glucose administration. • This problem can result in death if electrolyte levels are not carefully monitored. • The increased need for various minerals and electrolytes seen with diarrhea, ostomies, fistulas, vomiting, and other gastrointestinal losses can be met via TPN. • Metabolic and nutritional factors should be

evaluated for each patient receiving TPN. • Metabolic monitoring can include determination of serum or urine glucose levels (or both) several times daily and electrolyte levels daily until tolerance is established. • Other necessary laboratory tests include magnesium, phosphorus, calcium, bilirubin, SGOT, SGPT, alkaline phosphatase, blood urea nitrogen, and creatinine assays.

Coagulation monitoring is performed daily until the goal TPN rate is reached, as are triglyceride level determinations to determine the patient's ability to clear lipids before and after lipid administration. • Nutritional monitoring should include daily fluid balance evaluation, daily weight, nitrogen balance determinations as needed, and testing for visceral protein status once per week. • Institutional guidelines should be followed for monitoring TPN. • A typical initiation plan may progress as follows: (1) check all laboratory test results before starting TPN and all other related information; (2) initiate TPN at 1 L at a final concentration needed to meet the patient's needs; (3) monitor tolerance to TPN initiation as outlined (i.e., through laboratory tests); and (4) increase to the goal TPN rate. • Ongoing adjustments should be expected throughout the course of TPN administration.

When calculating amounts of specific nutrients when ordering TPN, the following are taken into account: (1) all macronutrients and micronutrients are based on patients' individual needs; (2) fluid (water) is provided at a volume of 25–50 ml/kg, depending on age, renal status, and other pertinent factors; (3) dextrose solutions are available in 5–70% solutions, and amino acids are available in 3–10% solutions; and (4) lipids come in 500-ml bottles, with 10% solutions containing 550 kcal and 20% solutions containing 1000 kcal (minimal fat needs of 2–4% of the kilocalories as essential fatty acids can be met with weekly administration of lipids).

The benefit of using perioperative nutrition remains controversial, with various studies showing conflicting results. • It seems at this time that 7–10 days of perioperative nutrition for patients with severe malnutrition may help reduce the risk of postoperative complications and morbidity associated with malnutrition. • Patients diagnosed with severe malnutrition (decreased visceral and somatic protein stores) and decreased oral intake before surgery who are not ready to undergo surgery and for whom oral or enteral feedings are not an option should be fed intravenously. • When delay in feeding does not seem logical for those with a suspected postoperative need for TPN, administration should be considered.

ANSWERS:
Question 29: A
Question 30: C
Question 31: B

32. Refeeding syndrome is characterized by which of the following electrolyte abnormalities?

A. Hyponatremia, hypokalemia, and hypercalcemia

B. Hyperphosphatemia, hypokalemia, and hypocalcemia

C. Hypokalemia, hypomagnesemia, and hypophosphatemia

D. Hypocalcemia, hyponatremia, and hypomagnesemia

Ref.: 34–37

COMMENTS: There are three areas of complication with use of TPN: (1) mechanical problems secondary to obtaining and continuing central venous access, (2) metabolic problems, and (3) nutritional complications.

Several *mechanical complications* may occur with TPN. • Pneumothorax may occur in as many as 4% of patients with elective access. • The incidence is usually higher in emergency situations

Table 8-2. Electrolyte Amounts for Total Parenteral Nutrition for Adults

Electrolyte	Recommended Amount/Day	Typical Amounts/L
Sodium	60–120 mEq	20–50 mEq
Potassium	60–120 mEq	20–50 mEq
Calcium	0–15 mEq	5 mEq
Chloride	60–150 mEq	20–50 mEq
Acetate	80–120 mEq	30–50 mEq
Phosphorus	20–40 mmol	5–15 mmol
Magnesium	0–25 mEq	5–8 mEq
Other typical additives:		
MVI 12 multivitamin formula	10 ml	
Trace element formula	5 ml	
Heparin	As needed	
Insulin (regular Humulin)	As needed	

and in nutritionally depleted patients. • Artery injury, air embolism, brachial plexus injury, thoracic duct injury, lymphatic injury, catheter embolus, venous thrombosis, and poor catheter position, among other problems, are possible mechanically related complications. • Catheter-related sepsis can be expected at a rate of 2–5%. • The rate of line sepsis is 20–30%. • Important steps to help prevent line infections include appropriate skin preparation before an operative procedure, appropriate maintenance of the central line, frequent catheter changes, careful use of multiple-lumen catheters, and appropriate antibiotic and thrombolytic treatment if sepsis develops.

A number of *metabolic complications* may result from TPN. • Standard use of vitamins and trace element solutions has eliminated the problem of deficiency states seen with extended TPN during the early stages of its usage. • Excess glucose can (1) increase blood glucose levels and induce hyperosmolar nonketotic coma; (2) lead to dehydration; (3) lead to lipogenesis with subsequent hepatic abnormalities (e.g., fatty liver); and (4) increase CO_2 production, which may compromise respiratory function. • Because rebound hypoglycemia can occur with discontinuation of TPN, weaning to 50 ml/hr before complete discontinuation is important. • Treatment for hyperglycemia in TPN patients is typically the addition of regular (not long-acting) insulin to the parenteral solution, with stringent monitoring of ACCU-CHECKS or serum blood glucose levels. • Critically ill patients with large fluctuations in blood glucose levels benefit from combination of regular insulin in the TPN and sliding-scale coverage with regular insulin to control what the dosage in the TPN cannot. • Fat deficiency can occur if fat is not provided at least twice weekly to meet essential fatty acid requirements. • Clinical signs of essential fatty acid deficiency include dry skin, poor wound healing, and hair loss. • Hepatic toxicity and benign transient liver function test result abnormalities can occur. • Gut atrophy and bacterial translocation can occur with gut disuse. • Depletion of or excess vitamins and minerals can cause unwanted deficiencies or elevated levels of nutrients (e.g., hyper- or hypokalemia and hyper- or hypophosphatemia). • Refeeding syndrome results when glucose is administered quickly to an individual with poor nutrient intake before TPN, the result being that glucose moves into the cells rapidly to be utilized and those nutrients required for metabolism of glucose rapidly follow to the intracellular spaces. • Subsequent rapid serum depletion of magnesium, phosphorus, or potassium develops. • Careful monitoring of the results of initial TPN administration is key. • Immunologic impairment due to large doses or rapid lipid administration has been shown to occur. • It is thought that, once the lipoprotein lipase system becomes overloaded, the reticuloendothelial system helps rid the body of excess amounts of lipids, causing neutrophils to become lipid saturated, affecting their ability to function. • Therefore, careful monitoring of lipid levels through triglyceride level determinations is important.

Nutritional complications of TPN include overfeeding and underfeeding. • Careful assessment and monitoring of the patient's nutritional status help ensure appropriate feeding regimens.

ANSWER:
Question 32: C

---

33. Which of the following statements regarding pro-inflammatory cytokines is/are not true?

A. They can induce behavioral changes.

B. They can increase energy release by accelerating the REE.

C. They can decrease energy release by slowing the REE induced by injury.

D. They can create shifts in mineral metabolism.

Ref.: 38

COMMENTS: See Question 34.

---

34. Immune-enhancing formulas (IEFs) are currently being investigated to improve immune function. Which nutrients have been provided in these formulas?

A. Glutamine

B. Arginine

C. ω3-Fatty acids

D. ω6-Fatty acids

E. All of the above

F. None of the above

Ref.: 39

COMMENTS: The production of cytokines and their effects on injury response are of growing interest for their potential application in nutritional management. • Cytokines are small messenger proteins, or glycoproteins, produced by T cells and macrophages in immune response to invasion. • At the cellular level, cytokines react to a stress signal, usually an antigen, responding to such stresses as surgery, sepsis, burns, or trauma, and can affect cells locally or systemically to mediate the immune response. • Once produced, the cytokine binds to a cell surface receptor, which allows for activation of mechanisms in the target cells. • Macrophages, hematopoietic cells, T cells, and B cells allow for cytokine binding. • The cytokines in turn allow for the coordination of the immune response via the following substances: interleukins (ILs), interferons (INFs), tumor necrosis factors (TNFs), and colony-stimulating factors (CSFs). • Pro-inflammatory cytokines have been researched in depth and have been shown to produce some of the vast metabolic changes that occur during injury. • Pro-inflammatory cytokines include tumor necrosis factor-alpha (TNF-α), interferon-gamma (IFN-γ), interleukin-1 (IL-1), and interleukin-6 (IL-6). • The presence of pro-inflammatory cytokines has been shown to influence the following metabolic and nutritional responses to stress: (1) behavioral changes, such as increased sleep and decreased oral intake and physical activity; (2) glucose metabolism, including increased glucose oxidation and gluconeogenesis; (3) protein metabolism, with increased whole-body protein turnover, muscle protein degradation, acute-phase protein synthesis, and amino acid oxidation; (4) lipid metabolism changes, such as hypertriglyceridemia, increased hepatic triglyceride synthesis, and decreased lipolysis; (5) increased energy release via accelerated REE and increased body temperature; (6) hormone release, including increase of corticosteroids, glucagon, and growth hormone, and a decrease in thyroxine; and (7) shifts in mineral metabolism. • The body's immune response tries to counteract these stresses with the anti-inflammatory cytokines (IL-4, IL-10, IL-11, and IL-13). • These counter-response cytokines are not well understood, and there are ongoing investigations to define their functions. • Current research in this area of immunology is focused on measuring and manipulating cytokine levels in specific disease states and on how nutritional and medical therapies can influence cytokine levels for better treatment outcomes by enhancing anti-inflammatory cytokine response to an injury.

IEFs are gaining popularity because of their potential to effect specific aspects of immune function. • They contain a variety of substances in various combinations, which include glutamine and arginine, along with short-chain fatty acids; ω3- and ω6-fatty acids; zinc; and vitamins A, C, and E in higher concentrations than in standard enteral formulas. • Guidelines from the United States Summit on Immune-Enhancing Enteral Therapy currently indicate that the following groups of patients may benefit from

IEF nutrition: (1) patients undergoing elective gastrointestinal surgery with moderate or severe malnutrition; (2) patients with blunt, penetrating torso trauma with an injury severity score ≥ 18 or an abdominal trauma index ≥ 20; (3) malnourished patients undergoing elective aortic reconstruction with known chronic obstructive pulmonary disease and an expected prolonged term of mechanical ventilation; and (4) nonseptic surgical or medical patients dependent on ventilator support who are at risk of infection. • Other patient populations that may benefit from IEFs have been identified, including those with existing malnutrition who are undergoing head and neck surgery and patients with third-degree burns over 30% of their body surface area. • Research in this area is ongoing.

ANSWERS:
Question 33: C
Question 34: E

35. Which of the following patients is a candidate for further work-up for gastric bypass surgery?

    A. A patient with a body mass index (BMI) of 36, with the obesity-related complication of hypertension

    B. A patient with a BMI of 31, currently starting oral weight-control medication

    C. A patient with a BMI of 40 with good family support and unsuccessful attempts at weight loss regimens

    D. A patient with a BMI of 42 with a history of failed gastric stapling

Ref.: 40

COMMENTS: See Question 36.

36. Which is true of the Roux-en-Y gastric bypass dietary regimen following surgery?

    A. A patient remains on orders to take nothing by mouth for 1 week to "jump-start" weight loss.

    B. Initial feedings of liquids are small, 30 ml at a time.

    C. High-calorie liquids are discouraged to avoid symptoms of dumping syndrome.

    D. Pureed foods are necessary for life to avoid adverse reactions.

Ref.: 41

COMMENTS: Bariatric surgery has emerged as a viable weight-loss method for patients with medically significant obesity and morbidly obese patients who are unable to accomplish or sustain weight loss. • Nutritional issues are complex in this population. • Historically, two types of surgical methods of promoting weight loss in morbidly obese patients include (1) surgeries that reduce caloric intake and (2) surgeries that limit nutrient absorption. • Currently, the surgical procedure of choice, the Roux-en Y gastric bypass, utilizes both of these mechanisms to promote weight loss.

Criteria for patient selection begins with classifying the degree of obesity. • Obesity can be classified on standardized tables based on weight for height measures. • However, for most practical purposes (e.g., for insurance reimbursement), BMI determination is the standard for obesity assessment. • BMI is a measure of obesity based on weight in kilograms per height in square meters. • Patients are categorized as follows: BMI of 25–29.9 kg/m² is **overweight**; BMI of 30–34.9 kg/m² is **obesity,**

Class I; BMI value of 35–39.9 kg/m² is **obesity, Class II**; and BMI of 40 kg/m² or greater is **extreme morbid obesity, Class III**. • Patients with extreme morbid obesity are candidates for surgical intervention. • Additional criteria for appropriate patient selection for Roux-en-Y gastric bypass include failure at previous attempts to lose weight, mental stability, cognitive ability to understand the scope of surgery and necessary dietary changes, and potential and current health problems complicated or caused by obesity. • A patient with a BMI greater than 35 with chronic or life-threatening obesity-associated co-morbidities (e.g., hypertension, diabetes, or heart disease) can also be considered a surgery candidate.

A team approach to the patient's care should be undertaken before and after surgery. • Initial screening and comprehensive follow-up are important factors in success. • Once the weight criterion is met, the screening process is initiated. • Dietary history, dietary evaluation, and dietary instruction from a dietitian are essential for assessment of compliance of dietary regimens and education for the overall postoperative nutritional course. • Patients are expected to lose 50–60% of their presurgery weight. • Therefore, numerous postoperative nutritional complications are possible. • Malnutrition, vitamin and mineral deficiencies, weight-loss failure, dehydration, anemia, and dumping syndrome may occur. • Gastrointestinal problems may include nausea, constipation, abdominal pain, marginal ulcers, incisional hernias, vomiting, diarrhea, gallstones, gastritis, and intestinal obstruction. • The nutritional complications that can occur with these gastrointestinal problems are numerous.

Oral feeding resumes on postoperative day 1 with small volumes of water. • A 3-day progression from clear liquids to pureed foods is recommended, with small-volume feedings of 30–60 ml at each feeding. • The diet eventually returns to regular foods given in small, frequent meals, with the following general instructions: (1) stop eating when full; (2) chew food well, to a pulplike consistency; (3) avoid high-calorie liquids, especially those with ice cream; and (4) mealtimes should last 30 minutes. • Because of the bypass of 90% of the stomach, entire duodenum, and a small portion of the jejunum, supplemental nutrient recommendations are necessary. • A multivitamin, vitamin B12, calcium, and in some instances iron, are typically prescribed.

ANSWERS:
Question 35: A, C, D
Question 36: B, C

REFERENCES

1. Van Way CW III: Basic nutrition, energy stores, and body composition. In: Van Way CW III (ed) *Handbook of Surgical Nutrition.* Lippincott, Philadelphia, 1992.
2. Harris RA: Carbohydrate metabolism. Major metabolic pathways and their control. In: Devlin TM (ed) *Textbook of Biochemistry with Clinical Correlations.* John Wiley, New York, 1986.
3. Stipanuk MA (ed): *Biochemical and Physiological Aspects of Human Nutrition.* Saunders, Philadelphia, 2000.
4. Compher C, Seto RW, Lew JI, et al: Dietary fiber and its clinical applications to enteral nutrition. In: Rombeau JL, Rolandelli RH (eds) *Clinical Nutrition: Enteral and Tube Feeding,* 3rd ed. Saunders, Philadelphia, 1997.
5. Souba WW, Hershkowitz K, Austgen TR, et al: Glutamine nutrition: theoretical considerations and therapeutic impact. *J Parenter Enteral Nutr* 14:237S–243S, 1990.
6. Fisher JE: Metabolism in surgical patients: protein, carbohydrate, and fat utilization by oral and parenteral routes. In: Townsend CT (ed) *Sabiston Textbook of Surgery: The Biological Basis of Modern Surgical Practice,* 16th ed. Saunders, Philadelphia, 2001.
7. Matthews DE, Fong Y: Amino acid and protein metabolism. In: Rombeau JL, Caldwell MD (eds) *Clinical Nutrition: Parenteral Nutrition,* 2nd ed. Saunders, Philadelphia, 1993.

8. National Research Council, Food and Nutrition Board: *Recommended Daily Allowances*, 10th ed. National Academy Press, Washington, DC, 1989.

9. McGarry JD: Lipid metabolism. I. Utilization and storage of energy in lipid form. In: Devlin T (ed) *Textbook of Biochemistry with Clinical Correlations*. John Wiley, New York, 1986.

10. Shanbhogue LK, Paterson N. Effect of sepsis and surgery on trace minerals. *J Parenter Enteral Nutr* 14:287–289,1990.

11. Barton RG: Nutrition support in critical illness. *Nutr Clin Pract* 9:127–139, 1994.

12. Russell MK: Serum proteins and nitrogen balance: evaluating response to nutrition support. *Support Line* 17:3–8, 1995.

13. Jeejeebhoy KN: Nutritional assessment. *Gastroenterol Clin North Am* 27:347–369, 1998.

14. Daley BJ, Bistrian BR: Nutritional assessment. In: Zaloga G (ed) *Nutrition in Critical Care*. Mosby Year Book, St. Louis, 1994.

15. American Dietetic Association: ADA's definition for nutrition screening and assessment. *J Am Diet Assoc* 94:838–839, 1994.

16. Trujillo EB, Robinson MK, Jacobs DO: Nutritional assessment in the critically ill. *Crit Care Nurs* 19:67–78, 1999.

17. Charney P: Nutrition assessment in the 1990's:Where are we now? *Nutr Clin Pract* 10:131–139, 1995.

18. Cerra FB: How nutrition intervention changes what getting sick means. *J Parenter Enteral Nutr* 14(Suppl):1966–1995, 1990.

19. Shopbell JM, Hopkins B, Shronts EP: Nutrition screening and assessment. In: Gottschlich MM, Fuhrman MP, Hammond KA, et al (eds) *The Science and Practice of Nutrition Support: A Case Based Core Curriculum*. Kendall/Hunt Publishing, Dubuque, IA, 2001.

20. Chiolera R, Revelly J, Tappy L: Energy metabolism in sepsis and injury. *Nutrition* 45S–51S, 1997.

21. Smith MK, Lowry SF: The hypercatabolic state. In: Shils ME, Olson JA, Shike M, et al (eds) *Modern Nutrition in Health and Disease*. Williams & Wilkins, Baltimore, 1999.

22. Makk LJ, McClave SA, Creech PW, et al: Clinical application of the metabolic cart to the delivery of TPN. *Crit Care Med* 18:1320–1327, 1990.

23. Matarese LE: Indirect calorimetry: technical aspects. *J Am Diet Assoc* 97(Suppl 2): S154–S160, 1997.

24. ASPEN American Society for Parenteral and Enteral Nutrition Board of Directors: Guidelines for the use of parenteral and enteral nutrition in adult and pediatric patients. *J Parenter Enteral Nutr* 17(Suppl):5SA–26SA, 1993.

25. Homann HH, Kemen M, Fuessenich MD, et al: Reduction in diarrhea incidence by soluble fiber in patients receiving total or supplemental enteral nutrition. *J Parenter Enteral Nutr* 18:486–490, 1994.

26. Williams MS, Harper R, Magnuson B, et al: Diarrhea management in enterally fed patients. *NCP* 13:225–229, 1998.

27. Kelly TW, Patrick MR, Hillman KM: Study of diarrhea in critically ill patients. *Crit Care Med* 11:7–9, 1994.

28. Kudsk KS, Croce MA, Fabian TC, et al: Enteral vs. parenteral feeding: effects on septic morbidity after blunt and penetrating trauma. *Ann Surg* 215:503–513, 1992.

29. Kudsk DA, Minard G: Enteral nutrition: In Zaloga G (ed) *Nutrition in Critical Care*. Mosby, St. Louis, 1994.

30. Zaloga G, Ackerman MH: A review of disease-specific enteral formulas. *Clin Issues Crit Care Nurs* 5:421–435, 1994.

31. Maillet JO: Calculating parenteral feedings: a programmed instruction. *J Am Diet Assoc* 11:1312–1323, 1984.

32. Bozzetti F, Gavazei C, Miceli R, et al: Perioperative total parenteral nutrition in malnourished gastrointestinal cancer patients: A randomized clinical trial. *J Parenter Enteral Nutr* 23:7–14, 2000.

33. The Veterans Affairs Total Parenteral Nutrition Cooperative Study Group: Perioperative total parenteral nutrition in surgical patients. *J Parenter Enteral Nutr* 325(8):525–523, 1991.

34. Solomon SM, Kirby DF: The refeeding syndrome: a review. *J Parenter Enteral Nutr* 14:90–97, 1990.

35. Brooks MJ, Melnik G: The refeeding syndrome: an approach to understanding its complications and preventing in occurrence. *Pharmacotherapy* 15(6):713–726, 1995.

36. Klein CJ, Stanek GS, Wiles CE: Overfeeding macronutrients to critically ill adults: metabolic complications. *J Am Diet Assoc* 98(7):795–806, 1998.

37. Apovian CM, McMahon MM, Bistrian BR: Guidelines for refeeding the marasmic patient. *Crit Care Med* 18(9):1030–1033, 1990.

38. Chang H, Bistrian B: The role of cytokines in the catabolic consequences of infection and injury. *J Parenter Enteral Nutr* 22:156–166, 1998.

39. Bower RH, Cerra FB, Bershadsky B, et al: Early enteral administration of a formula (Impact ®) supplemented with arginine, nucleotides, and fish oil in intensive care unit patients: results of a multicenter, prospective, randomized, clinical trial. *Crit Care Med* 23:436–449, 1995.

40. Shikora S: Surgical treatment for severe obesity: the state of the art for the new Millennium. *Nutr Clin Pract* 15:13–22, 2002.

41. Schauer P, Ikramuddin S, Gourash W, et al: Outcomes after laparoscopic Roux-en-Y gastric bypass for morbid obesity. *Ann Surg* 232(4):278–292, 2000.

CHAPTER 9

Morbid Obesity

Keith W. Millikan, M.D.

1. Morbid obesity can be defined by which of the following?

    A. 100 pounds over a person's ideal body weight

    B. 150 pounds over a person's ideal body weight

    C. 200 pounds over a person's ideal body weight

    D. Calculated body mass index (BMI) greater than 35–40 kg/m²

    E. Calculated BMI greater than 45–50 kg/m²

Ref.: 1, 2

COMMENTS: Metropolitan Life Insurance Company actuarial tables define **morbid obesity** as 100 pounds above the ideal body weight. This is the most commonly accepted definition of morbid obesity. • Since people vary in bone structure, the National Institutes of Health established that the guidelines for obesity would be based on the BMI. • The **BMI** is calculated by dividing weight in kilograms by height in meters squared. • Being overweight is defined as having a BMI of 25 kg/m², obesity a BMI of 30 kg/m², and morbid obesity a BMI of 40 kg/m² or 35 kg/m² with a concomitant obesity-related morbid condition.

ANSWER:
A, D

2. Which of the following are associated with morbid obesity?

    A. Coronary artery disease

    B. Type I diabetes mellitus

    C. Sleep apnea

    D. Reduction in life expectancy

    E. Asthma

Ref.: 1, 2

COMMENTS: Obese patients have an increased risk of coronary artery disease. • As BMI increases above 25 kg/m², mean blood pressure and total cholesterol levels increase, while high-density lipoprotein levels decrease. • Women with a BMI greater than 29 kg/m² have a significantly increased incidence of myocardial infarction. • Obese patients are at risk for developing type II adult-onset diabetes mellitus. • Obstructive sleep apnea and hypoventilation obstructive syndrome are common in the morbidly obese. • The most significant finding in morbidly obese patients is that individuals between 20 and 40 years of age have a 12-fold reduction in life expectancy.

ANSWER:
A, C, D

3. Which of the following statements regarding morbid obesity and bariatric surgery during the 1990s is/are not true?

    A. More than 1 million Americans were morbidly obese.

    B. The annual rate of bariatric surgery tripled.

    C. The mean age of patients undergoing bariatric surgery was approximately 40 years.

    D. Gastric bypass rates increased, while use of gastroplasty decreased.

    E. The proportion of procedures performed in female versus male patients did not change.

Ref.: 3

COMMENTS: The prevalence of obesity in the United States is increasing. • More than 1 million patients in the United States are morbidly obese, as defined by the National Institutes of Health. • From 1990 to 1997, the national annual rate of bariatric surgery more than doubled, from 2.7 to 6.3 per 100,000 adults. • The majority of the surgeries were gastric bypass. • Gastroplasty use declined. • The mean age of patients undergoing bariatric procedures is approximately 40 years. • Females comprised 82–86% of all patients undergoing bariatric procedures during the 1990s. • This proportion did not significantly change during the decade.

ANSWER:
B

4. According to the National Institutes of Health 1991 Consensus Statement, which of the following are criteria for the surgical treatment of morbid obesity?

    A. BMI over 40 kg/m²

    B. Failure of established weight-control programs

    C. More than 100 pounds over ideal body weight for height

    D. Severe comorbidities of obesity with a BMI over 35 kg/m²

    E. Patients of all ages

Ref.: 4

COMMENTS: The 1991 National Institutes of Health Consensus Development Panel on gastrointestinal surgery for severe obesity recommended using BMI, defined in terms of body weight (in kilograms) divided by height (in meters squared), rather than ideal body weight from the 1983 Metropolitan Life Insurance Company tables. • The panel stated that patients whose BMI exceeds 40 kg/m^2 are potential candidates for surgery if they strongly desire substantial weight loss because obesity severely impairs the quality of their lives. • The panel also agreed that patients may be considered for surgery if experienced clinicians judged them to have a low probability of success with nonsurgical measures, such as established weight-control programs. • Most insurance companies consider patients eligible if they are 100 pounds over ideal body weight.

The consensus panel also stated that, in certain instances, less severely obese patients (with BMIs between 35 and 40 kg/m^2) also may be considered for surgery. • Included in this category are patients with high-risk comorbid conditions, such as life-threatening cardiopulmonary problems (e.g., severe sleep apnea, pickwickian syndrome, and obesity-related cardiomyopathy) or severe diabetes mellitus. • Other possible indications for patients with BMIs between 35 and 40 kg/m^2 include obesity-induced physical problems that interfere with lifestyle (e.g., joint disease that would be treatable if the patient were not obese and body-size problems that preclude or severely interfere with employment, family function, and ambulation).

The recommended age for surgery is between 18 and 62 years. • Children and adolescents have not been sufficiently studied to allow a recommendation for surgery for them, even with a BMI over 40 kg/m^2.

ANSWER:
A, B, D

5. Which of the following statements regarding the dietary management of morbid obesity is/are true?

   A. Hospital-supervised and psychiatric behavioral modification programs have documented long-term weight loss success for the morbidly obese.

   B. The incidence of recidivism in the morbidly obese after dietary manipulation is nearly 50%.

   C. In 1992, the National Institutes of Health Technology Assessment Conference stated that dietary management of severe obesity failed to provide evidence of long-term efficacy.

   D. Drug therapy using a combination of phentermine and fenfluramine (Fen-phen) has no ill side effects.

   E. Drugs that block fat absorption or suppress appetite are effective for long-term weight loss therapy.

Ref.: 1

COMMENTS: Hospital-supervised, psychiatric behavioral modification, commercial organization, commercial diet, protein-sparing fast, and diet pill programs exist for the morbidly obese. • Unfortunately, no dietary approach has achieved uniform long-term success rates. • The incidence of recidivism after dietary manipulation in the morbidly obese reaches 95%. • The National Institutes of Health Technology Assessment Conference concluded in 1992 that dietary management of severe obesity with or without behavioral modification fails to provide evidence of long-term efficacy. • Use of phentermine and fenfluramine is associated with development of pulmonary hypertension and cardiac valve damage. • Agents such as orlistat, which blocks fat absorption, and sibutramine, an appetite suppressant, provide only modest weight loss and are inadequate therapies for the morbidly obese.

ANSWER:
C

6. During the 1960s, what was the first operation to become popular for the treatment of morbid obesity?

   A. Duodenal switch

   B. Proximal intestine resection

   C. Gastric bypass

   D. Gastroplasty

   E. Jejunoileal bypass

Ref.: 2

COMMENTS: Resection of the stomach or small intestine was recognized to provide weight loss as early as the late nineteenth century. • In 1945, increased fat loss was demonstrated in the stools of dogs after distal small bowel resection. • In the 1950s, resection of 50–70% of the proximal small intestine was shown to result in normal nutritional balance. • The first clinical trials of obesity surgery were conducted in 1955 but abandoned because the procedure, jejunal-transverse colon intestinal bypass, produced severe metabolic disturbances, liver failure, and protein-calorie malnutrition. • The procedure was modified by anastomosing the proximal jejunum to the distal ileum, with the bypassed segment of small bowel anastomosed to the colon. • Known as the jejunoileal bypass, this procedure was popular in the 1960s and was very effective for weight loss. • However, because of significant associated early and late complications, the jejunoileal bypass was abandoned. • Gastroplasty and gastric bypass procedures were developed later to avoid the significant complications associated with jejunoilial bypass.

ANSWER:
E

7. Match the early or late complication of the jejunoileal bypass with its cause or causes.

   A. Liver cirrhosis   a. Rapid weight loss

   B. Rheumatoid arthritis   b. Chelation of calcium with bile salts

   C. Cholelithiasis   c. Absorption of bacterial overgrowth products

   D. Osteoporosis   d. Protein-calorie ~~manipulation~~ malnutrition

   E. Kidney stones   e. Increased oxalate absorption from colon

      f. Malabsorption of bile salts

Ref.: 1

COMMENTS: The jejunoileal bypass is associated with numerous early and late complications. • The most serious complication is cirrhosis of the liver due to either protein-calorie malnutrition or absorption of degradation products from bacterial overgrowth in the bypassed intestine. • A rheumatoid arthritis syndrome is also caused by bacterial products from the bypassed intestine. • Rapid weight loss and malabsorption of bile salts increase cholelithiasis due to decreased cholesterol solubility. • Hypocalcemia is frequent, since calcium chelates with bile salts, leading to severe osteoporosis. • Kidney stones form as a result of increased oxalate absorption from the colon, where oxalate is normally bound to calcium.

• Intractable, malodorous diarrhea with potassium and magnesium depletion and metabolic acidosis is also common. • Bacterial overgrowth also can lead to vitamin K deficiency, intestinal nephritis, pneumatosis intestinalis, and bypass enteritis.

ANSWERS:
A-c, d; B-c; C-a, f; D-b; E-e

8. Routine preoperative testing for morbid obesity surgery should include which of the following?

 A. Arterial blood gas determinations

 B. Cardiac stress testing

 C. Chest x-ray

 D. Polysonographic studies

 E. Pulmonary function testing

Ref.: 1, 2

COMMENTS: Routine preoperative testing in preparation for a general anesthetic is modified in morbidly obese patients under certain circumstances. • Patients with no history of cardiopulmonary problems and a normal electrocardiogram require no further cardiac testing. • However, patients with severe hypertension, previous admissions for congestive heart failure, and/or a history of coronary artery disease should undergo cardiac stress testing and echocardiographic studies in conjunction with consultation with a cardiologist. • Patients with a normal chest x-ray, normal arterial blood gas levels, and no history of respiratory problems do not require any further pulmonary testing. • Any history suggesting sleep apnea or hypoventilation syndrome necessitates consultation with a pulmonologist and most likely polysonographic studies to rule out sleep apnea and pulmonary function testing to rule out hypoventilation syndrome.

ANSWER:
A, C

9. A multidisciplinary evaluation requires which of the following health care professionals?

 A. Endocrinologist

 B. Psychologist

 C. Dietician

 D. Pulmonologist

 E. Gastroenterologist

Ref.: 1, 2, 4

COMMENTS: Although hypothyroidism is rarely a cause of morbid obesity, thyroid function testing is usually done before surgery. • Because Cushing's disease may cause severe obesity, cortisol levels should be determined before surgery. • Since diabetes is also common in morbidly obese patients, fasting blood glucose determinations are recommended. • If endocrine problems are encountered during the evaluation, an endocrinologist may be consulted, but such a consultation is not required for all patients.

Psychological stability is a prerequisite for morbidly obese surgical patients. • The ability to conform to dietary regulations and to follow up, in both the short and the long term, are paramount to the success of obesity surgery. • Therefore, a psychological consultation is recommended to determine psychological stability before surgery. • Intelligence testing and self-assessment evaluations

have not been correlated with the long-term success of morbid obesity surgery.

Evaluation of a patient's eating habits, past diet failures, and ability to conform to the post–obesity surgery diet is best handled by a dietician. • A dietician will also aid in the supplementation of vitamins, calcium, iron, and protein in the postoperative period.

Pulmonary problems are common in morbidly obese patients, but in the absence of abnormal arterial blood gas values, abnormal chest x-ray results, and a history of sleep apnea or hypoventilation syndrome, pulmonary consultation is not required.

The patient's history must be carefully taken to rule out active ulcer disease, which is a contraindication to morbid obesity surgery. • An upper gastrointestinal barium examination or testing for *Helicobacter pylori* should be ordered if peptic ulcer disease is suspected. • If the results of either test are positive, upper endoscopy is recommended. • Routine consultation with a gastroenterologist is not necessary.

ANSWER:
B, C

10. Which of the following is/are currently acceptable operations for weight loss in morbidly obese patients?

 A. Jejunoileal bypass

 B. Duodenal switch

 C. Roux-en-Y gastric bypass

 D. Vertical banded gastroplasty

 E. Laparoscopic gastric band

Ref.: 1, 2

COMMENTS: Most surgeons believe that jejunoileal bypass patients should have their bypasses reversed because of the numerous early and late complications associated with the procedure, most notably biliary cirrhosis. • Jejunoileal bypass is no longer recommended for morbid obesity. • Biliary pancreatic diversion procedures, of which the duodenal switch is becoming most popular, are currently considered for super morbid obesity (BMI > 50 kg/m^2) or when gastroplasty or gastric bypass have failed. • The Roux-en-Y gastric bypass is currently the most popular procedure performed in the United States for morbid obesity. • Gastroplasty is popular in Europe and Canada and is recommended for patients with a history of duodenal ulcer disease. • Long-term results with gastroplasty are inferior to those of gastric bypass when amount and maintenance of weight loss are compared. • Gastric banding was recently approved in the United States and has shown early weight loss results comparable to those of other weight loss procedures. • No long-term results are available for gastric banding.

ANSWER:
B, C, D, E

11. Metabolic weight loss surgery for morbid obesity can be divided into which of the following categories?

 A. Gastric restriction

 B. Malabsorptive

 C. Malabsorptive and gastric restriction

 D. Colonic bypass

 E. Soft tissue resection (panniculectomy)

Ref.: 1, 2

COMMENTS: Surgery for morbid obesity patients can be divided into three categories: gastric restriction, malabsorptive procedures, and a combination of the two. • Examples of gastric restriction procedures are vertical band gastroplasty and gastric banding. • Both can be performed either through an open or a laparoscopic approach. • Malabsorptive procedures include the Scapinaro and the duodenal switch. • The procedures involve biliopancreatic bypass, which in effect causes malabsorption of nutrients. • These procedures are mainly reserved for super morbid obesity or patients who have failed with other weight loss procedures. • These procedures mainly are performed through an open approach. • The Roux-en-Y gastric bypass is both gastric restrictive and malabsorptive. • The procedure can be performed both laparoscopically and through a traditional open approach. • No procedure has been described involving colon bypass for weight loss in morbidly obese patients. • Skin and subcutaneous resections (panniculectomy) are usually performed in patients with morbid obesity after weight loss has occurred or for recurrent infections (panniculitis) but not for the purpose of achieving weight loss.

ANSWER:
A, B, C

12. Which of the following are acceptable technical components of the Roux-en-Y gastric bypass?

   A. Stapled but not transected gastric pouch

   B. Stapled and transected gastric pouch

   C. Silastic ring placed above the gastrojejunostomy

   D. 75-cm Roux-en-Y limb

   E. 150-cm Roux-en-Y limb

Ref.: 5

COMMENTS: In the past, most surgeons performed an open gastric bypass with a horizontally placed stapled line, without gastric transection, and a gastrojejunostomy above the staple line. • Because of reports of staple-line dehiscence (2–15%), surgeons have adopted a vertically oriented staple line with gastric transection. • The incidence of gastrogastric fistula is less than 1% with this technique. • Incorporation of a silastic ring in the upper gastric pouch has been proposed to prevent late stretching of the outlet stoma beyond the diameter of the ring. • However, band erosion has been reported with this technique. • Since no prospective long-term benefit has been reported with the silastic ring, most surgeons performing gastric bypass have not adopted its routine use.

The standard length of the Roux limb in gastric bypass surgery is 75–100 cm. • A 150- to 200-cm length has been introduced for patients with BMI greater than 50 kg/m^2. • The longer limb apparently provides greater malabsorption than do the shorter limbs. • However, this increased malabsorption has not resulted in late metabolic sequelae notably different from those resulting from using shorter Roux limb lengths.

ANSWER:
B, C, D, E

13. What is the 5-year mean excess weight loss after gastric bypass surgery?

   A. 30–40%

   B. 40–50%

   C. 50–60%

   D. 70–80%

   E. 80–90%

Ref.: 5

COMMENTS: Weight loss after gastric bypass generally peaks from 65 to 80% of excess weight loss between 12 and 18 months postoperatively. • Some degree of recidivism occurs between 3 and 5 years after gastric bypass. • Large clinical studies of gastric bypass patients demonstrate a 5-year mean excess weight loss of 50–60%.

ANSWER:
C

14. Intraoperative complications during laparoscopic or open gastric bypass surgery include which of the following?

   A. Bleeding

   B. Bladder injury

   C. Bowel injury

   D. Stapling mishaps

   E. Pulmonary embolism

Ref.: 5, 6

COMMENTS: Complications that occur during gastric bypass operations can be divided into three categories: (1) bleeding, (2) inadvertent injury to the gastrointestinal tract, and (3) stapling mishaps. • The incidence of intraoperative complications in one series of 1426 consecutive operations performed over 20 years was 1.4%. • Major bleeding episodes are usually iatrogenic. • Transoral placement of a stapling anvil can cause esophageal perforation during laparoscopic bypass. • Injury to the esophagus can also occur during manipulation of the gastroesophageal junction during open or laparoscopic approaches. • Injuries to the jejunum can occur from dissection or use of staplers during creation of the Roux-en-Y limb. • Misfiring of stapling devices during creation of the gastric pouch can cause injury to the cardia, obstruct the gastroesophageal junction, and sometimes incorporate the nasogastric tube. • No bladder injuries have been reported in laparoscopic or open series. • Pulmonary embolus is a complication seen in the early postoperative period but has not been reported as an intraoperative event.

ANSWER:
A, C, D

15. Early postoperative complications of Roux-en-Y gastric bypass include which of the following?

   A. Pulmonary embolism

   B. Gastrointestinal leak

   C. Small-bowel obstruction

   D. Wound dehiscence

   E. Marginal ulcer

Ref.: 5

COMMENTS: Pulmonary embolism is the leading cause of perioperative death among bariatric surgical patients. • The incidence of pulmonary embolism is reported to be 1–2%, as is the incidence of gastrointestinal leakage. • Persistent tachycardia and progressive tachypnea are the commonest early signs of pulmonary embolism. • Small-bowel obstruction within the first several weeks after surgery may occur in 1–2% of patients. • Most patients can be treated with tube decompression, which is most successfully accomplished using fluoroscopically guided nasogastric tube placement. • Early reports regarding patients undergoing laparoscopic procedures found obstruction at the jejunojejunostomy, due to obstruction of the Roux-en-Y limb by misplaced staple lines, higher than for patients undergoing open surgery. • The incidence of fascial dehiscence in large series approximates 1%. • Skin incisions also dehisce if staples are removed within the first week after surgery. • Marginal ulceration after gastric bypass occurs in 3–10% of patients but is almost always seen more than 30 days after surgery and is considered a late complication.

ANSWER:
A, B, C, D

16. Metabolic sequelae of Roux-en-Y gastric bypass include which of the following?

    A. Vitamin B_{12} deficiency

    B. Folate deficiency

    C. Iron deficiency

    D. Hypercalcemia

    E. Hyperproteinemia

Ref.: 5

COMMENTS: Since iron absorption occurs primarily in the duodenum, malabsorption of ingested iron is the primary cause of post–gastric-bypass iron deficiency. • Vitamin B_{12} deficiency after gastric bypass is the result of failure to cleave food-bound B_{12} from its protein moiety in the upper gastric pouch. • Crystalline B_{12} is absorbed in the distal ileum. • The cause of folate deficiency is unknown, but inadequate dietary intake is probably the commonest cause. • Deficiencies in any of these micronutrients can result in anemia. • Because these deficiencies are common, daily prophylactic multivitamin and mineral supplements are recommended for all patients who have gastric bypass. • Calcium is also absorbed in the duodenum and is commonly found to be deficient. • Oral calcium supplementation is recommended for all gastric bypass patients, and is particularly important for women, to prevent osteoporosis. • Hypoproteinemia may also occur in the gastric bypass population, and close monitoring of dietary intake should occur under the supervision of a nutritionist during the first year after gastric bypass.

ANSWER:
A, B, C

17. In comparing laparoscopic to open approaches for Roux-en-Y gastric bypass, laparoscopic approaches have been shown to be associated with which of the following?

    A. Shorter patient hospital stay

    B. Higher anastomotic leakage rate

    C. Similar wound-related complications

    D. Similar anastomotic stricture rates

    E. Similar weight loss rates 1 year after surgery

Ref.: 6

COMMENTS: In a randomized, prospective study comparing laparoscopic to open gastric bypass, the median length of hospital stay was shorter for laparoscopic patients (3 versus 4 days). • The rate of postoperative anastomotic leakage was similar in the two groups (1–2%). • Wound-related complications, such as infection (10.5 versus 1.3%) and incisional hernia (7.9 versus 0%), were commoner after open gastric bypass. • Late anastomotic stricture was less frequent after open gastric bypass (2.6 versus 11.4%). • Weight loss at 1 year was similar in the two groups.

ANSWER:
A, E

18. Vertical-banded gastroplasty has which of the following components, results, and/or complications?

    A. A stapled opening is created 7 cm from the gastroesophageal junction.

    B. A single application of staples is made between the stapled opening and the angle of His.

    C. A 11.5-cm strip of polypropylene is wrapped around the stoma on the lesser curvature and sutured to the stomach.

    D. Weight loss is similar to that attained with Roux-en-Y gastric bypass.

    E. Severe gastroesophageal reflux can occur.

Ref.: 1, 2

COMMENTS: Vertical-banded gastroplasty is a procedure in which a stapled opening is made in the stomach with the stapling device 5 cm from the cardioesophageal junction. • Two to four applications with a 90-mm stapling device are made between this opening and the angle of His. • A 1.5- by 5-cm strip of polypropylene mesh is wrapped around the stoma on the lesser curvature and sutured to itself but not to the stomach. • Prospective, randomized studies comparing vertical-banded gastroplasty to gastric bypass demonstrated significantly less weight loss for patients undergoing vertical-banded gastroplasty. • Among the reasons considered for the failure to maintain long-term weight loss with vertical-banded gastroplasty are staple-line dehiscence, enlargement of the gastric pouch, increased rate of emptying of the gastric pouch over time, and change of diet to high-caloric soft foods and liquids. • Vertical-banded gastroplasty may be associated with severe gastroesophageal reflux, which is resolved after conversion to gastric bypass.

ANSWER:
E

19. Postoperative complications and outcomes of vertical-banded gastroplasty include which of the following?

    A. Outlet stenosis

    B. Band erosion

    C. Greater than 1% mortality rate

    D. Malabsorption syndrome

    E. Greater than 5% reoperation rate

Ref.: 2

COMMENTS: Postoperative complications of vertical-banded gastroplasty include leakage (0.6%), wound infection (1.5%), staple-line dehiscence (2–7%), outlet stenosis (2.5–8.0%), band erosion (1–2%), and a 30-day mortality rate of less than 1%.

• Because vertical-banded gastroplasty only eliminates the reservoir function of the stomach and does not bypass any part of the gastrointestinal tract, malabsorption syndromes do not occur. • Five to 36% of patients require reoperation for inadequate weight loss, outlet stenosis, band erosion, or staple-line dehiscence.

A N S W E R :
A, B, E

20. Components of the biliopancreatic bypass without a duodenal switch include which of the following?

A. Subtotal gastrectomy

B. A 50-cm common channel of ileum for food and biliopancreatic secretions

C. "Sleeve" gastrectomy

D. Preservation of the vagus nerves

E. Preservation of the pylorus

Ref.: 2

COMMENTS: During a biliopancreatic bypass, a subtotal gastrectomy is performed, leaving a proximal gastric remnant of 200–500 ml. • The ileum is transected 250 cm proximal to the ileocecal valve. • The distal ileal limb is anastomosed to the gastric pouch. • The biliopancreatic or proximal limb is anastomosed end to side to the distal ileum, 50 cm proximal to the ileocecal valve. • This results in a 50-cm common channel between the two limbs. A modification of this technique is the biliopancreatic bypass with a duodenal switch. • The greater curvature of the stomach is resected to create a lesser curvature gastric sleeve ("sleeve gastrectomy"). • The sleeve gastrectomy maintains the integrity of the vagus nerves. • The duodenum is transected 5 cm distal to the pylorus. • The ileum is transected 250 cm proximal to the ileocecal valve, and the distal ileal limb is anastomosed end to end to the proximal duodenum. • The biliopancreatic limb is anastomosed end to side to the distal ileum 100 cm proximal to the ileocecal valve, resulting in a 100-cm common channel between the two limbs.

A N S W E R :
A, B

21. In comparing the biliopancreatic bypass and duodenal switch procedures, which of the following statements is/are true?

A. Both procedures are commonly performed in the United States.

B. Duodenal switch is associated with greater excess body weight loss.

C. Hypoventilation and obstructive sleep apnea improve with both procedures.

D. Calcium and iron homeostasis is improved with duodenal switch.

E. Both procedures are associated with significant rates of protein malnutrition.

Ref.: 2

COMMENTS: Biliopancreatic bypass and biliopancreatic bypass with a duodenal switch are performed routinely in Italy and Canada but not in the United States. • Excess body weight loss has been reported to be about 75% for each procedure. • Both procedures have been reported to result in significant improvement of

hypoventilation and obstructive sleep apnea syndrome. • A study comparing 457 patients undergoing biliopancreatic bypass with duodenal switch to 233 patients undergoing biliopancreatic bypass revealed that revision rates were lower and calcium and iron homeostasis were improved in patients undergoing biliopancreatic bypass with duodenal switch. • Both procedures resulted in a significant rate of protein malnutrition.

A N S W E R :
C, D, E

22. The laparoscopic gastric band procedure may have which of the following components?

A. Creation of a 30-ml virtual pouch

B. Suture fixation of both the anterior and posterior stomach walls to completely embed the band

C. A perigastric approach

D. A pars flaccida approach

E. A combined perigastric and pars flaccida approach

Ref.: 7

COMMENTS: The laparoscopic gastric band procedure involves the creation of a very small initial pouch of <15 ml (the "virtual pouch"). • Posterior dissection is performed above the peritoneal reflection of the bursa omentalis. • At this level, the stomach wall is naturally fixed to the crura, and there is no need for posterior wall suturing. • Suture fixation of the anterior wall is performed to embed the silicone band completely. • At least four gastrogastric sutures are needed. • The balloon (band) is partially or completely deflated during the operation to prevent a tight stoma due to postoperative edema. • The initial surgical technique employed a perigastric approach, with dissection of the lesser curvature close to the stomach wall. • The perigastric approach is technically difficult, which led surgeons to try a pars flaccida approach in which the neurovascular bundle of the lesser omentum is not separated from the stomach wall and trapped inside the band. • The pars flaccida approach is easier to perform than the perigastric approach, is associated with a lower risk of gastric prolapse, and has become widely used. • A combined technique also has been described, consisting of an initial pars flaccida dissection, which is finally converted to a perigastric placement of the band.

A N S W E R :
C, D, E

23. What is the commonest complication of the laparoscopic band procedure?

A. Gastric prolapse

B. Band erosion

C. Port problems

D. Gastric necrosis

E. Cholelithiasis

Ref.: 8, 9

COMMENTS: Gastric prolapse or slippage has been the commonest problem associated with laparoscopic gastric banding. • A study of a series of 1120 patients revealed 125 episodes in the first 500 patients (25%) and 28 episodes in the last 600 patients (4.7%). • Almost all of the instances were posterior prolapse and reflected the placement of the band across the apex of the lesser sac, a feature of the perigastric approach. • Erosion of the band into the lumen occurred in 34 (3%) of 1120 patients. • Tubing breaks or other problems with the access port occurred in 61 (5.49%) of the 1120 patients. • Tubing breaks are generally easily repaired because the port is in a subcutaneous position. • Other problems are uncommon. • Gastric necrosis is very rare. • In a series of 400 patients, only 1 case was reported. • In the series of 1120 patients, symptomatic gallstone disease led to cholecystectomy in 55 patients (5%).

ANSWER:
A

24. At 2–3 years after laparoscopic gastric banding, what is the expected mean excess weight loss?

   A. 10%

   B. 25%

   C. 50%

   D. 75%

   E. 85%

Ref.: 10, 11

COMMENTS: Laparoscopic adjustable gastric banding is a beneficial operation in terms of excess weight loss. • In a prospective study of 500 consecutive patients, excess weight loss was 42.8, 52, and 54.8% after 1, 2, and 3 years, respectively. • The mean BMI decreased from 44.3 to 34.2, 32.8, and 31.9 kg/m² after 1, 2, and 3 years. • A study of 625 patients revealed that the median excess weight loss after 1, 2, and 3 years was 45.8, 49.9, and 47.4%, respectively. • Median BMI decreased from 40.1 to 31.6, 31.8, and 32 kg/m² after 1, 2, and 3 years, respectively. • These studies and others confirm that the expected excess weight loss is approximately 50% at 2–3 years after surgery.

ANSWER:
C

25. What is the commonest indication to revise a vertical-banded gastroplasty or a gastric bypass?

   A. Inadequate weight loss

   B. Gastric outlet obstruction

   C. Acid reflux

   D. Stomal ulceration

   E. Protein malnutrition

Ref.: 2

COMMENTS: Insufficient weight loss is the commonest indication to revise a vertical-banded gastroplasty or a gastric bypass. • Inadequate weight loss is usually due to a staple-line dehiscence or an outlet dilation. • Unique complications requiring revision unrelated to inadequate weight loss are acid reflux after vertical-banded gastroplasty and marginal (stomal) ulceration after gastric bypass. • Acid reflux usually responds to medical therapy, and revisions to gastric bypass are reserved for refractory cases. • Stomal ulcers develop following gastric bypass after construction of a large gastric pouch and an increased concentration of parietal cells. • Stomal ulcers usually respond to medical therapy. • Persistent stomal ulcers require truncal vagotomy, reduction of gastric pouch size to 50 ml, and revision gastroenterostomy. • Protein malnutrition occurs after biliopancreatic bypass, not gastric bypass or vertical-banded gastroplasty.

ANSWER:
A

REFERENCES

 1. Greenfield L, Mulholland MW, Oldham KT, et al (eds): *Surgery: Scientific Principles and Practice*, 3rd ed. Lippincott Williams & Wilkins, Philadelphia, 2001.
 2. Townsend CM, Beauchamp RD, Evers BM, et al (eds): *Sabiston Textbook of Surgery: The Biological Basis of Modern Surgical Practice,* 16th ed. Saunders, Philadelphia, 2001.
 3. Pope GD, Birkmeyer JD, Fiwlayson SR: National trends in utilization and in-hospital outcomes of bariatric surgery. *J Gastrointest Surg* 6:855–861, 2002.
 4. National Institutes of Health Consensus Conference: Gastrointestinal surgery for severe obesity. *Am J Clin Nutr* 55:4875–6195, 1992.
 5. Brolin RE: Gastric bypass. *Surg Clin North Am* 81(5):1077–1095, 2001.
 6. Nguyen NT, Golman C, Rosenquist J, et al: Laparoscopic versus open gastric bypass: a randomized study of outcomes, quality of life, and costs. *Ann Surg* 234(3):279–291, 2001.
 7. Belachew M, Zimmermann JM: Evolution of a paradigm for laparoscopic adjustable gastric banding. *Am J Surg* 184:215–255, 2002.
 8. O'Brien PE, Dixon JB: Weight loss and early and late complications: the international experience. *Am J Surg* 184:425–455, 2002.
 9. Chevallier JM, Zinzindohove F, Elian N: Adjustable gastric banding in a public university hospital: prospective analysis of 400 patients. *Obes Surg* 12:93–99, 2002.
10. Sinsindohove F, Chevallier JM, Douad R, et al: Laparoscopic gastric banding: a minimally invasive surgical treatment for morbid obesity. *Ann Surg* 237(1):1–9, 2003.
11. Ceelen W, Walder J, Cardon A, et al: Surgical treatment of severe obesity with a low pressure adjustable gastric band. *Ann Surg* 237(1):10–16, 2003.

C H A P T E R 10

Wound Healing

George J. Kouris, M.D., and Gordon H. Derman, M.D.

1. Arrange the following events in the healing of an uncomplicated wound in proper sequence.

   A. Proliferation

   B. Inflammation

   C. Maturation

   Ref.: 1–3

COMMENTS: The process of wound healing is not a simple sequence of events but an array of simultaneously occurring metabolic and physiologic changes that are initiated at the time of injury and continue long after the process appears to have been completed. • Wound repair events are conceptually defined as inflammation, epithelialization, granulation, fibroplasia, and contraction. • The basic processes are similar for sutured wounds, which heal by primary intention, and wounds with tissue loss, which heal by secondary intention. • In general, the process of wound healing is divided into three overlapping phases: inflammation, proliferation, and maturation.

During **inflammation**, the capillary vessels become permeable to leukocytes and plasma proteins, which fill the wound with an inflammatory exudate of neutrophils, monocytes, and protein within hours. • Meanwhile, the wound epithelializes by 48 hr as basal epithelial cells multiply and fill in the wound surface. • On approximately the third day, fibroblasts appear in the wound in significant numbers, marking the beginning of the **proliferative** phase. • The proliferative phase is sometimes referred to as the fibroplasia phase because it is then that the fibroblasts begin to multiply and release collagen and interstitial matrix. • Meanwhile, endothelial cells begin to proliferate and form new vessels. • Wound contraction, carried out by myofibroblasts, also occurs at this time. • After approximately 3 weeks, the fibroblasts and macrophages gradually disappear from the wound, and the relatively acellular collagen begins a continuous process of remodeling and **maturation**.

ANSWER:
B, A, C

2. Which of the following statements regarding the inflammatory phase of wound healing is/are true?

   A. It begins 5–6 hr after the wound event.

   B. Bradykinin causes vasoconstriction, which inhibits neutrophil migration to the healing wound.

   C. The complement component C5a and platelet factor attract neutrophils to the wound.

   D. The presence of neutrophils in the wound is essential for normal wound healing.

   Ref.: 1, 3, 4

COMMENTS: The inflammatory phase starts immediately after the wounding occurs. • After the injury, there is a transient period (about 10 min) of vasoconstriction followed by active vasodilatation. • These events are mediated by substances released secondary to the local tissue injury. • Vasoactive components such as histamine cause brief periods of vasodilatation and increased vascular permeability. • The kinins (bradykinin and kallidin) are released by enzymatic action of kallikrein, which is formed after coagulation cascade activation. • These components, in addition to those of the complement system, stimulate release of prostaglandins (particularly PGE and PGE_2), which work in concert to maintain more prolonged vessel permeability not only of the capillaries but of larger vessels as well. • In addition, these substances, particularly the complement component C5a and platelet-derived factors such as platelet-derived growth factor (PDGF), act as chemotactic stimuli for neutrophils to enter the wound. • Although neutrophils do phagocytize bacteria from a wound, results of studies involving clean wound healing show that healing can proceed normally without them. • Monocytes, however, must be present for normal wound healing because, in addition to their role in phagocytosis, they are required to trigger a normal fibroblast response.

ANSWER:
C

3. The inflammatory phase of wound healing represents an immediate defense mechanism activated in response to injury. Which of the following statements regarding events that take place during the inflammatory phase is/are true?

   A. The inflammatory phase of wound healing includes a hemostatic component to control bleeding and an inflammatory component for cellular chemotaxis.

   B. Hemostasis is initiated when the endothelium of damaged blood vessels and the exposure of collagen attract and promote platelet aggregation.

   C. Neutrophils are chemoattracted to the area of injury by compliment factors such as C5a and leukotriene B4.

D. Platelets are responsible for the release of numerous biologically active substances important to the inflammatory phase of wound healing.

Ref.: 1–3

COMMENTS: There are three phases of wound healing in response to tissue injury. • The immediate response to tissue injury is the **inflammatory phase** of wound healing. • This phase is an immediate defense mechanism that limits the extent of tissue injury. • The **proliferative phase** is a tissue repair phase that includes regeneration of tissue matrix, reepithelialization, and neovascularization. • The final phase is the **maturational phase,** in which tissue integrity is reestablished, tensile strength is optimized, and tissue edema is reduced. • Although the process of wound healing revolves around this general sequence, the individual phases overlap significantly.

The inflammatory phase of wound healing has two components. • The hemostatic component functions to control bleeding. • The disruption of the endothelium that occurs during tissue injury promotes platelet aggregation. • Platelets degenerate, and several types of storage granules are released: (1) α granules contain growth factors such as PDGF, transforming growth factor (TGF) β, and insulin-like growth factor 1. • The granules also contain several adhesive glycoproteins, such as fibronectin, fibrinogen, thrombospondin, and von Willebrand factor. • Platelets also contain serotonin in structures called dense bodies. • Serotonin promotes vasodilation and increased vascular permeability.

The second component of the inflammatory phase of wound healing is the inflammatory component, to which platelets and other circulating blood products are the major contributors. • The release of serotonin and histamine by the platelets increases vascular permeability, and leukocytes are chemoattracted to the site of injury. • Complement factors such as C5a and leukotriene B4 promote neutrophil adherence and chemoattraction. • As the neutrophils migrate into the wound, they begin to release hydrolases and proteases contained within their lysozomes. • Neutrophils are the first cells to enter the wound and scavenge cellular debris and bacteria. • Monocytes enter the wound later and differentiate into macrophages. • The monocytes clean debris and, more important, release a number of growth factors that activate endothelial cells, fibroblasts, and epithelial cells, a sequence of events essential for the formation of granulation tissue. • Hence, the inflammatory phase functions to control bleeding and remove necrotic tissue and bacteria from the wound.

ANSWER:
A, B, C, D

4. Which of the following statements regarding the proliferative phase of wound healing is/are true?

A. The formation of granulation tissue is an important component of the proliferative phase of wound healing.

B. Granulation tissue includes collagen, macrophages, hyaluronic acid, fibroblasts, and capillary endothelial cells.

C. Angiogenesis, fibroplasia, and epithelialization are key components of the proliferation phase of wound healing.

D. Both angiogenesis and fibroplasia are stimulated by platelet- and fibroblast-derived growth factors.

Ref.: 1–3

COMMENTS: The proliferative phase of wound healing provides the scaffolding necessary for repairing the wound. • Angiogenesis, fibroplasias, and epithelialization are the key components of this phase of wound healing. • The proliferative phase is characterized by the formation of granulation tissue.

Granulation starts with endothelial cell division and migration into the wound (angiogenesis), creating a rich network of capillaries. • The fibroblasts found in this granulation tissue also differentiate and migrate into the wound, moving along the previously deposited fibrin-fibronectin matrix (produced in the inflammatory phase). • As fibroblasts proliferate (fibroplasias), they synthesize a new extracellular matrix. • Both angiogenesis and fibroplasia are stimulated by platelet- and fibroblast-derived growth factors. • The initial granulation tissue is composed of collagen (secreted by fibroblasts), fibronectin, hyaluronic acid, macrophages, fibroblasts, and capillary endothelial cells.

Hyaluronic acid is a nonsulfated glycosaminoglycan. • Glycosaminoglycans, along with adhesion glycoproteins such as fibronectin, laminin, and tenascin, create scaffolding along which fibroblasts move and deposit collagen. • Collagen types I and III are the major collagen types in the wound matrix.

ANSWER:
A, B, C, D

5. Which of the following statements regarding epithelialization is/are true?

A. It produces a watertight seal of surgical incisions within 48 hr.

B. A reepithelialized wound develops hair follicles and sweat glands, as does normal skin.

C. It is a process normally inhibited by surface contact with other epithelial cells.

D. Disruption of normal healing, such as in a chronic wound, may produce malignancy.

Ref.: 1–4

COMMENTS: Migration of epithelial cells is one of the earliest events in wound healing. • Shortly after injury and during the inflammatory phase, basal epithelial cells begin to multiply and migrate across the defect, using fibrin strands as a support structure.

Meticulously coapted surgical incisions seal rather promptly and after 24 hr are protected from the external environment. • Epithelialization of larger separations in wounds requires a long time. • Early tensile strength is a result of blood vessel ingrowth, epithelialization, and protein aggregation. • If the wound is not under excessive tension, the absence of tension allows approximation until adequate collagen has been synthesized to provide significant structural strength. • After covering the wound, the epithelial cells keratinize. • The reepithelialized wound has no sweat glands or hair follicles, which distinguishes it from normal skin.

Control of the cellular process during wound epithelialization is not completely understood, but it appears to involve inhibition of surface contact with similar cells. • Derangements in the control of this process can result in epidermoid malignancy. • This condition has been observed particularly in wounds resulting from ionizing radiation or chemical injury, but it can occur in any wound when the healing process has been chronically disrupted. • For example, squamous cell carcinoma has been observed to develop in chronic burn wounds or osteomyelitis (Marjolin's ulcer).

ANSWER:
C, D

6. Which of the following statements regarding epithelialization is/are true?

A. Mitosis is the predominant event in the process of epithelialization.

B. If the basement membrane zone is intact, epithelialization proceeds more rapidly.

C. Epidermal cells migrate from the periphery of the wound, from the depth of epithelium-lined hair follicles and sweat glands, or from the basal layer of the epithelium in the skin.

D. Keratinocytes move by an actin-myosin contractile system.

Ref.: 1–3

COMMENTS: There are two major events in the process of epithelialization: migration and mitosis. • Migration is the dominant process and is independent of mitosis. • Keratinocytes responsible for epithelialization are derived from the basal layer of the epithelium in the skin as well as the hair follicles and sweat glands present at the wound edge. • The more superficial the wound, the greater the number of these cells present and the more rapid the process of epithelialization. • Epithelial cells lose their contact inhibition and begin to migrate. • They are able to secrete collagenases and proteases, which facilitate movement under the debris of the wound surface. • Migrating cells do not divide. • Additional cells are recruited in the basal layer of the skin at the wound edge.

Several growth factors stimulate keratinocyte migration and mitosis, including basic fibroblast growth factor (bFGF), PDGF, TGF-α, and epithelial growth factor (EGF). • Epidermal cells contain a cytoskeleton and move by an actin-myocin contractile system. • Epiboly is a process whereby keratinocytes at the leading edge of the migration pile up on top of one another and tumble forward over the top of the heap (in a leapfrogging fashion) to move forward. • Keratinocytes lay down laminin and type IV collagen to create a new basement membrane. • When epithelial integrity is restored, the cells become columnar and start to divide. • Keratin forms as the cells mature.

A N S W E R :
B, C, D

7. Which of the following statements regarding wound contraction is/are true?

A. Wound dehydration is important to normal healing and contraction.

B. The amount of collagen content is directly proportional to the rate of wound contraction.

C. Myofibroblasts are modified fibroblasts that contact contractile protein similar to muscle.

D. Skin grafting tends to increase wound healing by facilitating contraction.

E. Older individuals generally have less contraction and deformity of facial wounds than do children because they have more excess skin in this area.

Ref.: 1–3

COMMENTS: Experimental evidence suggests that movement or contraction of wound edges results primarily from the action of myofibroblasts, which are modified fibroblasts with characteristics of both fibroblasts and smooth muscle cells. • The hallmark of myofibroblasts is the expression of α smooth muscle, the most prevalent formation of actin present in vascular smooth muscle cells. • Wound dehydration is not responsible for contraction. • Although collagen is a dynamic substance undergoing constant change during the healing process, contraction is not related to collagen content and is not inhibited by suppression of collagen synthesis or its cross-linking.

While the signals that initiate and terminate the contraction process have not been fully elucidated, wound contraction is a reproducible biologic phenomenon. • It occurs in all wounds and does not always stop immediately with wound closure. • Closure of an open wound by skin grafting or with a flap significantly reduces the amount of contraction but does not entirely eliminate it. • Because young individuals tend to have less excess skin over the face and hands than do older individuals, the contraction of wounds in these areas can produce significant distortion and permanent deformities in younger patients, particularly in children.

A N S W E R :
C, E

8. Which of the following statements regarding the proliferative phase of wound healing is/are true?

A. The extracellular matrix is composed of both structural and adhesive proteins.

B. Fibronectin is a structural protein that inhibits fibroblast migration.

C. Fibroblasts produce both an extracellular matrix and a hydrated polysaccharide gel.

D. The hydrated gel permits diffusion of nutrients to the cells.

E. Laminin is an adhesive protein that facilitates epithelial cell anchoring.

Ref.: 1–4

COMMENTS: The proliferative, or fibroblastic, phase usually begins about the third to fourth day after injury. • It is during this phase that fibrous collagen protein is produced. • Mediators such as C5a, fibronectin (secreted by macrophages), FGF, and PDGF released during the inflammatory phase attract fibroblasts to the healing wound. • Fibroblasts begin to proliferate and produce both an extracellular matrix and a hydrated polysaccharide gel in which the matrix is embedded. • The matrix is composed of structural proteins such as collagen and elastin and adhesive proteins such as fibronectin and laminin. • The gel is composed of glycosaminoglycans (hyaluronic acid, chondroitin sulfate, keratin sulfate, and heparin sulfate) linked to proteoglycans. • The gel permits diffusion of nutrients to the cells, and the structural proteins collagen and elastin act as a framework. • Laminin facilitates epithelial cell anchoring, and fibronectin anchors the fibroblast, is chemotactic to macrophages, and facilitates phagocytosis. • By virtue of its ability to bind the fibroblast and the matrix, fibronectin provides a sort of scaffold along which the fibroblasts can migrate.

A N S W E R :
A, C, D, E

9. The maturation phase of wound healing is characterized by which of the following?

A. Increased net collagen deposition and decreased collagen degeneration

B. Increased hypertrophy and redness of the wound

C. Steady increase in type III collagen

D. Decreased hyaluronic acid and chondroitin sulfate compared to the proliferative phase

Ref.: 1–4, 6, 7

COMMENTS: In normally healing wounds, the maturation phase starts approximately 3 weeks after the injury. • By 6 weeks after injury, the rates of collagen deposition and degeneration are nearly balanced. • Thus, the net collagen content remains the same, but the collagen becomes progressively more organized in appearance. • The red, raised scar of the proliferative phase starts to flatten, with a concomitant decrease in redness and itching. • The amount of type III immature collagen, which is deposited during the proliferative phase, gradually decreases and is replaced by the more mature type I collagen. • The ratio of type I to type III collagen, 8:1, is approximately equal to that normally found in skin that has not been injured. • The intracellular matrix also changes to a more normal makeup. • The large number of fibroblasts that dominated during the proliferative phase decreases, as do the amounts of substances produced by these cells, including the glycosaminoglycans, hyaluronic acid, and chondroitin sulfate.

ANSWER:
D

10. Which of the following statements regarding the role of collagen in wound healing is/are true?

A. Thermal shrinkage temperature and solubility in saline solution are correlated with the age of the collagen.

B. Net collagen content increases for up to 2 years after injury.

C. Tensile strength of the wound increases gradually for up to 2 years after injury.

D. Tensile strength is the force necessary to break the wound.

Ref.: 1–3

COMMENTS: Collagen synthesis by fibroblasts begins as early as 10 hr after injury and increases rapidly, peaking by day 6 or 7 and then continuing more slowly until day 42. • Collagen continues to mature and remodel for years. • The solubility in saline solution and the thermal shrinkage temperature of collagen reflect the intra- and intermolecular cross-links, which are directly proportional to collagen age. • After 6 weeks, there is no measurable increase in the net collagen content. • However, synthesis and turnover are ongoing for life. • Historical accounts of sailors with scurvy (and thus impaired collagen production) who developed reopening of previously healed wounds illustrate this fact.

Tensile strength correlates with total collagen content for approximately the first 3 weeks of wound healing. • At 3 weeks, the tensile strength of skin is 30% of normal. • After this time, there is a much slower increase in the content of collagen until it plateaus at about 6 weeks. • Nevertheless, tensile strength continues to increase as a result of intermolecular bonding of collagen and changes in the physical arrangement of collagen fibers. • Although the most rapid increase in tensile strength is early during the first 6 weeks of healing, there is a slow gain for at least 2 years. • The ultimate strength, however, never equals that of unwounded tissue, reaching a level only 80% of original skin strength. • Tensile strength is measured as the strength per unit area of tissue. • It may be differentiated from burst strength, which is the force required to break a wound and is independent of area. • For example, in wounds of the face and back, the burst strengths are different because of differences in skin thickness, even though the tensile strengths may be similar.

ANSWER:
A, C

11. Which of the following statements regarding growth factors is/are true?

A. Growth factors act in an endocrine manner.

B. Paracrine effects involve activation of complement.

C. Autocrine effects involve same-cell stimulation via cell-surface receptors.

D. Intracrine effects involve same-cell stimulation via intracellular effects.

Ref.: 1–3

COMMENTS: The term *growth factor* refers to any substance that stimulates growth. • Growth factors act in a number of ways. • They may be **paracrine**, that is, produced by one cell and acting on an adjacent target cell. • They may be **autocrine**, secreted by a cell and then acting on cell-surface receptors on the same cell. • They may be **intracrine**, produced by a cell and staying active inside the cell. • Hormones are released by cells that act on a distant target.

In general, growth factors are named according to their tissue of origin or their originally discovered action. • Growth factors stimulate growth by interacting with specific membrane receptors. • This process initiates a series of events that ultimately lead to the stimulation of cellular division. • These intermediate events include a variety of second-messenger systems mediated by agents such as inositol triphosphate, diacylglycerol, and cyclic adenosine monophosphate.

ANSWER:
C, D

12. Which of the following statements is/are true?

A. Transforming growth factor β (TGF-β) may have immunosuppressive effects.

B. Transforming growth factor α binds to the same receptors as does transforming growth factor β.

C. EGF and keratinocyte growth factor (KGF) stimulate epithelial growth and keratinization, respectively.

D. Urogastrone and epidermal growth factor have similar effects on gastric secretion.

Ref.: 1–3, 6, 7

COMMENTS: TGF-β is produced by platelets, fibroblasts, endothelial cells, smooth muscle, keratinocytes, lymphocytes, and macrophages. • It exerts an autocrine effect, thereby enhancing its own production. • In the wound, it is produced primarily by platelets, macrophages, and fibroblasts. • It increases collagen synthesis by enhancing collagen and matrix component production by fibroblasts and inhibiting collagenase production. • It also enhances angiogenesis and is chemotactic for fibroblasts, monocytes, and macrophages. • It has been found to have a suppressive effect on a variety of immune activities. • Increased production has been demonstrated in a variety of cancers and may explain some of the immunodeficiencies in individuals with these malignancies. • Mammalian TGF-β exists in three isoforms. • Isoform 1 is the most abundant.

Epithelialization is directly stimulated by at least two growth factors: EGF and KGF. • EGF is released by platelets, macrophages, and keratinocytes and acts in an autocrine fashion, amplifying its own secretion. • It stimulates epithelial cell migration and mitosis and is a mitogen for fibroblasts and endothelial cells. • It also stimulates secretion of collagenase by fibroblasts, resulting in epithelial growth and keratinization. • EGF is the same substance as urogastrone, a peptide in human urine that inhibits gastric secretion. • TGF-α is closely related to EGF, acting via common receptors and having primarily the same function. • TGF-α also has an angiogenic effect on endothelial cells. • KGF is released by fibroblasts to stimulate keratinotype division and differentiation.

ANSWER:
A, C, D

13. Which of the following statements is/are true?

A. PDGF is released only by platelets.

B. PDGF is chemotactic for platelets.

C. FGF is produced by fibroblasts.

D. FGF is a potent angiogenesis factor.

Ref.: 1–3, 6, 7

COMMENTS: PDGF is released by platelets at the site of vascular injury and is also synthesized by macrophages, endothelial cells, and fibroblasts. • It is chemotactic for fibroblasts, neutrophils, macrophages, and smooth muscle, and it stimulates fibroblasts to synthesize noncollagenous extracellular matrix, such as glucoseaminoglycans, fibronectin, and hyaluronic acid. • PDGF also stimulates fibroblast secretion of collagenase and may stimulate contractions.

FGF is produced by endothelial cells and macrophages. • It has acidic and basic forms, whose actions are identical but whose strengths differ (basic FGF is 10 times stronger than acidic FGF). • It is a potent angiogenesis factor, stimulating endothelial cells to divide and make new capillaries. • It is chemotactic for keratinocytes and fibroblasts and may hasten wound contraction. • FGF is stored in an inactive form in the basement membrane of the skin, where it is released after injury.

ANSWER:
D

14. Which of the following statements regarding angiogenesis is/are true?

A. Division of vascular smooth muscle cells is the key first step.

B. Hypoxia of macrophages stimulates angiogenesis.

C. Migration precedes breakdown of basement membrane and is followed by cell division to form new vessels.

D. Endothelial cells release proteases, which allow breakdown of basement membrane, followed by migration and division to form new vessels.

E. Fibroblast growth factor releases substances that stimulate fibroblasts, thereby inhibiting angiogenesis.

Ref.: 1–4, 8

COMMENTS: An important aspect of wound healing during the proliferative phase is angiogenesis, which is a process of vessel growth in a previously avascular area. • The first step in angiogenesis is stimulation of endothelial cell proliferation. • A stimulated endothelial cell must first break through the basal lamina and into the perivascular space. • This process requires a protease enzyme. • The endothelial cell subsequently migrates and divides. • Vacuoles form in adjacent cells, which fuse to form capillary lumens. • Capillaries sprout from larger vessels in response to further angiogenic stimulation by local factors. • A variety of angiogenic factors can be isolated from diverse tissues. • The factors most relevant to wound healing originate from leukocytes.

• Examples of angiogenesis factors include FGF, TGF-β, and TGF-α. • The latter two stimulate endothelial cell proliferation in addition to angiogenesis. • Many conditions probably regulate angiogenesis, but some of the best evidence indicates that the angiogenic process is regulated by a macrophage response to local oxygen tension. • Hypoxia stimulates angiogenesis, whereas increasing the oxygen concentration in the tissues stops this activity.

ANSWER:
B, D

15. Which of the following statements regarding the division of vascular endothelial cells is/are true?

A. It depends on activation by growth factor in S growth phase.

B. It depends on activation by growth factors in G_1 growth phase.

C. Smooth muscle cells and endothelial cells depend on the same growth factors.

D. Fibroblast growth factor stimulates division of endothelial cells.

E. PDGF stimulates division of smooth muscle cells.

Ref.: 1–3, 8

COMMENTS: See Question 16.

16. Angiogenesis is key in which one or more of the following?

A. Development of cartilage

B. Maintaining chronic inflammatory states

C. Ulcer healing

D. Tumor growth

Ref.: 1–3, 8

COMMENTS: Normal vascular endothelial cells turn over physiologically at a low rate. • However, under conditions that promote angiogenesis, endothelial cells are activated to divide. • Such conditions include wound healing, tumor growth, revascularization following ischemia, chronic inflammation, hypoxia, and organogenesis. • Angiogenesis, or formation of new blood vessels, occurs when endothelial cells sprout from existing vessels. • First, the endothelial cells break down surrounding extracellular matrix with a variety of proteases. • The cells then migrate and form tubes. • Cell division is not required for these beginning steps of angiogenesis but is required for sustained blood vessel growth.

Whereas angiogenesis is key to maintaining chronic inflammatory states, ulcer healing, and tumor growth, cartilage contains *no* vessels. • This fact has led to the observation that antiangiogenesis growth factors exist in tissues.

Among the growth factors that stimulate endothelial cells to divide are FGF and macrophage-derived endothelial growth factor. • Smooth muscle cells but not endothelial cells are stimulated to divide by PDGF. • Growth factors activate cells to divide in the G_1 phase of the cell cycle. • The G_1 phase is the stage at which cells become competent to start doubling DNA and other macromolecules. • Such competence requires expression of growth factor receptors early in the G_1 stage.

ANSWERS:
Question 15: B, D, E
Question 16: B, C, D

17. Which of the following statements regarding tissue ischemia is/are true?

   A. Prolonged total ischemia followed by reperfusion is a main cause of the formation of oxygen-derived free radicals.

   B. Oxygen-derived free radicals are highly toxic chemicals that can cause cell death.

   C. The deleterious effect of free radicals is worsened by superoxide dismutase.

Ref.: 1–3, 9

COMMENTS: Because a variety of cells in healing wounds are actively dividing, there is some normal nucleic acid metabolism and catabolism. • The enzyme xanthine dehydrogenase type D is normally used to convert xanthine to uric acid as follows: xanthine $+ H_2O +$ nicotinamide-adenine dinucleotide (NAD) $\rightarrow$ type D uric acid $+$ methemoglobin reductase (NADH) $+ H^p$. • This enzyme (dehydrogenase type D) is transformed into type O during ischemia. • At the same time, ADP is catabolized to adenosine, inosine, hypoxanthine, and xanthine. • In the presence of a reperfusion injury after prolonged ischemia and when oxygen becomes available, the following process takes place: xanthine $+ H_2O + 2O_2 \rightarrow$ uric acid $+ 2O_2 + 2H^p$. • The superoxide free radicals (O_2) eventually also form hydroxyl free radicals (OH_2). • These oxygen-derived free radicals are extremely cytotoxic. • Superoxide dismutase is a scavenger of superoxide radical and prevents formation of hydrogen peroxide and hydroxyl free radical.

A N S W E R :
A, B

18. Which of the following statements regarding wound healing is/are true?

   A. Denervation has no effect on wound contraction or epithelialization.

   B. A bacterial count at a level of 100 organisms per square centimeter retards wound healing.

   C. Chemotherapy introduced 10–14 days after primary wound closure has little effect on the final status of a wound.

   D. Tissue ischemia is the main component of tissue damage after irradiation.

Ref.: 1–5, 10, 11

COMMENTS: Denervation has no effect on wound contraction or epithelialization. • Flap wounds in paraplegics heal satisfactorily when other factors, such as nutrition and temperature, are controlled.

   Subinfectious bacterial levels appear to accelerate wound healing and the formation of granulation tissue. • However, when the level reaches 100,000 organisms per square centimeter of wound, healing is delayed because of decreased tissue oxygen pressure, increased collagenolysis, and a prolonged inflammatory phase.

   Various chemotherapeutic agents have various effects on wound healing. • Most antimetabolic agents (e.g., 5-fluorouracil) do not delay wound healing, although agents such as doxorubicin have been shown to decrease it. • When chemotherapy begins 10–14 days after wound closure, little effect is noted on its final status, despite a demonstrable early retardation in wound strength.

   Tissue ischemia may not be the primary factor involved in chronic wound-healing problems associated with irradiation. • Such problems are most likely related to the changes within the nuclei and concomitant cytoplasmic malformation.

A N S W E R :
A, C

19. If a patient requires reoperation 1 month after a vertical midline abdominal incision has been made, which of the following procedures promotes the most rapid gain in strength of the new incision?

   A. A separate transverse incision is made.

   B. The midline scar is excised with a 1-cm margin.

   C. The midline incision is reopened without scar excision.

   D. The rate of strength gained is not affected by incision technique.

Ref.: 1–3

COMMENTS: When a normally healing wound is disrupted after approximately the fifth day and then reclosed, the return of wound strength is more rapid than with primary healing. • This is termed the **secondary healing effect** and appears to be caused by elimination of the lag phase present in normal primary healing. • If skin edges more than about 7 mm around the initial wound are excised, and thus the incision is through essentially uninjured tissue, the accelerated secondary healing does not occur.

A N S W E R :
C

20. Which of the following statements regarding scar revision is/are true?

   A. It should be performed within 3 months to minimize fibrosis.

   B. It should be performed earlier in children than in adults.

   C. It corrects undesirable pigmentation.

   D. It should be delayed approximately 1 year to allow maturation.

Ref.: 1–3

COMMENTS: Changes in pliability, pigmentation, and configuration of a scar are known as **scar maturation**. • This process continues for many months after an incision, and it is generally recommended that revision not be carried out for approximately 12–18 months because natural improvement can be anticipated within this period. • In general, scar maturation occurs more rapidly in adults than in children. • Most erythematous scars show little improvement after revision, and so surgery should not be undertaken for correction of undesirable scar color alone.

A N S W E R :
D

21. Match the connective tissue disorders in the left-hand column with the important characteristics listed in the right-hand column.

   A. Osteogenesis imperfecta   a. It may be due to defects in elastin

   B. Ehlers-Danlos syndrome   b. Ten types have been characterized

   C. Marfan's syndrome   c. It is due to a defect in gene for type-1 collagen

   D. Epidermolysis bullosa   d. Phenytoin may be helpful.

Ref.: 1–3

COMMENTS: Osteogenesis imperfecta is due to mutations in the genes for type I collagen. • There are four kinds of osteogenesis imperfecta, and each presents several problems to the surgeon.

• Bones tend to break with little stress. • The dermis is thin, and there is increased bruisability. • Scarring usually is normal, and skin has normal extensibility. • Children with osteogenesis imperfecta have an increased incidence of inguinal and umbilical hernias.

Ehlers-Danlos syndrome is a group of collagen disorders characterized by joint laxity, skin hyperextensibility and fragility, poor wound healing, and vascular rupture. • At least 10 types have been identified.

Marfan's syndrome patients characteristically have a tall stature, arachnodactyly, lax ligaments, myopia, scoliosis, pectus excavatum, and often dissecting aneurysms of the root of the ascending aorta. • Marfan's syndrome may be due to collagen structure defects or defects in elastin.

Epidermolysis bullosa is characterized by blistering and ulcerations. • It is thought to have several causes, including excessive fibroblast production of metalloproteases and abnormal adhesion of the intracellular matrix to the basement membrane of the epidermis. • Gastrointestinal tract wounds are affected, often leading to stenosis and stricture. • Dermal incisions are associated with blistering. • Phenytoin, which can decrease collagenase activity in the skin, has been used to treat these patients.

ANSWER:
A-c; B-b; C-a; D-d

22. Which of the following statements regarding wound healing is/are true?

    A. Vitamin A is a necessary cofactor in the hydroxylation of lysine and proline in collagen synthesis.

    B. High doses of vitamin C improve wound healing.

    C. Vitamin E is involved in the stimulation of fibroplasia, collagen cross-linking, and epithelialization.

    D. Massage, pressure, and silicone sheeting have been shown to flatten and soften scars.

    E. Scarlet red accelerates wound healing.

Ref.: 1–3

COMMENTS: Vitamin A is involved in the stimulation of fibroplasia and epithelialization • Although there has been no conclusive evidence of efficacy in humans, vitamin A has been shown to reverse the inhibitory effects of glucocorticoids on the inflammatory phase of wound healing and epithelialization in animal studies.

Vitamin C is a necessary cofactor in the hydroxylation and cross-linking of lysine and proline in collagen synthesis. • Deficiencies in vitamin C (scurvy) can lead to the production of inadequately hydroxylated collagen, which either degrades rapidly or never forms proper cross-links. • Doses higher than physiologic doses do not improve wound healing.

Vitamin E is applied to wounds and incisions by many patients. • There is no evidence to support the use of vitamin E in wound healing. • Large doses of vitamin E have been found to inhibit wound healing.

Massage, pressure, and silicone sheeting have been shown to soften scars. • Although the mechanism of action is not clearly understood, the clinical efficacy is apparent.

Scarlet red does not stimulate epithelial growth.

ANSWER:
D

23. Which of the following statements is/are true?

    A. Keloids contain an overabundance of fibroblasts.

    B. A hypertrophic scar extends beyond the boundaries of the original wound.

    C. Improvement is usually seen with keloid excision followed by intralesional steroid injection.

    D. An ideal scar will result from an incision placed perpendicular to the lines of natural skin tension.

Ref.: 1–3

COMMENTS: Keloid formation is caused by an imbalance between collagen production and collagen degradation and results in a scar that extends beyond the boundaries of the original wound. • The absolute number of fibroblasts is not increased. • The treatment of keloids is difficult. • There is usually some improvement seen with excision and intralesional steroid injection. • In unresponsive cases, excision and radiation treatment has been successful.

Hypertrophic scars contain an overabundance of collagen, but the dimensions of the scar are confined to the boundaries of the original wound. • Hypertrophic scars are often seen in the upper torso and across flexor surfaces.

Scar formation is affected by multiple factors, including the patient's genetic makeup, wound location, age, nutritional status, infection, tension, and surgical technique. • In planning surgical incisions, an effort to parallel natural tension lines will promote improved wound healing.

ANSWER:
C

24. Which of the following impairs epithelialization during wound healing?

    A. bFGF

    B. PDGF

    C. Isotretinoin

    D. Fibronectin

    E. EGF

Ref.: 1–3

COMMENTS: Isotretinoin (Accutane) impairs epithelialization. • It has anti-keratinization properties, which result in thinning of the stratum corneum. • It also impairs epithelial cell migration from skin appendages.

In contrast, several growth factors stimulate keratinocyte migration and mitosis. • These include bFGF, PDGF, and EGF. • Fibronectin and vitronectin both support epithelial cell migration.

ANSWER:
C

25. Match the collagen type with the appropriate location in the body?

    A. Type I   a. Predominant in the basement membrane
    B. Type II   b. Abundant in skin, tendon, and bone
    C. Type III   c. Found in hyaline cartilage
    D. Type IV   d. Found in the dermis and arteries
    E. Type V   e. Found in the cornea

Ref.: 1–3

COMMENTS: Type I collagen is located in skin, tendon, and bone. • Type II collagen is found in hyaline cartilage. • Type III collagen is found in the dermis and arteries. • Type IV collagen is

the predominant type of collagen found in the basement membrane.
• Type V is found in the cornea (in association with Type III).

ANSWER:
A-b; B-c; C-d; D-a; E-e

26. Quantitative tissue cultures for a patient with a stage III sacral pressure sore reveal 10^8 organisms per gram of tissue after operative dèbridement. What is the next most appropriate step in the management of the patient's wound?

A. Muscle flap coverage

B. Wound vac

C. Intravenous antibiotics

D. Repeat dèbridement

Ref.: 1–3

COMMENTS: The National Pressure Ulcer Advisory Panel has recommended a staging system for pressure sores that is useful in planning pressure sore treatment. • **Stage I** is represented by the presence of nonblanchable erythema of intact skin. • **Stage II** involves partial-thickness skin loss involving the epidermis or dermis. • Clinically, the ulcer presents as a blister, abrasion, or a shallow crater. • **Stage III** is full-thickness skin loss with involvement of the underlying subcutaneous tissue. • Stage III wounds may extend down to but not through the underlying fascia. • **Stage IV** represents full-thickness skin loss with extensive destruction or tissue necrosis to underlying structures, which may include muscle and bone.

Studies have shown that wounds with quantitative cultures revealing greater than 100,000 organisms per gram of tissue that undergo reconstruction with skin or even muscle flaps have significantly greater risk of complications, including infection, fluid accumulation, and wound dehiscence. • Similarly, a skin graft is unlikely to survive in an environment with such a high bacterial inoculate.

The wound vac system uses a sponge and an occlusive dressing connected to a suction apparatus in a closed system. • In large wounds, the wound vac may serve as a bridge to reduce wound size for definitive reconstruction. • It has been shown to be effective in reducing wound edema, controlling wound drainage, encouraging diminution of wound size, and facilitating granulation tissue formation.

Although studies show that wound vac therapy may reduce bacterial counts over a period of time, the most appropriate management of this patient is repeat dèbridement of the wound. • Intravenous antibiotics may be indicated to treat underlying osteomyelitis.

ANSWER:
D

27. Match the cell or protein involved in collagen synthesis in the left-hand column with the appropriate activity in the right-hand column.

A. Pro-α-chains
B. Tropocollagen
C. Propylhydroxylase
D. Procollagen peptidase
E. Fibroblasts

a. Formed by cleaving nonhelical portions of procollagen
b. Combine in a triple helix to form procollagen
c. Cleaves nonhelical portions of procollagen
d. Site of collagen synthesis
e. Responsible for hydroxylation of proline

Ref.: 1–3

COMMENTS: See Question 28.

28. Which of the following statements is/are true?

A. Lysyl hydroxylase is the rate-limiting enzyme responsible for α-chain polymerization.

B. Vitamin C deficiency causes decreased hydroxylation of proline.

C. Lyceal oxidase mediates lysyl-lysine bond formation.

D. β-Aminopropionitrile inhibits lyceal oxidase.

Ref.: 1–3

COMMENTS: Collagen is manufactured by the fibroblasts. • The single-strand pro-α-chains are made intracellularly on ribosomes. • They combine in a triple helix to form procollagen. • The molecule has its nonhelical portion removed by procollagen peptidase, creating tropocollagen, a molecule that contains three α-peptide chains in a right-handed helix. • It is then packed into secretory vesicles in the Golgi apparatus and secreted. • In the extracellular space, enzymatic cleavage of the telopeptide end of the molecule occurs, allowing it to form intra- and intermolecular cross-links.

While the molecule is still in the cell, before secretion, its proline molecules are hydroxylated by two dioxygenases: lyceal hydroxylase and propylhydroxylase. • Propylhydroxylase is a rate-limiting enzyme in collagen synthesis. • Its function depends on several cofactors, including iron, α-ketoglutarate, ascorbate, and oxygen. • Without these cofactors, there is insufficient hydroxylation, the α-chains cannot form a stable helix, and collagen cannot be exported out of the cell. • Ascorbate deficiency (scurvy) and hypoxia affect collagen synthesis at this level. • Collagen cross-linking occurs in the extracellular space. • Lysyl oxygenase is an enzyme responsible for this. • It mediates oxidation of lysine to form lysyl-lysine bonds. • This cross-linking can be prevented by β-aminopropionitrile, which inhibits Lysyl oxidase, and D-penicillamine, which prevents cross-link formation by directly binding to collagen substrate.

ANSWERS:
Question 27: A-b; B-a; C-e; D-c; E-d
Question 28: B, C, D

REFERENCES

1. Townsend CM, Beauchamp RD, Evers BM, et al (eds): *Sabiston Textbook of Surgery: The Biological Basis of Modern Surgical Practice,* 17th ed. Saunders, Philadelphia, 2004.
2. Schwartz SI, Shires GT, Spencer FC (eds): *Principles of Surgery,* 8th ed. McGraw-Hill, New York, 2004.
3. Mulholland MW, Lillemoe KD, Doherty GM, (eds) et al: *Greenfield's Surgery: Scientific Principles and Practice,* 4th ed. Lippincott, Williams & Wilkins, Philadelphia, 2006.
4. Simmons RL, Steed DL: *Basic Science Review for Surgeons.* WB Saunders, Philadelphia, 1992.
5. Basson MD, Burney RE: Defective wound healing in patients with paraplegia and quadriplegia. *Surg Gynecol Obstet* 155:9–12, 1982.
6. Peacock EE: Symposium on biological control of scar tissue. *Plast Reconstr Surg* 41:8–12, 1968.
7. Barbul A: Immune aspects of wound repair. *Clin Plast Surg* 17:433–442, 1990.
8. Folkman J: Angiogenesis. In: Verstraete M, Vermlen R, Lijnan R, et al (eds) *Thrombosis and Hemostasis.* Leuven University Press, Leuven, Belgium, 1987.
9. White MJ, Heckler FR: Oxygen free radicals and wound healing. *Clin Plast Surg* 17:473–484, 1990.
10. Robson MC, Stenberg BD, Heggers JP: Wound healing alterations caused by infection. *Clin Plast Surg* 17:485–492, 1990.
11. Rudolph R, Arganese T, Woodward M: The ultrastructure and etiology of chronic radiotherapy damage in human skin. *Ann Plast Surg* 9:282–292, 1982.

CHAPTER 11

Pharmacology

Robert L. Barkin, Pharm. D., F.A.C., M.B.A.

1. With regard to transfer of drugs across cell membranes, which of the following statements is/are true?

    A. Passive transport occurs solely through a process of diffusion, which is governed by concentration gradients across the membrane.

    B. The greater the lipid-water partition coefficient of a drug, the faster its diffusion across a membrane.

    C. The transport of ionized compounds or of inorganic ions across membranes is related to the transmembrane potential.

    D. Active transport of a drug against an electrochemical gradient is an energy-requiring process.

    Ref.: 1–9

COMMENTS: The crucial step in drug absorption, distribution, biotransformation, and excretion is the passage of the drug across a cell membrane. • This can occur through either passive or active transport. • Cellular membranes are approximately 80 Å thick and are composed of a bimolecular lipid layer in which proteins are embedded and integrated. • Aqueous channels of various size are interspersed throughout the membrane. • **Passive transport** can occur by diffusion across the membrane or by passage of the drug through the aqueous channels. • In the latter case, the drug must be small enough to pass through unhindered. • The size of the channels is site-specific. • Capillary endothelial cells have large channels (40 Å), whereas red blood cells and intestinal epithelium have smaller channels (4 Å) and therefore permit passage only of water, urea, and other small water-soluble molecules. • Passage through the channels is also governed by transmembrane concentration gradients and transmembrane potentials. • Passive diffusion through the membrane (not via the channels) is dictated by concentration gradients and the lipid-water partition coefficient of the drug. • The greater the partition coefficient, the more readily a drug diffuses across a membrane. • **Active transport** is responsible for the rapid transfer of many organic compounds and occurs against electrochemical gradients. • This process is mediated by membrane-based proteins, which form a complex with the drug being transported. • Active transport is an energy-requiring process that may be associated with sodium-potassium transport.

ANSWER:
B, C, D

2. Which of the following factors may modify drug absorption?

    A. Drug solubility

    B. Drug concentration

    C. Circulation to the site of absorption

    D. Area of the absorbing surface

    E. Local pH

    Ref.: 1–9

COMMENTS: In addition to lipid solubility and molecular size, many variables may influence the absorption of drugs. • One such variable is **solubility.** • Drugs given in aqueous solutions are more rapidly absorbed than those given in oil-like solvents, suspension, or solid form. • Similarly, drugs that are ingested or injected in high **concentration** are absorbed more rapidly than are drugs in solutions of low concentration. • Increased **circulation** at the site of administration enhances absorption of an administered drug (e.g., Fentanyl transdermal). • Increased local blood flow to the site of local injection may be brought about by massage or local application of heat. • Decreased blood flow, ischemia, vasoconstrictors, or shock may slow absorption. • The **surface area** of the absorbing surface to which a drug is exposed (injected, applied, or administered) is an important determinant of the rate of drug absorption. • For example, drugs are absorbed rapidly from a large surface area, such as the pulmonary alveolar epithelium. • The epithelium of the small bowel is capable of absorbing more drug than can the gastric epithelium. • The **local pH** has a direct bearing on whether a drug is absorbed, especially for weak organic acids and for bases. • In an acidic environment, a weak acid is more likely to exist in its nonionized form, which usually is lipid soluble and likely to diffuse across the cell membrane. • In such an environment, a weak base is found in its ionized form. • The distribution of a weak acid or a base is determined by its pKa and the pH gradient. • This relationship is demonstrated in the following example of an orally administered acid (HA) with a pKa of 4.4. • Gastric pH is 2.4, and plasma pH is 7.4. • The gastric mucosa is permeable only to the nonionized form (HA) of the acid, whose concentration is arbitrarily designated 1 (see the diagram). • In the plasma, pH − pKa = 3.0. • Therefore, the ionized form is 1000-fold more likely to be found. Similarly, in gastric juice the nonionized form is more likely to be found, which favors absorption of the weak acid from the stomach.

TOTAL
(HA + A⁻)

$$[1] \quad HA \xrightarrow{\hspace{1cm}} A^- \quad [1000] \quad 1001$$

PLASMA
pH = 7.4

```
┌─────────────────────────────────┐
│     LIPOID MUCOSAL              │
│     BARRIER                     │
└─────────────────────────────────┘
```

GASTRIC
JUICE
pH = 1.4

$$[1] \quad HA \xleftarrow{\hspace{1cm}} A^- \quad [0.001] \quad 1.001$$

$$HA \rightleftharpoons A^- + H^+$$

Nonionized   Ionized

WEAK ACID, pK_a = 4.4

ANSWER:
A, B, C, D, E

3. With regard to the administration of drugs through the gastrointestinal (GI) tract, which of the following statements is/are true?

   A. Sublingual administration, in comparison with absorption lower in the GI tract, may yield higher plasma-drug levels because it avoids the "first-pass" effect of the liver.

   B. Drugs administered through the rectum do not pass through the liver and avoid "first-pass" before entry into the systemic circulation.

   C. Weak acids are absorbed more easily in the stomach than are weak bases; the converse is true in the small intestine.

   D. The gastric absorption of most drugs is improved if gastric emptying is retarded.

   E. Altering gastric pH usually has a profound impact on drug absorption.

Ref.: 1–9

COMMENTS: Absorption of drugs through the GI tract occurs through simple diffusion across the epithelium. • The rate of such diffusion is proportional to the lipid solubility of the drug in question. • If the drug is a weak acid or a base, its **nonionized form is more lipid soluble**, and the pH in the GI tract becomes perhaps the major determinant of the rate of diffusion. • For example, weak acids, which are predominantly nonionized in the acidic gastric contents, are more readily absorbed from the stomach. • In contrast, weak bases are predominantly ionized in the pH of the gastric juice and are therefore not absorbed until they reach the small intestine. • If the gastric contents are made more alkaline, acidic compounds become ionized to a greater degree and may be more slowly absorbed. • At the same time, basic drugs become ionized to a lesser degree and may be more rapidly absorbed. • Changing the gastric pH, however, may produce a relatively minor effect because the absorption of most drugs occurs primarily from the intestine because of its greater surface area. • Absorption of drugs from the stomach may be delayed or reduced if gastric emptying is retarded.

"First-pass" metabolism usually occurs in the liver or gut wall after absorption from the oral route and before systemic circulation is achieved. • When drugs are administered sublingually, absorption from the oral mucosa is rapid, and a higher concentration in the blood may be achieved by this route than by absorption lower in the GI tract. • The drug in this instance is not subjected to possible destruction by GI secretions, and thus passage through the liver is minimized as well. • The overall result is that drug metabolism, or biotransformation, is less rapid.

Rectal administration of drugs is useful when any type of ingestion is difficult, as with vomiting or when the patient is comatose. • The drug does not pass to the liver (and thus avoids first-pass hepatic metabolism) before its entry into the systemic circulation. • For this reason, high serum levels may be obtained. • Rectal absorption, however, is often irregular and incomplete. • Moreover, many drugs cause irritation of the rectal mucosa.

ANSWER:
A, B, C

4. Match the route of drug administration in the left-hand column with the correct statements in the right-hand column.

   A. Intravenous   a. Not suitable for oily solutions or insoluble substances
   B. Subcutaneous   b. Prompt absorption from aqueous solution and slow from oily or repository preparations
   C. Intramuscular   c. Precluded during anticoagulant therapy
   D. Oral   d. Most convenient, safest, and most economical

Ref.: 1–9

COMMENTS: The major routes of parenteral administration of a drug are intravenous, subcutaneous, and intramuscular. • Impediments to absorption are circumvented by the **intravenous** injection of drugs in aqueous solution, and the desired blood concentration is subsequently obtained with accuracy and immediacy. • There are many disadvantages with the intravenous route. • Unfavorable side effects are more likely to occur than with other routes of administration. • As a rule, when administered intravenously, a drug must be injected slowly, and this route is not suitable for oily solutions or insoluble substances.

The **subcutaneous** route of administration can be used only for drugs that are not irritating to tissue. • Otherwise, sloughing may occur. • Absorption from a subcutaneously administered drug is prompt but slower than by the intravenous route from aqueous solutions. • Absorption is slow and sustained from repository preparations. • The parenteral solvent may be oil-like, or the dosage form may be converted to an ester (decanoate or enanthate, e.g., fluphenazine decanoate, haloperidol decanoate, or fluphenazine enanthate). • If slow absorption is desired, the drug can be suspended in an insoluble vehicle or incorporated in a vasoconstrictor agent. • The latter principle is used when epinephrine is combined with a local anesthetic. • In a similar manner, absorption may be even slower when the drug in the form of a pellet is implanted subcutaneously. • The subcutaneous route is not suitable for administration of large volumes of a drug.

Drugs in aqueous solution are rapidly absorbed after **intramuscular** injection. • Slow but even absorption from the intramuscular site results if the drug is injected in an oil-like solvent or is suspended in various repository vehicles. • Penicillin is often administered in this manner. • Substances that are irritating and cannot be administered subcutaneously can often be given intramuscularly. • The intramuscular route is precluded during anticoagulant therapy and may interfere with the interpretation of certain diagnostic tests (e.g., creatinine phosphokinase determination).

The **oral route** of administration is the most convenient, safest, and most economical. • Absorption, however, is variable and depends on many factors, such as lipid solubility, the pH in the GI tract, and whether the drug is stable in GI fluid.

A N S W E R :
A-a; B-b; C-b,c; D-d

---

5. With regard to the administration of drugs through the skin, which of the following statements is/are true?

A. The rate of absorption of a drug is proportional to its lipid solubility in both the epidermis and dermis.

B. Absorption occurs more readily through abraded or denuded skin.

C. Absorption is enhanced by suspending the drug in an oil-like solvent and rubbing the preparation into the skin.

D. Absorption is retarded by occlusive dressings, which accumulate moisture, and lower lipid solubility.

Ref.: 1–9

COMMENTS: Few drugs easily penetrate intact skin. • Those that are able to penetrate are absorbed because they are lipid soluble, since the epidermis behaves as a lipoid barrier. • The dermis, in contrast, is freely permeable to many solutes, and, as a result, systemic absorption of many drugs occurs through abraded or denuded skin. • Toxic effects can result from absorption through the skin of a highly lipid-soluble substance, such as a lipid-soluble insecticide in an organic solvent.

Absorption can be enhanced by suspending a drug in an oil-like or other enhanced vehicle and rubbing the resulting product into the skin. • This method of administration is known as **inunction**. • Occlusive dressings enhance absorption through the skin by retaining moisture, which causes maceration of the epidermis and breakdown of the lipoid barrier.

A N S W E R :
B, C

---

6. With regard to the distribution of drugs into the central nervous system (CNS) and the cerebrospinal fluid, which of the following statements is/are true?

A. Ionized and lipid-insoluble drugs are not distributed into the brain.

B. Entry of nonionized organic substrates is dependent on lipid solubility.

C. In a manner similar to that of other capillary endothelial cells, the brain endothelial cells restrict passage of drugs bound to plasma proteins.

D. The cellular barrier between the blood and the extracellular space is composed of capillary endothelial cells, astrocytic processes, and cells of the choroid plexus.

Ref.: 1–9

COMMENTS: The distribution of drugs into the CNS generally is restricted, since nonionized and **lipid-insoluble** drugs are largely excluded from entry into the brain. • Entry of the nonionized forms of weak acids and bases is somewhat restricted, but these substances can enter in proportion to their lipid solubility. • Drugs that are highly **lipid-soluble** enter the brain rapidly. • In contrast to other capillary endothelial cells, those of the brain restrict passage of drugs bound to plasma protein. • The cellular barrier between the blood and the extracellular space of the CNS is formed by the capillary endothelial cells, glial cell (astrocyte) processes, and cells of the choroid plexus.

A N S W E R :
A, B, D

---

7. With regard to the fact that many drugs are bound to plasma protein, which of the following statements is/are true?

A. Albumin is the plasma protein largely responsible for binding drugs.

B. Binding is usually irreversible.

C. Binding to plasma proteins is highly specific, that is, the binding locus is specific for a given drug.

D. Bound drug has enhanced glomerular filtration.

Ref.: 1–9

COMMENTS: The various body compartments in which a drug accumulates can serve as potential reservoirs for subsequent release of the drug. • In this way, the pharmacologic effects of the drug are prolonged. • These body compartments include plasma proteins and other extracellular reservoirs, such as GI tract secretions, cerebrospinal fluid, the aqueous humor of the eye, endolymph fluids, and joint fluids. • Drugs may also accumulate in intracellular reservoirs. • For example, the antimalarial agent quinacrine may be stored within hepatocytes. • Other drugs, such as tetracycline antibiotics and heavy metals, may be adsorbed into the framework of the bony matrix.

Many drugs are bound to plasma proteins, most notably to plasma albumin. • Binding to other proteins occurs to a much smaller extent. • Basic drugs bind to an acidglycoprotein. • Acid drugs bind to albumin. • The binding is usually reversible. • The degree to which a drug binds to albumin is highly variable. • Some lipid-soluble organic acids, such as penicillins and warfarin, are more than 90% bound. • A drug that is bound to plasma has limited activity in tissue and at the site of action because only the unbound "free fraction" of drug is in equilibrium across membranes. • Binding therefore also limits glomerular filtration of the drug. • Binding of drugs to albumin is nonselective. • Many drugs with similar physical and chemical properties compete with each other and with endogenous substances for the binding sites. • Competition for the binding sites may lead to displacement of one metabolite or parent compound by another. • This phenomenon explains why some drugs, such as the sulfonamides, increase the risk of bilirubin encephalopathy in newborns. • These medications displace unconjugated bilirubin bound to albumin. • The risk of an adverse effect is highest if the displaced drug has a limited volume of distribution, if elimination of the drug is also reduced, or if the displacing drug is administered in high dosage by rapid intravenous injection. • After displacement of a drug from the inactive protein (albumin)-binding site, there may be an increase in the plasma or serum concentration of the free unbound (active) drug, but it is not reflected in the total serum concentration.

A N S W E R :
A

8. With regard to hepatic microsomal drug metabolism system, which of the following statements is/are true?

    A. Microsomal enzymes are found within the mitochondria.

    B. The enzymes of this system catalyze conjugation, demethylation, oxidation, reduction, and hydrolysis of drugs (phase I, or asynthetic phase).

    C. Enzyme activity and susceptibility to induction among normal individuals may vary sixfold or more.

    D. Lipid solubility is an important requirement for a drug to be metabolized by this system.

    Ref.: 1–9

COMMENTS: The enzyme systems involved in the metabolism of many drugs are located in the hepatic endoplasmic reticulum. • When liver homogenates undergo centrifugation, fragments of this enzyme network are isolated in the portion called microsomes. • The endoplasmic reticulum resembles a canal system within the cellular cytoplasm and is involved in the intracellular transport of many substances. • It is in continuity with the cell membrane and the nuclear membrane, and it contains many small ribonucleoproteins called ribosomes, which render the surface of the reticulum rough. • The microsomal enzyme system is capable of catalyzing many chemical reactions, including conjugation, demethylation, oxidation, reduction, and hydrolysis. • Thereafter, large water-soluble molecules (e.g., glucuronic acid and sulfates) are attached to the drug by a phase II (synthetic phase) reaction, forming a water-soluble metabolite, which is often inactive and ready for renal excretion. • The conjugation reaction occurs with glucuronide. • Glucuronides constitute the major proportion of metabolites of many drugs, such as phenols, alcohols, and carboxylic acids. • Glucuronides usually are inactive and are secreted into the urine and bile. • Glucuronides that have been excreted into the bile subsequently may be hydrolyzed by intestinal or bacterial enzymes, and the liberated drug may be absorbed. • This enterohepatic cycling may prolong the action of the drug (and is altered when the gallbladder is removed). • The activity of the microsomal enzymes can be enhanced by many drugs and chemicals encountered in the environment. • A marked variation in enzyme activity can be seen among normal individuals, and these rates may vary sixfold or more. • This variation is termed genetic polymorphism and is more common at cytochrome P-450 2C and 2D6. • Enzyme activity and susceptibility to induction appear to be genetically determined.

Lipid solubility is an important requirement for a drug to be metabolized by the hepatic microsomal system. • A highly lipid-soluble drug penetrates the endoplasmic reticulum more easily, and its binding with cytochrome P-450 is enhanced.

A N S W E R :
B, C, D

9. With regard to an important group of oxidases in the microsomal system called mixed-function oxidases, which of the following statements is/are true?

    A. These enzymes require both reduced nicotinamide adenine dinucleotide phosphate (NADPH) and molecular oxygen.

    B. Cytochrome P-450 is a group of proteins constituting the terminal oxidase.

    C. Metabolism of many drugs is enhanced by carbon monoxide.

    D. The rate of drug metabolism by the mixed-function oxidases is determined solely by the concentration of cytochrome P-450.

    Ref.: 1–9

COMMENTS: The hepatic microsomal system contains an important group of enzymes, called mixed-function oxidases, that catalyze oxidative reactions. • The reactions catalyzed by these oxidases include N^- and O^- dealkalation, aromatic-ring and side-chain hydroxylation, sulfoxide formation, N oxidation, N hydroxylation, deamination of primary and secondary amines, and replacement of a sulfur by an oxygen atom (desulfuration). • These enzymes require both NADPH and molecular oxygen. • The NADPH functions as the primary electron donor, and the electron transfer involves the flavoprotein NADPH–cytochrome C reductase.

Cytochrome P-450 is the terminal oxidase of the mixed-function oxidase system. • It is so named because it absorbs light at 450 nm when exposed to carbon monoxide. • Oxidized cytochrome P-450 binds with a drug, and the resulting complex is reduced by the reductase. • The reduced complex then combines with molecular oxygen. • NADPH donates an electron and two hydrogen ions, and the subsequent products are the oxidized metabolite, water, and regenerated oxidized cytochrome P-450. • The metabolism of many drugs can be blocked by carbon monoxide.

The rate of drug biotransformation by the oxidase system is determined by several factors, including the concentration of cytochrome P-450, the proportions of the various forms of cytochrome P-450, and their affinities for the drug, the concentration of the reductase, and the rate of reduction of the drug–cytochrome P-450 complex. • The rate of metabolism of various drugs may be influenced by competing endogenous and exogenous substances. • These many factors are therefore responsible for the sometimes marked species, strain, and individual variations in drug metabolism by the microsomal system.

A N S W E R :
A, B

10. Induction of microsomal enzyme activity is associated with which of the following?

    A. Enhanced pharmacologic effects of drugs that are inactivated by the enzyme system

    B. Increased synthesis of cytochrome P-450, NADPH–cytochrome C reductase, and other enzymes

    C. Proliferation of the endoplasmic reticulum and increases in liver weight and hepatic blood flow

    D. Susceptibility to induction, which is highest in individuals who have undergone previous induction

    Ref.: 1–9

COMMENTS: Many drugs can competitively inhibit microsomal enzymes. • Of more importance is the ability of certain drugs, known as **enzyme inducers**, to increase the activity of the microsomal enzyme system. • When this occurs, metabolism of a subsequently administered new drug is increased, its pharmacologic effects are subsequently reduced, and its efficacy is thus diminished. • Induction of microsomal enzyme activity has been associated with proliferation of the endoplasmic reticulum and increases in liver weight, hepatic blood flow, and bile flow. • An increase in synthesis of RNA polymerase, cytochrome P-450, NADPH–cytochrome C reductase, and other enzymes involved in drug metabolism has been noted as well. • In humans, susceptibility to induction is genetically determined and is highest for individuals with the slowest drug metabolism before induction. • For this reason, the effect of induction may be minimal if the patient has previous induction. • After the inducing agent has been discontinued, induction wanes over a period of days or weeks, depending on the time course for accumulation or excretion of the inducing agent. • Among the drugs whose activity is altered by mixed-function oxidase inducers are birth control pills, warfarin, disopyramide, metronidazole, doxycycline, mexiletine, theophylline, verapamil, and quinidine. • As a group of drugs, the anticonvulsants are enzyme inducers.

Some medications eliminated by the liver inhibit certain metabolic pathways and are termed **enzyme inhibitors.** • This decrease, or inhibition, of enzymes in the liver reduces the rate of metabolism of the other medications, resulting in an elevated serum level and possibly a toxic effect, side effects, or adverse effects in medications with or without narrow therapeutic ranges. • Saturation of drug-metabolizing enzymes by two or more drugs that use the identical enzyme system results in a decreased metabolic rate for one or more of the competing drugs (e.g., fluoxetine and sertraline). • Some drugs bind to an enzyme system (e.g., cimetidine–cytochrome P-450) and inhibit the enzyme system. • Such enzyme inhibitors include cimetidine (not ranitidine), isonicotinic acid hydrazide (INH), ketoconazole, allopurinol, erythromycin, clarithromycin, monoamine oxidase inhibitors, disulfiram, and verapamil.

ANSWER:
B, C

11. A deep venous thrombosis develops in a 45-year-old man with a long history of seizures, for which he is taking phenobarbital. In this context, which of the following statements is/are correct?

   A. Phenobarbital may induce the microsomal enzyme systems.

   B. A higher dose of warfarin is required than if the anticoagulant were administered alone.

   C. Cessation of phenobarbital without adjusting the warfarin dose may lead to severe bleeding.

   D. Chronic alcohol ingestion should be discouraged because it impairs metabolism of phenobarbital and warfarin.

Ref.: 1–9

COMMENTS: Several hundred compounds are known to induce the microsomal enzyme system. • They are loosely classified in two types: those that resemble *phenobarbital* and those that resemble the *polycyclic hydrocarbons.* • In the latter category, the increase in drug metabolism is limited to fewer substrates than in the former. • Chronic administration of a drug may stimulate not only its own metabolism but that of other drugs as well. • Simultaneous administration of phenobarbital and warfarin results in lower plasma concentrations of warfarin and less anticoagulant effect than when warfarin is administered alone. • The desired therapeutic effect of the anticoagulant can be obtained if the dosage of warfarin is increased. • If the phenobarbital is discontinued after the desired therapeutic effect of the warfarin has been obtained, the plasma concentration and effect of warfarin subsequently increase, and severe bleeding may occur. • Thus, when drugs are administered simultaneously and one or more of them stimulate drug metabolism, the effects of the other drugs must be carefully monitored when the inducing agent is initiated and discontinued.

Environmental factors may also induce the microsomal system, including some vegetables, alcohol, exposure to insecticides, and chemicals in cigarette smoke. • Acute ingestion of alcohol may inhibit the microsomal enzyme system, although, during chronic ingestion, induction may occur. • Ethanol does not appear to stimulate its own metabolism because it is metabolized mainly by nonmicrosomal enzymes. • By inducing the microsomal system, however, ethanol can influence the metabolism of other drugs, and therefore its ingestion should be discouraged in such circumstances.

ANSWER:
A, B, C

12. Nonmicrosomal enzymes metabolize fewer drugs than do their microsomal counterparts. With regard to nonmicrosomal drug metabolism, which of the following statements is/are true?

   A. It occurs primarily in the kidney.

   B. Nonmicrosomal enzymes are capable of catalyzing all conjugations and some oxidations, reductions, and hydrolytic reactions.

   C. In contrast to the microsomal enzyme system, nonmicrosomal enzymes do not show interindividual variation in the rate of drug metabolism.

   D. None of the nonmicrosomal enzymes is inducible.

Ref.: 1–9

COMMENTS: Although nonmicrosomal enzymes metabolize fewer drugs than do microsomal enzymes, their function is nevertheless important. • Nonmicrosomal enzymes are found primarily in the liver, but they can also be found in plasma and other tissues, such as the GI tract. • Nonmicrosomal enzymes are capable of catalyzing all of the major chemical reactions involved in biotransformation of drugs. • For example, all conjugations other than glucuronide formation (which is catalyzed by the microsomal enzymes) as well as some oxidation, reduction, and hydrolysis of drugs are catalyzed by nonmicrosomal enzymes. • Examples of drugs metabolized by nonmicrosomal enzymes include aspirin, sulfonamides, allopurinol, isoniazid, and hydralazine. • Among normal individuals, there is wide variation in the rate of drug metabolism by nonmicrosomal enzymes. • As for the microsomal enzymes, this interindividual variation may be sixfold or greater. • None of the nonmicrosomal enzymes involved in drug metabolism is known to be inducible.

ANSWER:
D

13. With regard to the excretion of drugs, which of the following statements is/are true?

   A. The more polar a drug is in its administered state, the more likely it is to be excreted unaltered.

   B. The kidney is the most important organ for eliminating drugs and their metabolites.

   C. Most metabolites transported into bile are subsequently excreted in the feces.

   D. Excretion of drugs can also occur through sweat, saliva, and breast milk, but the proportion of these excretions to the total excretion is quantitatively unimportant.

Ref.: 1–9

COMMENTS: Drugs are eliminated from the body unchanged or as their metabolites. • The more polar a drug is in its administered state, the more likely it is to be excreted unaltered. • Lipid-soluble drugs and drugs that are less polar are not readily excreted until they are metabolized to more polar, less lipid-soluble compounds.

The kidney is the most important organ involved in the excretion of drugs. • Drug excretion involves three processes: glomerular filtration, active tubular secretion, and passive tubular reabsorption. • In addition to the kidney, there are other sites of drug excretion. • Drugs may be eliminated in bile and feces, by the pulmonary bronchial tree, and in sweat, saliva, and breast milk. • Many drug metabolites formed in the liver are subsequently excreted into the intestinal tract in bile. • Although many of these metabolites are excreted in feces, most are reabsorbed into the blood and subsequently eliminated through urine.

Excretion of drugs into sweat and saliva occurs in a manner similar to the process that takes place in the kidney, albeit in clinically small amounts. • Drugs pass through the epithelial cells of the glands, and active secretion of drugs across the duct of the gland may also occur. • Reabsorption of the drug from the secretion also occurs. • Drugs excreted in the saliva enter the mouth, where they are usually swallowed. • Their fate thereafter is similar to that of drugs taken by mouth. • The same principles apply to the excretion of drugs in breast milk. • The amounts excreted within breast milk are important, not because of the quantity, but because the eliminated metabolites are possible sources of unwanted medicinal effects in nursing infants.

ANSWER:
A, B, D

14. Match each term in the left-hand column with the appropriate definition in the right-hand column.

A. Potency   a. Pattern of effects associated with a drug allergy
B. Efficacy   b. Relationship between the effect of a drug and the dose required
C. ED_{50} c. Ability of a drug to achieve the desired result without untoward side effects
D. LD_{50} d. Dose of a drug required to produce a specified intensity of effect in 50% of individuals
E. Hyperreactive   e. Condition whereby a drug produces its usual effect at an unexpectedly low dose
F. Tachyphylaxis   f. Drug dose required to cause death in 50% of organisms
   g. Tolerance that develops rapidly after only a few doses of the drug

Ref.: 1–9

COMMENTS: Several terms describe the relationship between the dose of a drug and its effect. • If the intensity of a drug's effect is plotted against the dose of the drug, the location of the appropriate effect of a drug along the dose axis is an expression of the **potency** of a drug. • Potency is the dose of a drug required to bring about the desired effect. • Potency may be an unimportant characteristic of a drug. • Whether the effective dose is 1 μg or 100 mg matters little, as long as the quantity can be reasonably given to a patient and the drug can be administered safely at the appropriate dosage. • There is no justification for the view that the more potent of two drugs is clinically superior. • **Efficacy** is a drug's ability to achieve the desired result without untoward side effects. • If undesired effects limit dosage, the drug's efficacy is correspondingly limited, even though it may be inherently capable of producing a greater effect than another drug. • The dose of a drug required to produce a specified intensity of effect in 50% of individuals is known as

the median effective dose, or ED_{50}. • If death of an organism is the end sought, the median effective dose (which kills 50% of the organisms) is termed the median lethal dose, or LD_{50}. • When a drug produces its customary effect at an unexpectedly low dosage, the patient is said to be **hyperreactive**. • **Hypersensitivity** is used to describe a patient's allergic reaction to a drug. • **Tachyphylaxis** is tolerance that develops rapidly after only a few doses of a drug have been administered. • Reduced sensitivity should be described as immunity only if the acquired tolerance is the result of an immune reaction to that medication.

ANSWER:
A-b; B-c; C-d; D-f; E-e; F-g

15. Regarding lipid therapy, match the drugs in the left-hand column with the correct toxicities in the right-hand column.

A. Cholestyramine (bile salt resin)   a. Flushing
B. HMG-CoA (3-hydroxy-3-methyl-glutaryl-coenzyme A) reductase inhibitor   b. Significant drop in high-density lipoprotein (HDL) levels
C. Niacin   c. Rhabdomyolysis
D. Probucol   d. Bleeding

Ref.: 1–9

COMMENTS: Epidemiologic evidence has shown that elevated low-density lipoprotein (LDL) cholesterol levels and decreased HDL cholesterol levels are significant risk factors for coronary artery disease (CAD). • For each 1% lowering of LDL cholesterol levels, there is a 2% reduction in risk. • Diet only mildly reduces LDL levels, and exercise only moderately increases HDL levels. • Pharmacologic therapy is far more effective and has been shown to improve survival appreciably for patients with elevated LDL cholesterol levels. • Although all patients with CAD should undergo aggressive therapy to reduce LDL levels to 130 mg/dl or below, pharmacologic therapy has significant toxicity. • The bile salt resins, such as cholestyramine, decrease fat absorption, reducing vitamin K absorption, which can lead to hypoprothrombinemia and cause bleeding. • The HMG-CoA reductase inhibitors are the most effective therapy for hypercholesterolemia, although HMG-CoA inhibitors cause hepatic dysfunction and rhabdomyolysis in rare cases. • Niacin inhibits hepatic synthesis of cholesterol. • Its acute administration can lead to flushing, which can be blocked by the concomitant administration of aspirin. • Probucol also inhibits hepatic cholesterol synthesis and is especially effective for treating cholesterol deposits in the skin (xanthelasma) and xanthomas in tendons. • However, probucol can significantly reduce levels, which may worsen CAD progression over time.

ANSWER:
A-d; B-c; C-a; D-b

16. Which of the following statements regarding elevated arterial blood pressure is/are correct?

A. A patient with an acute rise in blood pressure in the operating room in excess of 220 mmHg may best be treated with a fast-acting, short–half-life agent.

B. Short-acting antihypertensive agents are optimal for chronic therapy.

C. The presence of renal artery stenosis can be determined by administration of captopril, an agent that precipitates acute azotemia.

D. In addition to being effective therapy for hypertension, angiotensin-converting enzyme (ACE) inhibitors can reduce proteinuria and prevent renal dysfunction from progressing in patients with type II diabetes.

Ref.: 1–9

COMMENTS: Hypertension is a highly prevalent disease, with a large portion of the population being untreated or partially treated. • Acute hypertensive crises are uncommon, but if untreated they can precipitate an acute myocardial infarction (MI) or stroke. • Agents should be used that can control blood pressure and be adjusted quickly for fluctuation in pressure. • It is inadvisable to reduce the blood pressure too rapidly in patients with severe hypertensive crises. • Sodium nitroprusside (a potent vasodilator) or esmolol (an ultra–short-acting β-blocker) are optimal agents. • Another agent, diazoxide, is given as a bolus and thus cannot be titrated to changes in arterial blood pressure. • ACE inhibitors, a frequently used class of antihypertensive agents, have the attribute of preventing congestive heart failure (CHF) development in patients after MI. • For patients with unilateral renal artery stenosis, ACE inhibitors can precipitate acute renal failure. • In fact, a short-acting ACE inhibitor, captopril, is used as a test for renal artery stenosis. • In addition to being effective antihypertensives, ACE inhibitors have been reported to prevent progression of renal dysfunction and proteinuria in patients with hypertension and type II diabetes.

For chronic treatment of hypertension, long-acting, once-a-day antihypertensive agents increase patients' compliance.

ANSWER:
A, C, D

17. Which of the following statements regarding gout is/are true?

A. Gout is due to underexcretion or overproduction of uric acid.

B. Probenecid is the therapy of choice for underexcretors.

C. Allopurinol should be administered to all patients with an acute gouty attack in order to decrease uric acid production.

D. Colchicine is a highly potent uricosuric agent.

Ref.: 1–9

COMMENTS: Gout is a familial metabolic disease characterized by recurrent episodes of acute arthritis due to depositions of monosodium urate in joints and cartilage. • Formation of uric acid calculi in the kidney may also occur. • Gout is associated with high serum levels of uric acid, a poorly soluble substance that is the major end product of purine metabolism. • Gout can be due to overproduction of uric acid or underexcretion of uric acid by the kidney. • The treatment of gout is aimed at relieving acute gouty attacks and preventing recurrent gouty episodes and urate lithiasis. • Therapy for acute attacks often starts with colchicine, an alkaloid with anti-inflammatory properties. • It binds to the intracellular protein tubulin, preventing its polymerization into microtubules and leading to inhibition of leukocyte migration and phagocytosis. • Colchicine also inhibits the formation of leukotriene B_4. • Whereas colchicine is indicated for acute gouty attacks, allopurinol, a xanthine oxidase inhibitor that blocks the oxidation of xanthine or hypoxanthine to uric acid, is indicated for chronic overproducers of uric acid. • The administration of allopurinol should never be initiated during an acute attack because it can worsen it. • Use of allopurinol should follow the administration of colchicine. • Probenecid is a uricosuric agent often used to enhance uric acid secretion in patients with elevated uric acid blood levels and undersecretion.

ANSWER:
A, B

18. Which of the following statements regarding CHF is/are true?

A. Inotropic therapy is the only way to treat CHF effectively.

B. Unloading therapy decreases cardiac output.

C. Unloading therapy increases cardiac output.

D. β-Blockers are always contraindicated for patients with CHF.

E. Acute heart failure can best be treated with fluids.

Ref.: 1–9

COMMENTS: Patients may have a decreased ejection fraction (EF), as is often the case following MI, or a normal EF and poor left ventricular (LV) compliance, as may be seen in hypertensive patients with LV hypertrophy. • Patients with CHF respond best to unloading therapy with ACE inhibitors, which increase cardiac output. • Digitalis and diuretics are supportive therapies, but only ACE inhibitors have been shown to reduce mortality rates. • Although they acutely decrease LV function over time, β-blockers improve the outcome for patients with severe LV failure. • Carvedilol, a β-blocker with α-receptor–blocking properties causing vasodilation, has also been shown to prolong life for patients with severe LV failure. • Patients with acute CHF unresponsive to digitalis and diuretics may need intravenous dobutamine, an inotropic β-agonist that dilates medium-to-large arteries, thereby unloading the heart. • Administration of fluids during acute CHF would increase the preload, worsening the patient's condition.

ANSWER:
C

19. Which of the following statements regarding cardiac arrhythmia is/are true?

A. Digoxin therapy in atrial fibrillation (AF) increases concealed conduction to the atrioventricular (AV) node and increases AV node refractoriness, slowing the ventricular response.

B. Quinidine, if given alone to patients with AF, can slow the atrial rate, decreasing concealed conduction at the level of the AV node. This, combined with the vagolytic effect of quinidine, can accelerate AV node conduction and thus permit high ventricular rates.

C. Ventricular premature contractions (VPCs) must always be treated by lidocaine acutely and antiarrhythmic agents chronically.

D. Intravenous amiodarone administration is not indicated, since the half-life of amiodarone is approximately 55 days.

Ref.: 1–9

COMMENTS: AF is a frequently encountered supraventricular arrhythmia. • The common causes of AF are hypertensive cardiovascular disease, mitral valve disease (mitral regurgitation or stenosis), CAD, and hyperthyroidism. • These conditions should be evaluated in patients with AF. • The first aim of therapy for patients with AF is to slow the ventricular response, permitting adequate time for cardiac emptying and filling. • Digoxin slows the ventricular response by increasing the AF rate. • More impulses bombard the AV node, making the node refractory, and so fewer impulses reach the ventricle, slowing the ventricular response. • This phenomenon is called *concealed conduction*. • Digoxin is often given before quinidine to block the AV node, since quinidine alone can cause an increase in the ventricular response by being vagolytic and decreasing concealed conduction by slowing the atrial rate. • The Cardiac Arrhythmia Suppression Trial found that administration of antiarrhythmic agents to suppress VPCs results in higher mortality rates than does placebo therapy. • Serious ventricular arrhythmias, such as ventricular tachycardia, can be treated by intravenous lidocaine, which is effective in 6–10% of cases, or intravenous amiodarone, effective in 30–50% of cases. • The long half-life of amiodarone is not relevant when the drug is given intravenously, when the time to action is measured in minutes.

ANSWER:
A, B

20. Regarding anticoagulation, match the drug in the left-hand column with the correct statement in the right-hand column.

A. Warfarin
B. Heparin
C. Aspirin
D. Recombinant tissue plasminogen activator (rTPA)

a. Prolongs the partial thromboplastin time
b. Antithrombin (thrombolytic)
c. Prolongs the prothrombin time
d. Irreversibly blocks the platelet cyclooxygenase enzyme pathway

Ref.: 1–9

COMMENTS: Pulmonary embolic and other thrombotic states contribute significantly to patient mortality. • Patients with acute ischemic syndromes, acute pulmonary embolus following hip surgery and other orthopedic procedures, or chronic AF should be anticoagulated. • Depending on the disease process and the underlying pathophysiologic state, various anticoagulants or thrombolytic agents may be employed. • Patients with venous disease or chronic prothrombotic states often receive chronic warfarin (Coumadin) therapy monitored by the prothrombin time. • Physicians try to keep the international normalized ratio (INR) between 2 and 3. • The risk/benefit ratio at this range is optimal. • Patients who have a repeated thrombotic episode on warfarin should be evaluated for a protein S or protein C deficiency. • Heparin is given intravenously for acute ischemic syndromes, immediately following a pulmonary embolism, and occasionally subcutaneously for patients who are placed on bed rest for prolonged periods. • The adequacy of anticoagulation with heparin is monitored using the partial thromboplastin time. • Aspirin is an antiplatelet agent that irreversibly blocks the cyclooxygenase enzymatic pathway in platelets. • Continuing the use of aspirin for patients with CAD just before and after surgery has been reported to improve outcome. • A new group of antithrombin agents are thrombolytic and cause disruption of a newly formed thrombus. • rTPA is an antithrombin with proven efficiency during the first 6 hr following acute MI, for patients with acute pulmonary embolus, or for those with a nonhemorrhagic cerebrovascular accident. • The time factor for rTPA administration places considerable urgency on the early detection and diagnosis of MI, stroke, and pulmonary embolus.

ANSWER:
A-c; B-a; C-d; D-b

21. Regarding cardiac angina, which of the following statements is/are true?

A. Nitrates as therapy work best when given continuously.

B. β-Blockers should be avoided for patients with a low EF (<40%).

C. Nifedipine, a dihydropyridine calcium-channel blocker, causes significant vasodilation and reactive tachycardia, which may worsen angina.

D. The antiplatelet action of aspirin reduces mortality rates for patients after MI.

Ref.: 1–9

COMMENTS: Anginal pain develops when the oxygen supply is less than the myocardial oxygen demand. • This situation may be due to decreased blood flow secondary to CAD or increased vasoconstriction, as is found most frequently in young women without coronary atherosclerosis. • **Nitrates** are first-line therapy administered sublingually, topically, or intravenously to avoid first-pass hepatic metabolism. • Since continuous administration of nitrates leads to tolerance and ineffectiveness, intermittent nitrate therapy is optimal. • **β-Blockers** are effective antianginal therapy. • They decrease myocardial work and thus oxygen consumption by slowing the heart rate. • The best results are seen with patients with a low EF (<40%), who experience reduced mortality rates after MI on β-blocker therapy. • **Calcium-channel blockers** are an alternative therapy to β-blockers for patients with asthma, severe CHF, or insulin-dependent diabetes with previous hypoglycemic reactions. • However, if the dihydropyridines are used alone, the vasodilation they produce can cause a reactive tachycardia, which increases oxygen consumption, worsening the angina. • Thus, nifedipine is often combined with a β-blocker to slow the heart rate, thereby preventing an increase in oxygen consumption. • Whereas angina is due to the imbalance of oxygen supply and demand, an acute MI is due to plaque rupture or platelet thrombus, initiating coagulation. • **Aspirin** therapy has been shown to prevent a first MI (primary prevention), and, for patients who have had a previous MI, it can be used to prevent a recurrence (secondary prevention).

ANSWER:
C, D

22. Cefazolin 1 g given intramuscularly or intravenously is used for surgical prophylaxis. Which of the following statements regarding cefazolin is/are true?

A. Cefazolin is used for prophylaxis against infections with gram-negative rods.

B. Cefazolin is used because it penetrates all tissues, including the CNS.

C. Cefazolin does not produce a positive Coombs' test result.

D. Cefazolin can be given less frequently than other first-generation cephalosporins.

E. Since cefazolin can inhibit aldehyde dehydrogenase, patients receiving it cannot tolerate alcohol.

Ref.: 1–9

COMMENTS: The spectrum of activity of first-generation cephalosporins is mostly against gram-positive cocci, including some species of β-lactamase–producing *Staphylococcus aureus*. • They may have some activity against *Escherichia coli* and *Klebsiella pneumoniae* in vitro. • Cefazolin penetrates all tissues well except the CNS. • Meningitis increases the ability of cefazolin to penetrate CNS tissues but not sufficiently for clinical use. • Cefazolin, like other cephalosporins, can produce a positive Coombs' test result. • This reaction appears to be nonimmunologic in nature. • A cephalosporin-globulin complex forms, coats the erythrocytes, and reacts with the Coombs' serum. • Since cefazolin has the longest half-life of the first-generation cephalosporins, it can be given less frequently than the other drugs. • Only cephalosporins that have the tetrazole-thiomethyl side chain (i.e., cefamandole, cefbuperazone, and cefotetan) inhibit aldehyde dehydrogenase.

ANSWER:
D

23. Postoperatively, a patient develops a low-grade fever, presumably due to an infection with *S. aureus*. Which of the following is appropriate therapy before specific laboratory test results are obtained?

   A. Penicillin G

   B. Nafcillin

   C. Cefotetan

   D. Vancomycin

   E. Erythromycin

Ref.: 1–9

COMMENTS: Staphylococci are gram-positive cocci. • Penicillin G, nafcillin, vancomycin, and erythromycin have a spectrum that covers *S. aureus*. • Cefotetan, a third-generation cephalosporin, is indicated for gram-negative sepsis. • A parenteral first-generation cephalosporin could be used. • Since most *S. aureus* in hospitals are resistant to penicillin G, it is not a good antibiotic choice, although it may still be used for community-acquired gram-positive infections. • Vancomycin should be saved for methicillin-resistant *S. aureus* (MRSA), and the infection in question has not been shown to be MRSA. • The best choice is a β-lactamase-resistant penicillin, such as nafcillin. • If an oral form is acceptable, oxacillin may be used. • Erythromycin may be used but usually is reserved for treatment if nafcillin does not work or if the patient is penicillin sensitive.

ANSWER:
B

24. True or false: Rofecoxib does not have to be discontinued before surgery for reasons of platelet effects.

Ref.: 1–9

COMMENTS: All platelet cyclooxygenase is COX I, not COX II. • Rofecoxib is only COX II. • Rofecoxib has no effect on platelet cyclooxygenase preoperatively, perioperatively, and postoperatively. • Rofecoxib use will not augment bleeding or effect platelet aggregation, platelet function, or bleeding time. • It is COX I sparing owing to COX II selection. • COX I, nonselective NSAIDS (i.e., ibuprofen, diclofenac, naproxen, or ketoprofen) markedly decrease platelet aggregation and prolong bleeding times within a few hours of administration. • Rofecoxib is not associated with excessive drug-induced intraoperative or postoperative bleeding.

ANSWER:
True

25. Which of the following statements concerning acetaminophen is false?

   A. It may be a central COX 3 inhibitor.

   B. It utilizes the cytochrome P-450 1A2 and 3A5 pathway for metabolism.

   C. It is safe to use chronically at doses exceeding 4000 mg.

   D. It possesses a hepatotoxic metabolite (NAPQUI).

   E. It may be prescribed for patients with diminished renal function.

Ref.: 1–9

COMMENTS: For acute pain management, short-term use of 4000 mg of acetaminophen is acceptable in selected patients. • However, chronic use at this dose may affect liver function test results. • Risk factors for hepatotoxic dysfunction from 4000 mg include a history of alcohol abuse and the fasting state, which deplete glutathione stores, and use of cytochrome P-450 1A2 and 3A5 inducers (e.g., barbiturates, INH, etc.). Postoperatively, this dose will mask febrile episodes.

ANSWER:
C

26. Which one of the following is an opioid associated with hyperreflexia, myoclonus, seizures, and anticholinergic effects?

   A. Morphine

   B. Butorphanol (Stadol)

   C. Meperidine (Demerol)

   D. Buprenorphine (Buprenex)

Ref.: 1–9

COMMENTS: Meperidine has a neurotoxic metabolite designated as normeperidine. • This metabolite may precipitate seizures, myoclonus, and hyperreflexia when given to patients with diminished renal function. • These side effects may occur at higher doses and with prolonged administration. • Normeperidine is a nonopioid metabolite and is not naloxone responsive or reversible. • Meperidine is anticholinergic and may lead to peripheral and central anticholinergic effects, unlike morphine, which produces miosis. • Meperidine causes mydriasis.

ANSWER:
C

27. Which one of the following is an oral opioid-acetaminophen combination associated with cardiotoxicity, pulmonary edema, and poor analgesia.

   A. Hydrocodone (Vicodin, Norco, etc.)

   B. Oxycodone (Percocet)

   C. Codeine (Tylenol with codeine)

   D. Propoxyphene N100 (Darvocet = N 100 has 650 mg of acetaminophen)

Ref.: 1–9

COMMENTS: Propoxyphene has a nonopioid cardiotoxic metabolite that may cause pulmonary edema. • This metabolite is not naloxone reversible. • Although euphoria is achieved with propoxyphene at therapeutic doses, the analgesia is less than that achieved by acetaminophen with codeine. • Propoxyphene is also a cytochrome P-450 inhibitor.

ANSWER:
D

28. True or false: Tramadol 37.5 mg/acetaminophen 325 mg (Ultracet) may be prescribed for acute postoperative pain.

Ref.: 1–9

COMMENTS: This combination is indicated for acute pain. • The analgesia is equivalent to codeine, hydrocodone, or oxycodone, often without producing prominent euphoria. • Tramadol has a binary mechanism of action, providing both an opioid agonist effect and a dual monoamine reuptake inhibitor (5HT serotonin, NE norepinephrine) effect. • The combination product has a half-life ($T_{1/2\,beta}$) of 7 to 9 hr and may be prescribed on an every 6-hr dosing schedule. • This product is not a controlled substance.

ANSWER:
True

29. A patient describes a sulfonamide allergy. The clinician is planning to use a Cox II inhibitor for this patient. Is it true or false that celecoxib (Celebrex) or valdicoxib (Bextra) may be used for analgesia or anti-inflammatory effects?

Ref.: 1–9

COMMENTS: Both of these Cox II agents are sulfonamides and cannot be used for a patient with a sulfonamide allergy. • Vioxx, a nonsulfonamide, may be used with this allergy-risk patient.

ANSWER:
False

30. An elderly patient with mild-to-moderate dementia requires postoperative analgesia. A long-acting opiate (>60 mg morphine per day equivalent) not in combination with an NSAID or acetaminophen is being considered because of its simplicity in dosing. The clinician is considering fentanyl, a transdermal 3-day opiate patch. True or false: This an appropriate choice.

Ref.: 1–9

COMMENTS: It is true that this choice is rational for simple administration for both the patient and the care giver. • The transdermal fentanyl patch only needs to be changed every 3 days. • Fentanyl reaches a steady state during application of the second patch (day 6). • The 25-mcg/μg patch is equivalent to 60–90 mg of oxycodone or morphine. • Following removal of the patch, the fentanyl level in the dermis or subcutaneous layer will clear by 50% after 17 hr.

ANSWER:
True

31. A patient has recently been prescribed warfarin because of the placement of a mechanical prosthetic valve. After surgery, the patient complains of joint pain and polymyalgias on morning rounds. True or false: Acetaminophen administration will resolve these complaints without further sequelae.

Ref.: 1–9

COMMENTS: A rare effect of warfarin therapy is skin necrosis. • Hemorrhage from any organ or tissue is also a potential consequence of warfarin therapy. • The patient's signs and symptoms are a function of both the extent of bleeding and the anatomic location. • Complications of hemorrhage may be manifested as paralysis, dyspnea, dysphagia, cephalalgia, chest pain, abdominal pain, and *joint pain*. • It should be noted that the INR for mechanical prosthetic valves is 3–4.5.

ANSWER:
False

REFERENCES

1. Hardman JG, Limbird LE, Molinoff PB, et al (eds): *Goodman and Gilman's the Pharmacological Basis of Therapeutics*, 9th ed. McGraw-Hill, New York, 1996.
2. Schatzberg AF, Nemeroff CB (eds): *Textbook of Psychopharmacology*, 2nd ed. American Psychiatric Press, Washington, DC, 1998.
3. Bennett DR (ed): *Drug Evaluations Annual*. Division of Drugs and Toxicology, Department of Drugs, American Medical Association, Chicago, 1992.
4. Ellenhorn MJ, Schonwald S, Ordog G, et al (eds*): Ellenhorn's Medical Toxicology: Diagnosis and Treatment of Human Poisoning*, 2nd ed. Williams & Wilkins, Baltimore, 1997.
5. Goldfrank LR, Flomenbaum NE, Lewin NA, et al (eds): *Goldfrank's Toxicologic Emergencies*, 6th ed. Appleton and Lange, Stamford, CT, 1998.
6. Parfitt K (ed): *Martindale: The Complete Drug Reference*, 32nd ed. Pharmaceutic Press, London, 1999.
7. McEvoy GK (ed): *AHFS Drug Information*. Authority of the Board of the American Society of Health-System Pharmacists and American Hospital Formulary Service, Bethesda, Maryland, 2003.
8. Wickersham RM (ed): *Drug Facts and Comparisons*. Facts and Comparisons, A Wolters Kluwer Company, St. Louis, 2003.
9. Leikin JB, Paloucek FP (eds): *Poisoning and Toxicologic Handbook*. Lexi-Comp, Hudson, OH, 2003.

CHAPTER 12

Anesthesia

James A. Colombo, M.D., and Kenneth J. Tuman, M.D.

1. During a tracheostomy, a flash is noted in the surgical field while using electrocautery. Which of the following is the correct sequence of steps in the management of the patient?

   A. Extinguish flames with saline solution or water; turn off all anesthetic gases, including O_2; and hyperventilate with 21% O_2 through the endotracheal tube (ETT).

   B. Extinguish flames with saline solution or water, turn off all anesthetic gases *except* O_2, and hyperventilate with 100% O_2 through the ETT.

   C. Stop ventilation; disconnect all anesthetic gas supply, including O_2; extinguish flames with saline solution or water; remove the ETT; mask-ventilate; and re-intubate.

   D. Extinguish flames with saline solution or water; remove all draping immediately; stop ventilation; disconnect all anesthetic gas supply including O_2; allow patient to awaken; and then extubate.

   E. Stop ventilation; disconnect all anesthetic gas supply, including O_2; extinguish flames with saline solution or water; and resume ventilation.

Ref.: 1

COMMENTS: Airway fires occur most often during laser airway surgery but can happen in any O_2-rich environment where igniting stimuli may exist. • Any combustible material, including polyvinyl chloride tubing, surgical drapes, and human tissue, can ignite. • Both the surgeon and the anesthesiologist should take the following steps simultaneously: stop all gas flow, including O_2; extinguish the fire with water or saline solution; and remove the ETT or any foreign body present in the airway (e.g., bronchoscope or gauze). • Mask-ventilation is performed until the trachea is re-intubated. • Then, bronchoscopy is performed to determine the extent of the airway damage and to remove any foreign bodies that may be present. • The trachea should be left intubated for at least 24 hr after an airway fire, and humidified gases should be administered through the ETT or tracheostomy tube. • The use of steroids is controversial and probably of no benefit.

ANSWER:
C

2. Effective management of gastric acid aspiration includes which of the following?

   A. Tracheal intubation and saline lavage of the lungs

   B. Prophylactic antibiotic therapy

   C. Prophylactic steroid therapy

   D. Tracheal intubation, suctioning, and controlled ventilation with positive end-expiratory pressure (PEEP) therapy

   E. Diuresis

Ref.: 1–4

COMMENTS: Gastric aspiration can be a fatal complication. • The severity of the injury is determined by the volume and pH of the gastric fluid aspirated. • Fluid with a pH less than 2.5 and a volume greater than 0.4 ml/kg (approximately 30 ml for an adult) is associated with a greater degree of pulmonary damage.

Initial treatment should begin with **intubation, suctioning** of aspirated fluid, **pH testing** of fluid (if readily available), and **positive-pressure ventilation** with PEEP. • The level of PEEP is determined by the ability to adequately oxygenate ($PaO_2 > 60$ mmHg), ideally with the fractional concentration of oxygen in inspired gas (FIO_2) below 60%. • Saline lavage is not indicated, since it has been shown to aggravate injury. • Prophylactic antibiotic and steroid therapy are also not indicated. • With the initiation of positive-pressure ventilation and the loss of fluid into the damaged lung parenchyma, patients are often intravascularly depleted. • Thus, empirical diuretic therapy is not appropriate.

Antibiotic therapy may be indicated in cases of aspiration involving patients receiving enteral feeding but are not indicated as a general prophylactic maneuver. • Steroid medications are not indicated in the initial stages of aspiration.

ANSWER:
D

3. A 30-year-old man undergoes repair of a hernia under spinal anesthesia. He calls the next day complaining of a headache that worsens with moving from a supine to a sitting position. He also has complaints of tinnitus. Initial treatment should include which of the following?

   A. Bed rest, increased fluid intake, and analgesics

   B. Urgent computerized tomographic (CT) scan of brain to check for increased intracranial pressure (ICP)

   C. Consultation with an anesthesiologist

   D. Placement of an epidural blood patch

Ref.: 1

COMMENTS: Postdural puncture headaches (PDPHs) are typically characterized by frontal or occipital cephalgia that worsens with sitting or standing and is usually relieved by assuming a supine position. • Initial treatment is conservative, with bed rest, fluids, and analgesics. • PDPH may be associated with neurologic findings. • Common complaints are tinnitus, diplopia, and decreased hearing acuity. • An epidural blood patch usually gives immediate relief of symptoms and is administered if conservative measures are ineffective in relieving severe symptoms after 24 hr. • Factors associated with an increased incidence of PDPH include young age, female gender, large (cutting) spinal needles, and the direction of needle insertion. • Insertion of a cutting bevel (Quinkie design) spinal needle in a direction nonparallel to the dural fibers (which are aligned in a vertical plane running cephalad to caudad) is believed to result in a higher incidence of PDPH. • Informing the anesthesiologist that a PDPH has occurred is helpful in guiding further treatment if it is required.

ANSWER:
A, C

4. For a trauma patient with suspected intracranial hypertension, which intravenous anesthetic agent(s) is/are contraindicated, even when mechanical ventilation is controlled?

A. Midazolam

B. Methohexital

C. Thiopental

D. Ketamine

E. Morphine

Ref.: 1, 2

COMMENTS: Benzodiazepines (midazolam), opioids (morphine), and barbiturates (methohexital and thiopental) decrease cerebral blood flow and the cerebral metabolic rate, which in turn decrease ICP. • Ketamine is an arylcyclohexylamine structurally related to phencyclidine. • Ketamine increases the cerebral metabolic rate and cerebral blood flow and therefore the ICP. • Hence, ketamine is contraindicated when intracranial hypertension is suspected.

ANSWER:
D

5. Intubation of a spontaneously breathing but obtunded patient with a closed head injury is best accomplished by which of the following?

A. Awake "blind" nasal intubation

B. Induction with thiopental, muscle relaxation with succinylcholine, and oral tracheal intubation while maintaining manual in-line axial cervical traction

C. Awake fiberoptic intubation

D. Tracheostomy

E. Awake rigid laryngoscopy

Ref.: 1, 3, 4

COMMENTS: Securing an airway in a trauma patient can be difficult. • Concurrent cervical injury should be suspected in a patient with a head injury. • All methods listed are acceptable for intubating this patient, but the best way to attenuate increases in ICP is via thiopental induction, which can decrease cerebral blood flow and the cerebral metabolic rate by 40–60%. • Succinylcholine causes small, transient increases in ICP (approximately 4 mmHg), which are offset by the ICP-reducing

effect of thiopental. • In addition, the muscle paralysis induced by succinylcholine prevents coughing, which can increase the ICP by 50–70 mmHg. • Nasal intubation carries the risks of damage to the cribriform plate when preexisting fractures are present, and epistaxis can cause airway compromise in an obtunded patient. • Blind intubation under these circumstances therefore is less desirable than are other methods of securing an artificial airway. • Tracheostomy should be performed whenever airway distortion prevents prompt intubation by other methods. • In some situations, tracheostomy is the appropriate initial approach to securing the airway.

ANSWER:
B

6. Use of succinylcholine should be avoided for which of the following patients?

A. Patients with 40% body surface area burns in need of emergency intubation 2 hr after injury

B. Patients with 40% body surface area burns in need of emergency intubation 5 days after injury

C. Patients arriving at the emergency room immediately after sustaining an acute spinal cord injury (T4 complete)

D. Children under 2 years of age

E. Patients with end-stage renal disease and normal serum electrolyte levels

Ref.: 1, 2, 5

COMMENTS: Succinylcholine is a depolarizing muscle relaxant. • It causes paralysis by depolarizing the motor endplate via repeated action potential generation. • This results in an efflux of potassium ions and a transient rise in extracellular potassium levels. • This increase is approximately 0.5 mEq/L in patients without neurologic deficits or severe muscular injury. • Since the number of motor endplates is markedly increased (i.e., sensitization) 3–5 days after neurologic or muscular injury, administration of depolarizing muscle relaxants, such as succinylcholine, at this time can cause large increases in extracellular potassium and cardiac arrest. • Therefore, succinylcholine should be used only in an acute setting (immediately after injury) for patients with burns or spinal cord injury, where such sensitization is not observed within the first 1–2 days of injury. • There are no contraindications to the use of succinylcholine in healthy children. • The presence of renal failure does not preclude the use of succinylcholine if serum potassium levels are within a normal range.

ANSWER:
B

7. Which of the following determine(s) spread of local anesthetics in the cerebrospinal fluid?

A. Contour of the spinal canal

B. Baricity of the local anesthetic

C. Patient's position

D. Anesthetic volume

Ref.: 1, 2

COMMENTS: Spinal anesthesia is accomplished by injecting a local anesthetic into the subarachnoid space. • The level of spread is determined primarily by the baricity of the solution and the patient's position. • **Baricity** is the density of the local anesthetic solution compared to the density of the cerebrospinal fluid at normal body temperature. • Local anesthetics are characterized as hyperbaric, hypobaric, or isobaric relative to cerebrospinal fluid. • Normal lumbar lordosis and thoracic kyphosis of the spine also play a role in determining the final anesthetic level. • The dose and specific type of local anesthetic agent used determine the **duration** of the resultant blockade, but not **spread**. • Relatively small volumes are utilized for spinal anesthesia and have little effect on the resultant neural blockade.

ANSWER:
A, B, C

8. Which of the following is/are true regarding malignant hyperthermia (MH)?

   A. The propensity to develop MH is a genetically transferred trait.

   B. MH can be triggered by all potent (halogenated) inhalational agents.

   C. MH can be triggered by succinylcholine.

   D. Hyperthermia is an early sign of MH.

Ref.: 1–5

COMMENTS: MH is a rare, potentially lethal condition. • A fulminant episode is characterized by muscle rigidity, fever, tachycardia, respiratory and metabolic acidosis, severe hypermetabolism, arrhythmias, and eventual cardiovascular collapse. • MH can occur minutes to several hours after the administration of triggering agents, such as succinylcholine or potent (halogenated) inhalation agents. • The earliest, most sensitive, and specific sign of MH is an unexplained rise in end-tidal CO_2 levels (with venous blood gas acidosis) followed by tachycardia, frequently with multifocal premature ventricular contractions. • *Temperature increases are a relatively late finding.*

   Treatment involves cessation of triggering anesthetics, administration of dantrolene, forced cooling of the patient, induction of saline diuresis to avoid renal dysfunction from myoglobinuria and widespread rhabdomyolysis, and monitoring of blood gas and potassium levels. • MH is genetically transmitted, probably as an autosomal dominant trait with variable penetrance. • Elevated serum creatinine phosphokinase levels can be seen in MH-susceptible patients, but this test is not useful for screening because of its poor specificity. • Avoidance of triggering agents for patients suspected of MH susceptibility is the safest and easiest method of treatment.

ANSWER:
A, B, C

9. The benefits of epidural anesthesia include all but which of the following?

   A. Lower incidence of dural puncture headache compared to spinal anesthesia

   B. Decreased mortality rate compared to general anesthesia in high-risk surgical patients

   C. Reduced incidence of deep venous thrombosis during lower-extremity surgery

   D. Improved short-term graft patency during lower-extremity arterial bypass procedures

   E. Better ability to titrate level of anesthesia than with spinal anesthesia

Ref.: 1–3

COMMENTS: The use of epidural anesthesia has greatly increased since the mid-1970s. • Local anesthetic injected into the epidural space crosses the dura, producing regional anesthesia and analgesia. • Reported benefits include a reduced incidence of deep venous thrombosis during lower-extremity surgery, better titratability than with spinal anesthesia, improved vascular graft patency up to 6 months after surgery, and decreased incidence of spinal headache. • Additional benefits include enhanced postoperative pain relief via continuous epidural administration of opioids or dilute concentrations of local anesthetics (or both), and the need for less general anesthetic when used intraoperatively as an adjuvant for major thoracic, abdominal, and orthopedic procedures. • However, the mortality rate for high-risk patients has not been shown to be different than observed with general anesthesia.

ANSWER:
B

10. All but which of the following statements regarding the toxicity of local anesthetics is/are true?

    A. Neurologic symptoms almost always precede those of cardiac toxicity.

    B. Site of injection is an important determinant of toxicity.

    C. Addition of 1:100,000 epinephrine solution allows for administration of higher doses of local anesthetics.

    D. Relative toxicity is procaine < lidocaine < bupivacaine < tetracaine.

    E. Pregnancy reduces the risk of toxicity because hormones induce resistance to local anesthetics.

Ref.: 1–3, 5

COMMENTS: Systemic toxicity from local anesthetics primarily involves the central nervous system (CNS) and the cardiovascular system. • **CNS toxicity** usually occurs at doses well below those that result in cardiovascular toxicity. • Manifestations of CNS toxicity include confusion, dizziness, tinnitus, somnolence, and seizures. • The seizures are thought to be due to blockade of inhibitory pathways in the cerebral cortex. • **Cardiovascular toxicity** is due to direct blocking effects on both cardiac and vascular smooth muscle and is usually manifested as cardiovascular collapse. • Ventricular arrhythmias and asystole are the commonest electrocardiographic findings.

   Systemic absorption of the local anesthetics is highly dependent on the vascularity of the injection site and the presence or absence of epinephrine. • Epinephrine causes vasoconstriction and allows a higher maximum dose of local anesthetic to be safely administered without toxicity. • Absorption of local anesthetics occurs most rapidly, with the highest serum levels, from the highly vascular intercostal space and is slowest, with the lowest serum levels, from local subcutaneous tissue infiltration.

   Pregnancy reduces the toxic threshold as well as the dose of local anesthetic needed for therapeutic purposes. • The enlargement of epidural veins seen with progressive enlargement of the uterus decreases the size of the epidural space and the volume of cerebrospinal fluid in the subarachnoid space. • The decreased volume of these spaces facilitates the spread of local anesthesia. • Biochemical changes of pregnancy, particularly progesterone, may also play a role in toxicity and spread of local anesthetics. • It has been shown to have potent sedative effects.

ANSWER:
E

11. Which of the following statements regarding propofol is not true?

   A. Induction and sedation doses for children are higher than those for adults, after adjusting for weight.

   B. Propofol is a white, milky emulsion that may be contraindicated for patients with egg allergy.

   C. Unlike other induction agents, propofol does not suppress the respiratory system.

   D. The incidence of nausea and vomiting is lower with propofol-based anesthesia than with thiopental/isoflurane anesthesia.

   E. Hemodynamic changes seen with equianesthetic doses are frequently greater with propofol than with thiopental.

Ref.: 1, 2, 6

COMMENTS: Propofol is a nonbenzodiazepine, nonbarbiturate intravenous anesthetic with hypnotic properties. • Stemming from its chemical structure as a substituted derivative of phenol, it is insoluble in water and is formulated as a 1% emulsion similar to parenteral lipid formulations. • Persons allergic to eggs may have allergies to this formulation. • Induction doses are higher for children and adolescents than for adults and should be reduced for elderly patients, hypovolemic patients, and those with poor cardiac reserve. • Propofol produces profound dose-dependent respiratory depression that frequently leads to apnea in patients premedicated with other sedatives. • After single-bolus administration, propofol is rapidly redistributed (in 2–8 min) and highly metabolized. • For this reason, it is most commonly administered by continuous intravenous infusion. • Emergence from anesthesia occurs rapidly after discontinuation of propofol, making it particularly suitable for short procedures. • Nausea and vomiting are seen less frequently with a propofol-based anesthetic than with thiopental/isoflurane anesthesia, but hemodynamic alterations are similar or even greater than those seen with equianesthetic doses of thiopental.

ANSWER:
C

12. Which of the following statements regarding midazolam is/are true?

   A. The degree of anxiolysis, sedation, or hypnosis achieved with midazolam depends on the percentage occupancy of the drug at the benzodiazepine-aminobutyric acid (GABA) receptor sites in the CNS.

   B. Midazolam is two to four times as potent as diazepam.

   C. Respiratory depression caused by midazolam is usually minor but can be greatly exacerbated by concomitant use of other sedatives or opioids.

   D. Midazolam has no active metabolites, making it ideal for use in outpatients.

Ref.: 1, 2, 6

COMMENTS: Midazolam differs from other benzodiazepines in both structure and solubility. • An imidazole side ring imparts stability and ease of rapid hepatic metabolism, and a water-soluble structure allows for painless injection. • Two active metabolites of midazolam exist and accumulate when continuous infusions are used. • Like other benzodiazepines, midazolam potentiates respiratory depression (often synergistically) when administered with other sedatives or opioids. • Benzodiazepines readily cross the placenta and have been associated with an increased incidence of cleft lip and palate formation when administered during the first trimester. • Safety later in pregnancy has not been definitively established.

ANSWER:
A, B, C

13. Which of the following statements regarding neuromuscular blockade by nondepolarizing agents is not true?

   A. Effects are prolonged by aminoglycosides.

   B. Vagolytic side effects occur with pancuronium.

   C. Nondepolarizing agents trigger MH.

   D. Vecuronium undergoes mostly hepatic metabolism.

   E. Train-of-four monitoring effectively predicts the degree of blockade.

Ref.: 1, 2, 6

COMMENTS: Nondepolarizing muscle relaxants currently in clinical use include pancuronium, vecuronium, atracurium, *cis*-atracurium, mivacurium, rocuronium, and doxacurium. • Nondepolarizing muscle relaxants interfere with transmission at the neuromuscular junction by competing with acetylcholine for available receptor sites. • These effects may be reversed by anticholinesterases, which prolong the half-life of acetylcholine to overcome the competitive inhibition of the muscle relaxant. • The effect of nondepolarizing agents can be prolonged by aminoglycosides, clindamycin, tetracycline and other antibiotics, hypothermia, hypercarbia, and magnesium. • Vagolytic activity is common with pancuronium and rocuronium but not with other agents. • Except for mivacurium (which is metabolized by plasma cholinesterase) and atracurium/*cis*-atracurium (which is metabolized by Hoffman elimination and nonspecific ester hydrolysis), metabolism of nondepolarizing agents occurs in the liver, with varying amounts of biliary or renal metabolism and excretion. • Train-of-four monitoring involves the administration of stimuli percutaneously to a peripheral nerve four times over 1 second and noting the distal muscular response. • If fewer than two of the stimuli result in muscle contraction, more than 95% of receptors are blocked.

ANSWER:
C

14. Which of the following statements regarding flumazenil is/are true?

   A. It is a benzodiazepine antagonist that acts by competitive inhibition at the benzodiazepine receptor in CNS tissue.

   B. It has been used successfully to reverse the clinical effects of hepatic encephalopathy.

   C. It is contraindicated for patients with suspected cyclic antidepressant overdoses.

   D. It reverses the respiratory depressant actions but not the sedative effects of all benzodiazepines.

Ref.: 1, 2, 6

COMMENTS: Flumazenil is a benzodiazepine-specific antagonist that competitively inhibits the activity of benzodiazepines at the benzodiazepine-receptor complex. • Flumazenil does *not* antagonize the CNS effects of GABAergic-acting drugs (ethanol, barbiturates, or general anesthetics), nor does it antagonize the effects of opioids. • Flumazenil antagonizes the sedation, impaired recall, psychomotor impairment, and ventilatory depression produced by all benzodiazepines. • Use of flumazenil is contraindicated for patients given benzodiazepines for life-threatening conditions (e.g., control of status epilepticus or ICP), patients showing serious signs of cyclic antidepressant overdose (due to an increased occurrence of seizures), and patients with known hypersensitivities. • Case reports have demonstrated remarkable improvement in encephalopathic changes associated with liver failure. • Flumazenil should not be used as the only agent for treating hepatic encephalopathy but may be helpful for patients resistant to conventional medical therapy.

ANSWER:
A, B, C

15. Mechanisms of heat loss during general anesthesia include which of the following?

A. Convection

B. Radiation

C. Conduction

D. Evaporation

E. All of the above

Ref.: 1, 2, 5

COMMENTS: Heat loss in the operating room (OR) is a complex problem involving all of the above mechanisms. • The contribution of each mechanism depends on the surrounding conditions in the OR. • **Radiative** losses are often cited as the largest contributor to heat loss in the OR. • Radiant energy is emitted by every body having a temperature greater than 0° K. • Radiation requires no medium for transport because it is electromagnetic. • Heat freely radiates from a body at a temperature of 37°C to a room at 25°C as long as the temperature gradient exists. • **Conductive** heat loss requires that bodies be in direct contact with each other. • Body heat is conducted to the OR table and other surfaces that come in contact with the patient. • Heat is lost from the body by **convection** when OR air, which is circulated at a speed of approximately 3 cm/s, passes over the body. • Finally, heat losses from latent heat of vaporization (**evaporation**) occur during mechanical ventilation with dry air, skin preparation with cold cleansing solutions, through sweating, and from large open wounds.

ANSWER:
E

16. With regard to pulse oximetric studies, which of the following is/are true?

A. Pulse oximetric analysis is considered a standard of care for all surgical procedures requiring general anesthesia.

B. Methemoglobinemia, sometimes observed with nitroglycerin toxicity, results in a displayed arterial oxygen saturation of 85%.

C. Oxygen saturation measurements may be artificially elevated in the presence of carboxyhemoglobin.

D. A standard pulse oximeter measures light absorption at four wavelengths.

Ref.: 1, 4, 6

COMMENTS: The use of pulse oximetric studies has led to marked improvement in the care and safety of patients not only in the OR but also in the postanesthesia care unit and the intensive care unit. • The concept of oximetry is based on **Beer's law**, which relates the concentration of a solute in suspension (in this case, hemoglobin) to the intensity of light transmitted through the solution. • Pulse oximetric analysis measures the oxygen saturation

only of pulsatile blood by using two wavelengths of light (red and infrared). • The ratio of the pulse-added absorbencies of these two wavelengths is determined by the arterial oxygen saturation.

Because both **oxyhemoglobin** and **carboxyhemoglobin** absorb red light similarly, the pulse oximeter reads the sum of the two hemoglobins, producing an artificially elevated reading of the oxygen saturation. • A direct measurement of saturation from an arterial blood gas sample is required to confirm the presence of carbon monoxide. • **Methemoglobinemia**, a disorder that may occur with nitroglycerin toxicity, results in a displayed oxygen saturation of 85%. • Methemoglobin does not absorb red light in the same manner as does oxyhemoglobin or deoxyhemoglobin. • The absorbance of red and infrared light by methemoglobin is nearly equal and results in a displayed saturation of approximately 85%. • Because ambient light can affect pulse oximeter readings, it is occasionally necessary to cover the probe to avoid artifactual readings.

ANSWER:
A, B, C

17. While transporting an intubated patient from the OR to the intensive care unit, the pressure gauge on a completely filled size E compressed-gas cylinder containing O_2 reads 2200 pounds per square inch (psi). How long can O_2 be delivered at a flow rate of 5 L/min from an E cylinder whose pressure gauge reads 1100 psi?

A. 60 s

B. 5 min

C. 60 min

D. 125 min

E. 220 min

Ref.: 1, 2

COMMENTS: A full E cylinder reading 2200 psi contains approximately 625 L of O_2. • **Boyle's law** states that, for a fixed mass of gas at a constant temperature, the product of pressure and volume is constant. • Boyle's law allows the estimation of the volume of gas remaining in a closed container by measuring the pressure within the container. • When the pressure gauge reads 1100 psi, the volume of gas in the cylinder is half that of a full cylinder (or about 625 L ÷ 2 = 312.5 L). • At a flow of 5 L/min, the cylinder in question will last approximately 1 hr. • This information is important when portable sources of oxygen are used during transport and diagnostic procedures remote from the OR.

ANSWER:
C

18. After administration of epidural anesthesia to the T3 dermatome of a patient with severe lung disease who is undergoing open cholecystectomy, which of the following is least likely to occur?

A. Increased heart rate

B. Decreased venous return

C. Decreased alveolar ventilation

D. Systemic hypotension

Ref.: 1, 2, 5

COMMENTS: On average, central neuraxial blockade to the T3 **sensory** dermatome is associated with **sympathetic** blockade two spinal segment levels higher and **motor** blockade two spinal segments lower. • Blockade of the cardiac accelerator nerves

(T1–T4) and unopposed vagal activity result in relative bradycardia despite hypotension caused by the reduction in venous return secondary to vasodilation. • In addition, motor nerve blockade of intercostal muscle function reduces alveolar ventilation and may precipitate respiratory embarrassment in a patient with underlying pulmonary disease, particularly if a significant fraction of intercostal muscle function is impaired.

ANSWER:
A

19. Which of the following is least likely to occur in conjunction with a surgically induced stress response?

   A. Increased metabolic rate

   B. Hypercoagulability

   C. Immune response suppression

   D. Increased secretion of adrenocorticotropic hormone

   E. Increased secretion of thyroid-stimulating hormone

Ref.: 7

COMMENTS: Current evidence suggests that many adverse perioperative events can be attributed to the effects of the stress response. • Somatic and/or visceral pain can trigger the systemic release of catecholamines and neuroendocrine hormones. • Hormones released in response to stress include growth hormone, adrenocorticotropic hormone, vasopressin, prolactin, cortisol, glucagons, and renin-angiotensin aldosterone. • In contrast, secretion of thyroid-stimulating hormone is decreased by the stress response. • The overall systemic effects of the stress response lead to increased metabolic activity, a hypercoagulable state, and a less effective immune response to infectious agents.

ANSWER:
E

20. Preoperative noninvasive testing for the presence of inducible myocardial ischemia would be most appropriate for which of the following patients?

   A. A healthy 60-year-old man without historical cardiac risk factors scheduled for a gastrectomy due to gastric carcinoma

   B. A patient with a history of myocardial infarction 1 year ago and good exercise tolerance undergoing a laparoscopic cholecystectomy

   C. A patient with diabetes and renal insufficiency undergoing an inguinal hernia repair

   D. A patient with limited exercise tolerance and diabetes undergoing a right hemicolectomy

Ref.: 1

COMMENTS: The need for preoperative cardiac testing is determined by assessing a patient's risk of perioperative cardiac complications and the likelihood that the surgical procedure will produce physiologic conditions that increase myocardial demands. • Good exercise tolerance is an important prognostic determinant and can mitigate the need for cardiac testing if patients have known stable cardiac disease and are undergoing intermediate-risk surgery. • Operations associated with large fluid shifts and/or high blood loss, along with vascular surgical procedures, are commonly cited as higher-risk operations. • Patients at risk for cardiac complications will benefit from perioperative β-blocker therapy, and

β-blockers should be given to all patients with cardiac risk factors unless contraindicated. • Patients at high risk for cardiac complications undergoing intermediate- to high-risk surgical procedures (in reference to cardiac outcomes) should undergo noninvasive assessment of cardiac performance and possibly invasive testing if noninvasive results suggest significant cardiac risk. • Since surgery in itself is not an indication for cardiac testing, the patient described in A needs no further cardiac workup.

ANSWER:
D

21. A 67-year-old woman is scheduled for a right hemicolectomy due to carcinoma of the colon. She has adult-onset diabetes and shortness of breath when climbing stairs. A 12-lead electrocardiogram shows signs of bradycardia with left bundle-branch block. The serum creatinine level is 2.1 mg/dL. What is the most appropriate next step?

   A. Conduct cardiac catheterization immediately.

   B. Proceed with surgery and evaluate risk status postoperatively.

   C. Administer an exercise electrocardiogram.

   D. Administer a dobutamine stress echocardiogram.

   E. Institute β-blockade.

Ref.: 1

COMMENTS: This patient has a number of intermediate risk factors for perioperative cardiac complications, including an elevated serum creatinine level, limited exercise tolerance, left bundle-branch block, and diabetes. • It is possible that perioperative risk can be altered by preoperative testing and subsequent interventions. • Provocative cardiac tests such as a dobutamine stress echocardiogram further stratify risk and help to identify patients who need further cardiac workup or interventions.

ANSWER:
D

REFERENCES

1. Rogers MC, Tinker JH, Covino BG, et al (eds): *Principles and Practice of Anesthesiology.* Mosby-Year Book, St. Louis, 1993.
2. Stoelting RK (ed): *Pharmacology and Physiology in Anesthetic Practice,* 2nd ed. JB Lippincott, Philadelphia, 1991.
3. Sabiston DC Jr (ed): *Textbook of Surgery, The Biological Basis of Modern Surgical Practice,* 15th ed. Saunders, Philadelphia, 1997.
4. Schwartz SI, Shires GT, Spencer FC (eds): *Principles of Surgery,* 7th ed. McGraw-Hill, New York, 1999.
5. O'Leary JP (ed): *The Physiologic Basis of Surgery,* 2nd ed. Williams & Wilkins, Baltimore, 1996.
6. Greenfield LJ, Mulholland M, Oldham KT, et al (eds): *Surgery: Scientific Principles and Practice,* 2nd ed. Lippincott-Raven, Philadelphia, 1997.
7. Fleisher LA, Eagle KA: Clinical practice: lowering cardiac risk in noncardiac surgery. *N Engl J Med* 345:1677–1682, 2001.
8. Eagle KA, Berger PB, Calkins H, et al: ACC/AHA guideline update for perioperative cardiovascular evaluation for noncardiac surgery, executive summary: a report of the American College of Cardiology/American Heart Association Task Force on Practice Guidelines. *Anesth Analg* 94:1052-1064, 2002.

C H A P T E R 13

Immunology

Theresa W. Ruddy, M.D., and Richard A. Prinz, M.D.

1. Which of the following statements regarding the immune response is/are true?

   A. The primary immune response is more intense and rapid than the secondary immune response.

   B. A cell-mediated immune response consists primarily of T lymphocytes.

   C. B lymphocytes are precursors of plasma cells, which produce antibodies.

   D. The immune response has three phases, the first being the establishment of memory.

   Ref.: 1–5

COMMENTS: The immune response is characterized by a series of reactions triggered by an immunogen, defined as any one of a number of substances capable of triggering an immune response. Immunogens include substances recognized as foreign, or "nonself" (e.g., virus, bacteria, and histoincompatible tissues), as well as substances that are "altered self," or "modified self" (e.g., most tumor antigens). All immune responses, whether primary or secondary, are characterized by three phases: (1) **cognitive phase** (recognition of nonself antigen); (2) **activation phase** (proliferation of immunocompetent cells or lymphocytes); and (3) **effector phase** (development of immunologic memory). • The **primary** immune response is the result of the first (or primary) exposure to a specific antigen. • The **secondary** response results from a second (or third or fourth) exposure to the same antigen. • It is more rapid and more intense than the primary response and is the result of the phenomenon of immunologic memory.

There are two basic types of immune responses: a **cell-mediated** immune response (cellular immunity), mediated primarily by T lymphocytes, and a **humoral** immune response, mediated primarily by B lymphocytes. • There are two major types of lymphocyte. • **B lymphocytes**, or **B cells**, differentiate into antibody-producing plasma cells after activation. • They develop in the fetal liver and the bone marrow. • B lymphocytes are precursors of the plasma cell and can be identified by specific antigen-binding sites on their surface. • Plasma cells produce antibodies that are found in serum and that may be transferred passively in the serum. • **T lymphocytes**, or **T cells**, mature in the thymus from multipotential cells derived from the bone marrow.

A N S W E R :
B, C

2. Which of the following statements regarding the immune system is/are true?

   A. T lymphocytes develop in the fetal liver and in the bone marrow.

   B. The thymus and bone marrow are primary lymphoid organs.

   C. The spleen is a secondary lymphoid organ, and lymph nodes are tertiary lymph organs.

   D. Only lymphocytes that differentiate into B cells express differentiation antigens on their cell surface.

   Ref.: 1–5

COMMENTS: See Question 3.

3. Which of the following statements regarding T cells is/are true?

   A. T cells finish development in the thymus and then migrate to the spleen and lymph nodes.

   B. The various types of T cells can be identified by the binding of specific monoclonal antibodies to antigens on the cell surface.

   C. Helper T cells can be activated to produce antibodies.

   D. Cytotoxic T cells can destroy target cells by recognizing foreign antigens on the target cell surface.

   Ref.: 1–5

COMMENTS: T lymphocytes (T cells) mature in the thymus, and B lymphocytes (B cells) mature in the fetal liver and the bone marrow. • The thymus, liver, and bone marrow are referred to as the **primary** lymphoid organs. • The T and B lymphocytes subsequently migrate to the **secondary** lymphoid organs: the spleen, lymph nodes, and dispersed lymphoid tissues found in the bronchus, urogenital tract, and gut (i.e., Peyer's patches).

Lymphocytes that differentiate into T cells and B cells express various clusters of antigens on their membranes. • All of the T cells express the differentiation antigen cluster designated CD3, whereas B cells express the differentiation antigen clusters CD19 and CD20. • The CD3+ T cells can be distinguished and subdivided further by the expression of additional differentiation antigens on the T-cell surface, indicating them to be cytotoxic T cells (CD3+/CD8+), suppressor T cells (CD3+/CD8+), helper/inducer T cells (CD3+/CD4+), and delayed-type hypersensitivity T cells (CD3+/CD4+).

Cytotoxic T cells are capable of destroying a target cell by recognizing a foreign or "modified-self" antigen and class I major histocompatibility complex (MHC) molecules on the target-cell surface. • **Suppressor T cells** tend to suppress the activity of other T and B cells. • **Helper T cells** stimulate B cells to differentiate into plasma cells that produce antibody, facilitate maturation of precytotoxic T cells, and stimulate macrophages to produce a nonspecific, delayed inflammatory response. • Delayed-type hypersensitivity T cells bring macrophages and other inflammatory cells to areas in which delayed-type hypersensitivity reactions occur through the production of various chemoattractant molecules known collectively as chemokines.

ANSWER:
Question 2: B
Question 3: B, D

4. Which of the following statements regarding the MHC is/are true?

A. The MHC is a gene cluster on chromosome 6 that codes for proteins important to the process of rejection.

B. Part of the MHC codes for some components of the complement cascade.

C. Class I antigens are coded for by the D region of the MHC.

D. Class II MHC with bound antigen is recognized by the CD8$^+$ cytotoxic T cell.

E. Class I antigens are expressed only on leukocytes.

Ref.: 1–5

COMMENTS: The MHC is a cluster of genes located on human chromosome 6. • A copy of each MHC comes from each parent. • There are three classes of the MHC. • **Class I** MHC products are coded for by genes in the A and B regions of the MHC and are called class I antigens. • Class I antigens are glycoproteins found in the plasma membrane of all nucleated cells and platelets. • The class I MHC with bound antigen is recognized by the cytotoxic (CD8$^+$) T cell, leading to lysis of the target cell. • **Class II** antigens are also transmembrane glycoproteins that are coded for by genes in the D region of the MHC. • The class II antigens are expressed on B lymphocytes, macrophages, monocytes, and dendritic cells. • The class II MHC with bound antigen is recognized by the CD4$^+$ helper T cell. • This activates the helper T cell, which stimulates the development of cytotoxic T cells or B cells. • **Class III** proteins are components of the complement cascade that are coded for in the MHC. • Expression of MHC products are important in "self" identification and therefore in the process of rejection.

ANSWER:
A, B

5. Which of the following statements regarding antibodies is/are true?

A. Antibodies are composed of a variable region, which interacts with the host, and a constant region, which interacts with an antigen.

B. Antibodies are composed of four polypeptide chains consisting of two heavy chains and two light chains stabilized by interchain and intrachain disulfide bonds.

C. Immunoglobulin G (IgG) is the largest antibody.

D. Immunoglobulin M (IgM) is the major antibody produced during the primary immune response.

Ref.: 1–5

COMMENTS: Antibodies are a type of serum protein produced by plasma cells. • They are made up of a variable region and a constant region. • The variable region (Fab) is able to bind specifically to an antigen. • The constant region (Fc) mediates functions such as complement fixation and monocyte binding. • Genetic recombination allows for the diversity of the variable region, enabling antibodies to bind many types of antigen. • Antibody molecules have the basic structure of four polypeptide chains consisting of two identical heavy chains and two identical light chains cross-linked by interchain and intrachain disulfide bonds (see diagram). • IgG functions as an opsonin by binding to phagocyte Fc receptors. • When complement concurrently interacts with phagocyte receptors, there is a greatly amplified phagocytic response. • The largest antibody is IgM, which is a pentamer consisting of five monomeric units. • IgM is located on B-cell membranes and functions as the earliest antigen receptor. • IgM is released and stimulates B-cell differentiation, along with production of other immunoglobulins.

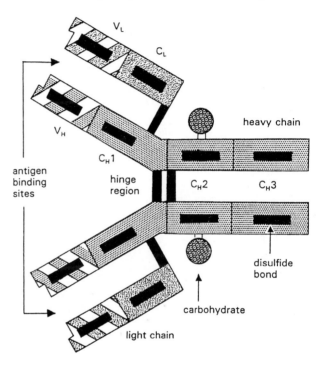

ANSWER:
B, D

6. Match each immunoglobulin in the left-hand column with the appropriate statement(s) in the right-hand column.

A. IgA   a. Binds mast cells
B. IgG   b. Major antibody of the secondary immune response
C. IgM   c. Most prevalent serum immunoglobulin
D. IgD   d. May bind complement
E. IgE   e. Found particularly in secretions
         f. Function unknown
         g. Mediates type I hypersensitivity reactions

Ref.: 1–5

COMMENTS: The five classes of antibodies are immunoglobulins A, G, M, D, and E. • They are distinguished by their heavy chains. • IgA is found in secretions and functions to protect mucous membranes. • IgG is the most prevalent serum immunoglobulin and the major antibody produced during the secondary immune response. • It is able to bind complement and function as an opsonin (an antibody that binds antigen to neutrophils and macrophages via the constant region). • IgM is a large antibody that is the major antibody produced during the primary immune response. • Like IgG, IgM can also fix complement. • IgD is found in minimal amounts, and its function is unknown. • IgE binds to mast cells and basophils. • After IgE binds antigen, it causes mast cells and basophils to release histamine and other substances that mediate type I hypersensitivity reactions.

A N S W E R :
A-e; B-b,c,d; C-d; D-f; E-a,g

---

7. Which of the following statements regarding immunogens is/are true?

   A. Immunogens have multiple antigenic epitopes, each of which may react with an antibody or T-cell antigen receptor specific for it.

   B. An antigen may be defined as any molecule recognized as foreign by the immune system.

   C. Immunogenicity is greater with a xenogeneic antigen than with a syngeneic antigen.

   D. Proteins are generally more complex than are nucleic acids and are therefore more immunogenic.

                                                          Ref.: 1–5

COMMENTS: An immunogen is any substance that can stimulate an immune response. • An antigen may be defined as any molecule recognized by the immune response. • Most immunogens have multiple antigenic epitopes, molecular structures that can react with the variable region of an antibody or the T-cell antigen receptor specific for that individual epitope. • Immunogenicity increases with increased grades of foreignness, complexity, and size. • **Foreignness** is greatest with a xenogeneic antigen (different species), less with an allogeneic antigen (same species, different genotype), even less with a syngeneic antigen (same species, same genotype), and least with an autologous (self) antigen. • **Complexity** is greatest with proteins, less with carbohydrates, and least with nucleic acids and lipids. • **Size** of more than 5000 daltons is generally required for a substance to be immunogeneic.

A N S W E R :
A, B, C, D

---

8. Which of the following statements regarding phagocytosis is/are true?

   A. Neutrophils are the major phagocytic cell within the tissue.

   B. Lysosomal granules require oxygen to destroy foreign particles.

   C. Chronic granulomatous disease results from a flaw in production of superoxide anions and, eventually, hydrogen peroxide in neutrophils.

   D. Once a monocyte migrates to tissue to become a macrophage, it loses all function except phagocytosis.

                                                          Ref.: 1–5

COMMENTS: There are two groups of phagocytic cells: mononuclear and polymorphonuclear. • **Monocytes** are mononuclear phagocytes that are derived from bone marrow and migrate to tissues, where they mature to become macrophages.

• **Neutrophils** are polymorphonuclear and are the major phagocytic cell within the tissue. • They circulate in the blood and migrate quickly to areas of inflammation.

During phagocytosis, a foreign particle is engulfed by part of the phagocyte to form a vacuole, or phagosome. • Lysosomal granules within the phagocyte bind with the phagosome to form a phagolysosome, where the foreign particle is destroyed through both oxygen-dependent and oxygen-independent mechanisms. • Oxygen-dependent mechanisms include formation of myeloperoxidase, superoxide anion, hydrogen peroxide, singlet oxygen, and hydroxyl radicals. • Oxygen-independent mechanisms include formation of cationic proteins, lysosomes, and proteinases. • In granulomatous disease, there is a flaw in the production of superoxide anions and hydrogen peroxide.

In addition to phagocytosis, macrophages break down, process, and present antigen to T and B lymphocytes. • They also secrete factors that facilitate clonal expansion of the antigen-specific lymphocytes. • Macrophages produce a wide variety of cytokines, including tumor necrosis factor (TNF), interferons, and interleukin-1 (IL-1).

A N S W E R :
A, C

---

9. Which of the following statements regarding nonspecific immune reactivity is/are true?

   A. Natural killer (NK) cells are large granular lymphocytes that do not express the T- or B-cell phenotype.

   B. NK cells require previous exposure to antigen to express cytotoxicity.

   C. NK activity is not restricted by the MHC.

   D. Interferon augments the activity of NK cells and macrophages.

                                                          Ref.: 1–5

COMMENTS: NK cells are large granular lymphocytes that do not express the T-cell– or B-cell–specific phenotype. • They mediate cytotoxicity toward a variety of targets, despite a lack of previous exposure to antigens from those targets. • NK-cell targets include cells infected with virus and "altered self" cells, such as tumor cells. • The cytotoxicity mediated by NK cells is not restricted by the MHC, and it can be greatly enhanced by various cytokines. • Interferons are glycoproteins synthesized by a variety of cells in response to viral infection. • They augment the activity of a number of cells, including macrophages and T cells, as well as NK cells.

A N S W E R :
A, C, D

---

10. Match the cell type in the left-hand column with the appropriate statement(s) in the right-hand column.

   A. T cells   a. Type of lymphocyte
   B. Macrophages   b. Provide some type of antitumor
                                  surveillance
   C. NK cells   c. Generated from culture of NK
                                  cells with interleukin-2 (IL-2)
   D. Lymphokine-activated   d. Used for anticancer
      killer cells   immunotherapy
   E. Tumor-infiltrating   e. Are NK cells sensitized by IL-2
      lymphocytes

                                                          Ref.: 1–5

COMMENTS: Lymphocytes include all T cells, B cells, NK cells, NK-derived lymphokine-activated killer cells, and tumor-infiltrating lymphocytes. • Macrophages and NK cells provide surveillance against foreign cells, including malignant cells. • Culture of NK cells with the cytokine IL-2 leads to the generation of lymphokine-activated killer (LAK) cells. • LAK cells possess augmented cytotoxicity against a broad array of tumor targets. • LAK cells show promise in animal models of tumor therapy. • In humans, LAK cells with IL-2 have shown minimal results against refractory renal cell carcinoma and melanoma. • Tumor-infiltrating lymphocytes are generated by culturing lymphocytes isolated from within disaggregated tumors with IL-2 for several weeks. • They have shown antitumor activity, and studies regarding their clinical use are ongoing.

ANSWER:
A-a,d; B-b; C-a,b; D-a,c,d,e; E-a,d

11. Which of the following statements regarding T-cell activation is/are true?

    A. Some antigens are processed and expressed on antigen-presenting macrophages.

    B. Antigen recognition is not specific, which allows clonal expansion and differentiation.

    C. Antigen expression requires the T cell to be MHC compatible with the antigen-presenting cell.

    D. T cells produce IL-1 in response to antigen presentation.

    E. Plasma cells are responsible for the synthesis of IL-2.

Ref.: 1–5

COMMENTS: When antigen enters a lymph node or the spleen, it may be first phagocytized by a macrophage, which processes the antigen and expresses it on the cell surface for presentation to B and T lymphocytes (see diagram). • Macrophages that do this are called **antigen-presenting cells.** • Other antigen-presenting cells include dendritic cells (a macrophage-like cell found in skin, lymph nodes, and other tissues) and a subset of B lymphocytes. • Recognition of

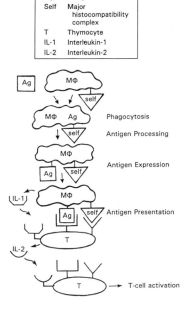

the antigen is highly specific and accomplished only by T-lymphocyte clones that have a receptor specific to that antigen. • When antigen is presented to the T cell, macrophages produce IL-1, T cells produce IL-2, and T cells increase expression of IL-2 receptor on the surface. • This activation by IL-2 causes T cells to proliferate. • Helper T cells interact with B cells to stimulate their differentiation into plasma cells that produce antibodies. • Plasma cells do not produce IL-2.

ANSWER:
A, C

12. Which of the following statements regarding interleukins is/are true?

    A. All interleukins will only up-regulate the immune system.

    B. Interleukin-8 (IL-8) is a neutrophil chemotactic factor.

    C. Interleukins are produced only by leukocytes.

    D. Interleukin-3 (IL-3) functions as a general hematopoietic growth factor.

Ref.: 1–5

COMMENTS: Interleukins are a group of cytokines that function in many various ways to up- and down-regulate the immune system. • IL-3 functions as a hematopoietic growth factor. • Interleukin-4 (IL-4), interleukin-6 (IL-6), and interleukin-10 (IL-10) are the interleukins that have known inhibitory functions. • IL-4 inhibits macrophage secretion of cytokines. • IL-6 inhibits TNF. • IL-10 inhibits monocyte/macrophage function and counteracts inflammatory cytokines. • IL-4, IL-6, and IL-10 also have a stimulatory function. • Interleukin-8 (IL-8) attracts neutrophils to the site of inflammation by movement through the vascular endothelium. • Interleukins are produced by a variety of cells, including macrophages and monocytes, T and B lymphocytes, mast cells, stromal cells of the thymus and bone marrow, fibroblasts, epithelial cells, and endothelial cells. • Most of the interleukins stimulate a particular or a few varieties of leukocytes.

ANSWER:
B, D

13. Which of the following statements regarding the cytokine IL-1 is/are true?

    A. The major cells that produce IL-1 are monocytes and macrophages.

    B. IL-1 leads to vasoconstriction and hypertension through stimulation of the hypothalamus.

    C. IL-1 may induce a fever.

    D. T-lymphocyte production of IL-2 is inhibited by IL-1.

    E. IL-1 may augment wound healing by increasing fibroblast proliferation and collagen synthesis.

Ref.: 1, 6

COMMENTS: Cells of the immune system cells are regulated by a variety of cytokines that are, in general, categorized according to their cell of origin. • One of these cytokines, IL-1, is a key regulator of inflammation, wound healing, and the immune response. • It is produced primarily by macrophages but is also produced by neutrophils, fibroblasts, NK cells, keratinocytes, endothelial cells, and vascular smooth muscle cells. • IL-1 can induce endothelial cells to produce prostaglandins, platelet-activating factor, and plasminogen activator, which can lead to vasodilation and hypotension by promoting endothelial leakage and intravascular thrombosis. • IL-1 directly stimulates the thermoregulatory center of the hypothalamus, inducing fever. • IL-1 stimulates the liver to produce several acute-phase proteins. • It plays a key role in joint inflammation by inducing synovial cells to produce prostaglandin E_2, collagenase, and phospholipase. • IL-1 mediates wound healing by activating basophils and eosinophils, stimulating neutrophil and macrophage activity, and locally increasing fibroblast proliferation and collagen synthesis. • IL-1 induces proliferation of T and B lymphocytes, IL-2 production, and expression of the IL-2 receptor. • IL-1 stimulates the release of other cytokines, including interferon, IL-3, IL-6, and colony-stimulating factors. • The effects of IL-1 on immunity are greatly amplified through stimulation of other cytokines. • IL-1 (along with TNF-α) are currently being studied as therapeutic agents for autoimmune disease, such as inflammatory bowel disease, psoriasis, and rheumatoid arthritis.

ANSWER:
A, C, E

14. Which of the following statements regarding IL-2 is/are true?

   A. The proliferation of T lymphocytes is inhibited by IL-2.

   B. IL-2 is produced by activated T lymphocytes.

   C. NK cell cytotoxicity is augmented by IL-2.

   D. Cytokine release by macrophages is inhibited by IL-2.

Ref.: 1, 6

COMMENTS: IL-2 was initially referred to as T-cell growth factor because it stimulated the proliferation of T lymphocytes in culture. • IL-2 is produced by activated T lymphocytes in response to presentation of antigen or IL-1. • It is also produced by NK cells. • IL-2 promotes the proliferation of activated T lymphocytes. • IL-2 stimulates B-cell proliferation and differentiation to plasma cells. • NK-cell proliferation and cytotoxic activity are augmented by IL-2. • IL-2 activates macrophages, leading to increased production of cytokines, including TNF and colony-stimulating factor. • IL-2 deficiency or IL-2 receptor deficiency leads to severe combined immunodeficiency.

ANSWER:
B, C

15. Which of the following statements regarding the complement cascade is/are true?

   A. Complement may be activated by immune complexes.

   B. The components C3a and C5a inhibit mast-cell release of granules.

   C. The components $C5b_{6,7,8,9}$ form a complex that causes cell lysis.

   D. The components C3a and C5a are chemotactic for macrophages and neutrophils.

Ref.: 1–5

COMMENTS: Complement components are mediators of inflammation and cell lysis. • The complement system is composed of 20 known proteins (C1, C2, C3a, C3b, ...), which are activated in a cascade mechanism. • The result is a small stimulus that leads to a greatly amplified effect. • The complement cascade is initiated by immune complexes (antigen bound to antibody) and by microbial products. • The initiator binds to the first component, C1. • Activated C3a and C5a act as chemotactic agents for macrophages and neutrophils. • Complement components are also anaphylatoxins in that they stimulate mast-cell degranulation, smooth muscle contraction, and increased vascular permeability. • Activated C5b initiates formation of the C5b-8 complex, which attaches to and lyses cell membranes.

ANSWER:
A, C, D

16. Which of the following statements regarding immunizations is/are true?

   A. Active immunization involves administration of either intact organisms or their component parts that are killed or biologically attenuated so that they are antigenic but do not produce disease.

   B. Passive immunization involves administration of an exogenous, immunologically active compound.

   C. The diphtheria-pertussis-tetanus (DPT) vaccine is an example of passive immunization.

   D. The Salk vaccine is an example of active immunization.

   E. RhoGAM is an example of a specific immunoglobulin administered for passive immunization.

Ref.: 1–5

COMMENTS: The two types of immunization are active and passive immunization. • **Active** immunization involves administration of intact organisms or their component parts that are killed or damaged so that they cannot cause disease but are still antigenic and cause an immune response. • **Passive** immunization involves administration of an exogenous, active component that provides immediate but only temporary specific immunity.

   One example of a bacterial vaccine currently used for active immunization is the DPT vaccine, which is a combination of inactivated diphtheria toxoid, heat-killed *Bordetella pertussis* organism, and inactivated *Clostridium tetani* toxoid. • Another example is the pneumovax vaccine. • Viral vaccines currently used for active immunization include the rubella, measles, mumps, poliomyelitis (Salk and Sabin vaccines), rabies, and hepatitis B vaccines.

   There are three types of passive immunization: antitoxin, immunoglobulin, and specific immunoglobulin. • **Antitoxins** are made from antiserum or neutralizing antibody specific for a given toxin, such as the *C. tetani* toxin. • **Immunoglobulin** is also referred to as gamma-globulin and is useful for maintenance of immunodeficient individuals. • RhoGAM, or Rh immunoglobulin, is an example of a **specific immune globulin.** • It is administered to Rh-negative women shortly after childbirth to prevent sensitization to Rh antibodies that cross the placenta from an Rh-positive infant to the mother during delivery.

ANSWER:
A, B, D, E

17. Match each type of hypersensitivity reaction in the left-hand column with the appropriate item(s) in the right-hand column.

   A. Type I   a. ABO incompatibility
   B. Type II   b. Contact dermatitis

C. Type III
D. Type IV

c. IgE bound to mast cells and basophils
d. Serum sickness
e. Anaphylaxis
f. IgG or IgM antibody reaction with cell-bound antigen
g. Tuberculin skin test

Ref.: 1–5

COMMENTS: Four types of hypersensitivity reactions have been defined. • They may be precipitated by both cell-mediated and humoral responses. • These reactions may lead to inflammation and tissue damage and may cause a wide variety of allergic and autoimmune diseases and conditions.

Type I (*immediate hypersensitivity*) reactions are initiated by antigens that react with IgE antibody. • They range from food allergy and hay fever to anaphylaxis. • Antigens include pollens, mold, danders, and food. • Binding of the antigen to IgE to mast cells or basophils results in release of a variety of mediators, including histamine, slow-reacting substance of anaphylaxis, serotonin, prostaglandins, and bradykinin. • Reactions vary in severity but generally include increased vascular permeability, increased secretions, and smooth muscle contraction. • They may clinically manifest as sniffling, sneezing, bronchoconstriction, angioedema, and even convulsions and death.

Type II reactions, also called *cytotoxic reactions*, result from the reaction of IgG or IgM antibodies with a cell-bound antigen. • The commonest example is the ABO and Rh incompatibility transfusion reaction, which leads to severe, almost immediate lysis of transfused red blood cells by anti-A or anti-B antibodies in the serum. • Although it does not cause immediate complement-mediated intravascular hemolysis, Rh incompatibility—caused by a reaction of the Rh antigen with anti-Rh antibodies—can be serious. • Other type II reactions include myasthenia gravis, resulting from autoantibodies to the acetylcholine receptors at the neuromuscular junction; Graves disease, in which autoantibodies against the thyroid-stimulating hormone receptor actually stimulate the thyroid; and idiopathic thrombocytopenic purpura, which results from antiplatelet antibodies.

Type III, or *immune-complex–mediated,* reactions result from deposition of the antibody-antigen complex from the circulation. • Classic immune-complex–mediated reactions include serum sickness, rheumatoid arthritis, and glomerulonephritis resulting from previous streptococcal infection, deposition of IgG-IgM complexes in the joints, deposition of immune complexes in the kidney, or systemic lupus erythematosus.

Type IV, or *delayed-type hypersensitivity,* reactions result from antigen stimulation of previously sensitized T cells, primarily CD4+ helper T cells. • The activated T cells then release cytokines and chemokines (chemoattractants), which result in the attraction and activation of other cells, particularly macrophages. • The classic clinical example is demonstrated by the tuberculin skin test, characterized by dermal induration due to lymphocyte and macrophage accumulation at the site of antigen injection, which develops over 48–72 hr. • Late hypersensitivity may play a role in the rejection of grafted tissues and organs. • The classic clinical example is contact dermatitis.

ANSWER:
A-c,e; B-a,f; C-d; D-b,g

18. Which of the following statements regarding TNF is/are true?

A. TNF is produced only by monocytes and macrophages.

B. TNF release is stimulated by endotoxin.

C. TNF is an anabolic stimulant to the host, resulting in deposition of fat.

D. TNF is responsible for cachexia associated with metastatic disease.

Ref.: 1, 6

COMMENTS: TNF is so named because of its ability to cause hemorrhagic necrosis in methylcholanthrene-induced sarcomas in mice. • TNF-α is produced primarily by monocytes and macrophages but also by neutrophils and NK cells. • TNF-β is produced by T and B lymphocytes. • TNF-α stimulates the activity of neutrophils and induces endothelial cells to produce IL-1 and synovial cells and fibroblasts to produce prostaglandin E_2 and collagenase. • TNF-α increases the procoagulant activity of endothelial surfaces, increases vascular permeability, degranulates neutrophils, and stimulates release of superoxides and arachidonic acid metabolites. • In gram-negative shock, endotoxin stimulates TNF-α release, which leads to hypotension, DIC, and even death. • TNF stimulates catabolism in muscle and fat cells, leading to an increase in anaerobic glycolysis, protein breakdown, and lipolysis. • It is largely responsible for cachexia associated with metastatic disease. • TNF-α also has a role in stimulating and mediating apoptosis.

ANSWER:
B, D

19. Which of the following statements regarding interferons is/are true?

A. Interferon-γ (INF-γ) is produced by macrophages.

B. Interferon production is inhibited by infection.

C. Interferons have a direct antiproliferative effect on cells.

D. Interferon-β (INF-β) is produced by fibroblasts.

E. Cytokine production by macrophages is inhibited by interferons.

Ref.: 1, 6

COMMENTS: Interferons are glycoproteins produced by a variety of cells in response to viral infection or other stimulants. • Interferons block viruses in two ways: through signaling pathways and by inhibition of translation machinery (protein synthesis). • There are three major classifications of interferons, based on their cells of origin: interferon-α (**INF-α**), produced mainly by macrophages; **INF-β**, produced by epithelial cells, fibroblasts, and macrophages; and **INF-γ**, produced by T lymphocytes and NK cells. • Interferons have a direct antiproliferative effect on cells but can also induce differentiation. • This explains their usefulness as anticancer agents, although some anticancer effects may also result from stimulation of the cytotoxic activity of macrophages, NK cells, and cytotoxic T cells. • Interferons stimulate a variety of cells to release other mediators and cytokines.

ANSWER:
C, D

20. Which of the following statements regarding chemokines is/are true?

A. Chemokines are high–molecular-weight molecules that are fixed to tissues.

B. Chemokines bind to specific receptors on leukocytes.

C. Chemokines are increased during an inflammatory event.

D. Some chemokines have been shown to protect cells against infection with HIV.

Ref.: 7

COMMENTS: A fundamental requirement for an effective immune response is the ability to recruit various kinds of immune cells to the site of an inflammatory or infectious event. • Studies conducted during the early 1990s identified a family of molecules, termed chemokines, that are responsible for this function. • Chemokines are low–molecular-weight cytokines that attract specific leukocyte populations to areas of inflammation and effect immune cell activation. • All members of the chemokine superfamily have four cysteine molecules linked by disulfide bonding.

The chemokines can be distinguished structurally by whether the first two cysteine molecules are adjacent (i.e., in a C-C sequence) or separated by an amino acid (i.e., in a C-X-C sequence). • The first chemokine to be identified was IL-8, a cytokine produced by activated monocytes and macrophages with chemoattractant effects on neutrophils. • By 1998, at least 30 chemokines had been identified and characterized as belonging to the C-C or C-X-C subgroups. • The ability of a chemokine to attract a specific leukocyte population is derived from the expression of a specific receptor for the chemokine on the leukocyte membrane. • To date, there are five recognized C-C chemokine receptors (designated CCR1–CCR5) and four recognized C-X-C receptors (designated CXCR1–CXCR4). • For example, the chemokine IL-8 is a C-X-C chemokine that binds to either the CXCR1 or the CXCR2 receptor on neutrophils. • The CXCR1 receptor is specific for IL-8, whereas the CXCR2 receptor binds IL-8 and other C-X-C chemokines.

Immune cell stimulation and activation often lead to increased production of specific chemokines and increased expression of the corresponding chemokine receptor(s) on leukocytes, needed at the site of the triggering event. • Chemokines for all of the major mononuclear and polynuclear leukocytes have been identified. • A highly provocative recent set of studies has also shown that the leukocyte tropism of HIV strains for monocytes and lymphocytes depends on the expression of specific monocyte- or lymphocyte-associated chemokine receptors. • Furthermore, specific chemokines have been shown to protect cells against infection with HIV.

ANSWER:
B, C, D

21. Which of the following statements regarding rejection of solid organ transplants is/are true?

A. Hyperacute rejection begins in the operating room with the reperfusion of the transplanted organ.

B. Liver transplants are especially susceptible to hyperacute rejection.

C. Most immunosuppressive medications are used to prevent chronic rejection.

D. The major cause of graft failure is acute rejection.

E. Recurrent infections in the transplanted organ can contribute to chronic rejection.

Ref.: 8

COMMENTS: There are three types of solid organ rejection, based on the timing of the rejection: hyperacute rejection, acute rejection, and chronic rejection. • The immunologic mechanism varies among these types of rejection.

Hyperacute rejection occurs immediately and is the result of preformed antibody that binds to the allograft on reperfusion of the organ in the operating room. • Hyperacute rejection is due to ABO incompatibility or a high titer of antidonor HLA I antibodies in the recipient. • For transplants of kidney, heart, pancreas, and lung, current protocols include preoperative testing for ABO incompatibility or HLA antibodies. • For reasons not completely elucidated, liver transplants are resistant to this process. • Liver transplants are performed without HLA matching and can be performed without ABO typing, although ABO type is usually matched.

Acute rejection occurs days to weeks following transplantation. • Since acute rejection is initiated by T-cell immunity, most medications for preventing and treating it are directed toward T-cell suppression. • Microscopically, acute rejection is characterized by a lymphocytic infiltrate, with plasma cells and eosinophils seen on tissue biopsy.

Chronic rejection occurs months to years after transplant and is the major cause of graft failure and mortality with all organ transplants. • There is loss of normal histologic structure, fibrosis, and atherosclerosis, with intergraft expression of certain cytokines. • Chronic rejection is the final common pathway of various insults, including repeated bouts of acute rejection, drug toxicity, chronic mechanical obstruction, recurrent infections, immunosuppressive noncompliance, and pretransplant organ issues such as ischemia time and organs of older donors. • There is no defined therapy for chronic rejection, but it is believed that a better understanding of cytokine-mediated atherosclerosis would help in the development of treatments and the prevention of chronic rejection.

ANSWER:
A, E

REFERENCES

1. Stites DP, Stobo JD, Fudenberg HH, et al: *Basic and Clinical Immunology.* Lange Medical Publications, Los Altos, CA, 1984.
2. Roitt I, Brostoff J, Male D: *Immunology.* CV Mosby, St. Louis, 1986.
3. Toledo-Pereyra LH: *Immunology Essentials of Surgical Practice.* PSG, Littleton, MA, 1988.
4. Myrvik QN, Weiser RS: *Fundamentals of Immunology.* Lea & Febiger, Malvern, PA, 1984.
5. Abbas AK, Lichtman AH, Pober JS: *Cellular and Molecular Immunology,* 3rd ed. WB Saunders, Philadelphia, 1997.
6. Staren ED, Essner R, Economou JS: *Seminars in Surgical Oncology.* Alan R Liss, New York, 1989.
7. Baggiolne M, Dewald B, Moser B: Human chemokines: an update. *Ann Rev Immunol* 15:675–705, 1997.
8. O'Leary JP: *The Physiologic Basis of Surgery,* 3rd ed. Lippincott, Williams & Wilkins, Philadelphia, 2001.

CHAPTER **14**

Transplant

S. Forrest Dodson, M.D.

1. Which of the following statements regarding kidney transplantation is/are true?

   A. The one-year actuarial survival rate for all patients is greater than 95%.

   B. The survival rate following transplantation appears to be improved only in diabetic patients.

   C. The primary cause of graft loss after 5 years is chronic rejection.

   D. Treatment of chronic rejection has improved significantly over the past 10 years.

   E. Treatment of renal failure with transplantation becomes cost effective at the end of the second transplant year.

   Ref.: 1–3

COMMENTS: From 1970 to 1990, the survival rate for patients following renal transplantation improved significantly, from 70 to 90%. During the past decade, the 1-year patient survival rate has continued to improve and is now greater than 95%. Diabetic patients have a less than 20% 5-year survival rate with dialysis and therefore represent the only group that has an improved survival rate following transplantation. Graft loss due to acute rejection has continued to follow a declining trend since the introduction of cyclosporine in the 1980s and tacrolimus in the 1990s. • However, the incidence of graft loss due to chronic rejection has not changed significantly over the past 10 years. • Despite improvements in immunosuppression and monitoring of opportunistic diseases, the 10-year survival rate after kidney transplantation is 44%, with most grafts being lost to chronic rejection. • Transplantation becomes cost effective when compared to dialysis at the end of the second year.

ANSWER:
A, B, C, E

2. Which of the following statements regarding kidney transplantation is/are true?

   A. Crossmatching is performed before kidney transplantation to prevent graft loss from chronic cellular rejection.

   B. A positive crossmatch is an absolute contraindication to cadaveric renal transplantation.

   C. Hyperacute rejection is responsive to additional immunotherapy.

   D. Routine screening of potential recipients using the panel reactive antibody (PRA) test can predict the presence of donor-specific antibodies.

   E. ABO incompatibility is an absolute contraindication to kidney transplantation.

   Ref.: 4–8

COMMENTS: Hyperacute rejection of a transplanted kidney generally occurs within minutes of reperfusion and is due to the presence of preformed immunoglobulin G (IgG) antibodies in the recipient's serum. • These antibodies attach to major histocompatibility antigens (HLA-A, HLA-B, and HLA-DR) on the donor vascular endothelium. • The test for donor-specific antibodies is called a **crossmatch** and is performed on all potential donors just before transplantation. • A **positive crossmatch** result is an absolute contraindication to cadaveric renal transplantation. • Crossmatching is performed to prevent the occurrence of hyperacute rejection, which is mediated primarily by complement-fixing antibodies. • Hyperacute rejection causes immediate loss of the graft and is not reversible.

Patients undergoing living-related renal transplantation with a positive crossmatch result can undergo treatment to remove the antibody (through plasmapheresis and/or administration of gamma globulin) and to prevent further antibody (anti-CD20) production. • If a subsequent crossmatch result is negative following treatment, living-related or -unrelated renal transplantation can be performed with an acceptable success rate. • Potential recipients of ABO-compatible renal allografts develop donor-specific HLA antibodies of the IgG class from antigen exposure due to transfusions, pregnancy, or previous transplants.

The presence of donor-specific antibodies can be predicted by periodically testing the reactivity of the recipient's serum to a panel of common A, B, and DR antigens and expressing the result as a percentage. • This test is referred to as the PRA, and patients who have a 90–100% PRA result routinely have donor-specific antibodies. • The higher the PRA result at the time of transplant, the more likely a patient is to have an episode of acute cellular rejection that is mediated primarily by T cells and is usually responsive to additional immunosuppression.

Previous recipients of ABO-incompatible allografts have had a high incidence of hyperacute rejection from preformed isoagglutinins, also of the IgG type, which attached to A and B antigens, also expressed by vascular endothelium. • However, success in Japan with ABO-incompatible donors and an increasing shortage of donors have resulted in recent evaluation of using ABO-incompatible renal allografts. • The combination of modern immunosuppression and the utilization of plasmapheresis to remove isoagglutinins has resulted in a 5-year survival rate of ABO-incompatible renal allografts of greater than 75%.

ANSWER:
B, D

3. Allocation of cadaveric renal allografts is dependent on which of the following?

   A. Time on hemodialysis

   B. HLA compatibility

   C. Recipient's age

   D. PRA results

   E. Region of transplant center

Ref.: 9

COMMENTS: Allocation of cadaveric renal allografts is dependent on the length of time the recipient has been on hemodialysis, HLA compatibility, PRA results, and the region of the transplant center. • Age is not a factor. • HLA antigens are inherited on chromosome 6, and, although multiple HLA antigens have been identified, kidney recipients and donors undergo tissue typing for only three antigens: HLA-A, -B, and -DR. • Since HLA-A, -B, and -DR antigens are inherited from each parent, usually as a codominant allele, offspring have two HLA-A antigens, two HLA-B antigens, and two HLA-DR antigens. • Siblings have a 25% chance of being HLA identical, a 50% chance of sharing one haplotype, and a 25% chance of being HLA dissimilar.

HLA matching for all six antigens has resulted in improved long-term outcome for both living-related and cadaveric renal transplants. • As a result, cadaveric organs that match for all six antigens are allocated nationwide. • If no six-antigen matches can be found for a cadaveric renal allograft, the organ is placed locally, with points given for the number of HLA matches, PRA results, and time spent on hemodialysis. • The benefit of allocating organs when the HLA match is fewer than six is questionable with modern immunosuppression. • The current system remains intact from years past, when only steroids and azathioprine (Imuran) were available.

ANSWER:
A, B, D, E

4. Which of the following best describes the preservation process for kidneys?

   A. Continuous pulsatile perfusion with solutions that mimic the intracellular electrolytes has proven to be superior to simple cold storage.

   B. Continuous pulsatile perfusion has reemerged over the past 5 years owing to the utilization of more high-risk donors.

   C. Simple cold storage allows for longer preservation time because of its simplicity.

   D. Simple cold storage is superior to continuous pulsatile perfusion when storage times are less than 24 hr.

Ref.: 10–14

COMMENTS: In the 1970s, hypothermic perfusion and preservation of kidneys began with the introduction of Euro-Collins solution, which mimicked the high-potassium, low-sodium environment of the intracellular electrolytes. • This solution allowed for simple cold storage of kidneys for up to 48 hr. • However, storage of extrarenal organs, such as the liver and pancreas, was limited to 8 hr. • The University of Wisconsin (UW) solution, introduced in the 1980s, was fortified with large, impermeable molecules to prevent cellular degradation due to hypothermia. • UW solution extended the cold-storage time for extrarenal organs up to 24 hr. • Initial trials with cold pulsatile perfusion using UW solution showed no significant improvement in long-term graft function when compared to simple cold storage of kidneys. • However, the rate of ATN was significantly lower for kidneys stored for longer periods (36–48 hr). • As a result, pulsatile perfusion has now resurfaced as the preferred method of storage for kidneys from high-risk donors, who may be older or whose kidneys may have been stored for a prolonged time. • In such cases, long-term graft function is presumed to be improved by preventing ATN with pulsatile perfusion.

ANSWER:
B

5. Two hours after transplantation with a kidney from a 60-year-old donor, a 30-year-old woman with lupus, a negative crossmatch result, a 10-hr cold ischemia time, and a pretransplant PRA result of 80% is producing no urine. What is the best course of action?

   A. Immediate renal flow scan to rule out arterial occlusion

   B. Immediate sonographic studies to verify vessel patency

   C. Immediate re-exploration

   D. Immediate administration of high-dose steroids to treat rejection

Ref.: 15

COMMENTS: The commonest cause of delayed graft function following kidney transplantation is ATN. • However, ATN is usually characterized by urine production in the range of 10–30 ml/hr which generally declines to 0–5 ml/hr over the first 24 hr. • Although surgical complications such as vascular thrombosis and ureteral obstruction are rare, they must be excluded for patients who present with anuria immediately following kidney transplantation.

The initial test of choice is a sonographic study to verify vessel patency; to exclude the presence of a fluid collection, due to a hematoma or a urinoma, that may be impinging on the graft; and to exclude arterial or venous obstruction due to kinking of one or both vessels. • If no flow in either of the vessels is seen during immediate sonographic imaging, re-exploration is indicated.

Early thrombosis of the graft may be salvaged in rare cases through immediate exploration and reimplantation. • Urinomas and hematomas should be evacuated. • The commonest source of bleeding is the arterial anastomosis. • Ureteral obstruction can be due to twisting of the ureter or, more commonly, stricturing at the anastomosis. • Occasionally, a ureter can be inadvertently connected to the peritoneum. • Reimplantation is warranted in all cases.

ANSWER:
B

6. Which of the following statements is/are true regarding the exocrine drainage of a pancreas allograft performed simultaneously with or following a kidney transplant?

   A. Elevation of plasma glucose levels is the first manifestation of pancreas rejection.

   B. Bladder drainage is preferred because it is associated with fewer complications.

   C. Most surgeons prefer enteric drainage because the incidence of complications attributed to bladder drainage, such as acidosis and urinary tract infections, can be avoided.

   D. Most surgeons prefer bladder drainage because the incidence of infections is reduced by avoiding contamination with enteric contents.

   Ref.: 16

COMMENTS: Since an elevated plasma glucose level is a late manifestation of rejection and is generally a precursor to graft loss, the results of fine-needle biopsy and/or a decreased urinary amylase level have been successfully used to detect early signs of rejection. • The incidence of conversion from bladder to enteric drainage was as high as 19% in one large series of patients studied because of the association of recurrent urinary tract infections and acidosis with bladder drainage. • Therefore, enteric drainage is the first choice of most centers for patients receiving a pancreas transplant either simultaneously with or following a kidney transplant. • The incidence of infections is the same with both techniques, and both require a similar level of skill. • Many large centers continue to use bladder drainage for solitary pancreas transplantation performed primarily to avoid progression of complications of diabetes. • Surgeons may choose bladder drainage for patients with a history of peritonitis or multiple abdominal surgeries.

ANSWER:
C

7. Of the following, which would exclude a patient from whole-organ pancreas transplantation?

   A. History of chronic renal failure with biopsy-proven Kimmelstiel-Wilson syndrome

   B. History of coronary artery bypass grafting

   C. History of diabetic neuropathy

   D. History of lower-extremity peripheral vascular disease

   E. None of the above

   Ref.: 16

COMMENTS: Selection criteria include diabetic patients with secondary complications of diabetes that do not preclude long-term survival. • Increasingly, data have shown that pancreas transplantation is able to arrest further development of early secondary complications of diabetes. • After pancreas-kidney transplantation, diabetic renal disease (Kimmelstiel-Wilson syndrome) in the transplanted kidney does not seem to recur. • Diabetic neuropathy is often reversed, as documented by increased nerve conduction velocity studies. • However, vascular disease of the lower extremities and coronary arteries is not reversed and significantly increases the surgical risk.

ANSWER:
E

8. Which of the following statements regarding secondary complications of diabetes and pancreas transplantation is/are true?

   A. Diabetic retinopathy generally improves after pancreas transplantation.

   B. Recurrence of diabetic nephropathy in renal allografts can be avoided.

   C. Diabetic neuropathy can improve after pancreas transplantation.

   D. Patients with advanced diabetic neuropathy have an improved survival rate after pancreas transplantation.

   Ref.: 16

COMMENTS: Successful pancreas transplantation was initially thought to be a potential cure for diabetic retinopathy and many of the other secondary complications of diabetes. • However, after pancreas transplantation, diabetic retinopathy can stabilize but generally does not improve. • Recurrence of diabetic nephropathy in renal allografts can be avoided by simultaneous kidney-pancreas transplantation. • Nerve regeneration has been shown to occur following pancreas transplantation, and diabetic neuropathy is the one secondary complication of diabetes that can actually improve. • This improvement may be associated with improved survival rates.

ANSWER:
B, C, D

9. Regarding liver transplantation for patients chronically infected with hepatitis C virus, which of the following statements is/are true?

   A. Post-transplant reinfection with hepatitis C virus occurs in all patients.

   B. Post-transplant reinfection with hepatitis C virus can be prevented with combination therapy with interferon and ribavirin and hyperimmunoglobulin.

   C. Post-transplant reinfection with hepatitis C virus causes cirrhosis in approximately 30% of patients at 5 years after liver transplantation.

   D. The clinical course of hepatitis C after reinfection is more virulent than that of the original infection.

   Ref.: 17–19

COMMENTS: Healthy individuals infected with the RNA virus hepatitis C usually develop cirrhosis or hepatocellular carcinoma over a 20–30-year period. • Patients chronically infected with hepatitis C virus undergoing liver transplantation are uniformly reinfected within a matter of days. • No therapy is effective in preventing reinfection. • Cirrhosis develops much earlier in the transplanted allograft, with approximately 30% of patients exhibiting cirrhosis on biopsy at 5 years following transplantation. • Combination therapy with interferon and ribavirin eradicates the recurrent infection in a small percentage of patients (approximately 5–10%) after transplantation. • Although studies have shown that the 3- and 5-year survival rates appears to be diminished by recurrence of the native infection, the overall results are acceptable, and hepatitis C remains an indication for liver transplantation.

ANSWER:
A, C

?

10. Regarding liver transplantation for patients chronically infected with hepatitis B virus (HBV), which of the following statements is/are true?

A. The rate of recurrence of hepatitis B after transplant is 50% at 5 years.

B. The use of the reverse transcriptase inhibitors lamivudine and adefovir can prevent recurrence in most patients.

C. The risk of reinfection with HBV depends on the status of the recipient's hepatitis B e-antigen and HBV DNA before transplantation.

D. Fulminant hepatic failure secondary to acute HBV infection is a contraindication to liver transplantation because of early recurrence of infection.

Ref.: 17, 20–22

COMMENTS: Before the availability of the reverse transcriptase inhibitors lamivudine and adefovir, liver transplantation for patients chronically infected with HBV had an unacceptably high rate of recurrence. • However, now patients undergoing transplantation for liver failure secondary to HBV infection have excellent outcomes, with a negligible rate of recurrence of the native infection. • Patients who test positive for e-antigen or for HBV DNA have an increased risk of recurrent infection. • Patients with fulminant hepatic failure secondary to HBV infection have the lowest risk of developing recurrent infection.

ANSWER:
A, B, C, D

11. Which of the following is/are used as induction agents given before or at the time of grafting?

A. Campath (Alemtuzumab)

B. Dacliximab (Zenapax)

C. Rapamycin (Rapamune)

D. Azathioprine (Imuran)

Ref.: 23–25

COMMENTS: See Question 12.

12. Which of the following is/are used as primary maintenance immunosuppressive agents?

A. Tacrolimus (Prograf)

B. Cyclosporine (Neoral, Sandimmune)

C. Mycophenolate (CellCept)

D. Rapamycin (Rapamune)

Ref.: 23–25

COMMENTS: Immunosuppression following solid abdominal organ transplantation generally begins with induction agents given before or at the time of grafting. • The three commonest induction methods are (1) T- and B-cell reduction with the cytolytic antibodies Thymoglobulin or Campath, (2) blockade of the interferon binding site (CD25 blockade) with one of two antibodies, either dacliximab (Zenapax) or basiliximab (Simulect), or (3) a steroid cycle with initial high doses of the maintenance agent, either cyclosporine or tacrolimus.

The induction phase is followed by maintenance immunosuppression, usually with either tacrolimus or cyclosporine. • Both of these two agents inhibit transcription of T-helper cells by interfering with calcineurin phosphatase, thus inhibiting cytokine production by the T cell. • The target level and dose of the maintenance agent is reduced as the risk of acute rejection gradually declines. • A third agent—either mycophenolate, rapamycin, or azathioprine (Imuran)—may be given in addition to tacrolimus or cyclosporine. • These agents are not as potent as tacrolimus or cyclosporine and can only rarely be used alone.

ANSWER:
Question 11: A, B
Question 12: A, B

13. Which of the following statements is/are true regarding the toxicities of immunosuppressive agents?

A. The calcineurin inhibitors cyclosporine, tacrolimus, and Rapamycin are nephrotoxic.

B. Both mycophenolate and rapamycin are toxic to the gastrointestinal system.

C. Tacrolimus has been associated with an increased incidence of post-transplant diabetes.

D. Both cyclosporine and tacrolimus can cause hirsutism and gingival hyperplasia.

E. Both cyclosporine and tacrolimus can cause aphonia (loss of speech).

Ref.: 24, 25

COMMENTS: All immunosuppressive agents have toxicities, which can be minimized by using various combinations of the agents at lower dosages. • Both of the calcineurin inhibitors, tacrolimus and cyclosporine, cause renal vasoconstriction, resulting in nephrotoxicity by reducing renal blood flow. • However, rapamycin is not nephrotoxic. • Rapamycin can cause thrombocytopenia and hypercholesterolemia. • Mycophenolate inhibits purine synthesis, which is essential for the proliferative responses of T and B cells to mitogens. • As a result, mycophenolate is primarily marrow toxic, but its usage is also frequently limited by its gastrointestinal side effects: gastroenteritis, causing diarrhea, flatulence, and bloating. • Mycophenolate is the only immunosuppressive agent that frequently causes toxicity to the gastrointestinal system. • Tacrolimus has been associated with an increase in post-transplant diabetes. • Only cyclosporine is associated with hirsutism and gingival hyperplasia. • Both cyclosporine and tacrolimus are neurotoxic and can cause tremors, seizures, dysphonia, and aphonia.

ANSWER:
C, E

14. Treatment of a lymphocele after kidney transplantation may include all except which of the following?

A. Percutaneous drainage to exclude urinoma regardless of symptoms

B. Percutaneous drainage with sclerosis

C. Prolonged external percutaneous drainage

D. Observation if asymptomatic

E. Laparoscopic internal marsupialization

Ref.: 15

COMMENTS: Lymphoceles following kidney transplantation are frequent, probably occur as a result of inadequate ligation of iliac lymphatics, and do not require intervention if asymptomatic. • However, if they present as a mass or cause ureteral obstruction, intervention is necessary, and initial treatment usually involves percutaneous drainage. • If the lymphocele recurs, most centers would place an external drain percutaneously using sonographic or computerized tomographic (CT) imaging. • If the lymphocele reaccumulates and becomes symptomatic after removal of the external drain, internal drainage by marsupialization is indicated. • This can be done in an open procedure or laparoscopically.

ANSWER:
A

15. Liver transplantation may be contraindicated for which of the following?

    A. Stage I hepatocellular carcinoma with cirrhosis

    B. Stage II hepatocellular carcinoma with cirrhosis

    C. A 30-year-old patient with liver failure and uncorrected pulmonary hypertension

    D. A 30-year-old patient with liver failure and hepatopulmonary syndrome

    E. A 30-year-old patient with liver failure and portal vein thrombosis

Ref.: 26, 27

COMMENTS: The list of patients waiting for liver transplantation is currently arranged by the model for end-stage liver disease (MELD) system. • The MELD system is based on points (0–40) calculated from a logarithmic formula that uses a patient's bilirubin, creatinine, and protime levels. • Patients also receive additional points for hepatocellular carcinoma and hepatopulmonary syndrome. • Patients whose imaging studies (CT, magnetic resonance, or sonographic) are consistent with clinical stage I or clinical stage II hepatocellular carcinoma receive additional points by the MELD system: 20 points for stage I and 24 points for stage II. • Stage I hepatocellular carcinoma is defined pathologically as a solitary tumor of less than 2 cm without vascular invasion. • Stage II hepatocellular carcinoma is defined pathologically as a solitary tumor smaller than 2 cm with vascular invasion, multiple tumors in one lobe smaller than 2 cm without vascular invasion, or a solitary tumor greater than 2 cm without vascular invasion. .

    The overall prevalence of pulmonary hypertension in the general population is 0.13%, although in patients with portal hypertension it is significantly higher, at 0.73%. • Patients with a normal pulmonary capillary wedge pressure and an elevated mean pulmonary arterial pressure, of 25 or more, have pulmonary hypertension by definition. • However, for patients with liver failure, pulmonary hypertension can be classified as mild (systolic pulmonary pressure <35), moderate (systolic pulmonary pressure 35–60), or severe (systolic pulmonary pressure >60). • Patients with untreated severe pulmonary hypertension who undergo liver transplantation are at a very high risk of cardiac death from right ventricular failure immediately following reperfusion. • Fortunately, treatment with prostacyclin (PGI₂) given by constant infusion can reduce the pulmonary pressures to a range where liver transplantation can be successful. • Liver transplantation may be contraindicated for patients with severe pulmonary hypertension unresponsive to prostacyclin. • For patients who do respond, prostacyclin can be gradually weaned following transplantation, and pulmonary pressures will remain normal.

Hepatopulmonary syndrome is essentially the opposite of pulmonary hypertension. • Pulmonary capillaries, which serve unoxygenated areas of the lung, respond to the liver disease by opening, causing a significant reduction in pulmonary systolic pressure and increasing the shunt fraction to as high as 10–20% (normal shunt fraction is 7%). • As a result, patients require increasing amounts of supplemental oxygen before undergoing transplantation. • However, transplantation is curative, and the shunt fraction is reduced to normal within 3–4 months after transplantation. • Portal venous thrombosis can be easily corrected by thrombectomy at the time of transplantation or with a superior mesenteric vein graft.

ANSWER:
C

16. Which of the following statements is/are true regarding cytomegalovirus (CMV) infection?

    A. Infection with CMV following kidney transplantation is the strongest predictor of poor long-term survival.

    B. The incidence of symptomatic CMV infection is declining owing to the utilization of screening tests.

    C. Patients at highest risk for developing CMV infection are those who test seropositive for CMV IgG.

    D. CMV infection is more likely to cause chronic allograft nephropathy than infection with BK virus.

    E. CMV infection can be indistinguishable from acute Epstein-Barr virus (EBV) infection.

Ref.: 28–30

COMMENTS: With the development of the very effective antiviral agent ganciclovir, acute rejection, not CMV infection, is now the strongest predictor of poor allograft survival. • The incidence of CMV infection is declining, probably due to very effective tests for viral load in the serum, such as CMV pp65 antigen and CMV DNA testing. • Patients who are at the highest risk for CMV infection are those who test seronegative for CMV IgG and who receive an allograft from a donor seropositive for CMV IgG. • CMV infection is usually an acute, systemic infection that can be become symptomatic in a variety of organ systems, resulting in gastritis, hepatitis, pneumonitis, retinitis, and marrow suppression. • CMV infection rarely involves only one organ and rarely causes chronic nephropathy. • BK infection is usually isolated to the kidney and its associated urinary system and causes chronic nephropathy if left untreated. • Acute infection with EBV usually causes inflammation of the gastrointestinal tract in the form of gastritis, enteritis, or colitis and is thus clinically similar to CMV infection. • The two can be easily distinguished by checking the serum viral loads with a quantitative CMV DNA and a quantitative EBV DNA testing. • In addition, biopsy specimens from inflamed gastrointestinal mucosa can be specifically stained for each virus.

ANSWER:
B

17. Biopsy results for an enlarged inguinal lymph node in a 40-year-old male 3 years after kidney transplantation are consistent with post-transplant lymphoproliferative disorder (PTLD). Which of the following statements is/are true?

    A. The use of antilymphocyte globulin is a risk factor for PTLD.

B. The disease is related to the recipient's immunity to EBV.

C. The disease is related to the recipient's immunity to CMV.

D. The disease is more common in children than in adults.

E. Administration of immunosuppressive agents should be tapered and administration of acyclovir or ganciclovir initiated.

Ref.: 31

COMMENTS: Post-transplant PTLD represents a spectrum of diseases related to EBV infection, including infectious mononucleosis, benign proliferation of B cells, and lymphoma. • In the transplant recipient, clones of EBV-transformed B cells are generated as a result of infection with EBV from the donor or personal contact. • Due to impaired immunity, transplant recipients unable to control the clonal expansion of EBV-infected B cells develop PTLD, which may be manifested as hyperplasia (an EBV-induced tumor) or neoplasia (lymphoma). • Risk factors for development of PTLD include the use of antilymphocytic globulin, EBV seronegativity, and CMV infection in a CMV-mismatched patient (donor positive for CMV IgG and recipient negative for CMV IgG). • The disease is more common in children than in adults. • Asymptomatic transplant recipients at risk or symptomatic recipients are surveyed for EBV infection by quantitative polymerase chain reaction (PCR) analysis of peripheral blood. • Patients with elevated serum levels of EBV are usually treated by decreasing the dosage of immunosuppressive agents and administering either acyclovir or gancyclovir. • Patients with hyperplastic tumors are usually treated by terminating administration of immunosuppressive agents and acyclovir or gancyclovir. • Patients with unresponsive hyperplastic tumors can be treated with the anti-B cell (anti-CD20) antibody Rituxan. • CHOP (cyclophosphamide, doxorubicin, vincristine, and prednisone) therapy is usually reserved for patients with lymphoma.

ANSWER:
A, B, C, D, E

18. True or false: Alcoholic liver disease is a contraindication for liver transplantation.

Ref.: 32

COMMENTS: Patients with alcoholic liver disease who are abstinent for more than 6 months and have good psychosocial support are considered good candidates for liver transplantation because of the low risk of alcohol recidivism. • Their long-term survival rate may be one of the highest as a group, since they are not as often subject to viral hepatitis and other progressive diseases that may recur in the transplanted liver.

ANSWER:
False

19. Which of the following is the most predictive of a patient's 1-year survival rate following liver transplantation?

A. Age of the recipient

B. Severity of the APACHE score before transplantation

C. Presence of an incidental hepatoma smaller than 4 cm

D. Use of antilymphocytic globulin

Ref.: 33

COMMENTS: The survival rate for patients after liver transplantation is directly related to the severity of the illness before transplantation. • Statistics show that patients who are well enough to be at home with liver disease at the time of transplantation have a 91.4% 1-year survival rate. • In contrast, patients who had been hospitalized have an 84.5% survival rate. • Those in an intensive care unit before transplantation have a 79.9% survival rate, and those on life support have a 69.7% survival rate.

ANSWER:
B

20. Donor organs for pediatric liver transplantation are acquired from which of the following?

A. Donor of similar size and habitus

B. Splitting of an adult cadaver liver and transplanting the appropriate segment

C. Resection of the left lobe or left lateral segment of a liver from an adult living donor

Ref.: 33

COMMENTS: Over the past 10 years, there has been a substantial expansion in the availability of donor grafts for pediatric liver transplantation. • Previously, many children died while waiting for an appropriately sized donor to become available. • Now, with the application of segmental liver resection techniques, full-size cadaver liver grafts can be reduced to the appropriate volume for pediatric recipients. • In addition, resection of the left lobe or the left lateral segment from a living adult donor can be performed, with comparable survival of the recipient and minimal risk to the donor.

ANSWER:
A, B, C

21. Six months after renal transplantation, a 56-year-old woman is admitted to the hospital with high fever, an elevated serum creatinine level, disseminated varicella skin lesions, and bilateral pulmonary infiltrates. Which of the following statements is/are true?

A. Bronchoscopic examination is unnecessary, since the diagnosis is obviously viral pneumonia.

B. At this stage, the patient does not need to be placed in isolation.

C. To avoid rejection, the immunosuppressive drug regimen should not be changed.

D. Intravenous acyclovir with or without hyperimmunoglobulin is the treatment of choice.

E. This is a potentially lethal condition.

Ref.: 1, 34

COMMENTS: Reactivation of herpes zoster (shingles) occurs in up to 15–30% of renal transplant recipients, usually during the first 6 months after transplantation. • Intravenous, followed by oral, acyclovir usually prevents systemic dissemination and leads to rapid healing of the skin lesions. • With such complications, administration of immunosuppressive agents should be drastically reduced to prevent death. • Respiratory isolation is necessary to prevent spread of infection to other patients. • Bronchoscopic examination is advisable to rule out superinfection with bacterial, fungal, or other opportunistic organisms. • Intravenous acyclovir with or without hyperimmunoglobulin (varicella zoster immunoglobulin) is the therapy of choice. • The acyclovir analogues famciclovir and valacyclovir are currently undergoing clinical trials.

ANSWER:
D, E

22. With respect to de novo post–renal-transplant diabetes mellitus, which of the following statement(s) is/are true?

A. It is more common in African-American recipients.

B. It is a side effect of cyclosporine and FK506 (Prograf) and is reversible after reduction of immunosuppressive therapy with these agents.

C. Risk factors include weight, age, and family history.

D. It has become less common since the introduction of tacrolimus and cyclosporine.

E. There is no association with steroid dosage.

Ref.: 1, 34

COMMENTS: Post-transplant diabetes mellitus (PTDM) is seen in 4–20% of renal transplant recipients. • Steroids, cyclosporine, and tacrolimus are diabetogenic. • There is a direct relationship between steroid dosage and the incidence of PTDM. • Tacrolimus-based immunosuppressive therapy was associated with an 18% incidence of new-onset PTDM in a recent multicenter trial, and it was decreased to 9% after reduction of steroid and tacrolimus doses. • Cyclosporine-based immunosuppressive therapy resulted in only a 4% incidence of new-onset PTDM. • Risk factors include age, obesity, family history of diabetes, and African-American race. • The potential mechanisms include decreased insulin secretion, increased insulin resistance, and a toxic effect of tacrolimus and cyclosporine on pancreatic β cells. • Only 25% of patients with PTDM develop persistent hyperglycemia, and 50% of patients in this group require continuous insulin therapy.

ANSWER:
A, B, C, E

23. With respect to hepatitis and *renal* transplantation, which of the following statements is/are true?

A. Hepatitis C is an absolute contraindication to organ donation.

B. All hepatitis B surface-antigen–positive patients are poor renal transplant candidates.

C. Hepatitis C–positive recipients have an extremely poor prognosis.

D. None of the above

E. All of the above

Ref.: 1, 34

COMMENTS: Patients with preexisting hepatitis C who have a moderate viral load measured with or without PCR testing, normal liver function, and minimal chronic active hepatitis found on liver biopsy are acceptable recipients for a renal transplant. • Donors with a similar profile may be acceptable for such a patient but not for a recipient who does not have hepatitis C. • Hepatic disease occurs in 7–24% of patients during the early post-transplant period and is the cause of late death in 8–28% of patients. • Hepatitis B and C are responsible for most of these deaths. • Hepatitis B surface-antigen–positive patients who have stable liver function and test negative for e-antigen do fairly well after renal transplantation and low-dose immunosuppressive therapy. • The replacement of

Imuran by cyclosporine has reduced the corticosteroid dose and improved the long-term outcome for these patients.

ANSWER:
D

24. Following transplantation, the incidence of primary nonfunction of the liver allograft ranges from 1 to 10%. Immediately after the liver transplantation procedure, which of the following is/are associated with this clinical syndrome in the liver allograft recipient?

A. Metabolic alkalosis

B. Hyperkalemia

C. Reduced mental status

D. Marked elevation in liver enzyme levels

E. Minimal bile output (if a T-tube biliary drainage catheter is in place)

Ref.: 35

COMMENTS: Primary nonfunction of a liver allograft is a poorly understood clinical syndrome associated with markedly abnormal function of the allograft (i.e., severe coagulopathy, acidosis, hyperkalemia, poor mental status, continued hyperdynamic cardiac function with high cardiac output, low system vascular resistance with liver failure, poor bile output, and usually renal failure). • Recipients with a normally functioning graft have marked metabolic alkalosis secondary to metabolism of the citrate component from banked blood replacement to bicarbonate by the liver graft during the immediate post-transplantation period. • Within the first 24 hr following liver transplantation, patients with normally functioning grafts return to normal cardiac hemodynamics from a hyperdynamic state. • The most specific pretransplantation predictor of primary nonfunction of the liver allograft is the amount of macrosteatosis (extracellular fat globules) in the liver allograft. • When more than 40–50% of the cross-sectional area of a liver biopsy specimen is macrosteatotic, the incidence of primary dysfunction may reach 50%. • Other purported predictors of this syndrome include high levels of vasopressor support in the donor and cold ischemia time. • Usually, potential liver donor grafts associated with these findings are not used. • The mechanism whereby the fat causes this clinical problem has not been clearly elucidated. • Although a variety of strategies have been attempted to ameliorate this syndrome, the only treatment is prompt retransplantation.

ANSWER:
B, C, D, E

25. Which of the following is/are the most significant clinical problem(s) associated with transplantation of the small intestine?

A. Inability to safely control acute rejection of the graft

B. High incidence of fatal lymphoproliferative disease (lymphoma)

C. High incidence of severe CMV infection

D. Shortage of donor organs

E. Severe clinical consequences of chronic graft-versus-host disease (GVHD) related to the large amount of lymphoid material associated with transplantation of the small-bowel allograft

Ref.: 36–38

COMMENTS: Small-bowel transplantation is likely the "last frontier" in solid organ transplantation. • In most large animal models, control of acute and chronic rejection of the transplanted small intestine has been extremely difficult. • The same has been true during the early clinical experience. • With the necessary marked increases in dosage for short-term and maintenance immunosuppressive therapy, the immunologic surveillance for cancerous lymphocytes is markedly degraded, leading to a high incidence of lymphoma (10–20%) in recipients. • In addition, with CMV in the "passenger" lymphoid material of the small-bowel allograft, in conjunction with high-dose immunosuppressive therapy, fatal, disseminated CMV infections are common despite long-term pharmacologic viral prophylaxis. • Some surgeons use only serologically CMV-negative donor intestine in CMV-negative recipients to avoid this often fatal complication. • With the current low demand for this developing procedure, the potential donors outnumber the candidates awaiting transplantation. • Because of the marked lymphoid load inherent in small-intestine transplantation and the findings in animal models, problems with GVHD (attack of host tissue by donor passenger lymphocytes, producing skin rashes and hemolysis of red blood cells) were anticipated. • A variety of strategies using γ irradiation of the donor graft and administration of a variety of antilymphocytic globulins to the donor were initially devised for clinical small-intestine transplantation. • It is surprising that, with no strategy for donor or recipient modification, GVHD is almost nonexistent.

A N S W E R :
A, B, C

---

26. With which of the following is/are acute rejection of the human small-bowel allograft associated?

   A. Increasing apoptosis of the crypts of the small-bowel graft

   B. Increasing lymphocytic infiltration of crypts of the small-bowel graft

   C. Increasing high volumes of diarrhea through the ostomy or the rectum

   D. Translocation of bacteria

   E. Endoscopic findings of ulceration of the graft mucosa

Ref.: 38

COMMENTS: Acute rejection of the small-bowel allograft is a clinical and pathologic diagnosis. • Usually, an episode of acute rejection is heralded by a nonspecific finding of a marked increase of diarrhea through the graft ostomy or the rectum. • Serial endoscopic monitoring of the graft demonstrates increasing ulceration and inflammation of the mucosa. • Serial endoscopic mucosal graft biopsies usually reveal a fairly distinctive progression of apoptosis of the crypts of the mucosa. • High-dose immunosuppressive therapy is required to preempt complete destruction of the graft and chronic allograft rejection. • Although these findings are fairly sensitive for diagnosing acute rejection, a CMV infection of the graft may produce similar findings. • Only careful review of the small-intestine graft biopsy results and serologic monitoring for CMV allow differentiation of these clinical problems. • Treatment of a CMV infection of the small-intestine graft is essentially the opposite of that for acute rejection: the infection is treated with some reduction in immunosuppressive dosage and an antiviral agent (e.g., ganciclovir). • Acute rejection of the small bowel usually results in severe translocation of bacteria and associated severe bacteremia. • These simultaneous events (high-dose immunosuppressive therapy and marked bacteremia) lead to a precarious clinical situation associated with septic shock and fatal multiple organ failure. • Clinical management of this common occurrence is one of the more difficult challenges in solid organ transplantation.

A N S W E R :
A, B, C, D, E

R E F E R E N C E S

1. Shapiro R: Outcome after renal transplantation. In: Shapiro R, Simmons RL, Starzl TE (eds) *Renal Transplantation.* Appleton & Lange, Stamford, Connecticut, 1997.
2. Cecka JM: The UNOS Scientific Transplant Registry, 1998. In: Terasaki PI, Cecka JM (eds) *Clinical Transplants.* UCLA Tissue Typing Laboratory, Los Angeles, 1998.
3. Schweitzer EJ, Wiland A, Evans D, et al: The shrinking renal replacement therapy "break-even" point. *Transplantation* 66:1702–1708, 1998.
4. Ting A: The lymphocytotoxic crossmatch test in clinical renal transplantation. *Transplantation* 35:403–407, 1983.
5. Bray RA: Flow cytometry crossmatching for solid organ transplantation. *Methods Cell Biol* 41:103–119, 1994.
6. Scornik JC, Brunson ME, Howard RJ, et al: Alloimmunization, memory, and the interpretation of crossmatch results for renal transplantation. *Transplantation* 54(3):389–394, 1992.
7. Karpinski M, Rush D, Jeffery J, et al: Flow cytometric crossmatching in primary renal transplant recipients with a negative anti-human globulin enhanced cytotoxicity crossmatch. *J Am Soc Nephrol* 12(12):2807–2814, 2001.
8. Tanabe K, Ishikawa N, Tokumoto T, et al: Role of anti-A/B antibody titers in results of ABO-incompatible kidney transplantation. *Transplantation* 70(9):1331–1335, 2000.
9. Iwaki Y: Histocompatibility testing and cross matching. In: Shapiro R, Simmons RL, Starzl TE (eds) *Renal Transplantation.* Appleton & Lange, Stamford, Connecticut, 1997.
10. Collins GH, Bravo-Shugarman MB, Terasaki PI: Kidney preservation for transplantation: initial perfusion and 30 hour ice storage. *Lancet* 2:1219–1222, 1969.
11. Belzer PO, Southard JH: Principles of solid organ preservation by cold storage. *Transplantation* 45:673–676, 1988.
12. Merion RM, Oh HK, Port FK, et al: A prospective controlled trial of cold-storage versus machine perfusion in cadaveric renal transplantation. *Transplantation* 50:230–233, 1990.
13. Polyak MM, Arrington BO, Stubenbord WT, et al: The influence of pulsatile preservation on renal transplantation in the 1990s. *Transplantation* 69(2):249–258, 2000.
14. Burdick JF, Rosendale JD, McBride MA, et al: National impact of pulsatile perfusion on cadaveric kidney transplantation. *Transplantation* 64(12):1730–1733, 1997.
15. Shapiro R: Complications of renal transplantation. In: Shapiro R, Simmons RL, Starzl TE (eds) *Renal Transplantation.* Appleton & Lange, Stamford, Connecticut, 1997.
16. Sutherland DER, Gruessner RWG, Dunn DL, et al: Lessons learned from more than 1,000 pancreas transplants at a single institution. *Ann Surg* 233(4):463–501, 2001.
17. Dodson SF, Issa S, Bonham A: Liver transplantation for chronic viral hepatitis. *Surg Clin North Am* 79(1):131–146, 1999.
18. Charlton M: Hepatitis C infection in liver transplantation. *Am J Transplant* 1(3):197–203, 2001.
19. Terrault NA: Hepatitis C virus and liver transplantation. *Semin Gastrointest Dis* 11(2):96–114, 2000.
20. Lo CM, Fan ST, Liu CL, et al: Prophylaxis and treatment of recurrent hepatitis B after liver transplantation. *Transplantation* 75(3 Suppl):S41–S44, 2003.
21. Lok AS: Prevention of recurrent hepatitis B post-liver transplantation. *Liver Transplant* 8(10 Suppl 1):S67–S73, 2002.
22. Villamil FG: Hepatitis B: progress in the last 15 years. *Liver Transplant* 8(10 Suppl 1):S59–S66, 2002.
23. Scott LJ, McKeage K, Keam SJ, et al: Tacrolimus: a further update of its use in the management of organ transplantation. *Drugs* 63(12):1247–1297, 2003.
24. Masri MA: The mosaic of immunosuppressive drugs. *Molec Immunol* 39(17–18):1073–1077, 2003.

25. Gourishankar S, Turner P, Halloran P: New developments in immuno-suppressive therapy in renal transplantation. *Exp Opin Biol Therapy* 2(5):483–501.

26. Budhiraja R, Hassoun PM: Portopulmonary hypertension: a tale of two circulations. *Chest* 123(2):562–576, 2003.

27. Scott VL, Dodson SF, Kang Y: The hepatopulmonary syndrome. *Surg Clin North Am* 79(1):23–41, 1999.

28. Helantera I, Koskinen P, Tornroth T, et al: The impact of cytomegalovirus infections and acute rejection episodes on the development of vascular changes in 6-month protocol biopsy specimens of cadaveric kidney allograft recipients. *Transplantation* 75(11): 1858–1864, 2003.

29. Tong CY, Bakran A, Peiris JS, et al: The association of viral infection and chronic allograft nephropathy with graft dysfunction after renal transplantation. *Transplantation* 74(4):576–578, 2002.

30. Li RM, Mannon RB, Kleiner D, et al: BK virus and SV40 co-infection in polyomavirus nephropathy. *Transplantation* 74(11):1497–1504, 2002.

31. Paya CV, Fung JJ, Nalesnik MA, et al: Epstein-Barr virus-induced post-transplant lymphoproliferative disorders: ASTS/ASTP EBV-PTLD Task Force and the Mayo Clinic Organized International Consensus Development Meeting. *Transplantation* 68(10):1517–1525, 1999.

32. Foster PF, Fabrega F, Karademir K, et al: Prediction of abstinence from ethanol in alcoholic recipients following liver transplantation. *Hepatology* 25:1469–1477, 1997.

33. Greenfield LJ, Mulholland MW, Oldham KT, Zilenock GB (eds): *Surgery, Scientific Principles and Practices*, 3rd ed. Lippincott Williams & Willkins, Philadelphia, 2005.

34. Morris PJ: *Kidney Transplantation: Principles and Practice*, 4th ed. WB Saunders, Philadelphia, 1994.

35. Williams JW: *Hepatic Transplantation*. Saunders, Philadelphia, 1990.

36. Putman P, Reyes J, Kocoshis S, et al: Gastrointestinal post-transplant lymphoproliferative disease in children after small intestinal transplantation. *Transplant Proc* 28:2777, 1996.

37. Abu-Elmagd K, Reyes J, Todo S, et al: Clinical intestinal transplantation: new perspectives and immunological consideration. *J Am Coll Surg* 186:512–525, 1998.

38. Sigurdsson L, Kocoshis S, Todo S, et al: Severe exfoliative rejection after intestinal transplantation in children. *Transplant Proc* 28:2783–2784, 1996.

CHAPTER 15

Critical Care

José M. Velasco, M.D.

1. With regard to cardiac output (CO), which of the following statements is/are false?

   A. CO alone is not an indicator of myocardial contractility.

   B. Ventricular end-diastolic volume (EDV), vascular resistance, and myocardial contractility determine stroke volume (SV).

   C. Arterial blood pressure alone is an accurate indicator of CO.

   D. CO varies directly with pulse rate up to 160 beats per minute in sinus rhythm, after which it decreases.

   E. Atrial contraction contributes up to 30% of the EDV.

   Ref.: 1, 2

COMMENTS: In simplest terms, CO is equal to the heart rate (HR) multiplied by the SV, which is equal to the EDV minus the end-systolic volume (ESV). • Therefore, CO = HR × (EDV − ESV). • The ejection fraction (EF) measures the percentage of EDV ejected during systole: EF = SV/EDV.

SV is a function of the extent of shortening of myocardial fiber, which depends on preload (initial volume), afterload (resistance to ventricular emptying), and contractility. • The relationship between diastolic filling and SV is governed by Starling's law, which states that, as muscle fiber length increases, so does the force of contraction. • Increasing fiber length stretches the sarcomere toward the optimal 2.2-µm length. • Therefore, CO alone is not an indicator of myocardial contractility.

EDV, vascular resistance, and myocardial contractility are the primary determinants of SV. • EDV is largely made up of passive ventricular filling during diastole. • Diastolic filling time shortens as the pulse rate increases to 160 beats per minute. • Beyond this rate, CO decreases. • Ventricular contractility depends on three interdependent variables: velocity of shortening, force of contraction, and length of displacement. • Atrial contraction contributes 15–30% of EDV, the so-called atrial kick. • Arterial blood pressure alone is not an accurate indicator of CO.

ANSWER:
C

2. Which of the following factors is/are not a determinant of CO?

   A. End-diastolic pressure

   B. Afterload

   C. Contractility

   D. Heart rate

   E. Ventricular interaction

   Ref.: 3

COMMENTS: The primary goal in the management of critically ill inpatients is to provide sufficient O_2 delivery to satisfy O_2 demand. • Oxygen consumption (VO_2) is initially dependent on oxygen delivery (DO_2). However, when oxygen delivery exceeds that which is necessary (the critical DO_2), VO_2 becomes delivery independent (Figure 15-1). • VO_2 is a reasonable estimate of adenosine triphosphate (ATP) turnover in the cells. • In clinical situations, the covariation of DO_2 and VO_2 usually represents efforts to deliver more O_2 in response to increased demand rather than O_2 supply dependence. • DO_2 can be optimized by increasing arterial oxygen content, increasing CO, or both. • The four factors that determine cardiac output are preload, afterload, contractility, and heart rate.

Preload is defined as end-diastolic sarcomere length, which is linearly related to EDV. • Left atrial pressure is correlated with left ventricular end-diastolic pressure in normal hearts. • Pulmonary capillary wedge pressure (PCWP) is a reflection of left atrial pressure and is commonly used as an index of preload. • The relationship between PCWP and EDV is not constant but is affected by changes in left ventricular compliance, wall thickness, heart rate, ischemia, and medications. • Ventricular interaction affects CO. • Shifts of the interventricular septum, normally slightly convex toward the right ventricle, may compromise ventricular filling. • **Afterload** is the impedance to ventricular ejection and is estimated by systemic or pulmonary vascular resistance. • An increase in afterload produces an increase in contractility (Anrep effect). • **Contractility** is an intrinsic property of the myocardium that is manifested as a greater force of contraction for a given preload. • All the available inotropic agents increase contractility by increasing intracellular calcium concentration and availability. • **Heart rate** may influence cardiac output in a number of ways. • Bradycardia and excessive tachycardia should be corrected. • An increase in heart rate affects preload and increases contractility (Bowditch phenomenon). • In general, preload must be optimized before afterload manipulation. • Inotropic agents should be used only after the other factors have been optimized.

ANSWER:
A

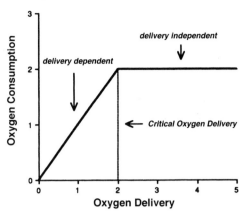

Figure 15-1 The relationship of oxygen consumption to oxygen delivery. As oxygen delivery increases, oxygen consumption becomes independent of delivery. (Adapted from Hill EP, Willford DC, Moore WY, et al: Oxygen transport and oxygen consumption vs. cardiac output at different haematocrits. *Perfusion* 2:39, 1987. Copyright by Edward/Hodder & Stoughton Educational.)

3. Which of the following mechanisms is/are the body's most important defenses in severe oxygen transport deficiency?

    A. Hyperventilation

    B. Reduction of VO_2

    C. Varying of the organ distribution of cardiac output

    D. Shift of the oxyhemoglobin dissociation curve

    E. Widening of the arterial-venous oxygen content difference

Ref.: 2

COMMENTS: See Question 4.

4. With regard to tissue utilization of oxygen, which of the following statements is/are true?

    A. The brain requires 15% of the resting CO and 20% of the total basal VO_2.

    B. The kidneys receive 25% of CO but can tolerate a reduction to one third of their normal blood flow for up to 1 hr.

    C. The heart extracts 70% of available oxygen from its arterial supply.

    D. During acute hypoxia, blood is preferentially shunted to the heart and brain.

    E. Arterial-venous oxygen difference is a measure of the extent to which blood flow matches the metabolic demand for oxygen.

Ref.: 2

COMMENTS: Increasing the proportion of CO to satisfy the continuous high requirements if the brain and heart for oxygen transport is crucial for survival during states of severe oxygen transport deficiency, such as cardiac arrest. • In general, organs with low oxygen extraction ratios tolerate decreased blood flow well. • Because the kidneys extract only 10% of oxygen available in the arterial blood supply, they tolerate decreased blood flow far better than does the heart or the brain. • Organs other than the heart tend to compensate for decreased blood flow by extracting more oxygen from their blood supply. • The extent of this extraction can be estimated by the arterial-venous oxygen content difference.

• Normally, the blood consumes only 25% of its total oxygen supply. • The normal mixed venous blood is 75% saturated, with a partial pressure of oxygen of 40 mmHg. • These values decrease in response to a fall in CO, which can be detected before changes in blood pressure, pulse rate, or central venous pressure (CVP) are noted. • Increased extraction is made possible by the relaxation of precapillary sphincters that enlarge the available capillary beds for oxygen exchange.

A N S W E R S :
Question 3: C, E
Question 4: A, B, C, D, E.

5. Which of the following factors can directly affect DO_2?

    A. Blood transfusions

    B. VO_2

    C. CO

    D. Fraction of inspired oxygen (FIO_2)

    E. Metabolic alkalosis

Ref.: 3, 4

COMMENTS: DO_2 is dependent on arterial oxygen content and CO:

$$CaO_2 = ([Hgb] \times 1.39)\,SaO_2 + (PaO_2 \times 0.0031)$$

where CaO_2 is the arterial oxygen content, [Hgb] is the hemoglobin concentration, SaO_2 is the arterial oxygen saturation, PaO_2 is the partial pressure of oxygen in arterial blood, 1.39 is the amount of oxygen in milliliters carried by each gram of fully saturated hemoglobin, and 0.0031 is the solubility of oxygen in plasma. • The factor ($PaO_2 \times 0.0031$) is usually insignificant. DO_2 is calculated according to the equation

$$DO_2 = CaO_2 \times CO \times 10$$

Oxygen consumption (VO_2) is calculated according to the equation

$$VO_2 = C(a{-}v)O_2 \times CO \times 10$$

where $C(a{-}v)O_2$ is the arteriovenous oxygen content. • Blood transfusions affect DO_2 by increasing the hemoglobin in blood, thereby increasing the CaO_2. • CO directly affects DO_2 delivery, and a change in FIO_2 changes the saturation in arterial blood. • VO_2 is dependent on DO_2 because inadequate DO_2 results in suboptimal VO_2, which in turn results in lactic acidosis. • Acid-base abnormalities do not directly affect DO_2 except in cases in which CO may be impaired by extremes of pH. • Changes in acid-base status have an effect on the oxygen pressure (PO_2) at which 50% of the hemoglobin is saturated (P_{50}, described in Question 6), causing increased or decreased affinity of oxygen at the tissue level. • This affects VO_2 but has no bearing on DO_2.

A N S W E R :
A, C, D

6. A 70-kg patient is admitted to the intensive care unit with a mean arterial pressure (MAP) of 50 mmHg, CVP of 8 mmHg, pulmonary artery occlusion pressure (PCWP) of 6 mmHg, CO of 7.0 L/min, hemoglobin level of 5 g/dl of pH 7.20, and PCO_2 of 52 mmHg. Which of the following values apply to this patient?

    A. P_{50} greater than 27

    B. Systemic vascular resistance (SVR) of 820 dyne sec/cm^{-5}

C. P_{50} less than 27

D. Shift of the hemoglobin dissociation curve to the left

E. Oxygen capacity of 8.85 ml/g

Ref.: 4

COMMENTS: O_2 forms an easily reversible combination with hemoglobin to yield oxyhemoglobin (Hgb-O_2). • From the hemoglobin dissociation curve, it can be seen that the amount of O_2 carried by hemoglobin increases rapidly up to a PO_2 of about 60 mmHg (Figure 15-2). • Above 60 mmHg, the hemoglobin dissociation curve flattens out, and there is a much smaller change in hemoglobin saturation for the same change in PO_2.

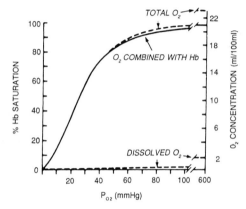

Figure 15-2 Hemoglobin dissociation curve (*solid line*) for pH 7.4, PCO_2 40 mmHg, and 37°C. The total blood O_2 concentration is also shown for a hemoglobin concentration of 15 g/100 ml of blood. (From West JB: *Respiratory Physiology: The Essentials*, 4th ed. Williams & Wilkins, Baltimore, 1990.)

Conversely, in the peripheral circulation, hemoglobin can release large amounts of O_2 with decreasing hemoglobin saturation and yet maintain a relatively high PO_2, which is needed to maintain a gradient for diffusion into the peripheral tissues. • The maximal amount of O_2 that can combine with hemoglobin is called the **O_2 capacity** (1.39 ml of O_2 can combine with each gram of hemoglobin). • In this patient, the O_2 capacity is $1.39 \times 5 = 6.85$. • The **O_2 saturation** is the actual amount of O_2 combined with hemoglobin divided by the O_2 capacity and then multiplied by 100. • Normal O_2 saturation is 97–100%. • O_2 content takes into account the amount of O_2 dissolved in plasma, which is 0.0031 ml O_2/dl blood/mmHg PO_2. • This factor is added to the O_2 capacity to yield the O_2 content.

The position of the hemoglobin dissociation curve is affected by a number of factors: carbon dioxide pressure (PCO_2), pH, temperature, 2,3-diphosphoglycerate (2,3-DPG) levels, cortisol levels, and aldosterone levels. • A shift to the right indicates that there is more unloading of O_2 at a given PO_2 in the tissue capillaries. • A leftward shift indicates decreased unloading of O_2 at a given PO_2 in the tissue capillaries. • Elevated PCO_2 and temperature and decreased pH cause a shift to the right. • The effect of elevated PCO_2, causing a shift to the right, is known as the Bohr effect and is presumably due to the effect of hypercarbia on pH. • ATP and 2,3-DPG lower hemoglobin affinity for O_2, causing a shift to the right. • The pH and 2,3-DPG have counterbalancing effects in that elevated pH causes increased formation of 2,3-DPG, and decreased pH causes decreased formation of 2,3-DPG. • Elevated cortisol and aldosterone levels cause a rightward shift. • The position of the oxyhemoglobin dissociation curve along the horizontal axis is characteristically termed the **P_{50}** value, which is the PO_2 at which

50% of the hemoglobin is saturated. • The normal value is approximately 27 mmHg.

The patient in question not only would have an elevated PCO_2, which would cause a rightward shift, but also metabolic acidosis secondary to low hemoglobin and low perfusion pressure. • A rightward shift would be expected, and the resultant P_{50} would be greater than 27. • The SVR in this patient is 480 dyne sec/cm^{-5}, as calculated by the formula: SVR = MAP – CVP/CO. • This value is compatible with a distributive type of shock in this patient, with a low SVR, a normal-to-low PAOP (PCWP), and a normal CO.

A N S W E R :
A

7. Which of the following is/are primarily responsible for increasing the CO of patients with acute mild-to-moderate normovolemic anemia?

A. Tachycardia

B. Increased contractility

C. Increased afterload

D. Decreased sympathetic nervous activity

E. Decreased blood viscosity

Ref.: 5

COMMENTS: DO_2 is maintained in patients with acute mild-to-moderate normovolemic anemia by a increased CO, compensating for a reduction in oxygen carrying capacity. • Decreased blood viscosity is primarily responsible for the increased CO, since it results in improved laminar flow. • In blood, viscosity depends on particulate concentration and flow. • A reduction in hematocrit by 50% produces an eightfold greater reduction in viscosity in the postcapillary venules compared to the aorta, thus facilitating disruption of cells in rouleau formation. • Because of decreased viscosity in acute normovolemic anemia, decreased afterload, improved preload, and increased contractility are observed. • Although increased cardiac sympathetic tone is seen during anemia, its direct effect on the heart is not primarily responsible for the increased CO.

A N S W E R :
E

8. Which of the following statements concerning radial artery cannulation is/are not true?

A. Performance of the Allen test is mandatory.

B. Arterial thrombosis is more common with catheters larger than 20 gauge and those left in place for 4 days or longer.

C. The incidence of infection is higher with catheters placed by surgical cutdown.

D. The catheter should be replaced every 3 days.

E. Intermittent flushing to keep the catheter free of clots is desirable.

Ref.: 4

COMMENTS: The radial artery is the site most frequently used for catheterization if the ulnar artery and palmar arterial arch are patent. • Therefore, the Allen test, which checks for ulnar collateral flow to the palm, should be performed before radial artery catheterization. • A normal test result consists of a palmar blush within 7 seconds after the ulnar artery is released. • The incidence of complications after arterial catheterization seems to be operator independent, unlike the case with pulmonary artery catheterizations. • Known risk factors include intermittent punctures, patient's age under 10 years, prolonged catheterization (>4 days), anticoagulant therapy, and the use of a catheter larger than 20 gauge or made of polypropylene rather than Teflon.

Most patients with arterial thrombosis remain asymptomatic. • Most thrombi (43%) are present at the time of catheter removal, and another 30% develop within 24 hr. • Damping of the arterial waveform may result from thrombosis. • If thrombosis is suspected, the catheter should be aspirated and not flushed forcefully. • Intermittent manual flushing with as little as 3 ml of fluid has been demonstrated to cause retrograde displacement of emboli from the radial artery cannula to the aortic arch and from there back into the cerebral circulation. • A higher incidence of thrombosis occurs within the first 24 hr when a surgical cutdown is performed (48 versus 23% with percutaneous placement), but the incidence of thrombosis at 1 week is the same for both methods of placement. • Brachial artery cannulation has a high incidence of embolic occlusion of the distal arteries (5–41%) and should therefore be avoided.

Infection remains the commonest complication. • Predisposing factors are prolonged catheterization, surgical cutdown, local inflammation, preexisting bacteremias, and failure to change the saline flush fluid, transducer, and flush tubing every 48 hr. • The need for intermittent arterial catheter replacement is not established and indeed is controversial. • Infected catheters are often colonized by gram-negative rods, *Enterococcus*, or *Candida*. • Povidone-iodine ointment should be used at the insertion site because of the increased risk of *Candida* infection. • Median nerve neuropathy has been associated with radial artery catheterizations because of compartment hypertension or nerve compression by blood.

ANSWER:
D, E

9. Which one of the following statements regarding arterial catheterization is/are true?

A. Aortic systolic pressure is lower than radial systolic pressure.

B. Aortic diastolic pressure is 10 mmHg higher than radial diastolic pressure.

C. Aortic MAP is slightly higher than radial MAP.

D. A blunted waveform is caused by small air bubbles in the tubing.

E. Underdamping causes systolic overshoot.

Ref.: 4

COMMENTS: The accuracy of a catheter-tubing-transducer system depends on its resonant frequency and damping characteristics. • In general, a lower damping coefficient requires a higher resonant frequency and vice versa. • The best frequency response for arterial pressure monitoring is achieved by using a good-quality transducer, the shortest length of noncompliant tubing, and an appropriately sized catheter. • A blunted waveform (overdamping) results in the underestimation of systolic pressure. • It is caused by use of compliant tubing, large bubbles in the tubing, kinking, and blood clots. • Underdamping causes systolic overshoot, which is seen with small air bubbles in the tubing and excessive lengths of noncompliant tubing. • The aortic MAP and diastolic arterial pressure are slightly higher than the radial MAP and diastolic arterial pressure. • However, the systolic pressure is consistently higher in the radial artery than in the aorta. • This discrepancy increases with distal progression, smaller arterial caliber, and age. • This is explained by the reflection of pressure waves from capillary beds, resulting in augmentation of systolic and reduction of diastolic values measured.

ANSWER:
A, C, E

10. In which of the following circumstances is a CVP reading a reliable guide in fluid management?

A. Chest radiograph consistent with pulmonary edema

B. Right ventricular diastolic pressure equal to the CVP

C. Mitral valve disease

D. Left ventricular EF of 0.40

E. Pulmonary hypertension

Ref.: 3

COMMENTS: Stroke volume requires optimization if shock states are to be corrected. • Stroke volume depends on preload, contractility, and afterload. • It is important to optimize preload first. • In the case of the left ventricle, preload is defined by left ventricular end-diastolic volume (LVEDV). • No bedside method that measures LVEDV is available. • Assessments of preload have included clinical indicators, CVP, PCWP, the use of volumetric catheters, echocardiographic studies, and duplex sonographic imaging. • The correlation between determinations of preload based on clinical assessment and those based on invasive monitoring is poor.

If CVP monitoring is to be used as a guide to fluid management, the right ventricular function must parallel the left ventricular function. • CVP and PCWP correlate well at low pressures, but as CVP increases to 8 mmHg or higher, its correlation with PCWP is unreliable. • Likewise, the correlation between PCWP and LVEDV is affected by changes in ventricular compliance, which occur frequently with critically ill patients. • For normal patients, right atrial pressure, right ventricular diastolic pressure, and CVP are equal. • CVP may be normal in the presence of left ventricular dysfunction and increase only after the dysfunction becomes severe, with resultant pulmonary congestion and rising right ventricular end-diastolic pressure. • CVP has been shown to have little correlation with left atrial pressure or PCWP in patients with valvular heart disease, pulmonary hypertension, and coronary artery disease with an EF of less than 0.5. • With critically ill patients, CVP is not well correlated with the PCWP. • CVP determination is useful for initial volume resuscitation and diagnosing right ventricular infarction and pericardial tamponade.

ANSWER:
B

11. With regard to interpreting CVP or PCWP measurements, which of the following statements is/are true?

A. They are best and most logically used when observing responses to volume and fluid infusion challenges.

B. Strict adherence to expected normal values is the best guideline for their use.

C. PCWP reflects the pulmonary capillary pressure (Pcap) within 1–2 mmHg in inflammatory states.

D. In the absence of pulmonary disease, PCWP is a reliable guide to left ventricular end-diastolic pressure.

E. If an acceptable wedge position cannot be obtained, the pulmonary artery systolic pressure is an acceptable indicator of left atrial pressure.

Ref.: 1–3

COMMENTS: CVP reflects filling pressures of the right ventricle, whereas PCWP reflects those of the left ventricle. • Elevated values reflect an inability of either ventricle to handle venous return. • Nonmyocardial factors that cause a rise in CVP include mechanical blockage or kinking of the catheter, vasoconstrictive drugs, positive-pressure ventilation, pneumothorax, flail chest, cardiac tamponade, and pulmonary embolism. • Nonmyocardial causes of elevated PCWP include pulmonary vascular disease, mitral valve incompetence, increased airway pressure, and increased pleural pressure. • Because of the interposed pulmonary vascular system, CVP is not always a reliable index of left ventricular function. • Left-sided pressures may rise sharply, and pulmonary edema may occur without a significant rise in CVP. • Both measurements are best used to assess the response to fluid challenges rather than to measure absolute normal values.

In the absence of an acceptable wedge position, the pulmonary artery diastolic pressure, not the pulmonary systolic pressure, can be an alternative indicator of mean left atrial pressure. • Pulmonary capillary pressure represents the hydrostatic pressure that drives the formation of edema in the lung. • Regardless of serum oncotic pressure and the efficiency of the lymphatic pump, edema occurs beyond a level of Pcap. • In normal lungs, with minimal pulmonary venous resistance, PCWP may predict Pcap within 1–2 mmHg. • However, in the presence of acute lung injury, hypoxia, and several vasoactive agents, cytokines have vasoconstrictive effects on either the arterial (serotonin) or the venous (histamine) side. • In such cases, the Pcap may be higher than the left atrial pressure. • Thus, PCWP may be used inaccurately as an endpoint during resuscitation of these patients, leading to further deterioration of O_2 transport.

ANSWER:
A, D

12. Which of the following criteria indicate(s) correct pulmonary artery catheter positioning?

A. Characteristic PCWP waveform

B. Mean pulmonary artery pressure (MPAP) less than mean PCWP

C. PO_2 of blood from a catheter in wedge position less than the PO_2 of systemic blood

D. Amount of air required for balloon inflation less than 0.7 ml

E. Continuous flush system

Ref.: 3, 6

COMMENTS: The characteristic waveform of the properly wedged pulmonary artery catheter reveals A and V waves and X and Y descents but no C waves. On the electrocardiogram (ECG), the A wave follows the QRS complex, and the V wave follows the T wave. • The absence of this waveform indicates improper pulmonary artery catheter positioning. • Because blood flows from the pulmonary artery to the left, the mean PCWP should always be less than the MPAP and less than or equal to the pulmonary artery diastolic pressure. • If MPAP were less than the mean PCWP, it would imply reverse flow through the pulmonary circuit. • Blood withdrawn through the wedged catheter should be fully oxygenated and have a higher PO_2 and lower PCO_2 than systemic arterial blood. • The obstruction to pulmonary blood flow during wedged positioning causes stasis of blood in the pulmonary circuit and allows longer capillary and alveolar exchange. • Patients who require high PEEP or have significant shunting of blood do not have as significant capillary-alveolar exchange because shunts cause a decrease in blood flow through the pulmonary capillaries.

Three functional lung zones based on the distribution of pulmonary blood flow and ventilation have been described (Figure 15-3).

• The position of the catheter tip should be located in zone 3 of the lung fields, which is the most posterior of the lung zones in a supine patient. • The importance of zone 3 is based on the dependent flow of blood in the pulmonary circuit when the patient is in the supine position and while venous pressure exceeds alveolar pressure, resulting in increased capillary blood flow. • The positioning of the pulmonary artery tip can be determined by a lateral chest radiograph. • Hypovolemia and positive end-expiratory pressure (PEEP) or continuous positive airway pressure (CPAP) increase the proportion of zones 1 and 2 in relationship to zone 3. • Positioning of the catheter in zone 1 or 2 should be suspected when the PCWP is greater than the pulmonary arterial diastolic pressure (PADP), when there are marked respiratory variations in the tracing, and whenever the PCWP increases by more than half of the increase in PEEP. • If the catheter tip is located in zone 1 or 2, PCWP reflects alveolar pressure, not left atrial pressure. • If less than 0.7 ml of air in the catheter balloon produces a PCWP tracing, the catheter is located too far distally, and complications usually follow. • The catheter should never be advanced unless the balloon is fully inflated (1.5 ml). • A continuous flush system is required for accurate pulmonary artery readings but does not indicate correct pulmonary artery catheter positioning.

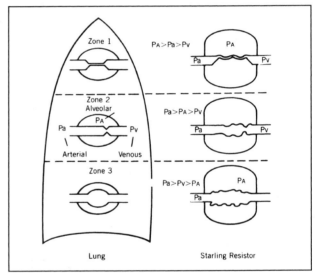

Figure 15-3 Pulmonary capillary bed has flow characteristics of Starling resistor where, when chamber pressure exceeds downstream pressure, flow is independent of downstream pressure. However, when downstream pressure exceeds chamber pressure, flow is determined by upstream-downstream difference. Alveolar pressure is the same throughout the lung. Pulmonary arterial pressure increases in the dependent regions of the lung. There may be a region at the top of the lung (zone 1) where pulmonary arterial pressure falls below alveolar pressure. Thus, zone 1 will occur wherever alveolar pressure exceeds pulmonary arterial pressure. This phenomenon may occur when pulmonary arterial pressure is decreased, as with hypovolemia, or when alveolar pressure is increased, as with application of positive end-expiratory pressure. Zone 1 produces an alveolar dead space. In zone 2, pulmonary arterial pressure increases and exceeds alveolar pressure. In zone 2, blood flow is determined by the difference between arterial and alveolar pressure. In zone 3, blood flow is determined by the arteriovenous difference. (From Bone RC: The treatment of severe hypoxemia due to the adult respiratory distress syndrome. *Arch Intern Med* 140:85, 1980. Copyright 1980, American Medical Association.)

ANSWER:
A

13. In which one or more of the following conditions does PADP not correlate with PCWP?

  A. Acute myocardial infarction

  B. Pulmonary hypertension

  C. Left ventricular dysfunction

  D. Severe chronic lung disease

  E. PADP of 17 mmHg and left atrial pressure of 10 mmHg

Ref.: 4

COMMENTS: PADP has been used to reflect PCWP and left ventricular filling pressures. • PADP reflects PCWP with reasonable accuracy for normal patients and those with acute myocardial infarction, left ventricular dysfunction, or chronic lung disease if no pulmonary vascular changes exist. • However, PADP exceeds PCWP for patients with tachycardia or pulmonary hypertension associated with acidosis, hypoxemia, pulmonary embolus, or pulmonary parenchymal disease. • PADP also reflects left atrial pressure when no pulmonary vascular hypertension exists. • PADP is usually 1–2 mmHg higher than PCWP and left atrial pressure. • PCWP has always been found to be superior to PADP for estimating left atrial pressure. • A difference between PADP and PCWP of more than 4–5 mmHg indicates elevated pulmonary vascular resistance.

ANSWER:
B, D, E

14. Which of the following statements regarding hemodynamic monitoring for critically ill patients is/are true?

  A. Right ventricular end-diastolic volume index (RVEDVI) correlates better than does PCWP with CO.

  B. RVEDVI is a better predictor of preload than is PCWP.

  C. Pulmonary artery catheter use improves outcomes for septic patients.

  D. EF is not a good index of ventricular contractility.

  E. At moderate-to-high levels of ventilatory support (PEEP 10–50 cmH$_2$O), there is a good correlation between PCWP and the cardiac index (CI).

Ref.: 7

COMMENTS: Critically ill patients exhibit great differences in right and left ventricular function. • PCWP has been considered a clinically relevant measure of left ventricular preload. • Yet measurement and interpretation of PCWP with mechanically ventilated patients for whom PEEP or inverse-ratio ventilation is used is difficult, particularly when variable left ventricular compliance exists. • The stroke volume index, calculated by dividing the CI by the heart rate, can be divided by the EF, yielding the RVEDVI. • Furthermore, a RVEDVI value of less than 140 ml/m^2 is a better predictor of the CI response to volume loading than is either CVP or PCWP when PEEP is used. • However, the values associated with the highest CI with critically ill patients vary from 80 to 160 ml/m^2, a range much too great to be used as an endpoint. • In addition, the correlation between RVEDVI determined by volumetric catheters and that measured by echocardiographic studies is poor. • Therefore, although RVEDVI is better correlated with CI than is PCWP, its use has not improved the clinical management of these patients. • Because the right ventricular EF depends greatly on the right ventricular afterload, increases in the pulmonary vascular resistance index reduce the EF, which is not a good index of right ventricular contractility. • End-diastolic volume is a more reliable indicator of ventricular preload than is filling pressure, especially for patients who require PEEP.

Objective evidence does not support the absolute value of pulmonary artery catheters in the initial management of all critically ill patients. • Available data indicate that their use results in improved outcomes in the following: aortic operations when large peripheral vascular resistance changes are foreseen, multiple-trauma patients with closed head or spinal cord injury, myocardial infarction accompanied by cardiogenic shock, and some pediatric patients with pulmonary hypertension. • Although pulmonary artery catheters are frequently used in other situations, such as sepsis or preoperatively to optimize DO$_2$ for patients with a history of myocardial infarction, evidence to support such use is uncertain at best.

ANSWER:
A, B, D

15. Which of the following factors are determinants of mixed venous oxygen saturation (SvO$_2$)?

  A. VO$_2$

  B. CO

  C. Hemoglobin concentration

  D. Arterial oxygen saturation (SaO$_2$)

  E. Myocardial VO$_2$

Ref.: 1, 2, 4

COMMENTS: SvO$_2$ is a measure of the oxygen saturation of blood in the pulmonary artery. • SvO$_2$ reflects the relationship between DO$_2$ and VO$_2$. • Under normal conditions, DO$_2$ is 2000 ml/min and VO$_2$ is 200 ml/min. • Usually, the arterial blood is fully saturated, and the saturation of mixed venous blood is 80%. • If the arterial blood is not fully saturated, the difference between the arterial and venous saturation corresponds to the O$_2$ extraction and to the DO$_2$/O$_2$ ratio. • The primary goal of management is to maintain the patient near the normal ratio of 5:1 and, if DO$_2$ fails, to intervene to avoid a critical level of 2:1. • When they are balanced— that is, when the critical DO$_2$ has been achieved—SvO$_2$ is normal. • When VO$_2$ is greater than DO$_2$, SvO$_2$ is decreased owing to increased demand for oxygen by peripheral tissue. • Because DO$_2$ is largely dependent on CO, hemoglobin concentration, and SaO$_2$, any factor affecting these values must be considered a cause of decreased SvO$_2$. • Blood returning from the periphery combines with coronary venous blood in the right atrium. • Myocardial VO$_2$ is not a major determinant of SvO$_2$ because the coronary blood flow is a small part of the total flow through the right ventricle.

ANSWER:
A, B, C, D

16. Which of the following conditions is/are associated with an elevated SvO$_2$?

  A. Septic shock

  B. Left-to-right shunt

  C. Distal migration of the oxymetric catheter

  D. Lactic acidosis

  E. Right-to-left shunt

Ref.: 4

COMMENTS: Mixed venous blood represents a perfusion-weighted average of blood draining from all the body's organ systems.

Values within the normal range of SvO_2 (0.68–0.77) suggest a balance between DO_2 and VO_2. • This balance indicates that the fraction of consumed oxygen delivered to the peripheral tissues is normal. • Four factors determine SvO_2: CO, hemoglobin concentration, SaO_2, and VO_2. Causes of elevated SvO_2 indicate an excess of DO_2 and VO_2 and are most commonly associated with septic shock and cirrhosis, in which there are abnormal distributions of blood flow with a low systemic vascular resistance and concomitant high CO. • In the septic state, high CO is also a result of the high catecholamine levels associated with sepsis. • A left-to-right intracardiac shunt causes an elevated SvO_2 but invalidates SvO_2 as an index of perfusion. • Other causes of elevated SvO_2 are hyperbaric oxygen therapy, states of low VO_2 (e.g., hypothermia, muscular paralysis, sedation, or coma), and cyanide toxicity. • In addition, high SvO_2 may indicate improper distal migration of the catheter. • Uncompensated changes in any of the four determinants of SvO_2 may result in a decrease in the measured value of SvO_2. • However, with a critically ill patient, the correlation between a change in an individual factor and a change in the SvO_2 is low. • A decrease in SvO_2 of more than 0.10 is likely to be of clinical significance regardless of the initial SvO_2. • A sustained decrease in SvO_2 of more than 0.10 does not explain the cause of the disparity in DO_2 and VO_2, and the clinician should analyze the individual factors (CO, hemoglobin concentration, SaO_2, and VO_2) that determine SvO_2 and affect the oxygen balance.

ANSWER:
A, B, C

17. With regard to complications associated with pulmonary artery catheterization, which of the following statements is/are true?

   A. Standby external pacemakers are recommended for patients with preexisting left bundle-branch block.

   B. Hemoptysis mandates immediate overinflation of the catheter balloon.

   C. To prevent pulmonary artery rupture, inflation of the catheter balloon should not exceed 75% of the balloon capacity.

   D. The occurrence of ventricular dysrhythmias while the right atrial pressure is being recorded suggests intracardiac catheter knotting.

   E. The rate of catheter-induced sepsis closely parallels the incidence of catheter colonization.

Ref.: 4

COMMENTS: The indications for the use of pulmonary artery catheters are in flux. • Their value for patients with sepsis or shock with hemodynamic instability is uncertain. • They may be useful in the management of patients unresponsive to the use of fluids and vasoactive agents. • Dysrhythmias occur in 12–67% of catheterizations but are usually self-limited, premature ventricular contractions. • Their incidence seems to be lower when patients are in the head-up and right lateral tilt position. • Complete heart block can develop in patients with preexisting left bundle-branch block. • Prophylactic pacing wire should be utilized with these patients. • Prophylactic lidocaine and full inflation of the balloon may prevent ventricular ectopy. • Any hemoptysis in patients with a pulmonary artery catheter suggests the diagnosis of perforation or rupture. • Mechanisms involved in pulmonary artery rupture include (1) overinflation of the balloon; (2) incomplete balloon inflation (<75%), forcing the exposed tip through the wall; and (3) pulmonary hypertension. • An "overwedge" pattern suggests eccentric balloon inflation, overdistention, or both. • If hemoptysis develops, the catheter should be pulled back with the balloon deflated.

• Massive hemoptysis necessitates placement of a double-lumen endotracheal tube and occlusion of the bronchus on the side of the rupture with a Fogarty catheter. • Emergency thoracotomy is needed. • Cooling, looping, or knotting of the catheter may occur in the right ventricle during insertion. • These situations can be avoided if no more of 10 cm of the catheter is inserted after a ventricular tracing is identified and before a pulmonary artery tracing appears. • Ventricular arrhythmias that occur while the right atrial pressure is being recorded suggest knotting. • Insertion of a guidewire into the catheter, followed by slow withdrawal of the catheter, may help to unknot the catheter. • Although catheter-related sepsis occurs in only up to 2% of insertions, bacterial colonization occurs in 5–35% of catheterizations. • Infections are more common when the catheter is left in place for more than 72 hr or when it is inserted via an antecubital vein.

ANSWER:
A, D

18. Regarding carbon dioxide (CO_2) kinetics, which of the following statements is/are true?

   A. The total amount of CO_2 produced is equivalent to the amount of O_2 consumed.

   B. The arteriovenous difference of CO_2 (a-vCO_2) is the same as that of oxygen.

   C. The end-tidal CO_2 and partial pressure of arterial CO_2 ($PaCO_2$) is identical.

   D. The end-tidal CO_2–arterial CO_2 gradient is an indirect measure of compression volume.

   E. All of the above

Ref.: 3

COMMENTS: The total amount of CO_2 produced by systemic metabolism is very close to the amount of O_2 consumed (200 ml/min). • The ratio between CO_2 produced and O_2 consumed is called the respiratory quotient and varies, depending on the energy sources. • The excretion of CO_2 is related to alveolar ventilation per minute. • Most of the blood CO_2 is present as bicarbonate. • The metabolically produced CO_2 is present as dissolved CO_2. • The a-vCO_2 is 4 ml/min, equivalent to the a-vO_2. • Even if 70–80% of the alveoli are collapsed, hyperventilation of the remaining alveoli can maintain normocarbia. • End-tidal CO_2 represents mixed alveolar gas that is in equilibrium with arterial blood. • Thus, the end-tidal CO_2 and the $PaCO_2$ should be identical. • When there is dead space, the alveoli are overventilated but minimally perfused, or some of the tidal gas represents inflation gas (e.g., resulting from positive-pressure ventilation with peak airway pressures >30 H_2O), then the end-tidal CO_2 is less than the $PaCO_2$. • Large gradients serve as an indirect measure of nonperfused alveoli or of compression volume.

ANSWER:
E

19. True or false: The alveolar-arterial oxygen gradient (A-aO_2) is useful as an early indicator of incipient respiratory failure.

Ref.: 1, 2, 4

COMMENTS: The partial pressure of oxygen in the atmosphere is 160 mmHg. • As this air is humidified in the upper airways, the partial pressure drops to 149 mmHg as a result of the effect of water vapor pressure at body temperature. • Ultimately, arterial blood leaves the pulmonary capillaries with an oxygen tension of 100 mmHg. • This blood is diluted by unsaturated blood from the bronchial and coronary circulation that empties into the left side of the heart. • The volume of this shunt is 3% of the output of the right side of the heart and results in an arterial partial pressure of 95 mmHg as blood enters the left ventricle. • The A-aO$_2$ is the difference between calculated alveolar and arterial oxygen pressures. • Assuming normal CO, an A-aO$_2$ below 350 mmHg corresponds to a shunt fraction of less than 15–20% at FIO$_2$ = 1. • When the inspired oxygen concentration is 100%, the normal A-aO$_2$ is 25–65 mmHg. • In circumstances causing serious venous admixture, this gradient may be more than 600 mmHg, resulting in an arterial partial pressure of oxygen (PaO$_2$) of 60 mmHg or less.

When the PaO$_2$ falls below 60 mmHg in a patient without previous lung disease or intracardiac defects, acute respiratory failure is diagnosed. • A PaO$_2$ below 30 mmHg is incompatible with life if allowed to continue for more than a few hours. • Several factors can cause such a drop in oxygen tension. • Perfusion of sections of the lung containing closed or nonventilated airways or alveoli causes shunting of unsaturated blood into the arterial circulation. • Injuries to pulmonary capillary endothelium or pulmonary vascular congestion leads to an increased diffusion distance for oxygen and collapse of alveoli. • Pulmonary surfactant is depleted by the resultant hypoxemia, furthering the insult. • As alveoli collapse, the lung volume is reduced, and an accompanying loss of compliance contributes to further shunting. • A number of insults can lead to this series of events, which is commonly known as adult respiratory distress syndrome (ARDS). • The use of PEEP helps correct this deficit by increasing the functional residual capacity (FRC) of the lung, increasing compliance and leading to alveolar reexpansion. • Nonrespiratory causes of an increased A-aO$_2$ include right-to-left intracardiac shunt and hyperthermia. • A decrease in PaO$_2$ with normal P(A-a)O$_2$ is seen with high altitude, decreased respiratory quotient, and central hypoventilation.

ANSWER:
True

20. With regard to the measurement of arterial blood gases and P(A-a)O$_2$, which of the following statements is/are true?

   A. Blood-gas analysis reports direct measurement of partial pressures of oxygen, carbon dioxide, and hemoglobin oxygen saturation (SO$_2$).

   B. Calculated SO$_2$ accurately parallels co-oximetric SO$_2$ measurement in critically ill patients.

   C. Iced arterial blood gas samples exhibit a 50% drop in oxygen tension within 1 hr.

   D. In healthy patients breathing room air, the P(A-a)O$_2$ varies between 10 and 15 mmHg.

   E. Radiographic changes usually precede abnormalities in A-aO$_2$.

Ref.: 2, 4

COMMENTS: The development of the Clark and Severinghaus electrodes during the 1950s made routine measurement of arterial and venous blood gases a standard procedure in the care of acutely ill patients. • Arterial blood samples should be procured under strict anaerobic conditions to prevent the presence of air bubbles. • In addition, placement of the sample in ice is necessary to reduce red blood cell metabolism. Iced, heparinized blood samples can be kept for 1 hr with only a 1% drop in oxygen tension. • Calculated SO$_2$ depends on assumptions based on direct measurement of the partial pressure of gases and a nomogram of the oxyhemoglobin

saturation curve, corrected for other factors. • In critically ill patients, direct determination of SO$_2$ by pulse oxymetric studies or oximetric catheters is preferred.

In patients breathing room air, the A-aO$_2$ represents an admixture of true shunting of blood and desaturation caused by a ventilation-perfusion (V/Q) imbalance. • When 100% oxygen is breathed, this P(A-a)O$_2$ gradient is caused by true shunting and perfusion of total nonventilated alveoli, thus eliminating the effects of alveolar-capillary diffusion barriers and V/Q imbalances. • When 100% oxygen is breathed, PaO$_2$ is slightly higher than 600 mmHg. • When mixed venous blood passes through the lung but does not come into contact with the alveoli, an absolute shunt exists, which is minimally improved by 100% oxygen. • Reduced ventilation results in a relative shunt, since it is less than the corresponding perfusion. • This shunt is a common cause of hypoxemia in acute and chronic respiratory insufficiency and can be corrected when a patient inspires 100% oxygen. • Increases in CO tend to minimize hypoxia and the A-aO$_2$ gradient that results from right-to-left absolute-relative shunt. • PEEP is used to improve lung function, but, by virtue of its potentially deleterious effect on cardiac function, it can accentuate hypoxemia. • Hence, pulmonary and cardiac function must always be assessed to evaluate arterial blood gases. • An increase in the P(A-a)O$_2$ on 100% oxygen is an early warning sign of deteriorating lung function. • This increase in gradient usually occurs before radiographic changes are evident.

ANSWER:
D

21. Which of the following conditions is/are usually associated with elevated dead space ventilation?

   A. Low CO

   B. Pulmonary embolism

   C. Pulmonary hypertension

   D. ARDS

   E. All of the above

Ref.: 4

COMMENTS: Carbon dioxide production and the dead space/tidal volume ratio (VD/VT) determine minute ventilation. • Patients whose VD/VT exceeds 0.6 usually require ventilatory support. • Small increases in VD/VT above 0.6 require large increases in minute ventilation to maintain a given arterial carbon dioxide pressure (PaCO$_2$). • The anatomic dead space includes the volume of the airways to the level of the bronchiole (150 ml). • The physiologic dead space also includes alveoli that are well ventilated but poorly perfused. • The commonest causes of increased dead space in critically ill patients are decreased CO, pulmonary embolism, pulmonary hypertension, ARDS, and excessive PEEP. • In dead-space ventilation, there is decreased blood flow to ventilated areas, which primarily affects carbon dioxide elimination. • Dead-space ventilation is defined as a high V/Q ratio. • Low CO, pulmonary embolism, and pulmonary hypertension directly cause decreased blood flow to the pulmonary vasculature. • In ARDS, some areas of lung are perfused but not ventilated. • Alveoli may be filled with secretions, exudate, blood, or edema, thereby increasing the shunt fraction. • Other areas of lung may be ventilated but not perfused, which accounts for the dead-space ventilation. • PEEP can cause dead-space ventilation by decreasing CO and by stenting open alveoli, which cause a collapse of surrounding capillaries, thereby decreasing alveolar perfusion.

ANSWER:
E

22. With regard to ventilatory mechanics, which of the following statements is/are true?

 A. The work of breathing at rest consumes 2% of total body oxygen consumption.

 B. The work of breathing may increase to 50% of total body oxygen consumption in postoperative patients.

 C. Chronic obstructive pulmonary disease (COPD) is associated with an increase in the work of breathing resulting from increased inspiratory work.

 D. Airway pressure reflects the compliance of the chest wall and diaphragm as well as that of the lungs.

 E. Compliance is measured as the change in volume divided by the change in pressure.

Ref.: 2

COMMENTS: The work of breathing at rest consumes 2% of total body VO_2. • The work of breathing can be markedly increased, up to 50% of the total VO_2, in postoperative patients because of increased airway resistance and decreased compliance of lung, chest wall, and diaphragm. • For patients with COPD, the work of breathing is increased because of increased expiratory work. • It can be assessed by preoperative pulmonary function testing and optimized by preoperative chest physical therapy, bronchodilators, and antibiotics if infection is present. • The proper use of volume-cycled ventilators and pressure-support ventilation can take over most of the work of breathing during the postoperative period. • Measuring airway pressure reflects the compliance of the chest wall and diaphragm as well as that of the lungs. • In relaxed patients this is of little importance, but in restless patients intraesophageal or intrapleural pressures provide a more accurate measure of compliance. • Compliance is defined as the change in pressure associated with each milliliter increase in lung volume. • In acute respiratory failure, decreased compliance is usually associated with decreased functional residual capacity. • Less compliant lungs need ventilatory management that maintains inflation of alveoli by the use of PEEP and recruits closed alveoli by elevating peak inspiratory pressures. • However, positive airway pressure may overdistend already ventilated alveoli. • Therefore, the peak inspiratory pressure should be kept below 40 cmH_2O. • In addition, tidal volume should be kept around 5 ml/kg to avoid volutrauma in patients with ARDS. • Changes in blood pH and carbon dioxide tensions reflect changes in patients' ventilation requirements. • The most useful variable in this regard is the end-expiratory carbon dioxide tension.

ANSWER:
A, B, D, E

23. Which of the following suggests the need for ventilatory support?

 A. Respiratory rate greater than 35 breaths per minute

 B. $PaCO_2$ greater than 60 mmHg

 C. Alveolar-arterial oxygen difference greater than 350 mmHg

 D. VD/VT greater than 0.6

 E. Shunt fraction greater than 5%

Ref.: 2, 3

COMMENTS: The indications for respiratory support include inadequate parameters of ventilation (respiratory rate >35, VD/VT >0.6, $PaCO_2$ >60 mmHg), oxygenation (A-a O_2 difference and PaO_2), and respiratory mechanics (vital capacity and inspiratory force). • In the absence of metabolic alkalosis or chronic hypercarbia, $PaCO_2$ greater than 60 mmHg is abnormal. • The pulmonary venous admixture (shunt fraction) can be defined as the amount of blood shunted around the lung as a fraction of the CO. • Shunt fraction is measured at the inspired oxygen concentration required to maintain adequate oxygenation (PO_2 60–70 mmHg). • A shunt fraction greater than 20% requires respiratory support.

ANSWER:
A, B, C, D

24. Which of the following characterizes ARDS?

 A. PaO_2/FiO_2 less than 300 mmHg

 B. Increased dead space ventilation and increased pulmonary compliance

 C. Hypoxemia with hypercarbia

 D. Bilateral interstitial infiltrates on chest x-ray that precede clinical abnormalities

 E. PCWP >18 mmHg

Ref.: 2, 4

COMMENTS: ARDS is a syndrome, not a disease process. • Because the lung has a limited response to injury, it is now recognized that there are many similarities in the pathophysiologic features and clinical presentation of acute lung injury after a variety of insults. • ARDS is seen with the systemic inflammatory syndrome and multiple organ failure, and it represents a common pathologic response. • This response includes an increase in capillary permeability, with interstitial edema and loss of alveolar architecture. • There is progressive hypoxemia, with increased pulmonary shunt fraction, decreased pulmonary compliance, and bilateral diffuse infiltrates not attributable to cardiac failure. • Criteria used to define ARDS include acute onset; PaO_2/FiO_2 less than 200 mmHg, bilateral infiltrates, and a PCWP <18 mmHg, or no clinical evidence of left atrial hypertension.

The lung response can be divided into an **exudative phase** (24–96 hrs, with leakage of proteinaceous fluid into the pulmonary interstitium and corresponding damage to the alveolar-capillary interface; an **early proliferative phase** (3–10 days), with proliferation of alveolar type II cells, cellular infiltration of the septum, and organization of hyaline membranes; and a **late proliferative phase** (7–10 days), with fibrosis of alveolar septum, ducts, and hyaline membranes. • The major criteria for the diagnosis of ARDS include hypoxia, which is relatively unresponsive to an increase in the inspired oxygen concentration; decreased pulmonary compliance (stiff lung); decreased functional residual capacity; increased dead-space ventilation; and a diffuse interstitial pattern seen on the chest x-ray. • It should be noted that the clinical and arterial blood gas abnormalities associated with ARDS may occur well before the radiographic changes are appreciated. • Similarly, clinical improvement may occur when the radiograph is still grossly abnormal. • In contrast to the classic picture of pulmonary failure, these patients are usually hypocarbic rather than hypercarbic. • To rule out other causes of pulmonary edema resulting from cardiogenic or hydrostatic causes, measurement of filling pressures is often required.

ANSWER:
D

25. Which of the following is/are thought to represent the common mechanisms in ARDS?

A. Neutrophil and macrophage activation

B. Injury to the alveolar-capillary interface

C. Endotoxemia

D. Platelet aggregation

E. Leukocyte–endothelial cell interaction

Ref.: 1–4

COMMENTS: See Question 26.

26. Which of the following may be associated with ARDS?

A. Gram-negative sepsis

B. Pulmonary aspiration

C. Excessive oxygen administration

D. Pancreatitis

E. Multiple trauma

Ref.: 1, 2

COMMENTS: ARDS was first described in 1967. • All the etiologic factors listed may be associated with ARDS. • Sepsis and gastric aspiration are most commonly associated with ARDS, but shock, major trauma, multiple transfusions, pancreatitis, drug overdose, pneumonia, and near drowning are also associated. • Four variables are associated with increased mortality rates in the setting of ARDS: presence of more than 10% bands, persistent acidemia, calculated bicarbonate level less than 20 mEq/L, and BUN level greater than 65 mg/dl. • Neither duration of mechanical ventilation nor level of static compliance is predictive of mortality rate. • Although a number of ventilatory and gas-exchange abnormalities coexist in ARDS, the final common pathophysiologic pathway is thought to be related to injury to the alveolar-capillary interface, which would allow intravascular fluid to leak into the interstitium and alveoli, resulting in increased extravascular lung water. • The mechanisms of acute lung injury are not precisely known. • The macrophage plays an important role in the release of cytokines and modulation of the host response. • Neutrophils accumulate in the pulmonary microvasculature in most patients with acute lung injury because of various chemotaxins, including C5a, lymphokines, leukotrienes, and immunoglobulins. • Neutrophils release granular substances, species of reduced oxygen, and arachidonic metabolites. • Disseminated intravascular coagulation and platelet aggregation often are found in these patients. • The fibrotic reaction may be due to endotoxin stimulation of connective tissue synthesis and alveolar macrophages. • Activation of endothelial cells in inflammatory states is divided into an early phase that leads to release of P-selectin, causing leukocyte adhesion, and a late phase induced by tumor necrosis factor (TNF) and interleukin-1 (IL-1). • TNF and IL-1 cause expression of adhesion molecules (E-selectin and interstitial and vascular adhesion molecules) as well as the conversion of the endothelial cell to a procoagulant phenotype. • Severity scoring and prognostic estimates are difficult. • Because death from ARDS is frequently due to nonrespiratory causes, measuring the severity of ARDS to predict death as an outcome may not be practical. • The severity of nonpulmonary organ dysfunction provides an additional estimate of prognosis: the more organ systems failing, the greater the mortality.

27. Which of the following treatments are appropriate for the management of virtually all cases of ARDS?

A. Mechanical ventilation

B. Albumin/furosemide

C. PEEP

D. Routine use of steroids

E. Routine use of broad-spectrum antibiotics

Ref.: 4, 8, 9

COMMENTS: Because the principal physiologic problem in ARDS is hypoxemia refractory to increasing FIO_2, the therapy is centered on the provision of mechanical ventilation to maximize oxygen delivery while minimizing lung injury. • PEEP is used to improve oxygenation and lung compliance. • PEEP should be optimized with the help of pressure-volume curves to facilitate the maintenance of open alveoli and the diffusion of oxygen into the pulmonary capillaries. • For a given FIO_2, the PaO_2 usually increases on administration of PEEP in cases of ARDS. • Excessive PEEP (>15 cm) can be hazardous because it may result in pneumothorax (barotrauma) and cause decreased venous return to the heart. • Overdistention of alveoli can be prevented by keeping the peak inspiratory pressure below 35 mmHg.

Newer ventilatory methods attempt to enhance alveolar recruitment, maintain alveolar patency throughout the respiratory cycle, maintain an SaO_2 of more than 90%, avoid dynamic hyperinflation (volutrauma), and reduce the risk of oxygen toxicity. • Spontaneous, augmented low-volume ventilation, using pressure support ventilation as a primary ventilatory support mode, directs flow to regions of low ventilation/perfusion. • It is supplemented by intermittent mandatory ventilation and PEEP. • The tidal volumes used are lower (5–8 ml/kg), accepting a lower PaO_2. • These newer modes of ventilation allow iatrogenic permissive hypercapnia.

Patients with ARDS have edematous, minimally compliant lungs that cause elevations in peak airway pressures to over 40 cm H_2O. • The elevated airway pressures contribute to further pulmonary injury by barotrauma, which causes further edema. • It is extremely difficult to both oxygenate and ventilate these patients. • Lower tidal volumes help reduce the barotrauma but result in an elevated $PaCO_2$ and a disturbed acid-base balance. • However, this disturbance is well tolerated by the patient as long as pH is maintained above 7.2. • At times, inverse-ratio ventilation is used to prolong the inspiratory phase. • Diuretics (in cases of obvious fluid overload and cardiac decompensation) and broad-spectrum antibiotics (in cases of established pulmonary infection or other sources of sepsis) may be useful for patients with ARDS. • Methylprednisolone in doses of 2–20 mg/kg/day has been used during the fibroproliferative phase of ARDS or when eosinophilia is found in the blood or bronchoalveolar aspirates. • However, the routine use of such drugs in the absence of these complicating factors has not been shown to be beneficial and should be avoided. • Fluid management is a long-standing controversy, particularly in hypoalbuminemic patients with acute lung injury or ARDS. • Recent data suggest that the combination of albumin/furosemide in patients with mild disease accelerates clearing of edema and shortens the length of the hospital stay. • However, there is no conclusive evidence that such therapy may work for patients with severe permeability problems.

A N S W E R :
A, C

28. With regard to patients on long-term ventilation, which of the following statements is/are true?

 A. Most patients on long-term ventilation have COPD, sepsis, ARDS, or refractory heart failure.

 B. The respiratory frequency/tidal volume ratio (f/VT) is greater than or equal to 105.

 C. Correction of underlying pulmonary and nonpulmonary complications best predicts successful weaning.

 D. An effective static compliance of more than 50 ml/cmH$_2$O and a dynamic compliance of more than 40 ml/cmH$_2$O are associated with improving gas exchange.

 E. Vital capacity of 12–15 ml/kg and peak inspiratory pressure less than 25 cmH$_2$O are appropriate guidelines for weaning.

Ref.: 3, 10

COMMENTS: Most surgical patients (90%) are weaned from mechanical ventilation in less than 1 week. • Conventional weaning criteria include (1) measurements of oxygenation by a pulse oximeter (best determined by arterial blood gases, with an SaO$_2$ >90% on any FIO$_2$ usually adequate for weaning), and (2) measurements of ventilation, such as a respiratory rate less than 24 breaths per minute, a PaCO$_2$ less than 50 mmHg, a peak inspiratory pressure below 30 cmH$_2$O, a tidal volume (VT) of at least 5–8 ml/kg, and a vital capacity double the VT value. • Failure to satisfy these conventional criteria is associated with unsuccessful weaning in as many as 63% of patients. • The rapid, shallow breathing test is performed by having the patient breathe room air for 1 minute as quickly as possible. • When the f/VT is less than or equal to 105, successful weaning occurs in 78% of patients. • Conversely, a f/VT greater than or equal to 105 is accompanied by a failure rate of 95%.

Clinical judgment and correction of underlying pulmonary and nonpulmonary complications continue to be the best guides to successful weaning. • In addition, helpful ventilation scores include an FIO$_2$ less than 40%, continuous positive airway pressure (CPAP) 3 cmH$_2$O, effective static compliance greater than 50 ml/cmH$_2$O, dynamic compliance greater than 40 ml/cmH$_2$O, ventilator minute ventilation less than 10 L/min, and triggered ventilatory rate less than 20 breaths per minute. • The duration of ventilatory support is not correlated with survival rates at discharge. • Forty-one percent of long-term ventilated patients survive. • Because of muscle atrophy, progressive ventilatory withdrawal designed to restore muscle function should be used. • Intermittent mandatory ventilation, pressure-support ventilation, and weaning by T-piece have been used effectively.

A N S W E R :
A, C, D, E

29. With regard to functional residual capacity (FRC), which of the following statements is/are true?

 A. FRC = residual volume (RV) + tidal volume (TV).

 B. Atelectasis occurs when the FRC is less than the closing volume (CV).

 C. FRC = expiratory reserve volume (ERV) + RV.

 D. FRC is increased by PEEP.

Ref.: 1, 2

COMMENTS: FRC is the volume of air in the lungs at the end of quiet exhalation. • It is equal to the sum of ERV and RV. • If the FRC falls too low, alveolar collapse ensues. • This volume is called the CV. • Early ambulation and incentive spirometry are used to support FRC above the CV in postoperative patients. • PEEP can increase the FRC in mechanically ventilated patients.

A N S W E R :
B, C, D

30. Which of the following is an appropriate definition of the shock state?

 A. Low blood pressure to maintain normal metabolic and nutritional functions

 B. Low CO to maintain normal metabolic and nutritional functions

 C. Shock index greater than 0.9 to maintain normal metabolic and nutritional functions

 D. Inadequate tissue perfusion to maintain normal metabolic and nutritional functions

 E. Abnormal vascular resistance to maintain normal metabolic and nutritional functions

Ref.: 1, 2

COMMENTS: The clinical state of shock can result from several mechanisms. • Cardiogenic shock is decreased CO and evidence of tissue hypoxia in the presence of adequate intravascular volume. • Furthermore, effective volemia may be decreased. Cardiogenic shock is diagnosed after documented myocardial dysfunction along with correction or exclusion of hypovolemia, hypoxia, and acidosis. • In addition, alterations in the vessels—either arteriolar resistance vessels or venous capacitance vessels—may also produce a distributive state, as is seen in septic shock. • Bleeding, reduction of extracellular fluid, or loss of plasma may cause a reduction in blood volume. • Neurogenic reflexes, spinal anesthesia, the end-stage of hypovolemic shock, or septic shock may bring about changes in the peripheral vascular resistance. • The final common pathway in all forms of shock, however, appears to be related to inadequate tissue perfusion. • Alterations in blood pressure may not adequately reflect the shock state. • High CO can be seen in many septic shock states. • The use of heart rate and mean arterial pressure as indicators of early shock possesses limitations posed by their variability and inaccuracy. • The use of the shock index (heart rate/systolic blood pressure) constituted an attempt to overcome the limitations of conventional vital signs. • However, its low sensitivity has limited its applicability.

A N S W E R :
D

31. Match each clinical situation in the left-hand column with the most appropriate treatment in the right-hand column.

A. Adequate volume status and hypotension refractory to inotropic agents	a. Inotropic agents
B. Distended neck veins, distant heart sounds, and equalization of pressures across the myocardium	b. Cardiac pacing
C. Hypotension, appropriate volume, and atrial fibrillation with ventricular response rate of 40	c. Fluid administration

Ref.: 1, 2

D. Hypotension and low right   d. Pericardiocentesis
   and left atrial pressures

E. Adequate volume, no   e. Intraaortic balloon
   mechanical defects,   counterpulsation
   and hypotension

Ref.: 1, 2, 3

COMMENTS: Cardiogenic shock may occur as a result of several mechanisms. • However, before assuming that hypotension is caused by a cardiogenic mechanism, one must be sure that there is adequate blood volume. • Therefore, a patient who is hypotensive with low right and left atrial pressures should undergo fluid administration as the initial management. • If cardiac performance improves with fluid administration, cardiogenic shock is probably not present. • If adequate filling pressures are attained and hypotension persists in the absence of mechanical defects, arrhythmia, and sepsis, a primary pump problem probably exists and should be managed with inotropic agents. • One form of cardiogenic shock is cardiac tamponade, which is seen in traumatized patients, postoperative cardiac patients, and patients suffering from uremia and certain malignancies. • Pericardial tamponade is manifested clinically with evidence of venous hypertension, and, on Swan-Ganz pressure determinations, there appears to be a trend toward equalization of pressures in the right and left sides of the heart. • Appropriate treatment is initial pericardiocentesis to relieve the intrapericardial pressure and allow adequate heart filling. • Abnormal heart rate and rhythm may alone produce cardiogenic shock, even if the myocardium contracts normally. • Tachyarrhythmias are frequently caused by atrial fibrillation or flutter and respond well to digitalis. • In the patient who is overdigitalized or hypokalemic, a very low ventricular rate in response to atrial fibrillation or flutter may result in hypotension and should be managed with cardiac pacing. • If, despite adequate blood volume, an appropriate heart rate, absence of a mechanical or valvular defect, appropriate administration of inotropic agents, and restoration of pressure and coronary blood flow, a patient remains in cardiogenic shock, support via intraaortic balloon counterpulsation may be needed. • Balloon counterpulsation is most beneficial in severe left ventricular dysfunction. • Patients with hemodynamic compromise secondary to right ventricular myocardial infarction require fluid resuscitation and inotropic support (dobutamine). • Any preload reducers must be avoided. • Afterload reducers in the presence of hypotension are not warranted.

ANSWER:
A-e; B-c; C-b; D-c; E-a

32. Regarding acute cardiac arrhythmias, which of the following are true?

   A. Arrhythmias are often provoked by electrolyte disturbances.

   B. Cardiac arrhythmias are detrimental when they reduce tissue perfusion or increase myocardial oxygen demand.

   C. The "three R" system (rate, rhythm, and QRS duration) best allows for quick classification of the arrhythmias.

   D. One of the first steps in evaluating an ECG is to identify the presence or absence of atrial activity (P waves), best seen in the inferior leads.

   E. All of the above.

Ref.: 1

COMMENTS: Various drugs, electrolyte disturbances, and cardiac ischemia often provoke arrhythmias. • Intracardiac catheter irritation and pacemaker dysfunction may also result in acute arrhythmias. • Hypokalemia, hyperkalemia, hypomagnesemia, acidosis, alkalosis, anemia, and hypoxemia all may exacerbate arrhythmic tendencies. • Cardiac arrhythmias are most detrimental when they reduce tissue perfusion or increase myocardial oxygen demand. • Management decisions must take into account a variety of factors affecting the patient's condition. • For example, tachyarrhythmias resulting in hypotension or angina should be treated immediately with drugs or cardioversion. • Acute intervention may not be necessary in patients with a history of well-tolerated arrhythmia. • The "three R" system (rate, rhythm, and QRS duration) allows for quick classification of various arrhythmias. • First, rate assessment permits the distinction of bradycardia (rate <60/min) from tachycardia (rate >100/min). • Sinus rhythm can be assessed by identifying atrial activity (regular P waves), which is best seen in the inferior leads (II, III, and aVF) on the electrocardiogram (ECG). • The presence or absence of P waves, the P wave morphologic pattern, and the relationship of the P wave to the QRS complex should be specifically examined. • Once the P wave has been characterized, ventricular activity (QRS complex) should be examined for regularity and morphologic features. • If the QRS complex is narrow (<0.12 sec), ventricular depolarization most likely occurs in response to normal atrioventricular conduction. • A wide complex QRS (>0.12 sec) suggests either an ectopic ventricular origin or aberrant supraventricular conduction. • If distinct P waves have been replaced with rapid, irregular waves and the QRS complex is irregularly irregular, atrial fibrillation is present. • Saw-tooth atrial activity suggests atrial flutter. • The lack of a QRS complex after each P wave suggests atrioventricular block. • The association of P waves and QRS complex suggests ventricular tachycardia.

ANSWER:
E

33. Which one of the following can define sinus tachycardia?

   A. Uniform P waves

   B. Gradual onset

   C. Fixed PR interval

   D. Regular rate

   E. All of the above

Ref.: 1

COMMENTS: The approach to sinus tachycardia is aimed at identifying the underlying cause. • The rate in sinus tachycardia is usually in the range of 100–180 beats per minute. • Sinus tachycardia is the normal physiologic response to exercise, fever, or hyperthyroidism. • Sinus tachycardia may also occur in association with anxiety, pain, hypovolemia, hypoxemia, and anemia. • Tachycardia decreases the period of diastolic filling and thus reduces ventricular filling. • However, the heart rate must exceed 200 beats per minute before one sees a decrease in CO in a normal heart. • When cardiac function is normal, there is generally little hemodynamic compromise from sinus tachycardia, since the heart rate rarely exceeds 180 beats per minute. • In patients with significant cardiac disease, whether coronary, myocardial, or valvular, a small increase in heart rate can greatly compromise CO. • In patients with symptomatic ischemia and/or infarction, β-blockers are the therapy of choice for rate reduction. • β-Blockers must be used cautiously in the setting of hypotension or underlying myocardial dysfunction because of the circulatory collapse that may ensue in these settings. • The following drugs may be used to control heart rate in the tachycardic patient, assuming that hypotension is not an issue: verapamil, digitalis, and procainamide.

ANSWER:
E

---

34. Which of the following is/are true regarding ectopic supraventricular tachycardias?

A. Multifocal atrial tachycardia most often occurs in association with obstructive lung disease.

B. Atrial fibrillation is a regular atrial rhythm with a single ectopic pacemaker focus.

C. Atrial flutter is a rhythm that usually arises in a localized region of re-entry outside the atrioventricular node or in a rapidly firing ectopic focus.

D. Both atrial fibrillation and atrial flutter eliminate the contribution of atrial contraction to CO.

E. None of the above.

Ref.: 1, 3

COMMENTS: Multifocal atrial tachycardia most often occurs in association with obstructive lung disease or metabolic dysfunction. • Unlike supraventricular tachycardia, atrioventricularis is the result of an ectopic tachycardia. • It is a rhythm with multiple foci of atrial ectopic activity. • Therefore, attempts to increase atrioventricular nodal refractoriness are ineffective. • Multifocal atrial tachycardia is recognized by irregularly irregular supraventricular QRS complexes, varying PR intervals, and the presence of at least three morphologically distinct P waveforms. • Verapamil may temporize or convert multifocal atrial tachycardia. • However, the definitive treatment is to reverse the underlying cause.

Atrial fibrillation is a chaotic atrial rhythm in which there is no single ectopic pacemaker to capture the atrium. • Atrial fibrillation is described as an irregularly irregular ventricular rhythm that can easily be confused with multifocal atrial tachycardia, sinus tachycardia, atrial flutter, or frequent premature atrial contractions. • There are no detectable P waves or effective atrial contractions because there is no organized atrial depolarization. • In atrial fibrillation, CO may fall by as much as 30% in patients with impaired ventricular function. • The acute therapy for atrial fibrillation is determined by the hemodynamic status of the patient. • Acute hemodynamic compromise requires synchronized cardioversion at 200–400 joules with a monophasic defibrillator (or 100–200 joules with biphasic one). • In hemodynamically stable patients, the initial therapy for atrial fibrillation is to slow the resting ventricular rate to less than 100 beats per minute. • Cardizem and/or digitalis is often effective in these patients. • Approximately 20% of patients with new-onset atrial fibrillation will appropriately correct with cardizem or digoxin alone. • If the heart rate remains rapid despite administration of cardizem and/or digoxin, verapamil, amiodarone, or β-blockers may be added. • In chronic atrial fibrillation, anticoagulation should be instituted for 4 weeks before attempts at rhythm conversion to minimize the risk of embolization.

Atrial flutter is a rhythm that is usually the result of organic heart disease. • Atrial flutter results from a localized region of re-entry outside the atrioventricular node or in a rapidly firing ectopic focus. • Because atrial flutter does not involve the atrioventricular node, atrial rates in atrial flutter are usually rapid (>250 beats per minute) and does not respond to vagal maneuvers. • Direct current cardioversion is the most effective method of restoring sinus rhythm. • Low energy levels (25–50 joules with a monophasic defibrillator and 12–25 with a biphasic one) are usually effective for flutter. • Because a large percentage of patients revert to flutter after cardioversion, it is best to use a digoxin prophylaxis.

ANSWER:
A, C, D

---

35. Regarding ventricular tachycardia, which of the following is/are true?

A. Ventricular tachycardia (VT) is defined as three or more consecutive ventricular beats occurring at a rate greater than 100 beats per minute.

B. VT is recognized by narrow QRS complexes.

C. The ECG hallmark of VT is atrioventricular dissociation.

D. VT may be initiated by a premature ventricular contraction (PVC).

E. All of the above.

Ref.: 1–3

COMMENTS: VT is defined as three or more consecutive ventricular beats occurring at a rate greater than 100 beats per minute. • The beats of VT are recognized by wide QRS complex with T waves of opposite polarity. • Atrioventricular dissociation is the ECG hallmark of VT. • This phenomenon results from the independent firing of the sinoatrial node and the ventricular focus. • Often, variation in the R-R interval is present. • VT results from the rapid firing of an ectopic ventricular pacemaker or electrical re-entry at the level of the Purkinje fibers. • VT may be initiated as a PVC. • In a hemodynamically compromised patient, VT is treated by synchronized cardioversion starting with 100 joules with a monophasic defibrillator (50 joules with a biphasic defibrillator), which may be increased to 360 joules with a monophasic defibrillator (200 joules with a biphasic defibrillator). • If the patient is hemodynamically stable, intravenous procainamide or amiodarone is the drug of choice. • A precordial thump may be attempted in witnessed VT.

ANSWER:
A, C, D

---

36. Match each clinical and ECG finding shown in the figure (A–E) with the most appropriate drug therapy.

a. Adenosine

b. Lidocaine

c. Digoxin, given intravenously, followed by quinidine or procainamide (Pronestyl)

d. Atropine, given intravenously

e. Quinidine followed by digoxin, given orally

f. No specific cardiac therapy

Ref.: 1, 2

COMMENTS: In **atrial fibrillation** (Figure part A), the rhythm is irregularly irregular without P waves and with narrow QRS complexes. • The treatment is intravenous digoxin given initially to control the ventricular rate, followed by quinidine or procainamide (Pronestyl) to convert the patient to sinus rhythm. • Giving quinidine first followed by digoxin orally is incorrect, because the rate may accelerate with quinidine if digoxin is not given first. • Lidocaine and atropine are not used in the treatment

A. Chest pain and dizziness;
heart rate, 100;
blood pressure, 140/70.

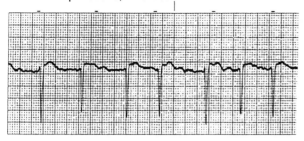

B. Asymptomatic.

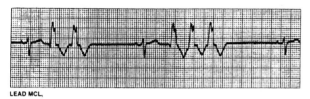

LEAD MCL,

C. Patient confused; heart rate, 50;
pressure, 90/65.

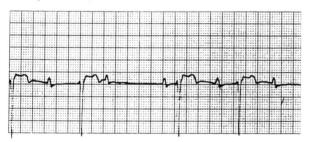

D. Dizziness; heart rate, 160;
blood pressure, 155/70.

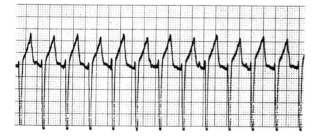

E. Sudden onset of coma.

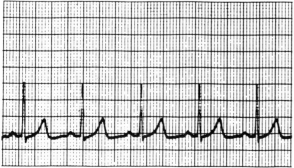

LEAD 2

of atrial fibrillation. • Adenosine is not used as a primary treatment of atrial fibrillation, although it is occasionally used as an adjunct to digoxin for rate control.

Ventricular tachycardia (Figure part B) is characterized by isolated PVCs and may not require treatment. • However, runs of more than three beats should prompt a search for treatable causes of arrhythmia. • Runs of six beats or more are more significant and can be treated with lidocaine, pending evaluation of potentially treatable causes of arrhythmia, such as hypokalemia, hypoxia, perioperative myocardial infarction, ischemia, and congestive heart failure. • Adenosine, atropine, and digoxin do not have a role in the treatment of ventricular tachycardia.

Second-degree atrioventricular block (Mobitz type I or Wenckebach block; Figure part C) is characterized by intermittently nonconducted P waves (a P wave without a QRS complex). • The figure shows a gradual PR interval prolongation followed by a nonconducted P wave. • Such prolongation of the PR interval is characteristic of Mobitz type I (or Wenckebach) second-degree block. • It is most often caused by excess vagal tones and responds to treatment with atropine. • If the patient is hemodynamically stable (i.e., with stable blood pressure and no evidence of congestive heart failure), no treatment is necessary. • In this case, however, the low systolic blood pressure and confusion indicate that therapy is warranted.

Supraventricular tachycardia (Figure part D) is characterized by a rapid, regular rate with narrow QRS complexes and absent or retrograde P waves. • Adenosine usually provides rapid conversion to sinus rhythm. • The primary side effect is hypotension, which may be managed by placing the patient in a Trendelenburg position. • Lidocaine and atropine have no role in supraventricular tachycardia. • Although digoxin may be used as a chronic or subacute therapy, adenosine is superior for immediate conversion. • The rhythm is **normal sinus** (Figure part E), and the patient does not require any specific cardiac therapy. • However, other causes of coma should be sought and treated. • For example, empiric therapy, such as intravenous glucose to treat possible hypoglycemia or naloxone (Narcan) to treat narcotic overdose, may be appropriate. • Other causes may be stroke, drug ingestion (intentional or accidental), or respiratory events causing hypoxia or hypercarbia.

ANSWER:
A-c; B-b; C-d; D-a; E-f

37. Regarding bradyarrhythmias, which of the following is/are true?

    A. Absolute bradycardia is a heart rate below 60 beats per minute.

    B. Relative bradycardia is a heart rate less than expected relative to an underlying condition or cause.

    C. The treatment sequence for symptomatic bradycardia is dopamine, atropine, and transcutaneous pacing.

    D. Atropine works by blocking the effects of vagal nerve discharges.

    E. Atropine is the drug of choice for Mobitz type II block.

Ref.: 1, 2, 3

COMMENTS: Bradycardia tends to reflect a noncardiogenic cause, such as vagal reflexes, hypoxemia, hypothyroidism, or drugs (β blockers, calcium channel blockers, or digoxin). Absolute sinus bradycardia is characterized by normal P wave features and 1:1 atrioventricular conduction at a rate less than 60 beats per minute. • Sinus bradycardia does not require treatment unless it causes hypotension or myocardial ischemia. • The treatment sequence for symptomatic bradycardia is as follows: (1) atropine 0.5–1.0 mg, (2) transcutaneous pacing if available, (3) dopamine 5–20 µg/kg/min, and (4) epinephrine 2–10 µg/min.

If bradycardia drops below the intrinsic rate of the ventricles (30–40 beats per minute), escape PVCs may occur. • Atropine works by blocking the effects of the vagal nerve. • Therefore, atropine is not indicated for third-degree heart block or Mobitz type II block. • Atropine may increase the atrial rate and produce an increased atrioventricular nodal block under such conditions. • Transcutaneous pacing is a class 1 intervention for all symptomatic bradycardias. • Dopamine should be used after the maximum dose of atropine is reached (0.04 mg/kg). • Moderate-dose dopamine therapy (5–10 µg/kg/min) has a β1- and α-adrenergic effect, resulting in enhanced myocardial contractility and increased CO, heart rate, and blood pressure. • High-dose dopamine therapy (10–20 µg/kg/min) had a predominately α-adrenergic effect, resulting in peripheral arterial and venous vasoconstriction. • Epinephrine is used if the patient has severe bradycardia with hypotension.

First-degree atrioventricular block is recognized by a prolonged PR interval (>0.2 sec). • It is generally physiologically unimportant but may signal drug toxicity or progressive disease of the conduction system. • There are two forms of second-degree atrioventricular block. • Mobitz type I (Wenkebach) block is characterized by sequential and progressive prolongation of the PR interval with periodic failure to transmit the atrial impulses. • The PR interval progressively lengthens and the RR interval shortens until QRS depolarization is blocked. • The sequence then repeats itself. • The site of blockage is generally within the atrioventricular node and may be the result of digitalis toxicity or intrinsic disease. • Mobitz type II block originates below the level of the atrioventricular node. • The PR interval remains constant. • In third-degree atrioventricular block, the atria and ventricles fire independently, usually at different rates. • Blockage of the atrioventricular node produces a narrow complex junctional rhythm at a rate of 40–60 beats per minute. • Infranodal atrioventricular block, which is associated with a wide QRS complex (> 0.10 sec), produces a slower heart rate (30–45 beats per minute). • Infranodal third-degree atrioventricular block needs to be treated with the immediate insertion of a transvenous pacemaker. • Pacemakers inserted distal to the atrioventricular node are inherently unstable.

ANSWER:
A, B, D

---

38. Match the antiarrhythmic agents in the left-hand column with their primary effect in the right-hand column.

Agent	Effect
A. Amiodarone	a. Prolongs repolarization in the atria and ventricles
B. Digitalis	b. Nonselective β blocker
C. Esmolol	c. Calcium-channel blocker that prolongs atrioventricular conduction
D. Propranolol	d. Prolongs atrioventricular conduction
E. Verapamil	e. Cardioselective β blocker

Ref.: 1–3

COMMENTS: **Amiodarone** prolongs repolarization in the atria and the ventricles and prolongs the QT interval. • It is a highly effective agent for both supraventricular tachycardia and ventricular arrhythmias. • It is indicated for ventricular and supraventricular arrhythmias that are unresponsive to conventional antiarrhythmic therapy. • Chronic administration is associated with several side effects, including pulmonary fibrosis, thyroid dysfunction, and crystalline deposits in the cornea. • It is contraindicated for torsades de pointes associated with prolonged QT interval and in association with drugs that prolong the QT interval.

Digoxin prolongs atrioventricular conduction and is a peripheral vasoconstrictor. • Since it is primarily excreted by the kidneys, careful monitoring is necessary in patients with impaired renal function. • It is indicated as maintenance therapy for atrial fibrillation and flutter. • Digitalis toxicity may result in atrioventricular block, junctional rhythms, and ventricular arrhythmias. • Its use is contraindicated for atrioventricular block, hypertrophic cardiomyopathy, and severe hypokalemia or hypomagnesemia.

Esmolol is a cardioselective β blocker that prolongs atrioventricular conduction and a peripheral vasodilator. • It is indicated for acute control of ventricular rate in PAT (paroxysmal atrial tachycardia), atrial fibrillation, and atrial flutter. • Bronchospasm has been reported in asthmatic patients. • Its use is contraindicated for atrioventricular block, hypotension, asthma, and severe systolic myocardial dysfunction.

Propranolol is a nonselective β blocker that blocks both β1 and β2 receptors. • It has a negative inotropic effect and causes peripheral vasodilation. • It is indicated for the acute control of sinus tachycardia, arrhythmias associated with thyroid storm, and atrial fibrillation and flutter. • Acute airway constriction may occur in asthmatic patients and patients with COPD. • It is contraindicated for atrioventricular block, hypotension, asthma, COPD, sick sinus syndrome, and severe systolic myocardial failure.

Verapamil is a calcium-channel blocker that prolongs atrioventricular conduction, produces peripheral vasodilation, and has negative inotropic effects. • It is indicated for the treatment of paroxysmal atrial tachycardia, atrial fibrillation and flutter, and multifocal atrial tachycardia (in the absence of hypotension). • It is contraindicated for atrioventricular block, hypotension, Wolff-Parkinson-White syndrome (because it can accelerate the ventricular response owing to shortening of the refractory period in accessory pathways), and patients with severe ventricular dysfunction who are on β blockers.

ANSWER:
A-a; B-b; C-e; D-b; E-c

---

39. Match each receptor on the left with one or more of its actions on the right.

A. α₁	a. Relaxes renal vascular smooth muscle
B. Dopamine-1	b. Stimulates myocardial contractility
C. β₂	c. Relaxes bronchial and vascular smooth muscle (skeletal muscle)
D. α₂	d. Inhibits uptake of norepinephrine at the sympathetic nerve terminal
E. Dopamine-2	e. Constricts venous vessels
F. β₁	f. Constricts vascular smooth muscle

Ref.: 4

COMMENTS: **Inotropic agents** increase cardiac contractility by increasing the concentration and availability of intracellular calcium. • The **phosphodiesterase inhibitor** milrinone blocks conversion of cyclic adenosine monophosphate (cAMP) to 5-AMP. • The higher concentration of cAMP results in increased calcium flux and increased calcium uptake by endoplasmic reticulum, which improves cardiac contractility and relaxation following contraction. • In vascular smooth muscle, the calcium uptake by the endoplasmic reticulum results in relaxation and subsequent vasodilatation. • This effect limits its use in hypovolemic shock unless it is combined with a vasopressor.

Catecholamines act by binding to adrenergic receptors. • Each type of receptor controls a particular cardiovascular function. • Epinephrine, norepinephrine, dopamine, and dobutamine are all catecholamines. • The α_1 receptor mediates arterial vasoconstriction by causing contraction of vascular smooth muscle, and the α_2 receptor induces constriction of venous capacitance vessels. • The β_1 receptor stimulates myocardial contractility, and the β_2 receptor causes relaxation of bronchial smooth muscle and relaxation of vascular smooth muscle in skeletal muscle beds. • The dopamine receptors cause relaxation of vascular smooth muscle. • The dopamine-1 receptor causes relaxation of renal and splanchnic vascular smooth muscle, and the dopamine-2 receptor inhibits uptake of norepinephrine at the sympathetic nerve terminal, resulting in prolonged action of norepinephrine at the mother end-plate. • The response to catecholamines is different in normal individuals from that in critically ill patients. • Receptor populations change over short periods of time, and up-regulation and down-regulation occur, depending on the disease state. • Because receptor numbers and affinities vary with the clinical setting, various and unexpected responses are seen. • It is important that catecholamines be administered for a predetermined effect. • If the effect is not attained with the particular catecholamine chosen, the dose should be adjusted or another agent used.

Dopamine stimulates dopamine receptors at infusion rates less than 5 µg/kg/ min and α_2 receptors at infusion rates as low as 2 µg/kg/min. • As the plasma concentration increases, dopamine selectively stimulates β-adrenergic receptors (5–10 µg/kg/min). • Further increases in the dopamine concentrations result in progressive α-adrenergic stimulation (10 µg/kg/min). • **Dobutamine** is a synthetic catecholamine that is a β_1-receptor stimulant at the usual dosage of 5–15 µg/kg/min. • At higher doses, tachycardia and vasodilation of vessels in the skeletal muscle bed occur as a result of β_2 stimulation. • Dobutamine increases CO, DO_2, and VO_2 in septic shock. • **Epinephrine** at low doses has α- and β_2-receptor activity (<0.02 µg/kg/min), whereas at higher doses it has α_1- and α_2-receptor activity (>0.02 µg/kg/min). • Epinephrine increases cardiac ectopic pacemaker activity, leading to dysrhythmias, and increases cardiac oxygen demand. • Its metabolic effects include increased renin production, hyperglycemia, and free fatty acid production. • **Norepinephrine** at low doses is a β_1- and β_2-receptor agonist and a potent chromotrope. • At higher doses, α_1- and α_2-receptor activity predominates, and the chronotropic effect diminishes. • Norepinephrine is a potent splanchnic and renal vasoconstrictor.

ANSWER:
A-f; B-a; C-c; D-e; E-d; F-b

40. Match the class of hemorrhage listed in the left-hand column with the initial changes in the right-hand column.

A. Class I	a. Decrease in systolic pressure
B. Class II	b. Tachycardia
C. Class III	c. Cold and pale skin, negligible urine output
D. Class IV	d. No changes

Ref.: 1–3

COMMENTS: Hemorrhagic shock is caused by an acute loss of the circulating blood volume. • In normal adults, the circulating blood volume is approximately 7% of the body weight, or approximately 5 L in a normal 70-kg man. • The response to hemorrhage has been divided into four classes. • **Class I** hemorrhagic shock consists of the loss of up to 15% of the circulating volume. • No measured changes occur with blood losses of this magnitude. • In **class II** hemorrhagic shock, which is defined as the loss of 15–30% of the circulating blood volume, tachycardia is noted, as is a decrease

in the pulse pressure. • This decrease in pulse pressure is generally related to an increase in the diastolic component, which in turn is related to elevation of catecholamines, produced by the neurohormonal response to shock. • **Class III** hemorrhagic shock is the loss of 30–40% of the total circulating volume. • At this stage, a consistent drop in systolic blood pressure occurs, and the degree of blood loss necessities a blood transfusion. • **Class IV** hemorrhagic shock consists of the loss of more than 40% of the circulating volume. • Symptoms include marked tachycardia and profound depression of the systolic blood pressure. • At this stage, tissue perfusion is significantly altered, urinary output is negligible, and the skin is cold and pale. • Tachycardia may not be seen in all hypotensive patients in shock, and bradycardia may be associated with improved outcomes.

ANSWER:
A-d; B-b; C-a; D-c

41. Which of the following statements accurately characterize(s) fluid shifts that occur during hemorrhagic shock?

A. The loss of intravascular volume is usually fully compensated by movement of extravascular interstitial fluid into the vascular space.

B. Intracellular fluid volume decreases as fluid shifts from the intracellular to the extracellular fluid compartment to compensate for the intravascular loss.

C. There is movement of interstitial fluid into the intracellular space even though full compensation of intravascular losses has not yet occurred.

D. There is a decrease in the transmembrane potential, resulting in increased sodium permeability and influx of sodium into the cell.

Ref.: 1, 2

COMMENTS: After acute hemorrhage, the extracellular fluid is depleted by two mechanisms. • The first mechanism consists of transcapillary refill, wherein the extracellular fluid replaces the circulating blood volume. • This transcapillary refill ultimately results in a reduction in the hematocrit. • In addition, the cell in shock is deprived of its energy-dependent moieties. • With severe hemorrhagic shock, there is an alteration in the transmembrane potential of cells (particularly muscle cells) associated with an alteration of the sodium-potassium pump, which is one of the energy-dependent moieties. • Because of a decrease in the efficiency of the sodium pump, sodium and fluid from the extracellular space leaks into the interior of the cell, and potassium leaks from the intracellular space into the extracellular space. • The cells thus become swollen with extracellular fluid. • The net effect of both of these mechanisms is a profound reduction in the functional extracellular fluid. • Thus, although the fluid that is lost in hemorrhagic shock is blood, the initial volume deficit experienced by the patient is a reduction in extracellular fluid.

ANSWER:
C, D

42. Regarding lactic acidosis, which of the following statements is/are true?

A. Type A lactic acidosis (Woods classification) is always a consequence of tissue hypoxemia associated with tissue hypoperfusion.

B. Type B lactic acidosis is always a consequence of tissue hypoxia associated with tissue hypoperfusion.

C. Lactate per se does not cause lactic acidosis.

D. The treatment of lactic acidosis requires administration of bicarbonate.

E. Serial lactate level determination may be a useful preoperative indication of circulatory shock.

Ref.: 1

COMMENTS: With the Cohen and Woods classification, lactic acidosis is divided into two major types: A and B. • Type A lactic acidosis is a consequence of tissue hypoxia associated with tissue hypoperfusion (e.g., from abnormal vascular permeability, left ventricular failure, and decreased CO) or of reduced arterial oxygen content ($PaO_2 < 35$ mmHg, e.g., from carbon monoxide poisoning, or severe anemia). • Type B acidosis is not associated with tissue hypoxemia and may be the result of liver disease, diabetes mellitus, drugs (e.g., acetylsalicylic acid or ethanol), or inborn errors of metabolism. • Anaerobic glycolysis produces lactate, ATP, and water but not lactic acidosis. • The acidosis associated with hyperlactacidemia is caused by hydrolysis of ATP, with release of hydrogen ions. • Gluconeogenesis from lactate produces hydrogen ions directly. • The treatment of lactic acidosis should be directed toward correction of the cause of acidosis. • Sodium bicarbonate has failed to improve the acid-base or hemodynamic state of these patients. • The presence of lactic acidosis represents the best objective determination of the presence and severity of circulatory shock. • In addition, both hypoxia and hypercapnia are important in this scenario.

ANSWER:
A, C, E

43. Regarding indexes of tissue perfusion, which of the following is/are true?

A. Normal cardiac index precludes tissue hypoxia.

B. Normal or high mixed venous oxygen saturation (SvO_2) precludes tissue hypoxia.

C. High plasma lactate levels always reflect hypoxia.

D. Supernormal oxygen delivery (DO_2) reverses tissue hypoxia.

E. There is supply dependence of oxygen consumption (VO_2) on oxygen delivery.

Ref.: 11

COMMENTS: When the oxygen needs of the body are not being met, oxidation of pyruvate is carried out anaerobically, leading to the creation of lactic acid. • Acidosis and elevated lactate levels can be detected in arterial blood only if capillary perfusion is sufficient to wash these products into the venous circulation. • Moreover, hypoxic and nonhypoxic mechanisms of lactic acid should be considered. • Gastric tonometric studies and measurement of intramucosal pH can assess regional perfusion before a generalized low flow state is manifested. • Thus, in some shock states, peripheral arterial pH may not accurately reflect intracellular pH.

Oxygen consumption is physiologically dependent on DO_2 below the critical DO_2 (4 ml/kg/min). • VO_2 is maintained constant as DO_2 decreases by progressive increases in the oxygen extraction ratio (O_2ER): $O_2ER = VO_2/DO_2$. • The critical O_2ER (0.6) is the ratio at the critical DO_2 below which the VO_2 decreases as the DO_2 decreases. • Incomplete reversal of tissue hypoxia and occult tissue hypoxia (in the gut) have been suggested as mechanisms of multiple organ failure. • One proposed reason for this is the concept of pathologic dependence of VO_2 on DO_2, characterized

by a greater critical DO_2, a lower critical O_2ER, and a greater VO_2 during the plateau phase. • However, when independent measurements are used, pathologic dependence is not found. • A change in DO_2 is not followed by a change in VO_2 unless the ratio is less than a low level of 2:1, in which case the VO_2 becomes supply dependent. • Randomized trials of supernormal delivery suggest that supernormal DO_2 could prevent but not reverse tissue hypoxia. • During hypermetabolism, supply dependence occurs at a ratio less than 2:1, but in these circumstances there is a higher than normal DO_2. • In patients with sepsis or ARDS, the critical ratio is closer to 3:1. • A decreased SvO_2 may indicate the presence of shock because the content of O_2 is lower than normal, indicating that insufficient oxygen is being delivered. • However, patients with cirrhosis and sepsis syndrome may have artificially elevated SvO_2 because of shunting of blood and/or cellular disorders of oxygen utilization.

ANSWER:
E

44. What is the correct management of the commonest acid-base imbalance seen in long-standing or severe hemorrhagic shock?

A. Intravenous sodium bicarbonate

B. Component blood therapy

C. Increased fluid administration

D. Vasopressors

E. Hyperventilation

Ref.: 2

COMMENTS: See Question 45.

45. With regard to fluid therapy in hemorrhagic shock, which of the following statements is/are correct?

A. Fresh whole blood is probably the best fluid to be administered for hemorrhagic shock.

B. With early acute hemorrhage, the hematocrit may be used as a reliable indicator of the total volume of blood loss and the requirements for transfusion.

C. Lactated Ringer's solution should be avoided in the management of shock because the lactate in it worsens the existing lactic acidosis.

D. Albumin is an excellent volume expander when blood is not available because most of it stays within the vascular space for relatively long periods of time.

E. Hypertonic saline therapy blunts neutrophil-mediated pulmonary injury.

Ref.: 1, 3, 12, 13

COMMENTS: Although the earliest acid-base balancing response during shock tends to be respiratory alkalosis due to tachypnea, it rapidly gives way to an increasingly severe metabolic acidosis as the hemorrhagic shock phase continues. • The underlying cause of this metabolic acidosis is inadequate tissue perfusion, which results in anaerobic metabolism and the liberation of lactic and pyruvic acids. • Thus, the appropriate treatment is to restore tissue perfusion by increasing intravenous fluids. • Treatment with intravenous sodium bicarbonate is not indicated in the normothermic shock patient unless the pH is less than 7.1. • When available, properly crossmatched fresh whole blood and a balanced electrolyte solution are the ideal replacement fluids for a patient in hemorrhagic shock. • This treatment replenishes not only the intravascular volume but also the red blood cells, thereby preserving the oxygen-carrying capacity of the blood. • In the absence of type-specific blood, type O Rh-negative (preferably with a low anti-A titer) can be administered as the "universal donor" blood. • Preparation of blood requires some time, and in an emergency when the vascular volume must be replenished quickly, lactated Ringer's solution may be administered at a rate as high as 2000 ml over a 45-minute period.

Failure of the patient to stabilize despite this rapid crystalloid administration is usually a sign of life-threatening, ongoing hemorrhage. • However, many patients do stabilize for variable periods during crystalloid administration, allowing proper preparation of type-specific blood. • In the normal patient with an average hematocrit, the sudden massive loss of blood that is characteristic of hemorrhagic shock does not immediately produce a drop in the hematocrit. • The drop in hematocrit is caused by the transcapillary refill of extracellular fluid that replaces the blood loss. • It is clear, therefore, that during the acute hemorrhagic shock process the initial hematocrit is not indicative of the total blood loss or of the need to transfuse blood. • Although lactic acidosis clearly occurs in states of hypoperfusion, the additional lactate present in lactated Ringer's solution does not appear to aggravate this metabolic situation.

Much research has been done on the relative value of other "volume expanders." • Although albumin has the theoretic advantage of being a protein, and therefore more likely to stay within the intravascular space, it has been found to rapidly equilibrate with all of the extracellular fluid compartment, and its value as a blood volume substitute is transient. • However, its use in acute critically ill patients with hypalbuminemia has been recently resurrected with reported improved outcomes. • Hypertonic saline infusion is an efficient means of resuscitation in hemorrhagic shock patients, thereby improving cardiac contractility, blood pressure, and tissue perfusion. • Moreover, hypertonic saline infusions seem to modulate leukocyte cytotoxicity. • This may explain the attenuation in the pulmonary edema and tissue injury frequently seen in those patients, in contrast to patients who develop ARDS after resuscitation with isotonic solutions. • Hypertonic saline infusions inhibit the cytokin-driven inflammatory response, resulting in lower serum levels of TNF-α and IL-6. TNF-α triggers up-regulation of neutrophil β_2 integrin expression and that of the corresponding endothelial ligand (ICAM-1).

ANSWERS:
Question 44: C
Question 45: A, E

46. Which of the following may be commonly seen as clinical manifestations of shock?

    A. Decreased core temperature

    B. Thirst

    C. Restlessness

    D. Apathy

    E. Vomiting

    F. Diarrhea

Ref.: 1, 2

COMMENTS: The clinical manifestations of shock are many and varied, depending on the cause and severity of the shock state. • The more obvious clinical manifestations are related to the sequelae of decreased circulating volume and include hypotension, tachycardia, and pale, cool skin. • A fall in the core body temperature, possibly caused by a lowered metabolic rate, is also seen. • In the injured patient suffering from hemorrhagic hypovolemia, thirst is commonly seen. • Obviously, administration of water by mouth in such circumstances may be hazardous. • Also, in patients with hemorrhagic hypovolemic shock, states of anxiety and restlessness resulting from tissue hypoxia may be seen initially and may give way to apathy and somnolence as central nervous system perfusion falls. • Nausea and vomiting from hypovolemic shock are commonly seen. • However, diarrhea is uncommon, and in fact intestinal ileus may be a common sequela of shock.

ANSWER:
A, B, C, D, E

47. Which of the following biochemical changes may be seen in patients in shock?

    A. Hyperglycemia

    B. Negative nitrogen balance

    C. Hyperlacticacidemia

    D. Metabolic alkalosis

    E. Hyperkalemia

Ref.: 2

COMMENTS: Shock almost invariably produces stimulation of the adrenal medullary output of epinephrine, stimulation of the pituitary-adrenocortical axis, induction of a low-flow state, and occasionally specific organ failure. • These events in turn result in the relatively common biochemical changes seen in states of hemorrhagic shock. • Increased circulating levels of epinephrine and cortisol result in glycogenolysis and frequently sustained hyperglycemia, as well as a change to a catabolic state, resulting in a negative nitrogen balance. • The low-flow state caused by hypovolemia results in decreased oxygen delivery to skin and muscle, among other organs, and an obligatory change in the metabolism of those organs from aerobic to anaerobic. • This is usually associated with significant metabolic acidosis, resulting in part from the excess production of lactic acid. • One of the compensatory mechanisms in hemorrhagic shock is the renal retention of sodium and water at the expense of increased potassium excretion. • However, the intracellular stores of potassium are sufficient that hypokalemia is virtually never seen, even during maximal renal compensation. • If hypoperfusion of the kidney persists for any significant length of time, the characteristic biochemical findings of renal failure, including metabolic acidosis and hyperkalemia, are seen.

ANSWER:
A, B, C, E

48. Match the ventilator modes on the left with the appropriate characteristics on the right.

    A. Intermittent mandatory ventilation (IMV)   a. Bronchopleural fistulas

    B. Pressure-support ventilation (PSV)   b. Limits peak airway pressures

    C. Airway pressure-release ventilation (APRV)   c. Muscle atrophy

    D. Pressure-targeted assist-control ventilation (A/C)   d. Decreases total work of breathing

E. Inverse-ratio ventilation e. Delivered breath high volume
   (IRV)   and high pressure

F. High-frequency   f. Excessive gas trapping
   ventilation (HFV)

D. High-level PS (5–50 cmH$_2$O) can be used as a stand-alone ventilatory support mode.

E. PS makes spontaneous breathing more comfortable for ventilator-dependent patients.

Ref.: 4, 10

Ref.: 3

COMMENTS: IMV combines a preset number of mandatory breaths of predetermined tidal volume (Vt) and spontaneous breaths. • Minute ventilation is the sum of patient-initiated (high pressure, low volume) and ventilator-generated (high pressure, high volume) breaths. • This combination has been associated with dynamic hyperinflation (volutrauma) and barotrauma. • Addition of PEEP, often more than 15 cmH$_2$O, increases the potential for barotrauma. • IRV has been primarily used for patients with acute lung injury or neonatal respiratory distress syndrome. • The inspiratory time is extended beyond the normal inspiratory/expiratory (I:E) ratio of 1:2 to as high as 4:1, potentially reducing risk of barotrauma by improving gas exchange at lower levels of peak distending pressures. • However, no benefit has been demonstrated in ARDS patients. • Furthermore, IRV can seriously compromise hemodynamics, requires heavy sedation, and may lead to muscle atrophy. • Extending the I:E ratio can be accomplished with PCV or with volume-controlled ventilation. • With PCV, the maximal airway pressure is preset; the Vt may not remain constant throughout the cycle owing to variable resistance, in contrast to volume-controlled ventilation; and the inspiratory flow is initially high but then decreases as alveolar pressure rises. • This decelerating flow pattern generates greater shear forces than does a constant inspiratory flow at the beginning of inspiration. • At the end, it generates lesser shear forces. PSV is used during stable support periods and for weaning. • It decreases the total work of breathing. • The patient must have an intact respiratory drive. • PSV can be used alone or in combination with IMV. • APRV is a pressure-controlled, time-triggered, pressure-limited, time-cycled ventilation that allows spontaneous breathing during the cycle and minimizes lung expansion. • Continuous positive airway pressure is maintained until the time-release valve opens, allowing the pressure in the system to fall to a lower level functional residual capacity (FRC). • The goal of APRV is to reduce peak airway pressures, thus minimizing barotrauma and volutrauma. • However, APRV has potential drawbacks in cases of severe airway obstruction. • It needs further evaluation for use in patients with low compliance. • HFV uses a small Vt at high frequencies. • It is useful during airway endoscopy and in cases of tracheobronchial fistula. • This technique has shown no advantages over conventional ventilation in cases of ARDS. • With A/C ventilation, every breath taken by the patient is supported. • Excessive work of breathing occurs in cases of inadequate peak flow or inspiratory sensitive setting. • Pressure-targeted A/C ventilation may result in inadequate minute ventilation. • When this form of ventilation is properly functioning, the patient on A/C performs no work, leading to muscle atrophy.

ANSWER:
A-e; B-d; C-b; D-c; E-f; F-a

49. Regarding pressure support (PS), which of the following statements is/are false?

A. The inspiratory pressure is terminated when a certain inspiratory flow minimum is reached.

B. It controls the ultimate inspiratory flow and tidal volume.

C. Pressure-volume (P-V) characteristics with pressure-supported breathing improve muscle efficiency during weaning.

COMMENTS: PS is a pressure-triggered, pressure-targeted, flow-cycled mode of ventilation. • It is used as a ventilatory mode during stable ventilatory support and for weaning. • PS can shift the work of breathing from the patient to the ventilator. • The flow delivery pattern of a PS-assisted breath synchronizes with spontaneous breathing patterns better than does the fixed pattern of a volume-assisted breath. • The inspiratory pressure is held consistent through servo control of delivered flow and is terminated when an inspiratory flow minimum is reached. • The patient controls ventilatory timing and sets the inspiratory flow and tidal volume. • During the weaning process, PS changes muscle work characteristics to a more normal P-V configuration, thereby facilitating gradual load return to patients during the weaning process. • During weaning, PS of the patient's breathing facilitates synchronization with ventilatory pattern reflexes, thus producing more physiologic muscle reloading as a stand-alone mode. • High-level PS (5–50 cmH$_2$O) provides ventilatory support to patients who have a reliable ventilatory drive and stable or improving lung mechanics.

ANSWER:
B, D

50. Concerning auto-PEEP, which one or more of the following is/are true?

A. Auto-PEEP can be caused by increased airway resistance and expiratory flow limitations.

B. Auto-PEEP is easily detected by the ventilator manometer.

C. Auto-PEEP is best managed by prolonging the expiratory time.

D. Auto-PEEP can be offset by applying external PEEP up to 50% of the auto-PEEP.

E. Auto-PEEP is best managed by increasing the tidal volume.

Ref.: 4

COMMENTS: Auto-PEEP is due to gas trapping at the end of expiration. • This increases the work of breathing, decreases effective alveolar ventilation, and subjects the patient to a higher risk of volutrauma and compromised hemodynamics. • In mechanically ventilated patients, increased expiratory resistance can cause auto-PEEP. • Risk factors include obstructive airway disease, minute ventilation requirements greater than 10 L/min, high ventilator rates with lower tidal volume, or low inspiratory flow rates. • Auto-PEEP is more reliably detected by graphic flow displays. • Alternatively, auto-PEEP can be measured by the end-expiratory occlusion technique or by an esophageal balloon pressure reading. • Even if intrinsic PEEP exists, the ventilator water manometer cannot detect it. • Auto-PEEP is best treated by prolonging the expiratory time and reducing the inspiratory time. • In the volume-cycled ventilatory mode, expiration can be prolonged by decreasing the respiratory rate, decreasing the tidal volume, or increasing the flow rate. • Minute ventilation should be minimized and bronchodilator therapy optimized. • Application of PEEP up to 10–15 cmH$_2$O but not exceeding 80–85% of auto-PEEP can decrease the work of breathing needed to initiate inspiratory flow. • Switching the patient from pressure triggering to flow triggering can be helpful as well.

ANSWER:
A, C

---

51. Which of the following is/are associated with inaccurate estimation of hemoglobin saturation of oxygen (SaO_2) by pulse oxymetric analysis?

   A. Carboxyhemoglobin

   B. Dark pigmentation

   C. Septic syndrome

   D. Nail polish

   E. Nitrite intoxication

Ref.: 4

COMMENTS: Pulse oximetric analysis is based on placing a pulsating arterial vascular bed between a diode and a light detector (spectrophotometer with plethysmographic characteristics). • It detects the oxygenated part of hemoglobin *available* for carrying oxygen (SaO_2), as opposed to the percentage of *total* hemoglobin that is oxygenated (% $HgbO_2$). • An elevated carboxyhemoglobin level causes overestimation of SaO_2 by pulse oximetric analysis because its absorption coefficient is similar to that of oxygenated hemoglobin. • Inaccurate readings are associated with the following: dark-pigmented skin, low-flow states, nail polish, vital dyes, ambient light, anemia, changes in oxyhemoglobin dissociation curve, and cardiac arrhythmias.

ANSWER:
A, B, C, D, E

---

52. With regard to the use of vasopressors and vasodilators in the management of hemorrhagic shock, which of the following statements is/are true?

   A. Vasopressors usually result in an elevation of the blood pressure.

   B. Vasopressors achieve their goal of blood pressure support primarily through inotropic effects.

   C. Dopamine given in low-to-moderate doses may provide inotropic and chronotropic support to the heart as well as enhance renal blood flow.

   D. In general, the use of vasopressors in hemorrhagic shock is discouraged.

   E. Vasodilators should be employed early in the management of hemorrhagic shock to promote tissue perfusion.

Ref.: 1, 4

COMMENTS: The use of vasopressors in the management of hemorrhagic shock has been somewhat controversial, but the general tendency is toward avoidance of their use. • Although they are effective in raising the blood pressure in patients in hemorrhagic shock, they do it primarily through increasing peripheral vascular resistance, which further reduces tissue perfusion (thus aggravating the principal problem in hemorrhagic shock). • Various vasopressors work through various mechanisms, depending on their relative α- and β-receptor stimulation effects. • Dopamine is an attractive vasopressor in that it provides

beneficial inotropic and chronotropic support to the heart while selectively enhancing renal blood flow through its peripheral β-adrenergic effects. • Even so, dobutamine, dopamine, and the other vasopressors should probably be avoided during the initial management of hemorrhagic shock because the principal deficit is one of effective circulating blood volume and poor tissue perfusion. • There is some evidence suggesting that after a proper circulating blood volume has been restored or if volume correction does not correct hypotension, the positive inotropic and chronotropic effects of vasopressors on the heart may lead to further improvement in a patient's status. • Because dopamine is not always successful, even at high doses, norepinephrine in combination with volume expansion is indicated initially, particularly if the mean systemic pressure is less than 60 mmHg or there is evidence of organ dysfunction. • Vasodilators have a theoretic advantage of promoting tissue perfusion by reducing peripheral vascular resistance. • However, this would be appropriate only once an effective circulating blood volume had been established, and the use of vasodilators for initial management of hemorrhagic shock should be avoided.

ANSWER:
A, C, D

---

53. Match each drug in the left column with one of the statements in the right column.

   A. Intravenous morphine a. Torsades de pointes
   B. Haloperidol b. Requires analgesic for pain
   C. Diazepam c. Pain management in shock
   D. Propofol d. Choice for hepatic failure
   E. Lorazepam e. Short-term sedation

Ref.: 2

COMMENTS: Perhaps paradoxically, pain is not a common problem among patients suffering from hypovolemic shock. • However, when pain is significant, administration of small intravenous doses of morphine is probably the preferred method of management. • Haloperidol has been associated with torsades de pointes, particularly in patients with a prolonged QTc (>500 msec) on the electrocardiogram. • Diazepam is a short-acting sedative, but it is metabolized in the liver. • Lorazepam does not require extensive hepatic metabolism. • Propofol possesses anxiolytic, sedative, and hypnotic activities, but it is not an analgesic.

ANSWER:
A-c; B-a; C-e; D-b; E-d

---

54. A 24-year-old woman undergoes a laparotomy for a class IV injury to the liver and during the procedure undergoes transfusion with 12 units of cold, stored, packed red blood cells. Despite appropriate treatment of the liver injury, there is persistent bleeding from the raw surface of the parenchyma. In addition to aggressive resuscitation, administration of which of the following is initially most appropriate?

   A. Calcium chloride

   B. Fresh-frozen plasma

   C. Platelets

   D. Correction of hypothermia

   E. Heparin

Ref.: 1, 14

COMMENTS: Hypothermia, acidosis, and coagulopathy are frequently encountered in the trauma patient. • Massive transfusion is defined as the administration of more than 10 units of blood or more than one blood volume of the patient within 24 hr. • The known associated complications include electrolyte and acid-base abnormalities, changes in hemoglobin-oxygen affinity, hypothermia, coagulopathy, and dysfunction of various organs. • A number of studies have documented a drop in the platelet count after massive transfusion. • In addition, platelet aggregation with ADP and collagen are noted to be depressed for up to 4 days after the transfusion. • Further studies analyzing the effect of routine prophylactic platelet transfusions in such patients have failed to document any advantage unless the patient has nonmechanical bleeding. • Moreover, platelet transfusion is not harmless. • It results in ultrastructural pulmonary lesion-platelet aggregates within microcapillaries, degeneration of endothelial and alveolar cells, and protein exudate in the interstitium. • Despite low levels of factors V and VIII in blood stored for 14–21 days, dilutional coagulopathy is rare. • In some patients, dilutional effects of massive transfusion can lead to bleeding complications. • Recommendations to combat this situation have included prophylactic administration of 1 or 2 units of fresh-frozen plasma for every 2–10 units of transfused blood. • Actually, the continued bleeding is often secondary to the underlying disease process. • Initially, a transient dilutional coagulopathy may be related to the duration of hypotension. • No correlation has been demonstrated between the coagulation factors and the incidence or degree of bleeding complications. • It can reasonably be concluded, therefore, that the routine administration of fresh-frozen plasma is of little value in patients undergoing massive transfusions.

The indications for administration of calcium should be based on hemodynamic considerations because lowering the ionized calcium level by citrate to a level that blocks coagulation could lead to death from myocardial dysfunction and decreased peripheral vascular resistance. • Hypothermia decreases clearance of citrate from the blood, thereby allowing a marked reduction in ionized calcium. • Because blood products are stored between 1 and 6C, rapid transfusion of these products leads to hypothermia, which in turn brings about a decrease in citrate metabolism, the hepatic clearance of drugs, and synthesis of acute-phase reactive proteins. • The clotting system is impaired because of a decreased ability to form stable clots and a decreased production of clotting factors. • Blood warmers, warm saline lavage, blankets, and heated inspired gases are useful adjunctive measures to prevent hypothermia. • Heparin is not indicated as the initial step in such a situation.

ANSWER:
D

55. Regarding renal function during states of hemorrhagic shock, which of the following statements is/are true?

A. The blood flow to the kidneys, like that to the brain, is maintained until late in the course of hemorrhagic shock.

B. Renal ischemia longer than 10 minutes produces irreversible renal damage in most patients.

C. Fractional excretion of sodium (FeNa) is more than 1–2% in most patients.

D. Alteration in the BUN level is as sensitive a measure of renal function as is creatinine and creatinine clearance.

E. Furosemide does not effectively protect against acute renal failure (ARF).

Ref.: 1, 15-19

COMMENTS: Although the kidneys are clearly "vital" organs, blood flow to them is quickly diminished in states of shock in favor of the brain and heart. • Most kidneys tolerate ischemia for up to 15 minutes with full return of function. • Longer periods of ischemia lead to escalating degrees of renal injury. • Numerous parameters can be followed when monitoring the extent of renal damage sustained during hemorrhagic shock, including urine output, BUN levels, creatinine levels, and creatinine clearance.

The BUN level is a less reliable measure of renal function (i.e., glomerular filtration rate [GFR]) than is the plasma creatinine (PCr) level because the BUN level is affected by variables other than the GFR alone. • BUN levels will increase with high-protein diets, tissue breakdown, enhanced catabolism, and exposure to medications such as corticosteroids. • Normally, urea is passively reabsorbed in the proximal tubule. • States of enhanced proximal tubule reabsorption, such as volume depletion and congestive heart failure, will therefore cause a rise in the BUN level out of proportion to the change in GFR and PCr. • In this setting, there is no renal parenchymal damage, and the true GFR may be stable or minimally changed. • Creatinine is a product of skeletal muscle metabolism and dietary protein intake. • Its production is relatively constant, and therefore the plasma concentration is stable. • It is less dependent on the variables that affect BUN and thus is a better reflection of a true change in the GFR. • Creatinine clearance is derived from a 24-hr urine collection or calculated using a formula such as the Crockroft-Gault formula:

$$(140 - age \times weight~[kg]) \div 72 \times PCr~(\times 0.85~for~females)$$

This formula estimates the GFR more accurately than does the measurement of BUN alone, but often it is not necessary. • Usually, following the PCr level is enough to monitor disease severity and changes in the GFR. • Determining whether an increase in the BUN and PCr levels (decrease of the GFR) represents renal parenchymal damage, such as acute tubular necrosis (ATN) or a prerenal cause, is essential when evaluating ARF. • The FeNa in the urine (U),

$$[UNa \times PCr \div PNa \times UCr] \times 100,$$

is the most accurate method for making this distinction, since it measures sodium handling directly. • In states of reduced effective circulating volume (e.g., volume depletion, congestive heart failure, etc.), there is enhanced proximal sodium reabsorption in order to protect intravascular volume. • The FeNa measures the percent of filtered sodium excreted in the urine. • A value less than 1% is consistent with a prerenal form of ARF, while a value greater than 1–2% suggests the presence of ATN. • Urine sodium concentration, on the other hand, is dependent on the rate of water reabsorption. • A water-avid patient with prerenal ARF may therefore have a urine sodium concentration greater than 20–40 mEq/L. • The FeNa eliminates this confounding variable. • Obviously, the ideal management of a patient in hemorrhagic shock is prompt restoration of effective circulating volume and systemic pressure. • Although capable of increasing urine output, furosemide, a loop diuretic, may worsen renal function by causing hypovolemia.

ANSWER:
E

56. Which of the following is not consistent with ATN?

A. Oliguria

B. FeNa greater than 1–2%

C. Urine osmolality less than 300 mOsm/L

D. Creatinine clearance greater than 125 ml/min

E. Sodium wasting is an appropriate response to ATN

Ref.: 1, 3, 4, 19–21

COMMENTS: ATN is characterized by a rise in plasma creatinine concentration (decrease in creatinine clearance or GFR), by a urine volume that is reduced (oliguric) or normal, by changes in the urinalysis, and by a FeNa greater than 1–2%. • Oliguria (urine output <500 ml/24 hr) is a frequent but not an absolute feature of ATN. • Whether oliguria occurs may depend on the severity of renal injury and/or the relative reabsorption of filtrate at the tubular level. • Even if a patient's GFR falls to 10 L/day (normal, 180 L/day), a urine output of 1–2 L/day would still will be normal as long as 8–9 L of filtrate was reabsorbed. • In cases of well-preserved tubular function, as in prerenal forms of ARF, FeNa is low, consistent with the sodium-avid state. • As tubular dysfunction progresses, the ability of nephrons to reabsorb sodium is disrupted, and a greater percentage of the filtered sodium is excreted in the urine. • As a result, the FeNa will be greater than 1–2%, reflecting inappropriate sodium wasting by altered tubular function. • However, as ATN becomes established, the high FeNa reflects an appropriate response to volume expansion and maintenance of normal sodium balance. • In a patient with a GFR of 20 L/day and a plasma sodium concentration of 150 mEq/L, the filtered sodium load is 3000 mEq/day (20×150). • A FeNa of 2.5% ($75 \div 3000$) will be required to maintain stable sodium balance, assuming an intake of 75 mEq/day of sodium. • Loss of urinary concentrating ability is an early feature of ATN. • A urine osmolality of less than 350 mOsm/L is consistent with ATN, while an osmolality greater than 500 mOsm/L suggests a prerenal cause of ARF. • However, lower values can be seen during prerenal ARF, limiting the value of this test as a sole indicator of tubular function. • A creatinine clearance of 125 ml/min represents normal renal function.

ANSWER:
D

57. A 62-year-old diabetic patient with rest pain is admitted for evaluation of his peripheral arterial system. He has chronic renal failure (CRF) with a serum creatinine of 5.0 mg/dl. Which of the following agents is/are not indicated to avoid contrast nephropathy?

A. Calcium-channel blocker

B. Hydration with diuretics

C. Mannitol and saline hydration

D. Acetylcysteine given only after contrast exposure

E. All of the above

Ref.: 3, 22–31

COMMENTS: Radiocontrast agents can lead to a reversible form of ARF. • The pathogenesis is not well established. • Renal vasoconstriction and direct tubular toxic effects of the contrast are two proposed mechanisms of injury. • Risk factors for developing contrast nephropathy include underlying chronic renal failure with a PCr greater than 1.5 mg/dl, diabetic nephropathy with renal insufficiency, congestive heart failure, multiple myeloma, and large contrast volume. • The risk is minimal in patients with normal renal function, including patients with diabetes. • Renal failure is nonoliguric and transient in most cases. • Severe renal failure requiring short- or long-term dialysis is rare and is most likely to occur in patients whose baseline creatinine level is greater than 4 mg/dl. • Saline volume expansion in the pre- and post-contrast period is the only preventive measure consistently shown to be of benefit. • Hydration with furosemide may increase the risk of contrast nephropathy when compared to saline alone. • Furthermore, the use of saline solution and mannitol does not add any benefit over the use of saline alone. • Calcium-channel blockers given to minimize renal vasoconstriction after contrast exposure have not been conclusively shown to prevent renal failure. • The role of nonionic contrast agents is not clearly defined. • Studies seem to support the use of iso-osmolar nonionic agents in high-risk patients, especially those with diabetes. • There are conflicting data on the role of acetylcysteine in the prevention of contrast nephropathy. • Given its relatively safe side effect profile and the few series supporting its use, acetylcysteine use can be justified, particularly in high-risk patients. • A rational approach to preventing contrast nephropathy among high-risk patients, such as the patient in question, would include acetylcysteine (600 mg PO bid the day before and the day of contrast exposure), saline volume expansion, and an iso-osmolar nonionic contrast agent. • The latter may be more important for patients with renal dysfunction and diabetes.

ANSWER:
E

58. Regarding the systemic inflammatory response syndrome, which of the following statements is/are true?

A. Invariably associated with infection

B. Body temperature above 38 or under 36°C

C. Tachypnea (>20 breaths per minute) or hyperventilation ($PaCO_2$ < 32 mmHg)

D. Leukocytosis (>12,000 cells/mm³) or leukopenia (<4000 cells/mm³)

E. Heart rate greater than 90 beats per minute

Ref.: 32–34

COMMENTS: Sepsis is a clinical response arising from infection, although a similar response may arise in the absence of infection and is termed the systemic inflammatory response syndrome. • All of the characteristics listed may be present in the systemic response to a wide variety of insults, not only to infection. • Noninfectious causes include pancreatitis, ischemia, multiple trauma, hemorrhagic shock, immune-mediated organ injury, burns, and the exogenous administration of mediators of the inflammatory process (e.g., TNF or the cytokines interleukin [IL]-1, -6, and -8). • When this syndrome is the result of confirmed infection, it is termed sepsis. • Septic shock is defined as sepsis-induced hypotension persisting despite adequate fluid resuscitation, along with manifestations of organ dysfunction and hypoperfusion abnormalities. • Septic shock is a distributive form of shock that results in a severe decrease in systemic vascular resistance associated with a normal or elevated CO. • In addition, abnormalities of cardiac performance, including decreased ejection fraction and ventricular dilatation, are characteristic of septic shock.

ANSWER:
B, C, D, E

59. Which of the following cytokines is/are known mediators of systemic inflammatory response syndrome?

A. IL-1

B. IL-4

C. Transforming growth factor β (TGF-β)

D. IL-2

E. Tumor necrosis factor α (TNF-α)

Ref.: 4

COMMENTS: See Question 60.

60. Which of the following is/are correct regarding cytokines in the pathophysiology of sepsis?

A. Elevated circulating phospholipase A_2 is not predictive of lethal multiple organ failure.

B. Serum levels of cytokines have greater biologic meaning than do tissue levels.

C. Elevated IL-6 levels are most consistently correlated with death in severe sepsis.

D. Circulating protein C levels are not predictive of outcome in septic patients.

E. Nitric oxide synthase inhibition improves survival in models of sepsis.

Ref.: 4, 34

COMMENTS: Experimental and clinical studies have demonstrated that the physiologic and metabolic effects of TNF and endotoxin (lipopolysaccharide) are nearly identical. • IL-1 has been shown to have metabolic effects similar to those of TNF. • However, TNF-α, IL-1, and other cytokines have dual beneficial and adverse effects, depending on the amount, timing, and anatomic locus of production. • TNF is thought to play an important role, but it is variably detected in the blood of patients with sepsis. • Cytokines are low—molecular-weight proteins produced by activated monocytes or macrophages. • Cytokines are involved in the differentiation, proliferation, and immunoregulatory function of various cells, including lymphocytes and macrophages. • Multiple organ failure is a systemic disorder of immunoregulation, inflammatory damage, endothelial dysfunction, and hypermetabolism. • Stimulation of mononuclear cells, neutrophils, and endothelial cells leads to an inappropriate regulation of endogenous inflammatory mediators, such as cytokines (IL-1, -6, and -8), platelet-activating factor, nitric oxide, and eicosanoids. • One source of cytokines is the tissue macrophage, where these substances may have local paracrine effects; cytokines at tissue levels may be of greater importance than the variable serum levels. • Anti-inflammatory cytokines (TGF-β, IL-4, IL-10, and granulocyte colony-stimulating factor) and IL-1 receptor antagonist constitute some of the host efforts to limit excessive reaction to endotoxemia. • TNF and IL-1 activate phospholipase-1. • Circulating phospholipase-1 is highly predictive of death in patients with peritonitis. • Endotoxin may damage the endothelium, but most of its effects can be facilitated by its association with an acute-phase reactant lipopolysaccharide, leading to activation of nuclear factors and increased cytokine production.

The physiologic responses of TNF are nearly identical to the responses of lipopolysaccharide. • TNF can cause fever or hypothermia, tachycardia, elevated CO, and decreased systemic vascular resistance. • In higher concentrations, TNF can cause hypotension, circulatory collapse, and acidosis. • Hormonal response from elevated TNF concentrations includes elevations in catecholamines, cortisol, and glucagon. • Oxygen consumption and carbon dioxide production also increase in response to elevated TNF. • IL-1 can cause fever and leukocytosis, increased production of acute-phase reactants, increased muscle catabolism, and other events that occur in sepsis. • Reciprocal interaction among cytokines, complement, and coagulation systems occur in multiple organ failure.

• TNF down-regulates thrombomodulin in the endothelial cell, which impairs activation of protein C. • This phenomenon may explain the strongly predictive value of this protein serum level. • There is a strong correlation between elevated levels of IL-6 and mortality rates in patients with multiple organ failure.

Nitric oxide plays an unclear role in sepsis. • Excess nitric oxide synthesis within the endothelium during the late phase of septic shock is a primary contributor to the loss of vascular tone and hypotension. • Nitric oxide synthase inhibitors (*N*-methyl arginine) allows reduced levels of pressors but definitive proof is lacking. • ATP-MgCl may restore nitric oxide synthase, thus restoring endothelium-dependent vasodilatation.

ANSWERS:
Question 59: A, E
Question 60: C

61. Which of the following treatment modalities may be appropriate in the management of a patient in severe septic shock?

A. IL-1 receptor antagonist

B. Aggressive volume administration

C. Vasopressor therapy

D. Mechanical ventilation

E. Steroids

Ref.: 1, 2

COMMENTS: Of the various forms of "shock," septic shock is probably the most difficult to manage. • In many instances, the source of sepsis may not be immediately apparent, and therefore correction of the underlying infectious process may be delayed. • Appropriate antibiotic therapy for recognized or presumed infections is clearly central to the ultimate resolution of septic shock. • While this is occurring, support of the patient's cardiopulmonary status is frequently warranted. • In most cases of septic shock, peripheral vasodilatation leads to pooling of the blood volume and a need for aggressive fluid administration initially. • Toxins produced in many infections are inhibitory to myocardial contractility. • Thus, once adequate volume has been achieved, inotropic agents (e.g., dobutamine) may be warranted. • Dopamine is one of the preferred agents in that it provides inotropic and chronotropic support for the heart while augmenting renal blood flow when given in low to moderate doses. • Norepinephrine has been used with success, provided volume restoration has been started. • Sepsis is one of the common predisposing factors in the development of ARDS, and as a consequence many patients in septic shock require mechanical ventilation. • The use of pharmacologic doses of corticosteroids is somewhat controversial, but large prospective trials have shown no benefit and possible detriment. • Clinical trials conducted with agents that target the initiating toxins and mediators have shown no change in outcome.

ANSWER:
B, C, D

62. With regard to multiple organ failure, which of the following statement is/are false?

A. Sepsis is the major risk factor.

B. Injury to the microvascular endothelium is uniformly present.

C. Neutrophil-mediated injury is dependent on adherence to the microvascular endothelium.

D. The high concentration of xanthine oxidase in ischemic endothelial cells prevents generation of toxic oxygen radicals.

E. Increase in the gastrointestinal barrier is often present.

Ref.: 3, 34

COMMENTS: Sepsis is the major risk factor in the development of multiple organ failure. Injury to the microvascular endothelium causes a generalized inflammatory state. • Early recognition and adequate treatment are essential if serious ischemia-reperfusion injury and multiple organ failure are to be prevented. • Several components of the immune defense system are involved. • Neutrophil-mediated injury is dependent on adherence to the endothelium and neutrophil aggregation. • Both are mediated by the glycoprotein complex CD11/CD18, to which monoclonal antibodies can be directed. • The endothelial cell exposed to ischemia is subject to a depression of ATP levels, accompanied by an increased xanthine oxidase/xanthine dehydrogenase ratio, which generates toxic oxygen radicals upon reperfusion. • Pharmacologic prevention of tissue injury following ischemia is based on enzyme inhibition and O_2 radical scavengers. • The most effective short-term protection is hypothermia. • Arachidonic acid metabolites are leukotrienes and prostacyclines. • Platelet-activating factor, produced by various inflammatory cells, causes microvascular injury through ischemia and stasis. • Breakdown of the intestinal mucosal barrier may allow the ongoing bacterial translocation and stimulation of the immunoinflammatory reaction. • Measurement of intragastric pH by tonometric studies may facilitate early detection of regional tissue hypoxia and optimization of resuscitation.

ANSWER:
E

63. Match the nutritional components in the left-hand column with the corresponding immunologic characteristics in the right-hand column.

A. Arginine   a. Decrease in prostaglandin E_2 and leukotriene B
B. Nucleotides   b. Decreased T-cell–mediated immunity, decreased IL-2 production, and increased susceptibility to infections resulting from lack of this nutrient in diet
C. ω-3 Fatty acids c. Gut major fuel source
D. Glutamine   d. Nitric oxide production

Ref.: 35

COMMENTS: All the nutrients listed play an important role in the process of modifying immune function. • **Arginine** increases protein synthesis and IL-2 production, induces secretion of anabolic hormones, enhances guanyl and adenyl cyclase activity, increases total CD-4 cells, and is responsible for nitric oxide production essential for optimal lymphocyte DNA synthesis. • Animals fed diets without purines and pyrimidines (**nucleotides**) have shown a decrease in T-cell–mediated immune response, decreased IL-2 production, and increased susceptibility to *Staphylococcus* and *Candida* infections. • Administration of **ω-3 fatty acids** is thought to reverse the immunosuppression caused by excessive production of prostaglandin E_2 and leukotriene B. • **Glutamine** is a nonessential amino acid involved in the production of ammonia and ketoglutarate. • It contributes an amide group for nucleotide synthesis. • Enterocytes use it as a preferential fuel source. • Glutamine deficiency in the stressed state is thought to result in

an alteration of the gut mucosal barrier, which in turn may continue the systemic inflammatory response.

ANSWER:
A-d; B-b; C-a; D-c

64. Which of the following factors decrease(s) the rate of bacterial translocation in the gastrointestinal tract?

A. Parenteral nutrition

B. Glutamine-enriched total parenteral nutrition

C. Septic shock

D. Addition of fiber to an elemental diet

E. Prolonged ileus

Ref.: 35

COMMENTS: Several investigators have shown an increase in intestinal mucosal permeability to bacteria and bacterial products (bacterial translocation) following hemorrhagic shock, sepsis, or lipid A infusion, although the gastrointestinal tract is grossly intact. • This breakdown of the mucosal barrier has been implicated in the pathophysiology of multiple organ failure. • The susceptibility of the splanchnic circulation to hypoperfusion, the high concentration of xanthine oxidase, and the presence of enteric flora enhance this theory. • Several factors are known to increase the rate at which bacterial translocation occurs: hemorrhagic shock, septic shock, bacterial overgrowth, prolonged ileus, bowel manipulation, parenteral nutrition, and antibiotic use. • Prolonged ileus and antibiotic use are probably predisposing factors to bacterial overgrowth. • It has been demonstrated that enterocytes of the gut mucosa preferentially use the amino acid glutamine and ketone bodies as respiratory fuel. • Furthermore, enteral and parenteral formulas that contain glutamine and/or ketone bodies (β-hydroxybutyrate and acetoacetate) promote bowel mucosal growth and probably decrease the rate of bacterial translocation. • Villous atrophy, decreased secretion of immunoglobulin A, decreased cellular immunity, bacterial overgrowth, and decreased barrier function with bacterial translocation have been associated with parenteral rather than enteral nutrition.

ANSWER:
B, D

65. A patient involved in a motor vehicle accident is found to have a thoracic spine fracture (T-6) and paraplegia. The patient is hypotensive with a systolic blood pressure of 70 mmHg and is bradycardic. The patient is breathing comfortably. Which of the following would be appropriate initial treatment?

A. Fluid administration

B. Steroid administration within 24 hr of injury

C. Immediate intubation

D. α-Agonist administration for spinal cord injury above T-4

E. Nasogastric tube placement

Ref.: 4, 36

COMMENTS: Neurogenic shock results from a loss of balance between vasodilatory and vasoconstrictor influences in the arterioles and venules. • Common causes include sensory stimulation, such as severe pain, exposure to unpleasant events or sights, high spinal anesthesia, and traumatic spinal cord injury. • Since the heart receives sympathetic input, there is a difference between injuries above T-4 and one below T-4. • The former depresses cardiac function and decreases venous return. • Bradycardia is caused by the sympathectomy of spinal insult above the level of T4, with no capacity for compensatory tachycardia. • Clinical characteristics include a blood pressure that is often low, as in other forms of shock. • However, the pulse rate is usually slower than normal, and the skin is flushed, warm, and dry. • A reduction in CO is found, secondary to decreased blood return to the heart because of the increased capacitance of the arterioles and venules. • The treatment of milder forms of neurogenic shock consists of removing the nociceptive stimulus. • Neurogenic shock resulting from high spinal anesthesia can usually be treated with a vasopressor such as ephedrine or phenylephrine, each of which increases CO by direct effects on the heart and by increasing peripheral vasoconstriction. • The treatment of neurogenic shock secondary to spinal cord injury is usually more complicated, not only because of more prolonged hypotension but also because of the question of coincident hypovolemic shock resulting from associated injuries. • Such patients often require ventilatory support because of decreased spontaneous respiration and loss of accessory muscles for breathing. • Aggressive fluid therapy should be instituted early under continuous cardiovascular monitoring. • Persistent hypotension necessitates recognition of possible hemorrhagic shock. • A vasopressor such as ephedrine or phenylephrine may be needed. • If the injury is below T-4, a pure α-agonist may aggravate reflex bradycardia. • Thus, a drug with mixed chronotopic and inotropic effects (e.g., norepinephrine or dopamine) is preferred. • A nasogastric tube should be inserted because these patients develop gastric atony, dilatation, and hypersecretion. • Although the administration of steroids remains controversial, their usefulness for a blunt spinal cord injury has been suggested when they are given within 8 hr of injury and their administration is extended for 48 hr. • Steroid use is optional. • Continued cardiac monitoring is necessary in patients with sinus bradycardia because they may develop cardiac pause, sinus arrest, asystole, and ventricular dysrhythmias.

ANSWER:
A, E

66. A 50-year-old trauma patient is admitted to the intensive care unit with a Glasgow Coma Score (GCS) of 8, unilateral posturing, intracranial pressure of 20 mmHg, and a systolic blood pressure of 70 mmHg. Accepted treatment of this patient includes which of the following?

   A. Fluid resuscitation to reach a cerebral perfusion pressure of 70 mmHg or above

   B. Mild hyperventilation to a $PaCO_2$ of 35 mmHg

   C. Transient moderate hypothermia

   D. Cerebrospinal fluid drainage for persistent elevated intracranial pressure

   E. All of the above

Ref.: 36, 37

COMMENTS: Traumatic brain injury is the leading cause of death in patients younger than 45 years. • As many as 75% of these patients have multiple trauma. • Correction of shock, hypoxemia, and elevated intracranial pressure constitute the mainstay in the management of these patients. • The brain has autoregulatory mechanisms to maintain a constant cerebral blood flow over a range of systemic pressures. • Cerebral perfusion pressure (CPP) is the difference between mean arterial pressure (MAP) and the intracranial pressure. • The normal range for MAP is 80–100 mmHg, and

the range for ICP is 5–10 mmHg. • Thus, the normal range for CPP is 70–95 mmHg. • Maintaining a minimum CPP of 70 mmHg and an ICP of 20 mmHg or lower improves outcome. • Initial management is directed at improving oxygenation and tissue perfusion. • If the goal of a CPP of 70 mmHg cannot be met with ICP control and adequate preload, then vasopressors or inotropes should be used. • An intraventricular catheter or an intraparenchymal probe should be inserted to monitor ICP in patients with a GCS of 8 or less and an abnormal CT scan; in patients with a GCS of 8 or less and a normal CT scan but with at least two of the following: age older than 40 years, unilateral or bilateral posturing, or a systolic blood pressure less than 90 mmHg; and in patients with a GCS greater than 8 at the discretion of the neurosurgeon, such as patients being operated on for other injuries. • The treatment threshold for ICP is 20–25 mmHg, although no prospective randomized trial has been done to demonstrate an improvement in survival.

In addition to all measures aforementioned, analgesia and sedation are crucial in the management of patients with brain injury. • Neuromuscular blockade may be indicated in refractory intracranial hypertension, but its use should be of short duration due to an increased incidence of pneumonia, renal failure, and muscle weakness secondary to muscle necrosis. • Osmotherapy with agents such as mannitol works through numerous mechanisms, including osmotic, hemodynamic, and cytoprotective means. • However, its use also is associated with serious side effects. • Thus, close hemodynamic monitoring is mandatory. • Hypothermia is used in the management of severe traumatic brain injury despite the lack of conclusive evidence supporting its use. • A recent study suggested that hypothermia is not beneficial in the management of these patients. • However, it continues to be used to treat these injuries.

ANSWER:
E

67. Which of the following regarding ventilator associated pneumonia (VAP) is/are true?

   A. The development of pneumonia is directly related to the length of ventilatory support

   B. Antibiotic treatment varies for early versus late VAP.

   C. The commonest organism associated with early VAP is pseudomonal species.

   D. Retrograde transmission of contaminated gastric contents to the oropharynx and subsequent aspiration predispose the patient to VAP.

   E. All of the above.

Ref.: 3, 38

COMMENTS: The development of pneumonia appears to be directly related to length of ventilatory support, and the risk is highest during the first 2 weeks of therapy. • The incidence is in the 20–25% range, and the mortality rate is higher than 30%. • Patients with COPD, burns, neurosurgical illnesses, ARDS, or witnessed aspiration or who are reintubated are at high risk for developing VAP. • The pathogenesis of VAP is thought to involve the aspiration of pathogenic organisms in quantities that overwhelm the local immune system of the patient. • Aspiration of contaminated gastric contents will predispose the patient to VAP. • Continuous enteral feedings, which promote alkalinization of the stomach, increase bacterial overgrowth and the incidence of VAP. • Gastroenteral feedings do not appear to predispose patients to a higher risk of pneumonia than do jejunostomy feedings. • Ulcer prophylactic agents that alter gastric pH may increase the incidence of VAP by increasing gastric pH and allowing for more bacterial colonization. • The risk of developing VAP may be reduced by avoidance of antacid therapies, nasogastric tube suctioning, and supine position and by ventilator circuitry changes every 24 hr. • Selective gut decontamination reduces the likelihood of colonization, but it does not reduce the incidence of nosocomial pneumonia. • Bacterial translocation via the portal system has not proved to be an etiologic factor in the clinical setting. • VAP can be classified as early (occurring within 4–7 days of intubation) and late (occurring after 7 days of ventilation). • This distinction is important because early VAP most often is caused by such organisms and *Streptococcus pneumoniae, Hemophilus influenzae,* and *Staphylococcus.* • These organisms are relatively easy to treat, as opposed to the difficult-to-treat organisms of late VAP: pseudomonal species, *Acinetobacter, Stenotrophomonas,* and methicillin-resistant *Staphylococcus aureus* (MRSA). • Empiric therapy usually consists of one or two agents with activity against gram-negative and gram-positive organisms. • Routine aspiration of bronchial aspirate through a wedged double-lumen catheter or bronchoalveolar lavage through a flexible bronchoscope should be performed at regular intervals.

ANSWER:
A, B, D

68. Regarding sepsis and septic shock in neutropenic patients with cancer, which of the following statements is/are true?

   A. Signs and symptoms of infection are ill-defined.

   B. TNF and C-reactive protein are extremely sensitive markers of infection.

   C. Granulocyte colony-stimulating factor (G-CSF) adjuvant therapy improves long-term survival.

   D. Recombinant human activated protein C therapy is associated with serious bleeding.

   E. Necrotizing enterocolitis mandates immediate left hemicolectomy.

Ref.: 39

COMMENTS: Infections and refractory malignancies are the commonest cause of death in cancer patients. • Early recognition and administration of polymicrobial antibiotic therapy is critical. • Often, fever is present in the cancer patient, but its relationship to an underlying infection is poor. • Moreover, common signs and symptoms of infection in these patients are poorly defined. • The cancer patient often has defects in the immune system, such as granulocytopenia, cell-mediated immunodeficiency, and humoral immunodeficiency. • This immune dysfunction predisposes these patients to certain bacterial, fungal, and viral infections. • Prompt diagnosis and treatment are therefore crucial for positive patient outcomes. • In neutropenic patients, elevated serum levels of IL-6 and Il-8 have been found to be associated with an increased likelihood of infection in these patients. • Studies evaluating other cytokines and acute-phase reactants as markers for early detection of infection in neutropenic patients are inconclusive.

   Treatment with adjuvant G-CSF to restore granulocytes appears promising in refractory fungal infection and necrotizing enterocolitis. • Recombinant activated human protein C adjuvant therapy has improved short-term survival rates in patients with multiple organ failure. • However, its use has been associated with bleeding complications. • Necrotizing enterocolitis is a recognized complication, especially in acute leukemia patients and patients undergoing chemotherapy for gastrointestinal malignancies. • It affects mainly the cecum and ascending colon. • It should be suspected in the granulocytopenic patient with high fever, abdominal pain, and diarrhea. • Urgent endoscopic evaluation is mandatory. • Polymicrobial intestinal flora are encountered commonly. • Contrast CT scan findings include bowel thickening, pneumoatosis intestinalis, and signs of perforated viscus. • Initial treatment consists of bowel rest, a combination of broad-spectrum antibiotics, vigorous fluid resuscitation, nutrition, and G-CSF. • Operative therapy is reserved for complications and should be deferred, if possible, until the granulocytopenia is resolved.

ANSWER:
A, D

69. A 45-year-old man is recovering from multiple organ failure following an operation for a perforated gastric ulcer. He has been afebrile for 48 hr and is off antibiotics. His white blood cell count is normal. Renal failure has resolved. His encephalopathy is improving, and his oxygenation is adequate on 30% oxygen and 5 cm PEEP. Attempts at weaning him off the ventilator have been unsuccessful. His negative inspiratory pressure is $-10 \, \text{cmH}_2\text{O}$. Neurologic examination shows a symmetric quadriparesis with facial sparing and depressed deep-tendon reflexes. A spinal tap fluid is normal. What is the most likely diagnosis?

   A. Guillain-Barré syndrome

   B. Myasthenia gravis

   C. Neuromuscular blockade

   D. Primary myopathy

   E. Critical illness polyneuropathy (CPU)

Ref.: 40

COMMENTS: See Question 70.

70. Which of the following statements is/are true concerning the condition described in Question 68?

   A. A nerve biopsy often shows demyelinization or inflammation.

   B. Failure to wean from the ventilator is due to phrenic nerve involvement.

   C. Corticosteroids are the treatment of choice.

   D. Serum antibodies against acetylcholine receptors are always present.

   E. Plasmapheresis is the initial treatment of choice.

Ref.: 40

COMMENTS: CPU is an axonal motor sensory neuropathy that accompanies sepsis with encephalopathy. • It is due to primary axonal degeneration, affecting motor fibers more than sensory fibers. • Frequently, it presents as failure to wean a patient from the ventilator, due to phrenic nerve involvement despite clinical improvement. • Symmetrical quadriparesis with facial sparing and depressed deep-tendon reflexes is characteristic. • Electromyography confirms the diagnosis. • Spinal fluid is normal, unlike in Guillain-Barré syndrome. • Facial involvement and detection of antibodies against acetylcholine is characteristic of myasthenia gravis. • Nerve biopsy shows axonal degeneration without demyelination or inflammation. • Treatment is supportive. • Corticosteroids are contraindicated.

ANSWERS:
Question 69: E
Question 70: B

71. In regard to pulmonary embolism (PE), which of the following is/are false?

A. Symptoms of early small to medium PEs are usually pulmonary in nature.

B. Ventilation perfusion (V/Q_2) abnormalities are present early after embolism, and shunt becomes the predominant mechanism for hypoxemia later.

C. Chest radiographic abnormalities are rarely present in most patients with PE.

D. More than one-third of patients with angiographic PE have negative leg study results for deep vein thrombosis (DVT).

E. Thrombolytic therapy has been shown to reduce mortality rates in comparison with heparin in patients with PE.

Ref.: 4

COMMENTS: The incidence of PE in the United States exceeds 500,000, with the prevalence of nonfatal PE approaching 20 per 1000 inpatients. • As many as two-thirds of these cases go undiagnosed. • Iliofemoral thrombosis appears to be the source of most clinically apparent emboli. • Predisposing factors include (1) prior embolism, (2) factors promoting stasis, (3) lower-extremity and pelvic operations and pelvic trauma, and (4) hypercoagulable states. • Many emboli are silent. Symptoms of small-to-medium emboli are usually pulmonary (i.e., dyspnea, chest pain, and cough). • Tachypnea and tachycardia are present as well. • Massive PEs often produce cardiovascular findings. • Pulmonary artery pressure tends to be increased but correlates poorly with the size of the embolus and may even be normal. • Even without infarction, radiographic abnormalities appear as diaphragmatic elevation, atelectasis, and effusion. • Although results of noninvasive leg studies for determination of DVT are negative in up to one-third of patients, their use in addition to clinical suspicion and lung screening could reduce the need for pulmonary angiography. • Angiography, however, is the definitive diagnostic technique for this disease. • A helical CT scan of the chest with infusion has shown excellent specificity. • Heparin therapy over 5–7 days with 4–5 days overlap with warfarin (Coumadin) constitutes the therapy of choice. • Coumadin should be continued for 6–12 weeks for calf vein and large-vein thrombosis. • Thrombolytic therapy has not been shown to reduce mortality rates in comparison with heparin in large prospective series.

ANSWER:
A, C, E

72. Which of the following precludes a diagnosis of brain death?

A. Uremia

B. Hypothermia below 32.2°C

C. Systemic blood pressure of 70/40 mmHg

D. Hypercarbia with a $PaCO_2$ greater than 60 mmHg with no respiratory response

Ref.: 3

COMMENTS: Brain death is the irreversible cessation of all functions of the brain, including the brain stem. • This condition must persist for a minimum of 6–12 hr unless there is no identifiable structural abnormality, in which case more prolonged observation is advisable. • A firm diagnosis requires exclusion of reversible causes of coma, such as sedation, hypothermia below 32.2°C, neuromuscular blockade, and shock. • The diagnosis is mainly clinical in a patient unresponsive to painful stimuli and with absent oculovestibular, corneal, and oculocephalic reflexes to ice-water calorics and a positive apnea test result. • Coma should be deep and fixed without response to external stimuli, including pain. • A confirmatory test, such as blood flow study, electroencephalography, or angiogram, is not obligatory, but it confirms brain death when performed 6 hr after the initial clinical tests. • Reversible causes of brain dysfunction that may confound the diagnosis must be identified and corrected. • They include drug intoxication, hypothermia (<32°C), hepatic encephalopathy, severe electrolyte disorder, hyperglycemia, uremia, and hypotension (mean arterial pressure <60 mmHg). • The corneal reflex and gag response should be absent. • The apnea test requires the following prerequisites: core temperature of 97.8°F (36.5°C) or more, systolic pressure of 90 mmHg or more, euvolemia, apnea, and normal oxygenation. • The patient is disconnected from the respirator while maintaining a supply of 100% oxygen. • If respiratory movements are absent and the $PaCO_2$ is more than 60 mmHg or there is a 20 mmHg increase in $PaCO_2$ above the baseline (if starting with >40 mmHg), the test result is positive. • If the mean arterial pressure drops below 60 mmHg or the patient desaturates, the test is terminated and the patient is connected to the ventilator. • If the $PaCO$ is less than 60 mmHg or if the increase is less than 20 mmHg, the patient should be given vasopressors and the test repeated later. • Up to 30% of brain-dead patients have a normal plantar response to pain.

ANSWER:
A, B, C

REFERENCES

1. Townsend CM, Beauchamp RD, Evers BM, et al (eds): *Sabiston Textbook of Surgery: The Biological Basis of Modern Surgical Practice,* 16th ed. Saunders, Philadelphia, 2001.
2. Schwartz SI, Shires GT, Spencer FC: *Principles of Surgery,* 7th ed. McGraw-Hill, New York, 1999.
3. Greenfield LJ, Mulholland MW, Oldham KT (eds): *Surgery: Scientific Principles and Practice,* 3rd ed. Lippincott, Williams & Wilkins, Philadelphia, 2001.
4. Civetta JM, Taylor RW, Kirby RR: *Critical Care.* Lippincott-Raven, Philadelphia, 1997.
5. Tuman KJ: Tissue oxygen delivery: the physiology of anemia. *Anesthesiol Clin North Am* 8:451–469, 1990.
6. West JB: *Respiratory Physiology; The Essentials,* 4th ed. Williams & Wilkins, Baltimore, 1990.
7. Gracias V: Pulmonary artery catheter consensus conference: consensus statement. *Crit Care Med* 25:910–925, 1997.
8. Martin GS, Mangialardi RJ, Wheeler AP, et al: Albumin and furosemide therapy in hypoproteinemic patients with acute lung injury. *Crit Care Med* 30:2175–2182, 2002.
9. Bidani A, Tzouanakis AE, Cardenas VJ, et al: Permissive hypercapnia in acute respiratory failure. *JAMA* 272:957–962, 1994.
10. Chad DC, Scheinburn DS: Weaning from mechanical ventilation. *Crit Care Clin* 14:799–817, 1998.
11. Levy MM: Pulmonary capillary pressure: Clinical implications. *Crit Care Clin* 12(4):819–839, 1996.
12. Vincent JL, Dubois MJ, Navickis RJ, et al: Hypoalbuminemia in acute illness: is there a rationale for intervention. *Ann Surg* 237:319–334, 2003.
13. Shields CJ, Winter DC, Manning BJ, et al: Hypertonic saline infusion for pulmonary injury due to ischemia-reperfusion. *Arch Surg* 138:9–14, 2003.
14. Eddy VA, Morris JA, Cullinane DC: Hypothermia, coagulopathy, and acidosis. *Surg Clin North Am* 80:845–854, 2000.
15. Levey AS: Measurement of renal function in chronic renal disease. *Kidney Int* 38:167–184, 1990.
16. Dossetor JB: Creatininemia versus uremia: the relative significance of blood urea nitrogen and serum creatinine concentrations in azotemia. Ann Intern Med 65:1287–1299, 1966.

17. Rose, BD: *Pathophysiology of Renal Disease*, 2nd ed. McGraw-Hill, New York, 1987.
18. Steiner RW: Interpreting the fractional excretion of sodium. *Am J Med* 77(4):699–702, 1984.
19. Miller TR, Anderson RJ, Linas SL, et al: Urinary diagnostic indices in acute renal failure: a prospective study. *Ann Intern Med* 89(1):47–50, 1978.
20. Anderson RJ, Linas SL, Berns AS, et al: Nonoliguric acute renal failure. *N Engl J Med* 296(20):1134–1138, 1977.
21. Dixon BS, Anderson RJ: Nonoliguric acute renal failure. *Am J Kidney Dis* 6(2):71–80, 1985.
22. Rudnick MR, Berns JS, Cohen RM, et al: Nephrotoxic risks of renal angiography: contrast media-associated nephrotoxicity and atheroembolism: a critical review. *Am J Kidney Dis* 24(4):713–727, 1994.
23. Barret BJ: Contrast nephrotoxicity. *J Am Soc Nephrol* 5(2):125–137, 1994.
24. Berns AS: Nephrotoxicity of contrast media. *Kidney Int* 36:730–740, 1989.
25. Rudnick MR, Goldfarb S, Wexler L, et al: Nephrotoxicity of ionic and nonionic contrast media in 1196 patients: a randomized trial. The Iohexol Cooperative Study. *Kidney Int* 47(1):254–261, 1995.
26. Solomon R, Weiner C, Mann D, et al: Effects of saline, mannitol, and furosemide to prevent acute decreases in renal function induced by radiocontrast agents. *N Engl J Med* 331(21):1416–1420, 1994.
27. Trivedi HS, Moore H, Nasr S, et al: A randomized prospective trial to assess the role of saline hydration on the development of contrast nephrotoxicity. *Nephron Clin Pract* 93(1):C29–C34, 2003.
28. Moore RD, Steinberg EP, Powe NR, et al: Nephrotoxicity of high-osmolality versus low-osmolality contrast media: randomized clinical trial. *Radiology* 182(3):649–655, 1992.
29. Tepel M, van der Giet M, Schwarzfeld C, et al: Prevention of radiographic-contrast-agent-induced reduction in renal function by acetylcysteine. *N Engl J Med* 343:180–184, 2000.
30. Shyu KG, Cheng JJ, Kuan P, et al: Acetylcysteine protects against acute renal damage in patients with abnormal renal function undergoing a coronary procedure. *J Am Coll Cardiol* 40:1383–1388, 2002.
31. Kay J, Chow WH, Chan TM, et al: Acetylcysteine for prevention of acute deterioration of renal function following elective coronary angiography and intervention: a randomized controlled trial. *JAMA* 289:553–558, 2003.
32. Parrillo JE, Parker MM, Natanson C, et al: Septic shock in humans: advances in the understanding of pathogenesis, cardiovascular dysfunction, and therapy. *Ann Intern Med* 113:227–242, 1990.
33. Bone RC, Sprung CL, Sibbald WJ: Definitions for sepsis and organ failure. *Crit Care Med* 20:724–726, 1992.
34. Khadaroo RG, Marshall JC: ARDS and the multiple organ dysfunction syndrome: common mechanisms of a common systemic process. *Crit Care Clinics* 18:127–141, 2002.
35. Hickey MS: Nutritional management of the critically ill patient. In: Weigelt JA, Lewis FR (eds) *Surgical Critical Care.* Saunders, Philadelphia, 1996.
36. King BS, Gupta R, Narayan R: The early assessment and intensive care unit management of patients with severe traumatic brain and spinal cord injuries. *Surg Clin North Am* 80:855–870, 2000.
37. Harris OA, Colford JM, Good MC, et al: The role of hypothermia in the management of severe brain injury: a meta-analysis. *Arch Neurol* 59:1077–1083, 2002.
38. Keenan SP, Heyland DK, Jacka MJ, et al: Ventilator-associated pneumonia. Prevention, diagnosis, and therapy. *Crit Care Clin* 18:107–125, 2002.
39. Safdar A, Armstrong D: Infectious morbidity in critically ill patients with cancer. *Crit Care Clin* 17:531–570, 2001.
40. Leijten FS, de Weerd AW, et al: Critical illness polyneuropathy: a review of the literature, definition and pathophysiology. *Clin Neurol Neurosurg* 96:10–19, 1994.

CHAPTER 16

Trauma

Mitchell Jay Cohen, M.D.

1. A 22-year-old man is brought to the emergency room after being involved in a motorcycle crash. He is combative, pale, and bleeding profusely from the nose and mouth and has a sizable scalp laceration. There is an obvious deformity of his right thigh. His vital signs are as follows: blood pressure 80/40, pulse 130 beats per minute, and respiratory rate 40 breaths per minute and labored. Which of the following initial management choices is correct?

A. Esophageal intubation, rapid infusion of lactated Ringer's solution through a central venous catheter, traction splint of extremity, and rapid suture of scalp laceration

B. Endotracheal intubation, rapid infusion of lactated Ringer's solution through percutaneous large-bore catheters, traction splint of extremity, rapid suture of scalp laceration, and exposure of the patient

C. Oxygen by mask, rapid infusion of lactated Ringer's solution through percutaneous large-bore catheters, pressure dressing on scalp wound, and exposure of patient

D. Cricothyroidotomy, rapid infusion of lactated Ringer's solution through percutaneous large-bore catheters, pressure dressing on scalp wound, traction splint of extremity, and exposure of patient

E. Open airway with jaw thrust maneuver, rapid infusion of lactated Ringer's solution through percutaneous large-bore catheters, rapid suture of scalp laceration, traction splint of extremity, and exposure of patient

Ref.: 1–3

COMMENTS: Upon their arrival in the emergency room, a primary survey is performed on all injured patients to identify and treat life-threatening injuries immediately. • The mnemonic *ABCDE* defines the specific, ordered prioritized initial evaluation. • *A* stands for *airway.* • Because of its urgency, assessment of the airway should be rapid and clinical. • With attention to cervical spine immobilization, the airway should be opened using a jaw thrust maneuver. • Gross trauma to the face or oropharynx may necessitate immediate surgical establishment of an airway. • Without significant facial or airway trauma, a patient should be intubated if airway occlusion, lack of ventilator drive, or mental status prevents protection of the airway.

B stands for *breathing.* After the airway is secured, ventilation and oxygenation must be assessed. • Physical examination should identify conditions such as tension pneumothorax, flail chest, pneumothorax, and massive hemothorax, which are impediments to

proper ventilation and oxygenation. • For a patient with tension pneumothorax, insertion of a 14-gauge catheter into the thorax at the second intercostal space at the midclavicular line can be lifesaving. • Defects in the chest wall greater than two-thirds the diameter of the tracheal lumen require occlusive dressing of the defect and a tube thoracostomy. • For unstable patients, rapid performance of bilateral needle decompression is indicated, based on clinical grounds alone. • Pulse oximetric analysis is used for continuous monitoring of hemoglobin oxygen saturation (SaO_2), and arterial blood samples are sent to the laboratory as soon as possible for measurement of blood gases. • All injured patients are given supplemental oxygen initially. • There should be a low threshold for instituting mechanical ventilation for patients with severely depressed mental status, unstable vital signs, or respiratory distress.

C stands for *circulation.* • Hemorrhagic shock is the commonest preventable cause of death in trauma patients. • The pulse is checked for quality, rate, regularity, and paradox. • A palpable distal pulse indicates a blood pressure of at least 80 mmHg. • Skin color and level of consciousness are indirect indicators of tissue perfusion. • Ashen gray coloring or mottling of the skin and agitation or decreased level of consciousness are indicators of at least a 30% total blood volume loss. • In addition, the systemic blood pressure usually remains normal owing to compensatory mechanisms until about a 30% total blood volume loss. • In younger patients, these compensatory mechanisms may maintain normal vital signs until much later, making a high index of suspicion and diligent resuscitation necessary. • Two large-bore peripheral intravenous catheters are used for initial resuscitation. • These are preferable to long central lines. • Once the initial ABCs have been performed, the primary survey quickly concludes with a rapid inspection for external sites of bleeding. • Direct pressure can control hemorrhage in most circumstances. • However, it rarely works on scalp lesions such as the one described in this patient. • Rapid suturing or stapling of the laceration is usually effective. • Peripheral vascular pulses are assessed and if lessened in a grossly deformed limb, gentle straightening or traction can be performed to attempt to regain a pulse. • Ultimately, unstable fractures of long bones are traduced and splinted.

D stands for *disability.* • A brief neurologic examination assessing pupillary reaction, level of motor and sensory responsiveness, and level of consciousness is performed. • *E* stands for *exposure.* • Complete disrobement of the patient is performed to facilitate thorough examination.

ANSWER:
E

2. A 22-year-old man suffers a gunshot wound to the abdomen, with injuries to the small bowel and stomach, which are repaired. He is discharged from the hospital. Six weeks after his injury, he continues to complain of intermittent left chest discomfort and shortness of breath. A chest x-ray is obtained (see the radiograph below). Diagnosis and treatment of this finding should include which of the following?

   A. Esophagogastroduodenoscopy (EGD)

   B. Computed tomograhic (CT) scan, UGI, and barium enema

   C. Observation until 3–6 months, followed by operative repair

   D. Repair through a thoracotomy

   E. Repair through a laparotomy

Ref.: 1–3

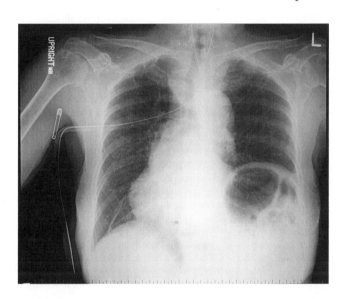

COMMENTS: The x-ray shows a diaphragmatic hernia, probably caused by a small, missed diaphragmatic injury. • All patients with penetrating abdominal injury should be examined for injury to the diaphragm on operative exploration. • Examination of the left diaphragm requires gentle retraction of the spleen downward. • The right diaphragm is approached by dividing the falciform ligament and applying firm downward pressure on the liver. • When an injury is found in the acute setting, it should be repaired if possible. • Small injuries of less than 2 cm can be closed with nonabsorbable suture in an interrupted horizontal mattress fashion. • Larger tears or tears with herniation of abdominal contents should be reduced and repaired using a running locked nonabsorbable suture. • Despite careful examination, patients may experience delayed herniation through diaphragmatic defects. • This situation occurs when an initially missed small injury grows and widens, ultimately causing chest pain and obstructive symptoms. • When delayed herniation is identified, a work-up including a CT scan, an upper gastrointestinal radiography series (UGI), and a barium enema is warranted. • Delayed injuries are more likely to be found on the left diaphragm. • Repair can be performed through a thoracotomy or laparotomy, depending primarily on the surgeon's preference. • A thoracotomy is useful for dissection of the often-dense adhesions found in hernias discovered after considerable delay. • Even so, hernias identified within 6–12 weeks (and sometimes longer) can safely be approached through a laparotomy.

ANSWER:
B, D, E

3. A 32-year-old woman leaps from the tenth floor of her apartment building in an apparent suicide attempt. The patient is brought to the emergency department with obvious head and extremity injuries. The primary survey reveals the patient to be completely apneic. By which method is a definitive airway provided for this patient immediately?

   A. Orotracheal intubation

   B. Nasotracheal intubation

   C. Cricothyroidotomy

   D. Fiberoptic intubation

   E. Needle cricothyroidotomy

Ref.: 1–3

COMMENTS: During the initial assessment of a multiple-trauma patient, establishment of the airway takes precedence over all other interventions. • With a patient who is totally apneic, an appropriate airway must be restored as rapidly as possible. • Orotracheal intubation can be accomplished rapidly and effectively even while the cervical spine is being protected. • Fiberoptic intubation, while appropriate in certain circumstances, cannot be performed quickly enough to be used with a totally apneic trauma patient. • Although it is operator dependent, nasotracheal intubation is more than 90% successful. • Since visualization of the vocal cords with a laryngoscope is unnecessary, there is no manipulation of the neck, making nasotracheal intubation the method of choice for patients with confirmed or suspected cervical spine injury. • To be successful, however, it is necessary that the patient have some spontaneous respirations. • Nasotracheal intubation is also contraindicated for patients with instability of the mid-face or suspected fracture of the cribiform plate. • Needle cricothyroidotomy with jet insufflation is useful for obtaining direct control of the airway in small children. • In adults, however, carbon dioxide retention occurs quickly because of the limited size of the placed "airway." • Cricothyroidotomy is reserved for emergency airway control in a patient with sufficient maxillofacial trauma or when attempts at orotracheal intubation have failed.

ANSWER:
A

4. A 24-year-old obese man is involved in an automobile fire. He shows evidence of inhalation injury, with carbonaceous sputum, an edematous oropharynx, and stridor. After attempted nasotracheal intubation, the patient remains hemodynamically stable, with an oxygen saturation of 97%. Before attempting orotracheal intubation, which of the following maneuvers is/are correct?

   A. Oxygenation via high-flow oxygen face mask

   B. Cricoid pressure

   C. Axial stabilization of the neck

   D. Preparation for possible cricothyroidotomy

   E. All of the above

Ref.: 1–3

COMMENTS: When a patient comes to the emergency room requiring intubation, initial care of the airway must include adequate suction and oxygenation with a face mask at high flow for spontaneously breathing patients or a bag-valve mask for others. • Positive-pressure ventilation should be administered before intubation to bring the SaO_2 near 100%. • It should be assumed that all trauma patients have a full stomach, and therefore cricoid pressure should be applied before and during intubation to compress the esophagus and prevent regurgitation. • It must also be assumed that patients who have sustained blunt trauma have a cervical spine injury. • Even patients with unobserved injuries must be treated as though they have a cervical spine injury until it has been determined that they do not. • Patients may be intubated without the administration of paralyzing agents. • Initial attempts should be made with sedation alone, preserving ventilatory drive if the initial intubation attempts fail. • When a paralyzing agent is needed, it is imperative that a cricothyroidotomy tray is at the bedside as well as a surgeon who is capable of performing the procedure.

A N S W E R :
E

---

5. A 56-year-old man hit by a car has multiple face lacerations, profuse bleeding from the nose and mouth, palpable deformity of the mandible, and left periorbital swelling and ecchymosis with impaired upward gaze. His respiratory rate is 40 breaths per minute. He is stridorous and anxious. Which of the following represents the correct order of initial evaluation and management?

   A. Supplemental oxygen, CT scan of the face and orbits, suturing of facial lacerations, and lateral cervical spine radiograph

   B. Nasotracheal intubation, posterior nasal packing, lateral cervical spine radiograph, and CT scan of the face

   C. Endotracheal intubation, posterior nasal packing, lateral cervical spine radiograph, and CT scan of the face

   D. Posterior nasal packing, endotracheal intubation, lateral cervical spine radiograph, and CT scan of the face

   E. Endotracheal intubation, posterior nasal pacing, lateral cervical spine radiograph, and plain radiograph of the face

Ref.: 1–3

COMMENTS: As for all injured patients, those with facial trauma require a systematic primary survey to secure the airway, breathing, and circulation. • Airway compromise is the foremost life-threatening complication of facial trauma. • Multiple mandibular fractures or combined maxillary, mandibular, and nasal fractures predispose the patient to developing acute airway obstruction due to posterior displacement of the tongue or soft-tissue swelling of the oropharynx. • Clinical signs such as stridor or profuse bleeding, decreased mental status, and low oxygen saturation are signs of impending airway compromise and indicate the need for prompt orotracheal intubation. • Often, with significant maxillofacial trauma, a surgically established airway in the form of a cricothyroidotomy is necessary. • Nasotracheal intubation is contraindicated. • After the airway is secure, life-threatening bleeding is controlled with direct pressure to open wounds. • Posterior packing or Foley balloon tamponade is usually successful in controlling nasopharyngeal bleeding. • All patients with facial trauma must be assumed to have a cervical spine injury. • Lateral cervical spine radiographs are necessary, and flexion-extension views should be obtained for patients with cervical tenderness. • Patients with altered mental status on whom a reliable examination cannot be performed should be kept in a cervical collar until it is determined that their cervical spine has not been injured. • Once airway and hemodynamic stability is obtained, a CT scan with thin (1.5- to 3-mm) sections in both axial and coronal views can best diagnose facial fractures and visualize anatomy. • Plain facial films have little use in this setting.

A N S W E R :
C

---

6. Regarding the patient in Question 4, which of the following is/are true?

   A. Repair of the facial fractures should be performed within 2–3 days, after the edema is decreased.

   B. If a CT scan is performed, Panorex imaging of the mandible is not indicated.

   C. In general, if a patient's mandibular fracture is reduced with a compression plate and screw fixation, the patient can resume eating sooner than if the fracture had been immobilized by intermaxillary fixation (IMF).

   D. Most fractures of the mandibular ramus, coronoid, and condyle are treated by complex internal fixation.

Ref.: 1–3

COMMENTS: Periorbital swelling and ecchymosis should alert the physician to the possibility of orbital fractures. • A thorough evaluation of vision papillary reaction and extraocular movements is crucial if permanent eye damage is to be avoided. • Impaired upward gaze and diplopia on upward gaze signify orbital floor fracture, with herniation of orbital contents into the maxillary sinus and associated inferior rectus entrapment. • This orbital blowout is well demonstrated on coronal views and three-dimensional reconstruction of the CT scan. • This finding mandates emergent surgical liberation of the herniated tissues and restoration of the orbital floor by plating the bone fragments or by autogenous bone grafting. • If entrapment is ruled out clinically and by CT scan, facial bone fractures may be repaired on an elective basis after the patient has been stabilized and life-threatening injuries have been cared for. • With mandibular injury, swelling and tenderness are usually present, but malocclusion is the most sensitive indicator of mandibular fracture. • Panorex provides a complete view of the mandibular body, angle, ramus, and condyles, which are often not well visualized on the CT scan. • The technique of IMF involves application of metal arch bars to the upper and lower dental arches. • Most mandibular fractures are immobilized by IMF for 6–8 weeks. • Frequent complaints by the patient include discomfort and weight loss secondary to inability to eat solid food. • Compression plates are technically unforgiving and more difficult to place, necessitating precise alignment, but they have the advantage of allowing patients to resume eating at a much earlier stage. • Most fractures of the ramus, coronoid, and condyle are treated with IMF alone.

A N S W E R :
C

---

7. A 44-year-old man suffers a gunshot wound to the abdomen. He is hemodynamically stable. Upon exploration, his injuries are found to include two small-bowel injuries 7 cm apart, each with destruction of 70% of the bowel wall, and a through-and-through injury to the ascending colon with destruction of 30% of the bowel wall. How should these injuries be managed?

   A. Resection and anastomosis of the small-bowel injuries and primary repair of the colon injury

   B. Primary repair of both small-bowel injuries and primary repair of the colon injury

   C. Primary repair of the small-bowel injuries, primary repair of the colon injury, and creation of a diverting ileostomy

   D. Resection of the small-bowel injuries and exteriorization of the colon injury as a colostomy

Ref.: 1–3

COMMENTS: The treatment of colon injury has progressed significantly since World War II. • Historically, all colon injuries were treated by diversion. • During World War II, there was even a decree by the surgeon general that no primary repairs were to be performed, no matter the degree of injury. • However, with the progression of surgical technique, resuscitative and critical care, and antibiosis, many colon injuries can be repaired primarily. • Selection of patients for primary repair or resection and primary anastamosis versus diversion depends on the stability of the patient. • Hemodynamically stable patients with injuries that involve destruction of less than 50% of the circumferential bowel wall and no vascular destruction can undergo primary repair. • Patients with destruction of more than 50% or vascular disruption of the circumferential bowel wall can undergo primary resection and anastomosis without diversion if they are hemodymically stable (i.e., with no sustained pre- or intraoperative hypotension and systolic blood pressure >90), have minimal associated injuries injury severity score (ISS) (<25 and Flint grade <11), and have no peritonitis. • Patients with more severe injuries should undergo resection and diversion or have the injury exteriorized as a colostomy. • Such colostomies can be reversed in as little as 2 weeks, provided the patient's condition has stabilized and other injuries do not prevent further surgical intervention. • Small-bowel injuries can be treated with segmental resection or primary repair and rarely, if ever, require exteriorization or diversion.

ANSWER:

A

8. A 47-year-old woman is brought to the trauma unit after a motor vehicle crash. She is alert but confused. Her eyes open on command, and she moves all extremities on command. She complains of headache and neck and left leg pain. Her airway is intact, and her breathing and vital signs are normal. She has a large frontal scalp hematoma. Cervical spine, chest, pelvic, and left femur radiographs are normal. While a cervical spine series is being performed, she is noted to become much more lethargic, moving only to pain. Which of the following pathologic conditions is likely to be present?

A. Subdural hematoma

B. Epidural hematoma

C. Cerebral contusion

D. Diffuse axonal injury

Ref.: 1–3

COMMENTS: Acute epidural hematoma is associated with arterial bleeding from the middle meningeal artery. • Clinically, there is commonly a lucid interval, followed by sudden neurologic deterioration. • Immediate CT scanning of the head is indicated to identify the site of the lesion and assess the degree of mass effect. • Operative evacuation of the hematoma is indicated if significant mass effect is noted, if there is a midline shift of more than 5 mm, or if there is neurologic deterioration. • Subdural hematoma is the commonest traumatic mass lesion of the head, occurring in approximately 20–40% of severe head injuries. • This lesion is usually due to shearing of venous sinuses and occurs between the dura and arachnoid layers. • Operative evacuation is necessary if mass effect is present. • Intracerebral hematomas most commonly occur in the subfrontal and anterior temporal regions of the brain. • They have the potential to cause significant mass effect, requiring evacuation. • Intraoperative sonographic studies are useful for ascertaining the location of clots and ensuring complete removal. • Diffuse axonal injury is generally a diagnosis of exclusion.

• Patients with severe head injury whose CT scan does not reveal significant lesions or those who remain vegetative or severely disabled despite rapid evacuation of mass lesions are given the diagnosis. • Currently, supportive care and optimization of cerebral perfusion pressure are the only treatments, and the prognosis for these patients is grim.

ANSWER:

B

9. A 27-year-old man is brought by ambulance after sustaining a blow to the head. Upon arrival in the emergency room, he is breathing spontaneously, has stable vital signs, opens his eyes only to pain, mumbles his words, and withdraws only to painful stimulus. His pupils are equal, round, and reactive to light. Which of the following is/are indicated in the initial evaluation and stabilization period?

A. CT of the head

B. Endotracheal intubation and hyperventilation

C. Intracranial pressure monitoring

D. Emergency burr hole on the right side

E. A, B, and C

Ref.: 1–3

COMMENTS: Brain injury is the commonest cause of death in trauma victims, accounting for about half of the deaths on the scene. • A neurologic assessment is performed by assessing papillary response and the Glascow Coma Scale (GCS). • The GCS evaluates eye opening, verbal response, and motor response; objectively measures the severity of injury; and guides therapeutic interventions. • A score of 13–15 indicates no to mild head injury. • A score of 9–12 indicates moderate head injury. • These patients require urgent head CT scan and admission to the hospital, with frequent neurologic evaluations. • A score of 8 or less reflects a severe head injury. • Such patients require intubation to stabilize and protect the airway. • Hyperventilation, which causes cerebral vasoconstriction and a reduction in intracranial pressure (ICP) was popular during the 1970s. • However, it may also exacerbate cerebral ischemia, and its effects are transient and difficult to predict. • Thus, it is no longer recommended as a first-line treatment for head-injury patients. • The current recommendation is for the use of mild hyperventilation only when necessary to control the ICP. • It should be discontinued as soon as possible. • CT scanning of the head should be performed as soon as the cardiopulmonary status of the patient has been stabilized. • CT scans can accurately image intracranial hematomas and contusions, subarachnoid and intraventricular hemorrhage, and skull fractures. • If the CT scan identifies a surgically correctable lesion, as discussed in the previous question, it should be treated accordingly. • Nonsurgical management of these patients involves supportive care in the intensive care unit and aggressive maintenance of cerebral perfusion pressure, which is defined as the mean arterial pressure minus the ICP. • Intracranial pressure monitors are routinely inserted in patients with severe head injuries and no surgically correctable lesions. • Ventriculostomy allows drainage of cerebrospinal fluid and cerebral compliance measurements. • It may be performed in the emergency room or the intensive care unit. • The normal ICP is about 10 mmHg, and treatment is warranted when the pressure climbs to or above 20 mmHg. • Initial therapy includes intravenous sedation and possibly paralysis. • When this fails, mild hyperventilation and osmotic diuretics may be used. • The purpose of osmotic diuretics is to dehydrate and shrink the normal brain tissue when the blood-brain barrier is intact, reducing the ICP. • Serum sodium

levels and serum osmolality should be checked regularly.
• Optimal sodium levels are 140–145 mEq/L, and optimal serum
osmolality is 295–310 mOsm/L. • The typical loading dose for
mannitol is 1 g/kg, followed by 0.25 g/kg intravenously every 4 hr.
• Recently, emphasis has been placed on aggressive colloid and
isotonic crystalloid fluid infusion and vasopressor therapy to maintain a cerebral perfusion pressure (CPP) of at least 60–70 mmHg.
• Despite aggressive efforts, the mortality rate for patients with
severe head injuries is 30–50%, and a large proportion of survivors
have significant neurologic deficits. • Burr holes are used only in
exceptional circumstances and should be placed on the side of the
largest pupil in comatose patients with decerebrate or decorticate
posturing whose condition does not respond to medical therapy.

ANSWER:
E

10. Regarding cervical spine injury, which of the following statements is/are true?

A. C1 (atlas) fractures are usually caused by an axial load and
involve a blowout of the ring.

B. Hangman's fractures are unstable and best treated by
operative spinal fusion.

C. Type II odontoid fractures are considered stable.

D. Anterior spinal subluxation with bilateral facet dislocation
is rarely associated with a complete spinal cord injury.

Ref.: 1–3

COMMENTS: Any patient sustaining an injury above the clavicles
produced by a high-speed motor vehicle crash or a head injury resulting in an unconscious state must be suspected of having a cervical
spine injury and must be immobilized with a cervical collar and back-
board until screening radiographic studies are performed and
fractures or dislocations are excluded. • C1 burst fractures (Jefferson
fractures) are caused by axial loading and often result in widening of
the spinal canal. • When isolated, they are considered stable and are
treated with a rigid cervical collar. • Hangman's fractures involve the
posterior elements of C2 and are usually caused by extension and distraction. • These fractures are unstable, and the treatment is traction
for displacement, followed by 3 months of immobilization in a halo.
• Odontoid fractures are divided into three types. • Type I fractures
involve the odontoid above base and are considered stable. • Type II
fractures occur at the base and are usually unstable. • Fractures with
less than 5 mm of displacement can be treated with 3 months of
immobilization in a halo, whereas those with greater displacement
generally require posterior fusion of C1 and C2 or screw fixation of
the anterior odontoid process. • Type III odontoid fractures extend
into the vertebral body and are treated with a rigid collar or a halo.
• Anterior subluxation of the cervical spine can occur with faced
fracture, unilateral or bilateral facet dislocation, or bilateral perched
facets. • Most bilateral facet fractures or perched facets result in
complete cord injury, whereas unilateral dislocations can produce
incomplete injury or no neurologic deficits.

ANSWER:
A

11. A 22-year-old man has a stab wound along the anterior border
of the sternocleidomastoid muscle 1 cm superior to the cricoid
cartilage with penetration of the platysma. There are no other
findings. The vital signs are normal. Which of the following
management choices is/are correct?

A. Admit the patient to the intensive care unit to observe
closely for airway obstruction and expanding hematoma.

B. Perform carotid arteriographic examination. If the findings
are normal, observe the patient.

C. Perform carotid arteriographic examination, a barium swallow, and rigid esophagosopic examination. If the findings
are normal, observe the patient.

D. Formally explore the neck to determine whether the platysma
is penetrated.

E. Perform carotid arteriographic examination, a barium
swallow, and flexible esophagoscopic examination. If the
findings are normal, observe the patient.

Ref.: 1–3

COMMENTS: For purposes of managing penetrating neck trauma,
the neck is divided into three zones (see the figure). • Zone I
extends from the clavicle to the cricoid cartilage, zone II from the
cricoid cartilage to the angle of the mandible, and zone III from the
angle of the mandible to the base of the skull. • Zone II neck
injuries may involve major vascular laryngotracheal or pharyngoesophageal structures. • A careful history and physical examination
are essential, even though the findings on physical examination
may be be normal in as many as 30% of patients with such injuries.
• Management of unstable or symptomatic patients with penetrating zone II neck injuries should include securing the airway, avoiding nasogastric intubation, and mandatory operative exploration.
• Other absolute indications for formal exploration of anterior
neck injuries include persistent hemorrhage, pulsatile or expanding
hematoma, coma, and stroke. • Also included are respiratory indications such as crepitation, dysphonia, palpable laryngeal injury,
stridor, hemoptysis, and tracheal tenderness. • Digestive indications are dysphagia, hematemesis, crepitation, and odnophagia.
• Management of asymptomatic zone II injuries includes a thorough
diagnostic work-up, including arteriographic, esophagographic,
rigid esophagoscopic, and possibly broncoscopic examination.
• Exploration is recommended if the platysma is penetrated.
• Four-vessel arteriographic study is the gold standard for assessing
carotid and vertebral arteries in the neck. • If an injury is identified,
cerebral blood flow should also be assessed to ensure perfusion
from the contralateral side in case arterial ligation is necessary.
• Injury to the larynx and/or trachea is usually manifested with
physical findings. • If respiratory tract injuries remain in question,
laryngoscopic and broncoscopic studies can be performed. • CT
scanning is also excellent for diagnosing laryngeal injury. • The
most difficult diagnosis to establish is that of esophageal injury.

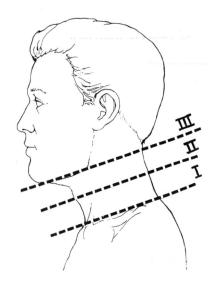

• In one study, investigators estimated the sensitivity of physical examination, esophagram, and esophagogastroduodenoscopy (EGD) to be 80, 89, and 89%, respectively. • However, the combination of esophagoscopic and rigid esophagoscopic examination identified all esophageal injuries. • Thus, a complete work-up of esophageal injury involves performance of both a barium swallow and a rigid esophagoscopic examination. • Since flexible esophagoscopic studies are associated with a false-negative rate of more than 50%, they should not be included as part of the evaluation.

ANSWER:
C, D

12. A 27-year-old woman is brought to the emergency room awake and alert after sustaining a gunshot wound to the neck. The wound is anterior to the origin of the sternocleidomastoid muscle at the angle of the mandible. The patient is asymptomatic. Which of the following management choices is/are correct?

   A. Cervical spine radiographic studies

   B. Mandatory neck exploration

   C. Four-vessel angiographic studies

   D. Rigid esophagoscopic examination

   E. Contrast esophagographic examination

Ref.: 1–3

COMMENTS: See Question 13.

13. Soon after the patient in Question 12 arrives in the emergency room, left hemiparesis and aphasia develop. At this time, which of the following treatments should be provided?

   A. Continued observation and implementation of selective management protocol

   B. Repair of carotid artery injury

   C. Ligation of injured carotid artery

   D. Repair of vertebral artery injury

Ref.: 1–3

COMMENTS: The management of patients with penetrating trauma to the neck requires the skills of a surgeon capable of performing vascular, general surgical, and otolaryngolic procedures. • The management of carotid artery injuries is somewhat controversial. • Physical examination alone cannot be relied on to diagnose carotid artery injuries. • For patients with no neurologic deficit preoperatively, every effort should be made to repair carotid artery injury. • Repair may include the use of a temporary shunt and vein grafting. • Patients with mild neurologic deficit, as defined by paresis of an extremity, should undergo repair of the carotid artery. • Carotid artery ligation may also be employed for patients who are unstable or in whom heparinization is impossible. • It has been shown that a neurologic deficit develops in only 20% of adults as a result of carotid artery ligation. • Injuries to the internal jugular vein should be repaired if the patient's condition allows and the injuries are amenable to repair. • The internal jugular vein can be ligated unilaterally without adverse consequences, and this treatment is advised for unstable patients. • Esophageal and hypopharyngeal injuries should be débrided and repaired primarily if possible. • If the damage is extensive or the injury has been present for more than 12 hr, it may be advisable to perform cutaneous esophagostomy for purposes of feeding and drainage, with a planned second-stage

procedure once sepsis subsides. • All esophageal repairs must be adequately drained externally because anastomotic leakage occurs in as many as 20% of patients. • Simple laryngeal or tracheal injuries can be repaired with mucosa-to-mucosa apposition. • Vertebral artery injuries may lead to fatal hemorrhage but almost never cause neurologic sequelae. • Angiographic studies can accurately locate the site of injury. • If there is a patent vertebral artery on the contralateral side, proximal and distal embolization may be performed safely and effectively by invasive radiologic technique. • If this procedure is unsuccessful or unavailable, surgical exploration is performed, and the proximal portion is exposed at the C1–2 interspace and ligated.

ANSWERS:
Question 12: A, C, D, E
Question 13: B

14. Regarding neck injuries, which of the following statements is/are true?

   A. The internal jugular vein may be ligated unilaterally without unfavorable sequelae.

   B. Unilateral ligation of the common carotid artery results in a neurologic deficiency in 80% of cases.

   C. Esophageal injuries should be drained externally only when extensive devitalization is present.

   D. Tracheostomy is indicated when dealing with most laryngeal or tracheal injuries.

   E. Injuries to the thyroid gland must be drained externally.

Ref.: 1–3

COMMENTS: The management of patients with penetrating trauma to the neck requires the skills of a surgeon capable of performing vascular, general surgical, and otolaryngolic procedures. • The management of carotid artery injuries is somewhat controversial. • Physical examination alone cannot be relied on to diagnose carotid artery injuries. • In patients with no neurologic deficit preoperatively, every effort should be made to repair a carotid artery injury. • Repair may include the use of a temporary shunt and vein grafting. • Patients with mild neurologic deficit, as defined by paresis of an extremity, also should undergo repair of the carotid artery. • Carotid artery ligation may also be employed for patients who are unstable or in whom the repair is technically impossible. • It has been shown that a neurologic deficit develops in only 20% of adults as a result of carotid artery ligation. • Injuries to the internal jugular vein should be repaired if the patient's condition allows and the injuries are amenable to repair. • The internal jugular vein can be ligated unilaterally without adverse consequences, and this treatment is advised for unstable patients. • Esophageal and hypopharyngeal injuries should be débrided and repaired primarily if possible. • If the damage is extensive or the injury has been present for more than 12 hr, it may be advisable to perform cutaneous esophagostomy for purposes of feeding and drainage, with a planned second-stage procedure once sepsis subsides. • All esophageal repairs must be adequately drained externally because anastomotic leakage occurs in as many as 20% of patients. • Simple laryngeal or tracheal injuries can be repaired with mucosa-to-mucosa apposition. • Cartilage fragments should be sutured in place to provide support for the airway. • If cartilage is lost or shattered, a flap created from strap muscles can be used to provide airway support. • A tracheostomy is performed for most patients with such injuries to allow edema to subside and to assess for stricture formation. • Thyroid gland injuries can be managed by débridement, hemostasis, and adequate external drainage with excellent results.

ANSWER:
A, D, E

15. A 30-year-old man suffers a stab wound to the right mid-infraclavicular region. He had a weak pulse in the ambulance 10 minutes ago and now arrives in the emergency department with no palpable pulse or obtainable blood pressure. His pupils are reactive. The initial surgical approach involves which of the following?

A. Median sternotomy

B. Right-sided cervical incision

C. Right-sided clavicular incision

D. Right-sided anterolateral thoracotomy

E. Left-sided anterolateral thoracotomy

Ref.: 1–3

COMMENTS: Approximately 5% of patients admitted to level I trauma units are either in extremis or without signs of life. • Patients in extremis are in profound shock with respiratory depression and mental obtundation. • Emergency department thoracotomy is not indicated for patients in arrest after blunt trauma, owing to extremely low success rates. • However, it may be lifesaving in patients in extremis or arrest after penetrating trauma. • Clear indications include (1) severe post-injury hypotension with suspicion of cardiac tamponade or thoracic hemorrhage, (2) cardiac arrest with signs of life, and (3) recent arrest after penetrating trauma (within 20 min), followed by performance of cardiopulmonary resuscitation. • Relative indications include severe hypotension or arrest secondary to intra-abdominal vascular injury or pelvic bleeding. • The first procedure to be performed is a left anterolateral thoracotomy. • This is true even if the site of bleeding is in the right chest or abdomen. • Once the chest is entered, the aorta is cross-clamped to preferentially perfuse the heart, lungs, and brain. • Next, the pericardium is opened to release potential tamponade, and open cardiac massage is instituted. • Internal defibrillation may be necessary. • The left-sided thoracotomy can then be carried across the sternum to the right side to gain control of the suspected injury. • Combined salvage rates from several series are 37% if the patient had vital signs upon admission, 6.5% if the patient had signs of life, and 3% if the patient had neither. • It should be noted that protocols vary widely, and the performance of emergency department thoracotomy remains controversial.

ANSWER:
E

16. Assume that the patient in Question 15 is hemodynamically stable but that no pulse can be found in the right upper extremity. Angiography shows a mid-clavicular right subclavian thrombosis. The initial surgical approach involves which of the following?

A. Median sternotomy

B. Right-sided clavicular incision

C. Right-sided cervical lesion

D. Right-sided anterolateral thoracotomy

E. Left-sided anterolateral thoracotomy

Ref.: 1–3

COMMENTS: If a patient is hemodynamically stable and is suspected of having a great-vessel injury, an angiogram should be obtained. • The choice of incision is based on the site of injury. • The patient in Question 15 has suffered a subclavian thrombosis on the right side. • The optimal approach is a right-sided clavicular incision with subperiosteal resection of the medial half of the clavicle. • Extension to a median sternotomy may be necessary to expose the innominate artery. • The right common carotid artery can be entirely exposed through a right cervical incision. • The distal left common carotid artery can be exposed through a left cervical incision. • Proximal exposure requires extension to a median sternotomy. • The distal left common carotid artery can be exposed through a left cervical incision, but the proximal artery requires extension to a median sternotomy. • The distal left subclavian artery can be approached via a horizontal clavicular incision. • Proximal control requires a left anterolateral thoracotomy, or trapdoor incision, to expose the proximal left carotid artery and left innominate vein. • Trapdoor incisions are formed by combining the horizontal clavicular median sternotomy and anterolateral thoracotomy incisions. • In unstable patients with suspected mediastinal injury, median sternotomy is the incision for best exposure. • If subclavian artery injuries are suspected and there is active hemorrhage, control is most easily obtained via anterolateral thoracotomy on the side of injury.

ANSWER:
B

17. A 47-year-old man who has been involved in a high-speed, head-on motor vehicle crash arrives at the emergency department. His vital signs are stable, and he has multiple rib fractures and a femur fracture. A portable frontal radiograph of the chest has been obtained (see the figure). Which of the following is/are more appropriate for further evaluation?

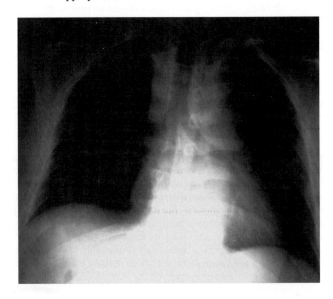

A. Admission for observation and a second chest radiograph for 6–8 hr

B. Immediate aortography

C. CT scan of the chest with contrast infusion

D. Immediate left anterolateral thoracotomy

E. B and C

Ref.: 1–3

COMMENTS: Ninety percent of aortic transections are fatal at the accident scene. • Most of the patients who survive and arrive at the hospital with vital signs have few or no signs or symptoms indicating the presence of aortic transection. • Thus, a high index of suspicion is necessary. • The mechanism of injury is a sudden deceleration that leads to the development of shear forces between the mobile aortic arch and the fixed descending aorta. • These shear forces lead to intimal disruption at the ligamentum arteriosum distal to the left subclavian artery, which is the first point of fixation. • Any patient who has sustained a significant deceleration injury, such as in an automobile crash at more than 30 mph or a fall of more than 30 feet, should be considered at risk for an aortic transection. • Physical findings of chest injury or tenderness should heighten the suspicion. • The most reliable finding on a chest radiograph indicating a potential aortic transection is widening of the superior mediastinum by more than 8 cm. • Other radiographic findings, in approximate decreasing order of frequency, include indistinct or obscured aortic arch, rightward nasogastric tube and tracheal deviation, depressed left main-stem bronchus, apical pleural cap, abnormal aortic contour, left hemothorax, and wide left and right paraspinal line. • Because only 20% of patients with positive findings on chest radiograph have an aortic injury, further diagnostic testing is required to establish a diagnosis. • Helical CT scanning with intravenous contrast media has been found to have a sensitivity and specificity of 100 and 90%, respectively, for mediastinal hematoma and 87 and 99%, respectively, for aortic injury. • However, arch aortography remains the most reliable test for locating and diagnosing aortic injury and should be performed liberally based on clinical suspicion. • Either a routine aortography or a screening CT scan, followed by aortography if the findings on CT scan are positive, should be performed. • Emergent operation is indicated to repair this injury because more than half the patients suffer rupture of the contained injury and die within the first 24 hr after the accident if it is not repaired. • Operative treatment of thoracic aortic injury entails approximately a 15% mortality rate and an 8% incidence of paraplegia. • Thoracotomy without diagnostic tests is not warranted in this situation.

ANSWER:
E

18. A 44-year-old man suffers a gunshot wound to the left thigh, which results in an arterial injury to the superficial femoral artery. His injury is repaired within 4 hr of the injury with a saphenous vein interposition graft. At the end of the operation, he had good distal pulses and was neurologically intact. Five hours later, he experiences increasing leg pain distant from the site of injury, pain with passive flexion and extension of the calf muscles, numbness in the left foot, and palpable but diminished pulses distal to the repair. What is the next step in the care of this patient?

   A. Return to the operating room for a revision of the repair

   B. Angiogram

   C. Heparin bolus and drip to maintain a partial thromboplastin time of approximately 55

   D. Four-compartment fasciotomy

   E. Below-the-knee amputation

Ref.: 1–3

COMMENTS: Even though this patient was diagnosed and treated within 4 hr of the injury, there were still substantial ischemia and soft-tissue injury to the leg. • Compartment syndrome results from swelling caused by ischemic reperfusion injury in the nonexpansible fascial compartments of the leg. • The symptoms include (in order of presentation) pain out of proportion or distant from the injury, severe pain on passive flexion and extension of the calf muscles, paresthesias in the affected leg, and diminished or absent distal pulses. • Normal compartment pressures range from 5–20 mmHg. • Elevated pressures, which can be measured by a transducer attached to a needle, are defined as 30 mmHg or above. • Treatment of compartment syndrome is immediate four-compartment fasciotomy, which can be performed through two incisions. • Fasciotomy should be performed at the time of vascular or orthopedic repair or for any patient who manifests any of the above-mentioned signs or who has elevated compartment pressures.

ANSWER:
D

19. A 22-year-old woman presents with a single stab wound to the left fifth intercostal space in the midclavicular line. She is anxious, has a blood pressure of 70/40, a pulse of 130 beats per minute, and a respiratory rate of 34 breaths per minute. There is no jugular venous distention, the trachea is in the midline, and there are muffled heart tones and decreased breath sounds on the left. Which of the following is/are possible diagnoses?

   A. Pericardial tamponade

   B. Massive left hemothorax

   C. Tension pneumothorax

   D. Flail chest

   E. A, B, and C

Ref.: 1–3

COMMENTS: See Question 20.

20. Regarding the patient in Question 19, which of the following initial management choices is correct?

   A. Pericardiocentesis, subxiphoid pericardial window, and needle decompression of the left and right chest and bilateral chest tubes

   B. Pericardiocentesis, subxiphoid pericardial window, and needle decompression of the right chest and left chest tube

   C. Pericardiocentesis, subxiphoid pericardial window if pericardiocentesis results are positive, and needle decompression of the left chest and left chest tube

   D. Transthoracic echocardiogram, chest x-ray, and left chest tube

   E. Emergency department thoracotomy

Ref.: 1–3

COMMENTS: All of the possible thoracic injuries listed following Question 19 are life-threatening and must be identified and treated during the primary survey of the trauma victim. • The triad of systemic hypotension, distended neck veins, and muffled heart tones is known as Beck's triad and is useful for diagnosing **pericardial tamponade**. • However, these findings often are not evident, even in the presence of severe, acute tamponade, particularly if the patient is hypovolemic. • Other signs of pericardial tamponade include pulsus paradoxus and the "water bottle" sign on the chest radiograph. • If the diagnosis of pericardial tamponade is suspected, diagnostic maneuvers should be selected on the basis of test availability and stability of the patient. • Transthoracic echocardiographic study is an excellent diagnostic test but is often unavailable and should be avoided in a hypotensive, shocky patient such as the one described in Question 19. • For patients with hypotension unresponsive to fluid resuscitation, pericardiocentesis is the procedure of choice, since it can be both diagnostic and temporarily therapeutic. • Aspiration of as little as 20–30 ml of blood may decrease intrapericardial pressure to allow more adequate ventricular filling. • A subxiphoid pericardial window can then be established under local anesthesia in the emergency department. • For patients in extremis, emergency department thoracotomy and pericardotomy may be lifesaving. • Once pericardial tamponade has been diagnosed and relieved, the patient should receive vigorous fluid resuscitation and expedient operative intervention.

A **massive hemothorax** is defined as more than 1500 ml of blood within the pleural space. • Massive hemothorax, which may cause hypotension and decreased breath sounds over the affected side, requires a chest radiograph and prompt tube thoracostomy. • **Tension pneumothorax** may mimic pericardial tamponade because both conditions inhibit filling of the right ventricle. • Pericardial tamponade inhibits filling by elevating intrapericardial pressure, whereas tension pneumothorax causes shifting of the mediastinum and obstruction of venous return. • Before placement of a left tube thoracostomy, placement of a 14-gauge needle in the second intercostal space at the midclavicular line will temporarily relieve the tension. • Patients with **open pneumothorax** are in respiratory distress secondary to total collapse of the affected lung and have an obvious "sucking" chest wound, which is not present in this patient. • Likewise, patients with **flail chest** present with paradoxical motion of the chest wall and respiratory failure. • Systemic hypotension is not usually associated with isolated flail chest. • Endotracheal intubation and mechanical ventilation are the initial measures taken to circumvent this life-threatening condition.

ANSWER:
Question 19: E
Question 20: C

21. Which of the following modalities is the most important for identifying a patient who will suffer complications from myocardial contusion?

A. Serial creatine phosphokinase (CPK) isoenzyme determinations

B. Electrocardiographic (ECG) studies

C. Echocardiographic studies

D. Gated ventricular angiographic studies

E. Spiral chest CT scanning

Ref.: 1–3

COMMENTS: The reported incidence of myocardial contusion ranges from 1 to 76%. • This wide range indicates the lack of a widely acceptable definition for myocardial contusion and the lack of a reliable standard for its diagnosis. • Myocardial contusion results from extravasation of blood and fluid into the myocardium, which causes reduced local coronary microcirculation. • Diminished perfusion in these areas may lead to tissue necrosis and infarction, even though no abnormalities of coronary artery flow exist. • Hypotension or hypovolemic shock may further compromise coronary perfusion. • Classic symptoms of significant myocardial contusion are limited to angina-like pain. • The commonest cause of early death after myocardial contusion is arrhythmia, usually ventricular tachycardia or ventricular fibrillation. • Serious arrhythmias can be produced by conduction abnormalities, including premature ventricular contractions, bundle-branch block, supraventricular

tachycardia, junctional rhythm, and heart block. • The first 24 hr after injury is the time period when patients are at greatest risk for the occurrence of these arrhythmias. • CPK isoenzyme level determinations have been advocated as useful in the diagnosis of myocardial contusion. • However, there is a poor correlation between elevated CPK levels and conduction abnormalities. • Echocardiographic study has never been shown to be superior to ECG as a predictor of arrhythmia. • Gated ventricular angiographic study is a nuclear medicine study that calculates right- and left-ventricular ejection fraction and quantification of ventricular function. • A number of investigations have shown that most "clinically significant" cardiac contusion injuries are revealed via ECG changes obtained in the emergency setting.

ANSWER:
B

22. A 52-year-old bank manager is an unrestrained driver involved in a high-speed motor vehicle crash against a bridge abutment. The paramedics report a bent steering wheel. Upon arrival in the emergency department, the patient has multiple fractures on both sides of the chest. The patient is profoundly tachypneic and confused, and pulse oximetric analysis reveals marked hypoxia. Paradoxical motion of the central portion of his chest is noted. Which of the following initial management choices is correct?

A. Stabilization of the flail segment by supporting it with sandbags

B. Stabilization of the flail segment by taping or strapping

C. Operative stabilization of the flail segment

D. Intubation and pressure-controlled ventilation

E. Intubation and volume-controlled ventilation

Ref.: 1–3

COMMENTS: In patients with flail chest, the bony and cartilaginous continuity of the thoracic cavity has been disrupted. • This loose segment creates a paradoxical motion as the patient attempts to breathe. • The most significant injury in these patients is not the flail itself but rather the underlying pulmonary contusion. • Therefore, treatment of patients with flail chest should be directed toward the underlying pulmonary contusion. • In patients who are unable to maintain satisfactory ventilation or those who have significant hypoxia, intubation and mechanical ventilation constitute the appropriate treatment. • Because of the presence of pulmonary contusion and associated decreased lung compliance, pressure-controlled ventilation may not deliver sufficient tidal volume. • However, volume-controlled ventilation ensures that adequate tidal volumes are delivered to the patient. • Vigorous respiratory therapy and pain control can obviate the need for routine intubation. • Thoracic epidural anesthesia and intercostal nerve blockade are useful adjuncts. • Few patients have a localized fracture amenable to direct operative stabilization.

ANSWER:
E

23. Regarding open pneumothorax wounds, which of the following statements is/are true?

A. If the chest wall opening is one-third the diameter of the trachea, inspired air passes preferentially through the chest wall defect into the pleural cavity.

B. A flutter-valve type of dressing may be used temporarily if formal surgical closure cannot be immediately performed.

C. Tube thoracostomy is not indicated for such an injury because the pleural cavity already freely communicates with the atmosphere.

D. Ventilation by the contralateral lung is unaffected by this injury because the two sides are separated by the mediastinum.

Ref.: 1–3

COMMENTS: An open pneumothorax, or "sucking" chest wound, occurs when major chest trauma produces a defect in the chest wall through the parietal pleura. • If the defect is more than two thirds of the diameter of the trachea, air passes preferentially through the chest wall with each respiratory effort, resulting in effective ventilation and hypoxia. • The initial management includes covering the defect with an occlusive dressing tape on three sides to allow a flutter-valve effect. • This type of dressing acts as a barrier to entry of air into the pleural cavity during inspiration but allows air to escape on expiration. • If the air does not escape freely, it may turn an open pneumothorax into a tension pneumothorax. • Thus, tube thoracostomy at a separate site from the open wound is mandatory. • Most of these wounds then require operative closure of the chest wall defect. • Intermittent shifts of the mediastinum during respiration can cause ineffective ventilation in the contralateral lung, impaired venous return because of bending of the vena cava, and cardiac arrhythmias.

ANSWER:
B

24. A 24-year-old man is an unrestrained driver in a motor vehicle crash. The patient remains hypoxic despite administration of oxygen. He has bilateral chest tenderness. A chest x-ray shows bilateral infiltrates. Which of the following is the most likely diagnosis?

A. Bilateral pneumonia

B. Adult respiratory distress syndrome (ARDS)

C. Aspiration pneumonia

D. Atelectasis

E. Pulmonary contusion

Ref.: 1–3

COMMENTS: Pulmonary contusion results from direct damage to the lung parenchyma from external trauma and can be caused by penetrating wounds, blunt trauma to the chest wall, or blast injury. • Pulmonary contusion appears on the chest x-ray as an infiltrate and represents diffuse parenchymal hemorrhage in the involved lobe or segment of lung. • As a rule, the infiltrate of pulmonary contusion is apparent on the initial chest film. • The other causes of lung infiltrate do not appear so quickly. • Subsequent appearance of infiltrate should suggest a diagnosis of aspiration atelectasis or pneumonia. • The hemorrhage of pulmonary contusion can continue for several hours after the injury, with progression of the infiltrate on the radiograph. • Hemoptysis is a common but not constant finding with contusion. • When pulmonary contusion is caused by penetrating injury, the pulmonary infiltrate surrounds the site of lung perforation and spreads circumferentially around the injury site. • If a major vasculature structure is injured near the hilum, massive hemorrhage into the lung and the bronchial tree may occur, resulting in substantial hemoptysis. • Most pulmonary

contusions are benign because pulmonary blood flow is under low pressure in the right side of the heart circuit, and bleeding generally stops by itself, with flow diverted to normal lung channels. • Blunt thoracic trauma is often associated with serious lacerations of the lung parenchyma secondary to direct injury to the chest wall, fracture of ribs, and tearing of the visceral pleura when the lung is compressed against a closed larynx, as in popping a balloon. • Manifestations of these injuries are pneumothorax, hemothorax, or hemopneumothorax. • Aspiration of gastric contents usually does not produce immediate radiographic changes and is manifested by abundant tracheobronchial secretions or bile in the tracheobronchial tree. • ARDS and atelectasis are not apparent on initial x-ray films.

ANSWER:
E

25. A 40-year-old man is brought to the emergency department with a single stab wound to the left chest in the seventh intercostal space in the anterior axillary line. His vital signs are normal, and he has bilateral normal breath sounds. On abdominal examination, no tenderness or mass is noted. An upright chest x-ray film shows no sign of hemothorax or pneumothorax. Regarding this patient's further management, which of the following statements is/are true?

A. The absence of a hemothorax or a pneumothorax indicates that the pleural cavity was not entered during the injury.

B. The absence of a hemothorax or a pneumothorax effectively rules out significant intra-abdominal injury.

C. If this patient is to have general anesthesia, he must first undergo a left-sided tube thoracostomy.

D. Further evaluation must be carried out for a possible intra-abdominal injury.

Ref.: 1–3

COMMENTS: Patients with penetrating trauma can have violation of the pleural cavity without the development of a hemothorax or pneumothorax. • A hemothorax or pneumothorax may develop later as a compilation of a penetrating injury of the chest, especially if the patient is given positive-pressure ventilation during general anesthesia. • It is therefore advisable to perform prophylactic left-sided tube thoracostomy in this patient before positive-pressure ventilation is initiated. • For asymptomatic patients with a stab wound to the chest and normal findings on initial chest x-ray films, an additional upright film should be obtained 6 hr after the first to rule out delayed hemothorax or pneumothorax. • If findings on the additional film are normal, it can safely be concluded that no injury has occurred, and the patient may be discharged. • On moderate expiration, the diaphragm rises to the level of the fifth intercostal space on the left and the fifth rib on the right. • As a consequence, injury to intra-abdominal organs or the diaphragm alone can occur with any penetrating injury of the lower chest. • In a wound medial to the midaxilary line and below the level of the nipples, a diagnostic peritoneal lavage should be performed to rule out penetration of the diaphragm. • A count of 10,000 red blood cells per high-power field has a high sensitivity for diaphragmatic injury. • If there is any evidence of diaphragmatic injury, the injury should be repaired either through a thoracotomy if there are other associated injuries in the chest or through a laparotomy if only diaphragmatic injury is suspected.

ANSWER:
C, D

26. A 28-year-old woman is an unrestrained driver in a motor vehicle crash. She has stable vital signs and left upper quadrant tenderness but no signs of peritonitis. What is the next step in management?

A. Exploratory laparotomy

B. Diagnostic peritoneal lavage

C. Admission for observation

D. CT scan of the abdomen and pelvis

E. Abdominal sonographic studies

Ref.: 1–3

COMMENTS: For evaluation of blunt abdominal trauma, the physical examination is neither sensitive nor specific for injury. • However, signs of peritonitis are an absolute indication for exploratory laparotomy. • Further testing to rule out intra-abdominal injury should be performed on all patients with abdominal pain or tenderness, an altered level of consciousness (GCS <14), spinal cord injury, or unexplained hypotension. • Intra-abdominal injury should also be excluded in all patients undergoing general anesthesia for surgery of extra-abdominal injuries within the observation period. • The diagnostic modalities available to the physician include diagnostic peritoneal lavage (DPL), CT scanning, and abdominal sonographic study focused assessment with sonography in trauma (FAST). • DPL was introduced in 1965 and has been the standard for evaluating blunt abdominal trauma. • It has an accuracy rate as high as 98% and a complication rate of less than 1%. • The pitfalls of DPL are lack of specificity, leading to a high rate of nontherapeutic laparotomy, and an inability to evaluate the retroperitoneum. • For these reasons, CT scanning with intravenous and oral and rectal contrast has become the diagnostic test of choice to evaluate stable patients after blunt abdominal trauma. • It can identify specific solid-organ injuries, thereby allowing nonoperative management. • It provides excellent assessment of renal perfusion and the retroperitoneum and pelvis. • Pitfalls of CT include the difficulty of diagnosing hollow viscus injury and duodenal injury. • In unstable patients, the danger of transportation and the time required to perform the scan preclude its use. • FAST sonographic studies allow quick visualization and triage of the unstable patient in the emergency department. • Sensitivity is reported to be as high as 96% and specificity as high as 97% for detecting intra-abdominal fluid and pericardial effusion. • FAST remains a poor study for diagnosing hollow viscus injury.

ANSWER:
D

27. A 37-year-old patient undergoes a trauma laparotomy and splenectomy after being involved in a high-speed automobile crash. Along with his abdominal injury, he suffers from a moderate closed head injury requiring prolonged intubation. Regarding postoperative nutrition, which of the following statements is/are correct?

A. Because of the likelihood of postoperative ileus, he should receive total parenteral nutrition (TPN) for 7 days before enteral feeding is attempted.

B. Because of his closed head injury, he should receive TPN for 7 days before enteral feeding is attempted.

C. He should receive early enteral feeding through a jejunostomy tube placed at the time of his laparotomy.

D. He should receive early enteral feeding into the stomach via a nasogastric tube or duodenum via a Dobhoff tube.

E. No attempt at nutritional support should be attempted until the patient is extubated.

Ref.: 1–3

COMMENTS: Over the past 20 years, significant advances have been made in the nutritional support of severely injured patients. • A severely injured patient such as the one described becomes profoundly hypermetabolic and catabolic. • This catabolism causes mobilization of amino acids from lean body protein, which can be attenuated by early feeding. • Scientific evidence for early feeding exists to show that patients whose caloric requirements are matched by day 7 have fewer septic complications, less loss of lean body mass, and lower ultimate mortality rates. • Enteral feeding is superior, since it prevents gastrointestinal mucosal atrophy, decreases bowel wall permeability and subsequent bacterial translocation, and decreases the likelihood of peritoneal sepsis and abscess formation. • TPN also improves the patient's outcome but does not provide these benefits. • Contrary to previous belief, abdominal surgery and closed head injury are not contraindications to early enteral feeding. • Furthermore, studies have shown that these patients tolerate pre- and post-pyloric feeding equally. • Early gastric feeding should be instituted with awareness that early gastroparesis or ileus may cause feeding to be intermittently stopped and adjusted while approaching caloric goals. • Only patients who cannot achieve their nutritional goal by day 7 should be given supplemental TPN. • Surgical placement of feeding access should not be attempted in acutely injured patients but may be considered later if a patient requires long-term tube feeding.

ANSWER:
D

28. A 25-year-old woman is the driver of an automobile involved in a high-speed motor vehicle accident. She is 30 weeks pregnant. She complains of abdominal pain but does not have peritoneal signs. Her vital signs are stable. Which of the following should be included in the work-up of this patient?

A. CT scanning

B. Sonographic studies

C. Arteriography

D. Diagnostic peritoneal lavage

E. B and D

Ref.: 1–3

COMMENTS: Trauma is the leading cause of death in women of childbearing age. • The commonest cause of fetal death in such situations is maternal death. • For this reason, all initial resuscitative efforts are directed toward the mother. • The approach to an injured pregnant patient is the same as to a nonpregnant one. • Knowledge of the physiologic processes throughout the progression of pregnancy is needed to best understand a pregnant patient's response to trauma. • During the second trimester, the mother's cardiac output reaches 7 L/min and remains at this level for the term of pregnancy. • Blood volume may increase by as much as 50%, a normal hematocrit being 32–36%. • Because of the elevated blood volume, pregnant patients can have a 30–35% blood volume loss without clinical signs of hypovolemia. • During pregnancy, systolic and diastolic blood pressures are 5–15 mmHg lower than normal because of the drop in systemic vascular resistance normally found in pregnancy. • If blood pressure is elevated, eclampsia and pre-eclampsia must be considered. • Diagnostic procedures for the seriously injured pregnant patient must be performed aggressively because cardiovascular resuscitation and stability are essential for fetal survival. • The fetus should also be assessed by physical examination as well as by continuous fetal monitoring. • Sonographic study is a valuable adjunct for assessing not only the fetus and uterine contents but also the interperitoneal contents. • Peritoneal lavage should be performed using the open technique, cephalad to the uterine fundus. • Indications for laparotomy are similar for pregnant and nonpregnant patients. • CT scanning is generally not indicated for the work-up of pregnant trauma patients because it entails increased radiation exposure. • Nevertheless, if a CT scan is warranted, it can and should be performed. • Arteriography exposes the patient to even higher doses of radiation and is indicated only when hemodynamic instability secondary to pelvic fracture warrants its use.

ANSWER:
E

29. Regarding the diagnosis and treatment of injuries in a pregnant patient, which of the following statements is/are true?

   A. As pregnancy progresses, the blood volume decreases and the blood pressure, hematocrit, and calculated bicarbonate concentration increase.

   B. Pregnant patients are at high risk for the development of disseminated intravascular coagulation (DIC).

   C. Amniotic fluid analysis is an unreliable test for determining the viability of the fetus.

   D. A pregnant patient should be positioned on her right side when being transported and evaluated.

   E. Patients who require celiotomy for intra-abdominal injuries should undergo cesarean section even if the uterus is uninjured.

Ref.: 1–3

COMMENTS: Pregnancy causes physiologic and structural changes sufficient to alter the signs and symptoms of injury as well as the results of diagnostic laboratory tests. • The blood volume increases by 50%. The blood pressure, hematocrit, and bicarbonate concentration decrease; the pulse and plasma volume increase. • Pregnant patients are at higher risk for DIC because of premature separation of the placenta or amniotic fluid embolism, which necessitates termination of the pregnancy. • Because pressure on the vena cava by the pregnant uterus reduces venous return to the heart, it is best if these patients are kept on the left side if possible. • If the patient needs to be supine, the right hip should be elevated and the uterus manually displaced to the left side. • Aspiration of amniotic fluid enables determination of the lecithin/sphingomyelin ratio (2:1) and detection of the ephosphatidylglycerol level, both of which indicate fetal pulmonary maturity. • In most cases of direct uterine trauma, a cesarean section is required. • Other indications include worsening fetal distress, DIC, inability to deliver vaginally, and the need to decompress the uterus to address major abdominal vessel injuries. • In general, the noninjured uterus should be left intact during celiotomy for other conditions. • The mother can usually deliver vaginally even if she has pelvic fractures.

ANSWER:
B

30. A 30-year-old man is ejected from his automobile after a head-on collision at high speed. He has sustained a pelvic fracture and undergoes exploratory laparotomy because of grossly

positive findings on supraumbilical open peritoneal lavage. On exploration, a contained pelvic hematoma and an expanding central abdominal hematoma are noted. Which of the following is/are included in the appropriate management of this patient?

   A. Observation of both hematomas

   B. Exploration of both hematomas to clarify the underlying pathologic condition

   C. Exploration of the central hematoma after obtaining proximal and distal vascular control, and observation of the pelvic hematoma

   D. Observation of the central hematoma and exploration of the pelvic hematoma after application of external fixators

Ref.: 1–3

COMMENTS: The hallmark of retroperitoneal injury is the retroperitoneal hematoma, which may be visualized on CT scan or encountered on surgical exploration. • Retroperitoneal hematomas are classified into three zones, depending on their location. • Zone I is defined as the central medial portion of the retroperitoneum and includes the duodenum, pancreas, and major abdominal vascular structures. • In general, all zone I hematomas require exploration regardless of the mechanism of injury. • Zone I hematomas can be classified as supramesocolic and inframesocolic. • Supramesocolic hematomas should be explored after obtaining proximal and distal vascular control by reflecting all left-sided viscera to the midline (Mattox maneuver). • Injury to the aorta or the celiac, mesenteric, or proximal renal arteries should be suspected. • Inframesocolic hematomas most commonly result from injuries to either the infrarenal aorta or the infrarenal vena cava. • Exposure is obtained by opening the midline retroperitoneum or reflecting the right-sided viscera cephalad (Catell maneuver). • Zone II is lateral to the psoas muscle above the iliac crest and below the diaphragm, incorporating the kidneys and retroperitoneal colon and its mesentery. • Hematomas caused by penetrating trauma should be explored. • Zone II hematomas after blunt trauma should not be opened if they are nonexpanding or nonpulsatile and if there are no urologic indications, such as nonvisualization of the kidney or extravasation of urine. • In stable patents with hematuria or suspected renal injury, preoperative CT scanning should be performed to define the hematoma and assess renal excretion. • Up to 95% of patients with blunt perirenal hematomas can be treated without operation. • Zone III hematomas arise in the pelvis and are the commonest retroperitoneal hematoma associated with blunt trauma. • In patients with blunt trauma, the hematoma should not be explored. • Hematomas caused by penetrating trauma often expand rapidly as a result of iliac vessel injury. • Control of the infrarenal aorta and inferior vena cava proximally and the iliac vessels distally should be established before the hematoma is opened. • Patients with pelvic fractures and exsanguinating hemorrhage need immediate operation, but operative control of pelvic bleeding is seldom successful, and pelvic packing is usually necessary.

ANSWER:
C

31. A 30-year-old man undergoes an exploratory laparotomy for a gunshot wound to the right upper quadrant. A hematoma is present in the area of the portal triad. An injury to the common bile duct is discovered, with a loss of more than 50% of the circumference of the wall of the duct. Further exploration reveals incomplete transection of the portal vein.

Which one of the following is the appropriate management of these injuries?

A. Ligation of the portal vein, débridement of the duct, and primary anastomosis with a stent

B. Resection of the portal vein with end-to-end anastomosis, débridement of the duct, and primary anastomosis with a stent

C. Venous interposition repair of the portal vein and Roux-en-Y choledochojejunostomy without a stent

D. Lateral venorrhaphy and Roux-en-Y choledochojejunostomy with a stent

E. Lateral venorrhaphy and ligation of the common bile duct with formation of a cholecystojejunostomy

Ref.: 1–3

COMMENTS: Hematomas in the portal triad must be explored. • While injuries to the extrahepatic biliary tract are uncommon, most are penetrating. • Associated intraperitoneal injuries are the rule and determine the surgical treatment and eventual outcome of patients with bile duct injury. • Most associated injuries involve the liver (78%) and major vascular structures (32%). • Repair of the extrahepatic bile duct depends on the condition of the patient. • Stenting of the duct, rather than repair, may be appropriate in a hemodynamically unstable patient. • In this situation, a second operation in a scarred field is necessary. • If the injury to the duct involves less than 50% of the circumference of the wall, primary repair with a stent brought out and away from the anastomosis is indicated. • Construction of a Roux-en-Y choledochojejunostomy with a stent brought from the anastomosis is indicated for more complex injuries. • If the diagnosis cannot be established on the basis of exploration, which may be the case with injuries to the intrapancreatic portion of the bile duct, an intraoperative cholangiogram should be performed via a needle into either the gallbladder or the bile duct. • The danger of repairing injuries to the bile duct is the development of a stricture at the site of repair, since the blood supply to the bile duct comes primarily from the vessels that run parallel to the duct. • The key principles in the management of ductal injuries are débridement, repair without tension, mucosal apposition of the edges, and knowledge of duct blood supply. • Although not mandatory, stents provide decompression and ready access for cholangiography. • All anastamoses of the bile duct should be externally drained because of the 10% incidence of leaks. • Portal vein injuries are treated by lateral venorrhaphy. • Ligation of the portal vein is compatible with survival in up to 50% of patients and can be appropriate in an unstable hypothermic patient with extensive destruction of the vein. • Postoperatively, these patients need massive fluid replacement because of bowel edema and sequestration of fluid in the splanchic bed.

ANSWER:
D

32. Regarding duodenal injuries, which of the following statements is/are true?

A. The most frequent site of injury is the second portion of the duodenum.

B. During abdominal exploration for blunt trauma, a retroperitoneal hematoma in the area of the duodenum does not need to be explored, provided it is small and the peritoneum overlying the hematoma is intact.

C. Approximately 75–85% of all duodenal injuries can be managed by simple débridement and closure.

D. When dealing with associated pancreatic injuries, it is not possible to resect the entire head of the duodenum without devascularizing the associated duodenum.

E. All of the above

Ref.: 1–3

COMMENTS: Duodenal injuries are associated with high rates of morbidity and mortality. • Blunt injuries are associated with a higher mortality rate as a result of diagnostic delay. • The commonest site of injury is the second portion of the duodenum, followed in decreasing order by the third, fourth, and first portions. • The preoperative diagnosis of duodenal injury is challenging. • Since the early signs and symptoms are nonspecific, blunt duodenal injuries are often manifested late with signs or peritonitis and sepsis. • CT scans may identify the injury by subtle findings of retroperitoneal air or fluid, thickening of the duodenum, or contrast extravasation. • Intraoperatively, the lesser sac should be opened and the periduodenal area inspected for blood and bile. • All central medial retroperitoneal hematomas should be explored and the duodenum kocherized to inspect for injury. • Seventy-five to 85% of duodenal injuries can be adequately dealt with by simple débridement and closure. • Segmental resection with end-to-end anastomosis is possible in all parts of the duodenum except the second portion.

In cases of duodenal injuries involving 75% of the circumference of the second portion, large tissue loss, devascularization, or delayed repairs in inflamed tissues, the following techniques should be used to aid in protecting the repair. • Buttressing the repair may be accomplished with omentum or a serosal patch from a loop of jejunum. • Diversion of gastric contents is accomplished by pyloric exclusion or duodenal diverticulization. • The addition of tube decompression to simple closure or to gastric diversion is controversial. • Retrograde jejunostomy is preferred over lateral tube duodenostomy because of lower fistula rates. • Pancreaticoduodenectomy is reserved for cases that involve massive tissue destruction and devascularization of the pancreaticoduodenal complex and is necessary in less than 3% of duodenal injuries. • A "trauma Whipple" should be undertaken only in very rare circumstances with a stable, resuscitated patient.

ANSWER:
E

33. Regarding duodenal hematomas, which of the following statements is/are true?

A. The common presentation is of a high small-bowel obstruction occurring 12–72 hr after abdominal trauma.

B. Patients with duodenal hematomas generally have peritonitis due to perforation.

C. An upper gastrointestinal radiographic series can demonstrate extravasation of contrast into the retroperitoneum.

D. Conservative management should be undertaken even with associated periduodenal injuries.

E. Operative management to provide feeding access is frequently necessary.

Ref.: 1–3

COMMENTS: Duodenal intramural hematomas generally result from blunt upper abdominal trauma. • The mechanism of injury is thought to be a force that crushes the third portion of the duodenum against the vertebral column. • This causes disruption of submucosal vessels and the development of an enlarging hematoma that occludes the duodenal lumen. • In general, the patient has signs of proximal small-bowel obstruction, including nausea, vomiting, and upper abdominal pain with significant tenderness. • The signs and symptoms usually develop 12–72 hr after the trauma episode. • Once associated injuries are ruled out, a barium swallow should be performed. • The demonstration of a coiled spring or stacked coins appearance confirms the diagnosis. • This study must be undertaken to ensure that there is no extravasation of contrast. • Conservative management, including nasogastric decompression, electrolyte repletion, and parental nutrition is likely to be successful in 75–85% of cases. • The process of resorption may take as long as 4 weeks. • If no resolution occurs over this period, surgical intervention is almost certainly necessary. • The operation can include evacuation of the intramural hematoma, with careful inspection of the mucosa for areas of disruption, and reapproximation of the seromuscular coat or the performance of a gastrojejunostomy. • The overall prognosis is excellent.

ANSWER:
A

34. The upper abdomen of a 42-year-old man strikes the steering wheel during a motor vehicle accident. Because of positive findings on peritoneal lavage, he undergoes an exploratory laparotomy, at which time transection of the pancreas at the neck is found. Which of the following is the most appropriate management of this injury?

A. Distal pancreatectomy with oversewing and drainage of the proximal pancreatic stump

B. Roux-en-Y pancreaticojejunostomy to the distal pancreas with oversewing and drainage of the proximal pancreatic stump

C. Primary repair and drainage of the pancreatic duct

D. Whipple operation

E. Total pancreatectomy

Ref.: 1–3

COMMENTS: Blunt pancreatic injuries are usually associated with liver, spleen, and/or duodenal injuries and are quite difficult to diagnose preoperatively. • Initially, patients have nonspecific signs and symptoms. • With time, they may develop nausea, vomiting, abdominal distention, upper abdominal pain, and increased fluid requirement. • Although the initial amylase level is unreliable even if elevated, demonstration of persistent or rising hyperamylasemia signifies pancreatic injury. • CT scanning of the abdomen with contrast is a poor means of diagnosing pancreatic injury initially. • However, delayed scans may identify free abdominal fluid, pancreatic edema, or even necrosis. • High suspicion of pancreatic injury warrants operative exploration. • Eighty percent of pancreatic injuries are secondary to penetrating trauma, almost all being diagnosed during exploratory laparotomy. • Care must be taken to thoroughly explore all hematomas within the lesser sac or at the root of the bowel mesentery. • The operative management of pancreatic injuries centers on débridement or resection of devitalized tissue, assessment and treatment of the pancreatic duct, and adequate external drainage. • Lacerations of the capsule can be repaired with nonabsorbable sutures without compromising the duct. • For pancreatic wounds with an intact duct, drainage of the area suffices. • Soft closed suction drains are preferred to Penrose or sump drains. • Careful exploration of the duodenum requires adequate kocherization and careful search for bile staining, swelling, or edema. • If the main pancreatic duct is injured to the left of the mesenteric vessels, a distal pancreatectomy and splenectomy with drainage of the proximal stump are appropriate. • The remaining proximal duct stump is closed with suture ligature. • Stapling devices such as a TA 55 may be used across the parenchyma. • The injury described in this question is the typical blunt pancreatic injury that results from a crushing abdominal blow against the vertebral body. • This should be treated by distal pancreatectomy. • Splenic preserving distal pancreatectomy has been found to add 50 minutes to operative time and can be a technically challenging addition. • Hence, it should be attempted only in very stable patients. • Roux-en-Y pancreaticojejunostomy to the distal pancreas with oversewing of the proximal pancreatic stump entails high morbidity rates, including a high leak rate, and is a technically difficult operation. • The Whipple procedure, a total pancreatectomy, should be reserved for injuries that involve extensive devitalization of the duodenum and head of the pancreas.

ANSWER:
A

35. Which of the following is/are indications for resection of a segment of small bowel?

A. Loss of more than 20% of the bowel wall

B. Two injuries in a segment

C. Compromise of the blood supply of a segment

D. Injuries within 40 cm of the ileocecal valve

E. Injuries within 40 cm of the ligament of Treitz

Ref.: 1–3

COMMENTS: Small-bowel injuries can be surprisingly lethal if not dealt with promptly. • There is a 3–7% mortality rate when blunt small-bowel injuries are treated more than 24 hr after the trauma. • Most small-bowel injuries are secondary to penetrating trauma and are found during the routine abdominal exploration. • During a laparotomy for abdominal trauma, the small bowel and its mesentery must be inspected completely from the ligament of Treitz to the ileocecal valve. • Blunt trauma can give rise to small-bowel injuries by one of three mechanisms: a sudden deceleration that causes shear forces to develop near a point of fixation, a crushing force that traps the small bowel against the vertebral body, or a blow to a fluid-filled loop of small bowel that causes a burst injury. • Isolated jejunal or ileal injuries frequently do not cause peritonitis immediately because the succus entericus that is spilled is chemically neutral and relatively sterile. • It is only when wetter bacterial growth begins to occur over a period of hours that peritoneal signs develop. • Aggressive use of peritoneal lavage can help diagnose these injuries. • A white blood cell (WBC) count of more than 500 WBCs/dl indicates the need for surgery, but findings on lavage may be negative with a small-bowel injury if the lavage is performed less than 4 hr from the injury. • Findings on CT scan are often unreliable, subtle, and nonspecific. • Most small-bowel injuries are managed by débridement and primary closure in one or two layers oriented transversely. • The indications for segmental resection include (1) loss of more than 50% of the bowel wall, (2) multiple injuries in a short segment that preclude primary repair or where time can be saved by resecting the segment, or (3) any compromise of the blood supply to a segment of small bowel. • Mesenteric hematomas require exploration if they are large (72 cm) and expanding or at the root of the mesentery.

ANSWER:
C

36. Which of the following is/are appropriate steps in managing rectal injuries?

A. Presacral drainage

B. Proximal, completely diverting colostomy

C. Irrigation of the distal segment with saline solution

D. Débridement and primary repair of the rectal injury

E. A, B, and D

Ref.: 1–3

COMMENTS: Rectal injuries continue to be a challenging problem facing the trauma surgeon. • The mortality rates average 10–15% and are a reflection of the particularly dangerous soilage that occurs in the pelvis, which is a relatively hypovascular area and thus poor in combating sepsis. • A high index of suspicion and prompt proctoscopic examination are necessary for diagnosing these injuries in a timely manner. • Any blood on the examining finger and any penetrating injury that crosses the midline in the pelvis warrants rigid proctoscopic examination. • There are three principles in the management of rectal injuries. • First, a proximal diverting colostomy is formed. • Classic teaching is to form a double-barrel colostomy, although a generously opened loop colostomy probably functions just as well. • Second, presacral drains are inserted through a curvilinear incision midway between the anal verge and the coccyx. • The surgeon must take care to dissect the entire retrorectal space and ensure that the drains are placed high enough to communicate with the rectal injury. • For most civilian injuries, passive drains suffice. • However, if there is extensive contamination or devitalization, active suction drainage is preferable. • Drains are removed after 5 days in the absence of significant drainage. • Third, débridement and primary repair of the rectal injury itself is performed, if it is accessible. • This can be accomplished transperitoneally for high rectal injuries (9 cm or more above the anal verge) or transanally for low rectal injuries (5 cm or less above the anal verge). • Midrectal injuries are sometimes inaccessible. • Distal irrigation has not been shown to be beneficial in civilian injuries. • It has, however, been shown to decrease morbidity and mortality rates in military-type, high-velocity injuries.

ANSWER:
E

37. Regarding colon injuries, which of the following statements is/are true?

A. They are reliably diagnosed by CT scanning.

B. Exteriorization of the repaired segment is recommended.

C. Colon lacerations are preferentially treated by resection.

D. Hematomas of the colonic mesentery should not be opened unless they are expanding.

E. They are associated with an intra-abdominal abscess rate of 5–15%.

Ref.: 1–3

COMMENTS: Colon injuries occur in about 18% of penetrating abdominal trauma cases and remain an important source of morbidity and mortality. • There continues to be a 5–15% rate of abscess formation, regardless of the operation performed, and about a 1–2% rate of fistula formation, which is most often associated with primary repair. • Colon injury may be suspected in patients with abdominal trauma and peritoneal signs or positive findings on lavage. • However, most are discovered during routine abdominal exploration for gunshot or stab wounds. • Free air can be demonstrated on chest radiographs in only 10% of these patients. • CT scanning of the abdomen with intravenous, oral, and rectal contrast is advocated to rule out colon injury in patients with stab wounds to the flank. • However, since the accuracy is only about 85%, these patients must be followed clinically for at least 24 hr. • During the trauma laparotomy, care must be taken to explore all hematomas involving the wall of the colon or the mesocolon to identify relatively occult perforations. • The surgical options for repair of colon injury include primary repair; resection and primary anastomosis; resection and end colostomy with mucous fistula or Hartmann's pouch; and exteriorized repair. • Colostomy formation has been the standard of care since the 1950s, although primary repair has assumed an increasing role during the last 15 years. • Exteriorized repair (which includes closure of the perforation, mobilization of the colon, and exteriorizing that segment) is associated with increased wound complications and fistula formation and is seldom used today. • Early studies advocated primary repair for colon injury only when patients were explored within 6 hr of injury, were hemodynamically stable, had minimal soilage, required less than 6 units of blood transfusion, and had no medical problems. • More recent data suggest that *all* colon injuries may be repaired primarily without an increase in morbidity or mortality rates, but this method is still controversial. • Most agree that primary repair should be performed on colonic lacerations not necessitating resection. • For injuries of the right colon requiring resection, ileocolostomy can be performed with an anastomotic leak rate of less than 5%. • For descending and sigmoid colon injury requiring resection, end colostomy should be considered, since colocolostomy in this setting has resulted in anastomotic leak rates of up to 20%.

ANSWER:
E

38. Regarding splenic trauma, which of the following statements is/are true?

A. Splenorrhaphy should be considered as the first line of operative treatment for all patients with blunt splenic injury.

B. The risk of postsplenectomy sepsis increases each year after removal of the spleen.

C. Splenic wound breaking strength is less than that of uninjured splenic tissue 3 weeks after splenorrhaphy.

D. A major disadvantage of splenic salvage is increased need for blood transfusion.

E. Nonoperative management of blunt injury is successful in 25% of eligible adult patients.

Ref.: 1–3

COMMENTS: The spleen is the most commonly injured organ following blunt trauma. • Splenic injuries are classified as follows: class I, capsular tear; class II, lacerations not extending to the hilum; class III, open lacerations extending into the hilum; and class IV, shattered spleen. • Splenectomy is the gold standard for definitive management of splenic injury, although the splenectomized state has been shown to predispose patients to overwhelming sepsis for encapsulated organisms, which carries a mortality rate of more than 50%. • Postsplenectomy sepsis occurs more frequently during the first 5 years of life, and the risk is greatest during the first 2 years after removal of the spleen. • To avoid this risk, which occurs in 0.026–1.0% of postsplenectomy patients, emphasis has been placed on splenic salvage. • Operative salvage of the spleen is successful in at least 50% of patients. • The highest success rate is in patients with grade I and II injuries, which often require only direct-pressure, hemostatic agents and simple splenic suture. • Suturing of the splenic parenchyma, mesh wrapping, and anatomic resection are used for grade III and IV injuries. • Wound healing studies of class II splenic injuries show that the wound breaking strength equals that of uninjured splenic tissue by 3 weeks after splenorrhaphy. • Compared to splenectomy, splenorrhaphy results in an increased need for blood transfusion, with its associated infectious complications and transfusion reactions. • This point must be taken into consideration when choosing the operation. • Splenorrhaphy should not be undertaken when there is life-threatening hemorrhage from the spleen, when there are multiple injuries in an unstable patient, or when the surgeon is not familiar with the appropriate techniques. • Nonoperative observation is indicated in stable patients without associated hollow viscus or other injuries and who do not require more than 2 units of blood during the initial 48 hr. • After blunt trauma, nonoperative splenic salvage is successful in 85% of eligible children and 70% of adults.

ANSWER:
D

39. Which of the following is/are contraindications to nonoperative management of splenic trauma?

   A. Blunt splenic trauma

   B. Penetrating splenic trauma

   C. Unconscious patient

   D. Associated hepatic injury

   E. Pediatric patient

Ref.: 1–3

COMMENTS: Preservation of all or most of the injured spleen, rather than splenectomy, has become the preferred treatment in many patients with splenic trauma. • Splenic preservation may take the form of splenorrhaphy, partial splenectomy, or nonoperative management and observation of splenic injury. • Nonoperative therapy for splenic trauma is the preferred management for most pediatric and adult patients and has been successful in approximately 90% of cases. • Nonoperative treatment should be undertaken only in selected patients. • It is not indicated for patients with penetrating trauma because of the exceedingly high incidence of associated injuries, such as to the colon and diaphragm, necessitating operative repair. • According to strict selection criteria, more than 60% of adult patients may be eligible for nonoperative management. • The first and foremost contraindication to nonoperative management is hemodynamic instability. • Hemodynamic instability in the presence of abdominal trauma indicates the need for emergent laparotomy. • With patients who are hemodynamicaly stable, continued transfusion requirements also necessitate laparotomy. • The patient should have a documented splenic injury on CT scan. • Associated hepatic injuries can also be treated with close nonoperative management and should not be considered a contraindication. • Unconscious patients can be monitored but, because of the lack of ability to follow them clinically, they should have a lower threshold for operative exploration.

ANSWER:
B, C

40. A 22-year-old man has an exploratory laparotomy for a gunshot wound to the abdomen, at which time a through-and-through injury to the infrarenal inferior vena cava is encountered. Which of the following is/are included in the appropriate management of this patient?

   A. Primary repair if the resultant stenosis will not exceed 50% of the lumen

   B. Packing for tamponade and no specific repair once hemostasis is achieved

   C. Ligation of the infrarenal inferior vena cava

   D. Synthetic or native vein patch graft

Ref.: 1–3

COMMENTS: Injuries to the inferior vena cava most often result from gunshot wounds to the abdomen. • A major determinant of survival is hemorrhagic shock, which is associated with a mortality rate of 80%. • Inferior vena cava injuries are diagnosed by complete exploration of retroperitoneal hematomas and a high index of suspicion. • The Catell maneuver, involving mobilization of the right colon and small-bowel mesentery, provides rapid exposure of the entire infrarenal inferior vena cava. • Proximal and distal control of bleeding is most easily achieved by direct pressure on the inferior vena cava above and below the injury. • If enough room can be dissected, encirclement and application of vascular clamps can be achieved but is often not necessary and can limit exposure for the repair. • Primary venorrhaphy is the simplest, quickest method of repair and can be accomplished with a running nonabsorbable monofilament suture. • A resultant stenosis of up to 50% of the cross-sectional area is acceptable. • A saphenous vein patch or other bovine synthetic patch should be used if more than 50% stenosis will result from a primary venorrhaphy. • Synthetic graft material should be avoided if there is concomitant bowel injury, which is usually the case. • For patients who are unstable, the infrarenal inferior vena cava can be ligated, but significant morbidity and late complications occur in more than 50% of patients. • Therefore, this technique should be used only as a lifesaving measure. • Ligation must never be used to treat suprarenal inferior vena cava injuries. • Tamponade of the inferior vena cava without definitive repair will likely lead to delayed bleeding and hematoma or pseudoaneurysm, and any lifesaving packing should be followed by definitive treatment with ligation or repair.

ANSWER:
A, C, D

41. During laparotomy, an actively bleeding injury in the right lobe of the liver is found. Which one of the following five sequences of maneuvers to control the bleeding is correct?

Maneuver	Sequence
1. Perihepatic packing and closure of the abdomen	A. 3, 5, 4, 2, 1
2. Pringle maneuver	B. 5, 3, 2, 4, 1
3. Temporary compression and packing	C. 3, 4, 2, 5, 1
4. Hematotomy and selective vascular ligation	D. 2, 3, 4, 5, 1
5. Right hepatic artery ligation	E. 3, 2, 4, 5, 1

Ref.: 1–3

COMMENTS: See Question 42.

42. Regarding liver trauma, which of the following statements is/are true?

A. Nonoperative treatment is considered the treatment of choice for stable patients with isolated hepatic trauma.

B. Temporary compression of the hepatoduodenal ligament may be performed for up to 90 minutes without causing ischemic damage.

C. Contained subcapsular hematomas discovered in the operating room should always be explored.

D. For deep lacerations that are actively bleeding, the finger fracture technique is rarely successful.

E. Liberal use of intraoperative packing, rapid abdominal closure, and secondary resuscitation in the intensive care unit has led to increased mortality rates in patients with grade IV and V hepatic injuries.

Ref.: 1–3

COMMENTS: More than two thirds of liver injuries are simple (grade I and II). • More than half of them have stopped bleeding by the time exploration is performed. • This finding and the widespread use of CT scanning in stable patients has prompted a growing interest in nonoperative treatment of hepatic trauma. • Currently, nonoperative treatment of stable patients with isolated hepatic or splenic and hepatic trauma is the treatment of choice. • Electrocautery, topical hemostatic agents, and simple suture hepatorrhaphy can effectively control minor liver injuries found on operative exploration. • Contained subcapsular hematomas discovered in the operating room should not be explored. • Complex injuries not involving the vena cava are almost always controlled by incorporating a variety of techniques. • Upon entering the abdomen, temporary compression and perihepatic packing with laparotomy pads are performed to stop hemorrhage. • The addition of temporary occlusion of the hepatoduodenal ligament (Pringle maneuver) may be necessary at this time. • Studies have documented a warm ischemic time of up to 60 minutes (from a Pringle maneuver) without untoward effects. • Once hepatic bleeding is temporarily controlled, the rest of the abdomen is inspected. • The packs are then removed from the liver, and any superficial bleeding vessels are point-ligated with absorbable suture. • For deep lacerations, the finger fracture technique is successful in all but the most severe cases. • Nonviable tissue is then débrided, and an omental graft is tacked to the liver. • This omental tacking aids in combating sepsis, sealing dead space, and sealing small bile leaks. • The use of closed suction drains allows the elimination of blood, perihepatic fluid, and bile, and these drains should be placed after repair of grade III, IV, and V injuries. • Right or left hepatic artery ligation is used on rare occasions when previous techniques fail to control hemorrhage. • Selective embolization by an interventional radiologist has been reported in more stable patients but remains controversial. • For patients who are in extremis or those with exsanguinating liver hemorrhage that cannot be controlled with other measures, perihepatic packing may be necessary. • The liver is tightly packed with laparotomy pads to provide vector forces to approximate tissue planes. • The abdomen is rapidly closed with towel clips and a steridrape, and the patient is transferred to the intensive care unit for warming, secondary resuscitation, maximization of oxygen delivery, and correction of coagulopathy. • Once the patient is stabilized, usually within 24–48 hr, he or she is returned to the operating room for repair and closure. • Liberal use of intraoperative packing has decreased the mortality rate from more than 80% to fewer than 50% for these patients.

ANSWERS:
Question 41: E
Question 42: A

43. True or false: Right or left hepatic artery ligation is poorly tolerated.

Ref.: 1–3

COMMENTS: Right or left hepatic artery ligation is used on rare occasions when previous techniques fail to control hemorrhage. • Although ligation of one branch of the hepatic artery appears to be associated with minimal long-term morbidity, its use in hypotensive patients may produce hepatic ischemia. • Enthusiasm for hepatic lobectomy has waned since the early 1970s because of the associated high mortality rate and because hemostasis can usually be obtained by less aggressive techniques.

ANSWER:
False

44. A 37-year-old man is brought to the emergency department after a motorcycle crash. His airway is intact; his respiratory rate is 35 breaths per minute, his heart rate is 130 beats per minute, and his blood pressure is 90/55 after 2 L of crystalloid resuscitation. He has a tender abdomen, clear chest radiograph, and butterfly-type pelvic fracture. Which one of the following is the most appropriate next step?

A. CT scan of the abdomen

B. Diagnostic peritoneal lavage (DPL)

C. Application of MAST garments

D. Application of external pelvic fixator

E. Emergent exploratory laparotomy

Ref.: 1–3

COMMENTS: Pelvic fractures may be a source of exsanguinating hemorrhage. • A systematic approach with simultaneous evaluation and resuscitation is necessary. • The commonest pelvic fractures associated with hemorrhage are the butterfly, or straddle, fracture, which is fracture of all four pubic rami; the open-book fracture, which is diastasis of the symphsis pubis of more than 2.5 mm; and the vertical shear fracture, a fracture of both anterior and posterior elements with vertical displacement of one hemipelvis of 1 cm or more. • In all cases of hypotension and significant pelvic ring fractures, intra-abdominal bleeding must be ruled out. • CT scanning is contraindicated for unstable patients. • DPL should be performed using an open supraumbilical approach. • Grossly positive aspiration signifies the need for emergent laparotomy. • If the findings on DPL are negative, angiography should be considered for evaluation and possible embolization of pelvic bleeding. • Hypotensive patients with microscopically positive DPL findings should first undergo angiography for potential embolization of arterial bleeding in the pelvis, following by exploratory laparotomy. • Hypotensive patients with microscopically positive DPL should first undergo angiography for potential embolization of arterial bleeding in the pelvis, followed by exploratory laparotomy. • Likewise, an unstable patient with a complex pelvic fracture who continues to show bleeding after lapatoromy should be taken emergently to the angiography suite for embolization. • Placement of an external fixation device is considered early in patients with pelvic ring fractures and hemodynamic instability. • Anterior pelvic fixation acts by decreasing pelvic volume, allowing tamponade to occur, and decreasing movement of the fractured elements, allowing hemostasis to occur. • The fixation is ideally used for temporary stabilization for 5–7 days, followed by definitive internal fixation. • Studies have shown that the use of anterior pelvic external fixation during the resuscitation period decreases the transfusion requirements and mortality rates.

• Exsanguinating hemorrhage unresponsive to resuscitation or angiographic control requires immediate exploration and surgical control of the bleeding. • Pelvic packing is an effective last resort but requires a return to the operating room for pack removal.

ANSWER:
B

45. Which of the following is/are indications for emergent angiography in hemodynamically unstable patients with a pelvic ring fracture?

   A. Patients with grossly negative findings on DPL

   B. Patients with microscopically positive findings on DPL

   C. Patients with grossly negative findings on DPL and continued bleeding necessitating more than 8 units of packed red blood cells during the first 24 hr

   D. Stable patients with an expanding pelvic hematoma

Ref.: 1–3

COMMENTS: In hemodynamically unstable patients with no other intra-abdominal injury, control of pelvic retroperitoneal bleeding takes priority. • Aggressive resuscitation and blood and factor replacement is mandatory. • Most pelvic bleeding is self-limiting. • However, when the patient continues to be hemodynamically unstable, angiography is considered the diagnostic and therapeutic procedure of choice. • Approximately 20% of patients with high-risk pelvic fractures who require more than 4 units of blood have pelvic arterial bleeding, which can be managed by embolization. • Angiography is also indicated for patients with pelvic fractures who are hemodynamically unstable with grossly negative findings on DPL or microscopically positive findings on DPL and those who remain unstable after exploration and control of intra-abdominal bleeding, especially when a pelvic hematoma is identified intraoperatively. • If a rapidly expanding hematoma is found at the time of operation and resuscitation requirements preclude closing the abdomen and taking the patient for angiography, intraoperative angiography may be considered. • If intraoperative angiography is not available, the hematoma should be opened and ligation of arterial and major venous bleeding attempted. • Pelvic packing may be lifesaving.

ANSWER:
A, B, C

46. Which of the following is/are appropriate management of an open pelvic fracture with a perineal wound?

   A. Diverting colostomy and distal irrigation only if there is an associated rectal injury

   B. Diverting colostomy and distal irrigation, regardless of the presence of a rectal injury

   C. Bowel rest and TPN

   D. Laparotomy and peritoneal and pelvic irrigation

   E. Primary suture closure of the open perineal wound after débridement and irrigation

Ref.: 1–3

COMMENTS: The mortality rate associated with an open pelvic fracture is reported to be as high as 50%. • Early death is largely the result of uncontrollable hemorrhage or concomitant head and thoracic injuries. • Late death usually is caused by sepsis. • Steps designed to avoid perineal and pelvic sepsis include diversion of the fecal stream by a colostomy and washout of any stool that is present in the distal colon and rectum. • A concomitant rectal injury must be examined and dealt with appropriately by a diverting colostomy. • The rectal tear may be repaired if exposure does not require extensive mobilization of the proximal rectum and it is possible to irrigate the distal rectum clean. • Presacral drains should be placed if the injury is associated with a perineal laceration. • The perineal wound should be adequately débrided and irrigated frequently, with the patient under general anesthesia if necessary, and packed open for continued wound care.

ANSWER:
B

47. A 30-year-old man is brought into the emergency room after being involved in a Jet Ski crash. His vital signs are stable. He is found to have bilateral pubic rami fractures on portable pelvic x-rays. He is unable to void urine freely. Which of the following should be the next step?

   A. Wait for the patient to void urine freely before attempting transurethral bladder catheterization.

   B. Initially attempt gentle transurethral bladder catheterization, but stop if resistance is encountered.

   C. Obtain a urethrogram before attempting transurethral bladder catherization.

   D. Insert a suprapubic cystostomy tube.

   E. Obtain a CT scan of the pelvis with three-dimensional reconstruction.

Ref.: 1–3

COMMENTS: Genitourinary injuries are frequently associated with pelvic fractures, especially bilateral pubic rami fractures. • The membranous portion of the urethra is particularly at risk for transection in male patients. • Inability to void is one of the classic signs of urethral transection or trauma. • Other signs are blood at the urethral meatus, a freely movable or high-riding prostate on rectal examination, and scrotal or perineal hematoma. • If any of these signs are present or there is significant anterior pelvic fracture, a urethrogram should be obtained to exclude an injury before transurethral catheterization is attempted. • If no injury is identified, a Foley catheter is inserted, and a cystogram may be obtained if bladder injury is suspected. • If a complete urethral injury is present, suprapubic cystostomy is necessary to provide urinary drainage in the acute setting, followed by delayed repair. • Likewise, a partial urethral tear, as seen on a contrast examination, is managed by a bridging catheter left in place for at least 3 weeks or suprapubic cystostomy, followed by delayed repair. • If the tear is allowed to heal over a catheter, a voiding cystourethrogram is obtained upon removal.

ANSWER:
C

48. Which of the following statements is/are true regarding renal trauma?

   A. A CT scan is inferior to an intravenous pyelogram (IVP) for evaluating renal function.

   B. Any extravasation after blunt renal injury is an indication for surgical exploration.

   C. On routine exploration of a patient with splenic rupture after blunt trauma, if a nonexpanding perinephric hematoma is encountered it should be opened.

D. Before opening a perineal hematoma, vascular control of the renal artery and vein must be established.

Ref.: 1–3

COMMENTS: The diagnosis and management of renal trauma varies, depending on the mechanism of injury: blunt or penetrating. • The most sensitive indicator of renal injury after blunt trauma is hematuria. • In hemodynamically stable patients without gross hematuria, the incidence of renal injury is less than 1%. • The presence of gross hematuria should prompt further radiologic evaluation. • IVP and CT scanning with intravenous infusion reliably demonstrate major renal injuries, specifically extravasation of contrast (including collecting system disruption) and nonfunction (from thrombosis, vascular disruption, or shattered kidney). • CT scanning clearly defines the extent of minor renal injuries and the degree of hemorrhage. • Indications for operation on isolated blunt renal trauma include clinical or CT evidence of ongoing hemorrhage, major collecting system disruption, unresolving extravasations, and severe hematuria. • Renal parenchymal injuries and minor lacerations of the collection system generally heal without complications. • The presence of extravasation is not an absolute indication for surgical exploration. • Up to 95% of blunt renal trauma can be successfully managed nonoperatively. • Penetrating renal trauma is generally identified on routine exploration. • All perinephric hematomas secondary to penetrating trauma should be opened. • Conversely, after blunt trauma, only expanding or pulsatile hematomas should be opened, unless preoperative testing revealed major collecting system disruption or nonfunction. • There is disagreement on whether vascular control should be established before opening Gerota's fascia, the argument being that vascular control decreases the rate of nephrectomy and minimizes bleeding. • In fact, initial vascular control has no bearing on overall blood loss, does not increase the nephrectomy rate, and decreases operative time by approximately 1 hr. • Furthermore, in situations when a rapidly expanding hematoma is crossing the midline or in a patient who is hemodynamically unstable, the swiftest maneuver to gain control of the renal pedicle is via the lateral approach. • Upon exploration of the kidney, all hematomas should be evacuated and the kidney evaluated for venous, arterial, and collecting system injury. • If a collecting system injury is in question, methylene blue dye may be given intravenously and its excretion in the defect sought after infusion. • All nonviable tissue is removed, all bleeding points are secured with 4-0 absorbable suture, and the collecting system is closed with 4-0 absorbable sutures so that it is watertight. • The parenchyma is then covered with capsular coaptation or omental packing. • Retroperitoneal drains are placed, especially if a collecting system injury is present.

ANSWER:
C

49. An 18-year-old male is brought to the trauma unit after suffering a gunshot wound to the abdomen. There is one wound 2 cm to the left of the umbilicus, and plain abdominal x-rays show a retained missile lodged in the right iliac spine. The patient's pulse is 100 beats per minute, and his blood pressure is 110/60 after initial resuscitation. What is the proper order of events during the laparotomy?

A. Inferior midline incision, examination for and repair of hemorrhage, four-quadrant packing, control of spillage from viscus injury, and definitive repair of encountered injuries

B. Xiphoid to pubis midline incision, four-quadrant packing with laparotomy pads, control of massive hemorrhage, control of gross bowel spillage, and definitive repair of encountered injuries

C. Xiphoid to pubis midline incision, control of gross bowel spillage, control of massive hemorrhage, four-quadrant packing with laparotomy pads, and definitive repair of encountered injuries

D. Inferior midline incision, four-quadrant packing with laparotomy pads, control of massive hemorrhage, control of gross bowel spillage, and definitive repair of encountered injuries

Ref.: 1–3

COMMENTS: Although trauma laparotomies vary, depending on the injuries encountered, a systematic approach can limit morbidity, maximize time available for definitive repair, and ensure that no injuries are missed. • Any laparotomy should begin with a surgical preparation from chin to knees. • Even with the patient described in this question, in whom the injury is likely to be limited to the abdomen, preparing the chest allows for exploration there if needed and, in the event of traumatic arrest, allows for left lateral thoracotomy. • In addition, if vascular control or vein for vascular repair is necessary, preparing the legs allows for both. • Once the incision is made, gross hematoma is evacuated and the abdomen tightly packed with laparotomy pads in four quadrants. • Doing so allows for temporary tamponade of bleeding and limiting of viscus spillage. • After packing and time for anesthesia to stabilize the patient, the laparotomy pads are removed quadrant by quadrant, beginning in the quadrant with the least likelihood of injury. • Hence, if the injury is likely in the lower left quadrant, pads in the right upper quadrant are removed, first working around the abdomen and examining the most severely injured area last. • With each removal, a quick assessment is made of injuries encountered. • Major hemorrhage and gross bowel spillage are quickly ligated and stitched. • No attempt should be made at definitive repair of injuries until the entire abdomen has been unpacked and all gross hemorrhage and spillage have been controlled. • Once the abdomen has been unpacked, a more thorough exploration can be undertaken and definitive repair of encountered injuries performed.

ANSWER:
B

50. A 26-year-old man sustains a gunshot wound to the right thigh. There are two wounds. One wound is on the anterior lateral aspect of the thigh and another on the posterior medial aspect. There is minimal bleeding from the anterior wound, the patient's vital signs are stable, and plain x-ray films reveal no orthopedic injuries or retained missile. The patient has good distal pulses and is neurologically intact in the injured leg. What is the proper management for this patient?

A. Observation for 24 hr and discharge

B. Immediate discharge

C. Angiogram

D. Delayed angiogram within the next 24 hr

E. Operative exploration

Ref.: 1–3

COMMENTS: When approaching an extremity gunshot wound, one should have a high index of suspicion for vascular injury. • A quick but thorough history and physical examination are the first steps in diagnosing injury. • Traditionally, signs of vascular injury are divided into hard signs and soft signs. • Hard signs include expanding hematoma, pulsatile bleeding, loss or change in distal pulses, thrill or bruit, and significant neurologic change. • Any hard sign warrants immediate operative exploration. • Soft signs include nonexpanding hematoma, nonpulsatile bleeding, and minor neurologic changes. • Soft signs warrant an urgent angiogram to evaluate for and define any arterial injury. • A positive angiogram necessitates operative exploration and repair. • Along with hard and soft signs, wounds in anatomic proximity to vessels warrant attention. • There exists significant controversy concerning these proximity wounds. • Traditionally, these wounds were all explored for injury, but this resulted in negative findings in up to 80% of cases. • Many centers and authors have advocated angiogram within the first 12–24 hr for proximity wounds. • These proximity angiograms are positive in only 2–5% of cases, which limits their usefulness. • Furthermore, many of the positive angiograms show only intimal damage, which does not necessitate repair. • Because of this, many centers have abandoned proximity angiograms and choose to observe these patients for 24 hr.

A N S W E R :
A

---

51. Regarding focused abdominal sonographic studies for trauma (FAST), which of the following statements is/are true?

    A. FAST is a useful imaging modality for visceral injury or perforation.

    B. Five hundred milliliters of free intraperitoneal fluid is necessary for a positive FAST scan.

    C. In patients with multiple injuries, FAST is equivalent to DPL at diagnosing intraperitoneal hemorrhage.

    D. FAST can accurately grade abdominal solid-organ injury.

    E. C and D.

Ref.: 1–3

COMMENTS: FAST has been rapidly adopted by many centers as a primary adjunct for diagnosing blunt abdominal trauma. • FAST consists of rapid abdominal ultrasound to identify free abdominal fluid as evidence of hemoperitoneum. • FAST can be performed in 3–4 min and has been shown to have a sensitivity of 73–88%, a specificity of 98–100%, and an accuracy of 96–98%. • A minimum of 200 ml of fluid must be present for a positive result. • In terms of reliability, FAST is equivalent to DPL for diagnosing intraperitoneal hemorrhage. • Despite the benefits of FAST, it is a poor test for diagnosing visceral injury. • It is also a poor test for grading the degree of solid-organ injury. • For these reasons, it is often used in conjunction with CT scanning for evaluating blunt abdominal trauma.

A N S W E R :
C

---

52. Regarding ureteral injuries, which of the following statements is/are true?

    A. A significant ureteral injury from penetrating abdominal trauma can safely be excluded if no red blood cells are seen on microscopic urinalysis.

    B. An IVP is indicated for any patient with penetrating abdominal injury near the course of the ureter.

    C. The procedure of choice for injuries of the lower third of the ureter near the bladder is primary repair over a stent with external drainage.

    D. An excretory urogram after ureteral repair may be omitted only if the patient is asymptomatic.

Ref.: 1–3

COMMENTS: Hematuria is an unreliable indicator of ureteral injury, since it is absent in up to 30% of cases. • A multiple-film **IVP** accurately establishes the diagnosis more than 90% of the time and should be performed in patients with suspected ureteral injury who are managed nonoperatively. • A "one-shot" large-bolus IVP may be obtained in the emergency department preoperatively or in the operating room to provide some clues as to the extent of renal injury and, more important, document function of the contralateral kidney. • IVP cannot be used to evaluate the ureters. • Most ureteral injuries are found on routine abdominal exploration for concomitant intra-abdominal injuries. • Any missile track through the retroperitoneum must be explored, and the ureter should be mobilized and inspected for injury. • A questionable injury may be assessed intraoperatively by injection of contrast medium through a catheter inserted in the urethral orifice via the bladder or by injection of indigo carmine dye intravenously. • Principles of repair include adequate mobilization and débridement. • It should be noted that the blood supply to the ureter is medial in the upper two thirds and lateral below the pelvic brim. • Most injuries to the proximal two thirds of the ureter are amenable to **ureteroureterostomy** incorporating spatulation and oblique anastomosis with fine absorbable interrupted sutures. • Renal mobilization may be added to obtain a tension-free anastomosis. • Injuries to the lower one third of the ureter are best treated by **reimplantation** into the bladder. • Boari flap and psoas bladder hitch are techniques that aid in obtaining a tension-free ureterocystostomy. • **Ileal interposition** and **renal autotransplantation** are more advanced techniques that are rarely necessary. • Unstable patients may be managed by **ligation** of the ureter proximal to the injury and insertion of a nephrostomy tube. • This may be followed by delayed reconstruction. • Retrograde ureterograms should be obtained in all patients for proper follow-up.

A N S W E R :
B

---

53. Regarding peripheral arterial injuries, which of the following statements is/are true?

    A. All patients with peripheral arterial injuries have diminished or no pulses distal to the injury.

    B. If the injury cannot be repaired primarily, prosthetic material should be used.

    C. All patients with posterior knee dislocations should undergo popliteal arteriography.

    D. Evidence of compartment hypertension is a contraindication to arteriography.

    E. After insertion of an interposition graft, completion angiography is unnecessary if distal pulses are present.

Ref.: 1–3

COMMENTS: Peripheral arterial injuries may be a source of substantial morbidity and disability if not appropriately managed. • About 20% of patients with serious arterial injuries have normal pulses distal to the site of the injury. • Consequently, any penetrating injury that threatens the path of a major artery should be carefully evaluated. • The ankle brachial index (ABI) should be determined bilaterally for lower extremity injuries. • An ABI of less than 0.9 on the injured side raises suspicion of injury and should prompt further work-up. • Most peripheral arterial injuries are caused by penetrating trauma, and certain blunt injuries are associated with a high incidence of vascular damage. • The latter include posterior knee dislocation, supracondylar femoral or humeral fractures, and first or second rib fractures. • These injuries traditionally indicate the need for arteriography. • The only contraindications to arteriography are exsanguinating hemorrhage, limb-threatening ischemia, and compartmental hypertension. • In these cases, immediate surgical intervention must be undertaken. • The principles of surgical repair of major vascular trauma include proximal and distal control of the injured vessel and repair of major venous and arterial injuries, since ligation of major draining veins can increase venous pressure and cause decreased arterial inflow, leading to thrombosis. • Venous repair should be attempted first in these cases. • An intraluminal shunt is placed in the artery to avoid limb ischemia during the venous repair. • This procedure is also frequently necessary to allow stabilization of associated fractures. • The damaged vessel is sharply débrided, mobilized, and reanastomosed end to end if possible. • Otherwise, an interposition graft is placed. • Autogenous greater saphenous vein is the conduit of choice. • When autogenous vein is not available, a synthetic graft may be used for both arterial or venous repair, although long-term patency rates are lower. • Synthetic grafts should be avoided for contaminated wounds if possible. • About 75% of local repairs and 50% of interposition grafts are patent during the early postoperative period. • Completion arteriography should be performed to evaluate the repair, visualize the runoff, and ensure that there are no concomitant injuries. • Finally, adequate soft-tissue coverage is required to protect the site of vascular repair.

A N S W E R :
C, D

54. An 18-year-old factory worker suffers a traumatic amputation of all four digits of his dominant hand in a bacon slicer. Which of the following methods should be used to transport the amputated fingers with the patient?

   A. Placed in a clean plastic bag and packed in Dry Ice

   B. Placed in a plastic bag, sealed, and placed in a larger plastic bag filled with water at 37°C

   C. Wrapped in sterile gauze

   D. Placed in a sealed plastic bag in a cooling chest filled with crushed ice and water

Ref.: 1–3

COMMENTS: Successful reattachment of amputated parts depends on a number of factors. • Upper-extremity reattachments are more successful than are lower-extremity reattachments, and younger patients are better candidates than older ones. • In addition, sharp amputations are more likely to be successfully reattached than are amputations caused by blunt mechanisms. • It is important, therefore, that the amputated part be recovered, if possible, and transported with the patient. • Such parts may well remain viable for 4–6 hr at room temperature but can remain viable for up to 18 hr if they are cooled. • Because it is important not to allow the amputated part to freeze, it should not be placed in Dry Ice. • Therefore, it is recommended that the amputated part be placed in a sterile, sealed plastic bag and transported in an insulated cooling chest filled with crushed ice and water.

A N S W E R :
D

R E F E R E N C E S

1. Townsend CM, Beauchamp RD, Evers BM, et al (eds): *Sabiston Textbook of Surgery, The Biological Basis of Modern Surgical Practice*, 17th ed. Saunders, Philadelphia, 2004.
2. Brunicardi FC, Andersen DK, Billiar TR, et al (eds): *Schwartz's Principles of Surgery*, 8th ed. McGraw-Hill, New York, 2004.
3. Mullholland MW, Lillemoe KD, Doherty GM, et al (eds): *Greenfield's Surgery: Scientific Principles and Practice*, 4th ed. Lippincott, Williams & Wilkins, Philadelphia, 2006.

CHAPTER 17

Burns

Laura Moore, M.D.

1. Select the true statements regarding the epidemiology of a burn injury.

   A. Burn injury is the second leading cause of trauma-related deaths.

   B. Ninety-five percent of all burn-related deaths occur in house fires.

   C. Two thirds of all burn injuries occur at home, with electrical burns being the commonest.

   D. Pediatric and geriatric burn injuries require investigation to rule out abuse or neglect.

   E. Most burn injuries are preventable.

Ref.: 1–3

COMMENTS: Each year nearly 2 million Americans seek medical attention for burn injuries. • These burns range in severity from mild scald burns occurring while cooking to extensive full-thickness burns with associated traumatic injury. • Burn injury is the second leading cause of trauma deaths. • Approximately 75% of burn deaths occur as the result of house fires. • Deaths due to burn injury tend to occur in a bimodal pattern either immediately after the burn or many weeks later as a result of complications related to sepsis and multiple organ failure. • Nearly two thirds of all burns occur in the home, with scald burns being the commonest type of burn injury. • Burn injuries in the pediatric and elderly population are often abuse related. • As a result, all burns occurring in these patient populations must be investigated for potential abuse. • Like other trauma-related injuries, burns are generally preventable. • Recent efforts aimed at community education and prevention have decreased the number and severity of burn-related injuries.

A N S W E R :
A, D, E

2. Which of the following statements regarding burn depth is/are true?

   A. First-degree burns are characterized by erythema, pain, and blistering of the skin.

   B. Second-degree burns involve the epidermis and dermis of the skin.

   C. Third-degree burns are characterized by erythema, pain, bullae, and moisture from fluid extravasation.

   D. Fourth-degree burns involve muscle or bone.

   E. Third-degree burns blanch to the touch.

Ref.: 1–3

COMMENTS: Burn depth is important when evaluating a patient for surgical procedure and long-term rehabilitative care. • **First-degree** burns involve only the epidermis (Fig. 17-1), most commonly result from prolonged exposure to ultraviolet light or minor flashes, and are characterized by painful blanching and erythema without blisters. • They usually heal within 2–3 days. • These burns are physiologically unimportant and not considered when calculating the total body surface area (TBSA) burned. • **Second-degree** (partial-thickness) burns involve the epidermis and the varying depths of dermis (see the figure). • They most commonly result from contact with hot liquids, flashes of flame, or exposure to chemicals. • These burns are divided into three subtypes: superficial, deep, and indeterminate. • *Superficial partial-thickness* burns affect the epidermis and superficial level of the dermis and are recognized by severe pain, moist erythema, and characteristic bullae formation. • These burn wounds heal within 2 weeks by re-epithelialization from the skin appendages (hair follicles and sweat glands). • *Deep partial-thickness* burns affect the deeper layer of dermis and destroy most of the skin appendages. • They are recognized by their dark-red or mottled yellow-white appearance and decreased pinprick sensation. • These burn wounds usually require skin grafting because re-epithelialization is unlikely or occurs slowly. • In *indeterminate partial-thickness* burns, the depth of burn is difficult to assess at the time of admission. • A variety of techniques have been used to determine depth, including fluorescein and indocyanine green fluorometry, laser Doppler flowmetry, thermography, ultrasonography, nuclear magnetic resonance imaging, and light reflectance, but none of these methods is accurate. • These burns should be observed over a period of 10 days to 2 weeks to predict the need for skin grafting. • **Third-degree** (full-thickness) burns involve coagulation necrosis of all skin elements down to the subdermal plexus (see Fig. 17-1). • They are usually caused by flame, immersion scalds, high-voltage electricity, or exposure to concentrated chemicals. • The burns are anesthetic, pearly white, charred, or parchment-like, and thrombosed veins may be seen through the eschar. • These wounds necessitate excision of eschar and skin grafting. • Circumferential full-thickness burns in the extremities do not always require escharotomy. • Use of Doppler sonographic studies has increased the accuracy of perfusion assessment in these circumferential burns and has reduced the need for escharotomy by as much as 50%. • **Fourth-degree** burns involve tissues other than the skin, such as muscle or bone.

ANSWER:
B, D

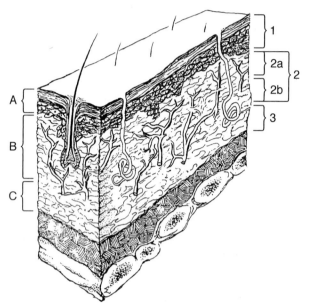

Figure 17-1 Various depths of burns. Layers of skin: A, epidermis; B, corium (dermis); C, subcutaneous fat. Depth of burn: 1, first degree; 2, second degree (2a, superficial; 2b, deep); 3, third degree. (Adapted from Greenfield LJ, *Surgery: Scientific Principles and Practice*, 2nd ed, Lippincott-Raven, New York, 1997, Chapter 12, reproduced with kind permission.)

3. A 33-year-old woman involved in a house fire sustains burns to bilateral lower extremities, anterior torso, genital area, and her entire left arm. Approximately what percentage of the TBSA is burned?

   A. 45%

   B. 64%

   C. 36%

   D. 72%

   E. 54%

*Ref.:*1–3

COMMENTS: Estimation of the extent of the burn is important when determining the fluid requirements, calorie requirements, and outcome (mortality and morbidity). • The initial triage to the appropriate level of medical care is determined primarily by the extent of injury. • It is usually described in terms of the percentage of TBSA involved. • The "rule of nines" (Fig. 17-2), developed as a guideline to estimate the size of burn injuries in adults, describes the percentage of body surface represented by various anatomic areas as follows: the entire head and neck 9%; each entire upper extremity 9%; the upper part of the anterior trunk 9% and the lower part 9%; the upper part of the posterior trunk 9% and the lower part 9%; the anterior part of each lower extremity 9% and the posterior part 9%; and the perineum and genitalia 1%. • For small burns, the area defined by patient's hand represents approximately

1% of the TBSA. • The rule of nines is not applicable to infants and children because they have proportionally larger heads and smaller legs than do adults.

ANSWER:
B

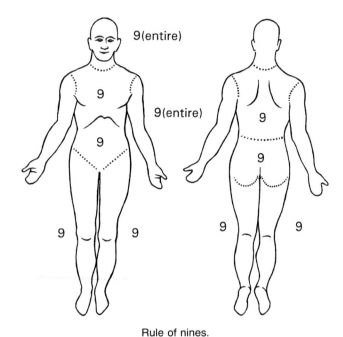

Rule of nines.

Figure 17-2 Rule of nines.

4. According to American Burn Association criteria, which of the following patients should not be referred to a burn center?

   A. A 30-year-old woman with an 8% partial-thickness burn to her right back and flank.

   B. A 42-year-old man with a 3% scald burn to his face and neck.

   C. A 2-year-old girl with 12% partial-thickness burns to bilateral lower extremities.

   D. A 65-year-old man with a history of diabetes mellitus and alcoholism with a 15% partial-thickness burn to his right arm and torso.

   E. A 36-year-old man with 20% partial-thickness burns to his torso and upper extremities sustained during a high-speed motor vehicle collision.

Ref.: 1, 2

COMMENTS: According to American Burn Association guidelines, the following injuries require transfer to a burn center: (1) partial-thickness burns greater than 10% of the TBSA; (2) burns that involve the face, hands, feet, genitalia, perineum, or major joints; (3) full-thickness burns in any age group; (4) electrical burns, including lightening injury; (5) chemical burns; (6) inhalation injury; (7) burns in any patient with preexisting medical disorders that could complicate management, prolong recovery, or affect mortality rate; (8) any patient with burns and concomitant trauma (such as fractures) in which the burn injury poses the greatest risk of morbidity or mortality (in such cases, if the trauma poses the greater immediate risk, the patient may be initially stabilized in a trauma center before being transferred to a burn center); (9) burned children in hospitals without qualified personnel or equipment for the care of children; and (10) burns in patients who will require special social, emotional, or long-term rehabilitative intervention.

ANSWER:
A

5. Which of the following is not a pathophysiologic feature of thermal injury?

A. Increased capillary permeability due to the direct effect of heat and the liberation of vasoactive mediators

B. Increased pulmonary vascular resistance during the immediate postburn period

C. Elevated thyronine (T_3) and thyroxine (T_4) levels

D. Elevated interleukin-6 (IL-6) level

E. Decreased immunoglobulin G (IgG) level

Ref.: 1–3

COMMENTS: Immediately following thermal injury, loss of fluid from the vascular compartment has been attributed to an increase in microvascular permeability due to the direct effect of heat and liberation of humoral factors and cytokines such as histamine, thromboxane A_2, free oxygen radicals, leukotrienes, platelet-activating factor, and interleukins (IL-1, IL-6, and IL-8) from damaged tissues. • Pulmonary vascular resistance increases during the postburn period, and pulmonary edema is rare during fluid resuscitation, even when large volumes of fluid are infused. • The early postburn period is characterized by elevated levels of glucagon, cortisol, and catecholamines and decreased levels of T_3 and T_4. • The IgG level is decreased after burn injury and gradually returns to normal within 2–4 weeks.

ANSWER:
C

6. A 45-year-old man weighing 70 kg sustains second- and third-degree burns to 50% of the TBSA with inhalation injury. Resuscitation is initiated according to the Parkland formula. Which of the following best represents the initial intravenous fluid rate for this patient?

A. 437.5 ml/hr
B. 625 ml/hr
C. 875 ml/hr
D. 732 ml/hr
E. 1000 ml/hr

Ref.: 1, 2

COMMENTS: The Parkland formula is used to estimate the fluid requirements for resuscitation during the first 24 hr after a burn injury. • The patient's response should determine the actual volume administered. • The formula is based on the weight of the patient in kilograms and the percentage of the TBSA burned. • The formula is as follows: 4 ml × patient's weight in kilograms × % TBSA. • The number derived from this formula represents an estimate of the total fluid requirements for the first 24 hr. • Half of this fluid volume is given over the first 8 hr, and the other half is given over the second 16 hr. • For the patient described

in this question, the calculations of the fluid requirements are as follows:

$$4 \text{ ml} \times 70 \text{ kg} \times 50\% \text{ TBSA} = 14{,}000 \text{ ml}$$

$$14{,}000/2 = 7{,}000 \text{ ml over the first 8 hr, } 7{,}000 \text{ ml over second 16 hr}$$

$$7{,}000/8 = 875 \text{ ml/hr for 8 hr}$$

$$7{,}000/16 = 437.5 \text{ ml/hr for 16 hr}$$

These amounts represent guidelines, but the volume infused should be tailored to each individual patient based on his or her response to resuscitation. • Urine output is the most reliable indicator of burn resuscitation in the first 24 hr. • The goal of resuscitation should be a urine output of 0.5 ml/kg/hr in adults and 1.0 ml/kg/hr in children up to 30%. • The infusion rates should be adjusted on an hourly basis to achieve this goal.

ANSWER:
C

7. The patient described in Question 6 undergoes resuscitation according to the Parkland formula. Five hours into the resuscitation, the patient is found to be oliguric. Which of the following would be the next stage in the treatment of this patient?

A. 40 mg of intravenous furosemide
B. Initiation of renal dose dopamine
C. Placement of a Swan-Ganz catheter
D. Renal sonographic studies
E. Increased rate of lactated Ringer's solution infusion

Ref.: 1, 2

COMMENTS: As mentioned in the Comments following Question 6, the Parkland formula provides an estimation of fluid requirements based on the patient's weight and percentage of TBSA burned. • However, the patient's response to the resuscitation is what ultimately determines the fluid requirements. • The Parkland formula is based on body surface area, and it can underestimate additional fluid requirements for patients with concomitant inhalation injury by 40–50%. • Other situations in which the Parkland formula may underestimate fluid requirements are electrical injury, postescharotomy, and alcohol intoxication. • During the first 24 hr after burn injury, oliguria is a result of hypovolemia and should be treated with fluid replacement. • Diuretics are almost never indicated during resuscitation. • Because plasma volume changes are independent of plasma colloid content during the first 24 hr after a burn, colloid-containing fluid resuscitation is of little benefit during this time. • Colloid should be avoided until capillary integrity is restored.

ANSWER:
E

8. Match the topical agent with its characteristics. More than one characteristic may apply.

Topical Agents	Characteristics
A. Sodium mafenide (Sulfamylon)	a. Does not penetrate eschar
B. Silver nitrate 0.5% solution	b. Good penetration of eschar

C. Silver sulfadiazine (Silvadene)

   c. Causes hyperchloremic metabolic acidosis
   d. Methemoglobinemia is a side effect
   e. Can cause transient leukopenia
   f. Causes pain on application
   g. Leaches electrolytes, causing hyponatremia and hypokalemia

Ref.: 1, 2

COMMENTS: The use of clinically effective topical antimicrobial agents has significantly decreased the incidence of invasive burn wound infection and improved the survival of burn patients. • Topical antimicrobial agents act by limiting microbial proliferation in the burn wound until burned tissue can be surgically excised. • **Sodium mafenide (Sulfamylon)** cream, an 11% suspension, is bacteriostatic and readily diffuses through the eschar. • It provides broad-spectrum antimicrobial coverage against most gram-positive and -negative species. • However, it does not provide coverage against methicillin-resistant *Staphylococcus aureus* and offers little antifungal activity. • Sulfamylon is painful on application, and 7% of patients develop hypersensitivity reactions. • It is a potent inhibitor of carbonic anhydrase, with resultant hyperchloremic metabolic acidosis. • **Silver sulfadiazine (Silvadene)** cream is a 1% suspension and is the most commonly used topical agent in burn care. • Like Sulfamylon, it is bacteriostatic and provides broad-spectrum antimicrobial coverage but poorly penetrates the eschar and is painless on application. • Besides poor penetration of eschar, its disadvantages include development of neutropenia, thrombocytopenia, and bacterial resistance and ineffectiveness against some gram-negative bacteria that can be seen several days after initiating therapy. • A **0.5% silver nitrate solution** has broad antimicrobial activity, similar to that of Silvadene. • It is painless on application and does not penetrate eschar. • Side effects include staining of all materials with which it comes in contact (including the patient's skin); leaching of electrolytes, with resultant hyponatremia, hypocalcemia, and hypokalemia; and, infrequently, methemoglobinemia resulting from nitrate-reducing bacteria within the burn wound.

ANSWER:
A-b,c,f; B-a,d,g; C-a,e

9. Which of the following statements regarding the metabolism of burn patients is/are true?

  A. Postburn hypermetabolism is mediated by catecholamine release.

  B. IL-1 and IL-6 levels are elevated in burn injuries and enhance the hypermetabolic response by increasing oxygen consumption.

  C. Elevated core and skin temperature and lower core-to-skin heat transfer are manifested in postburn hypermetabolism.

  D. Blood flow to the muscles in the burned limb increases.

  E. The burn wound preferentially utilizes glucose by anaerobic glycolytic pathways despite increased blood flow to the wound.

Ref.: 1–3

COMMENTS: The metabolic response after burn injuries is related to the extent of burn and is biphasic. • The **ebb** phase begins immediately after injury and is characterized by hypotension, decreased intravascular volume, poor tissue perfusion, and generalized hemodynamic instability. • Histamine, activated complement factors, oxidants, and prostanoids appear to be the major mediators of the ebb phase of the injury response. • During this phase of hypometabolism, metabolic expenditure is decreased and total body oxygen consumption is below normal levels. • Following resuscitation, the **flow** phase of physiologic response starts, wherein cardiac output is restored to normal, usually 24–48 hr after the burn injury. • The metabolic rate begins to rise between the fifth and tenth postburn days and plateaus at levels of 2.0–2.5 times that for an uninjured individual. • This postburn hypermetabolism is manifested by increased oxygen consumption, elevated cardiac output and minute ventilation, increased core temperature, wasting of lean body mass, and increased urinary nitrogen excretion. • Catecholamines (principally norepinephrine) are the major endocrine mediators of the hypermetabolic response. • Recent studies implicate IL-1 and IL-6, tumor necrosis factor, and probably interferon-α in postburn hypermetabolism. • The core temperature, skin temperature, and core-to-skin heat transfer are higher during postburn hypermetabolism because of increased heat production. • Blood flow to the wound increases markedly, exceeding by more than 10 times the blood flow to an equivalent area of uninjured skin. • Blood flow to the muscle in the burned area remains unchanged. • The burn wound utilizes glucose mainly by the anaerobic glycolytic pathway, with no significant change in oxygen consumption compared with that in unburned tissue.

ANSWER:
A, B, E

10. Which of the following can minimize metabolic expenditure in burn patients?

  A. Nursing the patients at ambient temperature below 30°C

  B. Adequate analgesia and sedation

  C. Early excision of the burn and complete wound closure

  D. Early diagnosis and treatment of infection

  E. Use of β-adrenergic blockers

Ref.: 1, 2

COMMENTS: Metabolic expenditure can be minimized by modifying the stressful stimuli. • Central thermoregulation is altered in burn patients, with an upward shift of the temperature of maximal comfort and least metabolic expenditure. • This zone of thermal neutrality is approximately 31–33°C. • Nursing of burn patients at ambient temperatures above 30°C to minimize cold stress has been shown to diminish the metabolic rate. • Pain accentuates metabolic expenditure, and controlled administration of analgesics and sedatives reduces the metabolic rate. • Laboratory studies have shown that early excision and complete wound closure reduce postburn hypermetabolism. • Systemic infection accentuates erosion of body mass, and metabolic expenditure in burn patients can be minimized by early diagnosis and treatment of infection. • Catecholamines are the major endocrine mediators of the postburn hypermetabolic response. • It has been shown experimentally but not clinically that pharmacologic blockade of β-receptors but not α-receptors substantially reduces the intensity of hypermetabolism.

ANSWER:
B, C, D, E

11. Which of the following statements regarding nutrition for burn patients is/are true?

  A. Caloric requirements can be estimated at 25 kcal/kg/day plus 40 kcal/%TBSA/day.

B. Burn patients typically require 1–2 g/kg/day of protein.

C. A calorie/nitrogen ratio of 200:1 is optimal for burn patients.

D. Total parenteral nutrition use is not associated with increased morbidity or mortality rates.

Ref.: 1, 2

COMMENTS: Understanding the hypermetabolic response and its impact on the nutritional demands of burn patients is a critical aspect of burn care. • The metabolic demands of burn patients can increase to 200% those of baseline. • In response to this increased demand, the body mobilizes carbohydrate, fat, and protein stores. • This increased metabolic demand quickly depletes the body's stores and requires exogenous nutritional support to prevent malnutrition. • Caloric requirements can be estimated using several available formulas. • One commonly used formula is the Curreri formula. • According to the Curreri formula, one can estimate the caloric requirements of burn patients by giving 25 kcal/kg/day plus 40 kcal/%TBSA/day. • Another formula multiplies the caloric requirements derived by the Harris-Benedict equation by a factor of 2. • The multiplication by a factor of 2 takes into account the estimated 200% increase in metabolic demand seen in burn patients. • It is important to note that these formulas only provide estimates of the caloric requirements. • Monitoring of nutritional laboratory test results (prealbumin and transferrin level determinations), nitrogen balance, daily weights, and immune function are all useful in determining the actual caloric requirements of individual patients. • Generally, burn patients require 1–2 g/kg/day of protein and should have a calorie/nitrogen ratio of 100:1 or less. • Calories may be delivered either enterally or parenterally. • Both methods are associated with a unique set of complications. • However, as a general rule, only patients who cannot tolerate enteral feedings are given parenteral nutrition.

ANSWER:
A, B

12. Which of the following statements regarding invasive burn wound infection is/are true?

A. Invasive wound infection is common in burns larger than 30% TBSA.

B. It is characterized by conversion of a partial-thickness burn to a full-thickness burn.

C. Definitive diagnosis can be made if quantitative culture of the biopsy specimen recovers more than 10^5 organisms per gram of tissue.

D. Incidence of *Candida* wound infection has increased owing to topical antimicrobial chemotherapy.

E. Topical antimicrobial agents have markedly decreased the incidence of invasive burn wound infection.

Ref.: 1, 2

COMMENTS: All burn wounds become contaminated with a patient's endogenous flora or with the organisms resident in the treatment facility. • Bacterial proliferation may occur beneath the eschar at the viable-nonviable interface, resulting in subeschar suppuration and separation of the eschar. • In a few patients, microorganisms invade the underlying viable tissue, producing invasive burn wound sepsis. • The incidence of invasive burn wound infection is higher in patients with multisystem organ failure or burns over more than 30% of the TBSA. • Gram-negative bacteria, primarily *Pseudomonas* species, are the commonest causative organisms. • Topical chemotherapy has markedly decreased the incidence of invasive bacterial burn wound infection, but the incidence of fungal wound infection has increased. • *Candida* species is the commonest fungus colonizing burn wounds but rarely causes burn wound sepsis. • Invasive burn wound infection is characterized by conversion of a second-degree burn to a full-thickness burn, focal dark-brown to black discoloration of the wound, and unexpectedly rapid eschar separation. • Invasive burn infection can be definitively diagnosed by wound biopsy, and the single most important criterion is the presence of microorganisms in unburned, viable tissue. • The presence of more than 10^5 organisms per gram of tissue is highly suggestive but not diagnostic of invasive burn wound infection.

ANSWER:
A, B, D, E

13. Select the true statements regarding infection in the burn patient.

A. Infection is the most frequent cause of death in burn patients.

B. Cell-mediated immunity is not altered in major burn injuries.

C. Hematogenous pneumonia is the most common pulmonary infection in burn patients.

D. Diminished granulocyte chemotaxis is an important factor in burn infection.

E. Suppurative thrombophlebitis can be a major source of sepsis.

Ref.: 1–3

COMMENTS: The incidence of invasive burn wound infection has been significantly reduced owing to topical antimicrobials, but infection in other organs and tissues is still common and is the most frequent cause of death in burn patients. • Bronchopneumonia has replaced hematogenous pneumonia as the commonest form of pulmonary infection in burn patients. • The decrease in the incidence of invasive burn wound infection has significantly reduced the incidence of hematogenous pneumonia. • Suppurative thrombophlebitis is also a major source of sepsis in burn patients and can occur in any previously cannulated peripheral or even central vein. • In major burns, a high incidence of infection is due to destruction of the mechanical barrier of the skin and global immunosuppression. • Circulating phagocytes, principally neutrophils and macrophages, demonstrate major alterations in function. • Granulocytes exhibit diminished chemotaxis and decreased bactericidal activity due to intracellular elevation of 3,5-cyclic AMP. • Cell-mediated immunity is also impaired after major burn injury, as evidenced by prolonged skin allograft survival.

ANSWER:
A, D, E

14. Which of the following statements regarding administration of antibiotics to burn patients is/are true?

A. Prophylactic systemic antibiotics are indicated for patients with extensive burns.

B. With invasive burn wound sepsis, systemic antibiotics should not be administered before culture and sensitivity results are available.

C. Positive wound culture results should be treated with systemic antibiotics.

D. Antibiotics effective against anaerobic organisms are always indicated for burn wound sepsis.

E. Subtherapeutic serum antibiotic levels are common in burn patients.

Ref.: 1, 2

COMMENTS: Prophylactic antibiotics have no role in the treatment of burns, and their use results in emergence of multiple antibiotic-resistant organisms. • Antibiotics should be used only for a documented infection or presumed sepsis. • Positive wound culture results do not necessarily indicate infection but reflect the organism likely responsible if infection is present. • For patients with invasive burn wound sepsis, administration of systemic antibiotics should be instituted before culture and sensitivity results are available, with the choice of antibiotics based on the sensitivity patterns of microbial flora resident in the burn center, as determined by the microbial surveillance program. • The antibiotic regimen is adjusted as necessary when culture and sensitivity results are available. • Anaerobic infection almost never occurs in burned patients, but anaerobic coverage is indicated rarely in patients with severe muscle necrosis or associated intra-abdominal infection. • Burn patients have altered pharmacokinetics of antibiotics, especially those predominantly excreted by the kidneys, resulting in lower serum levels when the usual recommended dosage is employed.

ANSWER:
E

15. Which of the following statements regarding burn wound excision is/are true?

   A. Excision is indicated for deep partial-thickness and full-thickness burn wounds.

   B. Early excision and closure of burn wounds have been shown to reduce the incidence of invasive burn wound infection, shorten the hospital stay, reduce pain, and improve functional recovery.

   C. Excision should be performed after successful fluid resuscitation.

   D. Tangential excision involves sequential excision of the eschar down to bleeding, viable tissue.

   E. Excision of more than 10% of the TBSA as a single procedure is associated with significant morbidity rates.

Ref.: 1, 2

COMMENTS: Excision is indicated for deep partial-thickness and full-thickness burn wounds. • Early excision and closure of burn wounds decrease the incidence of invasive burn wound infection, shorten the hospital stay, reduce pain, and improve functional recovery. • Excision should be performed after successful fluid resuscitation. • The two most common techniques of excision include tangential excision and fascial excision. • Tangential excision involves sequential excision of the eschar down to bleeding, viable tissue using a guarded dermatome. • Intraoperative hemorrhage may be profuse with tangential excision, so the excision should be limited to a maximum of 20% of the TBSA, 2 hr of operating time, or blood loss equivalent to the patient's blood volume. • Fascial excision is usually performed for very deep full-thickness burns and involves excision of eschar above the deep fascia.

ANSWER:
A, B, C, D

16. Match the items in the two columns.

Skin Coverage	Component Characteristics
A. Biobrane	a. No antimicrobial properties
B. Integra	b. Use complicated by accumulation of exudate, with associated increased risk of wound infection
C. Allograft	c. Wound closure with dermal component
D. Xenograft	d. Provides all normal functions of the skin
	e. May leave dermal equivalent
	f. Provides complete closure of the wound

Ref.: 1

COMMENTS: The advent of synthetic and biologic dressings has provided an alternative to the standard antimicrobial ointments and soaks. • Synthetic and biologic dressings offer the advantage of minimizing pain associated with dressing changes and decrease evaporative wound losses. • Unlike traditional antimicrobial dressings, the synthetic and biologic coverings do not inhibit epithelialization of the burn wound. • **Biobrane** is a synthetic covering made of silicone and collagen. • It is placed over partial-thickness burns while the underlying wound re-epithelializes, or it can be placed over the excised bed of full-thickness burns that are awaiting autografting. • The sheet becomes adherent to the wound within 24–48 hr. • Biobrane has no antimicrobial properties. • Its use is complicated by the accumulation of exudate under the dressing, with a resultant increased risk of wound infection. • **Integra** is a synthetic covering that consists of a collagen matrix with an outer silicone layer. • It is applied to the excised burn wound, and the collagen matrix integrates into the dermis of the wound. • After 2 weeks, the outer silicone layer is removed, and autograft is placed over the integrated collagen layer. • Integra is used for the closure of full-thickness burns and in reconstructive burn surgery. • Like Biobrane, Integra lacks antimicrobial properties and can increase the risk of invasive burn wound infection. • Allograft and xenograft are both biologic dressings that provide complete closure of the burn wound. • **Allograft** is derived from human cadaver donors, and **xenograft** is derived from swine donors. • Both are applied to the excised burn wound in the same manner as autograft. • They mimic the normal barrier and immunologic function of the skin. • Over time, they are rejected by the normal host immune mechanisms and slough off.

ANSWER:
A-a,b; B-a,c,f; C-a,d,e,f; D-a,f

17. Which of the following statements regarding burn wound closure is/are true?

   A. Split-thickness autograft is contraindicated if wound culture results are positive for β-hemolytic streptococci.

   B. Xenograft is the most frequently used and effective biologic dressing when an autograft is not available.

   C. Allograft dressings promote bacterial proliferation.

   D. Cultured autologous keratinocyte sheets can be used for permanent wound coverage with good results.

   E. Dermal substitutes provide better temporary wound coverage than do biologic dressings.

Ref.: 1–3

COMMENTS: The goal of burn wound care is timely, definitive closure. • After excision, the wound is immediately covered with a split-thickness autograft. • A split-thickness autograft is contraindicated if the surface bacterial count is more than 10^5 organisms per square centimeter of wound surface or β-hemolytic streptococci are cultured from the wound. • For large burns, closure of the wound is limited by available autograft. • Therefore, a biologic dressing such as cadaver cutaneous homograft (also called allograft) or xenograft (commonly porcine skin) is used for temporary wound closure. • The homograft is the dressing of choice when an autograft is not available and is the most frequently used biologic dressing. • Cutaneous homograft limits bacterial proliferation in the burn wound; prevents wound desiccation; promotes maturation of granulation tissue; prevents exudative protein and red blood cell loss; decreases wound pain; diminishes evaporative water loss, thus decreasing heat loss; and promotes maturation of granulation tissue. • Xenograft is less effective as a biologic dressing and allows survival of greater numbers of subgraft bacteria, presumably because such tissue is not vascularized by the host. • Cultured autologous keratinocyte sheets have been used for definitive coverage of extensive burn wounds, but these wounds are susceptible to microbial lysis, mechanical trauma, and development of wound contraction and scar formation. • Clinical experience with dermal substitutes such as Biobrane (collagen gel dermal analogue plus a Silastic epidermal analogue) and acellular allodermis has been limited, and their beneficial effects over biologic dressing have not been established.

ANSWER:
A

---

18. Select the true statements regarding inhalation injury.

A. Inhalation injury should be suspected in any patient with a history of closed-space smoke exposure, wheezing, hoarseness, singed nasal hairs, or carbonaceous sputum.

B. Bronchoscopy is the most reliable modality in the diagnosis of inhalation injury.

C. The separation of ciliated epithelial cells from their underlying basement membrane is a hallmark of inhalation injury.

D. Maintaining an open airway and maximizing gas exchange are key components of management.

Ref.: 1–3

COMMENTS: Inhalation injury is a major cause of morbidity and mortality in burn patients. • It should be suspected in any patient with a history of closed-space smoke exposure. • Other indicators of inhalation injury include wheezing, hoarseness, the presence of carbonaceous sputum, and/or singed nasal hairs. • The presence of carbonaceous sputum is the most specific sign of inhalation injury. • The work-up of suspected inhalation injury should include a carbon monoxide level determination. • A normal carbon monoxide level does not exclude the presence of inhalation injury, but an elevated level reflects the presence of a significant inhalation injury. • Bronchoscopy is the most reliable modality for the diagnosis of inhalation injury. • The presence of mucosal erythema, blebs, ulceration, bronchorrhea, and/or carbonaceous material are all indicators of inhalation injury. • Another diagnostic study for detecting inhalation injury is ^{133}Xe ventilation-perfusion lung scanning. • These scans have a diagnostic accuracy of 90% when used alone and 96% when combined with bronchoscopic examination.

The respiratory compromise seen in inhalation injury is related to the increased bronchial blood flow, with resultant interstitial edema and impaired gas exchange. • The release of inflammatory mediators results in increased capillary leak. • The ciliated epithelial cells lining the airways separate from their basement membranes, resulting in the formation of exudate, which eventually forms fibrin casts. • These fibrin casts lead to diminished airway diameter during exhalation (ball-valve effect) with resultant barotrauma. • Other components of inhalation injury include (1) reactive bronchospasm from aerosolized irritants; (2) small-airway occlusion, initially from edema and subsequently from sloughed endotracheal debris and loss of the ciliary clearance mechanism; and (3) microatelectasis from the loss of surfactant. • Maintaining an open airway and maximizing gas exchange are the key components in the

management of airway injury. • Intubation should be initiated early and helps to facilitate aggressive pulmonary toilet, which is essential in these patients. • Pulmonary infection is the most frequent cause of morbidity and mortality after an inhalation injury.

ANSWER:
A, B, C, D

---

19. A 36-year-old electric company employee is brought to the emergency department after sustaining a high-voltage electrical injury while working on a transformer. On primary survey, he is noted to have a cutaneous full-thickness burn on his right hand and a full-thickness burn on his right heel. Initial evaluation of the patient should include which of the following?

A. Electrocardiogram

B. Radiographic evaluation of the spinal column

C. Flexible bronchoscopy

D. Bladder catheterization

E. Lower-extremity angiograms

Ref.: 1–3

COMMENTS: Approximately 5% of all burn injuries are the result of electrical injuries. • Tissue damage is due to conversion of electrical energy to thermal energy. • Electricity causes injury by direct contact, conduction, arc, and secondary ignition. • Electrical injuries are generally classified into two types: low voltage and high voltage. • **Low-voltage** injuries usually result from exposure to household currents ranging from 110 to 220 volts. • These injuries result in thermal injury with little or no effect on the deeper tissues. • **High-voltage** (>1000 volts) injuries result in significant tissue damage. • Patients with high-voltage injury require a complete trauma evaluation, cardiac monitoring because of the high frequency of cardiopulmonary arrest and arrhythmia, serial evaluation of extremities involved for compartment syndrome, and urine monitoring for myoglobinuria. • Tetanic contractions of the paravertebral muscles can cause axial spine fractures. • Because of this, all patients with high-voltage electrical injury should have spinal immobilization followed by radiologic evaluation of the spinal column to assess for fractures. • The risk of acute renal failure is high in electrical burn patients because of myoglobinuria from muscle injury and underestimation of the fluid requirement due to misleadingly small cutaneous lesions overlying an area of devitalized tissue. • As a result, these patients must be aggressively resuscitated with alkalinization of the urine by administering intravenous sodium bicarbonate. • This therapy prevents the precipitation of myoglobin pigments within the renal glomeruli. • The goal of fluid resuscitation of these patients is a urine output of 2 ml/kg/hr, and the amount of intravenous fluid should be adjusted throughout the resuscitation phase to achieve this goal. • The presence of elevated compartment pressures represents a surgical emergency and must be treated with fasciotomy of the involved compartment to prevent limb loss and worsening myoglobinuria. • Complications following electrical injury include polyneuritis, quadriplegia, hemiplegia, transverse myelitis, cataracts, liver necrosis, intestinal perforation, focal pancreatic necrosis, and focal gallbladder necrosis. • An increased incidence of cholelithiasis has been reported to occur within 2 years of electrical injury. • Lightning injury, an unusual form of electrical injury, commonly produces immediate cardiopulmonary arrest due to electrical paralysis of the brain stem, and burns are characteristically superficial and exhibit a serpiginous and arborizing pattern.

ANSWER:
A, B, D

20. Which of the following statements regarding chemical injuries is/are true?

    A. Immediate wound care involves application of a neutralizing agent.

    B. Acid burns cause liquefaction necrosis.

    C. Alkali burns produce deeper injuries than do acid burns.

    D. Hydrofluoric acid burns may result in life-threatening hypocalcemia.

    E. Coal tar burn is best treated with immediate application of a petroleum-based ointment.

Ref.: 1, 2

COMMENTS: Chemical burns frequently result from accidental exposure to household agents. • The extent of damage caused by chemical exposure is related to the chemical nature of the substance, the concentration of the chemical, and the duration of exposure. • Burns resulting from chemical exposure cause a thermal injury from the energy produced during the reaction of acids and bases with the skin. • Tissue injury is also caused by protein denaturation, oxidation, and tissue desiccation. • Immediate wound care is essential. • Irrigation with copious amounts of water or saline solution will dilute or remove the chemical agent, thereby minimizing further damage and absorption. • As a general guideline, all significant chemical exposures should be irrigated with 15 to 20 L of water or saline solution. • The application of a neutralizing agent may generate heat and increase the amount of tissue damage and is therefore contraindicated. • An acid burn causes coagulation necrosis of tissue, and the coagulated tissue acts as a barrier for further acid penetration. • In contrast, an alkali burn causes liquefaction necrosis. • Thus, there is no barrier of coagulated tissue, resulting in more invasive injury. • Hydrofluoric acid, an occupational hazard, is a highly corrosive acid that produces deep-tissue injury. • The hydrogen ions of hydrofluoric acid produce coagulation necrosis, and free fluoride ions cause liquefaction and penetrate deeply to form salts with calcium and magnesium. • The formation of calcium salts diminishes serum calcium levels and may result in life-threatening hypocalcemia. • Administration of calcium gluconate is the most effective treatment for relieving pain and terminating the invasive tissue destruction. • Calcium gluconate reacts with hydrofluoric acid to form inactive calcium fluoride and can be used by local application as a gel, a local injection, or regional intravenous perfusion. • Hot coal tar causes direct thermal injury. • Immediate cooling of tar with cold water is the most important treatment, and any attempt to remove the adherent tar may accentuate the cutaneous injury. • After cooling, adherent tar should be covered with petroleum-based ointment to solubilize the tar and facilitate removal.

ANSWER:
C, D

21. Select the true statements regarding postburn sequelae.

    A. All second- and third-degree burns produce permanent scarring.

    B. The incidence of hypertrophic scar formation is less after excision and skin grafting than with wounds that heal spontaneously.

    C. Hypertrophic scars are best treated by early excision and wound closure.

    D. Burn scar hypopigmentation and irregularities can be significantly improved by dermabrasion and thin split-thickness skin grafting.

    E. Basal cell carcinoma is the most common carcinoma in an old burn scar.

Ref.: 1, 2

COMMENTS: All second- and third-degree burns produce permanent scarring. • Hypertrophic scar formation, one of the most troublesome sequelae of cutaneous burns, typically develops in deep partial-thickness and third-degree burns that heal spontaneously. • Hypertrophy after excision and skin grafting occurs less frequently and is dependent on the time from injury to excision, the anatomic part involved, and the surgical technique employed. • Hypertrophic scars are best treated with elastic garments until the scar matures (3–6 months in adults and up to 4 years in children), followed by excision and skin grafting of the residual scar. • Many burn wounds heal with hypopigmentation and irregular scar formation, which can be significantly improved by dermabrasion and thin split-thickness skin grafting. • Malignancy is a rare complication in unstable burn scars and is referred to as a Marjolin's ulcer. • The latent period for malignant change ranges from 1 to 75 years, with a mean of approximately 35 years. • Although basal cell carcinoma has been described in old burn scars, it is exceedingly rare, and most Marjolin's ulcers are squamous cell carcinomas.

ANSWER:
A, B, D

REFERENCES

1. Schwartz SI, Shires GT, Spencer FC, et al (eds): *Principles of Surgery*, 7th ed. McGraw-Hill, New York, 1999.
2. Sabiston DC Jr: *Textbook of Surgery*, 15th ed. Saunders, Philadelphia, 1997.
3. Greenfield LJ: *Surgery: Scientific Principles and Practice*, 2nd ed. Lippincott-Raven, New York, 1997.

CHAPTER 18

Surgical Infections

David M. Simon, M.D., Wahab Brobbey, M.D., and Miguel Madariaga, M.D.

1. A patient comes to the hospital with 2 weeks of fever, chills, cough, and right-sided pleuritic chest pain. The patient has been otherwise healthy and does not take any medication. He does not have any allergies. He has traveled recently to Texas. His physical examination revealed an icteric young man with a fever of 102°F (38.9°C) and tender hepatomegaly. There are decreased breath sounds in the right lower lobe. A computed tomographic (CT) scan of the chest and abdomen reveals a mass in the right lobe of the liver compatible with an abscess. Which of the following empiric antibiotic therapies should be used?

A. Ampicillin, gentamicin, and clindamycin

B. Levofloxacin and gentamicin

C. Vancomycin, clindamycin, and amikacin

D. Piperacillin/tazobactam and metronidazole

E. Imipenem and clindamycin

Ref.: 1

COMMENTS: The patient has a liver abscess, and the two possible causes are bacterial or amebic. • The symptoms of both may be similar, and clinical differentiation between them is usually not possible. • If the abscess is close to the diaphragm it may produce cough, pleuritic chest pain, or pain radiating to the right shoulder. • Diagnosis can be made by requesting serologic studies for ameba or by obtaining an aspirate of the fluid collection. • Before identifying the etiologic agent, the empiric antimicrobial treatment must cover polymicrobial bacterial infection (including aerobic gram-negative rods and anaerobes) as well as *Entamoeba histolytica*.

Gentamicin and levofloxacin have good coverage for gram-negative organisms. • Clindamycin and metronidazole cover anaerobes. • In addition, metronidazole is the antimicrobial of choice for *E. histolytica*. • Imipenem and piperacillin/tazobactam cover both gram-negative organisms and anaerobes. • The best combination in this case is piperacillin/tazobactam and metronidazole. • When using piperacillin/tazobactam or imipenem, it is not necessary to add additional "anaerobic coverage." In this case, metronidazole is added only for its amebicidal activity.

ANSWER:
D

2. A patient with recurrent duodenal ulcer is referred for surgical consultation. He has been having recurrent abdominal pain for the last 2 years. Fifteen months ago, an upper endoscopy showed a duodenal ulcer. The patient was treated with ranitidine and his condition improved, but the symptoms recurred. Before considering surgery, the clinician repeated an upper endoscopy. A *Campylobacter*-like organism (CLO) test result was positive. The clinician decided to treat the patient with a combination of two antibiotics and proton-pump inhibitors for 2 weeks. Which of the following tests to assess eradication of *Helicobacter pylori* should be performed after completion of treatment.

A. Urea breath test

B. CLO test

C. Biopsy and culture

D. Serum antibody (by ELISA)

E. Stool antibody test

Ref.: 2

COMMENTS: Surgery in the treatment of peptic ulcers is indicated only in the following circumstances: intractable hemorrhage, perforation, and obstruction. • The patient does not have any of these conditions, and *H. pylori*, the most important pathophysiologic factor for the development of duodenal ulcer, was never adequately treated. • The treatment options for *H. pylori* are numerous, but they must always include an H2-blocker or a proton-pump inhibitor plus at least two antibiotics. • The antibiotics most commonly used are amoxicillin, clarithromycin, and metronidazole. • Bismuth-containing regimens have also been used. • Depending on the combination used, the length of treatment varies from 2 to 4 weeks.

Methods of diagnosing *H. pylori* can be divided into two categories: invasive and noninvasive. • Biopsy and the CLO test require an endoscopy, while all the other tests do not. • Like the CLO test, the urea breath test takes advantage of the ability of *H. pylori* to split urea. • However, the urea breath test only requires the patient to "blow," whereas the CLO test is conducted on a piece of tissue. • The serologic test for *H. pylori* antibody is useful but of limited value in determining the success of therapy. • There is no stool "antibody" test for *H. pylori*, but there is a stool antigen test, which is as sensitive as the urea breath test.

Since there is no need to repeat an endoscopy in this patient, the clinician must consider the relative merits of the noninvasive methods. • Because antibody test results may remain positive after treatment, the best choice is the urea breath test, which determines the presence of live *H. pylori*.

ANSWER:
A

3. A woman is recovering well after surgery for appendicitis complicated by secondary peritonitis. Cefazolin (Ancef) was given perioperatively. On her third day of hospitalization, urine culture reveals *Candida* spp. and *Enterococcus faecalis*. The patient has remained afebrile since surgery, and her vital signs are stable. Her physical examination reveals an intubated young woman who is awake and calm. Her abdomen is soft and nontender. She has a urinary catheter in place. Her white blood cell count is 5.4 with a normal differential count. Urinalysis revealed many white blood cells, many epithelial cells, and many bacteria. Which of the following is the best treatment for this woman?

A. Resume cefazolin.

B. Start fluconazole and vancomycin.

C. Start amphotericin B and linezolid.

D. Start amphotericin B bladder washes and vancomycin.

E. There is no need for antimicrobials.

Ref.: 1

COMMENTS: A positive culture result does not always indicate infection or need for treatment. • Urinary catheters predispose to urinary tract infections. • However, infections generally produce symptoms such as fever, abdominal pain, dysuria, frequency, and leukocytosis. • This patient has contaminated urine (many epithelial cells) with colonization by several microorganisms. • There is no need to treat her. • It may be advisable to change or remove her catheter and repeat a urinanalysis and urine culture. • When more than one organism is seen in the urine, it is most likely a contaminated sample.

A N S W E R :
E

4. A 10-year-old boy who recently immigrated from Mexico has had a 2-day illness characterized by fever, odynophagia, dysphagia, and drooling at the mouth. Physical examination reveals a toxic child with a temperature of 102°F (38.9°C), tachycardia, and tachypnea. There is mild tenderness in the submandibular area and few palpable lymph nodes. The suspected diagnosis is epiglottitis, which is confirmed with a CT scan of the neck. Blood culture results are positive. What kind of organism will likely be seen on the Gram's stain?

A. Gram-positive cocci in pairs and chains

B. Gram-positive cocci in clusters

C. Slender gram-negative rods

D. Gram-negative coccobacilli

E. Spirochetes

Ref.: 1

COMMENTS: The patient has acute epiglottitis, most likely due to *Haemophilus influenzae* type B, which is recovered from the blood in up to 100% of cases. • Classically, the patient is a 2- to 4-year-old boy with a short history of fever, irritability, dysphonia, and dysphagia, which can occur at any time of the year. • However, the widespread use of *H. influenzae* type B vaccine in developed countries has led to a marked decline in invasive disease due to this organism. • The disease is still common in developing countries. • *Haemophilus* are gram-negative coccobacilli.

A N S W E R :
D

5. A 68-year-old woman is admitted to the hospital for neurosurgery after being found comatose at home. The patient lives alone, but her neighbor states that she has been "acting strangely" for the last several weeks. No additional history is available. Magnetic resonance imaging (MRI) of the brain reveals evidence of focal cerebritis and enlarged ventricles, with enhancement of the basilar meninges. A chest radiograph shows upper lobe consolidation. Results of a rapid human immunodeficiency virus (HIV) test are positive. The patient is taken to the operating room for placement of a ventricular drain. After surgery, which type of isolation is needed?

A. Standard precautions

B. Airborne precautions

C. Droplet precautions

D. Contact precautions

E. Reverse isolation

Ref.: 3

COMMENTS: This HIV-infected patient has evidence of meningitis, cerebritis, and upper lobe pneumonia. • The unifying diagnosis is pulmonary and cerebral tuberculosis. • This patient requires airborne precautions.

A variety of infection control measures are implemented to decrease the risk of transmission of microorganisms in hospitals. • Standard precautions are used for the care of all patients. • Hand washing between patient contacts and the use of barrier protection, such as gloves, gowns, and masks, to minimize exposure to potentially infectious body fluids (e.g., blood, feces, wound drainage, etc.) are important components of standard precautions and all infection-control programs.

In addition to standard precautions, airborne precautions are used for patients with known or suspected illness transmitted via small airborne droplets (≤5 μm). • Tuberculosis, measles, smallpox, and varicella (chickenpox) are examples of diseases requiring airborne precautions. • Because these organisms can be dispersed widely by air currents and may remain suspended in the air for long periods of time, they necessitate special air handling and ventilation. • Patients requiring airborne precautions are placed in "negative pressure" rooms, and all persons entering the room require an N-95 mask.

In addition to standard precautions, droplet precautions are used for patients with suspected or proven invasive disease due to *H. influenzae* and *Neisseria meningitidis* (e.g, pneumonia, meningitis, or sepsis) or other respiratory illnesses, such as diphtheria, pertussis, pneumonic plague, influenza, mumps, and rubella. • Droplets produced by these illnesses are usually generated by coughing but are larger than the droplets described above (>5 μm), travel only short distances (<3 feet), and do not remain suspended in air. • Patients require a private room, and persons entering the room require a surgical mask.

In addition to standard precautions, contact precautions apply to specific patients infected or colonized with epidemiologically important organisms spread by direct contact with a patient or contact with items in the patient's environment. • These organisms may demonstrate antibiotic resistance and include methicillin-resistant *Staphylococcus aureus* (MRSA), vancomycin-resistant *S. aureus* (VRSA), vancomycin-resistant enterococci (VRE), and multidrug-resistant gram-negative bacilli. • Enteric pathogens such as *Clostridium difficile* and skin infections such as impetigo (group A streptococci), herpes simplex, and scabies also require contact precautions.

A N S W E R :
A, B

6. A diabetic patient has been discharged recently from the hospital after an intracranial bleed. He is readmitted for aspiration pneumonia. His condition rapidly deteriorates, with hypotension and multiorgan dysfunction. Which of the following treatments is/are contraindicated?

   A. Volume resuscitation

   B. Antibiotics

   C. Activated protein C

   D. Intensive insulin therapy for hyperglycemia

   E. Low-dose hydrocortisone

   Ref.: 4

COMMENTS: Severe sepsis is defined by multiorgan dysfunction with or without shock and is due to a generalized inflammatory and procoagulant response to infection. • Efforts to improve the outcome using anticytokine therapy along with antibiotics and supportive care have until recently not been associated with improved survival. • Recently, a randomized, double-blind, placebo-controlled, multicenter trial evaluating recombinant activated protein C demonstrated a survival benefit in patients with severe sepsis. • However, activated protein C treatment was associated with an increased risk of bleeding and is contraindicated for patients with recent hemorrhagic stroke. • Fluid resuscitation and antibiotics are mainstays in the treatment of sepsis. • Intensive insulin therapy that maintains serum glucose levels at 80–110 mg/dl reduces morbidity and mortality in critically ill patients. • The mechanism is unknown, but it is possible that correcting hyperglycemia may improve neutrophil function. • The use of corticosteroids for sepsis remains controversial. • High doses of corticosteroids may in fact worsen outcomes by increasing the frequency of secondary infections. • However, low doses of corticosteroids may be beneficial for septic patients who may have "relative" adrenal insufficiency despite elevated levels of circulating cortisol. • Although the issue is controversial, the use of low-dose hydrocortisone is not contraindicated in this patient.

ANSWER:
C

7. A patient who develops angioedema after the administration of penicillin is scheduled for a craniotomy to ablate a seizure focus. Which of the following choices is/are appropriate for antibiotic prophylaxis?

   A. Cefazolin from the time of surgery and then for 7 days

   B. No antibiotic prophylaxis

   C. Vancomycin at the time of induction and then for 3–5 days

   D. Vancomycin at the time of induction

   E. Vancomycin and gentamicin at the time of induction

   Ref.: 5, 6

COMMENTS: The degree of wound contamination (clean versus contaminated procedure) combined with host factors (e.g., diabetes, advanced age, obesity, immunodeficiency, and nutritional status) and procedure-related factors (e.g., presence of foreign material and degree of trauma to host tissues) determine the overall risk for the development of surgical site infection (SSI). • Despite state-of-the-art aseptic technique, bacterial contamination of the surgical wound is inevitable. • Microorganisms that colonize the skin, such as *S. aureus,* coagulase-negative staphylococci, and streptococci, are the commonest wound pathogens, particularly during clean procedures. • SSI associated with contaminated procedures are frequently polymicrobial and are due to the normal flora of the entered viscus (i.e., coliforms and anaerobic bacteria associated with colonic procedures). • Prophylactic antibiotics are clearly indicated for most clean-contaminated and contaminated procedures and effectively decrease the rate of SSI. • Antibiotic prophylaxis of clean surgery remains controversial in certain cases. • However, when bone is incised, as in craniotomy, sternotomy, and placement of orthopedic hardware, antibiotic prophylaxis has proven efficacy in decreasing the incidence of SSI. • Antibiotics selected for clean procedures must have excellent activity against skin microorganisms. • Cefazolin is the usual choice. • However, as in this case, severe penicillin allergy prevents the use of other β-lactams, including cephalosporins and the carbepenems. • Vancomycin is the usual alternative. • Studies have demonstrated that clindamycin and trimethoprim/sulfamethoxazole may also be effective prophylactic agents for neurosurgical procedures. • The timing of antibiotic administration is critical and for best results should be given within 30 minutes of surgical incision. • Redosing during a prolonged procedure is recommended to maintain serum concentrations. • The duration of antibiotic prophylaxis following surgery remains a source of disagreement, although administration of antibiotics beyond 24 hr is rarely indicated.

ANSWER:
D

8. Endocarditis prophylaxis is recommended for which of the following patients?

   A. A patient with mitral valve prolapse without murmur undergoing rigid bronchoscopy

   B. A patient with a history of rheumatic fever with normal cardiac valves undergoing prostatic biopsy

   C. A patient with a prosthetic aortic valve undergoing endoscopic retrograde cholangiography for biliary obstruction

   D. A patient with severe hypertrophic cardiomyopathy undergoing tympanostomy tube insertion

   E. A patient previously treated for streptococcal endocarditis undergoing tonsillectomy

   Ref.: 7

COMMENTS: Although the incidence of endocarditis following most procedures in patients with underlying cardiac disease is low, certain patients are considered to be higher risk, primarily based on poorer prognosis if endocardial infection occurs. • The overall risk of endocarditis is determined by type of cardiac lesion and type of procedure known to be associated with significant bacteremia. • Individuals at highest risk for endocarditis are those who have prosthetic cardiac valves, a previous history of endocarditis, or complex cyanotic heart disease. • Moderate-risk cardiac lesions include hypertrophic cardiomyopathy, mitral valve prolapse with mitral insufficiency, and valvular disease secondary to rheumatic fever. • Patients considered at high or moderate risk for endocarditis undergoing bacteremia-producing procedures—such as endoscopic retrograde cholangiopancreatography (ERCP), sclerotherapy for esophageal varices, esophageal stricture dilatation, tonsillectomy, bronchoscopy with a rigid bronchoscope, prostate surgery, and cystoscopy—probably benefit from antibiotic prophylaxis. • However, antibiotic prophylaxis is not indicated for procedures such as endotracheal intubation, tympanostomy tube insertion, and urethral catheterization in the same patients. • The American Heart Association recommendations summarize the current approach to endocarditis prevention and provide specific antibiotic recommendations.

ANSWER:
C, E

9. A patient has HIV infection. His last CD4 count was 50 cells/mm³, and his viral load was 100,000 copies per milliliter. He comes to the hospital with sudden onset of right hemiparesis. He has been afebrile. A CT scan and an MRI of the brain show multiple ring-enhancing lesions in the left cerebral hemisphere. The *Toxoplasma* IgG antibody test result is positive. He has received pyrimethamine and sulfadiazine for 12 days. Neurologically, the patient is stable. Which of the following is the next best step?

A. Repeat an MRI of the brain.

B. Continue the same antibiotic therapy for an additional 10 days and reassess.

C. Switch treatment to pyrimethamine and clindamycin and reassess if the patient clinically does not improve after another 10–14 days.

D. Add corticosteroids to the treatment regimen.

E. Perform a positron emission tomographic (PET) or single photon emission computed tomography (SPECT) scan.

Ref.: 29

COMMENTS: Up to 90% of HIV-infected patients with advanced disease (CD4 <100 cells/mm³) with multiple ring-enhancing lesions and a positive *Toxoplasma* IgG antibody test result have cerebral toxoplasmosis. • Empiric treatment with pyrimethamine, sulfadiazine, and folinic acid is recommended. • Most patients with central nervous system (CNS) toxoplasmosis respond rapidly to this therapy, with nearly 90% of patients demonstrating neurologic improvement at 2 weeks. • Radiographic improvement occurs at a slower pace, with approximately 50% improvement on repeat MRI of the brain occurring within 3 weeks of initiating treatment. • For patients who do not improve by 2 weeks, a brain biopsy is indicated. • Although lymphoma is the most likely alternative diagnosis in AIDS patients with CNS lesions, up to 25% of brain biopsy specimens reveal toxoplasmosis. • Thallium 201 (SPECT) or PET may provide useful information, since a "cold" lesion revealed by SPECT or hypometabolic lesions seen by PET scanning are consistent with infection. • However, false-positive and -negative results can occur with these functional imaging studies. • Pyrimethamine plus sulfadiazine or clindamycin are considered first-line therapy for toxoplasmosis. • The addition of corticosteroids may be useful for treatment of increased intracranial pressure. • However, this anti-inflammatory effect may make interpretation of clinical and radiographic responses difficult.

ANSWER:
A

10. Which of the following statements regarding the collection of blood cultures is/are true?

A. The optimal timing for drawing a blood culture is approximately 1 hr before the onset of fever.

B. Blood collected via intravascular devices for culture should be paired with blood obtained by peripheral venipuncture.

C. At least two sets of blood cultures should be obtained for any patient with suspected bacteremia.

D. A minimum of 10 ml of blood should be collected for each set of cultures.

E. All are correct.

Ref.: 8

COMMENTS: Early studies demonstrated that rigors and fever often follow bacteremia by 30–90 minutes. • Since circulatory phagocytes are generally effective in removing bacteria from the bloodstream, collection of blood culture should occur as early as possible in the course of a febrile episode. • Good data document that two or three sets of blood cultures containing at least 10 ml of blood per set are adequate for demonstrating most episodes of bacteremia or fungemia. • After adequate skin antisepsis, peripheral venipuncture sites are preferred for blood collection for culture. • Central venous catheters are frequently used for blood collection but should be paired with a peripheral blood draw to aid in the interpretation of a positive test result. • A positive blood culture result obtained from intravenous catheters combined with a negative result from a blood culture obtained from a peripheral site may represent only colonization of the line and not true bacteremia.

ANSWER:
E

11. Which of the following statements regarding anaerobic bacterial infections is/are true?

A. Anaerobic bacteria are common inhabitants of skin and mucous membranes.

B. *Bacteroides* spp. are the commonest isolates in intra-abdominal anaerobic infections.

C. If appropriate cultures are obtained, anaerobes are found in over 75% of intra-abdominal abscesses.

D. Proper treatment of anaerobic infections consists of surgical drainage, débridement of necrotic tissue, and appropriate antibiotic therapy.

E. All of the above are true.

Ref.: 1

COMMENTS: Anaerobic bacteria are normal inhabitants of the skin, mucous membranes, and gastrointestinal tract. • In fact, anaerobic bacteria outnumber aerobic organisms by more than 10:1 in the oral cavity and by more than 1000:1 in the colon. • Therefore, it is not surprising that anaerobes are cultured from up to 90% of intra-abdominal abscesses. • The commonest pathogens in this group are *Bacteroides* spp. *Bacteroides fragilis* is an important co-pathogen in the pathogenesis of intra-abdominal abscesses. • As with most serious infections, proper treatment involves appropriate drainage of abscesses and débridement of devitalized tissue when present, as well as appropriate antibiotic therapy. • Antibiotics with excellent broad-spectrum anaerobic activity include the carbapenems (imipenem, meropenem, and ertapenem), β-lactam/β-lactamase combinations (ampicillin/sulbactam, ticarcillin/clavulanate, and piperacillin/ tazobactam), and metronidazole. • Although the second-generation cephalosporins (i.e., cefoxitin and cefotetan) and clindamycin also have anaerobic coverage, over the past decade an increase in resistance among *Bacteroides* to these agents has been observed. • For example, as many as 30% of *B. fragilis* isolates are resistant to clindamycin.

ANSWER:
E

12. Which of the following statements regarding methicillin-resistant *S. aureus* (MRSA) is/are true?

   A. MRSA is a common nosocomial pathogen, but it can also be detected in the community.

   B. The treatment of choice is vancomycin.

   C. MRSA is more virulent than methicillin-sensitive *S. aureus*.

   D. Hospitalized patients colonized with MRSA require contact isolation.

   E. Treatment of surgical patients with intranasal mupirocin decreases wound infection rates due to this bacteria.

Ref.: 10–12

COMMENTS: Staphylococci are the commonest cause of nosocomial infections in surgical patients. • Recent reports suggest that carriage of MRSA into the community has increased, and more infections with this organism are being seen among persons without health care-associated risks (nosocomial risks).

At the beginning of the antibiotic era, *S. aureus* was susceptible to penicillins. • Resistance developed to penicillin via β-lactamase production, and new antibiotics were discovered, including the penicillinase-resistant penicillins (methicillin, oxacillin, nafcillin, etc). • MRSA is by definition methicillin-resistant. • Methicillin is not used in clinical practice because it induces interstitial nephritis, but it is still used in the laboratory to differentiate methicillin-susceptible *S. aureus* (MSSA) from MRSA. • Vancomycin or linezolid can be used to treat MRSA. • *S. aureus* strains with intermediate susceptibility to vancomycin (VISA) and vancomycin-resistant *S. aureus* (VRSA) have been reported in the United States.

Although some studies suggest that there is a significant increase in mortality from infections caused by MRSA compared to MSSA, the increased death rate is most likely due to comorbidities and not to differences in virulence between MSSA and MRSA. • Hospitalized patients colonized with MRSA require contact isolation to avoid the spread of the bacteria to other patients. • A recent prospective, randomized, placebo-controlled study showed that intranasal mupirocin did not significantly reduce *S. aureus* surgical site infections. • However, it did significantly reduce the rate of all nosocomial *S. aureus* infections among the patients who were *S. aureus* carriers.

ANSWER:
A, B, D

13. Which of the following statements is/are true?

   A. The use of a disinfectant in the preparation of skin for surgery is a standard of care.

   B. Sterilization of the skin is achieved by using antiseptics such as povidone-iodine.

   C. Hydrogen peroxide is an excellent antiseptic that may be used for cleansing of surgical wounds.

   D. Hexachlorophene is the antiseptic of choice in preparing skin for surgery.

   E. None of the above is true.

Ref.: 13

COMMENTS: The safety of modern surgery is enhanced by the ability to reduce the number of bacteria in the vicinity of the operative field. • An **antiseptic** is a chemical agent that either kills or inhibits the growth of pathogenic organisms. • By custom and law, this term refers only to agents applied to the body. • A **disinfectant** is a chemical used on inanimate objects to kill pathogenic organisms. • Antiseptic and disinfectant chemicals do not kill all organisms. • Sterilization, on the other hand, is the process of killing all microorganisms (bacteria, viruses, parasites, fungi, and spores). • This can be achieved through pressurized steam, dry heat, chemicals, or radiation.

Commonly used antiseptics for skin cleansing include chlorhexidine, hexachlorophene, iodine compounds, alcohol, and hydrogen peroxide. • Povidone-iodine (Betadine) is available as a 10% solution, and at that dilution it is considered both safe and effective for use in contaminated traumatic wounds. • In contrast, povidone-iodine surgical scrub (Betadine scrub) and hexachlorophene (pHisoHex) may be harmful to tissues and may increase infection rates when used in wounds. • In addition, hexachlorophene can be neurotoxic and teratogenic if absorbed through the skin. • Peroxide is a cytotoxic agent that may damage newly formed epithelium and should not be used in granulating wounds.

ANSWER:
E

14. Which of the following statements regarding hand hygiene is/are true?

   A. Health-care workers (HCWs) should clean their hands with an antiseptic-containing agent before and after each contact with a patient.

   B. The use of soap and water for hand washing is required when hands are visibly soiled with blood or body fluids.

   C. Adherence to hand hygiene guidelines by HCWs is generally good.

   D. Alcohol-based hand rubs are inferior to antimicrobial soaps for hand decontamination.

   E. Vancomycin-resistant enterococci (VRE) and MRSA are frequently isolated from hands of HCWs.

Ref.: 14

COMMENTS: Hand washing by HCWs may be the single most effective measure for preventing nosocomial infection. • The spread of bacteria, particularly antibiotic-resistant organisms, such as MRSA and VRE, from contaminated HCWs to patients is well documented. • Despite recommendations to wash hands before and after all contacts with patients, adherence to such policies by HCWs has been poor. • Although hand washing with soap and water is required when hands are visibly soiled with blood, the widespread use of alcohol-based hand rubs by HCWs between patient contacts may decrease spread of resistant bacteria to patients. • Alcohol-based products are superior to antimicrobial soaps for standard hand decontamination. • Alcohol-based hand rubs have the broadest spectrum of antimicrobial activity among available hand hygiene products, and their use results in rapid reduction in microbial skin counts. • The ability to make these rubs available at the entrance to patients' rooms, at the bedside, or in pocket-sized containers to be carried by HCWs may improve compliance with hand-hygiene policies. • The Centers for Disease Control has recently published guidelines for hand hygiene in heath-care settings that include recommendations for hand-washing antisepsis, hand-hygiene techniques, and surgical hand antisepsis.

ANSWER:
A, B, E

15. Which of the following statements regarding tetanus prophylaxis is/are true?

  A. A patient has a minor, clean wound. His second tetanus shot was 4 years ago. He requires a dose of tetanus toxoid. Antitetanus immunoglobulin is not required.

  B. A patient has a minor, clean wound. He has never received tetanus vaccine. He requires both tetanus toxoid and antitetanus immunoglobulin.

  C. A patient has a dirty wound. He completed three tetanus shots when he was a child but has not had a tetanus booster in 20 years. He is immune and does not require additional toxoid or antitetanus immunoglobulin.

  D. A patient has a dirty wound. He does not remember when and how many tetanus shots he received in the past. He requires a toxoid dose. Antitetanus immunoglobulin is also required.

Ref.: 15

COMMENTS: Approximately 100 cases of tetanus occur in the United States annually. • Tetanus occurs in nonimmune individuals after a penetrating injury is inoculated with spores of *Clostridium tetani*. • With appropriate local anaerobic conditions, these spores germinate and produce a neurotoxin, tetanospasmin, which is responsible for the signs and symptoms of tetanus. • The majority of cases of tetanus occur in older adults (age > 60 years) who have waning immunity. • The need for active immunization with tetanus toxoid and/or passive immunization with human tetanus immunoglobulin depends on the nature of the wound and the immune status of the patient. • Tetanus toxoid and immunoglobulin are indicated for patients with dirty (tetanus-prone) wounds who have received fewer than three doses of tetanus toxoid in the past or whose immunization status is unknown. • Dirty wounds include wounds contaminated with feces, saliva, or soil and wounds related to punctures, gunshots, crush injury, burns, or frostbite. • Tetanus toxoid is indicated only for patients with dirty wounds who have received three doses of toxoid more than 10 years ago and have not received a booster within 5 years of the injury. • Patients with clean, minor wounds require tetanus toxoid if they have received fewer than three doses of toxoid less than 10 years ago and have not received a booster or the patient's immune status is unknown. • Immunocompromised patients receiving chemotherapy or hematopoietic stem cell transplant (HSCT) recipients may be at increased risk for tetanus. • HSCT recipients begin reimmunization with tetanus toxoid 12 months posttransplant.

A N S W E R :
A, D

16. Match each agent in the left-hand column with one or more mechanisms of antimicrobial action in the right-hand column.

  A. Carbapenems   a. Impairment of bacterial DNA synthesis
  B. Aminoglycosides   b. Inhibition of cell wall synthesis
  C. Quinolones   c. Disruption of ribosomal protein synthesis
  D. Cephalosporins   d. Disruption of cell wall cation homeostasis
  E. Vancomycin   e. Disruption of cytoplasmic membrane

Ref.: 30

COMMENTS: All the antimicrobial agents listed are **bactericidal** (i.e., their associated mechanisms of action result in bacterial death).

• **Bacteriostatic** agents (e.g., tetracyclines, chloramphenicol, erythromycin, clindamycin, and linezolid) act by preventing bacterial growth but do not result in bacterial death. • They work primarily through inhibition of ribosomal protein synthesis. • Both carbapenems and cephalosporins are β-lactam antibiotics and hence have a similar mode of activity. • Enzymes located within the bacterial cytoplasmic membrane are responsible for peptide cross-linkage. • These enzymes are called penicillin-binding proteins (PBPs) and are the site at which β-lactam drugs bind. • This binding interferes with bacterial cell wall synthesis, eventually resulting in cell lysis. • Gram-negative bacteria contain a variable number of various PBPs. • Each β-lactam antibiotic has various affinities for the various PBPs. • Vancomycin is a glycopeptide that also inhibits bacterial cell wall synthesis and assembly. • Vancomycin complexes to cell wall precursors, preventing elongation and cross-linkage, making the cell susceptible to lysis. • This antibacterial activity is limited to gram-positive organisms. • Aminoglycosides bind irreversibly to the 30S bacterial ribosome and interfere with protein synthesis. • For this to take place, they must penetrate the cell wall, which occurs optimally under aerobic conditions. • Unlike other antibiotics that inhibit protein synthesis, aminoglycosides are bactericidal. • This feature is secondary to their disruptive effect on calcium and magnesium homeostasis within the cell wall. • Quinolones inhibit topoisomerase II (DNA gyrase) and topoisomerase IV, impairing DNA synthesis in bacteria. • Appreciation of the mechanism of action of antimicrobials may have a bearing on the selection of alternative therapies when bacterial resistance to the drug of choice develops.

A N S W E R :
A-b; B-c,d; C-a; D-b; E-b

17. Which of the following statements concerning cephalosporins is/are correct?

  A. Cefazolin (Ancef) is a reasonable choice for nosocomial urinary tract infection.

  B. Cefoxitin monotherapy is effective for the treatment of hospital-acquired intra-abdominal sepsis.

  C. Ceftriaxone is effective against *Pseudomonas aeruginosa*.

  D. Cefepime is effective against enterococci.

  E. All of the above are false.

Ref.: 1

COMMENTS: Cephalosporins are chemically similar to penicillins and have similar mechanisms of action and toxicities. • Because cephalosporins are more stable in the presence of bacterial β-lactamases, they have a broader spectrum of antibacterial activity than do penicillins. • Cephalosporins are loosely classified into four major groups, or generations, based mainly on the spectrum of antimicrobial activity. • In general, first-generation cephalosporins have better coverage for gram-positive organisms, and later generations exhibit improved activity against gram-negative bacteria. • Cefazolin (Ancef) is a first-generation cephalosporin that has good coverage for gram-positive cocci. • It also covers some community-acquired gram-negative bacteria, such as *Escherichia coli*, but its gram-negative coverage is not adequate, and resistance to it is common. • Ancef is not appropriate treatment for nosocomial urinary tract infection. • Cefoxitin is a second-generation cephalosporin that has demonstrated efficacy in the treatment of intra-abdominal, pelvic, and gynecologic infections. • These infections generally are due to facultative gram-negative bacilli and anaerobic organisms, especially *Bacteroides fragilis*. • However, approximately 15% of *B. fragilis* isolates may be resistant. • Nosocomially acquired organisms, such as Enterobacteriaceae and *S. aureus,* may be resistant to cefoxitin, making cefoxitin monotherapy a poor choice for nosocomial intra-abdominal infections. • Ceftriaxone is a third-generation cephalosporin widely used for community-acquired pneumonia and meningitis. • It has excellent coverage against *Streptococcus pneumoniae.* • This cephalosporin does not cover *P. aeruginosa,* but other third-generation cephalosporins, such as ceftazidime, do. • Cefepime is a fourth-generation cephalosporin that combines the spectrum of first- and third-generation cephalosporins. • This agent has broad activity against Enterobacteriaceae, *P. aeruginosa,* and methicillin-susceptible *S. aureus.* • However, cefepime has poor activity against enterococci and *B. fragilis.*

ANSWER:
E

18. Adverse events associated with the use of quinolones include which of the following?

   A. Tendinitis and possible tendon rupture

   B. Seizures

   C. Arthropathy in children

   D. *C. difficile* colitis

   E. Narrowing of the QT interval

Ref.: 1

COMMENTS: The quinolones are antibiotics that exert their bactericidal effect by inhibiting topoisomerase II (DNA gyrase) and topoisomerase IV, impairing DNA synthesis. • These antibiotics have a broad spectrum of activity covering many gram-positive cocci, but they are not active against MRSA, and some of them, such as ciprofloxacin, may not adequately treat infections due to *S. pneumoniae,* gram-positive bacilli (anthrax), and many gram-negative species. • Gatifloxacin and moxifloxacin have anaerobic activity. • Most quinolones also have activity against *Mycobacterium tuberculosis* and atypical respiratory pathogens such as *Mycoplasma pneumoniae, Chlamydia pneumoniae,* and *Legionella* spp. Adverse effects of quinolones include gastrointestinal intolerance, antibiotic-associated colitis, cutaneous reactions, hepatotoxicity (trovafloxacin was withdrawn from the market for this reason), QT interval prolongation (leading to ventricular arrhythmias), and Achilles tendon rupture. • Quinolone use is generally avoided in children, because animal studies suggest that these drugs cause cartilage erosion. • However, children receiving quinolones have rarely experienced joint symptoms, which appear to be reversible. • Results of MRI studies performed to identify subclinical cartilage damage have been negative.

ANSWER:
A, B, C, D

19. Which of the following is/are characteristic of aminoglycosides?

   A. Active against a broad spectrum of gram-negative aerobes and useful for synergy against some gram-positive cocci

   B. No emergence of resistant bacterial strains

   C. Narrow margin between therapeutic and toxic blood levels

   D. Nephrotoxicity, ototoxicity, and neuromuscular paralysis

   E. Excellent activity in abscesses where gram-negative organisms are involved

Ref.: 1

COMMENTS: Until the mid-1980s, aminoglycosides were the only reliable empiric treatment for serious gram-negative infections. • However, the introduction of third-generation cephalosporins, extended-spectrum penicillins, carbapenems, and quinolones has reduced the frequency of use of aminoglycosides. • The aminoglycoside mechanism of action involves irreversible binding to the 30S bacterial ribosome. • However, aminoglycosides must first penetrate the cell wall, and, since this step is oxygen dependent, it does not occur under anaerobic conditions. • For this reason, aminoglycosides have no activity against anaerobic bacteria or facultative bacteria in an anaerobic environment (e.g., an abscess). • Aminoglycosides are useful against gram-negative aerobes, including *P. aeruginosa,* and they are effective as synergistic agents (usually in combination with a β-lactam or vancomycin) against *Staphylococcus epidermidis, S. aureus,* and enterococci. • Resistance to aminoglycosides does occur. • Selection of an aminoglycoside should be based on local patterns of resistance. • Aminoglycosides are difficult to use clinically because of their low ratio of therapeutic-to-toxic level. • Monitoring serum concentrations of aminoglycocides is usually required for safe and therapeutic blood levels. • The two major toxic side effects are nephrotoxicity and ototoxicity. • The ototoxicity, both auditory and vestibular, is potentially more significant because it is nonreversible and cumulative. • The auditory toxicity affects response to the higher frequencies, making early detection difficult. • The nephrotoxicity is usually a dose dependent, reversible, acute tubular necrosis, producing nonoliguric renal failure. • Paralysis can occur after aminoglycoside administration and is due to inhibition of presynaptic release of acetylcholine and postsynaptic blockade of acetylcholine receptors at the neuromuscular junction. • Neuromuscular blockade is a rare but potentially lethal event. • This risk is increased in patients receiving tubocurare, succinylcholine, or similar agents and in patients with myasthenia gravis. • This effect is reversible with intravenous administration of calcium carbonate.

ANSWER:
A, C, D

20. Which of the following statements regarding secondary peritonitis is/are true?

   A. It usually occurs as a result of perforation of an intra-abdominal viscus.

   B. Carbapenems, aminoglycosides, and fourth-generation cephalosporins have equal efficacy in treatment studies.

   C. Increased age, cancer, cirrhosis, and systemic illness are factors that increase the mortality rate.

   D. Sequestration of bacteria within fibrin clots leads to intra-abdominal abscess formation.

   E. The most common bacteria cultured from the abdomen is *E. coli.*

Ref.: 1, 9

COMMENTS: Secondary peritonitis usually occurs as a result of perforation of an intra-abdominal viscus: perforated peptic ulcer, appendix, or diverticulum or penetrating gastrointestinal trauma. • The infection is polymicrobial, with facultative aerobes and anaerobes acting synergistically. • One study revealed an average of 2.5 anaerobes and 2 facultative aerobes identified per case of secondary peritonitis. • *E. coli* is the commonest isolate in culture. • *Bacteroides* spp. are the commonest anaerobes cultured from abdominal infections. • About 10^{12} bacteria reside in the colon per gram of feces, with 90% of these bacteria being anaerobic organisms. • Any process that impairs immunologic function or is associated with general debilitation increases mortality. • Age, cancer, hepatic cirrhosis, and the presence of a systemic illness have been shown to increase mortality. • One of the defense mechanisms of the peritoneal cavity is the production of fibrin to sequester bacteria to limit systemic spread. • This sequestration leads to the formation of intra-abdominal abscesses that generally require drainage for cure. • Treatment of secondary peritonitis requires surgical intervention for removal of the source of infection and eradication of residual bacteria with systemic antibiotics. • Antibiotic selection should include agents with broad-spectrum coverage for facultative aerobes, gram-negative bacilli, and anaerobes. • Carbapenems are a good empiric choice for treatment. • Aminoglycosides and fourth-generation cephalosporins lack anaerobic activity.

ANSWER:
A, C, D, E

---

21. For which of the following are perioperative antibiotics indicated?

A. Perforated appendix

B. Open fracture of the humerus

C. Mastectomy

D. Traumatic colonic perforation

E. Elective cholecystectomy

Ref.: 9

COMMENTS: Surgical wounds can be classified according to the risk of infection. • Clean wounds are defined as nontraumatic in origin. • There is no evidence of inflammation encountered during surgery and no breaks in surgical technique occur. • There must also not be a breach of the respiratory, alimentary, or genitourinary tract. • A good example of a clean surgical wound is a mastectomy wound. • Generally, antibiotic prophylaxis is not needed for such procedures. • However, in cases of clean-contaminated or contaminated wounds, the use of perioperative antibiotics is indicated. • A clean-contaminated wound is a nontraumatic wound in which a minor break in surgical technique occurs or in which the respiratory, gastrointestinal, or genitourinary tract has been entered without significant spillage. • Examples include transection of the appendix or cystic duct in the absence of acute inflammation or entrance into the biliary or genitourinary tract without evidence of infected bile or urine. • Some debate exists regarding antibiotic prophylaxis for elective open and laparoscopic cholecystectomy. • Several studies suggest that wound infection rates are similar among patients whether they receive prophylactic antibiotics or not. • However, patients considered at high risk for infectious complications, including patients 60 years of age or older, those undergoing procedures with evidence of acute inflammation, common bile duct stones, or jaundice likely benefit from perioperative antibiotics. • Patients who have had previous biliary tract operations or ERCP should also receive perioperative antibiotics. • Contaminated wounds include traumatic wounds (e.g., open fractures) and wounds from operations involving a major break in surgical technique, such as gross spillage from the gastrointestinal tract or entrance into the genitourinary or biliary tract in the presence of acute infection. • This category also includes dirty wounds, defined as old traumatic wounds with devitalized tissue, and those involving existing clinical infections, such as perforated appendix.

ANSWER:
A, B, D

---

22. Match the skin lesion in the left-hand column with the etiologic microorganism in the right-hand column.

A. Purpura fulminans   a. *N. meningitidis*
B. Ecthyma gangrenosum   b. *Staphylococcus. aureus*
C. Painless chancre   c. *Bacillus anthracis*
D. Impetigo   d. *P. aeruginosa*
                    e. *Streptococcus pyogenes*
                     (group A streptococci)

Ref.: 1

COMMENTS: The appearance and distribution of skin lesions during a febrile illness can provide important clues to the cause of infection. • Purpura fulminans occurs in the setting of overwhelming sepsis and disseminated intravascular coagulation. • The meningococcus or *S. pneumoniae* are the usual pathogens, although invasive group A streptococci and *S. aureus* can produce similar skin changes. • The confluence of petechial and purpural lesions produces extensive hemorrhage and necrotic patterns over the trunk and extremities. • Ecthyma gangrenosum develops in the setting of *Pseudomonas* bacteremia. • Painless, round lesions with indurated borders and necrotic centers develop from initial bullous lesions. • Cutaneous anthrax is characterized by the development of a chancreform lesion at the site of incubation with spores from *B. anthracis*. • After a short incubation period (1–3 days), a painless papule develops, enlarges, and then vesiculates with surrounding nonpitting edema. • Bloodstream invasion may occur and is associated with high mortality rates. • Impetigo is a contagious superficial infection of the skin. • The skin lesions begin as vesicles that rapidly pustulate and rupture. • The purulent discharge dries and creates the crusts that characterize this disease. • *S. aureus* and/or group A streptococci are usually cultured from these lesions.

ANSWER:
A-a,b,e; B-d; C-c; D-b,e

---

23. Which of the following statements regarding clostridial infections is/are true?

A. The presence of clostridial organisms in a surgical or traumatic wound warrants immediate antibiotic administration and surgical intervention.

B. The oxidation-reduction potential in contaminated tissues is a significant factor in the development of a clostridial infection.

C. Despite the potentially fulminant course of clostridial infections, the skin overlying clostridial cellulitis may not be discolored or edematous.

D. Clostridial myonecrosis (gas gangrene) should be treated with immediate surgical debridement, antibiotics, and hyperbaric oxygenation.

E. A frozen section of soft tissue without polymorphonuclear infiltrates rules out the diagnosis of clostridial myonecrosis.

Ref.: 1

COMMENTS: Clostridial organisms are ubiquitous and are a common contaminant of traumatic wounds. • In most wounds, however, the high oxidation-reduction potential of the surrounding healthy tissues prevents colonization and invasion of these tissues. • In such cases, the presence of clostridia is clinically insignificant. • When colonization with clostridia occurs in the presence of necrotic tissue, their proliferation and invasion of other tissue can occur, leading to clostridial cellulitis. • This form of clostridial infection is confined to the superficial fascial planes, and, although it may spread rapidly, systemic effects may be mild and the skin of normal color. • Clostridial myonecrosis occurs when the deeper muscular compartments are invaded, usually by *Clostridium perfringens*. • The inaccessibility of systemic antibiotics to this ischemic, necrotic tissue, coupled with the low oxidation-reduction potential of such wounds, permits rapid dissemination of the clostridia through the muscular compartments. • Symptoms of clostridial myonecrosis are variable: pain out of proportion to the physical examination findings; systemic toxicity; a rapidly spreading zone of cellulitis; bronzing of the skin; and a thin, watery, brown discharge. • Gram's staining reveals large numbers of gram-positive rods and an absence of neutrophils. • In the appropriate clinical setting, an innocuous appearance of the postoperative wound does not exclude the possibility of clostridial sepsis. • Therapy should include immediate surgical débridement and antibiotic therapy (penicillin G plus clindamycin). • Adjuvant hyperbaric oxygen treatment may be helpful, but it has not been evaluated in a randomized, controlled trial.

ANSWER:
B, C, D

24. Which of the following statements regarding diabetic foot infections is/are true?

A. Foot infection occurs more frequently in diabetic than in nondiabetic patients.

B. The saline injection-aspiration method is the preferred method for obtaining reliable cultures.

C. Diabetic foot infections are commonly polymicrobial.

D. Osteomyelitis of the foot is frequently encountered in patients with a long history of diabetes and neuropathic ulcers.

E. Bone scan is the method of choice for diagnosing foot osteomyelitis in diabetics.

Ref.: 1

COMMENTS: Diabetic patients have more infections of the lower extremities because of risk factors such as vascular insufficiency, decreased sensation, hyperglycemia, and impairment of the immune system, particularly neutrophil dysfunction. • The most reliable results of culture are obtained by deep-tissue biopsy of the infected foot. • Diabetic foot infections commonly are polymicrobial. • Although gram-positive aerobic cocci are the most commonly isolated species, anaerobic bacteria and aerobic gram-negative bacilli are also frequently isolated. • These various microorganisms act synergistically in initiating and perpetuating infection. • Because of this synergy and the decreased perfusion secondary to vascular impairment, these infections may necessitate higher than normal doses of antimicrobial agents to achieve therapeutic antibiotic tissue levels. • In addition to antibiotics, early incision and drainage of abscess with débridement of devitalized tissue, immobilization, and supportive care are important in the total management of the diabetic foot. • In the presence of significant vascular insufficiency, revascularization of the distal lower extremity may improve healing and prevent amputation. • Radioactive studies using technetium 99 (bone scan) or gallium citrate or indium-labeled leukocyte scans have poor specificity and should not routinely be performed. • Results of these studies are difficult to interpret in the presence of chronic ulcers and bone degeneration from chronic neuropathy. • MRI has become the radiographic study of choice for diagnosing osteomyelitis.

ANSWER:
A, C, D.

25. Which of the following clinical situations or laboratory results require(s) systemic antifungal therapy?

A. A single positive blood culture result obtained from an indwelling intravascular catheter

B. *Candida endophthalmitis*

C. Oral candidiasis

D. *Candida* isolated from a drain culture in a patient who recently underwent surgery for colonic perforation

E. None of the above

Ref.: 1

COMMENTS: Candidemia is associated with significant morbidity (e.g., endocarditis, septic arthritis, and ophthalmitis) and mortality (approximately 40%). • The management of candidemia, particularly in patients with intravascular devices, remains controversial. • Although some patients—usually immunocompetent patients—spontaneously clear the bloodstream with removal of the intravascular device, other patients—particularly those who are immunosuppressed—have disseminated disease and require systemic antifungal therapy. • There are no accurate diagnostic tests or methods for selecting high-risk patients to determine which patients require systemic antifungal therapy. • Therefore, all patients with at least one positive blood culture result for *Candida* should be treated with an antifungal agent. • All nonsurgically implanted lines should be removed, and, if continued central venous access is required, a new line should be placed at a new site (not exchanged over a guide wire). • Some would attempt to sterilize the bloodstream without removal of tunneled catheters or subcutaneous ports. • However, in cases of persistent candidemia or septic shock, these devices should also be removed. • Amphotericin B or fluconazole appear to have similar efficacy for treatment of candidemia. • Voriconazole and caspofungin are new antifungal agents that are also effective against *Candida*. • These agents may be particularly useful for nonalbican species such as *Candida krusei* or *Candida glabrata,* which are less susceptible to fluconazole. • All patients with candidemia should be evaluated for manifestations of disseminated disease, such as ocular involvement or osteomyelitis. • *Candida* identified from a surgical drain most likely represents colonization and does not require systemic antifungal therapy. • Mucocutaneous candidiasis can be treated with local nystatin or clotrimazole.

ANSWER:
A, B

26. Which of the following statements regarding antifungal agents is/are true?

A. Voriconazole is at least as effective as amphotericin B against invasive aspergillosis.

B. Intravenous voriconazole is relatively contraindicated in patients with renal failure.

C. Voriconazole causes irreversible visual changes.

D. Caspofungin is at least as effective as amphotericin B for the treatment of invasive candidiasis and, more specifically, candidemia.

E. Caspofungin is effective in the treatment of cryptococcal meningitis.

Ref.: 16, 17

COMMENTS: Voriconazole is a broad-spectrum triazole that is active against *Aspergillus* spp. Voriconazole is a selective inhibitor of the fungal cytochrome P-450 system utilized in the production of ergosterol for cell membrane synthesis. • A randomized trial comparing voriconazole with amphotericin B for primary therapy of invasive aspergillosis showed that initial therapy with voriconazole led to better responses and improved survival. • The survival rate at 12 weeks was 70.8% in the voriconazole group and 57.9% in the amphotericin B group, and voriconazole resulted in fewer severe side effects than did amphotericin B. • In patients with a creatinine clearance rate of less than 50 ml/min, voriconazole should be given orally (not intravenously), since the intravenous vehicle (cyclodextrin) may accumulate and cause liver failure. • Patients receiving voriconazole may experience episodes of visual changes, which are reversible. Caspofungin is an echinocandin with an antifungal spectrum that includes *Candida* spp. and *Aspergillus* spp. but not *Cryptococcus neoformans*. • Caspofungin inhibits the synthesis of β-(1-3)-D-glycan, an essential component of the cell wall present in susceptible organisms. • A recent study showed that the clinical outcome with caspofungin was similar to that with amphotericin B for the primary treatment of invasive candidiasis and candidemia.

ANSWER:
A, B, D

27. Match each clinical characteristic or agent in the left-hand column with the correct infecting organism or organisms in the right-hand column.

A. Fibrosing mediastinitis	a. *Candida albicans*
B. Amphotericin	b. *Nocardia asteroides*
C. Intertrigo	c. *Actinomyces israelii*
D. Brain abscess	d. *Cryptococcus. neoformans*
E. Pelvic mass	e. *Histoplasma capsulatum*

Ref.: 1, 18

COMMENTS: Amphotericin B remains an important agent for the treatment of systemic mycotic infections, including candidiasis, mucormycosis, cryptococcosis, histoplasmosis, coccidiodomycosis, sporotrichosis, and aspergillosis. • Amphotericin B is a fungicidal agent. • Binding of amphotericin B to ergosterol in fungal cell membrane alters permeability, with leakage of intracellular ions and macromolecules leading to cell death. • Adverse events such as infusion reactions and nephrotoxicity are common with the conventional (deoxycholate) form of the drug. • New lipid formulations of amphotericin B have been developed and are associated with a reduction in toxicity without sacrificing efficacy. • Newer triazoles (voriconazole and posiconazole) and echinocandins (caspofungin, micafungin, and anidulafungin) are emerging as alternative broad-spectrum antifungal agents. • Histoplasmosis is predominantly a pulmonary infection caused by *H. capsulatum*, a dimorphic fungus, endemic to the Mississippi and Ohio River valleys and along the Appalachian Mountains. • Histoplasmosis has been associated with massive enlargement of the mediastinal lymph nodes due to granulomatous inflammation. • During the healing process, fibrotic tissue can cause postobstructive pneumonia or constriction of the esophagus or the superior vena cava, producing dysphagia and/or superior vena cava syndrome. • Actinomycosis is caused by a group of gram-positive higher-order bacteria that are part of the normal flora found in the oral cavity, gastrointestinal tract, and female genital tract. • Typically, infections due to *Actinomyces* spp. occur often after disruption of mucosal surfaces and lead to oral and cervical disease, pneumonia with empyema, and intra-abdominal or pelvic abscesses. • Intrauterine device placement has been associated with pelvic abscess due to this organism. • Sinus tract formation is common as these organisms extend, unrestricted, through tissue planes. • High-dose penicillin and surgical drainage are generally required

for cure. • *Nocardia* spp., another higher-order bacteria, are found in soil, organic matter, and water. • Human infection occurs after inhalation or skin inoculation. • Chronic pneumonia can occur, usually in immunocompromised patients. • Skin lesions and brain abscesses are common with disseminated infection.

Prolonged treatment with sulfonamides in combination with other antibiotics is required for cure. • *C. neoformans* causes meningitis and pulmonary disease. • Infection is common in the setting of immunodeficiency, e.g., organ transplantation, autoimmune deficiency syndrome (AIDS), but may also occur in immunocompetent hosts. • *C. albicans* is a common inhabitant of the mucous membranes and the gastrointestinal tract. • Intertrigo is one form of cutaneous candidiasis that occurs in skin folds, where a warm moist environment exists. • Vesiculopustules develop, enlarge, and rupture, causing maceration and fissuring. • Obese and diabetic patients are at risk of developing candidal intertrigo. • Local care including nystatin powder is usually effective.

ANSWER:
A-e; B-a,d,e; C-a; D-b; E-c

28. Which of the following statements is/are correct regarding spontaneous bacterial peritonitis (primary peritonitis) in a cirrhotic patient?

A. Infection is usually polymicrobial.

B. Ascitic fluid culture results are always positive.

C. The most likely pathogenic mechanism is translocation from the gut.

D. Five days of antibiotic treatment may be adequate.

E. Infection-related mortality has declined to less than 10%.

Ref.: 19, 20

COMMENTS: Spontaneous bacterial peritonitis (SBP) is a monomicrobial infection. • Enteric gram-negative rods account for 60–70% of episodes of SBP. • *E. coli* is the most frequently recovered pathogen, followed by *Klebsiella pneumoniae*. • Streptococcal species, including pneumococci and enterococci, are also important pathogens. • Ascitic fluid culture results are negative in many cases, but inoculation of blood culture bottles at the bedside yields bacterial growth in approximately 80% of cases. • SBP most likely develops from the combination of prolonged bacteremia secondary to abnormal host defense, intrahepatic shunting, and impaired bactericidal activity of ascetic fluid. • Transmural migration of gut flora and transfallopian spread of vaginal bacteria to the peritoneal space may also occur. • Initial antimicrobial treatment should include coverage against aerobic gram-negative organisms. • A third-generation cephalosporin, such as cefotaxime or ceftriaxone, is a reasonable choice. • Duration of antibiotic treatment is unclear. • Two weeks has been suggested, but shorter courses (5 days) may have similar efficacy. • Although the in-hospital mortality rate approaches 40%, infection-related mortality has declined significantly (10%). • Unfortunately, the probability of recurrence is 70% at 1 year with 1- and 2-year survival rates of 30% and 20%, respectively.

ANSWER:
D, E

29. Which of the following patients with cirrhosis benefit(s) from prophylactic antibiotic therapy to decrease risk of SBP?

A. Patients awaiting liver transplantation

B. Patients hospitalized with acute gastrointestinal bleeding

C. Patients with ascitic fluid protein levels of less than 1g/100 ml

D. Patients who have recovered from a previous episode of SBP

E. All of the above

Ref.: 20

COMMENTS: Randomized trials have demonstrated that secondary prophylaxis with oral norfloxacin 400 mg/day or trimethoprim/sulfamethoxazole five times per week decreases the risk of recurrent SBP from 68% to 20%. • However, overall mortality in these patients is unchanged compared to patients not receiving secondary prophylaxis. • Another observation is that long-term quinolone use has been associated with the development of infection due to quinolone-resistant bacteria. • Approximately 30–40% of patients with cirrhosis hospitalized for acute gastrointestinal bleeding develop infection during hospitalization. • Norflaxocin (400 mg twice a day for 7 days) decreased the incidence of infective episodes due to gram-negative bacteria. • The risk of SBP increases tenfold in patients with an ascitic fluid protein concentration less than 1g/100 ml fluid. • Norfloxacin 400 mg a day during hospitalization decreases the incidence of SBP in these patients as well. • Patients hospitalized awaiting liver transplantation likely have one of the risk factors for SBP, as described in the Comments for Question 28, and therefore may benefit from antibiotic prophylaxis. • Active infection is a contraindication for liver transplantation.

A N S W E R :
E

30. Which of the following is/are important risk factors for the transmission of HIV to the surgeon after a percutaneous injury?

A. Source patient has advanced HIV infection with a CD4 T-cell count of <50 cells/mm³.

B. Surgeon sustains deep puncture injury.

C. Visible blood was present on sharp object causing the injury.

D. Injury from a device that had entered a blood vessel of the source patient before injury.

E. All of the above.

Ref.: 29

COMMENTS: The risk of HIV transmission after percutaneous exposure to HIV-infected blood is about 0.3%. • The risk is influenced by several factors, including depth of the injury and the presence of undiluted blood on the device causing injury. • Exposure to blood from patients in the terminal stages of AIDS, which likely reflects high titers of circulating virus, also increases the risk to HCWs. • Although no prospective study demonstrating benefit from postexposure prophylaxis with antiretroviral agents has been completed, a retrospective case control study suggests that, in those who received zidovudine prophylaxis after exposure, the odds of HIV infection were reduced significantly (by approximately 80%). • Postexposure prophylaxis, which now includes at least two antiretroviral agents, should be started immediately (within 72 hr) for high-risk injuries.

A N S W E R :
E

31. A 32-year-old HIV-positive intravenous drug user is admitted to the hospital following a seizure. Examination reveals a right

pronator drift. An MRI study of the brain reveals two ring-enhancing lesions. Which of the following diagnoses should be considered?

A. Progressive multifocal leukoencephalopathy (PML)

B. Glioblastoma multiforme

C. Toxoplasmosis

D. Lymphoma

E. Bacterial endocarditis

Ref.: 29

COMMENTS: With the widespread use of highly active antiretroviral therapy, the incidence of neurologic disease among HIV-infected individuals has declined. • Major HIV-related CNS diseases include AIDS-dementia complex, meningitis, myelopathy, opportunistic infections (e.g., cryptococcosis, PML due to JC virus, cytomegalovirus [CMV], herpes, and toxoplasmosis), and neoplasms (primary CNS lymphoma). • For patients with advanced HIV disease (CD4 T-cell count <100 cells/mm³) who have focal neurologic disease and ring-enhancing lesions on brain imaging, the two major diagnostic considerations are toxoplasmosis and primary CNS lymphoma. • PML is also a possibility in AIDS patients, but CNS lesions are usually not associated with cerebral edema. • One should also consider non-HIV-associated conditions, including primary brain tumors such as glioma and bacterial brain abscess, which may occur in the setting of bacterial endocarditis and intravenous drug abuse. • Current management recommendations for HIV patients with focal brain lesions include approximately 2 weeks of empiric therapy for toxoplasmosis, followed by brain biopsy if radiographic or clinical deterioration occurs.

A N S W E R :
B, C, D, E

32. During an emergency appendectomy, a surgical resident sustained an injury from a contaminated hollow-bore needle with spontaneous bleeding. Which one of the following blood-borne organisms is most likely to be transmitted, assuming the patient was infected with all of them?

A. HIV

B. Hepatitis B

C. Hepatitis C

D. Malaria

E. Syphilis

Ref.: 1

COMMENTS: All the organisms mentioned are potentially transmissible through the exposure described above. • After a significant exposure to blood-borne pathogens, the risk is about 30% for acquiring hepatitis B, 3% for hepatitis C, and 0.3% for HIV. • Malaria and syphilis may be acquired through blood transfusion, and acquisition through a needle-stick is theoretically possible. • Because of the high risk associated with hepatitis B exposure, it is recommended that all HCWs be vaccinated against hepatitis B. • In the event that a nonimmune HCW is exposed to hepatitis B, it is recommended that he or she receive hepatitis B immunoglobulin within 7 days of the exposure and also start a vaccination series. • Postexposure prophylaxis with antiretroviral drugs may be indicated after exposure to

HIV-infected blood. • There is no postexposure prophylaxis available against hepatitis C.

ANSWER:
B

33. A 68-year-old man with a history of diabetes, hypertension, and peripheral vascular disease has been diagnosed with persistent *Salmonella* bacteremia. The patient's only complaints are fever and back pain. A transesophageal echocardiogram was normal. Which of the following tests should be recommended to confirm the clinical suspicion?

   A. CT scan of the chest and abdomen

   B. Duplex ultrasound of the lower extremities

   C. Explorative laparotomy

   D. Bone marrow culture and stool culture

   E. No need to confirm diagnosis

Ref.: 1

COMMENTS: The patient has persistent bacteremia without evidence of cardiac involvement. • However, an endovascular infection, such as an infected aortic atherosclerotic aneurysm, is a likely diagnosis in this patient. • *S. aureus* and *Salmonella* spp. are common pathogens infecting preexisting atherosclerotic vessels. • MRI, CT scanning, and sonographic studies may reveal the presence of an aneurysm but often may not provide adequate preoperative detail. • Nuclear studies, such as gallium- or indium-labeled leukocyte scans, may help localize intra-arterial infection, but they have low sensitivity (<30%). • Although antibiotic therapy is needed in this disease, the vascular lesion is rarely sterilized, and aneurysmal enlargement with rupture is the rule. • A high index of suspicion is required for early diagnosis, since mortality rates exceed 80% if rupture recurs. • If possible, perioperative angiography is usually performed to better delineate the extent of the aneurysm and operative approach.

ANSWER:
A

34. Therapy for a person infected with HIV and a CD4 T-cell count below 50 cells/mm^3 may include which of the following?

   A. Two nucleoside reverse transcriptase inhibitors and one protease inhibitor

   B. Two nucleoside reverse transcriptase inhibitors and one nonnucleoside reverse transcriptase inhibitor

   C. Trimethoprim/sulfamethoxazole

   D. Azithromycin once a week

   E. All of the above

Ref.: 22

COMMENTS: Further understanding of the pathogenesis of HIV infection, combined with an increase in the number of available antiretroviral agents, has made treatment of HIV-infected individuals more complex. • The decision to initiate antiretroviral therapy is based on a patient's prognosis, which is best determined by plasma HIV RNA (viral load) and CD4 T-cell count. • Most experts agree that patients with CD4 T-cell counts of less than 200 cells/mm^3, regardless of plasma HIV RNA values, should receive antiretroviral therapy. • Current guidelines recommend considering treatment of asymptomatic HIV-infected adults who have CD4 T-cell counts

less than 350 cells/mm^3 and/or HIV RNA counts of greater than 55,000 copies/ml. • Combination therapy employing more than three antiretroviral agents demonstrates a more durable suppression of HIV replication and preservation of immunologic function than does single or dual drug therapy. • Effective antiretroviral regimens include two nucleoside reverse transcriptase inhibitors (zidovudine, lamivudine, stavudine, didanosine, abacavir, or tenofovir) plus a protease inhibitor (indinavir, nelfinavir, amprenavir, lopinavir, ritonavir, or atazanavir) or a nonnucleoside reverse transcriptase inhibitor (efavirenz or nevirapine). • Failure of a multidrug regimen may be due to poor adherence or development of drug-resistant virus. • Resistance testing may provide guidance for antiretroviral drug selection in treatment-experienced patients. • Another important aspect of care of patients with AIDS is the use of prophylaxis against common opportunistic infections. • Trimethoprim/sulfamethoxazole is recommended for prophylaxis against *Pneumocystic carinii* when the CD4 T-cell count is less than 200 cells/mm^3. • *Mycobacterium avium* complex infection is a late complication in AIDS patients with CD4 T-cell counts lower than 50 cells/mm^3 and can be prevented using weekly azithromycin.

ANSWER:
E

35. A surgical resident sustains a needle stick with a hollow-bore needle contaminated with blood of a patient who is hepatitis B antigen positive. The resident completed a series of three hepatitis B vaccines 1 year ago, but his antibody response was not checked. Which of the following statements describes the management of this case?

   A. There is no need to do anything, since the source does not have active hepatitis B infection.

   B. The resident needs a booster of hepatitis B vaccine.

   C. The resident should receive hepatitis B immunoglobulin immediately.

   D. The resident should receive hepatitis B immunoglobulin (HBIG) and a hepatitis B vaccine booster immediately.

   E. The resident needs to be tested for anti-hepatitis B antibody immediately. If the test result is negative, then proceed as in alternative D.

Ref.: 23

COMMENTS: HCWs who sustain injuries from needles contaminated with blood containing hepatitis B virus have a risk as high as 62% of developing serologic evidence of hepatitis B infection. • The source patient is hepatitis B antigen positive, which is an indication of active hepatitis B infection. • The resident has been vaccinated against hepatitis B, but his immune status is unknown and should be determined. • If the resident is anti-hepatitis B antibody positive, no intervention is necessary. • However, if he is anti-hepatitis B antibody negative, HBIG (which can be given up to 7 days after the exposure) and a hepatitis B vaccine booster should be administered. • If the resident was never vaccinated, then he should immediately receive HBIG and begin hepatitis B vaccination series.

ANSWER:
E

36. A patient with AIDS who has never been treated with anti-retroviral therapy is admitted to the hospital after 2 weeks of

fever and with postprandial right upper quadrant pain. His serum alkaline phosphatase level is elevated, and a sonographic gallbladder study reveals thickened gallbladder walls, with pericholecystic fluid but no evidence of gallstones. Which of the following organisms may be responsible for this clinical syndrome?

A. Cytomegalovirus (CMV)

B. Cryptosporidium

C. *Campylobacter* spp.

D. *Toxoplasma gondii*

E. *Rhodococcus equi*

Ref.: 29

COMMENTS: Patients with HIV infection are prone to acalculous cholecystitis and other cholangiopathies, such as papillary stenosis, biliary strictures, and sclerosing cholangitis. • This patient has a syndrome consistent with acalculous cholecystitis. • Organisms responsible for this entity in HIV patients include CMV, *Cryptosporidium, Isospora, Salmonella* spp., *Campylobacter* spp., and enteric gram-negative bacteria. • Patients may have mild right upper quadrant pain, but fulminant gangrenous cholecystitis may also occur. • Sonographic studies reveal a thickened gallbladder wall or pericholecystic fluid. • HIDA-technetium scan results are abnormal. • Cholecystectomy is required. • Papillary stenosis, biliary strictures, and sclerosing cholangitis can be diagnosed by ERCP. • Although certain pathogens have been associated with these conditions (e.g., CMV, *Cryptosporidium*, Microsporidia, and *Mycobacterium avium* complex), medical therapy has not been shown to be effective. • Biliary stenting or sphincterotomy may be effective. • The other organisms mentioned can infect patients with HIV infection. • Toxoplasmosis is associated with cerebritis and brain abscesses. • *Rhodococcus equi* causes cavitary pneumonia.

ANSWER:
A, B, C

37. Concerning anorectal surgery in patients infected with HIV, which of the following statements is/are true?

A. Wound healing is dismal in both symptomatic and asymptomatic HIV patients.

B. Up to one third of wounds in patients with symptomatic AIDS may take more than 6 months to heal.

C. Most symptomatic AIDS patients undergoing sphincterectomy are at higher risk than asymptomatic HIV patients of developing partial incontinence by the operation.

D. Surgical morbidity rates are correlated with CD4 T-cell counts.

E. Most common lesions are anal condylomata and painful ulcers. The majority of these anal ulcers yield negative culture and biopsy results.

Ref.: 24, 31

COMMENTS: Anorectal disease is a common indication for surgical intervention in patients infected with HIV. • Wound healing following anorectal surgery in HIV-positive patients appears to be dependent on the preoperative CD4 T-cell count. • A distinction can be made between HIV-negative patients, asymptomatic HIV patients, and patients with symptomatic HIV disease. • In the first two categories, wound healing occurs within the usual 6 weeks following the operation. • Patients with symptomatic HIV disease, particularly those with low CD4 T-cell counts (<200 cells/mm^3) may experience poor healing. • Only 12% heal within the first month, and 34% may take longer than 6 months to heal. • Furthermore, if sphincterectomy is performed, some impairment of continence may occur postoperatively. • Since anorectal surgery in a symptomatic HIV-positive patient may be followed by prolonged wound healing and functional impairment, a thorough evaluation of potential risk factors and, if possible, determination of HIV status are advised before proceeding with anorectal surgery in individuals at high risk of being infected. • Most anorectal lesions in patients with HIV infection are anal condylomata (43%), of which 10% are associated with anal intraepithelial neoplasia. • Also common are painful ulcers (32%), most of which were idiopathic, but 20% are associated with active herpes virus infection.

ANSWER:
B, C, D, E

38. Which of the following previously healthy patients scheduled for surgery should undergo HIV antibody testing?

A. A 35-year-old man seen for removal of a lipoma in the anterior triangle of the neck. Routine preoperative complete blood count reveals a white cell count of 4,500 cells/ml with normal differential, hemoglobin of 13•g/dl, and platelets of 81,000/ml.

B. A 40-year-old man seen for inguinal hernia repair. Physical examination reveals white, adherent, nonremovable plaques in the lateral aspect of his tongue.

C. A 28-year-old woman seen for breast lump removal who develops a painful vesicular rash following the T8–T10 dermatomes on the right side.

D. A 20-year-old man undergoing nephrectomy for living-related transplantation.

E. All of the above.

Ref.: 1

COMMENTS: Several risk groups have been identified in whom HIV testing is indicated. • These groups include persons with sexually transmitted diseases and persons in high-risk categories, such as injected drug users, homosexual and bisexual men, hemophiliacs, patients with active tuberculosis, and pregnant women. • Donors of blood or organs should be tested. • Certain clinical or laboratory findings also should prompt HIV testing. • These findings include idiopathic thrombocytopenia, oral hairy leukoplakia, reactivation varicella zoster involving more than one dermatome, unexplained oral candidiasis, persistent vulvovaginal candidiasis, and herpes simplex virus infection resistant to treatment.

ANSWER:
E

39. Which of the following statements about HIV-positive patients with gastrointestinal bleeding is/are correct?

A. The commonest cause of lower gastrointestinal bleeding is CMV colitis.

B. Ganciclovir therapy prevents rebleeding in patients with documented CMV disease.

C. Kaposi's sarcoma is the commonest AIDS-associated cause of upper gastrointestinal bleeding.

D. Upper gastrointestinal bleeding is usually secondary to infection.

E. Lower gastrointestinal bleeding is more common than upper gastrointestinal bleeding.

Ref.: 25

COMMENTS: Gastrointestinal bleeding is a relatively infrequent complication in HIV-infected individuals. • Upper gastrointestinal bleeding is more frequent than lower gastrointestinal hemorrhage and is usually unrelated to HIV infection (e.g., due to peptic ulcer disease, esophageal varices secondary to portal hypertension, or a Mallory-Weiss tear). • However, in patients with advanced HIV infection, AIDS-associated causes, such as Kaposi's sarcoma, become more common. • CMV infection can produce disease at all levels of the gastrointestinal tract and is the commonest cause of colitis and lower gastrointestinal hemorrhage in AIDS patients. • Ganciclovir is effective therapy for CMV disease of the gastrointestinal tract and prevents recurrent hemorrhage. • Significant bone marrow suppression with neutropenia is a frequent side effect of ganciclovir therapy. • In stable patients, endoscopy with biopsy is the initial diagnostic procedure of choice for HIV-infected patients with gastrointestinal bleeding.

ANSWER:
A, B, C.

40. Which of the following statements about the epidemiology of tuberculosis in the United States is/are true?

A. The incidence of tuberculosis has declined in the last decade.

B. Tuberculosis in foreign-born individuals currently accounts for the majority of tuberculosis cases in the United States.

C. Extrapulmonary tuberculosis is rarely infectious and poses minimal public health risk.

D. The source of infection for most persons at risk are patients with adult pulmonary tuberculosis.

E. HIV infection is the greatest known risk factor for reactivating latent tuberculosis infection.

Ref.: 26

COMMENTS: During 2002, a total of 15,078 tuberculosis cases were reported in the United States, representing a 43.5% decline from 1992. • Declines since that time have occurred in all age groups, racial and ethnic populations, and regions of the United States. • However, rates of tuberculosis in two groups— U.S.-born non-Hispanic blacks and foreign-born persons—now account for nearly 75% of tuberculosis cases in the United States. • The usual mode of transmission is airborne and, in the absence of concurrent pulmonary disease, patients with extrapulmonary tuberculosis are not infectious. • Adult pulmonary tuberculosis is defined by a positive sputum culture result and often also a positive smear for AFB, especially if the disease is cavitary. • HIV infection is the greatest known risk factor for reactivating latent tuberculosis infection. • The estimated risk of developing tuberculosis for an HIV-infected tuberculin-positive individual is 7–10% per year.

ANSWER:
A, C, D, E

41. A patient with a hereditary hemolytic anemia requires a splenectomy. Which of the following measures is least important in preventing or controlling future infections?

A. Pneumococcal immunization

B. *H. influenza* type B immunization

C. Quadrivalent meningococcal immunization

D. Immediate administration of antibiotics if it is presumed that the patient has sepsis

E. Education of the patient and family about increased risk of infections

Ref.: 1

COMMENTS: Pneumococcal immunization is uniformly recommended for asplenic patients. • The vaccine should be given 2 weeks before the splenectomy or at the time of discharge in the event of an emergency procedure. • *H. influenza* type B vaccination should be given to all asplenic individuals who did not receive the immunization during childhood. • Meningococcal vaccine is usually not given to asplenic hosts because of the short duration of protection. • Meningococcal vaccine administration to asplenic individuals traveling to high-risk areas or to teens or young adults who may be attending college or joining the military should be strongly considered. • Immediate administration of antibiotics primarily to treat encapsulated bacterial pathogens (e.g., pneumococci and *Haemophilus* spp.) in patients with suspected postsplenectomy sepsis is mandatory and may be lifesaving. • Patients and relatives usually do not have knowledge of the potential risks after splenectomy. • They should be educated on those matters. • Patients should preferably wear a bracelet or other kind of medical device informing of their status.

ANSWER:
C

42. Which of the following statements regarding CMV infection and solid-organ transplantation (SOT) is/are true?

A. Symptomatic infection occurs 2–6 months post-transplantation.

B. Patients being treated for acute rejection are at increased risk of developing symptomatic CMV infection.

C. Transmission can occur through the donor organ.

D. Reactivation of latent infection is associated with the greatest risk of developing severe disease.

E. CMV infection may be associated with premature atherosclerosis in cardiac transplant patients.

Ref.: 32

COMMENTS: CMV is the most important pathogen affecting solid organ recipients. • Symptomatic CMV disease may develop in as many as 50% of allograft recipients, usually 2–6 months post-transplant. • CMV-seronegative recipients who are primarily infected are at greatest risk of developing severe CMV disease. • Primary infection can occur through the donor organ, unscreened blood products, or intimate contact with a viral shedder. • Reactivation of latent infection is less likely to cause severe disease. • Patients receiving OKT3/ALG therapy for acute rejection also appear to be at risk of developing CMV disease. • In addition to clinical disease directly attributable to CMV infection,

CMV has indirect immunomodulatory activity. • Symptomatic CMV infections are associated with an increased incidence of bacterial infections and opportunistic infections such as aspergillosis and *Pneumocystis carinii* pneumonia. • In heart transplant patients, acute rejection and accelerated atherosclerosis are associated with CMV infection.

ANSWER:
A, B, C, E

43. Which of the following is the commonest infectious complication in patients with multiple trauma?

    A. Pneumonia

    B. Urinary tract infection

    C. Sinusitis

    D. Intravascular catheter-related bacteria

    E. CNS infection

    Ref.: 1

COMMENTS: Nosocomial pneumonia is the leading cause of morbidity and mortality in trauma patients, with an incidence of up to 44%. • Urinary tract infections are also very common and are usually catheter associated. • Sinusitis is recognized as a source of fever in trauma patients who are at risk because of the use of nasotracheal and nasogastric tubes, nasal packing, and facial fractures. • Intravascular device-related bacteremia due to *S. aureus* and coagulase-negative staphylococci is another major cause of infectious complications in patients with trauma, especially because of emergency conditions during placement, proximity to wounds, and frequent manipulations of the catheter. • CNS infections may occur in trauma patients, but they are infrequent even in patients with head trauma and cerebrospinal fluid leakage.

ANSWER:
A

44. Which of the following statements regarding necrotizing pancreatitis is/are true?

    A. It develops in up to 30% of patients with acute pancreatitis.

    B. Infection is the main determinant of prognosis.

    C. Surgical débridement should be undertaken once infected necrosis is diagnosed.

    D. Percutaneous drainage has proven efficacy in the management of infected pancreatic necrosis.

    E. Carbapenems and quinolones have equal efficacy in preventing infection.

    Ref.: 33

COMMENTS: Necrotizing pancreatitis develops in 20–30% of patients with acute pancreatitis. • Diagnosis can be made using contrast-enhanced CT. • Infected necrosis is the most feared complication of severe acute pancreatitis, since the mortality rate is triple that of noninfected pancreatic necrosis. • Infected necrosis develops in 30–70% of patients with acute necrotizing pancreatitis and accounts for approximately 80% of deaths related to acute pancreatitis. • Antibiotic prophylaxis or treatment should begin immediately once necrotic pancreatitis is diagnosed. • Imipenem/cilastatin, a carbapenem, has been shown to reduce the incidence of pancreatic infection and produced results superior to those achieved with a quinolone in one prospective, randomized trial. • However, the addition of metronidazole, an agent with excellent coverage against anaerobic bacteria, to a quinolone may be as effective as imipenem/cilastatin in preventing pancreatic infection. • Patients with acute necrotizing pancreatitis who fail to improve despite antibiotics should undergo CT-guided fine-needle aspiration of necrotic areas and/or abnormal fluid collections for culture. • Immediate surgical intervention is mandatory for patients with proven infected necrosis. • Percutaneous drainage of necrotic areas generally is ineffective treatment for infected necrosis.

ANSWER:
A, B, C

45. A 28-year-old man who sustained closed head trauma in a motor vehicle accident a month ago comes to the emergency department with a 3-day history of progressive headache, fever, and confusion. His wife reports the recent onset of clear drainage from his left nare. His physical examination reveals a fever of 102°F (38.9°C), a stiff neck, and no rash. Which of the following statements concerning the patient is/are true?

    A. He most likely has bacterial meningitis secondary to *S. aureus*.

    B. Antiretroviral prophylaxis has been beneficial in preventing bacterial meningitis after head trauma.

    C. Empiric antibiotics should include an extended-spectrum cephalosporin and vancomycin.

    D. Corticosteroid administration with antibiotics may improve the outcome.

    E. He requires immediate surgical intervention for repair of cerebrospinal fluid leakage.

    Ref.: 27, 36

COMMENTS: The patient likely sustained a basilar skull fracture and a dural rent, with subsequent development of a dural fistula from the subarachnoid space and nasal cavity or paranasal sinuses. • Cerebrospinal fluid rhinorrhea may occur and can easily be diagnosed by detecting the presence of β_2-transferrin in nasal secretions. • Among patients with known basilar skull fracture, approximately 10% develop cerebrospinal fluid rhinorrhea. • Of those patients, up to 30% develop bacterial meningitis. • *S. pneumoniae* is the commonest pathogen (65% of cases). • Other organisms, such as *H. influenzae, N. meningitidis,* and *S. aureus,* account for the remaining cases. • Empiric treatment should include an extended-spectrum cephalosporin (ceftriaxone, cefotaxime, or cefepime) and vancomycin, since the incidence of β-lactam-resistant pneumococci is increasing. • Prophylactic antibiotics have no proven benefit and may predispose to meningitis due to antibiotic-resistant gram-negative bacteria. • A recent prospective study demonstrated a survival advantage among patients with pneumococcal meningitis who received corticosteroids before or at the time of antibiotic administration. • Spontaneous closure of the dural fistula is less likely in patients with delayed presentation of cerebrospinal fluid leakage with meningitis, and surgical repair is indicated. • Diagnostic studies to identify the site of the fistula and treatment of any CNS infection should be completed before surgical intervention.

ANSWER:
C, D

46. A 25-year-old man who recently returned from Southeast Asia has developed a large painful swelling in the right inguinal area. He admits to unprotected sex during his visit and had developed a small painless ulcer on the penis, which healed without a scar 2 weeks ago. Physical examination reveals a fever of 102°F (38.9°C) and firm right inguinal adenopathy with areas of fluctuance. Which of the following is/are appropriate in the management of this patient?

A. Obtain an incisional biopsy specimen of the inguinal nodes.

B. Perform serologic tests for *Chlamydia trachomatis*, syphilis, and HIV.

C. Start oral doxycycline 100 mg twice daily for 21 days.

D. Perform a CT scan of the chest and abdomen for staging of the disease.

E. None of the above.

Ref.: 1

COMMENTS: Few sexually transmitted diseases are characterized by inguinal lymphadenopathy with or without associated ulcers involving the genitalia. • These diseases include lymphogranuloma venereum (LGV), syphilis, granuloma inguinale, chancroid, and sometimes herpes simplex. • The presentation of this patient is classic for LGV, which is caused by *C. trachomatis* serovars L1–L3. • LGV has three stages. • Initially, there is a small, painless ulcer that heals without scarring, followed (days to weeks) by discrete inguinal lymphadenopathy that is usually unilateral (in two thirds of cases). • The swollen lymph nodes may coalesce to form abscesses and sinus tracts if untreated. • Incisional biopsy is contraindicated in these patients because of the potential for sinus tract formation. • Healing can occur without treatment as hardened inguinal masses develop and slowly involute. • Relapse occurs in approximately 20% of untreated patients. • The disease, which is endemic in Southeast Asia, Africa, India, South America, and the Caribbean Islands, is diagnosed by serologic testing and resolves with doxycycline. • The differential diagnosis of inguinal lymphadenopathy in this age group includes the sexually transmitted diseases mentioned above and sometimes lymphoma, but a CT scan is clearly not warranted at this stage.

ANSWER:
B, C

47. Which of the following statements regarding hepatitis C virus (HCV) infection are true?

A. Prevalence of HCV infection is higher among HCWs than in the general population.

B. Chronic HCV infection occurs in 75–85% of patients after acute infection.

C. Hepatic failure due to chronic HCV infection is the commonest indication for liver transplantation.

D. Pegylated interferon plus ribavirin is effective therapy for the majority of patients with chronic HCV infection.

E. Factors associated with the development of cirrhosis include male gender, alcohol use, and coinfection with HIV.

Ref.: 1, 28

COMMENTS: Persons with acute HCV infection typically are asymptomatic (60–70%) or have mild clinical illness. • Fulminant hepatitis is rare. • Chronic HCV infection develops in approximately 75–80% of persons with acute HCV infection. • Cirrhosis develops in 10–20% of chronically infected individuals, usually after more than 20 years of infection. • Liver failure due to chronic HCV infection has become the leading indication for liver transplantation. • Increased alcohol use, male gender, HIV coinfection, and HCV genotype 1 are associated with severity of liver disease. • Hepatocellular carcinoma can be a late complication in 1–2% of patients with cirrhosis. • Antiviral therapy is recommended for individuals at increased risk for progressive liver disease, as demonstrated by persistently elevated serum transaminase levels, detectable HCV RNA levels, and moderate inflammation revealed in liver biopsy specimens. • The combination of pegylated interferon and ribavirin is the most effective regime to date.

However, up to 60% of patients receiving this treatment fail to achieve a sustained virologic response. • Predictors of poor response include HCV genotype 1 (commonest genotype in the United States), more extensive fibrosis observed in liver biopsy specimens, and high baseline HCV RNA levels. • Adverse events (e.g., bone marrow suppression and fatigue) are common and significant, leading to discontinuation of combination therapy in 20% of patients. • The prevalence of HCV infection is highest in injected drug users and patients undergoing hemodialysis. • Overall, nearly 2% of the U.S. population has persistent HCV infection. • Although transmission of HCV to HCWs occurs after approximately 3% of needle-stick exposures from HCV-infected patients, the prevalence of HCV infection among HCWs, including surgeons, is similar to that of the general population.

ANSWER:
B, C, E

48. Which of the following markers is/are clinically useful for predicting progression to AIDS among persons infected with HIV-1?

A. CD4 T-cell count

B. p24 antigen level

C. HIV-1 RNA plasma viral load

D. Serum neopterin level

E. Serum β₂-microglobulin level

Ref.: 1

COMMENTS: HIV plasma viral load strongly predicts the rate of decrease in CD4 T lymphocytes and progression to AIDS and death. • Progression to AIDS within 6 years occurs in 80% of HIV-infected individuals with viral loads of greater than 30,000 copies/ml, compared to 55.2%, 31.7%, 16.6%, and 5.4% for individuals with viral loads of 10,000–30,000, 3001–10,000, 501–3000, and less than 500 copies/ml, respectively. • The baseline viral load is a stronger predictor of progression of disease and outcome than is the CD4 T-cell count. • However, the combination of HIV load and CD4 T-cell count gives the best prognostic estimate for HIV-infected individuals. • CD4 T-cell count reflects the degree of immunocompromise and is most useful for determining the risk of opportunistic infection. • The normal CD4 T-cell count is greater than 600 cells/mm³. • Symptomatic HIV infection usually begins when CD4 T-cell counts fall below 350 cells/mm³. • Opportunistic infections, such as *P. carinii* pneumonia, occur when CD4 T-cell counts fall below 200 cells/mm³. • Without antiretroviral treatment, the median time from infection to the development of AIDS is approximately 11 years. • The p24 antigen represents one of the major core proteins of HIV. • It can be detected during the acute phase of HIV infection and during late symptomatic disease. • Serum neopterin produced by macrophages stimulated by interferon and β₂-microglobulin levels reflect lymphocytic turnover. • Although both may be found in HIV-infected individuals, neither is specific for HIV infection.

ANSWER:
A, C

49. Which statements about *M. tuberculosis* treatment and prophylaxis are true?

   A. Two-drug therapy with insoniazid (INH) and rifampin (RIF) for 9 months is standard therapy for active pulmonary tuberculosis.

   B. Treatment failure can be due to drug resistance or nonadherence.

   C. HIV-infected individuals require prolonged therapy for active tuberculosis.

   D. INH prophylaxis for latent tuberculosis infection is given for at least 12 months.

   E. INH prophylaxis should be given to individuals with recent conversion from purified protein derivative (PPD)-negative to PPD-positive status.

Ref.: 34

COMMENTS: Recent Centers for Disease Control guidelines recommend that all patients with active pulmonary tuberculosis receive four-drug therapy consisting of INH, RIF, pyrazinamide, and ethambutol for the initial 2 months of treatment. • For patients with drug-susceptible tuberculosis and negative sputum test results after 2 months of therapy, treatment can be completed with 4 months of INH and RIF. • Extrapulmonary disease requires 6–9 months of treatment, except for meningitis, which is treated for 1 year. • HIV-infected individuals are treated similarly to non-HIV infected patients with tuberculosis. • However, significant drug-drug interactions may occur with antiretroviral agents and tuberculosis drugs that may alter therapeutic decisions.

Treatment failures are generally due to nonadherence by patients to multidrug regimens. • Currently, local health departments have directly observed therapy programs to improve compliance with and completion of antituberculosis medication regimens. • Another cause of treatment failure is infection due to multidrug-resistant strains of *M. tuberculosis*. • Conditions associated with a higher rate of resistance include tuberculosis among those known to have higher prevalence of drug resistance, such as Asians or Hispanics and previously treated individuals; persistence of culture-positive sputum after 2 months of therapy; and known exposure to drug-resistant tuberculosis.

Certain individuals are at considerable risk of developing active tuberculosis once infected (latent tuberculosis infection). • Tuberculosis skin testing (Mantoux/PPD) is useful in identifying latent tuberculosis infection in high-risk individuals. • Three cut points have been recommended for defining a positive tuberculin reaction: greater than 5 mm, greater than 10 mm, and greater than 15 mm of induration. • Persons considered at highest risk (>5 mm of induration) include individuals with HIV infection, recent contacts of tuberculosis case patients, and organ transplant patients. • Individuals also at risk (>10 mm induration) include injected drug users, residents of nursing homes and prisons, hospital employees, and recent immigrants from countries with high tuberculosis prevalence. • These individuals who are at considerable risk of developing active tuberculosis once infected should receive 9 months of INH therapy.

ANSWER:
B, E

50. A 50-year-old woman with a history of severe dilated cardiomyopathy and left ventricular assist device (LVAD) placement is admitted to the hospital with fever and *S. aureus* bacteremia. Which of the following statements regarding LVAD-associated infection is/are true?

   A. LVAD-associated infection is a common event, occurring in up to 50% of LVAD recipients.

   B. LVAD-associated bacteremia is a contraindication to cardiac transplantation.

   C. The majority of LVAD-associated infections occur within 1 month of implantation.

   D. Gram-positive bacteria are responsible for most of LVAD-associated bacteremias.

   E. Optimal duration of antibiotic therapy for LVAD-associated bacteria is poorly defined.

Ref.: 35

COMMENTS: LVAD implantation has become an effective means of treating severe heart failure in patients awaiting cardiac transplantation. • Unfortunately, device-related infection is common and occurs in nearly 50% of LVAD recipients. • Localized infections involving the drive line exit site or LVAD pocket occur but are frequently associated with bacteremia. • The majority (60%) of LVAD-associated infections occur within 30 days of implantation. • Gram-positive bacteremia accounts for more than 75% of infections, with staphylococci being the most frequent blood isolate. • Although short courses of systemic antibiotics for localized infections may be curative, the optimal duration of antibiotic therapy for LVAD associated bacteremia is unclear. • Relapse is common, and, generally, systemic antibiotics should be continued through transplantation.

Transplantation is not contraindicated for patients with recent LVAD-associated bacteremia. • Post-transplantation outcomes, such as length of hospitalization and 1-year survival rates, are not different among infected and noninfected LVAD patients.

ANSWER:
A, B, D, E
C

REFERENCES

1. Mandell GL, Bennett JE, Dolin R: *Principles and Practice of Infectious Diseases*, 5th ed. Churchill Livingstone, Philadelphia, 2000.
2. Suerbaum S, Michetti P: *Helicobacter pylori* infection. *N Engl J Med* 347(15):1175–1186, 2002.
3. Garner JS: Guidelines for isolation precautions in hospitals. *Infect Control Hosp Epidemiol* 17(1):53–80, 1996.
4. Bernard GR, Vincent JL, Laterre PF, et al: Efficacy and safety of recombinant human activated protein C for severe sepsis. *N Engl J Med* 344(10):699–709, 2001.
5. American Society of Health-System Pharmacists: ASHP therapeutic guidelines on antimicrobial prophylaxis in surgery. *Am J Health Syst Pharm* 56(18):1839–1888, 1999.
6. Barie PS: Surgical site infections: epidemiology and prevention. *Surg Infect* (Suppl 1):9–21, 2002.
7. Dajani AS, Taubert KA, Wilson W, et al: Prevention of bacterial endocarditis: recommendations by the American Heart Association. *JAMA* 277(22):1794–1801, 1997.
8. Magadia RR, Weinstein MP: Laboratory diagnosis of bacteremia and fungemia. *Infect Dis Clin North Am* 15(4):1009–1024, 2001.
9. Sabiston DC Jr: *Textbook of Surgery*, 15th ed. Saunders, Philadelphia, 1997.
10. Perl TM, Cullen JS, Wenzel RP, et al: Intranasal mupirocin to prevent postoperative *Staphylococcus aureus* infections. *N Engl J Med* 346:1871–1877, 2002.

11. Salgado CD, Farr BM, Calfee DP: Community-acquired methicillin-resistant *Staphylococcus aureus:* a meta-analysis of prevalence and risk factors. *Clin Infect Dis* 36:131–139, 2003.

12. Centers for Disease Control and Prevention: Vancomycin-resistant *Staphylococcus aureus:* Pennsylvania. *Morbid Mortal Wkly Rep* 51: 931, 2002.

13. Abrutyn E, Goldmann DA, Scheckler WE (eds): *Infection Control: Reference Service*, 2nd ed. Saunders, Philadelphia, 2001.

14. Boyce JM, Pittet D: Guidelines for hand hygiene in healthcare settings: recommendations of the Healthcare Infection Control Practices Advisory Committee and the HICPAC/SHEA/APIC/IDSA Hand Task Force. *Morbid Mortal Wkly Rep* 51(RR-16):1–45, 2002.

15. Centers for Disease Control and Prevention: Diphtheria, tetanus, and pertussis: recommendations for vaccine use and other preventive measures. *Morbid Mortal Wkly Rep* 40(RR-10):1–28, 1991.

16. Mora-Duart J, Betts R, Rotstein C, et al: Comparison of caspofungin and amphotericin B for invasive candidiasis. *N Engl J Med* 347:2020–2029, 2002.

17. Herbrecht R, Denning DW, Patterson TF, et al: Voriconazole versus amphotericin B primary therapy of aspergillosis. *N Engl J Med* 347:408–415, 2002.

18. Garrett HE Jr, Roper CL: Surgical intervention in histoplasmosis. *Ann Thorac Surg* 41:711–722, 1986.

19. Bhuva M, Ganger G, Jenssen D: Spontaneous bacterial peritonitis: an update on evaluation, management and prevention. *Am J Med* 97:169–175, 1994.

20. Such J, Runyon BA: Spontaneous bacterial peritonitis. *Clin Infect Dis* 27:669–674, 1998.

21. Sande MA, Volberding P: *Medical Management of AIDS*, 6th ed. Saunders, Philadelphia, 1990.

22. Dybul M, Fauci AS, Barlett JG, et al: Panel on clinical practices for treatment of HIV: guidelines for using antiretroviral agents among HIV-infected adults and adolescents. *Ann Intern Med* 137:381–433, 2002.

23. U.S. Public Health Service: Updated U.S. Public Health Service guidelines for the management of occupational exposures to HBV, HCV, and HIV and recommendations for postexposure prophylaxis. *Morbid Mortal Wkly Rep* 50(RR-11):1–52, 2001.

24. Yuhan R, Orsay C, Delpino A, et al: Anorectal disease in HIV-infected patients. *Dis Colon Rectum* 41:1367–1370, 1998.

25. Chalasani N, Wilcox CM: Gastrointestinal hemorrhage in patients with AIDS. *AIDS Patient Care Standards* 13:343–346, 1999.

26. Centers for Disease Control and Prevention: Trends in tuberculosis morbidity: United States, 1992–2002. *Morbid Mortal Wkly Rep* 52:217–220, 222, 2003.

27. de Gans J, Van de Beek D: Dexamethasone in adults with bacterial meningitis. *N Engl J Med* 347:1549–1556, 2002.

28. Centers for Disease Control and Prevention: Recommendations for prevention and control of hepatitis C virus infection and HCV-related chronic disease. *Morbid Mortal Wkly Rep* 47(RR-19):1–39, 1998.

29. Dolin R, Masur H, Saag MS: *AIDS Therapy*, 2nd ed. Churchill Livingstone, Philadelphia, 2003.

30. Katzung BG: *Basic and Clinical Pharmacology*, 8th ed. McGraw-Hill, New York, 2001.

31. Beck DE, Wexner SD: *Fundamentals of Anorectal Surgery*. McGraw-Hill, New York, 1992.

32. Simon DM, Levin S: Infectious complications of solid organ transplantations. *Infect Dis Clin North Am* 15:521–549, 2001.

33. Baron TH, Morgan DE: Acute necrotizing pancreatitis. *N Engl J Med* 340:1412–1417, 1999.

34. Centers for Disease Control and Prevention: Treatment of tuberculosis, *Morbid Mortal Wkly Rep* 52(RR11):1–77, 2003.

35. Argenziano M, Catenese KA, Moazami N, et al: The influence of infection on survival and successful transplantation in patients with left ventricular assist devices. *J Heart Lung Transplant* 16:822–831, 1997.

36. Chawdhury MH, Tunkel AR: Antibacterial agents in infections of the central nervous system. *Infect Dis Clin North Am* 14:391–408, 2000.

CHAPTER 19

Transmissible Diseases and the Surgeon: Prevention and Management

Daniel J. Deziel, M.D.

1. Which of the following is/are not standard precautions for reducing the spread of transmissible diseases?

   A. Hand washing before contact with a patient

   B. Hand washing after glove removal

   C. Wearing gloves during contact with a patient

   D. Negative-pressure air flow

   E. Eye protection

Ref.: 1

COMMENTS: Standard, or universal, precautions are designed to prevent spread of transmissible disease by contact with blood, body fluids, or any other potentially infected material. • These precautions apply to *all* patients *all* of the time. • Hand washing is fundamental and should be performed before and between each contact with a patient and after glove removal. • Gloves are worn when contacting a potentially contaminated area. • Surgical masks and eye protection are required if mucous membrane or eye exposure is possible. • Gowns are part of standard precautions when more extensive blood or fluid exposure may occur. • Specific engineering controls for airflow and processing are integral to preventing spread of certain airborne pathogens and as such are not a component of basic standard precautions. • Specific procedures for infection control are mandated by federal regulatory agencies. • Surgeons and all health care workers must be familiar with the specific infection control policies and procedures established at their places of work.

ANSWER:
D

2. Wearing a surgical mask when examining a patient with influenza is an example of which type of precaution?

   A. Standard precaution

   B. Airborne precaution

   C. Droplet precaution

   D. Contact precaution

Ref.: 1

COMMENTS: In addition to **standard precautions**, specific **transmission-based precautions** have been developed to reduce disease spread. • Transmission-based precautions are based on the mode of transmission of certain organisms. • **Airborne precautions** are designed to combat spread by droplet nuclei, which are small (<5 μm) airborne particles that can stay suspended in the air for up to 1 hr. • Tuberculosis, measles, and varicella infection are examples of diseases spread by droplet nuclei. • Prevention requires specific respiratory protection not provided by a standard surgical mask. • Droplets are larger particles that convey organisms when the mucous membranes (nose, mouth, and conjunctiva) are contaminated. • Droplets, unlike droplet nuclei, do not stay suspended and travel up to about 3 feet. • **Droplet precautions** include use of a standard surgical mask and eye protection. • Numerous organisms can be transmitted by droplets, including influenza, *Haemophilus influenzae*, mumps, rubella, Group A streptococcus, meningococcus, and mycoplasma. • **Contact precautions** are for organisms spread by direct surface-to-surface contact. • Gloves and gowns are worn at all times, since everything in contact with the patient is potentially contaminated. • Typical organisms or circumstances requiring contact precautions that a surgeon is likely to encounter include vancomycin-resistant enterococcus, *Clostridium difficile,* methicillin-resistant *Staphylococcus aureus*, wounds with group A streptococcus, condyloma, undiagnosed diarrhea, and multidrug-resistant organisms. • The surgeon must be familiar with the policies and procedures regarding transmission-based precautions at his or her particular institution.

ANSWER:
C

3. Which of the following by-products of surgical energy sources has been proven capable of transmitting viral infection to surgeons?

   A. Electrocautery smoke

   B. Laser plume

   C. Ultrasonic scalpel vapor

   D. None of the above

Ref.: 2

COMMENTS: The potential infectivity of the smoke, plume, aerosol, or vapor produced by surgical energy sources has long been a concern. • These products have been demonstrated to contain various biologic components with potential for pathogen transmission. • To date, the only clinically proven transmission to surgeons has involved human papilloma virus (HPV) during laser ablation of anogenital condylomata. • However, investigators have detected viable bacteria, viruses, virions, bacteriophages, viral genes, and intact strands of viral DNA in laser plume. • Electrocautery smoke is thought to be a less probable route of disease transmission than laser plume, although intact virions have been demonstrated to be present in it. • Relatively little is known about the infectivity of the by-product of the ultrasonic scalpel. • It has been described as a cool aerosol, which is considered to have a higher chance of conveying infectious material than does a higher-temperature aerosol. • Measures to avoid potential exposure during surgical ablation of infected tissues include the use of high-filtration masks and smoke evacuators.

ANSWER:
B

4. Which type of hepatitis virus has a DNA genome?

    A. Hepatitis A

    B. Hepatitis B

    C. Hepatitis C

    D. All of the above

    E. None of the above

Ref.: 3

COMMENTS: Five viruses (hepatitis A, B, C, D, and E) are recognized as causes of acute hepatitis. • They have some similar and some dissimilar features in how they are transmitted and in the potential consequences of infection. • Hepatitis B virus (HBV) contains partially double-stranded DNA. • All of the other types are RNA viruses. • Hepatitis A, C, and E viruses contain single-stranded RNA. • Hepatitis D (δ hepatitis) is an incomplete virus or virus particle with a small, circular RNA. • It must coexist with HBV to replicate and produce infection. • The diagnosis of hepatic viral infection and determination of disease status depends on the detection of viral proteins encoded by these genomes or the presence of antibodies to them.

ANSWER:
B

5. Worldwide, which of the following is the commonest mode of transmission of hepatitis C virus (HCV)?

    A. Fecal-oral

    B. Sexual

    C. Parenteral

    D. Vertical (childbirth)

Ref.: 3, 4

COMMENTS: HCV is primarily spread by the parenteral routes. • Sexual transmission can also occur but is less common than with HBV. • Injected drug use currently accounts for most HCV transmission in the United States. • Injected drug use leads to HCV transmission by direct transfer of infected blood on shared needles

or syringes and by contamination of drug preparation equipment. • Blood transfusions were an important method of spread before the availability of screening. • Routine testing of donors for evidence of HCV infection was initiated in 1990, and multiantigen testing was implemented in 1992, reducing the risk for infection to 0.001% per unit transfused.

ANSWER:
C

6. What is the prevalence of HCV infection in the United States?

    A. 0.2%

    B. 2%

    C. 10%

    D. 20%

Ref.: 4, 5

COMMENTS: The prevalence of HCV infection in the United States is approximately four times greater than the prevalence of human immunodeficiency virus (HIV) infection. • The rate among health care workers, including general, orthopedic, and oral surgeons, is no higher. • As would be expected, some populations have a much higher prevalence, including hemophiliacs (60–90%), injected drug users (60–90%), and chronic hemodialysis patients (up to 60%).

ANSWER:
B

7. The clinical course of the majority of patients with HCV infection is characterized by which one of the following?

    A. Acute constitutional symptoms and jaundice

    B. Acute fulminant hepatic failure

    C. Development of chronic hepatitis

    D. Progression to cirrhosis

    E. Development of hepatocellular carcinoma

Ref.: 3, 4

COMMENTS: The incubation period for HCV is about 5–10 weeks. • Most acute infections are asymptomatic. • About 25% of patients may have constitutional symptoms and elevated aminotransferase levels. • Fulminant, acute hepatic failure is rare. • Infection with HCV is particularly serious, however, because 85% of patients will develop chronic hepatitis. • Over years, patients with chronic HCV can progress to cirrhosis (20%), liver failure (10%), and hepatocellular carcinoma (1–5%). • Chronic HCV may be associated with more severe or progressive liver disease in patients with concurrent hepatopathy, especially alcoholics. • Chronic HCV is now the leading indication for liver transplantation. • In comparison, only about 10% of individuals with HBV develop chronic infection.

ANSWER:
C

8. Which of the following blood tests confirms HCV infection?

    A. Detection of HCV RNA

    B. Detection of HCV surface antigen

C. Detection of HCV antibodies by enzyme immunoassay

D. Detection of HCV antibodies and alanine amino transferase (ALT) levels of 500–1000

Ref.: 4

COMMENTS: The screening test for HCV is an immunoassay for anti-HCV antibodies. • While results are positive in 90% of patients with HCV, the predictive value of the test is limited when the prevalence of infection is low. • In addition, anti-HCV antibodies may not be detectable for 18 weeks following exposure. • Their presence does not differentiate the state of infection. • Qualitative reverse transcriptase-polymerase chain reaction (RT-PCR) for detection of HCV RNA is confirmatory. • Infection may also be confirmed by a recombinant immunoblot assay for HCV antibody.

ANSWER:
A

9. What is the approximate probability of transmission of HCV to a health care worker through a needle-stick injury from an infected source?

A. 0.5%

B. 5%

C. 30%

D. 50%

Ref.: 3, 4

COMMENTS: See Question 10.

10. What is the approximate probability of transmission of HIV to a health care worker through a needle-stick injury from an infected source?

A. 0.3%

B. 3%

C. 10%

D. 30%

Ref.: 4, 6

COMMENTS: Health care workers are at risk of contracting transmissible viral disease when stuck by needles with contaminated blood or by mucosal membrane exposure to blood or other bodily fluids. • The risk of documented seroconversion is approximately 3–10% for HCV and 0.3% for HIV after needle-stick injury. • The risk of HBV infection after needle-stick injury is 5–30%. • The percentage risk of HCV following mucous membrane or other cutaneous exposure is not defined. • The risk of HIV with mucous membrane exposure is about 0.1%. • When an exposure occurs, the infected area should be thoroughly washed with soap and water. • The source should be tested for infection with HBV, HCV, and HIV. • The risk of contracting HIV infection is greatest with hollow needles, deep intramuscular injury, or when the exposure involves a greater amount of virus (i.e., from a larger amount of blood or a source with late-stage HIV infection).

ANSWERS:
Question 9: B
Question 10: A

11. Which of the following clinical conditions is indicated by the presence of antibodies in the serum against hepatitis B surface antigen (anti-HBs) and hepatitis core antigen (anti-HBc) in the absence of hepatitis B surface antigen (HBsAg)?

A. Active acute infection with HBV

B. Normal response to vaccination with the hepatitis B vaccine

C. Chronic active hepatitis due to HBV

D. Recovery with subsequent immunity following acute hepatitis B

E. Asymptomatic chronic carrier of HBV

Ref.: 3, 6

COMMENTS: The pattern of negative HBsAg, positive anti-HBs, and positive anti-HBc assay results is seen during the recovery phase following acute hepatitis B and clearance of HBsAg from the liver. • This antibody pattern may persist for years and is not associated with liver disease or infectivity. • Vaccination with the hepatitis B vaccine (genetically manufactured HBsAg particles without HBcAg or HBV DNA) is associated with the development of anti-HBs antibody alone. • Active, ongoing infection with HBV, whether acute hepatitis, chronic active hepatitis, or asymptomatic chronic carrier state, is manifested by the presence of HBsAg and anti-HBc in the serum.

ANSWER:
D

12. A nonimmune surgical resident is stuck by a contaminated needle from an HBs-Ag–positive source. Which of the following is the correct initial treatment?

A. Interferon

B. Vaccination against HBV

C. Hepatitis B immunoglobulin (HBIg)

D. Vaccination plus HBIg

Ref.: 3

COMMENTS: The best method of preventing occupational HBV infection is to vaccinate all health care workers at risk if they do not have natural immunity from previous infection. • When exposure occurs, the affected area should be immediately and thoroughly washed with soap and water. • The source is tested for HBV, HCV, and HIV. • If the source tests positive for HBV, nonimmune individuals are given HBIg for passive prophylaxis and are vaccinated. • If a previously vaccinated individual incurs a needle injury, titers should be checked and a dose of vaccine given if titers are not detected. • Interferon is not used for prophylaxis following acute exposure but may be useful for some patients with chronic HBV or HCV infection.

ANSWER:
D

13. The operating surgeon is stuck with a needle while performing an elective repair of an abdominal aortic aneurysm on a patient who is found to be HCV antibody positive. Which one of the following measures may be appropriate?

A. Administration of interferon and ribavirin if the surgeon has HCV RNA detected 3 weeks later

B. Administration of HCV vaccine and immunoglobulin if the surgeon is HCV antibody negative

C. Administration of HCV immunoglobulin alone if the surgeon is HCV antibody positive

D. Administration of HCV immunoglobulin if the surgeon is initially HCV antibody negative but converts to HCV antibody positive at 6 weeks

Ref.: 4

COMMENTS: There is no vaccine or passive immunotherapy available for HCV. • When occupational exposure occurs, immediate measures are to thoroughly wash the contaminated area with soap and water and to evaluate the source for HBV, HCV, and HIV if the status is unknown. • The exposed individual should be tested for HBV antibody at baseline and again in 6–12 weeks. • Symptomatic acute illness occurs in only 20–30% of patients. • For this reason, some recommend routine testing for HCV RNA 2–3 weeks postexposure. • There are no proven or standard recommendations for prophylactic treatment following exposure from a positive source. • Interferon and ribavirin may be given.

ANSWER:
A

14. A surgical scrub nurse is inadvertently stuck by a needle from an HIV-positive patient. Which of the following statements regarding postexposure prophylaxis is true?

A. Combined therapy with nucleosides and protease inhibitors is generally well tolerated.

B. Combined drug therapy should not be started until source infection is confirmed by Western blot.

C. Combined drug therapy should be started immediately.

D. Single-drug therapy is indicated unless the source has a high viral load.

Ref.: 4, 7

COMMENTS: Most occupationally acquired HIV infection has been documented in nurses or laboratory technicians. • Postexposure drug prophylaxis should be initiated as soon as possible, ideally within 2 hr. • In cases where the status of the source is unknown, standard serologic testing (enzyme immunoassay and Western blot) is indicated, but results may take several days. • A rapid HIV test can now give results within 1 hr. • However, serologic test results may be negative in infected individuals for 3–12 weeks following virus acquisition. • The decision to start postexposure drug prophylaxis must therefore consider any known risk factors that the source may have, regardless of serologic results. • Postexposure prophylaxis consists of multidrug therapy with a combination of nucleosides and protease inhibitors. • Adverse side effects are frequent and sometimes severe. • Recommendations for postexposure prophylaxis continue to evolve.

ANSWER:
C

15. Which of the following markers is the most clinically useful for following the course of a person infected with HIV?

A. Viral load

B. CD4 count

C. Serum neopterin

D. Serum β_2-microglobulin

E. p24 antigen level

Ref.: 7

COMMENTS: The CD4 cell count, although somewhat imperfect, is the most useful determination for following the course of an HIV infection. • The normal CD4 cell count is approximately 800–1200 cells/mm^3. • Symptomatic disease usually begins when the CD4 count falls below 300–400 cells/mm^3. • Opportunistic infections begin to occur when the CD4 cell count is less than 200 cells/mm^3. • The time course of this CD4 cell count decline is prolonged and may take more than 10 years. • Direct quantification of virus load with plasma viremia shows increasing viral titers as the disease progresses. • β_2-Microglobulin is shed into the serum in HIV-infected patients and reflects increased lymphocyte turnover. • Neopterin is produced by macrophages stimulated by interferon. • Although both are found in increasing amounts as HIV infection progresses, neither of these two determinations is specific for HIV infection, and they are generally used in a research setting. • The determination of p24 antigen is specific for HIV but not very sensitive.

ANSWER:
B

16. The chance of an HIV-infected individual's transmitting infection best correlates with which of the following?

A. CD4 cell count

B. Viral load

C. Absolute lymphocyte count less than 1000/mm^3

D. Active opportunistic infection

Ref.: 4, 8

COMMENTS: Blood measurements of viral load reflect the risk of HIV disease transmission by any route: parenteral, sexual, or perinatal. • The risk of acquiring HIV infection through occupational exposure also correlates with the viral load in the source. • Both viral load and CD4 cell count reflect the stage of disease, in that patients with late viral infection have low CD4 levels and high viral counts. • Opportunistic infections are also more prevalent as CD4 counts fall and immunodeficiency worsens. • Clinical AIDS is defined in patients with positive HIV serologic findings when CD4 counts are less than 200/mm^3 or when one of a number of defined associated conditions exists. • The list of these AIDS-defining conditions includes specific opportunistic infections, neoplasms, and degenerative conditions.

ANSWER:
B

17. A 36-year-old man with HIV infection and a CD4 cell count of 500/mm^3 has an incarcerated groin hernia. In addition to universal precautions, which one of the following is recommended?

A. Avoidance of prosthetic mesh

B. Disposable surgical instruments

C. Prophylactic trimethoprim/sulfamethoxazole

D. All of the above

E. None of the above

Ref.: 4

COMMENTS: Beyond universal precautions that are used for all patients, there are no specific recommendations regarding the preoperative or intraoperative management of patients with HIV infection. • Operative treatment should be according to the surgical condition and antiretroviral drug therapy according to the status of the HIV disease. • Prophylactic antibiotics or prosthetic materials are used based on the same indications as for non-HIV–infected individuals. • Trimethoprim/sulfamethoxazole is used for prophylaxis of *Pneumocystis carinii* pneumonia in patients with clinical AIDS but has nothing to do with surgical prophylaxis. • Standard surgical instruments and sterilization techniques are appropriate. • The use of disposable instruments is often convenient and simple when performing minor procedures outside of the main operating room.

ANSWER:
E

18. Which of the following is the most frequent type of pathologic condition leading to abdominal surgery in patients with AIDS?

    A. Acute appendicitis

    B. Kaposi's sarcoma

    C. Gastrointestinal (GI) lymphoma

    D. Opportunistic infection

    E. Immune thrombocytopenia

Ref.: 6, 9

COMMENTS: Approximately 10–20% of HIV-infected patients develop abdominal or GI symptoms that warrant surgical evaluation. • A wide array of pathologic conditions may be encountered in these patients, and the illness may or may not be related to HIV infection. • An emergency laparotomy may be indicated for GI bleeding, obstruction, perforation, peritonitis, or trauma. • Elective procedures may have diagnostic, therapeutic, or supportive intent. • Approximately two thirds of known HIV-infected patients undergoing laparotomy are found to have HIV-related disease. • Among these diseases, opportunistic infections (cytomegalovirus [CMV] and *Mycobacterium avium intracellulare* [MAI]) are the commonest, followed by neoplastic disease (lymphoma and Kaposi's sarcoma), and HIV-related thromobocytopenia. • The general surgeon must be mindful, however, that acute surgical conditions unrelated to HIV infection are present in one third of patients with known HIV disease and a surgical abdomen.

ANSWER:
D

19. A patient with AIDS has right upper quadrant pain, fever, and elevated alkaline phosphatase levels. Ultrasound examination demonstrates nondilated, thickened bile ducts. There are no gallstones. Which of the following organisms is the most likely cause?

    A. HCV

    B. CMV

    C. Cryptosporidia

    D. MAI

Ref.: 3, 4, 6

COMMENTS: AIDS-associated cholangiopathy is a condition characterized by pain and cholestasis with bile duct stenosis, similar to the clinical picture seen with sclerosing cholangitis. • The condition may be idiopathic or associated with opportunistic biliary infection, most commonly with cryptosporidia. • Other infectious causes include CMV, microsporidia, and cyclospora. • Treatment is with antimicrobial drugs and relief of mechanical obstruction, usually by endoscopic methods (sphincterotomy, dilatation, and stenting). • Hepatic disease and elevated levels of liver enzymes are common in patients with HIV infection, particularly those with late-stage disease. • Patients often have coexisting chronic HBV or HCV infection. • A multitude of opportunistic infections may affect the liver, including MAI, CMV, and *Candida albicans*. • These patients may have a clinical presentation similar to those with cholangiopathy but do not have the ductal changes detected on ultrasound or endoscopic retrograde cholangiographic studies.

ANSWER:
C

20. The operative mortality rate for laparotomy in patients with AIDS has most closely been associated with which one of the following?

    A. Total lymphocyte count less than 1000 cells/mm^3

    B. CD4 cell count less than 500/mm^3

    C. Active opportunistic infection

    D. Duration of HIV infection

    E. Emergency operation

Ref.: 9

COMMENTS: Prognostic factors in AIDS patients undergoing abdominal operations have not been extensively analyzed. • The cumulative operative mortality rate following major abdominal procedures is approximately 20%. • Most deaths are related to the patient's underlying disease and not to specific operative complications. • Emergency operations have been associated with higher mortality rates than have elective procedures, particularly for patients with intestinal perforations due to opportunistic infections such as CMV or MAI. • However, there is no convincing evidence that patients with HIV infection without AIDS-defining criteria have an inordinate risk of death or complications after abdominal surgery.

ANSWER:
E

21. Which of the following is the commonest manifestation of GI bleeding in HIV patients?

    A. Upper GI bleeding due to CMV

    B. Upper GI bleeding due to duodenal ulcer

    C. Lower GI bleeding due to CMV

    D. Lower GI bleeding due to *C. difficile*

Ref.: 6

COMMENTS: GI bleeding in HIV infected individuals is usually related to a complication of HIV infection. • Lower GI bleeding is twice as common as upper GI bleeding. • Lower GI bleeding is usually caused by colitis of infectious origin (CMV, MAI, bacteria, or herpes simplex). • Upper GI bleeding is related to Kaposi's sarcoma or lymphoma approximately 50% of the time. • CMV-induced ulcers do occur in the upper GI tract, but not as frequently as in the lower GI tract. • Colonoscopy or esophagogastroduodenoscopy is the diagnostic procedure of choice in stable patients.

ANSWER:
C

22. Laparotomy is performed for pneumoperitoneum on a 26-year-old, HIV-positive man who has been hospitalized with abdominal pain and intractable diarrhea. He has a 2-cm cecal perforation, and the colon is dilated throughout. Select the most appropriate therapy.

 A. Suture repair of perforation and drainage

 B. Suture repair of perforation and diverting ileostomy

 C. Abdominal colectomy with ileostomy and Hartmann's procedure

 D. Ileocecal resection with primary anastamosis

Ref.: 6, 10

COMMENTS: Infection of the GI tract with CMV is one of the commonest causes of intestinal perforation in HIV-infected patients and is an AIDS-defining condition. • Diagnosis is based on demonstration of intranuclear inclusion bodies on biopsy. • Initial treatment is with antiviral agents and support. • Surgery is indicated for perforation, bleeding, or obstruction from stricture formation. • CMV perforations are most frequently ileocolic in location. • They can be in the small intestine, stomach, or duodenum. • Operative management of colon perforations is by resection without anastomosis. • Determination of the extent of resection has various considerations, but since the entire colon is typically involved, total abdominal colectomy is often advisable. • Such patients are often desperately ill, and appropriate and timely surgical intervention and aggressive support are necessary for survival.

ANSWER:
C

23. A 30-year-old, HIV-positive man has an infected right lower quadrant incision following appendectomy for acute appendicitis. His CD4 count is 400/mm^3. Which of the following organisms is most likely responsible?

 A. *Candida* spp.

 B. *Escherichia coli*

 C. CMV

 D. Methicillin-resistant *S. aureus*

Ref.: 4

COMMENTS: Postoperative abdominal wound infections in HIV-positive patients are usually caused by the same bacterial organisms seen in HIV-negative patients. • Defense against these bacteria is not dependent on cell-mediated immunity. • The overall risk of these wound infections is not necessarily higher than in non-HIV patients, although patients with any type of advanced systemic disease would be expected to be more vulnerable. • The unusual systemic opportunistic infections to which immunocompromised patients are susceptible are not postoperative pathogens. • *Candida* infections, although common, are usually superficial mucosal problems and not deep infections. • The patient described in this question has a CD4 cell count that is only modestly depressed.

ANSWER:
B

24. Concerning anorectal disease in HIV-positive patients, which of the following is true?

 A. Idiopathic anal ulcers are typically lateral in location.

 B. Herpes simplex virus (HSV) is the commonest cause of proctitis in sexually active homosexual men.

 C. Infection with human papilloma virus predisposes to rectal lymphoma.

 D. Anal squamous cell cancer occurs more frequently in patients with CMV.

Ref.: 10

COMMENTS: Idiopathic anal ulcers are easily distinguishable from anal fissures. • The latter are usually located in the anterior or posterior midline and are associated with edematous skin tags. • HIV-related anal ulcers frequently are multiple, lateral in location, deep, and not always associated with skin tags. • Biopsy is advised for histologic examination, as is viral culture and acid-fast staining. • The pathogens sought are CMV, HSV, MAI, and HIV. • A dark field examination should be done to exclude the presence of syphilis. • Biopsy is also done to exclude malignancy. • HSV is second to gonococcus as a cause of proctitis in sexually active homosexual men. • The treatment usually has been symptomatic with oral analgesics, lidocaine ointment locally, and sitz baths. • Acyclovir administered orally and topically has been effective in lengthening the asymptomatic period, promoting healing, and shortening the period of virus shedding. • Within the GI tract, the rectum is the second-commonest site for lymphoma, following the stomach. • Most lesions are non-Hodgkin's lymphomas, 70% of which are high-grade B-cell type. • They usually present as extraluminal, diffuse processes initially diagnosed incorrectly as abscesses. • Treatment consists of multiagent chemotherapy, with a median survival of less than 12 months. • Squamous cell cancer of the anus occurs more frequently in homosexual and bisexual men than in heterosexuals. • This phenomenon is thought to be due to infection with human papilloma virus.

ANSWER:
A

25. A 45-year-old man with HIV infection is evaluated for a persistently symptomatic posterior anal fissure with associated edematous tags. His CD4 count is 100/mm^3. Which of the following statements regarding surgical treatment is true?

 A. Wound healing is unaffected by stage of HIV disease.

 B. Internal anal sphincterotomy is unlikely to cause incontinence.

 C. Internal anal sphincterotomy is contraindicated in HIV-positive patients.

 D. Operative morbidity is correlated with CD4 count.

Ref.: 10

COMMENTS: Anorectal surgery in HIV-positive patients should be approached with caution and concern regarding wound healing during the postoperative period. • A distinction should be made among HIV-negative patients, asymptomatic HIV-positive patients, and patients with AIDS. • In the first two categories, wound healing can be expected to occur within the usual 6 weeks following the operation. • A patient with symptomatic HIV disease, particularly those with CD4 cell counts less than 200/mm^3, may have very poor healing. • Only 12% are healed within the first month, and one third may take longer than 6 months to heal. • Furthermore, if a sphincterotomy is performed, most patients will have some impairment of continence postoperatively. • In light of these factors, a thorough evaluation of potential risk factors and, if possible, determination of HIV status are advised before proceeding with anorectal surgery in groups at high risk of being infected. • CD4 counts have been shown to be correlated with morbidity. • Sixty-five percent morbidity rates have been seen in patients with CD4 counts of less than 200/mm^3, compared with 7% morbidity rates in patients with counts greater than 200/mm^3. • In summary, cautiously performed anorectal surgery in an asymptomatic HIV-positive patient is appropriate. • Anorectal surgery in a patient with AIDS, however, may be followed by prolonged wound healing and functional impairment.

A N S W E R :
D

26. A 32-year-old, HIV-positive injected drug user is admitted following a seizure. Examination reveals a pronator drift. A computed tomographic (CT) scan with intravenous contrast shows two ring-enhancing lesions. Which of the following statements is true?

    A. Neurologic symptoms are unrelated to AIDS.

    B. Toxoplasmosis is the most likely diagnosis.

    C. Primary central nervous system lymphoma is the most likely diagnosis.

    D. Biopsy should be performed on all enhancing lesions in HIV patients.

Ref.: 7

COMMENTS: Ten percent of AIDS patients experience a neurologic symptom as the first sign of their illness, and 40% of AIDS patients eventually develop one or more neurologic deficits. • Major HIV-related central nervous system (CNS) diseases include HIV encephalopathy, meningitis, myelopathy, opportunistic infections (progressive multifocal leukoencephalopathy caused by papovavirus CMV, herpes, toxoplasmosis, and cryptococcosis), neoplasms (primary CNS lymphoma), and cerebrovascular complications. • *Toxoplasma gondii*, the protozoan that causes toxoplasmosis, accounts for 50–70% of focal brain lesions in these patients and is the commonest cause of focal enhancing lesions on CT. • Ten to twenty-five percent of focal lesions are CNS lymphomas. • Primary CNS lymphoma is a rare intracranial tumor in the general population, accounting for only 1.5% of primary brain tumors. • However, it is significantly more common in HIV patients, even compared to other immunosuppressed populations. • Current management recommendations for HIV patients with focal brain lesions include 2–3 weeks of empiric treatment for toxoplasmosis, followed by biopsy if the radiologic or clinical condition deteriorates.

A N S W E R :
B

27. Select the true statement regarding splenectomy in HIV-infected patients.

    A. It is associated with a 30% risk of overwhelming postsplenectomy infection.

    B. Splenectomy may accelerate progression to AIDS.

    C. A laparoscopic approach is contraindicated.

    D. HIV-associated thrombocytopenia is the primary indication.

Ref.: 4, 6, 11

COMMENTS: Approximately 10–20% of patients with asymptomatic HIV disease develop thrombocytopenia similar to but immunologically distinct from classic idiopathic thrombocytopenic purpura. • Initial treatment with corticosteroids produces a response in most (80%) patients. • Those who fail to respond or who relapse when steroid use is tapered are appropriate candidates for splenectomy. • Splenectomy yields a favorable result in 80% of patients. • Neither the morbidity of splenectomy nor the risk of overwhelming postsplenectomy infection appears to be increased in HIV patients. • Likewise, there is no evidence that the absence of the spleen worsens HIV disease. • In fact, it has been suggested that splenectomy may actually slow disease progression in some patients. • Other occasional indications for splenectomy in HIV-related conditions include opportunistic infections, abscesses, and malignancies.

A N S W E R :
D

28. A 50-year-old homeless man is admitted to the hospital with fever, cough, and bloody sputum. A chest x-ray demonstrates a right upper lobe infiltrate. Which one of the following measures is appropriate?

    A. The patient should wear a surgical mask and be admitted to a private room.

    B. The patient should wear a particulate filter respirator and be admitted to a private room.

    C. The patient should wear a surgical mask during transport and be admitted to a private negative-pressure room.

    D. The staff should be required to wear gowns while in the patient's room.

Ref.: 1

COMMENTS: Airborne precautions (see Question 2) are necessary to reduce the exposure of staff and other patients to individuals with suspected pulmonary or laryngeal tuberculosis (TB). • Early recognition of patients at risk for TB is critical, including patients with possible symptoms of TB and those at higher risk of active disease. • Typical symptoms include persistent cough, bloody sputum, fever, night sweats, and weight loss. • A chest x-ray may show a cavitary lesion or upper lobe infiltrate. • Individuals at higher risk include the homeless, elderly, known contacts of TB cases, injected drug users, foreign-born individuals, and patients with HIV infection, renal failure, malignancy, or immunosuppression. • The largest-growing proportion of new TB cases is in the HIV and immunosuppressed population. • A person with suspected TB must have his or her face covered with a surgical mask during transport and should be admitted to a private negative-airflow room equipped with engineering controls specifically designed to reduce airborne exposure. • Precautions must be implemented promptly for any suspected case and should not be delayed to wait for confirmation by acid fast bacteria (AFB) culture results, which may take weeks. • Staff entering the patient's room must wear special particulate filter respirators (fit testing required) or equivalent respirator systems. • The use of appropriate respiratory equipment for protection of health care individuals is mandated by the Occupational Safety and Health Administration (OSHA) and the National Institute of Occupational Safety and Health (NIOSH).

A N S W E R :
C

29. Bronchoscopy is to be performed on the patient described in Question 28. Which of the following statements is correct?

    A. Endoscopy staff should wear a powered air-purifying respirator (PAPR) during bronchoscopy.

B. Endoscopy staff should take prophylactic isoniazide (INH) for 3 days after the procedure.

C. Bronchoscopy should be performed under general anesthesia with endotracheal intubation.

D. Bronchoscopy should be deferred if the patient's tuberculin skin test result is positive.

Ref.: 1

COMMENTS: Health care providers are at increased risk of exposure to TB during cough-inducing or aerosolizing procedures, such as bronchoscopy, endotracheal intubation, or suctioning. • Respiratory protection requires use of a particulate filter respirator or a **PAPR.** • The latter device provides filtered air to a hood that is worn. • Use of a PAPR may be recommended when prolonged exposure is possible, such as during bronchoscopy. • The risk of infection depends on the concentration of droplet nuclei and the duration of exposure. • The diagnosis of pulmonary TB is made presumptively, based on tuberculin skin test and chest x-ray results and confirmed by AFB smear and culture results. • Bronchoscopy is indicated for diagnosis of patients with undiagnosed pulmonary infection and for the exclusion of cancer, regardless of skin test results.

A N S W E R :
A

30. Which of the following statements is true regarding drug therapy for *Mycobacterium tuberculosis?*

A. INH prophylaxis is indicated for all persons who convert from PPD negative to PPD positive.

B. A multidrug regimen is standard treatment for active TB.

C. A multidrug regimen is standard treatment for all PPD-positive individuals.

D. INH prophylaxis is indicated for 4–6 weeks after occupational exposure.

Ref.: 6, 12

COMMENTS: Exposure to *M. tuberculosis* is determined by skin testing. • Fewer than 10% of exposed individuals develop infection. • Skin testing is performed at least annually in health care workers. • The majority of PPD-positive individuals have old exposures. • When PPD test results are positive, however, a chest x-ray and sputum for AFB smear and culture are obtained. • INH prophylaxis is indicated for persons under age 35 with positive skin test results and those over age 35 with high-risk conditions (i.e., HIV, injected drug use, contact with a known TB source, from a medically underserved population, foreign born, or with an abnormal chest x-ray result). • Duration of prophylaxis is 6–12 months. • Active pulmonary TB is diagnosed by sputum AFB smear and/or culture analysis. • The standard treatment for active disease involves a multidrug regimen with INH, rifampin, and other drugs (pyrazinamide, ethambutol, or streptomycin) for months. • Surgical therapy (usually resection) is occasionally necessary for patients who fail medical therapy or develop persistent problems, such as residual lung cavity or destruction, bronchiectasis, or hemoptysis.

A N S W E R :
B

31. A 65-year-old man has fever, abdominal pain, a 20-pound weight loss, and ascites. Paracentesis yields cloudy fluid containing more than 500 white blood cells/L (mainly lymphocytes) and 3.0 g/dL of protein. Cytologic test results are negative for malignant cells, and AFB smear analysis is negative. Which of the following is the least likely diagnosis?

A. Hepatic cirrhosis

B. Bacterial peritonitis

C. Tuberculous peritonitis

D. Peritoneal neoplasm

Ref.: 4, 6

COMMENTS: Tuberculous peritonitis is a relatively infrequent manifestation of TB in the United States but has become recognized somewhat more commonly, along with the increased frequency of tuberculous infection, in certain higher-risk populations. • Typical symptoms are fever, weight loss, and abdominal pain. • Ascites may be impressive or absent. • Affected patients will have a positive skin test result but usually have not had clinically significant pulmonary disease. • Characteristics of the ascitic fluid that accumulates with tuberculous peritonitis are a high white blood cell count (>500/L) of predominately lymphocytes and a high protein content (>2.5 g/dl). • AFB smear results are not usually positive, and AFB culture results are positive less than one half of the time. • Diagnosis is usually made by peritoneal biopsy, and this situation is well suited to laparoscopic evaluation. • Treatment is with antituberculosis drugs. • Therapeutic surgery may be indicated for intestinal obstruction or fistula. • In fact, small-bowel stricturoplasty was first introduced for the treatment of tuberculous strictures. • Ascites caused by bacterial peritonitis is also manifested by a high white blood cell count (polymorphonuclear leukocytes predominate) and protein content. • Peritoneal malignancy may also be manifested by a high cell count (especially red blood cells) and high protein level. • Cytologic studies are not always diagnostic, particularly with primary peritoneal malignancies (e.g., mesothelioma). • In contradistinction to these conditions, the ascites associated with hepatic cirrhosis is manifested by lower white blood cell counts (<300/L) and protein content (<2.5 g/dl).

A N S W E R :
A

32. A 32-year-old woman develops watery diarrhea, cramping, and fever 3 days after an elective sigmoid colon resection for cancer. Results of a stool assay for *C. difficile* cytotoxin are positive. When examining the patient, which of the following precautions is most appropriate?

A. The clinician should wear a gown and gloves during proctoscopic examination.

B. All visitors should wear a mask, gown, and gloves.

C. The patient should be placed in isolation with no visitors.

D. Perform gas sterilization of the stethoscope after abdominal auscultation.

Ref.: 1, 6

COMMENTS: *C. difficile* is a gram-positive, spore-forming anaerobic bacillus. • It produces a toxin that causes pseudomembranous colitis in patients who have had their intestinal flora altered by antibiotics. • Since *C. difficile* can be spread by direct contact, transmission-based contact precautions are appropriate (see Question 2). • These measures include wearing gloves when contacting anything on the patient or in the room and a gown as well if a greater amount of contamination is possible. • Hands should be thoroughly washed after the gloves are removed. • The stethoscope must be cleaned, but an alcohol pad will suffice.

ANSWER:

A

REFERENCES

1. Rush University Intranet: <http://iris.rush.edu/frontpage/trainindex.html>
2. Barrett WL, Garber SM: Surgical smoke, a review of the literature: is this just a lot of hot air? *Surg Endosc* 6:979–987, 2003.
3. Greenfield LJ, Mulholland MW, Oldham KT et al. (eds): *Surgery: Scientific Principles and Practice,* 3rd ed. Lippincott, Williams & Wilkins, Philadelphia, 2001.
4. Cameron JL: *Current Surgical Therapy,* 7th ed. Mosby, St. Louis, 2001.
5. Centers for Disease Control: Recommendations for prevention and control of hepatitis C virus and HCV-related chronic disease. *Morbid Mortal Wkly Rev* 47(RR-19):1–39, 1998.
6. Townsend CM, Beauchamp RD, Evers BM, et al (eds): *Sabiston Textbook of Surgery: The Biological Basis of Modern Surgical Practice,* 17th ed. WB Sounders, Philadelphia, 2004.
7. Centers for Disease Control: Public Health Service guidelines for the management of health care worker exposures to HIV and recommendations for postexposure prophylaxis. *Morbid Mortal Wkly Rev* 47(RR-7):1, 1998.
8. Centers for Disease Control: 1993 Revised classification system for HIV infection and expanded surveillance case definition for AIDS among adolescents and adults. *MMWR* 41:1–19, 1992.
9. Deziel DJ, Hyser MJ, Doolas A, et al: Major abdominal operations in acquired immunodeficiency syndrome. *Am Surg* 56:445–450, 1990.
10. Beck DE, Wexner SD: *Fundamentals of Anorectal Surgery.* McGraw-Hill, New York, 1992.
11. Tsoukas CM, Bernard NF, Abrahamowicz M, et al: Effect of splenectomy on slowing human immunodeficiency virus disease progression. *Arch Surg* 133:25–31, 1998.
12. Pust RE: Tuberculosis in the 1990s: resurgence, regimens and resources. *South Med J* 85:584–593, 1992.

CHAPTER 20

Surgical Technology

Edward F. Hollinger, M.D., Ph.D.

1. A 74-year-old man presents complaining of 24 hr of gross melena. His initial hemoglobin level is 6.8 g/dl. Upper gastrointestinal (GI) endoscopy fails to reveal any source of bleeding. Lower GI endoscopy is attempted but is unable to adequately visualize the mucosa because of gross blood in the lumen. Which of the following tests would be reasonable next steps to localize the source of the GI bleed?

   A. Computerized tomographic (CT) scan of the abdomen and pelvis with oral (PO) and intravenous (IV) contrast

   B. Nuclear medicine scan with radiolabeled red blood cells (RBCs)

   C. Nuclear medicine scan with radiolabeled sulfur colloid (SC)

   D. Magnetic resonance imaging (MRI) of the abdomen and pelvis with IV contrast

   E. Angiography

   Ref.: 1

COMMENTS: See Question 2.

2. What are the approximate slowest bleeding rates that can be visualized by nuclear medicine (radiolabeled sulfur colloid or RBCs) and angiography?

   A. 0.01 and 1 ml/min, respectively

   B. 0.1 and 0.5 ml/min, respectively

   C. 1 and 5 ml/min, respectively

   D. 1 and 0.01 ml/min, respectively

   E. 0.5 and 0.1 ml/min, respectively

   F. 5 and 1 ml/min, respectively

   Ref.: 1

COMMENTS: Endoscopy is typically the preferred initial imaging modality for evaluating GI hemorrhage. • However, it can be limited by poor visualization, especially in the unprepped lower GI tract, and inability to reach the affected areas (e.g., the proximal colon or small bowel). • Both angiography and nuclear medicine scintigraphy can localize the site of an active GI bleed. • Angiographic localization generally requires active bleeding rates of at least 0.5 ml/min to visualize IV contrast extravasating into the bowel lumen. • Selective mesenteric angiography can determine the specific arterial blood supply of the hemorrhage site. • In the upper GI tract, temporary embolization with Gelfoam can be performed with a low risk of bowel ischemia. • However, because of poorer collateral supply, embolizing arteries in the lower GI tract is associated with an increased risk of localized bowel ischemia. • Nuclear medicine techniques using radiolabeled sulfur colloid or autologous RBCs can identify slower bleeds, to a minimum of about 0.1 ml/min. • Multiple scans over several hours also can identify slow or intermittent bleeds. • However, the interpretation of nuclear medicine scans is more difficult because only the radioactive tracer, not normal bowel, is visualized. • Both of these techniques can localize bleeding but, unlike endoscopy, cannot characterize the lesion responsible for hemorrhage.

ANSWERS:
Question 1: B, C, E
Question 2: B

3. In well-studied animal models of the arterial response to balloon injury, what is the basic sequence of events leading to myointimal hyperplasia following balloon distention of the vessel wall?

   A. Vessel spasm, local thrombosis, and scarring

   B. Smooth muscle cell (SMC) death, leukocyte infiltration, and fibrosis

   C. Local extravasation of growth factors due to increased permeability and SMC hypertrophy

   D. Platelet degranulation, migration of adventitial fibroblasts, and collagen deposition

   E. Platelet degranulation, SMC proliferation, migration, and matrix deposition

   Ref.: 2, 3

COMMENTS: Balloon distention injury of a normal muscular artery sets in motion a complex response. • The delicate endothelium is denuded, exposing the underlying collagenous tissue to the blood. • A carpet of platelets adheres, and their degranulation releases a host of local mitogens, including serotonin, transforming growth factor β, and platelet-derived growth factor (PDGF). • These compounds have many local effects, the most important of which may be to direct migration of SMCs from the media across the internal elastic lamina in the area of subintimal damage. • Platelets act as an important mediator, as evidenced by the fact that thrombocytopenic animals develop little intimal hyperplasia following balloon injury. • Both mechanical stretching and release of intracellular and matrix-derived factors, including those of the fibroblast growth factor (FGF) family, cause the normally quiescent SMCs to undergo a wave of cell division. • Proliferation peaks at 48 hr and declines to near baseline at 4 weeks. • Migration into the inner portion of the artery also takes place during this period and is essential for development of intimal hyperplasia (IH). • Proliferation and deposition of matrix material in the intima by SMCs that have left the arterial media is the final step in generating a thick, potentially obstructive neointima. • It should be noted that the muscular artery of a young animal is different from a diseased, plaque-laden, stenotic vessel in an aged human. • Although a variety of pharmacologic treatments reduce IH following balloon injury in animal models, in human clinical trials only platelet adherence blockade (a monoclonal antibody against glycoprotein [GP] IIb/IIIa) has been shown to reduce restenosis rates following coronary angioplasty.

ANSWER:
E

4. What are the mechanisms of the immediate increase in flow channel diameter following balloon dilatation in atherosclerotic arteries?

   A. Molding of soft atheroma to the "imprint" of the balloon

   B. "Stretching" of the nondiseased portion of the artery around the plaque

   C. A dissection of artery wall and plaque, with subsequent distention and late healing

   D. Displacement of the plaque radially through the vessel wall

   E. Displacement of the plaque axially into a less diseased portion of the artery, where obstruction is no longer critical

Ref.: 4, 5

COMMENTS: The mechanism of action of balloon angioplasty probably varies from lesion to lesion, depending on the physical characteristics of the plaque and artery. • However, a human study of iliac angioplasty using intravascular ultrasonography (IVUS) to assess mechanisms showed dissection of the plaque away from the artery wall, creating new arterial extension and enlarging the previous flow channel occurring in each case. • To a lesser extent, stretching of the free wall and compression of the plaque itself also played a role in luminal enlargement. • Subsequent studies using IVUS have differed mainly in terms of the proportional enlargement due to dissection versus plaque compression and arterial wall stretching. • It may be that "plaque fracture," as it is termed, with creation of an expanded flow channel in the area of dissection between plaque and vessel wall, is necessary for a good result. • In clinical terms, this is likely in larger arteries with plaques that are focal and concentric rather than diffuse and eccentric.

ANSWER:
B, C

5. Which of the following is/are true regarding intracoronary stents?

   A. Stent deployment is limited to large vessels (>5 mm in diameter).

   B. The most important factor in optimizing stent efficacy is deployment with minimal residual luminal stenosis.

   C. Stent placement is contraindicated in the setting of acute myocardial infarction (MI).

   D. Coated stents have not been shown to be superior in preventing in-stent stenosis.

   E. Poststenting care should include antithrombotic therapy.

Ref.: 6–8

COMMENTS: Stents increasingly are being used to address two major limitations of percutaneous transluminal coronary angioplasty (PTCA): restenosis and acute or threatened vessel closure. • Stents can be characterized by their deployment method (balloon-expandable versus self-expanding), design (tubular versus coil), length, coverings, and coatings (active versus passive). • Stents are typically deployed on balloon catheters using conventional PTCA guiding catheters and guide wires. • Newer, smaller predeployment stent sizes afford the option of radial artery catheterization in addition to the more typical femoral artery route. • The single most important factor in determining stent efficacy is deployment with only minimal residual luminal stenosis. • Suboptimal dilation occurs both because of inadequate balloon expansion and because of elastic recoil of the stented vessel. • High-pressure balloon pre- and poststenting dilation is typically used to avoid the former, while the latter is largely a factor of stent design and resistance. • Although early stents were limited to use in large (>3 mm) coronary arteries, newer stents can be used routinely in small (2.25–2.75 mm) vessels. • In particular, small-vessel stents are useful if results of balloon PTCA are suboptimal or in the setting of persistent residual stenosis. • A significant problem with coronary stents is restenosis. • Several approaches to in-stent restenosis have met with success. • Changes in stent design (thin struts), intracoronary γ or β irradiation, and coated stents that release antiproliferative drugs (e.g., sirolimus) have been demonstrated to decrease in-stent restenosis. • Finally, pretreatment with aspirin and clopidogrel and post-treatment with GP IIb/IIIa inhibitors can decrease complications and limit stent thrombosis.

ANSWER:
B, E

6. An 80-year-old man undergoes cardiac catheterization via the right femoral artery. The arteriotomy is closed using a percutaneous suture technique. Three days after discharge from the hospital, he comes to the emergency room complaining of pain and swelling in the right groin. Examination reveals a tender, pulsatile mass at the arterial puncture site. He is hemodynamically stable and has palpable distal pulses in the leg. Which of the following would best establish the diagnosis?

   A. Arteriography

   B. Needle aspiration

   C. Surgical exploration

   D. Observation

   E. Color duplex ultrasonography (US)

Ref.: 9

COMMENTS: See Question 8.

7. For the patient in Question 6, a 2.5-cm pseudoaneurysm of the common femoral artery is detected. Which of the following is most likely to be successful?

   A. Observation with restriction of activity

   B. Surgical exploration of the femoral artery

   C. Application of a sandbag to the site

D. US-guided compression of the pseudoaneurysm

E. US-guided thrombin injection into the pseudoaneurysm

Ref.: 9

COMMENTS: See Question 8.

8. While awaiting definitive therapy, the patient develops fevers and erythema at the arterial puncture site. Blood cultures reveal gram-positive organisms. Which of the following is/are indicated?

A. US-guided thrombin injection

B. Operative exploration and aneurysm repair with polytetra-fluoroethylene (PTFE) graft

C. IV antibiotics

D. Endovascular covered stent placement

E. Close observation with restriction of activity

F. Operative exploration with femoral artery ligation

Ref.: 9

COMMENTS: Localized swelling, hematoma, and pain occur frequently after removal of arterial catheters, especially if anticoagulation is necessary. • It is important to differentiate a hematoma from a pseudoaneurysm. • Doppler US is the most useful diagnostic modality, although CT scanning may be helpful if US is not available or is limited by local pain. • An arteriogram can delineate the vascular anatomy but entails the risk of additional injury from a second arterial puncture. • Aspiration of the mass is not indicated, since hemorrhage may ensue. • A complete distal neurovascular examination should be performed to identify impaired perfusion or neurologic compromise resulting from local compression.

In the past, small pseudoaneurysms (<6 mm) generally were treated with observation, with approximately an 80% rate of spontaneous thrombosis at short-term follow-up. • The introduction of US-directed compression of the psuedoaneurysm with a duplex probe allowed more immediate resolution of the aneurysm. • Local compression results in stasis and clotting of the aneurysm in more than two thirds of patients. • However, 20–60 minutes of compression is required, causing significant discomfort for the patient. • Results of local compression are also worse for large pseudoaneurysms and for patients undergoing anticoagulation. • The most successful technique is US-guided injection of 100 μm/ml of bovine thrombin into the pseudoaneurysm. • Injection continues until US examination reveals thrombosis of the false aneurysm, which usually occurs with the first thrombin injection. • Local thrombin injection is successful in more than 90% of patients with false aneurysms and generally is independent of aneurysm size or the use of anticoagulation. • The commonest complication of thrombin injection is thrombosis of the affected artery. • This is more common for small arteries, such as the brachial artery, and in pediatric patients.

An infected false aneurysm is manifested as a pulsatile mass accompanied by fever and sometimes sepsis. • Local signs of infection may be present if the graft is superficial. • Septic arteritis is more common when prosthetic material is present (e.g., percutaneous closure devices or grafts) and raises the risk of rupture because of weakening of the arterial wall. • The patient should be placed on bed rest, closely monitored, and started on IV antibiotics. • Management consists of operative exploration, beginning with obtaining proximal and distal control of the involved vessel. • The infected arterial segment should be resected and surrounding infected tissues widely débrided. • If collateral supply is sufficient to retain limb viability (as is usually the case with the femoral artery) arterial ligation, long-term IV antibiotics, and delayed revascularization are preferred. • If critical ischemia is present, extra-anatomic bypass

can be used to restore flow while avoiding the involved area. • For infected femoral pseudoaneurysms, obturator foramen bypass provides a means for revascularizing the leg while avoiding the infected tissue bed. • If primary repair of the artery is required, an autogenous graft (e.g., superficial femoral vein) should be used.

A N S W E R S :
Question 6: E
Question 7: E
Question 8: C, E, F

9. Regarding sentinel lymph node (SLN) biopsy, which of the following is/are true?

A. Accurate SLN biopsy requires preoperative injection of both isosulfan blue dye and a radioactive tracer.

B. An SLN is defined as the first lymph node (or nodes) to receive lymphatic drainage from a tumor at a given site. The histologic status of the SLN is hypothesized to be representative of the entire lymph node basin.

C. When using lymphazurin (isosulfan blue dye) for axillary sentinel node biopsy, the blue dye will be preferentially retained in the sentinel lymph node(s).

D. Preoperative lymphoscintigraphy is not advisable before SLN biopsy for melanomas of the head and neck.

E. Contraindications to SLN biopsy in breast cancer include previous axillary surgery, locally advanced tumors, or multicentric carcinoma and clinically positive axillas.

Ref.: 10–14

COMMENTS: Although much effort has been directed toward employing molecular, cellular, and biochemical markers to determine the prognosis and treatment of solid tumors, the presence or absence of lymph node metastasis remains the most powerful predictor of outcome for both malignant melanoma and breast cancer. • The concept of SLN biopsy is that there is a primary, or "sentinel," lymph node (or nodes) that tumor cells initially traverse before spreading to the full regional lymph node basin. • A tracer substance injected at the primary tumor site provides a road map to identify the SLN(s). • Then, careful examination of the SLN(s) is hypothesized to represent the status of the entire lymph node basin. • In clinical practice, SLN biopsy is employed both to decrease the extent of operation for selected patients (decreasing the number of nontherapeutic lymphadenectomies) and to increase the identification rate of occult lymph node metastases (increasing the accuracy of staging). • Evidence of a survival benefit for elective lymph node dissection in selected melanoma patients and immunohistochemical and reverse transcriptase-polymerase chain reaction (RT-PCR) detection of metastases in lymph nodes deemed negative by standard histopathologic studies implies that conventional techniques understage some patients. • Similar findings have been observed in studies of micrometastatic nodal disease in breast cancer.

SLN biopsy as an alternative to elective node dissection in melanoma was first proposed by D. L. Morton et al., who used blue dye injected around the primary melanoma site to identify the SLN. • Since then, others have advocated the use of radioactive colloid and a hand-held γ-probe counter with or without the use of blue dye. • The use of either technique or both in combination is generally acceptable at the present time for staging melanoma patients. • Most surgeons now advocate the use of preoperative lymphoscintigraphy in melanoma patients. • The discordance between predicting the location of the SLN based on physical examination and the location revealed by lymphoscintigraphy can be as high as 30%. • This is particularly true on the trunk, head, and neck. • Lymphoscintigraphy can demonstrate multiple

SLNs in the expected basin, SLNs in multiple nodal basins, and intrasite SLNs.

SLN sampling is an attractive alternative to axillary lymph node dissection (ALND) in breast cancer because the risk of lymphedema is significantly lower (3 versus 17% in one series). • The most significant remaining question is whether ALND confers a survival benefit compared to axillary sampling alone. • Two large trials, National Surgical Adjuvant Breast and Bowel Project (NSABP) B-32 (SLN alone or followed by ALND for SLN-negative patients) and American College of Surgeons Oncology Group trial Z0011 (completion of ALND versus observation for SLN-positive patients), are currently exploring this issue. • For axillary SLN biopsy, both lymphazurin (isosulfan blue dye) and radioactive colloid are efficacious. • Radioactive colloid is injected intraparenchymally or intradermally at least 30 minutes before the procedure. • It is preferentially retained within the SLN(s), with delayed drainage to subsequent nodes. • The optimal injection pattern for lymphazurin remains unclear. • It can be injected around the edge of the tumor or biopsy cavity, into the overlying skin, or in a circumareolar fashion. • Intraparenchymal peritumoral injection has a higher rate of visualization of mammary nodes than does intradermal injection. • Since the transit time of blue dye is rapid, it should be injected only several minutes before beginning the dissection. • Optimally, a blue lymphatic channel leading to the most proximal blue-stained node in the axilla should be located, since staining of distal, nonsentinel lymph nodes occurs frequently. • Multiple studies have demonstrated that the SLN is identified in 92–98% of cases, with an accuracy of greater than 95% in predicting the status of the remaining axillary nodes. • False-negative rates for axillary SLN biopsy range from 0–14%, with a regression toward 5% as the surgeon's experience increases. • Axillary SLN biopsy demonstrates a significant learning curve. • It is recommended that surgeons document their results and continue to perform axillary lymph node dissections until they consistently achieve SLN detection rates of greater than 90% and false-negative rates of less than 5%. • A number of studies suggest that the learning curve extends over 30 cases. • Contraindications to SLN biopsy include inflammatory, locally advanced, or large primary tumors (>5 cm), multicentric disease, previous axillary surgery with alteration of lymphatic drainage, and clinically suspicious axillary lymphadenopathy.

ANSWER:
B, E

10. Concerning the use of electrosurgical units during surgical incisions, which of the following statements is/are true?

   A. Coagulation current entails a higher risk of infection than does the scalpel.

   B. Coagulation current causes greater necrosis than does cutting current.

   C. Burns at the return electrode (grounding) site do not occur because of the direction of the electrocautery current.

   D. Bipolar cautery limits tissue destruction to the area between the electrodes.

   E. Tissue heating depends on electrocautery waveform, power setting, and contact area.

Ref.: 15–17

COMMENTS: See Question 12.

11. Concerning the effect of lasers, electrocautery, and scalpel on wound healing, which of the following statements is/are true?

   A. Electrocautery requires less time to construct cutaneous flaps than do the other modalities.

   B. The bursting strength of flaps created using the scalpel is greater than that of those constructed using electrocautery but not greater than those constructed using an Nd:YAG or CO_2 laser.

   C. Better hemostasis is achieved using electrocautery than using the scalpel.

   D. Less drainage is observed at 48 hr for flaps created using the scalpel compared to that using other modalities.

   E. Electrocautery significantly increases the risk of infection.

Ref.: 15–17

COMMENTS: See Question 12.

12. Match the following waveforms with the appropriate electrocautery settings.

   A. Coagulation

   B. Cut

   C. Blend

Ref.: 15–17

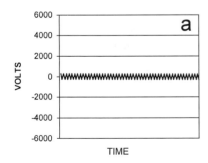

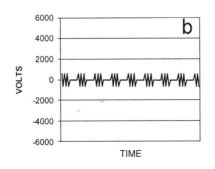

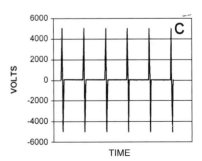

COMMENTS: In 1928, W. T. Bovie, in collaboration with H. • Cushing, developed the first commercially feasible electrosurgical unit. • Cushing warned "that the new instrument adds a complication to already complicated procedures." The advantages of rapid and meticulous hemostasis should be balanced against the hazards of tissue destruction. • Electrosurgical units develop local heat by electrical resistance to alternating current between 100 kHz and 10 MHz.

Tissue destruction depends on the power level and the specific waveform utilized. • A continuous sine wave "cutting" current (100% duty cycle) produces temperatures exceeding 1000°C, leading to instant vaporization and rapid dissipation of heat. • Use of this setting provides little conduction of heat for hemostasis. • Both "coagulation" and "blend" settings make use of a limited duty cycle, where the current is applied in brief bursts. • "Coagulation" typically uses an approximately 6% duty cycle, with current applied 6% of the time and damped the remaining 94%. • This facilitates conduction of thermal energy to surrounding tissues and improved hemostasis. • "Blend" settings are a mixture of "cut" and "coagulation" currents, typically with duty cycles of 40–75%. • Both "blend" and "coagulation" settings make use of higher voltages than does the "cut" mode, which can increase the risk of inadvertent arcing to surrounding structures. • "Coagulation" current causes more inflammation, necrosis, and abscesses than does scalpel use, but it provides a tool for constructing cutaneous flaps and achieving hemostasis more rapidly. • "Cutting" current is less destructive than is "coagulation" current but also less hemostatic. • A bipolar applicator produces tissue destruction nearly limited to the area between the electrodes, using any waveform. • Drainage is less and bursting strength greater for flaps created using sharp dissection compared to those achieved by other modalities. • Significantly less drainage is observed after 48 hr for flaps constructed using electrocautery than those created with a CO_2 laser.

ANSWERS:
Question 10: A, B, D, E
Question 11: C, D, E
Question 12: A-c; B-a; C-b

---

13. Match the following scenarios with the laparoscopic electrosurgery phenomenon.

A. The colon is injured when an arc occurs between an abraded spatula electrocautery shaft and the adjacent bowel.	a. Direct coupling
B. While using a hybrid trochar system (metal cannula with plastic retaining collar), a small-bowel thermal injury is noted in a loop of bowel near the trochar site, away from the operative field.	b. Capacitive coupling
C. After an uneventful laparoscopic cholecystectomy, a burn is noted on the patient's leg at the site of the electrosurgercal grounding pad.	c. Insulation failure
D. A blood vessel grasped with a laparoscopic dissecting forceps is cauterized by touching the activated hook electrocautery to the blade of the dissecting forceps.	d. None of the above

Ref.: 18–20

COMMENTS: Monopolar electrocautery provides a simple and convenient means of obtaining hemostasis during laparoscopic procedures. • However, early attempts to transition from bipolar electrocautery (used during early laparoscopic gynecologic procedures) to monopolar cautery resulted in several types of complications. • All result from the use of trochar cannulae to pass through the abdominal wall and the limited field of view afforded by

the laparoscope. • The physics principle that governs electrocautery is that current will seek the path of least resistance to ground. • Normally, this is the intended site of cautery at the tip of the instrument. • However, under certain conditions, cautery energy can be deposited at an unintended site and may result in inadvertent tissue damage.

Insulation failure occurs when small breaks in the insulated shaft of a laparoscopic instrument or cautery electrode allow current to pass to structures adjacent to the instrument shaft. • The site of tissue injury may not be within the field of view of the laparoscope. • This type of injury can be avoided by inspecting laparoscopic instruments before use and avoiding prolonged activation of the electrocautery without tissue contact.

Direct coupling occurs when the activated cautery electrode touches another conductive instrument that is in contact with tissue. • This is not necessarily a liability, since in both open and laparoscopic procedures tissue is routinely grasped with forceps for cautery. • However, inadvertent contact between conductive elements (e.g., the laparoscope) and the cautery electrode can result in injury. • Again, the limited field of view afforded by the laparoscope makes tissue injury more likely in laparoscopic than open procedures.

A capacitor is formed when two conductors are separated by an insulator. • Application of current to one conductor produces a coupled current in the other. • An insulated cautery electrode passing through a hybrid (metal trochar with a plastic collar) trochar system forms such a capacitor. • When high-voltage cautery modes are used (e.g., activating the cautery without touching tissue or high power settings during fulguration) 10–40% of the cautery energy can be capacitively transferred to the metal trochar. • If this trochar is in contact with bowel, injury can result. • If a low-power-density pathway to ground is provided (such as having the metal trochar in direct contact with the abdominal wall) the current is harmlessly returned via the grounding electrode. • Therefore, hybrid trochar systems should be used with caution.

Grounding pad burns generally result from improper initial application of the grounding electrode or the electrode's "pulling off" during the case. • If only a small portion of the electrode is in contact with the patient, the current density can be high enough to damage the skin. • Modern electrocautery units use active monitoring of the return electrode to decrease the risk of these injuries.

ANSWERS:
A-c; B-b; C-d; D-a

---

14. Which of the following statements is/are true with regard to the argon beam coagulator (ABC)?

A. The coagulator delivers a laser beam that coagulates tissue by a light reaction.

B. The depth of necrosis is related to the power setting of the argon beam.

C. The coagulator is useful for minimizing bleeding from raw surfaces of intestine.

D. The coagulator can be a useful adjunct to laparoscopic surgery.

Ref.: 21–23

COMMENTS: The ABC uses a radiofrequency range of energy across a jet of inert gas (argon) that provides a noncontact monopolar zone of necrosis. • It is most useful for aiding hemostasis with solid organs such as the liver, spleen, and kidney. • The depth of injury is proportional to the duration and energy delivered and the organ treated. • The depth of thermal injury to the spleen and liver ranges from 2 to 7 mm. • The absence of smoke and the no-touch technique make it particularly useful for laparoscopic application. • The ABC has demonstrated a clear advantage in the reduction of hyperplastic nasal turbinates, telangiectatic lesions in the nasal mucosa, and progressive papillomatosis of the larynx. • When used properly and with an understanding of its potential for inadvertent thermal injury, ABC can be safe and result in improved hemostasis; minimal depth of thermal injury; shortened duration of the procedure; decreased blood loss, edema, and ecchymosis; and the ability to more safely coagulate around neural tissue.

ANSWERS:
B, D

15. Which of the following statements is/are true with regard to the ultrasonic harmonic scalpel?

    A. The active blade vibrates at a frequency of 100,000 Hz.

    B. The time required for advanced laparoscopic procedures has been reduced when using the harmonic scalpel.

    C. Electrical energy generated by the scalpel is the mechanism for coagulation.

    D. Use of the harmonic scalpel is more cost-effective than use of clip appliers for dividing medium-sized blood vessels.

    E. The harmonic scalpel cannot injure adjacent structures because no heat is generated.

Ref.: 18, 29

COMMENTS: The harmonic scalpel uses mechanical energy rather than electrical energy to achieve hemostasis. • A piezoelectric element in the handpiece vibrates at a frequency of 55,000 Hz, and a laparoscopic extender carries the energy to the tissue. • The blade couples with the tissue and mechanically denatures protein, forming a coagulum that seals small vessels. • Prolonged application of the harmonic scalpel produces secondary heat that seals larger vessels. • Coaptation occurs at lower temperatures (50–100°C) than with electrocautery or lasers (150–400°C). • Low-power settings cause slower heating and more coagulation, and higher-power settings result in rapid but less hemostatic cutting. • The time required for procedures such as short gastric vessel division has been reduced, resulting in a shortened operating time for advanced laparoscopic procedures. • If one considers the shortened time for a procedure when using the harmonic scalpel and the cost of clip appliers when they are used for vessel ligation and division, the harmonic scalpel has also been shown to reduce the overall cost of advanced laparoscopic procedures. • The harmonic scalpel entails a lower risk of lateral thermal injury than does laser or electrocautery. • However, adjacent structures may still be injured by heat transmitted through tissues or by inadvertent contact with the active blade.

ANSWERS:
B, D

16. What is the fundamental tissue property measured by a CT scan?

    A. Atomic number

    B. Density

    C. Relative x-ray attenuation

    D. Hydrogen content

    E. Gray scale

Ref.: 18, 29

COMMENTS: See Question 17.

17. Rank the following in order of increasing Hounsfield units (HU).

    A. Water

    B. Muscle

    C. Air

    D. Cortical bone

    E. Lung

Ref.: 1, 25

COMMENTS: CT scanning is an imaging technique introduced in the early 1970s that generates cross-sectional images in the axial plane. • The CT image is mathematically reconstructed from multiple planar views (projections) acquired at different angles around the patient. • The image is a map of the relative linear attenuation of x-rays by the tissues traversed by the x-ray beam. • The amount of attenuation is determined by the number of atoms and electrons present in the tissue traversed. • The relative attenuation coefficient is expressed in HU (CT number). • HUs for several tissues are shown below. • By definition, the HU value for water is always zero and that for air is −1000. • Each CT slice is composed of multiple pixels. • The pixel size is determined by dividing the field of view by the number of pixels. • Each pixel is a two-dimensional representation of the volume element (voxel) of tissue in the patient. • The (three-dimensional) volume of the voxel is calculated by multiplying the pixel size by the slice thickness. • The brightness of each pixel in the CT image is proportional to the average attenuation coefficient of the tissues within that voxel. • Window width and level can be changed to optimize the visual display of CT images. • Window width is the difference between the maximum and minimum HU of the displayed image. • Window level represents the HU value of the pixel midway between displayed absolute black (minimum HU) and white (maximum HU). • Typical window and level settings for several examinations are shown below.

Tissue	Approximate HU Value
Air	−1000
Lung	−300
Fat	−90
Water	0
Muscle	50
Cortical bone	1000+

Examination Type	Window	Level
Head	80	40
Mediastinum	450	40
Lung	1500	−500
Abdomen	150	60

ANSWERS:
Question 16: C
Question 17: C, E, A, B, D

18. Concerning the use of US in clinical practice, which of the following is/are false?

    A. US has a frequency equal to that of human hearing (20 kHz).

    B. A 10-MHz transducer is ideal for scanning deep abdominal structures.

    C. The speed of US in blood is slower than that through air.

D. Hypoechoic tissues are less echoic, or darker, than surrounding tissue.

E. B-mode US is appropriate for scanning for gallstones.

Ref.: 1, 26, 27

COMMENTS: US is mechanical energy generated by a piezoelectric crystal and transmitted through a medium. • Higher frequency yields greater resolution but less depth of penetration. • Thus, deep structures require lower frequencies. • US has a frequency higher than that of human hearing (20 MHz). • Low-frequency probes (2 MHz) are used for imaging large body areas, such as the abdomen, especially in obese patients. • Mid-range probes (3–5 MHz) are used for general-purpose imaging. • High-frequency probes (7–10 MHz) are used for superficial small-parts scanning and vascular mapping.

The propagation velocity in tissue depends on the mechanical properties of the medium through which it travels. • In general, the stiffer and less compressible the medium, the faster the propagation velocity. • US travels more slowly through air (343 m/s) and faster through bone (3000 m/s). • For soft tissue, the speed of US is approximately 1540 m/s. • As US interacts with tissue, energy is lost by reflection, scattering, refraction, and absorption. • Refraction and absorption divert sound energy from the receiving transducer. • The commonest causes of artifacts are air, calcium, and reverberation.

The **A mode** is the amplitude mode and is used primarily for ocular imaging and echoencephalography. • The **B mode** is the brightness mode. • For real-time imaging, B-mode US is the most commonly used in clinical practice. • The **M mode**, or motion mode, is designed to study the heart. • The effectiveness of US is highly operator dependent.

ANSWERS:
A, B, *C*, E

19. The US images displayed below illustrate anatomic structures routinely seen during the performance of a breast US examination as well as a number of commonly encountered artifacts related to the real-time performance of a breast scan. Match the answer that most closely corresponds to the images shown.

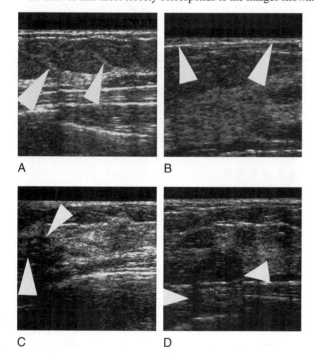

A   B

C   D

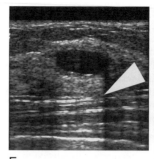 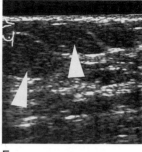

E   F

a. Subareolar ducts

b. Shadowing

c. Adipose tissue

d. Enhancement

e. Skin illustrating variable thickness

f. Cooper's ligaments

Ref.: 26

COMMENTS: During its formation, the breast develops within an envelope of connective tissue. • This envelope of fascia splits into an anterior and posterior layer surrounding the parenchyma. • The suspensory **Cooper's ligaments** of the breast tether the breast tissue to this bilaminar fascial envelope. • They are most clearly seen as bright, hyperechoic linear extensions arching toward and away from the anterior leaf of the superficial fascia at the dermal boundary.

The skin appears as a hyperechoic (bright) line at the top of the image. • It is thickest at the nipple-areolar junction (approximately 4 mm in depth) and thinnest at the periphery of the breast (approximately 2 mm in depth). • Careful assessment of the skin line during breast scanning can provide important clues, such as **skin of variable thickness** (e.g., a localized thickening), that may reflect changes in the parenchyma deep to that area. • A light touch on the transducer preserves these subtle differences.

A scan of the nipple-areolar area shows multiple hypoechoic (dark) structures in a rich connective-tissue latticework that is hyperechoic (bright). • The hypoechoic areas are ducts. • Depending on the orientation of the transducer to the scanned area, the ducts may appear in cross section, tangentially, or parallel. • The ducts converging at the nipple-areolar junction, or the **subareolar ducts**, are larger than those located peripherally. • Nipple discharge is often associated with an ectatic (i.e., markedly enlarged) duct. • US can be used effectively to locate and analyze an area that is often clinically difficult to detect.

Shadowing is an artifact generated by the interaction of tissue with the US beam. • The US pulse generated by the transducer travels in a straight line from this source into the tissue being scanned and then is returned. • The amplitude (strength of signal) of the returning echo is then displayed on the monitor in varying shades of gray, with their intensity dependent on the amplitude of the returning signal. • Shadowing is seen as a hypoechoic (dark) area immediately underneath the area of interest. • The shadowing itself results from a lack of return signal to the transducer. • This loss of signal can result from several interactions: the signal may be deflected away from the transducer; scattered within the focal lesion, with resultant diminution of the return echo; or simply converted to heat and dissipated. • Shadowing is seen in both benign and malignant conditions.

Enhancement is another useful artifact. • It is often called through-transmission and is seen on the monitor as a bright band extending below the area of interest. • Because of the lack of impedance to the US signal (i.e., reflection and scatter) in and through the area of interest, there is increased signal reception deep to the focal lesion. • The area of through-transmission appears correspondingly brighter than the areas immediately adjacent to this point. • Ultrasound pulses are reflected back to or away from the transducer by slight differences in acoustic impedance between one tissue type and another. • If an area is composed of tissue or fluid with approximately the same acoustic properties, the strength of the returning US signal is greater than that of the signal returning from the area adjacent to it.

Adipose tissue appears hypoechoic (darker) in relation to stromal tissue (hyperechoic). • Adipose tissue can appear around as well as within the breast parenchyma. • It is also seen immediately underneath the skin and is traversed by Cooper's ligaments. • By virtue of the contrast between the darker adipose tissue and brighter stromal network of the parenchyma, the anterior lobar contour is easily seen. • There is an additional retromammary layer of adipose tissue deep to the posterior surface of the breast lobe, but it is often not well developed and may be poorly visualized.

ANSWERS:
A-f; B-e; C-a; D-b; E-d; F-c

20. Breast US is used as a clinical tool to evaluate *mammographic* abnormalities, *clinically detected* abnormalities, and as an *adjunctive* means of evaluating "dense breasts" noted on mammography. Evaluation of a US-detected focal lesion includes an assessment of a lesion's contour, margins, and internal echo characteristics and the presence or absence of shadowing and enhancement. Match the lettered image with the most likely diagnosis.

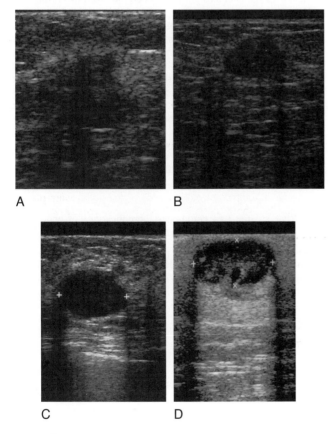

A B

C D

a. Cyst

b. Fibroadenoma

c. Breast cancer

d. Complex cyst

Ref.: 26

COMMENTS: Depending on the fluid characteristics within a **cyst** and the tension exerted on the cyst wall by hydrostatic pressure, the contours and internal echo pattern of a cyst may vary. • If the wall is tense, the cyst contours are round. • If not, the cyst may appear ovoid or even elongated. • However, the margins are always sharp and smooth, with bilateral edge shadowing. • If the fluid within the cyst is uniform, the cyst appears anechoic (black) and through-transmission (posterior enhancement) is present.

A classic fluid-filled cyst is uniformly anechoic (black). • In a **complex cyst**, the presence of internal echoes in what would otherwise appear to be a simple cyst may be due to more viscous liquid. • This is most commonly seen in long-standing cysts where proteinaceous material has been secreted into the cyst lumen. • Internal echoes within the cyst may also be generated by an intracystic papilloma or by reverberation artifact. • Because of the indeterminate nature of the internal echoes, fine-needle aspiration is required for diagnosis of complex cysts.

Fibroadenomas have many of the characteristics of a cyst. • Their smooth contour can result in bilateral edge shadowing, and the homogeneity of the tissue comprising a fibroadenoma often produces posterior enhancement. • These internal characteristics produce a homogeneous internal echo pattern that is hypoechoic. • Focal lesions thought to be potentially solid on US scans should be subjected to histologic or cytologic evaluation. • Medullary carcinoma, a solid lesion, may also appear indistinguishable from a fibroadenoma.

Breast carcinoma displays characteristic features on ultrasound examination. • Typically, the contour is jagged and irregular, and the desmoplastic response generated by the malignancy causes heterogenous and irregular internal echoes. • Because of the large degree of scattering and attenuation of the mixed tissue components, the area corresponding to the body of the tumor is hypoechoic. • Posterior shadowing can be irregular and does not disappear with a change of transducer angulation or increased transducer pressure. • Some breast cancers can have smooth contours, posterior enhancement, and other findings associated with benign conditions. • Careful and thoughtful analysis of each focal lesion is required.

ANSWERS:
A-c; B-b; C-a; D-d

21. Which of the following transducer positions is/are used as part of a focused assessment for the sonographic examination of the trauma patient (FAST) examination for abdominal trauma?

A. Transverse views of the supraumbilical region

B. Sagittal views of the subxiphoid region

C. Left upper quadrant, posterior axillary line

D. Transverse suprapubic view

E. Right upper quadrant, midaxillary line

F. Left upper quadrant, anterior axillary line

Ref.: 28

COMMENTS: Increasingly, US is being used as an extension of the physical examination in evaluating trauma patients. • A FAST scan may be included during the secondary survey portion of the Advanced Trauma Life Support protocol of the American College of Surgeons. • After placement of a nasogastric tube, but before placement of a Foley catheter, a 3.5-MHz transducer is used to assess for blood in the pericardial sac, Morison's pouch, pelvis, and splenorenal recess. • The examination is conducted rapidly (in 2–3 minutes) in sequence using four views: (1) a sagittal transducer orientation in the subxiphoid region to identify fluid in the pericardium; (2) a sagittal transducer orientation in the right midaxillary line between the eleventh and twelfth ribs to examine the liver, kidneys, diaphragm, Morison's pouch, and right paracolic gutter; (3) a sagittal transducer orientation at the left posterior axillary line between the ninth and tenth ribs to evaluate the kidney, spleen, splenorenal space, and left paracolic gutter; and (4) a transverse transducer orientation about 4 cm superior to the symphysis pubis oriented inferiorly to visualize the full bladder, rectouterine space, and both sides of the pelvis.

The FAST scan is particularly useful in identifying the need for laparotomy in hypotensive patients with blunt abdominal trauma. • Sensitivity, specificity, and negative predictive values of greater than 95% have been demonstrated. • US is less useful in detecting solid-organ injuries, with sensitivities of 44–90% and negative predictive values of 72–99%. • Serial FAST scans can assess for the development of hemoperitoneum following changes in the patient's condition.

ANSWERS:
B, C, D, E

22. Match the following structures with the upper-limit normal sizes on US or CT examinations.

A.	Gallbladder wall thickness	a.	1 mm
B.	Common bile duct diameter	b.	3 mm
C.	Common bile duct diameter after cholecystectomy	c.	6 mm
D.	Gallbladder anteroposterior diameter	d.	1 cm
E.	Pancreatic head short axis	e.	1.5 cm
F.	Pancreatic tail short axis	f.	2.5 cm
		g.	4 cm
		h.	6 cm

Ref.: 1, 29

COMMENTS: See Question 23.

23. Which of the following ultrasound findings are suggestive of acute cholecystitis?

A. An 8-mm thick gallbladder wall

B. A 1.2-cm diameter common bile duct (CBD)

C. Focal gallbladder tenderness

D. Multiple intraluminal triangular echoes

E. Fluid in the gallbladder fossa

Ref.: 1, 29

COMMENTS: US and CT imaging are very useful in evaluating pathologic conditions of the biliary system and pancreas. • The initial study of choice for evaluating right upper quadrant abdominal pain is US, which can confirm cholelithiasis and cholecystitis or suggest other causes of pain unrelated to the gallbladder. • The gallbladder should be examined for size, wall thickness, internal contents, edema, and habitus. • A thickened gallbladder wall (>3 mm) is commonly seen in acute cholecystitis. • However, pancreatitis, liver diseases such as hepatitis, ascites, and congestive heart failure also can cause gallbladder wall thickening. • Cholecystitis is suggested by focal gallbladder tenderness (sonographic Murphy's sign), increased gallbladder size (anteroposterior diameter >4 cm), impacted stones at the gallbladder neck or complex intraluminal echoes, and pericholecystic fluid collections. • US is more than 95% sensitive for gallstones, seen as an echogenic focus that may exhibit acoustic shadowing. • Gallstones may be mobile or fixed within the gallbladder. • Focal gallbladder tenderness is the most accurate finding for excluding acute cholecystitis. • Less than 10% of patients without focal tenderness have acute cholecystitis. • The presence of multiple intraluminal triangular echoes, yielding a "comet tail" appearance, is suggestive of adenomyomatosis.

A right upper quadrant US examination should include evaluation of the CBD and a survey for intrahepatic bile duct dilatation. • Normally, the diameter of the CBD is less than 6 mm. • For patients over 60 years old, 1 mm can be added to the normal diameter for each decade over 60. • The CBD normally dilates to 8–10 mm after cholecystectomy. • Nonvisualization of CBD stones does not exclude choledocholithiasis, since stones are visualized by US in only about one third of cases. • Intrahepatic duct prominence is also suggestive of biliary obstruction.

A right upper quadrant US examination also should include some assessment of the pancreas. • However, the patient's body habitus or overlying gas within the bowel can limit visualization of the pancreas. • The pancreas is better imaged with CT than with US. • The body of the pancreas is normally found anterior to the splenic vein, which provides a useful landmark during US imaging. • The normal short-axis diameter of the pancreas is 2.5 cm at the head and less than 1.5 cm at the tail. • The total size of the pancreas generally decreases with increasing age. • However, proper "proportions" of the pancreas should be maintained. • Focal enlargement suggests a pancreatic mass. • Many pancreatic CT protocols make use of water contrast to better image abnormalities in or near the duodenal wall, which can be missed if oral radio-opaque contrast is used. • Pancreatitis is suggested by pancreatic duct dilation or stricture, stranding of peripancreatic fat, diffuse pancreatic enlargement with loss of internal structure, and pancreatic or peripancreatic fluid collections. • However, a normal-appearing pancreas on CT does not exclude clinical pancreatitis.

ANSWERS:
Question 22: A-b; B-c; C-d; D-g; E-f; F-e
Question 23: A, C, E

24. What are the two commonest complications of endoscopic retrograde cholangiopancreatography (ERCP) with sphincterotomy?

A. Cholangitis   0.1%

B. Perforation   0.3%

C. Hemorrhage   2%

D. Pancreatitis   5%

E. Hepatic hematoma

Ref.: 18

COMMENTS: ERCP allows evaluation of the cause of CBD dilatation and provides therapeutic options. • Diagnostic ERCP directly visualizes the ampulla of Vater and allows radiographic imaging of the CBD and pancreatic duct. • Therapeutic options include biliary and pancreatic sphincterotomy, stone removal, biliary or pancreatic stenting, and internal drainage of pancreatic fluid collections such as pseudocysts. • Hyperamylasemia may be seen in up to 60% of patients after ERCP. • However, only about 5% of patients develop clinical symptoms of pancreatitis. • The exact cause of post-ERCP pancreatitis is unknown. • However, it is commonly attributed to increases in pancreatic duct pressure with extravasation of pancreatic enzymes from acini into the pancreatic parenchyma. • Post-ERCP pancreatitis is usually mild and responds to conservative management. • More severe cases may require aggressive management, including drainage of pseudocysts or operative pancreatic débridement and necrosectomy. • Hemorrhage may occur after endoscopic sphincterotomy but is clinically significant in less than 2% of patients. • Local bleeding can be treated with electrocautery or sclerosis with epinephrine. • Severe hemorrhage may require selective percutaneous embolization or operative exploration via a duodenotomy. • Biliary perforation occurs in approximately 0.3% of cases, usually as a result of an extended sphincterotomy. • Most patients respond to nonoperative management, including nothing-by-mouth status, nasogastric decompression, and broad-spectrum antibiotics. • Operative intervention (primary closure or omental patch with consideration of pyloric exclusion) should be undertaken if sepsis causes deterioration of the patient's condition. • Cholangitis (0.1% of cases) is more common in patients with pre-ERCP biliary obstruction or after stent placement.

ANSWERS:
C, D

25. Concerning the cardiopulmonary effects of pneumoperitoneum during laparoscopy, which of the following is/are true?

   A. Cardiopulmonary dysfunction occurs when the intra-abdominal pressure (IAP) reaches 20 mmHg or more in normovolemic patients.

   B. Positive end-expiratory pressure (PEEP) offsets the hemodynamic effects of pneumoperitoneum.

   C. Hypovolemia lowers the level of IAP needed to cause deleterious hemodynamic effects.

   D. Laparoscopic surgery prevents diaphragmatic dysfunction during the postoperative period for patients with chronic obstructive pulmonary disease (COPD).

   E. Increased IAP leads to increased concentrations of plasma renin, decreased venous return, and decreased intracavitary atrial pressures.

Ref.: 30, 31

COMMENTS: Intraabdominal hypertension may cause pulmonary and cardiovascular compromise when the IAP reaches 20–40 mmHg of pressure in normovolemic patients. • PEEP and IAP have additive effects on decreasing preload. • IAP hypertension results in elevated peak airway pressures, decreased pulmonary compliance and vital capacity, and increased alveolar dead space. • Although laparoscopic surgery has been associated with less derangement of pulmonary function and a lower incidence of postoperative pulmonary complications than has laparotomy, its use in patients with COPD may be deleterious. • The hemodynamic effects of increased IAP seem to be due to decreased cardiac output caused by decreased preload, increased systemic vascular resistance, and an abrupt increase in mean arterial pressure.

ANSWERS:
A, C

26. Which of the following insufflation gases for laparoscopic pneumoperitoneum has the greatest solubility in water?

   A. Carbon dioxide

   B. Nitrous oxide

   C. Helium

   D. Argon

   E. Air

Ref.: 18

COMMENTS: See Question 28.

27. Which of the following insufflation gases for laparoscopic pneumoperitoneum supports combustion?

   A. Carbon dioxide

   B. Nitrous oxide

   C. Helium

   D. Argon

   E. None of the above

Ref.: 18

COMMENTS: See Question 28.

28. Which of the following insufflation gases for laparoscopic pneumoperitoneum can cause hypercarbia and acidosis?

   A. Carbon dioxide

   B. Nitrous oxide

   C. Helium

   D. Argon

   E. None of the above

Ref.: 18

COMMENTS: The ideal insufflation agent for laparoscopy should be colorless, physiologically inert, nonexplosive when used with electrocautery, and nontoxic. • Low tissue solubility decreases loss of gas to absorption, while a high blood solubility reduces the risk of embolization after inadvertent injection of gas into the circulation. • Finally, the agent should be readily available, have a long shelf life, and be inexpensive. • Carbon dioxide, the most common insufflation agent, is highly water soluble but can cause hypercarbia and acidosis. • Following a long laparoscopic procedure, it can take several hours to completely eliminate the accumulated carbon dioxide and return the body's acid-base status to the preoperative state. • Carbon dioxide and the resultant acidosis can decrease cardiac contractility, increase CVP, and increase pulmonary artery pressures and pulmonary vascular resistance. • Central effects of carbon dioxide include sympathetic stimulation resulting in vasoconstriction and tachycardia. • Usually these changes are not clinically significant, but they can be important in patients with underlying cardiac or respiratory problems. • The other gases listed do not affect acid-base balance but have their own disadvantages. • Nitrous oxide does not alter pH status and may provide some local analgesia; however, it supports combustion in the presence of hydrogen or methane gas. • This raises the (at least theoretical) risk of explosion if cautery is used. • Helium also has no effect on pH balance, but its poor water solubility can lead to the development of postoperative subcutaneous emphysema. • Argon is physiologically inert, but porcine models have demonstrated a cardiac depressant effect following argon insufflation.

A N S W E R S :
Question 26: A
Question 27: B
Question 28: A

29. A mildly obese patient is undergoing laparoscopic cholecystectomy. The patient is anesthetized and endotracheal intubation performed. Because of difficulty obtaining adequate venous access, a left-sided internal jugular triple-lumen central venous catheter is inserted. A Veress needle technique is selected for obtaining pneumoperitoneum. Fifteen milliliters of 1% lidocaine solution is infiltrated at the umbilicus, the Veress needle inserted, and insufflation of CO_2 at 2.5 L/min begun. The abdomen begins to inflate in the expected fashion. However, the anesthesiologist notes a sudden decrease in end-tidal CO_2 followed by progressive hypotension. What is the most likely cause of the patient's instability?

    A. Malignant hyperthermia

    B. Anaphylactic reaction to lidocaine

    C. Decreased pulmonary ventilation resulting from elevation of the diaphragm by the pneumoperitoneum

    D. Carbon dioxide embolus

    E. Decreased venous return with pneumoperitoneum caused by preoperative volume depletion (dehydration)

    Ref.: 19, 32

COMMENTS: See Question 31.

30. Immediate treatment of the patient's instability is initiated. Which of the following should be performed?

    A. Immediately stop CO_2 insufflation and decompress the abdomen.

    B. Administer high-dose steroids and Benadryl.

    C. Extubate and immediately reintubate the patient to ensure correct endotracheal tube position.

    D. Stop inhalation anesthetic agents and administer 100% oxygen.

    E. Give a rapid IV fluid bolus of 2 L of 5% albumin solution via the central line.

    Ref.: 19, 32

COMMENTS: See Question 31.

31. Despite initial therapy, the patient's vital signs continue to deteriorate. Which of the following additional measures may be helpful?

    A. Place the patient in the left lateral decubitus position.

    B. Place the patient in the right lateral decubitus position.

    C. Aspirate the patient's central venous catheter.

    D. Perform emergent laparotomy.

    E. Place bilateral chest tubes.

    Ref.: 19, 32

COMMENTS: Gas embolism is a rare but potentially fatal complication of laparoscopy. • Venous CO_2 embolization can result from direct laceration of a major vein by the Veress needle or, less commonly, by systemic absorption of CO_2 at large raw tissue beds. • A significant gas embolus in the central venous circulation can cause a "gas lock" of the right ventricle, with pulmonary outflow obstruction or impaired venous return precipitating cardiovascular collapse. • An early sign of CO_2 embolus is a decrease in end-tidal CO_2 because of decreased lung perfusion relative to ventilation, resulting in increased physiologic dead space. • Other signs include elevated airway pressures because of bronchoconstriction, elevated central venous pressures, and cardiac arrhythmias. • A continuous "mill wheel" cardiac murmur caused by intercardiac gas may be heard with an esophageal stethoscope.

The most important immediate measure is to discontinue CO_2 insufflation and decompress the abdomen by releasing the existing pneumoperitoneum. • Stopping inhalational anesthetic agents and providing positive-pressure ventilation with 100% oxygen is also recommended. • The patient should be placed in the left lateral decubitus position. • If a central line is in place, it may be aspirated in an attempt to remove trapped gas. • Since the entrained CO_2 is rapidly absorbed, successful resuscitation is possible if the embolus is small and the condition is recognized quickly.

A N S W E R S :
Question 29: D
Question 30: A, D
Question 31: A, C

32. Laparoscopic splenectomy is performed for idiopathic thrombocytopenic purpura (ITP). How should the specimen be removed?

    A. Extending one of the port site incisions to accommodate the specimen

    B. Fragmenting the specimen and removing the pieces through a 12-mm port

    C. Placing it in a retrieval bag, fragmenting it, exteriorizing the bag through a port site, and removing it piecemeal

    D. Placing it in a retrieval bag and removing the intact specimen through a separate incision

    Ref.: 18

COMMENTS: Laparoscopic surgery must accommodate the need to remove specimens that are larger than the laparoscopic port sites. • There are a variety of techniques by which this may be accomplished, depending on the nature and size of the specimen and whether there is a need to preserve the specimen intact. • Potential routes for specimen removal include port sites, extended port site incisions, separate abdominal wall incisions, and transanal and transvaginal routes. • Use of a retrieval bag can minimize contamination and specimen loss and is particularly important if the specimen is infected, friable, or malignant. • Fragmentation of large solid specimens is appropriate to preserve the advantage of small laparoscopic incisions, provided an intact specimen is not required for pathologic evaluation. • Fragmentation is contraindicated if the lesion is potentially malignant. • When laparoscopic splenectomy is performed for ITP, it is standard to place the spleen in a sturdy retrieval bag, externalize the bag orifice at a port site, and then remove the spleen piecemeal. • Great care must be taken to avoid internal rupture of the spleen or of the bag, which can result in splenosis.

A N S W E R :
C

33. With regard to expanded polytetrafluoroethylene (PTFE; Gore-Tex) and polypropylene mesh (Marlex), which of the following statements is/are true?

    A. Expanded PTFE contains spaces smaller than 10 μm and may harbor bacteria.

    B. Expanded PTFE and polypropylene mesh are well tolerated without significant evidence of rejection.

    C. Polypropylene mesh and expanded PTFE incorporate into host tissue at equal rates.

    D. Polypropylene mesh and expanded PTFE come in both absorbable and nonabsorbable forms.

Ref.: 33

COMMENTS: Absorbable synthetic mesh materials include polyglycolic acid (Dexon), polyglactin (Vicryl), and carbon fiber mesh. • Nonabsorbable meshes include tantalum, stainless steel, polyester cloth (Dacron), polyester sheeting (Mylar), nylon mesh, Dacron mesh (Mersilene), acrylic cloth (Orlon), polyvinyl sponge (Ivalon), PTFE (Teflon mesh and cloth), expanded PTFE (Gore-Tex), polyvinyl cloth (Vinyon-N), and polypropylene mesh (Marlex and Prolene). • Polypropylene mesh, PTFE, Dacron, and Teflon mesh are well tolerated without significant evidence of rejection. • Any biomaterial that contains pores or spaces less than 10 μm in size cannot allow ingress of granulocytes to clear infection. • Consequently, these materials are associated with an increased chance of infection and sinus tract formation. • Expanded PTFE contains spaces smaller than 10 μm. • In contrast, polypropylene is made of widely spaced monofilament fibers. • Expanded PTFE has been shown to allow penetration of fibroblasts to a depth of only 10% at 3 years, whereas polypropylene mesh has complete incorporation of host tissue throughout the thickness of the biomaterial at 3 years.

ANSWERS:
A, B

34. Match each type of laser with the appropriate medium.

A. CO$_2$	a. Solid
B. Neodymium:yttrium aluminum garnet (Nd:YAG)	b. Gaseous
C. Argon	c. Electronic
D. Potassium titanyl phosphate (KTP)	
E. Diode	

Ref.: 34

COMMENTS: Several types of lasers have found application in medicine. • Primarily, they include the CO$_2$ laser, argon laser, KTP laser, and Nd:YAG laser. • Lasers are named for the medium used to produce light, that is, the medium stimulated by the energy source leading to release of the stored energy as photons (light). • These media may be gaseous, as in the case of the CO$_2$ and argon; solid, as in the case of the KTP or Nd:YAG laser; and even electronic, as in the case of the diode laser. • The wavelength of laser light produced depends on the medium used; lasers of different wavelength have dramatically different abilities to cut, coagulate, or vaporize tissue.

ANSWERS:
A-b; B-a; C-b; D-a; E-c

35. Which of the following characteristics affect the energy deposited in tissues by the laser?

    A. Laser power

    B. Laser beam diameter

    C. Duration of exposure

    D. Tissue color

    E. Color of the laser light

Ref.: 34

COMMENTS: Lasers produce their effects on tissue through absorption. • The absorbed light generates heat, resulting in tissue effects, which include cutting, coagulation, and vaporization. • A variety of factors regulate the effect of laser light on tissue: (1) the power of the laser (measured in watts); (2) the spot size, or diameter, of the laser beam contacting the tissue; (3) the duration of laser exposure; and (4) the degree of absorption of laser light, which is a function of tissue color and laser light color (which is a function of the laser's wavelength). • Power (watts) divided by spot size (in square centimeters) equals the **power density**. • Increased power density, as well as increased exposure time or tissue absorption, increases the local tissue effect. • To cut with a laser, one generally uses higher power with a small spot size (focused beam) for a short duration. • Optimal coagulation requires lower power but a larger spot size (defocused beam) and a longer lasing duration.

ANSWERS:
A, B, C, D, E

36. Match each type of laser with the appropriate phrase(s).

A. Nd:YAG	a. Fiberoptic laser
B. Argon	b. Deep coagulation
C. KTP	c. Superficial coagulation
	d. Useful for treating neovascular lesions in diabetic retinopathy
	e. Treatment of obstructing, nonoperable rectal cancer

Ref.: 34

COMMENTS: The Nd:YAG, argon, and KTP lasers are delivered via optical fibers. • When used as a free beam, the Nd:YAG laser generates significant coagulation. • The argon and KTP lasers are considered superficial photocoagulators but may also cut and vaporize without the extensive damage characterized by the free-beam Nd:YAG laser. • In contrast to the CO$_2$ laser, there is fair divergence of the Nd:YAG, argon, and KTP laser beams, which results in minimal tissue effect 2 inches or more from the tip. • When the tip is quite near (1–2 mm) the tissue, cutting results; when the tissue is several millimeters from the tip, vaporization results; and when the tissue is 1–2 cm from the tip, coagulation occurs. • Whereas the depth of tissue injury with the argon and KTP lasers varies between 0.5 and 2.0 mm, the free-beam Nd:YAG is highly absorbed in dark tissue and may result in tissue injury at 2–6 mm depth. • The argon laser is absorbed by pigments (e.g., hemoglobin and melanin), making it useful for procedures such as treatment of neovascular lesions in diabetic retinopathy and superficial vascular lesions such as telangiectasias or port-wine stains, but limiting its ability to coagulate an actively bleeding lesion. • Because the Nd:YAG laser causes deep tissue penetrance and coagulation, it has become the laser of choice for endoscopic palliation of nonoperable obstructing tumors of the respiratory and gastrointestinal tracts and for treatment of a bleeding lesion (e.g., an ulcer).

ANSWERS:
A-a,b,e; B-a,c,d; C-a,c

---

37. Match the following sutures with their absorption characteristics.

   A. Polyglycolic acid (Dexon) 14d

   B. Poliglecaprone 25 (Monocryl) 7d

   C. Surgical silk 1y

   D. Chromic catgut 7d

   E. Nylon 4y

   F. Polyglactin 910 (Vicryl) 14d

   a. Slow hydrolysis with approximately 10–15% strength loss per year

   b. Hydrolysis with approximately 50% strength remaining at 14 days

   c. Proteolysis with approximately 50% strength loss after 1 week

   d. Hydrolysis with approximately 50% strength remaining at 7 days

   e. Proteolysis with approximately 50% strength loss after 1 year

Ref.: 35–37

COMMENTS: Surgical sutures may be characterized by their composition (natural versus synthetic or monofilament versus braided), absorption characteristics, and absorption mechanism (hydrolysis or proteolysis). • Sutures are considered nonabsorbable if they retain most of their tensile strength after 60 days in body tissues. • Plain catgut suture, derived from sheep or cattle intestine, is absorbed in about a week. • Treatment of catgut with chromium delays proteolytic digestion. • Chromic catgut retains about 50–60% of its strength after 2 weeks and incites less tissue reaction than does plain gut. • Polyglycolic acid (Dexon) and polygalactin 910 (Vicryl) are composed of braided filaments of synthetic polymers. • Both are degraded by hydrolysis and retain nearly all their tensile strength for the first week. • About 50% of their strength remains at 2 weeks, with almost no strength remaining at 1 month. • Polyglyconate (Maxon) and polydioxanone (PDS) are monofilament polymers with strength comparable to that of braided absorbable sutures. • Approximately 50% of their strength remains at 4 weeks. • Poliglecaprone 25 (Monocryl) and polygalactin 910 (Vicryl Rapide) are synthetic sutures with characteristics similar to those of chromic catgut. • However, they are absorbed by hydrolysis and do not incite the inflammatory response seen with catgut. • They retain about 50% of their original tensile strength after 1 week. • Silk and nylon are classified as nonabsorbable, but both are slowly absorbed or digested. • The handling characteristics of silk remain the gold standard for suture materials, but silk incites significant inflammation. • Silk undergoes proteolysis, losing about half its tensile strength after 1 year, and often cannot be found after 2–3 years. • Nylon is a synthetic polymer available in both monofilament (Dermalon and Ethilon) and braided (Neurolon and Surgilon) forms. • It undergoes slow hydrolysis, with 10–15% of its tensile strength lost per year. • Metal sutures are nonreactive and have high tensile strengths but have poor handling characteristics.

ANSWER:
A-b; B-d; C-e; D-c; E-a; F-b

---

38. Which of the following is the most appropriate type of central catheter for a patient requiring long-term home parenteral nutrition?

   A. Tunneled, single-lumen catheter

   B. Tunneled, double-lumen catheter

   C. Single-lumen catheter with implanted port

   D. Double-lumen implanted port

   E. Nontunneled triple-lumen catheter

Ref.: 36

COMMENTS: A number of catheter devices are available for the purpose of providing long-term central venous access. • These catheters are typically indicated for administration of parenteral nutrition, chemotherapeutic agents, antibiotics, or other medications. • Selection of the most appropriate device must take into account the specific therapeutic needs, the estimated duration of therapy, and the concerns and capabilities of the individual patient. • The goal is to provide durable access for the necessary length of treatment with the lowest risk of complications, particularly catheter sepsis. • Multilumen catheters in general have been associated with higher infection rates than have single-lumen catheters. • Implanted ports are designed for intermittent cannulation and have been particularly useful for patients receiving cytotoxic chemotherapy for malignant disease. • They are convenient for patients because there is no externalized portion that requires attention. • However, implanted ports have been associated with higher rates of sepsis when used for home hyperalimentation.

ANSWER:
A

---

39. Which of the following infectious complications of an implanted Hickman central venous catheter require(s) catheter removal?

   A. Exit site infection

   B. Subcutaneous tunnel infection

   C. Bacteremia without local signs of catheter infection

   D. Septic thrombophlebitis

   E. All of the above

Ref.: 36

COMMENTS: The seemingly obvious response to a possibly infected central venous catheter would be to remove the catheter and treat the patient with antibiotics. • In clinical practice, the solution is often not so simple, since many patients have ongoing needs for central vascular access and may not have other readily available access sites. • There is also a spectrum of clinical severity of catheter infection, and infection sources other than the catheter may be responsible for the patient's symptoms. • Local infection at the catheter exit site can frequently be resolved without catheter removal. • Infections involving the subcutaneous tunnel are more problematic and more often necessitate catheter removal, although catheter salvage may still be possible. • If there is bacteremia without local evidence of infection, other sources should be sought. • Gram-positive bacteria infect vascular catheters more easily than do gram-negative bacteria. • Septic thrombophlebitis mandates immediate catheter removal.

ANSWER:
D

---

40. A patient with a subclavian Hickman catheter develops pain and swelling of the arm and neck. The catheter continues to function, and ongoing vascular access is required. What is the the most appropriate management?

   A. IV antibiotics and catheter removal

   B. Infusion of thrombolytic agents through the catheter

C. Systemic anticoagulation and catheter removal

D. Systemic anticoagulation without removing catheter

E. Immediate catheter removal

Ref.: 37

COMMENTS: Venous thrombosis is an important complication of long-term central vascular access catheters. • The diagnosis can often be confirmed by noninvasive Doppler US evaluation or venography. • Because the thrombosis typically forms in the vein distal to the catheter tip, it is not unusual for the catheter to continue to function. • Treatment requires systemic anticoagulation. • The catheter may be left in place, particularly for patients who require continued access and who may have limited alternative access sites. • If there is evidence of infected thrombosis, catheter removal and antibiotics are indicated.

ANSWER:
D

41. Which of the following is/are true regarding radiofrequency ablation (RFA) for liver tumors?

A. Frictional heating of tissues to temperatures greater than 60°C results in cellular death and necrosis.

B. Electrode localization is not as critical as needle placement for percutaneous ethanol injection.

C. Vaporization at the tip of the electrode is imperative for complete lesion ablation.

D. The "heat sink" effect refers to impaired heating of tissues close to adjacent structures, such as large blood vessels.

E. Lesions up to 6 cm in diameter can be treated with a single deployment of the RFA needle electrode.

Ref.: 38–40

COMMENTS: RFA makes use of high-frequency alternating current delivered by a needle electrode. • As ions in the tissue oscillate in response to the alternating electric current, friction produces heat. • At temperatures above 60°C, cellular death occurs, resulting in a zone of necrosis surrounding the electrode. • The RFA probe consists of an insulated needle with an uninsulated tip. • The tip of the probe may consist of an electrode array up to 4 cm in diameter. • The probe may be inserted percutaneously, laparoscopically, or via a limited laparotomy. • Correctly locating the electrode array within the tumor mass is critical to successful RFA. • US imaging commonly is used for guidance, although CT and MRI imaging have also been utilized. • Tumors larger than 3 cm usually require multiple deployments of the electrode. • Typically, the array is placed at the most posterior aspect of the tumor and then repositioned anteriorly at 2–2.5 cm intervals for subsequent treatments. • A margin of 1 cm of normal liver tissue around the lesion is typically included within the treatment volume.

Proper treatment planning, especially for larger lesions requiring multiple deployments, is critical to the success of RFA. • Adjacent structures, especially large blood vessels, can act as a "heat sink" by removing energy from local tissues. • This effect can result in dimpling of the treatment sphere near large vessels. • The rate of complications also increases when treating lesions near vital structures. • If the tip of the electrode is too hot, an insulating "char" can cause decreased energy absorption, reducing the treatment volume. • Current RFA systems measure the temperature and impedance at the tip of the electrode to decrease charring and maximize energy deposition within the treatment volume.

Complications of RFA include liver abscess, pleural effusion, skin burns, pneumothorax, and subcapsular hematoma. • Systemic complications, including renal insufficiency, can be reduced by aggressive preprocedure hydration. • Although clinical trials are still progressing, RFA appears to be at least as effective as percutaneous ethanol injection and cryoablation and may have a lower complication rate.

ANSWERS:
A, D

42. A patient previously diagnosed with inoperable lung cancer has face and neck swelling, severe headaches, and dyspnea on exertion. Which of the following can best be used to evaluate this patient's symptoms?

A. Duplex US imaging

B. Ventilation-perfusion radionuclide lung scan (VQ scan)

C. CT of neck and chest

D. Technetium 99m-labeled RBC scan

E. MRI of neck and chest

F. Arteriogram

G. Chest x-ray

Ref.: 41

COMMENTS: See Question 43.

43. Imaging confirms the presence of an obstructing lesion of the superior vena cava (SVC). Which of the following modalities can best be used to treat SVC syndrome arising from this patient's malignancy?

A. Anticoagulation

B. External radiation therapy

C. Aggressive diuresis

D. Thrombolysis and angioplasty

E. Thrombolysis, angioplasty, and stent placement

F. Surgical bypass

Ref.: 41

COMMENTS: SVC syndrome may result from benign or malignant causes. • Benign causes include tumors, inflammatory processes, trauma, vascular disease, and instrumentation of central veins (e.g., pacemakers and central lines). • Malignant causes are more common, accounting for more than 80% of reported cases. • As many as 3–5% of lung cancer patients may develop SVC syndrome during the course of their illness. • Clinical presentation may include face, neck, or upper extremity edema; headaches; dyspnea; cough; and voice changes. • Symptoms typically are progressive over several weeks, but acute presentation is also possible. • Physical examination findings may include jugular venous distention, facial and upper extremity edema, and prominent collateral veins. • The primary determinant of the severity of symptoms after SVC compromise is the development of collateral veins, especially the azygos system.

Although the diagnosis of SVC syndrome generally is suggested clinically, imaging is helpful both for confirming the diagnosis and for guiding therapeutic decision making. • Chest x-ray may demonstrate abnormalities such as hilar or mediastinal masses. • Duplex US imaging of the central veins usually reveals venous obstruction. • If normal venous waveforms are seen in the internal jugular, brachiocephalic, and subclavian veins, the presence of significant SVC obstruction is unlikely. • CT or MRI imaging of the thorax can be used to delineate the anatomy of the obstruction as well as to evaluate the underlying cause when it is not known. • Contrast venography with pressure measurements, while invasive, can be used to further evaluate the anatomy of the lesion and guide therapeutic decision making. • In cases where a previous tissue diagnosis has not been made, imaging should be used to facilitate biopsy of the obstructing mass.

Radiation therapy remains a first-line therapy for SVC syndrome caused by malignancy. • A total of 20–30 Gy is delivered. • Complete response rates of 15–60% and partial response rates of 50–90% have been demonstrated. • However, as many as one third of patients may have recurrence of SVC syndrome following radiation therapy. • Chemotherapy also may be used, but its use may be limited by side effects. • Recently, thrombolysis has been used for treatment of patients with acute SVC occlusion. • Clot lysis may open a channel through a completely occluded vessel, allowing placement of a wire across the lesion. • Balloon angioplasty can then be used to further widen the channel. • However, angioplasty alone frequently is associated with rapid recurrence or immediate reocclusion because of the elastic nature of most venous lesions. • Because it has the highest primary patency rate, combined thrombolysis, angioplasty, and stent placement can achieve relief of symptoms in over 90% of cases. • Subsequent restenosis can be treated with additional procedures.

The long-term patency of endovascular therapy for benign lesions is not well known. • Because of the long expected life span of patients with benign lesions, surgical bypass can provide an effective solution for SVC syndrome. • Bypass is usually performed via a median sternotomy from a patent vein above the obstruction to the right atrium using either autologous vein (often a spiral or panel graft from the saphenous) or a PTFE graft. • Five-year patency rates of up to 85% have been reported for surgical bypass. • Anticoagulation frequently is used as an adjunct to other modalities. • However, anticoagulation alone usually is not effective in treating SVC syndrome.

ANSWERS:
Question 42: A, C, E, G
Question 43: B, E

---

44. Which of the following can cause spuriously elevated pulse oximeter readings?

A. Hypotension (blood pressure of 60/40 mmHg)

B. Methemoglobinemia

C. Fingernail polish

D. Anemia (hemoglobin of 5 g/dl)

E. Hyperbilirubinemia

F. IV methylene blue

Ref.: 42

COMMENTS: Continuous bedside oximetry was introduced in the 1960s. • The first devices consisted of a phototransmitter and a photodetector situated on opposite sides of the earlobe. • Two major problems were encountered: readings varied with earlobe thickness and skin pigmentation, and the device could not differentiate between hemoglobin in arteries and veins. • Pulse oximetry was introduced in the mid-1970s. • These devices were calibrated to utilize only the portion of the transmitted light signals that demonstrated phasic changes in intensity. • This signal corresponds to the light transmitted through the (pulsatile) arteries. • Light of two wavelengths is used: 660 nm (red) and 940 nm (infrared). • At red

wavelengths, oxygenated blood reflects more light than does deoxygenated blood. • In the infrared portion of the spectrum, the opposite is true. • By comparing the transmission at both wavelengths, the fraction of hemoglobin in the oxygenated form (percent saturation) can be calculated.

At arterial saturations greater than 70%, pulse oximeter readings differ from co-oximetry (the gold standard) by less than 3%. • However, several conditions can cause erroneous pulse oximeter readings. • Both methemoglobinemia and carboxyhemoglobinemia can cause falsely *elevated* pulse oximeter measurements. • Therefore, co-oximetry (which utilizes four wavelengths of light rather than two) should be used when dyshemoglobinemia is suspected. • Skin pigments, such as melanin or bilirubin, usually do not result in significant alterations in pulse oximeter readings but may occasionally cause small false *reductions*. • Dark (blue or black) fingernail polish may cause a 3–5% false *reduction* in the oximeter reading. • Pulse oximeters have been shown to be accurate down to a blood pressure of 30 mmHg and a hemoglobin level of 3 g/dl. • Intravenous methylene blue (which is used to treat methemoglobinemia) may cause up to a 65% *decrease* in pulse oximeter measurements.

ANSWER:
B

REFERENCES

1. Grainger RG, Allison D: *Diagnostic Radiology: A Textbook of Medical Imaging*, 4th ed. Churchill-Livingstone, London, 2001.
2. Clowes AW, Kohler TR: Anatomy, physiology and pharmacology of the vascular wall. In: Moore W (ed) *Vascular Surgery: A Comprehensive Review*, 5th ed. Saunders, Philadelphia, 1998.
3. LeBoretin H, Plow EF, Topol EJ: Role of platelets in restenosis after percutaneous coronary revascularization. *J Am Coll Cardiol* 28:1643–1651, 1996.
4. Losordo DW, Rosenfield K, Pieczek A, et al: How does angioplasty work? Serial analysis of human iliac arteries using intravascular ultrasound. *Circulation* 86:1845–1858, 1992.
5. VanLankeren W, Gussenhoven EJ, vanderLugt A, et al: Intravascular sonographic evaluation of iliac artery angioplasty: what is the mechanism of angioplasty and can intravascular sonography predict clinical outcome? *Am J Roentgenol* 166:1355–1360, 1996.
6. Colombo A, Stankovic G, Moses JW: Selection of coronary stents. *J Am Coll Cardiol* 40:1021–1033, 2002.
7. Bermejo J, Botas J, Garcia E, et al: Mechanisms of residual lumen stenosis after high-pressure stent implantation: a quantitative coronary angiography and intravascular ultrasound study. *Circulation* 98:112–118, 1998.
8. Schomig A, Neumann FJ, Kastrati A, et al: A randomized comparison of antiplatelet and anticoagulation therapy after the placement of coronary-artery stents. *N Engl J Med* 334:1084–1089, 1996.
9. Cameron, JL: *Current Surgical Therapy*, 7th ed. CV Mosby, St. Louis, 2001.
10. Morton DL, Wen DR, Wong JH, et al: Technical details of intraoperative lymphatic mapping for early stage melanoma. *Arch Surg* 127:392–399, 1992.
11. Cochran AJ, Balda BR, Starz H, et al: The Augsburg Consensus. Techniques of lymphatic mapping, sentinel lymphadenectomy, and completion lymphadenectomy in cutaneous malignancies. *Cancer* 89:236–241, 2000.
12. McMasters KM, Giuliano AE, Ross ML, et al: Sentinel lymph node biopsy for breast cancer: the standard of care. *N Engl J Med* 339:990–995, 1998.
13. Cox CE, Pendas S, Cox JM, et al: Guidelines for sentinel node biopsy and lymphatic mapping of patients with breast cancer. *Ann Surg* 227:645–651, 1998.
14. Sener SF, Winchester DJ, Martz CH, et al: Lymphedema after sentinel lymphadenectomy for breast carcinoma. *Cancer* 92:748–752, 2001.
15. Gelman CL, Parroso EG, Britton CT, et al: The effect of lasers, electrocautery, and sharp dissection on cutaneous flaps. *Plast Reconstr Surg* 94:829–833, 1994.
16. Soballe PW, Nimbkar NV, Hayward I, et al: Electrocautery lowers the contamination threshold for infection of laparotomies. *Am J Surg* 175:263–266, 1998.

17. Harrell GJ, Kopps DR: Minimizing patient risk during laparoscopic electrosurgery. *AORN J* 67:1194–1205, 1998.
18. Scott-Conner CEH: *The SAGES Manual: Fundamentals of Laparoscopy and GI Endoscopy.* Springer, New York, 1998.
19. Arregui ME, Fitzgibbons RJ, Ketkhouda N, et al: *Principles of Laparoscopic Surgery.* Springer-Verlag, New York, 1995.
20. MacFadyen BV, Ponsky JL: *Operative Laparoscopy and Thoracoscopy.* Lippincott-Raven, Philadelphia, 1995.
21. Dowling RD, Ochoa J, Yousem SA, et al: Argon beam coagulation is superior to conventional techniques in repair of experimental splenic injury. *J Trauma* 31:717–720, 1991.
22. Gale P, Adeyemi B, Ferrer K, et al: Histologic characteristics of laparoscopic argon beam coagulation. *J Am Assoc Gynecol Laparosc* 5:19–22, 1998.
23. Go PM, Goodman GR, Bruhn EW, et al: The argon beam coagulator provides rapid hemostasis of experimental hepatic and splenic hemorrhage in anticoagulated dogs. *J Trauma* 31:1294–1300, 1991.
24. Laycock WS, Tru TL, Hunter JG: New technology for the division of short gastric vessels during laparoscopic Nissen fundoplication. *Surg Endosc* 10:71–73, 1996.
25. Webb WR, Brant WE, Helms CA: *Fundamentals of Body CT,* 2nd ed. WB Saunders, Philadelphia, 1998.
26. Wong DW: Endorectal ultrasonography for benign disease. In: Staren ED (ed), *Ultrasound for the Surgeon,* Lippincott-Raven, Philadelphia, 1997.
27. Case TD: Ultrasound physics and instrumentation. *Surg Clin North Am* 78:197–217, 1998.
28. Rozycki GS, Feliciano DV, Davis TP: Ultrasound as used in thoracoabdominal trauma. *Surg Clin North Am* 78:295–310, 1998.
29. Weissleder R, Wittenberg J, Harisinghani MG: *Primer of Diagnostic Imaging,* 3rd ed. CV Mosby, St. Louis, 2003.
30. Kraut EJ, Anderson JT, Safwat A, et al: Impairment of cardiac performance by laparoscopy in patients receiving positive end-expiratory pressure. *Arch Surg* 134:76–80, 1999.
31. Koivvusalo AM, Kellokumpu I, Sheenin M, et al: A comparison of gasless mechanical and conventional carbon dioxide pneumoperitoneum methods for laparoscopic cholecystectomy. *Anesth Analg* 86:153–158, 1998.
32. Joshi GP: Complications of laparoscopy. *Anesthesiol Clin North Am* 19:89–105, 2001.
33. Amid PK, Shulman AG, Lichtenstein IL: Selecting synthetic mesh for the repair of groin hernia. *Postgrad Gen Surg* 4:150–155, 1992.
34. Joffe SN: *Lasers in General Surgery.* Williams & Wilkins, Baltimore, 1989.
35. TeLinde RW, Thompson JD: *TeLinde's Operative Gynecology,* 8th ed. Lippincott, Baltimore, 1997.
36. Townsend CM, Beauchamp RD, Evers BM, et al (eds): *Sabiston's Textbook of Surgery, The Biological Basis of Modern Surgical Practice,* 16th ed. Saunders, Philadelphia, 2001.
37. Greenfield LJ, Mulholland MW, Oldham KT, et al (eds): *Surgery: Scientific Principles and Practice,* 2nd ed. Lippincott-Raven, Philadelphia, 1997.
38. McGahan JP, Brock JM, Tesluk H, et al: Hepatic ablation with use of radio-frequency electrocautery in the animal model. *J Vasc Interv Radiol* 3:291–297, 1992.
39. Lencioni RA, Allgaier HP, Cioni D, et al: Small hepatocellular carcinoma in cirrhosis: randomized comparison of radio-frequency thermal ablation versus percutaneous ethanol injection. *Radiology* 228:235–240, 2003.
40. Yeh KA, Fortunato L, Hoffman JP, et al: Cryosurgical ablation of hepatic metastases from colorectal carcinomas. *Am Surg* 63:63–68, 1997.
41. Schindler N, Vogelang RL: Superior vena cava syndrome: experience with endovascular stents and surgical therapy. *Surg Clin North Am* 79:683–694, 1999.
42. Marino PL: *The ICU Book,* 2nd ed, Lippincott, Baltimore, 1996.

CHAPTER 21

Principles of Laparoscopy

Daniel J. Deziel, M.D.

1. Which of the following is not an appropriate technique for placement of the initial abdominal trocar during laparoscopy?

   A. Blind placement after pneumoperitoneum with Veress needle

   B. Use of optical trocar without pneumoperitoneum

   C. Closed placement of trocar without pneumoperitoneum

   D. Open placement of Hasson cannula without pneumoperitoneum

   Ref.: 1

COMMENTS: There are closed and open techniques by which the initial trocar can be placed to gain access to the abdomen for laparoscopic operations. • One standard closed method involves initial establishment of a pneumoperitoneum through a Veress needle and subsequent "blind" placement of the trocar. • Critical to this approach is ensuring adequate insufflation of the peritoneal cavity before the trocar is placed. • Proper handling of the trocar during insertion is critical to the safety of any method. • An alternative closed technique uses specially designed optical trocars that allow the laparoscope to be positioned in the trocar as it is being inserted. • The tissues are spread or cut under videoscopic vision as the trocar is advanced, and a pneumoperitoneum is not required. • Open techniques utilize a cutdown and open the fascia and peritoneum under direct vision. • A blunt, noncutting Hasson trocar is then placed and secured with a conical sleeve before the pneumoperitoneum is established. • This is often considered the safest method. • Blind placement of a trocar without a safe pneumoperitoneum is not permissible.

ANSWER:
C

2. During introduction of a Veress needle, what is the first maneuver that should be performed to confirm intraperitoneal placement?

   A. Aspirate the needle.

   B. Perform a saline drop test.

   C. Flush the needle.

   D. Connect the insufflator and measure the pressure.

   Ref.: 1

COMMENTS: When using the Veress needle technique, free entry of the needle into the peritoneal cavity must be confirmed before insufflation begins. • Usually, two audible clicks can be heard as the needle traverses the fascia and then the peritoneum. • A 10-ml syringe is attached and aspirated to ensure that no blood, urine, or intestinal content is returned. • The drop test is confirmatory when the stopcock on the end of the needle is opened and saline solution in the needle hub is seen to flow freely into the abdomen. • The needle can likewise be flushed freely, and the instilled saline solution should not return when the needle is subsequently aspirated. • The insufflator should not be connected until free entry into the peritoneal cavity is verified.

ANSWER:
A

3. Select the most appropriate site for initial trocar placement for laparoscopic cholecystectomy in a patient with a midline incision from the pubis to the top of the umbilicus.

   A. Umbilical

   B. Suprapubic

   C. Left lower quadrant

   D. Right upper quadrant

   Ref.: 1

COMMENTS: The most appropriate site for placement of the initial trocar for a laparoscopic operation depends on a number of considerations: the operation to be done, the size and shape of the patient, the location of scars from previous operations, and the presence of such factors as organomegaly, hernias, or masses. • Often, but not invariably, the umbilicus will be the initial site of choice. • Alternative sites and nonmidline sites must frequently be used when the patient has had previous abdominal surgery. • An open technique for trocar placement is always advisable when alternative sites are used. • The area of a previous incision should be avoided. • Nonmidline sites should avoid important abdominal wall vessels and thus need to be at or lateral to the border of the rectus muscles.

ANSWER:
D

4. Which abdominal wall vessels are most typically visible laparoscopically?

   A. Superior deep epigastrics

   B. Inferior deep epigastrics

C. Superficial circumflex iliacs

D. Superficial epigastrics

Ref.: 1

COMMENTS: Bleeding from abdominal wall vessels is the most frequent complication of trocar placement. • To avoid this troublesome problem, the surgeon must be familiar with the typical anatomy of these vessels. • The abdominal wall is supplied by both superficial and deep vessels. • The most commonly injured vessels are the superficial epigastric and circumflex iliac vessels and the deep inferior and superior epigastrics. • The inferior deep epigastric vessels can be seen from the peritoneal aspect in the inguinal region as they ascend obliquely and medially toward the umbilicus to enter the rectus sheath. • Unfortunately, there are no reliable landmarks for the other deep vessels. • In thinner individuals, the superficial vessels can be transilluminated to identify their location, but this is not helpful in larger patients.

ANSWER:
B

5. Visceral injury can be avoided by use of which type of trocar?

A. Hasson cannula

B. Conical noncutting trocar

C. Trocar with safety shield

D. None of the above

Ref.: 1

COMMENTS: Injury to intra-abdominal viscera and major blood vessels can occur with trocars of any type, style, or design. • Only attention to the details of proper trocar insertion technique can minimize this risk. • There are many types of trocars available from various manufacturers, with many similarities but some differences. • The surgeon must be familiar with the correct operation and handling of whichever trocars are being used. • Any trocar should be checked before insertion to ascertain that it is properly engaged and that the stopcock is closed. • The skin incision must be large enough, and the surgeon must be careful to insert the trocar in the proper location and direction and to use the proper technique. • Secondary trocars should always be placed under direct laparoscopic vision.

ANSWER:
D

6. Which of the following insufflation gases should not be used with electrocautery?

A. Carbon dioxide

B. Nitrous oxide

C. Argon

D. Helium

Ref.: 1

COMMENTS: See Question 7.

7. Which of the following insufflation gases has the lowest risk of gas embolus?

A. Carbon dioxide

B. Nitrous oxide

C. Argon

D. Helium

Ref.: 1

COMMENTS: Carbon dioxide is by far the most widely used gas for insufflation during laparoscopic surgery. • It is readily available and relatively inexpensive. • It has a diffusion coefficient about 20 times that of oxygen, and therefore it is rapidly absorbed and has a low risk of gas embolism. • Since CO_2 does not support combustion, it can be used with electrocautery. • The primary disadvantage of CO_2 is that hypercarbia and acidosis can result from its use. • In some circumstances, alternative gases may be used. • Nitrous oxide does not produce acid-base disturbances and may be associated with less pain. • Hence, it has been used for procedures under local anesthesia. • However, it will support combustion. • Use of the inert gases argon and helium avoids acid-base problems, but these gases have low solubility and possibly entail a greater risk of gas embolism. • Argon may be associated with cardiac depression. • These gases are expensive and are generally not used.

ANSWERS:
Question 6: B
Question 7: A

8. Thirty minutes into a laparoscopic procedure, the visualization becomes poor. The insufflation monitor shows a pressure of 20 mmHg and a flow rate of 0 L/min. What is the most likely explanation?

A. Empty CO_2 tank

B. Insufflator malfunction

C. Improper insufflator settings

D. Inadequate muscle relaxation

Ref.: 1

COMMENTS: When the visualization inexplicably deteriorates during a laparoscopic procedure, the cause is often inadvertent loss of the pneumoperitoneum that has been maintaining the operative field. • There are numerous reasons why this can occur, particularly through leakage at trocar sites or through trocars. • Usually, this can be promptly detected and, if it is the cause, the insufflator flow should be set at the upper level. • In the situation described in this question, the intraperitoneal pressure is high, and there is no flow. • This indicates obstruction to flow, possibly along the insufflation tubing or at a closed trocar stopcock. • Another common cause for this circumstance is inadequate muscle relaxation. • This causes the intraperitoneal pressure to increase and the insufflator to automatically stop flow when the pressure exceeds the set limit. • The surgeon should check the insufflator before beginning the procedure to ensure that the pressure and flow settings are appropriate.

ANSWER:
D

9. During a laparoscopic Nissen fundoplication, the patient's end tidal CO_2 increases to 48 mmHg, and airway pressure rises. The blood pressure and heart rate are stable. What is the most appropriate treatment at this time?

A. Place a chest tube for a pneumothorax.

B. Immediately desufflate the abdomen.

C. Increase minute ventilation.

D. Convert to an open procedure.

Ref.: 1

COMMENTS: CO_2 diffuses across the peritoneum into the venous circulation, where it is carried to the lungs for alveolar elimination. • Hypercarbia may occur, and an increase in the expired CO_2 content is typical. • The mechanical effects of the pneumoperitoneum decrease diaphragmatic excursion and thoracic compliance and increase airway pressure. • To some degree, these effects can be anticipated in every laparoscopic procedure. • Usually, these changes can be compensated for by having the anesthesiologist increase the patient's minute ventilation. • Some patients, particularly those with more severe underlying cardiac or pulmonary disease, may not tolerate the chemical and mechanical effects of pneumoperitoneum well and may require conversion to an open procedure. • When a patient acutely and unexpectedly decompensates during a laparoscopic operation, the surgeon's first maneuver should be immediate release of the pneumoperitoneum.

ANSWER:
C

10. Which of the following body compartments is the largest reservoir for CO_2?

A. Bone

B. Skeletal muscle

C. Lungs

D. Peritoneum

Ref.: 1

COMMENTS: CO_2 is quickly absorbed during laparoscopic surgery, but not all of it can be promptly eliminated. • Body stores of CO_2 therefore increase throughout the course of an operation, with bone serving as the largest reservoir. • Stored CO_2 is not immediately eliminated when the procedure is over and the pneumoperitoneum has been evacuated. • Since it may take several hours to expel the CO_2, one should be cautious about premature extubation of a patient after an involved laparoscopic operation, particularly if the patient has underlying respiratory disease.

ANSWER:
A

11. Which of the following hemodynamic parameters does not increase during laparoscopy with a CO_2 pneumoperitoneum?

A. Mean arterial pressure

B. Cardiac index

C. Systemic vascular resistance

D. Pulmonary vascular resistance

Ref.: 1

COMMENTS: The observed physiologic consequences of a CO_2 pneumoperitoneum result from both the chemical effects of hypercarbia, with its attendant acid-base changes, and the direct mechanical effects of the increased intraperitoneal pressure. • Hemodynamic changes include a generalized increase in vascular resistance and, hence, an increase in cardiac afterload and a decrease in cardiac index. • The increase in afterload can increase myocardial oxygen demand and potentially represent an adverse situation for patients with cardiac disease.

ANSWER:
B

12. A 50-year-old woman is undergoing laparoscopic cholecystectomy with a CO_2 pneumoperitoneum. Shortly after the CO_2 is infused, her heart rate decreases to 40 beats per minute. What is the most likely cause of the bradycardia?

A. Gas embolism

B. Unrecognized bleeding

C. CO_2 pneumoperitoneum

D. Anesthetic drugs

Ref.: 1

COMMENTS: Cardiac arrhythmias are not uncommon during laparoscopic surgery and may occur in as many as one quarter to one half of patients. • These arrhythmias may involve tachycardia, premature ventricular contractions, or bradycardia, which is actually the most frequent. • Bradycardia has been attributed to the vasovagal effect when stretching the peritoneum. • It is recommended that gas insufflation be initiated at a slow rate so that the pneumoperitoneum develops gradually and the patient's tolerance can be assessed.

ANSWER:
C

13. Which of the following would be least appropriate for treatment of the patient described in Question 12?

A. Volume expansion

B. Atropine

C. Desufflation of the abdomen

D. Left lateral Trendelenburg position

Ref.: 1

COMMENTS: When a patient develops bradycardia during induction of the pneumoperitoneum, the appropriate measures are to desufflate the abdomen and administer intravenous fluid and atropine if necessary. • In the rare event of gas embolism, the patient should be positioned to prevent the gas from entering the right ventricular outflow tract: in the left lateral decubitus position with the head tilted down. • A central venous catheter may be used to aspirate the gas.

ANSWER:
D

14. Which of the following pulmonary changes would not be anticipated during laparoscopic surgery?

A. Increased airway pressure

B. Increased pulmonary capillary wedge pressure

C. Increased functional residual capacity

D. Decreased thoracic compliance

Ref.: 1

COMMENTS: The physiologic effects of a pneumoperitoneum can be detrimental to pulmonary mechanics and air exchange. • Functional residual capacity, thoracic compliance, and diaphragmatic excursion are decreased, while airway pressure and vascular resistance are increased. • The patient's respiratory status must be closely monitored throughout the procedure. • Adjustments in tidal volume and ventilatory rate can be made to compensate. • The surgeon should limit the intraperitoneal pressure and work at the lowest pressure that will provide safe exposure.

ANSWER:
C

15. A 60-year-old man is oliguric in the recovery room during the first hour following a laparoscopic colon resection. His blood pressure is 120/80, his heart rate 84 beats per minute, and his respiratory rate 12 breaths per minute. Which of the following is the least plausible explanation for his urine output?

   A. Hypovolemia

   B. Renal effects of pneumoperitoneum

   C. Ureteral injury

   D. Renal infarction

Ref.: 1

COMMENTS: Hypovolemia, with or without bleeding, must always be considered a potential cause of low urine output in a postoperative patient. • The physiologic consequences of the pneumoperitoneum may also contribute to early postoperative oliguria. • Renal blood flow is decreased, and the resulting decrease in the glomerular filtration rate may be substantial. • These effects may persist for some time afterward owing to elevations in serum renin and ADH levels. • Urine output is therefore not necessarily a good indicator of volume status immediately after a laparoscopic operation. • Obstruction of the Foley catheter is another easily diagnosable cause of low urine output. • Bilateral ureteral injury is extremely

rare but may occur. • There should be no reason to expect renal infarction in this situation.

ANSWER:
D

16. A normovolemic 20-year-old patient is undergoing laparoscopic appendectomy. Which of the following physiologic changes would be least likely with a CO_2 pneumoperitoneum at 12 mmHg?

   A. Decreased femoral venous flow

   B. Decreased systemic venous return

   C. Decreased renal blood flow

   D. Decreased glomerular filtration rate

Ref.: 1

COMMENTS: Potentially adverse mechanical effects of a pneumoperitoneum are related to the level of intraperitoneal pressure. • The surgeon should strive for the lowest pressure possible that will permit safe visualization and performance of the operation. • All of the hemodynamic changes listed occur as intraperitoneal pressure rises. • However, diminished venous return due to increased resistance to flow in the inferior vena cava would not be expected to be significant in an otherwise healthy resuscitated patient until the intraperitoneal pressure reaches 20 mmHg or higher.

ANSWER:
B

REFERENCE

1. Soper NJ, Swanstrom LL, Eubanks WS (eds): *Mastery of Endoscopic and Laparoscopic Surgery*, 2nd ed. Lippincott, Williams & Wilkins, Philadelphia, 2005.

C H A P T E R **22**

Principles of Ultrasound

Mark R. Edwards, M.D., and Daniel J. Deziel, M.D.

1. Which of the following most accurately represents the average speed at which ultrasound waves move through the human body?

A. 350 m/sec

B. 2000 m/sec

C. 500 cm/sec

D. 1540 m/sec

E. 800 m/sec

Ref.: 1

COMMENTS: Sound moves through biologic tissue at a speed that is dependent on tissue density. • Sound moves more slowly through less dense matter, such as air (330 m/sec), and more quickly through high-density material, such as bone (4050 m/sec). • The *average* speed of sound through human tissue is 1540 m/sec. • Since most soft tissues have a similar density and therefore sound passes through them at a similar speed, ultrasound machines are designed on the assumption that the speed of sound through soft tissues is 1540 m/sec.

ANSWER:
D

2. Which of the following terms is correctly defined as the "conversion of electrical to mechanical energy"?

A. Piezoelectric effect

B. Artifact

C. Impedance

D. Interference

Ref.: 1

COMMENTS: Ultrasound transducers contain crystals. • When a sound wave deforms one of the crystals, voltage is produced. • The corollary also is true: when a crystal has voltage applied to it, a sound wave is generated. • This is described as the piezoelectric effect and has practical applications to the field of ultrasonography. • Crystals used in ultrasound machines initially act as speakers that send out sound waves. • The returning sound

that is reflected back causes the crystals to vibrate and generate voltage.

ANSWER:
A

3. Concerning acoustic impedance, which of the following statements is/are true?

A. It can be amplified by increasing the gain on the ultrasound equipment.

B. It is influenced by the density of the tissue and the velocity of the sound wave.

C. It permits the operator to distinguish between two structures even if their densities are the same.

D. It is calculated by multiplying the amplitude of the waves by the density of the tissue.

Ref.: 1

COMMENTS: Diagnostic ultrasonography is centered on the analysis of sound waves that have been reflected back to the ultrasound transducer. • The fact that sound waves are reflected back is due to acoustic impedance, which can be loosely defined as the opposition to the passage of sound waves through tissue. • Acoustic impedance is dependent on the speed of sound in the tissue and the density of the tissue. • It can be calculated as acoustic impedance = density × velocity. • Increasing the gain on the machine does not affect any of these parameters.

ANSWER:
B

4. Which of the following are characteristics of higher-frequency transducers?

A. Poor penetration and good resolution

B. Good penetration and good resolution

C. Poor penetration and poor resolution

D. Good penetration and poor resolution

Ref.: 1

COMMENTS: See Question 6.

5. Which of the following relationships between frequency and wavelength is/are true?

A. Lower frequency, shorter wavelength

B. Lower frequency, longer wavelength

C. Higher frequency, longer wavelength

D. Higher frequency, shorter wavelength

Ref.: 1

COMMENTS: See Question 6.

6. Which of the following relationships between wavelength and depth of penetration is/are true?

A. Shorter wave length, shallow penetration

B. Shorter wave length, deeper penetration

C. Longer wave length, shallow penetration

D. Longer wave length, deeper penetration

Ref.: 1

COMMENTS: High-frequency transducers provide high-resolution images at the expense of tissue penetration. • In ultrasonography, three types of resolution exist: axial resolution, lateral resolution, and temporal resolution. • **Axial resolution** is the ability to distinguish one object from another object below it. • It is dependent on frequency. • By definition, a higher frequency means a shorter wavelength. • Since the depth of penetration is dependent on the wavelength, a higher frequency results in less tissue penetration. • **Lateral resolution** is the ability to differentiate two objects that are next to each other. • It is independent of frequency and dependent on the beam width. • **Temporal resolution** is the perception of real-time movement and is dependent on the frame rate.

ANSWERS:
Question 4: A
Question 5: B, D
Question 6: A, D

7. Match the terms in the left-hand column with the appropriate descriptions in the right-hand column.

A. Hyperechoic   a. Brighter than the surrounding tissue

B. Hypoechoic   b. Black

C. Isoechoic   c. Similar in appearance to surrounding tissue

D. Anechoic   d. Less dark than surrounding tissue

E. Echogenicity   e. Appearance of tissues and nearby structures determined by ultrasound

Ref.: 1

COMMENTS: A region in a sonographic picture where echoes are brighter than nearby structures is referred to as **hyperechoic**. • In contrast, **hypoechoic** areas appear darker than surrounding areas. • **Isoechoic** areas appear similar to surrounding structures, and **anechoic** areas appear black, without echoes, on a sonographic image.

• **Echogenicity** refers to the appearance of tissues relative to each other as determined by ultrasound studies.

ANSWER:
A-a; B-d; C-c; D-b; E-e

8. Which of the following is not an advantage of transabdominal ultrasound when compared to computed tomography (CT)?

A. Lower cost

B. Portability

C. Greater safety

D. Speed of examination

E. Independence of examiner

Ref.: 1

COMMENTS: Transabdominal ultrasound has several advantages compared to CT. • They include cost, portability, safety, and speed of the examination. • However, ultrasound examinations are operator dependent. • The quality of the images, or lack thereof, depends on the technical expertise of the person operating the ultrasound machine.

ANSWER:
E

9. Match each structure in the right-hand column with the most likely effect in the left-hand column.

A. Reverberation   a. diaphragm

B. Posterior enhancement   b. simple cyst

C. Mirror image   c. bullet

D. Comet tail   d. bone

Ref.: 1

COMMENTS: While the utility of ultrasound is unquestionable, problems with it do exist. • Artifacts are errors in ultrasound images that occur because the machine design is based on assumptions that are not always true. • **Reverberation** takes place when sound waves are trapped between two areas and the waves are forced to bounce back and forth. • Some of this trapped energy eventually returns to the transducer. • However, the temporal delay leads to an artifact in the image. • A reverberation artifact resembles a ladder, with hyperechoic areas representing the rungs. • Ultrasound images of fluid-filled structures, such as cysts, sometimes display an artifact known as **posterior enhancement**. • This artifact occurs because the ultrasound machine makes the assumption that sound waves are uniformly attenuated by tissue. • Fluids are efficient at transmitting sound waves. • As the sound travels through a cyst and reaches the tissue below it, the attenuation changes. • The ultrasound machine incorrectly interprets this change, and posterior enhancement is the result. • Posterior enhancement appears as a hyperechoic (bright) area below the fluid-filled structure. • When sound waves are reflected by a curved surface, such as the diaphragm or bladder, instead of by a flat surface, a **mirror-image** artifact may appear. • When the transducer sound waves strike a piece of metal, the metal can act as a bell and continue "ringing" for a longer time than the actual contact between the ultrasound wave and the metal object. • As this additional sound energy returns to the transducer, it is incorrectly interpreted as having come from a deeper location. • The result is a hyperechoic line extending from the metallic object that resembles a **comet tail.**

ANSWER:
A-d; B-b; C-a; D-c

10. Which of the following best describes the appearance of a stone in the gallbladder on an ultrasound image?

   A. A hyperechoic object with a halo sign

   B. Multiple mirror images

   C. A hypoechoic object within the gallbladder lumen

   D. A hyperechoic object with a posterior shadow

   E. An anechoic object with posterior enhancement

Ref.: 1

COMMENTS: The sonographic diagnosis of cholelithiasis is generally indicated by the presence of a mobile, hyperechoic, intraluminal object with posterior shadowing. • If these three criteria are not met, the diagnosis is less certain.

ANSWER:
D

11. Which of the following are sonographic characteristics of an inflamed gallbladder?

   A. Gallbladder distention

   B. Pericholecystic fluid

   C. Wall thickness of 2 mm

   D. Sonographic Murphy's sign

   E. Gallstones

Ref.: 1

COMMENTS: Gallbladder distention, pericholecystic fluid, sonographic Murphy's sign, and gallstones can all be present on a sonogram with the diagnosis of cholecystitis. • Gallbladder wall thickness is considered abnormal if it is greater than 3 mm.

ANSWER:
A, B, D, E

12. Which of the following characteristics of a malignant thyroid nodule is/are often present on sonographic images?

   A. Areas that are hypoechoic compared to the surrounding tissue

   B. Peripheral calcifications

   C. Irregular margins

   D. Absence of cystic areas

Ref.: 1

COMMENTS: Ultrasound has proven useful in the evaluation of thyroid carcinoma. • Thyroid cancers are seen as heterogeneous hypoechoic areas with irregular borders. • When microcalcifications are present (psammoma bodies), their location is the interior of the lesion, not on the periphery. • Cystic masses are usually not malignant.

ANSWER:
A, C, D

13. Which of the following is/are appropriate uses of the focused assessment with sonography in trauma (FAST) examination?

   A. Assessment of pleural effusion

   B. Assessment of peritoneal fluid following trauma in a pregnant patient

   C. Assessment of decreased in the hematocrit in a trauma patient (primary survey)

   D. Follow-up of a trauma patient with a solid organ injury (secondary survey)

Ref.: 1

COMMENTS: The FAST examination has become a vital component in the initial evaluation of trauma patients. • Currently, the primary focus of the FAST examination is to detect fluid presumed to be blood, but as time progresses, more advanced applications will undoubtedly arise. • The examination is completed quickly during a primary survey (of an unstable patient) or a secondary survey (of a stable patient) and focuses on detecting fluid in the pericardial space and dependent portions of the abdomen. • The examination is divided into three parts: cardiac, abdominal, and thoracic. • The cardiac examination consists of a sagittal view in the subxiphoid region. • The abdominal examination focuses on longitudinal views of the left and right upper quadrants and a transverse view of the pelvis. • The thoracic portion is an upward scan from the upper abdominal quadrants, which can detect pleural effusions or pneumothorax.

ANSWER:
A, B, C, D

14. Which of the following statements regarding the FAST examination is/are true?

   A. It can reliably evaluate the retroperitoneum.

   B. It can quickly detect the presence of pericardial fluid.

   C. It can assess the presence or absence of pleural effusion.

   D. It is useful in detecting a cardiac contusion.

   E. Is considered a replacement for CT scans.

Ref.: 1

COMMENTS: Despite the usefulness of the FAST examination, it does have limitations. • As described in Question 13, the FAST examination can quickly evaluate for the presence of both pericardial fluid and pleural effusion. • However, it does not evaluate the retroperitoneum and does not detect a cardiac contusion. • CT still has many practical applications with trauma patients and has not been fully replaced by the FAST examination.

ANSWER:
B, C

15. Regarding vascular arterial ultrasound imaging, which of the following statements is/are true?

   A. In Doppler ultrasound, the reflected wave returning to the transducer has the same frequency as the transmitted wave.

B. For Doppler ultrasound, the transducer should be held at a 90-degree angle to the body.

C. Arterial stenosis leads to decreased flow velocity.

D. Carotid endarterectomy can generally be carried out based on duplex imaging alone without the need for angiography.

Ref.: 1

COMMENT: Doppler ultrasound relies on the fact that the sound wave that has been reflected back to the transducer has a different frequency than does the transmitted wave. • If the transducer is held at a 90-degree angle while performing a Doppler ultrasound, regardless of the actual velocity in a blood vessel, the ultrasound machine will read zero velocity. • This is because the theoretical velocity is calculated by the equation *velocity = $\Delta f\ c/2f\ cos\ \theta$* (where c is the speed of sound in soft tissue, Δf is the change in frequency of reflected versus transmitted sound waves, f is the frequency of transmitted sound, and $cos\ \theta$ is the angle between the ultrasound and the direction of motion of the target). • Since the cosine of 90 degrees is zero, the theoretical velocity would be zero if the transducer is held at a 90-degree angle to the target. • Unless the arterial stenosis is so severe that the blood flow is completely impeded, the velocity increases in arterial stenosis. • Carotid ultrasound has proven very sensitive in detecting carotid stenosis. • This, coupled with the fact that carotid angiography is an invasive procedure, has lead to the frequent use of ultrasound as the sole imaging modality before performance of a carotid endarterectomy.

ANSWER:
D

16. Which of the following sonographic features is/are associated with a simple breast cyst?

A. Isoechoic

B. Hypoechoic

C. Anechoic

D. Posterior enhancement

E. Posterior shadowing

Ref.: 1

COMMENT: A simple cyst in the breast appears anechoic compared to the surrounding breast tissue. • Posterior enhancement artifact is also common for the reasons described in Question 7.

ANSWER:
C, D

17. Which of the following statements best describes the use of breast ultrasound imaging?

A. It should be used instead of breast biopsy.

B. It can be used to distinguish between cystic and solid masses.

C. It is considered a screening test to evaluate the entire breast.

D. It can be used to define microcalcifications.

Ref.: 1

COMMENTS: As the technology of breast ultrasonography has continued to improve, the modalities in which it is used have increased. • While breast ultrasound can aid in the performance of a breast biopsy and other interventional modalities, ultrasound images cannot replace the information that biopsy provides. • Breast ultrasound is employed in the workup of a palpable breast mass to aid in the differentiation of a cystic from a solid mass. • Breast ultrasound is employed early in the workup of breast lesions but is not a screening tool for the entire breast. • It is difficult to adequately characterize microcalcifications using breast ultrasound. • If suspicious calcifications are seen on mammography, a biopsy should be performed for a thorough evaluation.

ANSWER:
B

18. Regarding intraoperative ultrasound, which of the following statements is/are true?

A. It is very accurate in determining vessel encasement by tumor.

B. It necessitates the presence of a board-certified radiologist in the operating room.

C. It generally doubles the operative time.

D. It is less sensitive than CT in locating small pancreatic tumors.

Ref.: 1

COMMENTS: Intraoperative ultrasound imaging has become an important part of the evaluation of many diagnoses. • In addition to being a valuable tool for determining vascular encasement of tumor, intraoperative ultrasound has also proven useful for delineating small pancreatic tumors not well seen on CT. • For intraoperative ultrasound, a board-certified radiologist does not have to be present. • However, the surgeon performing this test should have sufficient training to be technically proficient in ultrasound imaging

ANSWER:
A

19. Which of the following statements concerning laparoscopic ultrasound imaging is/are true?

A. It results in more artifacts than does transabdominal ultrasound imaging.

B. It should not guide tumor resection.

C. It can detect only palpable hepatic tumors.

D. It has similar sensitivity and specificity to intraoperative cholangiography when used by experienced surgeons.

Ref.: 1

COMMENTS: Laparoscopy is being utilized in a growing number of situations, as is laparoscopic ultrasound imaging. • Laparoscopic ultrasound has been used to help assess the extent of tumor invasion and to guide resection. • It can also detect small, intraparenchymal tumors in organs such as the pancreas or liver. • In experienced hands, laparoscopic ultrasound can provide much of the same diagnostic information as intraoperative cholangiography.

ANSWER:
D

20. Endoscopic ultrasound imaging has proven useful for which of the following?

   A. Staging esophageal tumors

   B. Diagnosis of common bile duct stones

   C. Detecting portal vein invasion by pancreatic cancer

   D. Identifying small pancreatic tumors not seen by CT scan

Ref.: 1

COMMENTS: Endoscopic ultrasound imaging is useful for all of the applications described in this question.

ANSWER:

A, B, C, D

REFERENCES

1. Machi J, Staren ED: *Ultrasound for Surgeons*, 2nd ed. Lippincott, Williams & Wilkins, Philadelphia, 2005.

CHAPTER 23

Oncology

José M. Velasco, M.D., Tina J. Hieken, M.D., Katherine F. Baker, M.D., and Edward Kaplan, M.D.

A. Principles

Tine J. Hieken, M.D., and José M. Velasco, M.D.

1. Which the following statements regarding cancer in the United States is/are true?

A. Neoplastic disease is the leading cause of death.

B. One in four deaths is caused by cancer.

C. In general, the incidence of a given cancer parallels the death rate from the same cancer.

D. Age-adjusted cancer death rates increased in the 1990s regardless of gender.

Ref.: 1–3

COMMENTS: Cancer is second only to cardiovascular disease in 2000 as a cause of death in the United States (29.6% of all deaths). • Approximately 40% of Americans eventually will develop cancer. • The incidence of age-adjusted cancer death rates declined in the 1990s in nearly all populations. • Because the various forms of cancer are not equally deadly, the incidence of a malignancy differs from its death rate. • For some cancers, such as ovarian and esophageal cancer, the incidence and death rates are nearly equal, implying that most patients diagnosed with those cancers will die from them. • For other malignancies, such as breast and thyroid cancer, the incidence rate is much higher than the death rate, since many patients survive their cancer diagnosis. • Early detection has decreased the incidence and mortality of some cancers, such as cervical cancer, by the widespread use of Papanicolaou (Pap) smears. • Approximately 62% of people who develop cancer survive at least 5 years.

ANSWER:
B

2. Regarding carcinogenesis, which of the following statements is false?

A. Ionizing radiation has been associated with the development of thyroid cancer.

B. Exposure to asbestos has been associated with the development of nasopharyngeal cancer.

C. Promotion is a reversible process.

D. Benzene exposure has been associated with the development of acute leukemia.

Ref.: 2–5

COMMENTS: Carcinogenic agents may be chemical, physical, viral, or genetic and have in common the ability to induce malignant neoplasms.

Chemical carcinogens have been recognized for over 200 years. • The first description of a causal relationship between a carcinogen and the development of cancer was made in 1775, when Percival Pott described cancer of the scrotum in chimney sweepers. • Aromatic hydrocarbons isolated from coal tar were ultimately shown to be the causative agents. • Coal tar has been associated with cancer of the skin, larynx, and bronchus. • Exposure to β-naphthylamine, an aromatic amine used in the dye industry, has been associated with tumors of the urinary tract. • Benzene exposure has been associated with the development of acute leukemia and asbestos exposure with the development of mesothelioma. • Chemical carcinogens act via a multistep process. • The first step is **initiation**, during which the carcinogen reacts irreversibly with DNA to form a covalent adduct. • The reaction is nonenzymatic and therefore nonspecific. • The second step is **promotion**, which is a slow, reversible process in which initiated cells are stimulated by promoting agents to develop into cancer cells. • Promotion occurs during the latency period. • The third and final step is **progression**, which involves the maturation of cancer cells into a fully malignant tumor. • There is a characteristic **latency period** between the first exposure to a carcinogen and the development of a tumor. • The latency period is dose dependent.

Physical carcinogens include ionizing and ultraviolet radiation. • Both are associated with the development of skin cancer. • Ionizing radiation also may lead to the development of neoplasms of the thyroid, bone, and blood.

Viral carcinogens include both RNA and DNA viruses. • The RNA virus HTLV-1 is the causative agent of adult T-cell leukemia, and the RNA viruses HIV and HCV are strongly associated with cancer development as well. • Among the DNA viruses, the Epstein-Barr virus has been associated with Burkitt's lymphoma, nasopharyngeal cancer, and lymphoma, while papillomaviruses have been implicated in the development of cervical and skin cancers.

A N S W E R :
B

3. Regarding the progression of cells from normal to cancerous, which of the following is not true?

   A. *Dysplasia* describes cells with altered size, shape, and organization.

   B. In the absence of atypia or dysplasia, hyperplasia confers only a modest, if any, risk of cancer in a given tissue.

   C. All dysplastic tissues eventually progress to frank carcinoma.

   D. Metaplastic changes may be reversible.

Ref.: 2

COMMENTS: The development of cancer is a multistep process by which cells develop dysregulated growth. • Unregulated growth and dissemination of cells characterize malignancy. • Malignant transformation occurs after a series of alterations in a number of genes within a cell. • The progression of a cell from normal to malignant can be seen in a series of histologic "plasias." **Hyperplasia** is an increase in cell number associated with rapid growth rates. • It rarely leads to cancer in the absence of associated atypia or dysplasia. • Hyperplastic colonic polyps, for example, unlike their adenomatous counterparts, are not considered precancerous. • Hyperplastic breast tissue is associated with a slightly increased risk for the development of breast cancer but not nearly the fourfold increased risk that is seen with atypical hyperplasia. • **Metaplasia** is the reversible replacement of one mature cell type with another in an area in which it is not normally found. • It may be caused by chronic inflammation, such as squamous cell metaplasia to gastric columnar-type cells in the lower esophagus in a patient with chronic reflux esophagitis. • **Dysplasia** is a term used for epithelial tissues that contain cells altered in size, shape, and organization. • Dysplasia is classified as mild, moderate, or severe, depending on the degree of cell dedifferentiation. • Although some dysplastic tissues may develop into invasive cancers, not all do.

A N S W E R :
C

4. Regarding the biology of malignant neoplasms, which of the following statements is true?

   A. Most malignant neoplasms arise from a single cell that has undergone transformation to form a malignant clone.

   B. Cancer cells proliferate faster than normal cells, and the rate of proliferation increases as the tumor mass increases.

   C. Malignant cells are characterized by reversion to more primitive cell types, cellular monomorphism, and increased cohesion.

   D. Tumors double in size at least every 20 days, and, therefore, essentially all human neoplasms are clinically detectable within 1 year after the inception of neoplastic transformation.

Ref.: 2, 3

COMMENTS: Most cancers are believed to arise from a single cell that has undergone transformation to form a malignant clone, although some cancers (e.g., neurofibrosarcomas in von Recklinghausen's disease) may develop from multiple clones of cells.

• With the possible exceptions of leukocytes and intestinal mucosa cells, cancer cells generally proliferate faster than normal cells. • As such, the bone marrow and intestinal mucosa are often affected by anticancer therapies designed to take advantage of the rapid proliferative rate of malignant tissue. • A tumor's proliferative rate tends to decrease as the tumor size increases. • Changes characteristic of malignant cells include the production of various polypeptides and hormones not normally produced, reversion to a more primitive cell type, cellular pleomorphism, frequent mitoses, hyperchromatism, and the loss of contact inhibition. • Tumor doubling time may be used to assess the aggressiveness of a tumor. • A clinically detectable 1-cm tumor represents approximately 30 divisions and 1 billion cells. • Most tumors double in volume every 20–100 days, although this rate can vary widely from every 8 days to every 600 days. • Most tumors, therefore, are present at least 1 year, but some for very much longer, before they are clinically detectable.

A N S W E R :
A

5. With regard to the spread of neoplasms, which of the following statements is false?

   A. Metastatic cells enter the lymph nodes via the subcapsular space and later permeate the sinusoids of the node.

   B. Carcinoma in situ is a lesion with histopathologic characteristics of malignancy but without detectable invasion beyond the basement membrane.

   C. Lymphatic involvement is common with epithelial neoplasms, whereas most sarcomas metastasize hematogenously.

   D. The metastatic process is highly efficient, as evidenced by the fact that the number of circulating tumor cells correlates with the metastatic burden.

Ref.: 2, 5

COMMENTS: Carcinoma in situ is a neoplasm with cytologic characteristics of malignancy but without detectable invasion through the basement membrane of the epithelial layer. • There are essentially four mechanisms by which cancer cells disseminate: **tissue infiltration**, **lymphatic invasion**, **vascular invasion** (capillaries and veins frequently and arteries rarely), and **direct implantation**. • Metastatic cells generally enter lymph nodes via the subcapsular space. • Only later do the tumor cells permeate the sinusoids and gradually replace the parenchyma of the node. • Lymph nodes are commonly involved in epithelial neoplasms, whereas sarcomas rarely metastasize to them. • The **metastatic process** is highly inefficient. • In some animal tumor models, tumors may shed as many as 100 million viable cells into the bloodstream during their growth and yet produce few lung metastases. • It is estimated that less than 0.01% of highly metastatic tumor cells, injected intravenously, form new tumor foci. • To metastasize, a malignant cell must go through a complex multistep process, referred to as the **metastatic cascade** (see Question 6). • The elements of this cascade are the same via lymphatics and capillaries.

A N S W E R :
D

6. Regarding the metastatic process of cancer, which of the following is true?

   A. The first step is motility and invasion.

   B. The second step is transport.

C. The third step is arrest and extravasation.

D. All of the above are true.

Ref.: 2, 5

COMMENTS: The metastatic process, known as **metastatic cascade**, includes several steps. • The first step is **motility and invasion**. • Before a malignant cell can invade, it must detach from the parent tumor and pass into the lymphatic or venous system. • Activation of the "angiogenic switch" is associated with a dramatic increase in the metastatic potential of a given tumor.

The second step is **transport**. • Once in the lymphatic or venous system, the cell must circulate to the distant site of growth. • During this transport, the cell must survive a number of host defense mechanisms, such as destruction by antibodies, complement, natural killer cells, or macrophages. • In addition, the cell must survive a multitude of mechanical stresses, including turbulence in small blood vessels, poor nutrition, and widely variable oxygen levels.

The third step is **arrest and extravasation**. • Surviving tumor cells are arrested in the target lymph node or small blood vessels of the organ in question. • Precisely how the tumor cells attach to endothelial cells and then invade surrounding tissue is a subject of active investigation. • Attachment to the endothelial cells is mediated by cellular adhesion molecules (CAM), which include the I-CAM and M-CAM family (cadhedrins), integrins, cell-surface lectins, and lectin-binding glycoproteins. • Endothelial cells from small vessels of various organs express different levels of such molecules. • Such organ differences may help explain different patterns of organ preference seen in different metastasizing tumors. • After arrest, the tumor cells must move through the subendothelial basement membrane to invade the surrounding tissue. • To accomplish this, various proteolytic enzymes (plasminogen activator, metalloproteinases, and cathepsins) produced by the tumor cells digest the basement membrane. • Study of these molecules may facilitate the understanding, prediction, and prevention of metastases. • For example, cathepsin D is used as a prognostic indicator in breast cancer.

The final step is **establishment of new growth**. • The more primitive and autonomous a tumor is, the less dependent it is on normal growth factors and the more capable it is of forming new tumor deposits. • This phase is dependent on angiogenesis in the metastatic foci as well as evasion of specific and nonspecific immune responses.

ANSWER:
D

7. Regarding oncogenes and proto-oncogenes, which of the following statements is true?

A. Proto-oncogenes are proteins capable of inhibiting oncogenes.

B. Oncogenes are nucleic acid sequences unique to the viral genome.

C. Exposure to carcinogens causes insertion of oncogenes into the human genome.

D. Proto-oncogenes may be activated by mutation, amplification, or translocation.

Ref.: 2, 5

COMMENTS: A number of gene types may be altered during the development of cancer. • **Oncogenes** are genes that, when expressed, contribute to the development of malignancy. • **Proto-oncogenes** are genes found in normal tissues that, when activated by mutation,

amplification, or translocation, become oncogenes and may lead to transformation of the cell to a malignant phenotype. • Human tumors associated with germ-line activation of proto-oncogenes include medullary thyroid cancer (RET) and rare forms of familial melanoma (CDK4). • **Tumor suppressor genes** differ from oncogenes in that it is the loss of their expression that leads to the development of cancer. • Unlike oncogenes, a tumor suppressor gene must develop mutations in both alleles before it leads to a malignant phenotype. • The most commonly mutated tumor suppressor gene in human solid tumors is p53.

ANSWER:
D

8. Regarding monoclonal antibodies, which the following statements is false?

A. A monoclonal antibody is defined as an antibody with specificity against only one set of antigenic determinants.

B. Monoclonal antibodies have the ability to react with an indefinite number of antigenic determinants.

C. Monoclonal antibody hybridomas are made by fusing a plasma cell to a myeloma cell.

D. An idiotype is the antigenic determinant in the variable region of an antibody.

Ref.: 2, 3

COMMENTS: Hybridomas are created by fusing a plasma cell to a myeloma cell, thereby conferring the immortality of the myeloma cells on the plasma cell population. • Because the initial plasma cell is capable of synthesizing a monoclonal antibody with specificity against only one set of antigenic determinants (epitopes), the resulting hybridoma cell line produces an essentially limitless amount of that monoclonal antibody. • Because immunoglobulins are proteins, they may have antibodies against themselves. • The antibody against the immunoglobulin may bind specifically to an antigenic determinant in the variable region (a so-called idiotype). • An anti-idiotype is an antibody to the idiotype, which may suppress or augment the host's response to various antigens. • The potential applications of monoclonal antibodies include immunodiagnosis, immunotherapy, tests for follow-up after cancer treatment, and research.

ANSWER:
B

9. Which of the following statements is true?

A. The enzymes prostatic acid phosphatase, alkaline phosphatase, neuron-specific enolase (NSE), and CA 125 are important for staging certain cancers.

B. Lactic dehydrogenase (LDH) has little value as a tumor marker.

C. Prostate-specific antigen (PSA) is highly specific for prostate cancer and therefore is a useful screening marker for the disease.

D. The presence of an M protein in association with abnormal plasma cells is considered specific for multiple myeloma.

Ref.: 1–3

COMMENTS: Prostatic acid phosphatase, alkaline phosphatase, LDH, and NSE are enzymes whose levels may be elevated in association with certain malignancies. • The normal prostate secretes **prostatic acid phosphatase**. • Elevation of prostatic acid phosphatase levels in patients with prostate cancer indicates extension of tumor beyond the capsule, but the correlation between elevated levels and total body tumor burden is poor. • Therefore, prostatic acid phosphatase testing is not helpful for staging prostatic tumors. • **Alkaline phosphatase** consists of a number of isoenzymes produced by the liver, bone, and placenta. • Elevation of alkaline phosphatase levels in patients with malignancy usually indicates involvement of liver or bone by metastatic disease. • However, elevated alkaline phosphatase levels are nonspecific for malignancy because they are found in a number of benign disorders, including choledocholithiasis. • **Placental alkaline phosphatase** is a nonspecific marker that is normally made in the placenta. • It is elevated in a few patients with ovarian cancer and testicular seminomas. • **LDH** is an isoenzyme found in a number of normal organs. • Testing of LDH levels has proved valuable for monitoring patients with lymphoma and melanoma. • In lymphoma, elevated levels reflect tumor burden. • LDH is part of the American Joint Commission of Cancer (AJCC) staging system for classifying stage IV melanoma. • **NSE** levels are occasionally elevated in patients with small-cell neuroendocrine carcinoma of the lung. • Measuring the polypeptide chains of immunoglobulins has been valuable in patients with multiple myeloma or B-cell lymphoma. • In these cases, there is often asynchronous production of the polypeptide chains, the light chains being produced in excess of the heavy chains. • These proteins can be detected in blood or urine. • Electrophoresis demonstrates a distinct peak, indicating the presence of an **M protein**. • The presence of an M protein in association with abnormal plasma cells is considered specific for multiple myeloma. • **CA 125** is a tumor-associated antigen. • Testing of CA 125 levels is used primarily in patients with ovarian cancer. • Testing can be useful for monitoring treatment but is not useful as a diagnostic screening tool because CA 125 is produced by other tumors, lung and colon cancer, and in some patients with nonmalignant diseases, such as gynecomastia and cirrhosis. • **CA 15.3** is another tumor-associated antigen whose levels may be elevated in patients with breast, ovarian, and lung cancer. • Testing of CA 15.3 levels has been used in the past for monitoring breast cancer patients, but testing levels of CA 27.29, a more specific breast tumor marker, has largely supplanted it. • **CA 19.9** is a tumor-associated antigen whose usefulness seems to be in detecting pancreatic cancer. • **PSA** levels are elevated in patients with prostatic disease. • Although PSA testing is sensitive for the presence of prostatic disease, it is not specific for prostate cancer. • Elevated levels may also be seen in patients with benign prostatic hypertrophy. • Since PSA levels do correlate with the tumor burden in patients with prostate cancer, the test is useful for monitoring these patients.

ANSWER:
D

10. Regarding metastatic cancer, which of the following statements is true?

    A. Axillary lymph node dissection is essential for staging a sarcoma of the breast.

    B. Melanoma tends to metastasize first to the lung, brain, and gastrointestinal tract.

    C. Bone is frequently the site of metastasis for cancer of the breast and prostate.

    D. Primary brain cancers have a predilection for metastasis to the lung.

Ref.: 2

COMMENTS: In order to make rational decisions concerning therapy, it is necessary to understand the routes by which particular cancers spread. • In general, cancers are able to spread through four main routes: **direct invasion of adjacent tissues, lymphatic spread, hematogenous spread** via vascular embolization, and **implantation** in a serous cavity. • Metastasizing tumors often have a predilection for selected organ sites. • The reasons for this are not clearly understood and constitute an area of active investigation. • Some theories include the presence of essential growth factors in certain tissues needed for a particular tumor's growth and the interaction of tumor surface adhesion molecules with certain tissues, leading to the establishment of metastatic disease. • Understanding the behavior of a particular tumor is important for treatment planning. • Systemic therapy may play a significant role in the treatment of a cancer with a propensity for hematogenous spread, such as breast, colon, or lung cancers. • Systemic therapy may have a limited role in cancers that spread primarily by local invasion, such as brain neoplasms and tumors of the oral pharynx. • For tumors with a low proclivity for lymphatic spread, such as most types of sarcoma, lymph node dissection neither improves outcome nor aids in staging. • It is also necessary to understand the patterns of metastatic spread to make rational decisions concerning surveillance testing. • For example, there is little reason to obtain serial bone scans for surveillance of a tumor that does not tend to metastasize to bone.

ANSWER:
C

11. With regard to unknown primary tumors presenting as metastatic disease, match the site of metastasis in the left-hand column with the more likely possible site(s) of the primary tumor in the right-hand column.

A. Supraclavicular node	a. Breast cancer
B. Axillary lymph node	b. Melanoma
C. Ovarian metastasis	c. Prostate cancer
D. Bone metastasis	d. Colon cancer
E. Skin metastasis	e. Stomach cancer
	f. Ovarian cancer

Ref.: 2, 5, 6

COMMENTS: Usually the site of a primary tumor is known, although some cancers present as metastatic disease and the primary tumor is not readily apparent. • In fact, sometimes the site of the primary tumor may never be identified because the primary tumor is too small to be detected by standard methods or because of regression of the primary lesion before the metastases are identified. • Knowledge of likely sites of origin can direct the evaluation of metastasis of unknown origin.

ANSWER:
A-a,d,e,f; B-a,b; C-d,e; D-a,c; E-a,b

12. Which of the following statements is true?

    A. Granulocyte colony-stimulating factor (G-CSF) is used to ameliorate the thrombocytopenic effects of chemotherapeutic agents.

    B. Interleukin-2 (IL-2) is produced by natural killer (NK) cells.

    C. Tumor necrosis factors (TNF-α and TNF-β) are produced by NK cells.

    D. G-CSF, granulocyte/macrophage colony-stimulating factor (GM-CSF), and erythropoietin exert their effects on bone marrow.

Ref.: 2

COMMENTS: The underlying principle of biologic therapy (biologic response modifiers) for treatment of cancer is to augment the host's native immune responses and intensify tumor rejection responses. • A number of proteins have been found to be responsible for the growth and development of cells within the hematopoietic and lymphoid systems. • **Cytokines** are proteins produced and secreted by a cell. • Several of the key regulatory cytokines (i.e., interleukins and interferon-α [INF-α]) have been isolated, and some are currently in clinical use. • Others are undergoing further investigation. • **IL-2**, a lymphokine produced by activated T cells, can bind to a specific cell-surface receptor on activated T lymphocytes. • In addition to being a key factor in T-cell proliferation, it also activates **NK cells**. • IL-2 has been used extensively in clinical trials in patients. • It has single-agent activity (e.g., against melanoma and renal cell cancer) and is also used in combination with chemotherapeutic agents. • **IFN-α** has immune modulatory effects, including activation of NK cells, modulation of antibody production by B lymphocytes, and induction on the tumor cell surface of major histocompatibility complex (MHC) antigens. • **IFN$_{α2b}$** is approved for use as adjuvant treatment of node-positive melanoma patients. • **Tumor necrosis factors (TNF-α and TNF-β)** are produced by activated macrophages and have a wide variety of biologic effects. • They activate osteoclasts, act as growth factors for fibroblast, and have antiviral activity. • They also exert immunomodulatory effects, interacting with other cytokines and inducing surface MHC antigens. • TNF may have direct cytotoxic effects on cells and may have a role in the development of cancer cachexia. • Hematopoietic growth factors are playing an increasing role in ameliorating the deleterious effects of chemotherapy and in permitting dose-intense therapy. • **G-CSF** and **GM-CSF** have proliferative effects on bone marrow progenitor cells from which neutrophils are derived, modulating the effects of chemotherapy-induced neutropenia. • **Erythropoietin** promotes the proliferation of committed erythroid precursors and is used to treat anemia.

A N S W E R :
D

13. Which of the following options is/are appropriate for treatment of metastatic cancer?

   A. A Whipple procedure to relieve obstructive jaundice in a patient with adenocarcinoma of the head of the pancreas and multiple small metastatic lesions in the liver.

   B. Resection of three liver lesions, metastatic from a colorectal primary tumor, in the absence of another site of disease.

   C. Resection of two lung metastases from a sarcoma of the lower extremities in the absence of other metastatic disease.

   D. Radiation therapy for a painful hip lesion in a patient with diffuse bony metastases from prostate cancer.

Ref.: 2

COMMENTS: Treatment of metastatic cancer varies widely. • In most circumstances, the goal of treatment for metastatic disease is palliation, since cure is unlikely. • Decisions concerning appropriate treatment of metastatic disease must take into account multiple factors, including the natural history of the disease, number of metastatic sites, rate of tumor growth, history of previous response to therapy, the patient's overall physiologic condition, toxicity of the proposed treatment, likelihood of achieving a response to therapy, the quality of life with and without therapy, and the patient's desires. • Whereas aggressive therapy may be indicated for limited metastatic foci, such as surgical resection or ablation for hepatic metastasis from colorectal carcinoma, it may be reasonable simply to provide supportive care for a patient with multiple metastatic

sites, who has a history of failing multiple previous therapeutic regimens, or who is in a debilitated condition. • The two overriding goals of treatment for advanced cancer are to palliate symptoms and prolong life. • When evaluating options for palliation of symptoms, the side effects of the treatment should be less than the severity of the symptom it is purported to palliate. • Attempts to prolong life have generally been less than successful. • In some circumstances, the current therapeutic modalities (i.e., surgery, chemotherapy, biologic therapy, and radiation therapy) have been shown to improve survival with a reasonable quality of life. • A subset of patients with "oligometastatic" disease may enjoy significant disease-free survival and meaningful prolongation of life after ablative therapy.

A N S W E R :
B, C, D

14. With regard to clinical trials, which of the following statements is/are true?

   A. Phase II trials establish the maximum tolerated dose of an experimental agent.

   B. Comparing one group of patients receiving a given treatment with another that received a different treatment 10 years ago introduces observational bias into the study.

   C. Randomization into trials is done to ensure that each group of patients has a similar chance of achieving the desired outcome.

   D. An example of a phase I trial would be studying whether Herceptin plus docetaxel is effective in decreasing the size of metastases from breast cancer.

Ref.: 2, 5

COMMENTS: Clinical trials in oncology are an important method for bringing new therapies into clinical use in a rational and scientific way. • The essence of a clinical trial is the idea that, by examining how a given treatment affects a representative group of patients, generalizations can be made as to the applicability of the treatment to a broader group of patients with the disease. • The results are examined (**statistical analysis**) to determine the probability that, with a certain level of confidence in the observed outcome (**confidence interval**), the results could have been achieved by random variation or chance alone (***p* value**). • The surgeon must understand the basic premises of clinical trial designs to analyze critically the data from these studies and to make rational clinical decisions. • **Phase I trials** ask the question: "Is the new treatment safe and at what dose?" **Phase II trials** ask the question: "Is the new treatment effective in treating the disease in question?" **Phase III trials** ask the question: "Is the new treatment any better than our standard treatment?" It is phase III trials that often take the form of randomized, controlled clinical trials to minimize the chance that variations in treatment outcome are related to factors other than differences in treatment (**bias**). • Minimizing the sources of bias introduced into a study strengthens the study design and the evidence for its conclusions. • **Comparative control groups** are utilized to assess the efficacy of a new treatment against a control group receiving standard therapy. • The control group establishes the *expected rate* of outcome in the null hypothesis of no effect of the investigational intervention, and the intervention group gives the *observed rate* of this outcome with investigational treatment. • **Randomizing patients into treatment arms** ensures that patients in the treatment arms are equally likely to achieve a given outcome. • Randomizing patients into treatment arms and stratifying them for known prognostic factors accomplish this. • **Blinding investigators and patients** removes the possibility of observational bias that may occur with differences in how outcome observations are made in the control and intervention arms of a trial. • Blinding patients and investigators to which treatment was received, documenting all outcome observations for later verification by an independent blinded observer, and ensuring similar follow-up for the groups of patients can minimize observational bias. • **Concurrent comparison of intervention and control groups** eliminates the possibility of a chronologic bias, which may occur because changes in therapeutic and diagnostic capabilities over time may affect the outcomes. • **Analyzing data on an "intention to treat" basis** ensures comparison of randomized groups. • An analysis that examines the treatment patients actually received rather than the treatment they were supposed to receive does not compare the randomly assigned groups, which were supposed to ensure that each group had a similar chance of achieving the desired outcome. • There are multiple reasons why patients assigned to a particular treatment group may not actually receive the intended therapy. • The factors that affect failure to receive therapy are an important part of evaluating the experimental and control therapies.

ANSWER:
C

---

15. True or false: The penetrance of the APC gene is nearly 100%.

Ref.: 2, 6

COMMENTS: A number of cancer-susceptibility genes have been identified. • While commercial testing is available for several germ-line mutations, at the present time, routine testing of high-risk individuals should be limited to cases of adenomatous polyposis coli (APC), retinoblastoma (RBD), von Hippel's disease (VHL), familial medullary thyroid carcinoma, and multiple endocrine neoplasia (MEN) type II. • There is an as yet unproven benefit to testing for breast cancer (BRCA1 and 2), hereditary non-polyposis colon cancer (hMSH2, hMLH1, hPMS1, hPMS2, and hMSH6), and Li-Fraumeni syndrome (p53). • In all but APC gene (located on the long arm of chromosome 21; 5q21) mutations, the penetration is much less than 100%. • The decision to perform genetic testing is made by the patient after consultation with the physician and a genetic counselor to evaluate the risks and benefits of testing. • This field is evolving rapidly as new information accumulates and changes recommendations for prevention and surveillance. • However, the legal, ethical, and financial issues that arise have not been resolved yet.

ANSWER:
True

REFERENCES

1. Townsend CM, Beauchamp RD, Evers BM, et al (eds): *Sabiston Textbook of Surgery: The Biological Basis of Modern Surgical Practice*, 16th ed. Saunders, Philadelphia, 2001.
2. Schwartz SI, Shires GT, Spencer FC: *Principles of Surgery*, 7th ed. McGraw-Hill, New York, 1999.
3. Jemal A, Murray T, Samuels A, et al: Cancer statistics, 2003. *CA Cancer J Clin* 53:5–26, 2003.
4. Tannock IF, Hill RP: *The Basic Science of Oncology*, 2nd ed. McGraw-Hill, New York, 1992.
5. DeVita VT, Hellman S, Rosenberg SA: *Cancer: Principles and Practice of Oncology*, 6th ed. Lippincott, Williams & Wilkins, Philadelphia, 2001.
6. Saclarides TJ, Millikan KM, Godellas CS: Surgical oncology: an algorithmic approach. Springer-Verlag, New York, 2003.

B. Surgical Therapy

José M. Velasco, M.D.

1. Which of the following historical characteristics of a mass suggest(s) malignancy?

A. Sudden development of a painful, tender mass

B. Slow, progressive, painless growth of a mass

C. Sudden dramatic enlargement of a previously stable-sized mass

D. A mass that waxes and wanes in size with or without associated tenderness

Ref.: 1, 2

COMMENTS: The age of the patient and the location of a mass are important characteristics that raise or lower the index of suspicion that a mass may be malignant. • Other factors include the growth characteristics of the mass, the presence or absence of pain, and the presence or absence of associated inflammatory symptoms. • The growth characteristic most suggestive of malignancy is that of slow, progressive enlargement. • The sudden and dramatic enlargement of a previously stable-sized mass is usually caused by spontaneous or trauma-induced hemorrhage into the mass. • This is commonly seen in thyroid nodules. • A mass that waxes and wanes in size or is painful, especially when associated with tenderness, warmth, and erythema, usually suggests an inflammatory process. • The rapid onset of pain likewise suggests inflammation, whereas a more gradual onset of pain in a slowly enlarging mass suggests malignant invasion of adjacent structures, especially nerves. • There are, of course, many exceptions to these broad generalizations (e.g., inflammatory carcinoma of the breast or hemorrhage into a small thyroid cancer).

ANSWER:
B

2. Which of the following physical characteristics of a mass does not suggest malignancy?

A. Hard texture

B. Soft texture

C. Fixation to deeper structures

D. Pulling inward of overlying skin

E. Matted contiguous masses

Ref.: 1, 2

COMMENTS: Malignancies characteristically invade surrounding structures and, in many instances, incite a fibroplastic (scirrhous) host response within and around the tumor. • This leads to the hard texture characteristic of most epithelial malignancies and to the fixation of locally advanced cancers to deeper structures or overlying skin, the matting of contiguous lymph nodes, and the invasion of nerves. • Neural invasion causes pain or functional loss (e.g., vocal cord paralysis from recurrent laryngeal nerve invasion by thyroid cancer or facial nerve paralysis from parotid malignancies). • A rubbery feel can indicate a benign (e.g., breast fibroadenoma) or malignant (e.g., solitary or matted lymphoma nodes) process. • Well-circumscribed masses are usually benign because the invasiveness of malignancies usually makes their borders somewhat indistinct. • In most cases, the association of warmth, erythema, or both with a mass suggests a benign inflammatory condition.

ANSWER:
B

3. Which of the following eponyms is not used to describe a physical finding suggestive of metastatic or locally advanced malignancy?

A. Blumer's shelf

B. Virchow's node

C. Grey Turner's sign

D. Krukenberg's tumor

E. Sister Mary Joseph's sign

Ref.: 1, 2

COMMENTS: Part of the physical evaluation of a patient with a suspected malignancy involves the search for signs that suggest invasion of surrounding structures or distant spread. • **Blumer's shelf** (rectal shelf) is a hard, nodular ridge felt ventrally on digital rectal examination between the rectum and the uterus in a female or the rectum and the bladder in a male. • It signifies transcoelomic spread of an intra-abdominal cancer with implants in the deep pelvic peritoneal sac. • **Virchow's node** is a medially located left supraclavicular lymph node metastasis from an intra-abdominal primary site (most often gastric or pancreatic). • **Krukenberg's tumor** is an ovarian mass detectable on bimanual pelvic examination, ultrasonography, or computed tomography (CT) scan. • It signifies a "drop metastasis" or transcoelomic implantation of tumor on the ovary from another intra-abdominal primary site (classically gastric). • **Sister Mary Joseph's sign** is a periumbilical deposit of tumor within the abdominal wall secondary to an underlying intra-abdominal malignancy. • The precise pathophysiology of such tumor nodules is not agreed on, but they may be due to direct invasion through the abdominal wall by peritoneal tumor seeding or retrograde lymphatic or hematogenous tumor spread via the umbilical ligament. • **Grey Turner's sign** applies to the presence of flank ecchymosis, classically associated with hemorrhagic pancreatitis.

ANSWER:
C

4. Regarding the biopsy of a tumor mass, which of the following statements is true?

    A. Fine-needle aspiration biopsy enables definitive diagnosis of a malignancy only rarely, and it carries a significant risk of tumor seeding along the needle tract.

    B. Excisional biopsy is the favored procedure for large, deep, soft-tissue sarcomas of the extremities.

    C. Incisional biopsy involves removal of a small portion of a tumor, and it is useful for thyroid nodules so as not to compromise curative resection.

    D. Biopsy incisions for suspected cancers need not always be oriented in natural skin lines.

    E. Image-guided fine-needle biopsy of potentially resectable pancreatic masses has simplified the management of these tumors.

Ref.: 1–3

COMMENTS: Interpreting the results of **fine-needle aspiration (FNA) biopsy** of a tumor, a simple office procedure with minimal risk, requires the expertise of a cytopathologist. • Results positive for malignancy are highly accurate. • Negative results, especially from clinically suspicious lesions, should be viewed with caution and may warrant further investigation, usually with open biopsy. • Reports of needle-tract seeding from FNA biopsy are rare, and the clinical significance of the possibility of seeding is lessened by the fact that the area in question will likely be definitively resected or irradiated as part of the local therapy for the cancer. • However, image-guided fine-needle biopsy of potentially resectable pancreatic tumors should be avoided, since it has been associated with low yields and a definite risk of tumor seeding while not altering the course of therapy. • **Incisional biopsy**, best used for large tumors, involves removing of a small portion of a tumor through an open incision. • Negative results of an incisional biopsy of a clinically worrisome lesion must be viewed with caution because of the possibility of sampling error. • Biopsy incisions for suspicious lesions should be oriented in a manner that allows them to be easily encompassed in the planned resection incision, not necessarily in the natural skin lines. • Incisional biopsy is usually inappropriate for thyroid nodules because of the risks of bleeding and of seeding the neck wound with tumor cells. • Biopsy of thyroid nodules is generally performed preoperatively with FNA or core biopsies, or intraoperatively with total excision (usually by thyroid lobectomy). • **Excisional biopsy** is used for total removal of small masses (e.g., breast or subcutaneous nodules), frequently with a margin of normal tissue to avoid the need for re-excision. • It is usually inappropriate to perform a biopsy of large suspicious masses by marginal excision because the definitive wide re-excision may be unnecessarily debilitating, both cosmetically and functionally.

ANSWER:
D

5. With regard to the staging of cancer, which of the following statements is true?

    A. Assessment of the degree of local growth and regional (lymphatic) and distant (hematogenous) involvement of a cancer is mandatory when planning therapy.

    B. Open sampling of clinically suspicious regional lymph nodes before definitive surgical therapy is advisable to stage tumors adequately preoperatively.

    C. CT or magnetic resonance imaging (MRI) of the brain, chest, abdomen, and pelvis, along with radionuclide bone scans,

should be performed preoperatively in most patients with epithelial malignancy.

    D. Staging laparotomy for Hodgkin's disease is no longer an appropriate staging technique.

Ref.: 1–4

COMMENTS: The proper choice of therapy in cancer management depends on adequate knowledge of the local, regional, and distant extent of disease. • Therefore, all cancers must be clinically, radiographically, or surgically staged before definitive therapy. • The degree to which the oncologist relies on radiographic imaging techniques and surgical staging depends on the natural history of the cancer in question, the likelihood of metastasis to specific sites, and the cost, risk, and accuracy of the staging technique under consideration. • Careful clinical evaluation and routine laboratory testing, including a chest radiograph and chemistry profile, constitute the minimal accepted staging workup for most cancers. • Additional imaging techniques are of variable benefit, depending on the natural history of the cancer in question. • Total body scanning occasionally detects distant disease not previously suspected. • However, the prohibitive cost makes it unwise to use such an approach as a routine staging strategy. • Hodgkin's disease, when it presents confined to supradiaphragmatic or upper abdominal sites, remains an appropriate indication for a staging laparotomy in selected cases but only when therapy will be altered by the outcome. • This procedure, which involves splenectomy, liver biopsy, and sampling of intra-abdominal lymph nodes at multiple sites, can lead to changes in the staging of the disease that would influence therapeutic strategy in up to 30% of cases. • The risk of inappropriately treating these patients if surgical staging is not performed is thought to justify the small but acceptable risk of laparotomy. • The risk can be lessened further with the use of minimally invasive laparoscopic techniques. • In cases of cancers likely to spread to cervical, axillary, or groin lymph nodes, clinically suspicious nodes in the expected lymph drainage site generally warrant formal dissection of the area without prior surgical staging. • Preliminary open biopsy of these areas may compromise the subsequent definitive surgery, risk tumor spillage within these relatively poorly defined fascial compartments, and increase the likelihood of injury to the neurovascular structures in the area.

ANSWER:
A

6. Performing which the following operations would be inappropriate without first obtaining a biopsy specimen confirming the presence of cancer?

    A. Radical right hemicolectomy for an "apple core" narrowing of the ascending colon.

    B. Modified radical mastectomy for a clinically and mammographically obvious breast cancer with overlying "skin puckering."

    C. A pancreaticoduodenectomy for a large, hard mass in the head of the pancreas that produces painless jaundice.

    D. Parotidectomy for a 2-cm, slowly growing solid parotid mass without evidence of facial nerve dysfunction.

Ref.: 1–4

COMMENTS: Ideally, tissue confirmation of malignancy is obtained before radical surgical extirpation is performed. • In cases in which the tumor is easily accessible, either directly or endoscopically (e.g., breast tumors and tumors of the upper aerodigestive tract), it would be improper to perform radical surgery without tissue confirmation. • On occasion, however, a biopsy specimen is not easily obtained, carries unacceptable risk, complicates subsequent extirpative therapy, or would not alter the extent of the operation. • In such cases, it may be proper to proceed with definitive, curative surgical excision in the absence of a confirming biopsy specimen. • Colon lesions that are radiographically worrisome but colonoscopically inaccessible should be resected without histologic confirmation because colotomy and biopsy at the time of laparotomy risk both tumor spillage and stool contamination of the peritoneal cavity. • Even multiple transduodenal needle-aspiration biopsies may fail to prove the presence of pancreatic carcinoma because of sampling error. • If the surgeon believes that pancreaticoduodenectomy is an appropriate therapy for a mass at the head of the pancreas and if the clinical index of suspicion is high enough, proceeding without tissue confirmation may be appropriate, provided the patient gives informed consent. • Benign conditions have been found in up to 5% of the cases. • Parotid tumors, whether benign or malignant, are generally resected, with preservation of uninvolved branches of the facial nerve, and radiation therapy is given postoperatively for malignant lesions with close margins. • Preoperative histologic confirmation of malignancy in such cases would not alter the extent of resection. • In all of these cases, clinical judgment, enhanced by thorough knowledge of the tumor's natural history, enables the surgeon to make a proper risk-benefit assessment regarding the need for biopsy.

ANSWER:
B

7. Which of the following tumors requires resection of the largest margin of normal tissue around the clinically obvious tumor to achieve an acceptable likelihood of control at the local primary site. Assume that no other treatment modalities will be used.

   A. Adenocarcinoma of the colon

   B. Basal cell carcinoma of the skin

   C. Invasive breast cancer

   D. Squamous carcinoma of the distal esophagus

   E. Squamous carcinoma of the skin

Ref.: 1–3, 5

COMMENTS: See Question 8.

8. When determining how widely to resect a primary malignancy, which one or more of the following factors need not be considered?

   A. Location of tumor

   B. Capacity for contiguous spread through tissue planes

   C. Capacity for lymphatic dissemination

   D. Tendency for multifocal disease to be present within the organ in question

   E. Capacity for embolic interstitial spread

Ref.: 1–3, 5

COMMENTS: Proper surgical therapy of solid tumors (excluding myeloproliferative malignancies) requires careful consideration of the tumor's *local* growth behavior and invasiveness as well as its capacity for and pattern of *regional* (lymphatic) and *distant* (hematogenous) spread. • Cancers are known to spread by one or more of five pathways: (1) direct invasion through tissue planes,

(2) interstitial emboli, (3) via lymphatic channels to regional nodes, (4) systemically via lymphovenous connections or hematogenous (venous and occasionally arterial) routes, and (5) implantation within serosa-lined cavities (peritoneal, pleural, and pericardial spaces). • The extent of excision around a primary tumor is determined by the tumor's ability to invade locally through contiguous tissues or to spread embolically within the interstitium in the vicinity of the tumor but in a noncontiguous manner. • Pathophysiologically, the capacity of a tumor to invade and spread locally is related to its capacity for cellular multiplication, cellular migration, alteration of cellular adhesiveness, phagocytosis, and elaboration of cytotoxic and lytic substances. • The location of a tumor also has a bearing on the breadth of excision. • Risk-benefit considerations suggest that in certain circumstances tumors close to functionally or cosmetically important organs should be resected with a narrower margin to avoid injury to or loss of that organ, even if this adds slightly to the risk of local recurrence (e.g., a skin cancer close to the eye, in contrast to one in the middle of the back). • Proximity to bone, major motor nerves, or major vessels may also influence the decision for closer margins. • The breadth of local excision (e.g., mastectomy for breast cancer) is influenced by the multifocal or multicentric nature of some tumors. • Finally, the blood supply to the organ in question may have an impact on the extent of local excision. • Much more colon, for example, is resected than is needed to achieve free margins around the primary tumor because the mesenteric dissection requires ligation of the blood supply to large sections of the colon. • The local invasiveness of a tumor influences the breadth of excision needed to achieve local control. • *Basal cell carcinoma* rarely invades more than a few millimeters beyond its clinically evident border. • *Squamous cell carcinoma* of the skin spreads slightly more widely. • *Carcinoma of the colon* requires only a 1- to 2-cm margin around the primary site to achieve local control, although much more colon is usually resected to encompass regional nodes. • *Breast cancer* requires a significant margin of normal tissue around the primary site if local control is to be achieved without the use of radiation therapy. • *Esophageal and gastric cancers* have a propensity to spread in the submucosal plane as far as 10 cm from the primary site, and extremely wide margins are therefore required to clear the suspected areas of tumor infiltration. • The capacity of tumors to implant locally or to spread via lymphatics or blood vessels influences the ultimate disease-free survival rate, but the breadth of excision of the primary tumor is not likely to affect such aspects of tumor biology.

ANSWERS:
Question 7: D
Question 8: C

9. In which one of the following cases would regional lymph node dissection not be appropriate as part of the initial definitive surgical therapy?

   A. A T1 (<2 cm in diameter) squamous cell carcinoma of the anterior one third of the tongue

   B. A small (approximately 2 cm in diameter) exophytic adenocarcinoma of the cecum not associated with obstruction or bleeding

   C. An adenocarcinoma of the head of the pancreas, 2 cm in diameter, producing jaundice

   D. A Clark level IV, 1.6-mm thick, superficial spreading melanoma of the proximal anterior right thigh with a single, firm, enlarged right inguinal lymph node

   E. A high-grade myxoid lyposarcoma, 5 cm in size, located deep in the lateral aspect of the thigh

Ref.: 1–3, 5

COMMENTS: The decision to proceed with regional node dissection in these clinical cases is based on consideration of all of the concepts mentioned in Question 10. • (A) *Small cancer, anterior oral cavity*: The likelihood of nodal disease in such a small cancer is sufficiently low that it does not warrant risking the morbidity associated with a neck dissection. • (B) *Small exophytic colon cancer*: Proper staging of colon carcinoma requires mesenteric lymphadenectomy, which can be done with minimal additional risk. • (C) *Pancreatic cancer*: Removal of the regional nodes that drain the head of the pancreas leads to better staging and local control. • (D) *Advanced melanoma*: Clinically positive primary lymph node drainage areas should be dissected for melanoma (and other malignancies) in the absence of systemic disease. • Sentinel node biopsy, rather than a formal lymph node dissection, would be indicated as a first step on this patient if signs of advanced disease (clinically positive lymph node) are absent. • Elective lymph node dissection for melanoma remains controversial. • (E) *Pleomorphic liposarcoma*: Knowledge that liposarcomas, even aggressive ones such as that described, rarely metastasize to regional lymph nodes makes dissection of the nodes inappropriate, despite the relatively high likelihood that distant disease will develop in this case. • Had the tumor been located within a lymph node basin, then a lymph node dissection would have been needed to achieve clear margins.

ANSWER:
A, E

10. With regard to regional lymphadenectomy, which of the following statements is/are true?

  A. Anatomic lymph node dissection adversely affects the host's immune response and should be performed only in cases of clinically suspicious adenopathy.

  B. Regional lymph nodes act as a fairly effective barrier to the spread of epithelial malignancies beyond the local or regional site.

  C. A pathologically negative regional node dissection confers an approximately 95% likelihood that there has been no distant metastasis.

  D. The rationale for regional lymph node dissection is primarily therapeutic rather than prognostic.

  E. The risk of swelling and propensity for infection in an extremity must be considered when elective axillary or groin dissections are recommended.

Ref.: 1–3, 5

COMMENTS: The rationale for performing regional lymphadenectomy for epithelial malignancies is based on the desire to remove all tumor that may be present and to determine the metastatic potential of the tumor so as to predict prognosis and direct subsequent systemic therapy more accurately. • Risk-benefit decisions in this regard are related to the morbidity of the regional dissection contemplated, the likelihood (based on the characteristics of the primary tumor) that nodes are cancerous, and the degree to which prognosis or subsequent therapy will be altered by the information provided by the dissection. • From the standpoint of morbidity, removal of axillary and groin lymph nodes disrupts collateral venous and lymphatic channels and confers an increased risk of swelling in the associated extremity. • The propensity for infection after minor breaks in the skin in these extremities may be increased as a result of inadequate processing of antigenic information because of the absence of regional lymph nodes. • There is no clear evidence, however, that the patient's overall systemic immune response is adversely affected.

It was originally believed that regional lymph nodes acted as barriers to further spread of cancer and that systemic disease would be seen only after the regional nodes had become "choked" with tumor. • It is now recognized that this "barrier function" of regional lymph nodes is performed poorly, and, from a biologic standpoint, it is more appropriate to consider involvement of regional lymph nodes as a measure of the metastatic potential of the tumor. • Thus, regional lymph node dissections are as much for prognostic purposes and subsequent treatment planning as for therapeutic purposes, increasingly so in this era of broadening indications for adjuvant systemic therapy. • For example, in breast cancer, clinical trials (e.g., NSABP B-04) have shown that axillary lymph node dissection may be of prognostic value only insofar as survival does not appear to be influenced by whether the axillary lymph nodes are resected, irradiated, or observed until clinically positive and then removed.

Negative findings on regional node dissection do not guarantee against systemic disease, and the predictive value of such findings varies tumor by tumor. • For example, systemic disease in those with breast cancer develops relatively commonly (in up to 30% of patients) after negative regional lymph node dissections. • In cancers of the upper aerodigestive tract, however, systemic disease is rarely seen without previous cervical lymph node involvement. • Widespread acceptance of sentinel node biopsy techniques in the management of patients with skin and breast cancer has mandated a reassessment of otherwise previously accepted algorithms, particularly in the absence of clinical evidence of advanced disease.

ANSWER:
E

11. Assuming that there is no other evidence of disease, which one or more of the following cases of distant metastatic disease would be appropriately treated by surgical resection of the metastasis?

  A. A solitary 6-cm right-lobe liver metastasis from a sigmoid cancer resected 1 year earlier

  B. Three right-sided and one left-sided pulmonary metastases from a chondrosarcoma of the pelvis successfully treated 18 months earlier

  C. Three small metastases easily resectable with a left lateral segmentectomy from a node-negative infiltrating lobular carcinoma of the breast treated by mastectomy 3 years earlier

  D. Three small (<2 cm in diameter) superficial liver metastases (two in the right lobe and one in the left lobe) from a previously resected cecal cancer

  E. A solitary left-lobe liver metastasis, 3 cm in diameter, with associated involvement of portal lymph nodes from a splenic flexure colon carcinoma resected 2 years earlier

Ref.: 1–3, 5

COMMENTS: See Question 12.

12. With regard to the surgical management of distant metastases, which of the following statements is/are true?

  A. Liver resection for metastatic colon carcinoma should be reserved for solitary lesions less than 5 cm in diameter, with a long (>3 years) disease-free interval from the time of the initial surgery.

  B. The 5-year survival rate after liver resection for selected cases of metastatic colon carcinoma is approximately 25%.

C. Pulmonary resection for metastatic sarcoma is not warranted because of the propensity for sarcomas to disseminate widely and subclinically to other organ systems.

D. Resection of metastatic cancer is warranted if all gross disease from all sites of metastasis can be removed.

E. A solitary lung nodule in a patient with a history of melanoma successfully resected 2 years earlier should be treated with systemic therapy because of the high likelihood of additional subclinical systemic metastases.

Ref.: 1–3, 5

COMMENTS: Until the mid-1960s, surgical resection of distant metastatic disease was considered surgical heresy because of the generally held belief that patients so afflicted were incurable. • It has become clear, however, that in many instances distant metastatic disease is not necessarily a harbinger of widespread dissemination and that successful surgical resection may in fact lead to cure or at least long-term disease-free survival. • The decision to proceed with resection of distant metastases depends on the following factors: the likelihood that the true extent of disease is confined to what is clinically or radiographically apparent, the morbidity of the proposed operation, and the unavailability of more effective nonoperative methods of controlling the disease. • The clinical situations most successfully managed by surgical resection of metastatic disease have been colon cancer metastatic to the liver and sarcoma metastatic to the lung.

With colon cancer, liver resection should be considered when there is no extrahepatic metastatic disease and all of the apparent disease can be resected with free margins, preserving sufficient functional liver volume. • This may necessitate a formal lobar resection or may be accomplished by multiple wedge resections, depending on the size and location of the lesions. • A short disease-free interval between primary therapy and development of the metastases may reflect the biologic aggressiveness of the tumor but is not in itself a contraindication to liver resection. • Disease-free survival rates of 40% at 3 years and 25% at 5 years have been reported in a series of selected cases. • With the mortality rate for major liver resection in the range of <5% in competent hands, liver resection for limited metastatic colon cancer confined to the liver could be considered standard therapy. • Liver resection for metastases from other tumors has been reported, but successes are anecdotal, and such procedures are not considered standard therapy.

In the case of sarcomas, distant metastases are so frequently confined to the lungs that resection of the pulmonary involvement is reasonable, even in cases of multiple and bilateral metastases. • A solitary lung nodule appearing in a patient with a history of cancer is not necessarily a metastasis. • If the patient is a smoker, the likelihood that the solitary nodule represents a primary lung cancer (rather than a solitary metastasis) is approximately 50% and warrants careful evaluation and potentially curative resection. • Metastases to skin and subcutaneous tissue, bone, and mediastinal or retroperitoneal lymph nodes generally suggest a more disseminated process and are a relative contraindication to surgical therapy.

ANSWERS:
Question 11: A, B, D
Question 12: B

13. Regarding en bloc multiorgan resection for cancer, which of the following statements is not true?

A. En bloc resection of the breast, axillary nodes, pectoralis muscles, and internal mammary nodes improves survival from breast cancer but should not be done because of the morbidity associated with the procedure.

B. Total pelvic exenteration for extensive invasive rectal carcinoma can provide cure in up to 25% of selected cases.

C. Colon cancer invading the abdominal wall should be treated by en bloc resection of the colon tumor along with the involved abdominal wall.

D. A large right adrenal tumor invading the kidney and liver should be resected en bloc with the involved contiguous organs if technically possible.

Ref.: 1–4

COMMENTS: Many patients have probably been denied the opportunity for cure by surgeons unwilling to perform en bloc multiorgan resections when indicated. • The reluctance to proceed with such an operation is frequently based on the assumption that a large tumor invading contiguous organs is likely to have metastasized distantly and is therefore incurable. • On occasion, this assumption is erroneous because some tumors grow to a large size without evidence of distant metastasis as a result of their limited biologic potential to spread hematogenously.

The issues to consider before undertaking large multiorgan resections include the presumed distant metastatic potential of the tumor; the functional (or in some cases cosmetic) importance of the organs requiring resection; the capability of reconstructing the defects in soft tissue, bone, blood vessels, or hollow viscus; the ability of the patient to withstand the magnitude of the procedure contemplated; and the unavailability of other equally or more effective but less invasive modalities of therapy. • Cutting across gross tumor or "pinching off" the tumor to avoid resection of contiguous involved organs and relying on radiation therapy or systemic therapy to control gross residual disease is rarely successful and should be avoided in potentially curable situations.

The Urban procedure for breast cancer (case A) represents an appealing operative strategy from the standpoint of en bloc resection of the primary site and its major regional lymph node basins, but it has never been shown to enhance survival. • Total pelvic exenteration (en bloc resection of the rectum, the uterus in females, and the bladder, case B) is moderately disabling functionally because construction of both a colostomy and a urinary conduit is required. • However, it has been shown to provide long-term disease-free survival. • Cure is attainable in up to 25% of selected cases, and this procedure offers the best opportunity (especially when supplemented with pelvic irradiation) to achieve local control of extensively invasive rectal carcinoma. • Bulky but locally confined colon cancers are potentially curable if treated by en bloc multiorgan resection, including the abdominal wall (case C). • In case D (adrenal carcinoma), the only opportunity for cure would be with a resection that included an appropriate portion of the attached liver and the kidney. • In this location, it would likely be involvement of the vena cava that would limit resectability.

ANSWER:
A

14. With regard to cytoreductive (debulking) surgery, which of the following statements is true?

A. Adequate debulking of diffuse intra-abdominal ovarian adenocarcinoma followed by systemic chemotherapy offers the best opportunity for long-term survival and even cure.

B. After subtotal resection of a retroperitoneal sarcoma attached to the aorta, conventional radiation therapy is more effective if only 2 g, rather than 10 g, of tumor remains.

C. The effectiveness of radiation therapy in sterilizing residual tumor after incomplete resection is linearly and inversely related to the volume of tumor remaining.

D. In selected cases, cytotoxic chemotherapy is capable of sterilizing deposits of clinically detectable gross residual tumor.

Ref.: 1–4

COMMENTS: The effectiveness of radiation therapy, chemotherapy, or both for enhancing local control or improving survival after complete surgical resection of a solid tumor has been demonstrated in a number of clinical trials investigating a number of tumor sites. • It is generally believed that the less residual tumor there is to be treated by these adjunctive therapies, the more effective are the therapies. • This is not, however, a linear relationship. • In fact, effectiveness is frequently not seen unless the tumor has been reduced to microscopic residual volume. • One notable exception to this generalization is ovarian cancer, which frequently tends to disseminate widely to the visceral and parietal peritoneal surfaces of the abdominal cavity. • It has been shown that if the tumor can be "debulked," leaving no nodules larger than 2 cm, cytotoxic chemotherapy in many instances is effective in sterilizing the remaining tumor load, leading to long-term survival.

ANSWER:
A

15. Partial or complete resection of which of the following organs could be justified to prevent a future cancer?

A. Colon

B. Pancreas

C. Breast

D. Testicle

E. Thyroid

Ref.: 1–3

COMMENTS: On occasion, the risk that cancer will develop in an organ is sufficiently high that consideration is given to the prophylactic removal of part or all of that organ. • Risk-benefit considerations when proceeding to resection include the likelihood that cancer will develop, the functional or cosmetic disability caused by loss of the organ, and the morbidity associated with the surgical procedure itself. • Unfortunately, the likelihood that the cancer will be disseminated and incurable at the time of diagnosis if the organ is not prophylactically removed applies to most solid tumors, insofar as subclinical lymphatic or hematogenous spread can occur before the primary tumor becomes clinically evident.

Although pancreatic cancers are highly aggressive and usually incurable, prophylactic resection of this organ is not appropriate. • Regarding the colon, however, the polyposis syndromes (e.g., Gardner's syndrome and familial polyposis) and long-standing pancolonic involvement with ulcerative colitis confer such a high risk of future colon cancer that prophylactic proctocolectomy or a sphincter-preserving variation of that procedure should be considered. • A strong family history of breast cancer, especially when coupled with the presence of a mutation in the BRCA1 or BRCA2 gene, can be associated with a future risk of breast cancer that approaches 90%. • In such high-risk individuals, bilateral mastectomy reduces the risk by more than 90%, usually with an acceptable cosmetic result if reconstruction is performed. • Undescended testicles have a known association with subsequent development of testicular carcinoma, and many oncologists believe that if the testicles cannot be repositioned into the scrotum they should be resected. • Identification of the RET proto-oncogene in patients with a family history of medullary thyroid cancer or multiple endocrine neoplasia type II (MEN-II) syndrome is associated with a nearly

100% likelihood of development of medullary thyroid cancer. • Total thyroidectomy is being performed in patients as young as 5 years old with this proto-oncogene.

ANSWER:
~~B~~   A C D E

16. In which of the following circumstances would palliative surgery not be indicated?

A. Carcinoma of the body of the pancreas that produces severe back pain

B. A large gastric cancer obstructing the gastroesophageal junction, associated with two small liver metastases

C. A bleeding cecal cancer, 5 cm in diameter, with multiple liver metastases

D. Adenocarcinoma of the head of the pancreas with partial portal vein involvement

Ref.: 1–4

COMMENTS: All of these clinical scenarios represent disabling symptoms caused by cancers that are generally incurable. • In many instances, however, surgical resection may offer the best means of palliation for the patient. • Consideration of surgery as a palliative measure depends on the pathophysiologic mechanism of the symptom being produced, the likelihood that resection would be effective in alleviating the symptom, the likelihood of morbidity from the proposed surgical procedure, the availability of effective but less invasive palliative measures, and the life expectancy of the patient.

As a rule, tumors within a hollow viscus produce symptoms by obstruction or bleeding. • These are most effectively alleviated by resection or, in the case of obstruction, both resection and surgical bypass. • Radiation therapy can be effective in controlling bleeding and relieving obstruction, but the benefits are usually short-lived. • Mechanical stenting of obstructions such as those at the gastroesophageal junction, within the colon, and within the biliary tree can be effective. • However, it often requires multiple stent changes, can be associated with infection, and is generally not recommended for long-term use. • The bleeding cecal cancer would be best managed by resection, whereas that causing biliary obstruction would be best bypassed with a biliary-enteric anastomosis if long-term survival was anticipated. • Portal vein involvement by an adenocarcinoma of the head of the pancreas does not contraindicate pancreatic resection. • Skin ulcerations caused by recurrent cancer may be effectively managed with radiation therapy if bone invasion is not present. • For a patient with an ulcerated chest wall recurrence from breast cancer, the most effective palliative treatment would be a full-thickness chest wall resection. • The back pain associated with pancreatic cancer is usually due to tumor growth into the retroperitoneum and would not be relieved by pancreatectomy. • Selective celiac neural block is most effective in relieving this pain.

ANSWER:
A

17. Planned primary multimodality therapy results in improved survival or reduced morbidity of therapy in all but which of the following tumors?

A. Locally advanced squamous cell carcinoma of the pharynx

B. Infiltrating carcinoma of the breast

C. Wilms' tumor

D. Melanoma

E. Sarcoma of the extremities

Ref.: 1–4

COMMENTS: Although all of the major treatment modalities (surgery, radiation therapy, chemotherapy, and immunotherapy) have individually contributed to improved results in cancer therapy, the greatest impact on the management of cancer since the early 1970s has probably been the evolution of multimodality therapy. • In some cases, it has led to improved survival, exemplified dramatically by Wilms' tumor and testicular cancer. • In other cases, multimodality therapy has reduced morbidity while maintaining equivalent cure rates. • Locally and regionally advanced carcinoma of the pharynx, for example, has successfully been treated with combined modalities involving radiation therapy and chemotherapy, thereby avoiding the functional and cosmetic disabilities attendant to major resections in this area. • Tumorectomy, axillary dissection, and radiation therapy provide the same cure rate as does modified radical mastectomy for many breast cancers but with preservation of the breast. • The cure rates are further improved by the addition of adjuvant chemotherapy or hormonal therapy. • Limb preservation surgery (marginal resection of the tumor followed by radiation therapy) for sarcoma of the extremities offers, in selected cases, the same opportunity for local control and cure as does amputation. • Surgery remains the sole curative therapy for melanoma.

ANSWER:
D

18. Which of the following statements concerning sentinel lymph node biopsy is not true?

A. The technique utilizes injection of a vital blue dye and/or radioactive tracer to identify the sentinel node.

B. The sentinel node is the first draining node, from a particular location, in each basin.

C. There is only one sentinel node in each basin.

D. The technique is not useful in patients with suspicious palpable adenopathy.

Ref.: 1, 2, 4

COMMENTS: See Question 19.

19. In which of the following cases would sentinel node biopsy not be a reasonable option?

A. A 1.5-mm melanoma of the right thigh with a clinically negative groin

B. A 2-cm infiltrating ductal carcinoma of the right breast with a clinically negative axilla

C. A 1-cm infiltrating ductal carcinoma of the right breast with a 1.5-cm firm node in the right axilla

D. A 2.5-cm squamous cell carcinoma overlying the right calf

Ref.: 1, 2, 4

COMMENTS: Sentinel lymph node biopsy was first used in a patient with carcinoma of the penis. • Currently, it is widely utilized for melanoma and also for invasive breast cancer. • The indications for other malignancies that characteristically metastasize to regional lymph nodes, such as colon, lung, and selected cases of squamous cell cancer, are not well established. • The technique was first described utilizing injection of a vital blue dye at the primary tumor site, but radioactive tracers have also been used as effective localizing agents. • Some surgeons use a combination of the two techniques for more accurate detection of the nodes.

The sentinel lymph node, by definition, is the first draining node in a given regional lymph node basin, although often more than one sentinel lymph node can be found in a given basin. • Various lymph nodes within the same nodal basin may represent sentinel nodes, depending on the location of the primary tumor within the anatomic area served by that particular basin. • For instance, a breast cancer in the upper, outer quadrant may drain to a different sentinel node in the axilla than does a cancer in the lower, inner quadrant.

Sentinel node biopsy is likely best utilized in patients with early cancers that may not yet have lymph node metastases, thereby sparing patients a full lymph node dissection. • It therefore currently has no role in patients with palpable suspicious adenopathy. • Sentinel node biopsy would benefit a patient with a 1.5-mm melanoma, considered an intermediate-thickness lesion, and a patient with a 2-cm breast cancer. • Both of these patients have relatively low chances of metastasis to lymph nodes. • It would not be useful in a breast cancer patient with a suspicious palpable node in the axilla.

ANSWERS:
Question 18: C
Question 19: C

20. Regarding radiofrequency thermal ablation (RFA) of colorectal liver metastasis, which of the following statements is false?

A. Cryotherapy has a lower cost and overall lower morbidity than does RFA.

B. The size of the thermally ablated lesion is determined by the radiofrequency pulse and the probe dimensions.

C. Under ultrasound imaging, the ablated lesion appears as a hyperechoic area.

D. Following RFA, predictors of failure include an ablated zone smaller than the original tumor and a lack of progressive decline in lesion size thereafter.

E. RFA is contraindicated in the presence of uncontrolled extrahepatic disease.

Ref.: 6, 7

COMMENTS: Resection of primary and metastatic hepatic malignancies is the treatment of choice. • However, resection may be achieved in fewer than 25% of patients with primary hepatic malignancies and in fewer than 10% of those with colorectal metastatic disease. • RFA is becoming the most commonly used ablative modality because it allows greater preservation of parenchyma and it may be applied to multiple, bilobar lesions or in areas not technically amenable to resection (centrally located liver lesions). • In addition, it may be applicable in some high-risk patients with isolated hepatic recurrences or in combination with resection. • Cryotherapy is based on the cyclic application of low temperatures (−195°C) through a probe positioned in the tumor and cooled with circulating liquid nitrogen. • Cell destruction occurs by ice crystal formation, resulting in cellular dehydration, protein denaturation, and ischemia. • Recently, radiofrequency therapy increasingly has replaced cryotherapy as the ablative treatment of choice because of lower cost, smaller probes, and lower overall morbidity. • Initial local control appears to be the same, but long-term follow-up is needed.

RFA is based on the delivery of a high-frequency (460–500 kHz) alternating current, which results in tissue hyperthermia, leading to protein denaturation and cellular destruction. • A needle electrode is inserted in the tumor under ultrasound or CT guidance. • The temperature generated by the radiofrequency pulse and by the probe dimensions determine ablation size. • The power output of the generator is adjusted to keep the temperature at the tip of the probe between 95 and 105°C. • The heat generated is the difference between the heat generated by the current within the tissue and the heat lost through conduction and convection. • Convection is the main mechanism of heat loss from the lesion, which acts as a protective measure to prevent damage to vessel walls. • The biliary tract is at risk for thermal injury, and proximity of the tumor to major vessels may limit complete ablation. • The evolving ablated lesion appears on a sonogram as a hyperechoic area when the temperature reaches 90°C. • The ablated area is larger than the original tumor owing to ablation of surrounding normal parenchyma (about 1 cm). • The use of larger, expandable electron needle tips has allowed application of this modality to lesions larger than 5 cm, with initial encouraging results. • However, as mentioned earlier, long-term follow-up is required.

The criterion for successful lesion ablation is complete destruction, as assessed by the continuing decline in the size of the lesion following the initial increase at 1 week. • Ideally, the tumor must be a nodular type. • Laparoscopy allows treatment of lesions in difficult-to-reach areas, such as the dome of the liver or areas in close proximity to other organs. • Limited long-term follow-up data support the use of RFA for patients with disease confined to the liver, a maximum of 3–4 lesions, and a tumor size less than 5 cm.

ANSWER:

A

REFERENCES

1. Townsend CM, Beauchamp RD, Evers BM, et al (eds): *Sabiston Textbook of Surgery: The Biological Basis of Modern Surgical Practice*, 16th ed. Saunders, Philadelphia, 2001.
2. Schwartz SI, Shires GT, Spencer FC: *Principles of Surgery*, 7th ed. McGraw-Hill, New York, 1999.
3. Economou SG, Witt TR, Deziel DJ, et al: *Adjuncts to Cancer Surgery*. Lea & Febiger, Philadelphia, 1991.
4. DeVita VT, Hellman S, Rosenberg SA: *Cancer: Principles and Practice of Oncology*, 6th ed. Lippincott, Williams & Wilkins, Philadelphia, 2001.
5. Saclarides TJ, Millikan KM, Godellas CS: *Surgical Oncology: An Algorithmic Approach*. Springer-Verlag, New York, 2003.
6. Adam R, Hagopian EJ, Linhares M, et al: A comparison of percutaneous cryosurgery and percutaneous radiofrequency for unresectable hepatic malignancies. *Arch Surg* 137:1332–1340, 2002.
7. Siperstein A, Garland A, Engle K, et al: Local recurrence after laparoscopic radiofrequency thermal ablation of hepatic tumors. *Ann Surg Oncol* 7:106–113, 2000.

C. Radiation Therapy

Katherine F. Baker, M.D., and José M. Velasco, M.D.

1. Which part of the cell is thought to be the target of radiation damage?

   A. Mitochondria

   B. Nucleus

   C. Nucleolus

   D. Cytoplasm

Ref.: 1

COMMENTS: In most cell types, radiation causes the cells to lose reproductive integrity. • Experimental data are most consistent with the nucleus's being the critical target in the cell, specifically in the DNA of the chromosomes. • There is some evidence that the cell membrane may be another target by which irradiation may cause cell death, but the most critical target appears to be the nucleus.

ANSWER:
B

2. Which of the following beams would be appropriate for treating a skin cancer?

   A. Superficial (100 kV)

   B. Cobalt 60 (1.25 MV)

   C. X-rays from a linear accelerator (20 MV)

   D. Electrons (6 MeV)

   E. X-rays from a linear accelerator (6 MV)

Ref.: 2, 3

COMMENTS: See Question 3.

3. Which of the following beams would be appropriate for treating a rectal cancer?

   A. Superficial (100 kV)

   B. Cobalt 60 (1.25 MV)

   C. X-rays from a linear accelerator (20 MV)

   D. Electrons (6 MeV)

   E. X-rays from a linear accelerator (6 MV)

Ref.: 2, 3

COMMENTS: Low-energy x-rays or electrons are most commonly used for treating superficial lesions. • Superficial x-rays and electrons deposit most of their energy close to the surface, with the maximum dose at the skin surface with superficial x-rays and within a few centimeters of the skin surface with electrons. • Higher-energy x-rays, such as megavoltage x-rays, have a "skin-sparing" effect, by which much of the energy is deposited in deeper tissues. • The energy of electrons is deposited within a limited range, with higher-energy electrons having a greater depth of penetration. • Nearly all of the energy from a 6-MeV electron beam is deposited within the first 3 cm of tissue, making it an ineffective treatment for deeper tumors. • The dose from a superficial x-ray beam is also deposited near the skin surface, with a rapid drop in dose past the first few millimeters. • The megavoltage x-ray beams have a much greater depth of penetration and are useful for treating deep-seated tumors. • A 6-MV photon beam would be as effective for treating a deep tumor as would a higher-energy beam (such as 20 MV photons), but the higher-energy beam may spare more of the normal tissues, especially in a large patient. • Cobalt 60 treatment machines have relative skin-sparing properties, with the maximum dose deposited 0.5 cm below the skin surface. • While in the past cobalt 60 was used for deep-seated tumors, today linear accelerators have generally replaced cobalt 60.

ANSWERS:
Question 2: A, D
Question 3: C, E

4. Which of the following patients would have the most radioactivity in his or her body?

   A. A 47-year-old woman treated with 6-MV photons from a linear accelerator for a rectal cancer, 10 minutes after daily treatment.

   B. An 82-year-old man treated with 10 MV photons for a prostate cancer, 1 hr after daily treatment.

   C. A 52-year-old woman, 30 minutes after injection with radioactive technetium (^{99m}Tc) for a bone scan.

   D. A 75-year-old man treated with cobalt 60 x-rays for a larynx cancer, 10 minutes after daily treatment.

   E. A 73-year-old man treated with 13-MeV electrons for a lymphoma in the left neck.

Ref.: 4

COMMENTS: Patients receiving external-beam irradiation are not made radioactive by treatment. • Once the daily treatment is completed, there is no radioactivity in the patient's body. • A bone scan is performed by measuring the relative amounts of radioactivity in different areas of the body. • The radioactive technetium is preferentially taken up in bone and remains there until it undergoes radioactive decay.

ANSWER:
C

5. Regarding time-dose fractionation schedules in radiation oncology, which of the following statements is/are true?

   A. Delivering 25 Gy in five fractions is an example of hypofractionation.

   B. Delivering 1.15 Gy per fraction twice daily to 80.5 Gy over 7 weeks is an example of hyperfractionation.

   C. Accelerated fractionation reduces the overall length of a treatment course compared to standard fractionation.

   D. Delivering a higher total dose without risking more toxicity can compensate for longer treatment breaks.

   Ref.: 5–7

COMMENTS: Time-dose fractionation scheduling is an important consideration in radiation oncology. • The dose delivered, time for delivery, and how the dose is spread over time corresponds to local disease control and toxicity. • Assuming that 1.8–2.0 Gy per fraction is "standard fractionation," hypofractionation uses larger fraction sizes. • Often, the total dose is reduced to compensate for the increased risk of late normal tissue toxicity associated with large doses per fraction. • Today, hypofractionation is rarely used in the United States, although several series from Europe have been published using hypofractionation successfully in the preoperative setting.

Conversely, hyperfractionation delivers a higher total dose of radiation (10–15%) using a reduced dose per fraction, keeping the overall treatment time similar to that for standard fractionation. • The risk of late toxicity is reduced with smaller doses per fraction, and thus the total dose may be increased.

Accelerated fractionation reduces the total treatment length by delivering two or more treatments on some or all of the treatment days. • It is hypothesized that local tumor control may be improved because tumor cells do not have the same opportunity for regeneration throughout treatment if the total dose is delivered over a shorter period of time.

Long treatment breaks may adversely affect outcome because tumor cells may regenerate. • Compensating by increasing the total dose may increase the risk of toxicity to the surrounding normal structures.

A N S W E R :
A, B, C

6. Regarding cells damaged by radiation, which of the following statements is/are true?

   A. They are killed immediately.

   B. They may be able to struggle through one or two mitoses before dying.

   C. They may be able to divide with minimal alterations in cellular fashion.

   D. They may be unable to divide but remain physiologically functional, although reproductively sterile.

   Ref.: 1, 2

COMMENTS: Although some cells may die an intermitotic death following irradiation, most cells do not die until the time of cell division. • If there is enough time between doses of irradiation, some of the damage is repaired (this is called sublethal or potentially lethal damage). • Irradiation causes a delay in division even in cells that are not lethally damaged.

A N S W E R :
B, C, D

7. Regarding irradiation of normal tissues, the risk of long-term injury (late complications) depends on which of the following?

   A. Type and amount of tissue treated

   B. Total dose of radiation

   C. Amount of dose given with each daily fraction

   D. Whether a short treatment break is given during the course of therapy

   E. Severity of acute reactions during treatment

   Ref.: 2

COMMENTS: Late complications occur more often with high total doses of radiation and with high doses per fraction of treatment. • Small areas of normal tissue can tolerate relatively high doses of radiation, but the doses to large volumes or entire organs are limited. • For example, if both entire lungs are treated with doses of 2 Gy per fraction, the risk of fatal pneumonitis is high, even with total doses of only 15–20 Gy. • However, small areas of lung can be safely treated with total treatment doses of 70 Gy or more. • Some organs or tissues (e.g., kidney, liver, lungs, and lymphocytes) are much more sensitive to radiation than are others (e.g., muscle, bone, and peripheral nerve). • Spreading the treatment course over a long period of time or giving breaks from treatment during a course of irradiation decreases acute reactions but has little impact on late normal tissue complications. • The amount and severity of acute reactions do not predict the appearance of late normal-tissue injury.

A N S W E R :
A, B, C

8. Regarding intensity-modulated radiation therapy (IMRT), which of the following is/are true?

   A. IMRT utilizes inverse planning techniques to permit higher radiation doses with better dose conformity.

   B. Treatment errors resulting from discrepancies in patient setup or intrafractional organ motion (e.g., respiratory motion) are less critical with IMRT.

   C. IMRT enables relative sparing of normal structures located in close proximity to tumor volumes.

   D. IMRT does not require computer-based CT images.

   Ref.: 8–10

COMMENTS: IMRT relies strongly on computer technology, physicians, and physicists to deliver conformal radiation treatments. • Physicians delineate targets on computer-based CT or MRI images. • Computer-based inverse planning develops treatment plans with tight dose conformity around targets, allowing sparing of normal structures and dose escalation. • The complex technology is labor intensive and requires stringent quality assurance. • Accuracy in patient setup and target delineation, including consideration of organ motion, is critical, given the highly conformal dose distribution.

A N S W E R :
A, C

9. Which of the following is/are reasons for dose fractionation of radiation therapy?

   A. Tumors are able to repopulate between treatments.

   B. Normal cells are able to repair damage between treatments.

C. Tumor cells are redistributed through the cell cycle.

D. Tumors become less hypoxic.

E. Normal cells become less hypoxic.

Ref.: 1, 2, 11

COMMENTS: The primary reasons for dose fractionation of radiation therapy are repair, redistribution, reoxygenation, and repopulation. • Cells can recover from some damage caused by radiation, with 90% of the repair occurring within 2–6 hr. • Cells are more sensitive to radiation during the M and G_2 phases of the cell cycle and are more resistant during S and G_1. • Fractionation of the treatment allows more of the cells to progress through the cell cycle to more sensitive phases. • Tumors often contain hypoxic areas, which are relatively resistant to radiation. • With divided doses, some hypoxic tumor cells become more oxygenated as other tumor cells die and are removed. • Radiation causes some delay in repopulation, but, during a period of protracted radiation, both tumor cells and normal cells eventually begin repopulating.

A N S W E R :
B, C, D

10. Regarding planning a course of radiation therapy, all but which of the following factors determines the total dose of treatment?

    A. Type of surrounding normal tissues

    B. Histologic tumor type

    C. Size of the tumor

    D. Gender of the patient

    E. Total volume of tissue irradiated

Ref.: 2

COMMENTS: When a course of radiation therapy is given, the usual factors limiting the dose are the type and amount of normal tissue included in the treatment volume. • The general principle is to give a large enough dose to have a chance of curing the tumor but a low enough total dose to limit the risk of complications. • The type of tumor also influences the total dose because some tumors (e.g., seminomas and lymphomas) are much more sensitive to radiation and can be cured with lower doses than can other histologic types (e.g., epithelial tumors and sarcomas). • Because a dose of radiation kills only a proportion of cells, a large dose of radiation is required for large tumor burdens. • To control microscopic amounts of epithelial tumors, a total dose on the order of 45–50 Gy is required. • For tumors 2–3 cm in size, a dose of 70 Gy or more is necessary.

A N S W E R :
D

11. Regarding radiation therapy, which of the following statements is/are true?

    A. Malignancies such as leukemias and prostate cancer are relatively radioresistant, whereas those such as melanoma are more radiosensitive.

    B. Placement of intracavitary radiation sources plays a role in the treatment of uterine cancer.

    C. Pancytopenia, telangiectasias, pericarditis, and nephropathy are possible sequelae of radiation therapy.

D. Combination neoadjuvant treatment with chemotherapy and radiation is increasing the surgeon's ability to perform conservative surgery, resulting in organ preservation.

Ref.: 1, 2

COMMENTS: Radiation therapy is another method of locoregional control in cancer care. • It makes use of **ionizing radiation**, which is energy sufficiently strong to remove an orbital electron from an atom. • This radiation may have a particulate form, such as electrons, protons, or neutrons, or it may have an electromagnetic form, such as high-energy photons. • **Radiosensitivity** is the measure of susceptibility of cells to injury by ionizing radiation. • In general, the more frequently the cells divide, the more sensitive they are to the effects of radiation. • The effects of radiation in achieving cell damage may occur through impairing the cell's ability to replicate (reproductive death). • Radiation may also cause structural damage or injure cells through metabolic incapacitation independent of a cell's reproductive cycle (interphase death). • **Radioresistance** occurs when a cell becomes impervious to the damaging effects of ionizing radiation. • Radiation-induced cell kill can be modified by several factors, including oxygenation of the tumor, hyperthermia, and concomitant administration of chemotherapeutic agents. • The basic unit of radiation, known as the **gray (Gy)**, is the amount of energy absorbed (joules) per unit mass (kg). • This terminology has replaced the unit **rad**, used in the past (100 rad = 1 Gy; 1 rad = 1 cGy).

Normal tissues are able to tolerate specified amounts of radiation before short-term or long-term injury occurs. • Irradiation causes progressive changes in small vasculature and interstitial connective tissues. • **Early radiation-induced toxicity** may include fatigue, diarrhea, esophagitis, skin and mucosal reactions, and hematopoietic suppression. • **Late sequelae of irradiation** may appear months or years after treatment and may include chronic skin changes, strictures of the gastrointestinal tract, bone necrosis, nephritis or renal insufficiency, pulmonary fibrosis, and chronic pericarditis. • With the exception of fatigue, these sequelae develop as a consequence of the specific organs being irradiated. • Careful planning of radiation therapy and its delivery is necessary to minimize such sequelae.

Radiation therapy may be used as single-modality therapy (e.g., prostate cancer therapy), adjuvant therapy following surgical resection (e.g., for treatment of early-stage breast cancer), neoadjuvant treatment before definitive surgical resection (e.g., combined-modality treatment of esophageal or rectal cancers), or in combination with chemotherapy without the addition of surgical resection (e.g., treatment of some head and neck cancers). • **Brachytherapy** is a term used to describe radiation treatment in which the radiation source is in contact with the tumor. • Common examples of the use of brachytherapy include **low-dose-rate sources (LDR)**, used for treatment of uterine cancer, and **high-dose-rate sources (HDR)**, used for treatment of esophageal and lung cancers.

A N S W E R :
B, C, D

12. Regarding radiation absorbed dose (rad), which of the following statements is/are true?

    A. One rad is equal to 1 Gy.

    B. One rad is equal to 1 cGy.

    C. One gray of neutrons is equivalent in effectiveness to 1 Gy of x-rays.

    D. A single dose of 10 Gy of photons is equivalent in effectiveness to 10 Gy given in five fractions of 2 Gy each.

Ref.: 1, 3

COMMENTS: The old unit of measure for the absorption of energy per unit of matter or tissue was the rad. • Currently, the unit used internationally is the gray (Gy), which is defined as 1 joule of absorbed energy per kilogram of tissue. • The gray is equivalent to 100 rad (thus, 1 rad = 1 cGy). • The biologic effects of radiation depend not only on the total dose but also on the type of radiation and the relative biologic effectiveness (RBE). • Neutrons have a higher RBE than do photons (x-rays) by a factor of approximately 3. • One gray of neutrons causes three times the damage as 1 Gy of photons. • Fractionated doses of radiation are not biologically equivalent to the same dose given in a single fraction. • When the dose is fractionated, some of the damage caused by the radiation can be repaired before the next dose is given.

A N S W E R :
B

R E F E R E N C E S

1. Hall EJ: *Radiobiology for the Radiologist*, 3rd ed. JB Lippincott, Philadelphia, 1988.

2. Hendrickson FR, Withers HR: Principles of radiation oncology. In: Holleb AI, Fink DJ, Murphy GP (eds) *Clinical Oncology*. American Cancer Society, Atlanta, 1991.

3. Khan FM: *The Physics of Radiation Therapy*. Williams & Wilkins, Baltimore, 1984.

4. Johns HE, Cunningham JR: *The Physics of Radiology*. Charles C Thomas, Springfield, IL, 1983.

5. Thames HD: On the origin of dose fractionation regimens in radiotherapy. *Semin Radiat Oncol* 2:3–9, 1992.

6. Cox JD: Clinical perspectives of recent developments in fractionation. *Semin Radiat Oncol* 2:10–15, 1992.

7. Fowler JF: Brief summary of radiobiological principles in fractionated radiotherapy. *Semin Radiat Oncol* 2:16–21, 1992.

8. Eisbruch A: Introduction. *Semin Radiat Oncol* 12:197–198, 2002.

9. Low DA: Quality assurance of intensity-modulated radiotherapy. *Semin Radiat Oncol* 12:219–228, 2002.

10. Jaffray DA, Yan D, Wong JW: Managing geometric uncertainty in conformal intensity-modulated radiation therapy. *Semin Radiat Oncol* 9:4–19, 1999.

11. Withers HR: Biologic basis of radiation therapy. In: Perez CA, Brady LW (eds): *Principles and Practice of Radiation Oncology*, 2nd ed. JB Lippincott, Philadelphia, 1992.

D. Systemic Therapy

Edward Kaplan, M.D., and José M. Velasco, M.D.

1. Regarding small-cell lung cancer, which of the following statements is/are true?

   A. In general, small-cell lung cancer is not treated by surgical resection because it has often spread systemically at the time of diagnosis.

   B. Patients with limited stage small-cell lung cancer in whom the disease is confined to the chest and can be encompassed with radiotherapy can be cured with a combination of chemotherapy and radiotherapy.

   C. Patients who have limited stage disease and a complete clinical response to chemotherapy should receive prophylactic cranial irradiation (PCI) to treat occult metastatic disease and prolong overall survival.

   D. The syndrome of inappropriate antidiuretic hormone secretion (SIADH) and the Eaton-Lambert syndrome (a myasthenia-like syndrome) are paraneoplastic syndromes associated with small-cell lung cancer.

   Ref.: 1

   COMMENTS: Small-cell carcinoma of the lungs is associated with the early development of distant metastases. • A study of patients with small-cell lung cancer who underwent curative surgical resection and died within 30 days of surgery from non-cancer-related causes showed that at autopsy 70% had metastatic cancer. • Patients with limited-stage small-cell lung cancer can be cured with a combination of chemotherapy and radiotherapy, although the 5-year survival rate is only about 7%. • The role of PCI remains controversial. • Only patients who have a complete response to therapy at other sites of disease should be considered for PCI. • PCI decreases from 20 to 6% the likelihood that patients will later develop brain metastases, but such therapy does not increase overall survival. • SIADH and the Eaton-Lambert syndrome are strongly associated with small-cell lung cancer. • The presence of SIADH is not correlated with the stage of disease or prognosis. • The Eaton-Lambert syndrome is a myasthenia-like syndrome characterized by muscle weakness and fatigue that is most pronounced in the pelvic girdle and thighs. • In contrast to true myasthenia gravis, muscle strength improves with exercise. • Often, the symptoms of the Eaton-Lambert syndrome are alleviated following chemotherapy for small-cell lung cancer, but sometimes they worsen. • Guanidine may also be used as therapy.

   ANSWER:
   A, B, D

2. Regarding testicular cancer, which of the following statements is/are true?

   A. Metastatic, nonseminomatous testicular cancer can be cured with chemotherapy.

   B. Effective chemotherapy regimens for testicular cancer must include doxorubicin (Adriamycin).

   C. Failure of elevated markers to return to normal following chemotherapy for metastatic, nonseminomatous germ-cell tumors indicates persistent disease.

   D. Primary mediastinal seminomas have a higher cure rate either with radiotherapy or with chemotherapy than do nonseminomatous mediastinal tumors.

   Ref.: 2

   COMMENTS: Metastatic testicular cancer is curable in 70–80% of patients using a regimen of cisplatin, VP-16, and bleomycin. • Adriamycin does not have significant activity against testicular cancer. • Human chorionic gonadotropin-β (β-hCG) or α-fetoprotein levels (or both) are elevated in 85% of patients with metastatic nonseminomatous germ cell tumors. • About 40% of patients have an elevated α-fetoprotein level, and 75% an elevated β-hCG level. • Embryonal carcinomas can secrete both β-hCG and α-fetoprotein. • Choriocarcinomas are associated specifically with an elevation of β-hCG levels. • Yolk sac (endodermal sinus) tumors are associated with elevated α-fetoprotein and normal β-hCG levels. • The β-hCG level is elevated in about 10% of apparently pure seminomas, but the α-fetoprotein level should not be elevated in a pure seminoma. • If patients with a seminoma have elevated α-fetoprotein levels, they should be managed as if they had nonseminomatous disease. • Failure of these elevated tumor markers to return to normal strongly suggests the presence of residual or persistent disease. • In young men with midline tumors (retroperitoneal or mediastinal), the diagnosis of an extragonadal germ-cell tumor should always be considered, because this cancer is potentially curable. • Although primary mediastinal seminomas have a high cure rate, the cure rate for nonseminomatous extragonadal germ-cell tumors is less than 50%.

   ANSWER:
   A, C, D

3. Regarding the treatment of metastatic malignant melanoma, which of the following statements is/are true?

   A. Dacarbazine (DTIC) is the most effective single chemotherapeutic agent.

   B. Interferon-α results in objective response rates of about 50% and a 20–25% rate of long-term remission.

   C. Interleukin-2 (IL-2), combined with lymphokine-activated killer (LAK) cells, has demonstrated antitumor effects against advanced disease, but the toxic side effects can be severe.

   D. Patients having surgical resection for cutaneous malignant melanoma with a high risk of recurrence benefit from adjuvant treatment with IL-2b.

   Ref.: 1

   COMMENTS: DTIC is the most active single chemotherapeutic agent for metastatic melanoma, with response rates of 15–25%.

• As adjuvant chemotherapy, however, DTIC has not been shown to be beneficial. • The response rates to interferon-α are between 10 and 20% and are partial and short-lived. • IL-2 and LAK cell therapy has demonstrated antitumor activity, but the side effects include hypotension, oliguria, capillary leak syndrome, confusion, and arrhythmias. • IL-2b has been shown to improve the rates of disease-free survival and overall survival when used in the adjuvant setting for patients with cancerous lymph nodes. • Ongoing studies are aimed at determining the optimal dose and schedule.

A N S W E R :
A, C, D

4. Which of the following solid tumors is/are generally considered to be curable with chemotherapy?

A. Hodgkin's disease

B. Testicular cancer

C. Intermediate-grade non-Hodgkin's lymphoma

D. Low-grade non-Hodgkin's lymphoma

Ref.: 1

COMMENTS: Hodgkin's disease can be cured by a number of regimens of combination chemotherapy, including Adriamycin, bleomycin, vinblastine, and dacarbazine (ABVD); nitrogen mustard, vincristine (Oncovin), procarbazine, and prednisone (MOPP); or MOPP/ABV (Adriamycin, bleomycin, and vinblastine). • ABVD is the regimen used most commonly because of the high risk of developing myelodysplasia or acute myelogenous leukemia with MOPP. • Most metastatic **testicular cancers** are highly curable when treated with cisplatin-based regimens, such as the Einhorn regimen, which contains cisplatin, VP-16, and bleomycin. • **Intermediate-grade non-Hodgkin's lymphomas**, such as diffuse large-cell lymphoma, are curable with several regimens, including cyclophosphamide, doxorubicin (Adriamycin), and vincristine (Oncovin) (CHOP) and prednisone with or without rituximab. • The **low-grade non-Hodgkin's lymphomas** are highly responsive to chemotherapy, and patients can have a prolonged survival, often of many years. • In general, however, these diseases are not curable with chemotherapy. • Newer therapies utilizing monoclonal antibodies, such as rituximab (Rituxan) or tositumomab (Bexxar), may be changing the treatment paradigm for these lymphomas.

A N S W E R :
A, B, C

5. Patients who are positive for the human immunodeficiency virus (HIV) have an increased risk of developing which of the following malignancies?

A. Hodgkin's disease

B. Kaposi's sarcoma

C. High-grade non-Hodgkin's B-cell lymphomas

D. Acute nonlymphocytic leukemias

Ref.: 1

COMMENTS: The incidence of **Hodgkin's disease** does not appear to be increased in patients who are positive for HIV. • However, in such patients who simultaneously develop Hodgkin's disease, the malignancy may have an atypical presentation or distribution. • HIV-positive patients with Hodgkin's disease more frequently present with advanced stages of the disease

and with systemic symptoms. • **Kaposi's sarcoma** is clearly seen more often in HIV-positive patients and is an "AIDS-defining" illness. • It is interesting to note that the percentage of acquired immunodeficiency syndrome (AIDS) patients who develop Kaposi's sarcoma has been declining for several years. • **High-grade non-Hodgkin's B cell lymphomas** also are "AIDS defining": patients who are HIV-positive and develop these lymphomas are defined as having AIDS by the Centers for Disease Prevention and Control. • The prognosis for these patients is much poorer than that for patients who have the same lymphomas but do not have HIV infection. • **Acute nonlymphocytic leukemia** is not seen more frequently in HIV-positive patients.

A N S W E R :
B, C

6. Patients with Hodgkin's disease who are cured by chemotherapy can later develop which of the following side effects or complications?

A. Infertility in men

B. Acute nonlymphocytic leukemia

C. Non-Hodgkin's lymphomas

D. Hyperthyroidism

Ref.: 1

COMMENTS: More than 80% of men treated with MOPP chemotherapy develop azoospermia and testicular atrophy. • The ABVD regimen (Adriamycin, bleomycin, vinblastine, and DTIC [dacarbazine]) appears to be less toxic, with only about 35% of the patients developing azoospermia. • The incidence of secondary malignancies, such as leukemia or non-Hodgkin's lymphoma, is increased in patients who have been treated for Hodgkin's disease. • The combination of radiation therapy and alkylating agents increases the risk of developing leukemia even further than does chemotherapy alone. • At the National Cancer Institute, patients treated with MOPP alone had a 10-year actuarial risk of developing leukemia of less than 2%, whereas those who received chemotherapy and radiation therapy had a risk of 17%. • Hypothyroidism is seen more frequently in patients treated for Hodgkin's disease, but it is thought to be due to radiation scatter during radiotherapy rather than to chemotherapy.

A N S W E R :
A, B, C

7. Which of the following malignant lymphomas is/are T-cell lymphomas?

A. Human T-cell lymphotropic virus type 1 (HTLV-1)-related leukemia lymphoma

B. Mycosis fungoides

C. Burkitt's lymphoma

Ref.: 1

COMMENTS: In the United States, most malignant lymphomas are of B-cell origin, although several subtypes of non-Hodgkin's lymphomas do originate from T cells. • **HTLV-1-related leukemia lymphoma** is caused by the HTLV-1 retrovirus. • The disease is endemic in Japan and the Caribbean and presents with skin lesions and hypercalcemia. • Many patients have circulating cells with a characteristic cloverleaf appearance of the nucleus. • The prognosis is poor. • **Mycosis fungoides** is one manifestation of cutaneous T-cell lymphomas. • Patients often present with erythematous skin changes that may be misdiagnosed as eczema or some other dermatosis. • Indurated plaques may form, or patients may develop generalized erythroderma. • Circulating malignant cells with convoluted nuclei are called Sézary cells. • Often, cutaneous T-cell lymphoma has an indolent course. • Treatments include radiation therapy, topical chemotherapy, photochemotherapy, systemic chemotherapy, and interferon. • **Burkitt's lymphoma** is a B-cell malignancy. • It is most common in Africa, is nearly always associated with the Epstein-Barr virus, and has a characteristic chromosomal translocation (8:14). • Involvement of the mandible as well is more commonly seen in Africans.

ANSWER:
A, B

8. Match each malignancy in the left-hand column with its available systemic therapy in the right-hand column.

A. HER-2 positive metastatic breast cancer	a. Carboplatin and etoposide
B. Colon cancer, stage III (node positive)	b. Cisplatin, etoposide, and bleomycin
C. Node-positive, estrogen receptor (ER)-negative breast cancer	c. Doxorubicin (Adriamycin) and cisplatin
D. Postmenopausal, node-negative, ER-positive breast cancer	d. 5-Fluorouracil (5-FU) and leucovorin
E. High-grade sarcoma	e. Trastuzumab (Herceptin)
F. Small-cell lung cancer	f. Methotrexate, vinblastine (Velban), doxorubicin, and cisplatin (MVAC)
G. Invasive bladder cancer	g. Methotrexate, doxorubicin, ifosfamide, and dacarbazine (DTIC) (MAID)
H. Prostate cancer	h. Anastrozole (Arimidex)
I. Testicular cancer	i. Flutamide

Ref.: 1

COMMENTS: The range of active chemotherapeutic agents available for use has increased considerably during the past decade. • The treatment of a number of tumor types, including those listed in this question, has been enlarged by chemotherapy, hormone therapy, and monoclonal antibody therapy either as an adjuvant regimen or in the setting of metastatic disease.

Herceptin is a monoclonal antibody against the growth factor receptor *HER-2/neu.* • This receptor is overexpressed in approximately 25% of all breast cancers. • The receptor is also present on other epithelial malignancies, including lung, prostate, colon, ovarian, head and neck, and pancreatic cancers. • Studies are underway to determine the efficacy of Herceptin in the treatment of other cancers.

The effectiveness of 5-FU against metastatic *colon cancer* is significantly enhanced when it is given with folinic acid (leucovorin). • This combination reduces the rate of recurrence by one third when used as adjuvant therapy for node-positive (stage III) colon cancer. • Newer regimes, which add Oxaliplatin or Irinotecan to 5-FU and folinic acid, are used in metastatic disease and are being evaluated for adjuvant use.

Patients with node-positive, ER-negative *breast cancer* should be treated with adjuvant chemotherapy, no matter what the menopausal state of the patient. • Doxorubicin (Adriamycin) and cyclophosphamide constitute one of several effective adjuvant regimens. • Survival of postmenopausal women with node-negative breast

cancer is improved when they are treated with adjuvant hormonal therapy. • Anastrozole (Arimidex) has been recently approved for use as adjuvant treatment after it was demonstrated to have equal or better efficacy than Tamoxifen in the ATAC Trial, a large randomized multi-institutional study.

The combination of carboplatin and etoposide (VP-16) is probably as good as any of the other combinations for *small-cell lung cancer.* • It is also a useful combination for non–small-cell lung cancer, although newer agents such as paclitaxel or docetaxal have replaced VP-16.

Metastatic high-grade *sarcomas* are highly responsive to combination chemotherapy such as the MAID program. • Some studies even suggest a usefulness for this program in an adjuvant setting.

A similar situation has been found with cisplatin-based programs such as MVAC for *invasive bladder cancer.* • Flutamide (Eulexin) is an antiandrogen utilized with luteinizing hormone–releasing hormone (LH-RH) antagonist (goserelin or leuprolide [Lupron]) in place of orchiectomy for advanced *prostate cancer.*

Testicular cancer is highly curable with a combination of surgery and the Einhorn combination chemotherapy regimen of cisplatin, etoposide, and bleomycin.

ANSWER:
A-e; B-d; C-c; D-h; E-g; F-a; G-f; H-i; I-b

9. In which of the following ways can chemotherapy be effectively used in the treatment of cancer?

A. As induction or salvage treatment for advanced disease

B. As an adjuvant to the local or regional methods of treatment

C. As the primary treatment for patients presenting with localized cancer

D. By direct installation or site-directed perfusion of specific organs or body regions

E. All of the above

Ref.: 1

COMMENTS: Induction chemotherapy is drug therapy given as a primary treatment to patients who present with advanced or widespread cancer and, in most cases, when no alternative treatment exists. • This treatment can be *curative* (e.g., with leukemia, non-Hodgkin's lymphomas, Hodgkin's disease, and germ-cell neoplasms) or *palliative*, as for most solid tumors. • **Salvage** treatment is used for patients whose tumors fail to respond to the initial chemotherapy program and who are generally less likely to respond to alternative regimens. • **Adjuvant** chemotherapy is a systemic drug treatment after the primary tumor has been treated by surgical excision, irradiation, or both with the intent to cure. • The selection of appropriate regimens is based on experience in the treatment of patients with advanced stages of the same tumor type. • Success of this treatment probably depends on the sensitivity of "micrometastases" (clinically undetectable cancer) to the drug or drugs being given. • Adjuvant chemotherapy is considered the standard for improving the cure rate for many patients with colorectal and breast cancer and is being investigated for many other tumor types. • **Primary** chemotherapy, also referred to as neoadjuvant, prototherapy, or upfront chemotherapy, utilizes cytotoxic drugs to minimize or localize the cancer and thus improve the effectiveness of surgery and radiation therapy. • Such therapy has been shown to be beneficial with lung cancer, locally advanced breast cancer, bladder cancer, and head and neck cancer. • Preliminary studies have shown benefit with stomach and rectal cancer. • The treatment benefits may result from the destruction of micrometastases, thereby leading to downstaging of the tumor. • In addition, a response implies a decrease in the size and extent of the local tumor mass, influencing the extent of the subsequent surgical procedure or the necessary radiation field. • It has not been shown conclusively, however, whether such systemic therapy can indeed permit a diminution of local or regional therapy with maintenance of the cure rate. • Special uses of chemotherapy include the *perfusion* of organs (e.g., infusion for metastatic cancer in the liver, for primary hepatic tumors, or limb perfusion for sarcomas). • *Intrathecal* chemotherapy, via a lumbar puncture needle or into an Ommaya reservoir, can be used to treat carcinomatous meningitis or meningeal leukemia and lymphoma. • *Installation* chemotherapy into the pleural or pericardial space can control malignant effusion. • *Intraperitoneal* chemotherapy may be effective treatment for intraperitoneal carcinomatosis.

ANSWER:
E

10. Regarding the testing of new anticancer drugs, which of the following statements is/are true?

    A. Phase II drug trials determine the effectiveness of a National Cancer Institute group A drug in specific human tumors.

    B. Phase I drug testing utilizes laboratory animals exclusively.

    C. Group C drugs are those with proven effectiveness within a tumor type and are available for use, but they require special application for release by the National Cancer Institute on an individual basis.

    D. Phase III trials are usually randomized, comparing experimental therapeutic regimens with standard treatment.

Ref.: 1

COMMENTS: The average time from discovery of a new anticancer agent to its marketing is 10–12 years. • Preclinical trials utilize laboratory assays or animal studies exclusively. • Three or four phases of clinical testing or trials are undertaken before a new agent is released for clinical use. • **Phase I** determines the maximally tolerated dose (MTD) and outlines a toxicity profile. • Patients with any histologically confirmed, advanced malignancy not amenable to conventional forms of treatment are eligible. • **Phase II** utilizes the MTD from phase I studies to determine the effectiveness in patients with various tumor types. • **Phase III** utilizes agents that have demonstrated (variable) benefit against a particular tumor type in phase II trials and compares them in a randomized fashion with standard programs. • This may involve a combination of drugs rather than just single agents. • **Phase IV** involves the integration of drug therapy with the primary therapy (surgery, radiation, or both).

ANSWER:
A, C, D

11. Which of the following chemotherapeutic agents is/are known to cause nephrotoxicity?

    A. Cisplatin

    B. Carboplatin

    C. Ifosfamide

    D. Methotrexate

    E. Cyclophosphamide

    F. 5-FU

Ref.: 1

COMMENTS: **Cisplatin** is found to improve the outcome in a number of solid tumors, including cancer of the lung, head and neck, ovary, and bladder and germ-cell tumors. • The nephrotoxicity that has been associated with its use can be prevented or minimized with diuretics and vigorous saline hydration. • **Carboplatin** is better tolerated than is cisplatin and is being substituted for it in many of these diseases. • Whether it is as effective remains controversial. • Renal impairment is infrequent with carboplatin. • **Ifosfamide** and **cyclophosphamide** cause hemorrhagic cystitis but not nephrotoxicity. • **Methotrexate**, a folate antagonist, can cause dose-dependent renal toxicity from tubular deposition of the drug. • **5-FU** toxicity is usually manifested as stomatitis or diarrhea.

ANSWER:
A, D

12. Match each chemotherapeutic agent in the left-hand column with the appropriate characteristic and mode of action in the right-hand column.

    A. Methotrexate   a. Acts as an alkylating
                                     agent
    B. Cyclophosphamide   b. Is a plant alkaloid
    C. Doxorubicin (Adriamycin)   c. Is an antimetabolite
    D. Vincristine   d. Is an antitumor
                                     antibiotic

Ref.: 1

COMMENTS: **Methotrexate**, an antimetabolite that inhibits dihydrofolate reductase, maintains the intracellular pool of reduced folates. • This causes folate to accumulate intracellularly in an inactive form. • Ultimately, purine nucleotide synthesis is inhibited. • Administering a reduced folate, such as leucovorin, can reverse this effect. • Other commonly used antimetabolites include 5-FU, 6-thioguanine, and cytosine arabinoside. • **Cyclophosphamide** is an alkylating agent that interacts with DNA, causing continuing single- and double-strand breaks and a misreading of the DNA code. • As a group, the alkylating agents form positively charged carbonium ions that attach to electron-rich sites on nucleic acids and proteins. • Their primary cytotoxic effect is due to interaction with DNA. • The original alkylating agent was nitrogen mustard, still used to treat Hodgkin's disease. • Other alkylating agents include **melphalan**, used to treat multiple myeloma, and **chlorambucil**, used to treat chronic lymphocytic leukemia. • **Doxorubicin (Adriamycin)** is an antibiotic that has been found to have several antitumor mechanisms of action, including intercalation between DNA base pairs and the formation of free radicals. • Doxorubicin-induced cardiomyopathy is thought to be due to free-radical formation in the heart muscle. • **Vincristine** and **vinblastine** are plant alkaloids derived from the periwinkle plant, *Vinca rosea*. • Both drugs arrest mitosis in metaphase by binding to tubulin. • Vincristine causes minimal myelosuppression but can cause peripheral neuropathy. • Another commonly used plant alkaloid, **VP-16 (etoposide)**, is derived from the mandrake plant and inhibits a DNA structure enzyme, topoisomerase II.

ANSWER:
A-c; B-a; C-d; D-b

13. Regarding bone marrow transplantation, which of the following statements is/are true?

　A. It is not indicated for neuroblastoma because of the high frequency of bone marrow involvement.

　B. Immunosuppressive therapy is always necessary after bone marrow transplantation.

　C. Graft rejection occurs in about 30% of allogeneic bone marrow transplantations.

　D. ABO blood group compatibility is necessary for a successful allogeneic bone marrow transplantation.

　E. Graft-versus-host disease is not observed after syngeneic (identical twin) bone marrow transplantation.

　F. Patients older than 50 years of age are eligible for bone marrow transplantation.

Ref.: 1, 3

COMMENTS: Bone marrow transplantation is achieved by intravenous infusion of a small subset of hematopoietic cells called stem cells that can proliferate, differentiate, and mature after administration to the recipient. • The stem cells are always obtained from a living donor, either from the bone marrow using needle aspirations or from peripheral blood by apheresis. • There are three sources of stem cells: *autologous* (the patient's own marrow), *syngeneic* (marrow from an identical twin), and *allogeneic* (marrow from a donor not genetically identical to the recipient). • Allogeneic bone marrow donors are selected on the basis of HLA typing.

　Immunosuppressive therapy is not used for autologous and syngeneic transplantation, but it is required after allogeneic bone marrow transplantation because a tissue mismatch exists between donor and recipient. • Immunosuppression is achieved by administration of total-body irradiation, chemotherapy, or both before transplantation and by the use of immunosuppressive agents after transplantation. • With adequate immunosuppression, the risk of graft rejection is less than 5% in recipients of marrow from HLA-identical siblings and about 5–15% in patients receiving a T-cell–depleted marrow graft. • ABO incompatibility does not constitute a barrier to allogeneic bone marrow transplantation. • However, because a severe hemolytic reaction can be induced following marrow reinfusion from an ABO-incompatible donor, all erythrocytes should be removed from the graft before transplantation.

　Graft-versus-host disease, resulting from the presence of immunocompetent cells in the graft that react against the recipient's tissue, is the most serious complication of allogeneic bone marrow transplantation. • It is not seen with autologous or syngeneic bone marrow transplantation, in which donor and recipient are genetically identical. • Patients older than 50 years are frequently treated with an autologous marrow transplant. • Allogenic transplant carries a higher morbidity and mortality due to graft-versus-host disease with increasing age. • However, as immunosuppressive therapy and supportive care techniques improve, age limits are rising, especially at centers that perform many transplants. • The use of high-dose therapy and bone marrow transplantation is an accepted form of treatment for patients with stage IV neuroblastoma. • Patients with marrow involvement are candidates for an allogeneic transplant if a donor is identified or for an autologous bone marrow transplant using a purged autograft. • In the latter instance, the marrow is harvested only after bone marrow involvement is controlled with conventional-dose cytoreductive therapy.

A N S W E R :
E, F

14. With regard to monoclonal antibody therapy, which of the following statements is/are true?

　A. Monoclonal antibodies cannot be used with chemotherapy.

　B. Radiolabeled monoclonal antibodies are now commercially available.

　C. Responses to monoclonal antibody therapy are inferior to responses to chemotherapy.

　D. Monoclonal antibodies exhibit antitumor activity by multiple mechanisms.

　E. Treatment with monoclonal antibodies is palliative in nature.

Ref.: 1, 4–6

COMMENTS: Various monoclonal antibodies are approved and available for use in the systemic treatment of cancer. • Trastuzumab (Herceptin), a monoclonal antibody against the epidermal growth factor receptor HER-2/neu, is approved for treatment of metastatic breast cancer. • Rituximab (Rituxan), an antibody against the B-cell marker CD20, is used for treatment of low grade non-Hodgkin's lymphoma. • These antibodies can be used with chemotherapy. • Herceptin has been shown to increase response rates to both paclitaxel (Taxol) and *cis*-platinum. • Alemtuzumab (Campath) is a monoclonal antibody that targets the CD-52 antigen in chronic lympocytic leukemia cells. • It causes cell lysis by multiple mechanisms of action.

　Tositumomab (Bexxar) is the first commercially available radioimmunotherapy. • It is indicated for treatment of patients with CD20+ follicular non-Hodgkin's lymphoma. • Gemtuzumab ozogamicin (Mylotarg) is FDA approved for the treatment of patients with CD33+ acute myelogenous leukemia in first relapse. • About 26% of patients experience a response to this monoclonal antibody when used as a single agent. • Studies are ongoing evaluating its use in combination with chemotherapy. • These monoclonal antibodies are derived from mouse antibodies that have been chimerized to decrease the immunogenicity of the molecules by grafting the active regions onto human immunoglobulins.

　Responses to monoclonal antibodies have been as good or better than responses to standard chemotherapy in patients with similar treatment histories. • The response rate to Rituxan in patients with low-grade lymphomas has been 50–100%. • The response rate to Herceptin has been 11–15% in pretreated patients and 24% in chemotherapy-naive patients. • Furthermore, an additional 20–25% of patients treated with Herceptin have attained stable disease. • Historically, these results compare favorably to the results of chemotherapy. • Response duration seems better with monoclonal antibodies as well. • However, phase III studies randomizing chemotherapy against monoclonal antibody therapy have yet to be done.

　Although the mode of in vitro antitumor activity is not completely understood, several mechanisms have been postulated. • Complement-dependent cytotoxicity, antibody-dependent cell-mediated cytotoxicity, direct cytotoxicity, and competitive receptor binding that displaces or obstructs the receptor's ligand have been observed with these agents. • Thus far, antibodies have been used only for palliation, but studies are under way to determine whether Rituxan can increase the cure rate of intermediate-grade non-Hodgkin's lymphoma in combination with chemotherapy. • Similarly, Herceptin has been proposed as adjuvant treatment for breast cancer and adjuvant or curative treatment of other diseases.

A N S W E R :
B, D, E

15. Regarding prostate cancer, which of the following statements is false?

   A. If a patient's father had cancer of the prostate at age 50, his risk of developing prostate cancer is sevenfold.

   B. The current staging classification does not define hormone sensitivity in metastatic prostate cancer.

   C. Patients with stage A-1 prostate cancer require no further immediate treatment.

   D. Levels of prostate-specific antigen (PSA), as measured by a serum test for detecting prostatic carcinoma, may be elevated in patients with benign prostatic hypertrophy (BPH).

Ref.: 1, 7

COMMENTS: Patients with stage A-1 prostate cancer have small amounts of well-differentiated disease that is usually discovered incidentally during transurethral resection or by needle biopsy. • These patients require no further immediate treatment because the disease may not become a clinical problem for many years (cancer-related mortality rate 1.9%). • The PSA level may be elevated in the presence of BPH, but the elevation is only moderate. • A marked elevation in the PSA level is more likely to be due to prostate cancer. • More than 80% of patients with prostate cancer have no family history of the disease. • However, if the patient's father had cancer of the prostate, his risk increases fourfold if the onset was by age 70, fivefold if by age 60, and sevenfold if by age 50. • If two or more first-degree relatives have had cancer of the prostate, the risk increases five- to eightfold.

   The refined "ABCD" staging system for prostate cancer includes subtypes to reflect PSA and hormone sensitivity: D-0 = elevated PSA level; D-1 = pelvic lymph node involvement; D-1.5 = rising PSA level after failed local therapy; D-2 = metastatic disease; D-2.5 = rising PSA level after nadir level; D-3 = hormone refractory; D-3S = hormonally sensitive; and D-3I = hormonally insensitive.

ANSWER:
B

16. Regarding hormone-refractory prostate cancer, which of the following statements is/are true?

   A. Prostate cancer is considered hormone refractory when the PSA levels climb to twice its baseline during hormonal therapy.

   B. It is inappropriate to administer hormonal therapy to patients with localized disease who have a rising PSA level as the only evidence of disease progression.

   C. Luteinizing hormone–releasing hormone (LHRH) analogues (e.g., goreselin) should not be discontinued despite disease progression.

   D. Estramustine is highly effective as a single chemotherapeutic agent in prostate cancer.

Ref.: 1

COMMENTS: The most commonly accepted definition of hormone-refractory prostate cancer includes three progressive increases in PSA values. • Castrate serum testosterone levels must also be demonstrated. • Patients who initially present with localized prostate cancer and subsequently have a rise in their PSA level, even without evidence of obvious metastatic disease in the bone or elsewhere, will often be treated with hormone therapy. • If someone has been on LHRH analogues for prostate cancer and subsequently has a rise in PSA level or other signs of progressive disease, the LHRH analogue should be continued because flares of disease and associated symptoms have been observed when the LHRH agonist was discontinued. • This finding is likely because of testicular testosterone production recovery and subsequent flare in otherwise subdued hormone-sensitive disease. • Second-line hormonal manipulations include antiandrogen drug withdrawal, additional antiandrogen agents, estrogens, ketoconazole, and steroids. • Although historically chemotherapy was not considered useful in prostate cancer, many newer agents have been proving effective, especially when using PSA level drop as a response criteria. • Estramustine, although relatively ineffective by itself, is commonly used in combination with other chemotherapy agents. • Effectiveness has been reported with mitoxantrone and taxanes. • Novel modes of therapy include the use of gene or vaccine therapy, matrix metalloproteinase inhibitors, and anti-angiogenesis drugs against new molecular targets. • Because of the long natural history of prostate cancer, it is crucial that more patients be enrolled in these clinical trials.

ANSWER:
C

17. With regard to epithelial ovarian cancer, which of the following statements is/are true?

   A. Elevation of the serum CA 125 level may precede the appearance of clinically obvious recurrence by 2–7 months.

   B. Patients who are clinically free of disease following chemotherapy and then have negative findings on a second-look operation have a subsequent recurrence rate of approximately 5%.

   C. Taxol is commonly used in "front-line" combination treatment.

   D. Cisplatin given intraperitoneally results in better response rates and longer survival rates than when administered systemically.

Ref.: 1

COMMENTS: Elevation of CA 125 levels can precede by months the appearance of detectable recurrent ovarian cancer. • At present, however, testing for CA 125 levels is not specific enough to be used as a screening diagnostic test for ovarian cancer. • Following negative findings on a second-look operation for ovarian cancer, the recurrence rate is generally 15–20% or higher in some groups of patients. • Some have questioned the value of second-look operations because of the associated high recurrence rates despite "negative" findings and the poor prognosis in those with "positive" findings. • Taxol, a chemotherapeutic agent that disrupts mitosis and is extracted from the bark of the Pacific yew tree, has significant antitumor activity in ovarian cancer. • Taxol and cisplatin or carboplatin are considered appropriate therapy for stage III and IV ovarian cancer. • Current studies suggest a benefit with these drugs in maintenance therapy. • Cisplatin can be given intraperitoneally, but there is no convincing evidence that this route of administration has any therapeutic advantage over systemic administration. • For the present, therefore, intraperitoneal chemotherapy should be considered experimental.

ANSWER:
A, C

18. Regarding chemotherapy treatments for colorectal carcinoma, which of the following statement is/are true.

A. 5-FU remains the only chemotherapeutic agent approved by the FDA for colon cancer.

B. Adjuvant treatment of stage III colon cancer with 5-FU and folinic acid reduces local recurrence rates, but it does not improve survival.

C. Folinic acid confers a survival advantage to patients with metastatic colon cancer when it is used in combination with 5-FU.

D. Capecitabine is an oral drug that can be used in place of 5-FU in metastatic colon cancer.

Ref.: 1

COMMENTS: 5-FU has traditionally been the mainstay of treatment for metastatic colorectal carcinoma. • The addition of folinic acid significantly enhances its efficacy but does not impact survival. • Nonetheless, therapy with 5-FU and folinic acid does reduce recurrence rates when used as adjuvant therapy in node-positive (stage III) colon cancer. • Recently, two new agents, irinotecan and oxaliplatin, have been approved for metastatic colon cancer. • When used in combination with 5-FU and folinic acid, they significantly impact response and survival rates. • The combination of oxaliplatin with 5-FU (as bolus and infusion) and folinic acid was recently shown in European studies to improve survival when used as *adjuvant* treatment for both stage II and III colon carcinoma. • Standard practice guidelines in the United States still consider 5-FU and folinic acid as the appropriate adjuvant treatment for stage III and select stage II colon cancer patients. • Capecitabine (Xeloda) is a novel oral alternative to intravenous 5-FU. • It is absorbed through the intestinal tract, metabolized in the liver to 5'DFUR, and converted to 5-FU at the tumor site. • It is being used for metastatic colon cancer and being evaluated in other situations where 5-FU is considered the standard therapy.

ANSWER:
B, D

REFERENCES

1. DeVita VT, Hellman S, Rosenberg SA: *Cancer: Principles and Practice of Oncology,* 6th ed. Lippincott, Williams & Wilkins, Philadelphia, 2001.
2. Scher HI: Chemotherapy for invasive bladder cancer: neoadjuvant versus adjuvant. *Semin Oncol* 17:555–565, 1990.
3. Armitage J, Gale R: Bone marrow autotransplantation. *Am J Med* 86:203–206, 1989.
4. Hortobagyi G, Hung M: The role of the *HER-2* gene and its product in the management of primary and metastatic breast cancer. In: *American Society of Clinical Oncology 1998 Fall Educational Book.* American Society of Clinical Oncology. Alexandria, VA, 1998.
5. Horning S: Targeted therapy for B cell lymphoma. In: *Hematology 1998: American Society of Hematology Education Program Book.* American Society of Hematology, Washington, DC, 1998.
6. Cardarelli PM, Quinn M, Buckman D, et al: Binding to CD20 by anti-B1 antibody or F(ab) (2) is sufficient for induction of apoptosis in B-cell lines. *Cancer Immunol Immunother* 51:15–24, 2002.
7. Crawford ED, Blumenstein BA: Proposed substages for metastatic prostate cancer. *Urology* 50:1027–1028, 1997.

CHAPTER 24

Skin

Steven D. Bines, M.D.

1. Which of the following statements about skin structure is/are true?

   A. The epidermis is composed mainly of cells that provide specialized barrier functions.

   B. The Langerhans cells located in the dermis mainly provide a mechanical barrier to ultraviolet (UV) radiation.

   C. The basal cells in the basement membrane of the epidermis represent the least-differentiated form of keratinocyte.

   D. The number of melanocytes in the epidermis is constant among individuals of different skin color.

   E. Type II collagen represents 50% of the dry weight of the dermis.

   Ref.: 1–3

COMMENTS: The skin consists of two layers: the predominantly cellular **epidermis**, separated by the basement membrane from the deeper **dermis**, which is largely composed of structural proteins. • **Keratinocytes**, the main cell type in the epidermis, originate as the rapidly dividing, less-differentiated basal cells in the basal layer of the epidermis. • They travel upward, differentiate, and acquire keratohyalin granules. • These cells provide a protective mechanical barrier. • **Melanocytes**, of neuroectodermal origin, are present in the basal layer of the epidermis. • These cells have dendritic processes that transfer melanin pigment to neighboring keratinocytes via melanosomes. • The density of melanocytes is the same among people of various races. • Differences in the rate of melanin production, transfer, and degradation lead to variations in skin color. • **Langerhans cells**, which originate from the bone marrow and express class II major histocompatibility antigens, are the immunologic cells of the epidermis and act as antigen-presenting cells. • Collagen is responsible for the tensile strength of the skin and for about 70% of the dry weight of the dermis. • Type I collagen is the predominant type in adults, whereas early fetal dermis consists mostly of type III collagen.

ANSWER:
A, C, D

2. Which of the following statements regarding the physical properties of skin is/are true?

   A. Tension enables skin to regain its original shape after distortion.

   B. Elasticity is the property that resists stretching.

   C. The striae of Cushing's syndrome are caused by loss of tensile strength and elasticity.

   D. Langer's lines indicate the direction of elastic forces in the skin.

   E. None of the above is true.

   Ref.: 1–3

COMMENTS: Tension is the property of skin that resists stretching. • It is reduced in infants, the elderly, and patients with collagen disorders, such as Ehlers-Danlos syndrome. • Elasticity is the property that allows skin to regain its original shape after distortion. • It is decreased in the elderly and as a result of sun damage. • Elastic fibers in the skin are composed of branching proteins that can be stretched to twice their resting length. • The direction of the lines of tension varies anatomically. • In 1861, Langer described the direction of these lines of tension in the skin, a concept useful today. • Skin incisions are placed along these lines to reduce tension and the width of the resultant scar.

ANSWER:
C

3. With regard to percutaneous absorption of some materials, which of the following statements is/are true?

   A. The major barrier to diffusion is the stratum corneum.

   B. Electrolytes applied to the skin in aqueous solution are rapidly absorbed.

   C. Lipid-soluble substances are rapidly absorbed.

   D. Substances in gaseous form cannot penetrate the skin.

   E. Only trace amounts of drugs can enter the bloodstream from a patch application.

   Ref.: 1–3

COMMENTS: The skin allows selective absorption of some materials, enabling them to appear in detectable amounts in the blood. • This process is the physiologic basis for skin-patch pharmaceuticals. • Water is absorbed in vapor or liquid form. • Electrolytes applied in aqueous form are not absorbed, except in small quantities that enter via skin appendages. • Iodine may enter the blood by skin appendage absorption or by causing an increase in the negative charge of skin. • Lipid-soluble substances, particularly those that are partially water soluble, are rapidly absorbed.

• Phenol and steroid hormones rapidly penetrate the skin, whereas protein hormones do not. • Lipid-soluble vitamins, but not water-soluble vitamins, are rapidly absorbed. • With the exception of carbon monoxide, substances in gaseous form (e.g., oxygen, nitrogen, and carbon dioxide) easily penetrate the skin.

ANSWER:
A, C

4. Match each item in the left-hand column with the appropriate item in the right-hand column.

A. Contributes to the color of skin

B. Arteriovenous shunts

C. Causes vasoconstriction of cutaneous arteries and arterioles

D. Prolonged exposure to cold water

a. Sympathetic nervous system

b. Glomus bodies

c. Subpapillary plexus

d. Trench foot

Ref.: 1–3

COMMENTS: The blood supply to the skin is complex and capable of multiple vascular reactions. • Skin color and temperature depend on the amount of blood flowing through the subpapillary plexus, with flow increasing as ambient temperature rises. • Vertical vascular channels connect the subpapillary plexus to another horizontal plexus at the dermal-subcutaneous junction. • Cold produces vasoconstriction and pallor. • Prolonged cold causes paresis of skin capillaries and arteriolar dilatation, producing livid discoloration. • If, after prolonged exposure to ice-cold water, the skin is rapidly brought to normal temperature, reactive hyperthermia and even blistering may result (trench foot). • Arteriovenous anastomoses in the digital skin (glomus bodies) contribute to temperature regulation. • Dissipation of large amounts of body heat can occur via increased flow through these shunts. • Sympathetic stimulation of skin vessels causes vasoconstriction, whereas sympathectomy results in dilatation of small cutaneous arteries and arterioles, forming the basis of the therapeutic usefulness of sympathectomy.

ANSWER:
A-c; B-b; C-a; D-d

5. Match each item in the left-hand column with the appropriate item in the right-hand column.

A. Modulate cold sensation
B. Modulate sensitivity to warmth
C. Modulate sensation of pressure
D. Modulate tactile sensation
E. Modulate thermoregulation

a. Ruffini's endings
b. Krause's end-bulbs
c. Meissner's corpuscles
d. Pacinian corpuscles
e. Autonomic nerve fibers

Ref.: 1–4

COMMENTS: A variety of highly specialized structures are responsible for modulating the skin's various sensory functions. • The numbers of these structures vary with the region of the body. • **Pacinian corpuscles** are found in subcutaneous tissue, in the nerves of the palm of the hand and the sole of the foot, and in other areas. • Each of these corpuscles is attached to and encloses the termination of a single nerve fiber. • They are involved in the sensation of pressure. • **Ruffini's endings** are a variety of nerve endings in the subcutaneous tissue of the fingers and modulate sensitivity to warmth. • **Krause's end-bulbs** are formed by expansion of the connective tissue sheath of medullated fibers and are involved in the sensation of cold. • **Meissner's corpuscles**

occur in the papillae of the corium of the hands, the feet, the skin of the lips, and other areas concerned with tactile sensation. • **Autonomic fibers** that synapse to sweat glands and receptors in the vasculature govern thermoregulation.

ANSWER:
A-b; B-a; C-d; D-c; E-e

6. With regard to sweat secretion, which of the following statements is/are true?

A. There are three types of sweat gland: apocrine, eccrine, and holocrine.

B. The highest concentration of sweat glands is in the axilla.

C. Direct application of heat is the major stimulus for sweat formation.

D. Eccrine sweat is an ultrafiltrate of plasma.

E. Eccrine sweat glands are distributed over the entire body and produce aqueous sweat for thermal regulation.

Ref.: 1–3

COMMENTS: There are two types of sweat glands: eccrine glands and apocrine glands. • The **eccrine** glands secrete aqueous sweat, and the **apocrine** glands secrete a milklike substance. • Sweat glands are distributed over the entire body, the highest concentration per square inch being on the palms and soles. • Most sweat is the result of nervous stimulation carried over sympathetic nerves and mediated by acetylcholine. • Sweat is inhibited by atropine. • Hyperhidrosis is a condition of increased sweating that can be corrected by direct surgical excision or sympathectomy performed at the appropriate level. • The production of sweat is an active process. • Normally, sweat is hypotonic but can approach isotonic concentrations during high rates of production. • It is not a simple ultrafiltrate of plasma. • Sodium secretion in sweat parallels that of chloride, the concentration being less than that in plasma. • Potassium concentration in sweat approaches that in plasma. • Urea and ammonia are excreted in concentrations much higher than those in plasma. • Lactic acid is actively secreted and provides the skin with an acidic mantle. • With evaporative water loss, no electrolytes are lost, and the process is insensitive to atropine. • Total cutaneous water loss as the result of evaporation at rest without visible sweating is about 500–700 ml/day.

ANSWER:
E

7. With regard to hidradenitis suppurativa, which of the following statements is/are true?

A. It is an infection of apocrine glands, subcutaneous tissue, and fascia.

B. Staphylococci and streptococci are the predominant organisms isolated.

C. The axilla, areola, groin, perineum, and perianal and periumbilical areas are usually involved.

D. The lesions begin with slight subcutaneous induration and progress to suppuration and cellulitis.

E. Treatment can vary from improved hygiene to curettage and primary wound closure to radical excision with split-thickness skin grafting or open wound packing.

Ref.: 1–3

COMMENTS: Hidradenitis suppurativa is an acneiform infection involving the apocrine glands in several areas. • The presenting symptoms are suppuration and cellulitis or a chronic condition characterized by coalescing cutaneous nodules surrounded by fibrous reaction. • Treatment is individualized. • In some patients, cure is achieved with improved hygiene. • Some patients respond to high doses of tetracycline or topical antibiotics. • Occasionally, in extensive chronic cases, radical excision and reconstruction with split-thickness skin grafts, flaps, or open-wound packing is required.

A N S W E R :
A, B, C, D, E

---

8. Match each item in the left-hand column with the appropriate item in the right-hand column.

A. Cystic mass occurring over a tendon sheath	a. Epidermal inclusion cyst
B. Epidermal cell-lined cysts filled with keratin	b. Ganglion
C. Congenital lesion occurring in the midline	c. Dermoid cyst
D. Congenital coccygeal sinus	d. Pilonidal cyst
E. Cyst found most commonly on the scalp	e. Trichilemmal cyst

Ref.: 1–3

COMMENTS: A number of cystic lesions occur in the skin. • Complete excision of each of the lesions listed above is curative. • Otherwise, recurrence is common. • When infection is present, primary incision and drainage with secondary excision are preferred. • The diagnosis often can be determined from the history and location of the cyst. • **Epidermal inclusion cysts**, the most common type of cutaneous cyst, have a completely mature epidermis with a granular layer. • The creamy material in the center of these cysts is keratin from desquamated cells. • The wall of a **trichilemmal cyst**, the second most common type, does not have a granular layer and is often found on the scalp. • A **ganglion** consists of a wall of connective tissue filled with a collagenous material. • Ganglions commonly occur over the tendons of the wrist, hands, and feet and may be congenital, related to trauma, or a result of arthritic conditions. • **Dermoid cysts** are found along the body fusion planes and usually occur over the midline abdominal and sacral regions, over the occiput, and on the nose. • Malignant degeneration has not been reported. • **Pilonidal cysts** result from penetration of a congenital coccygeal sinus by an ingrown hair, which sets the stage for infection and cyst formation. • They are more common in males.

A N S W E R :
A-b; B-a; C-c; D-d; E-e

---

9. Match each lesion in the left-hand column with the appropriate clinicopathologic statement in the right-hand column.

A. Wart	a. Hypertrophy of epidermis
B. Keratosis	b. Viral etiology, contagious, and autoinoculable
C. Keloid	c. Dense accumulation of fibrous tissue
D. Lipoma	d. Occurs commonly on the back, between the shoulders, and on the back of the neck
E. Neuroma	e. May be associated with von Recklinghausen's disease

Ref.: 1–3, 5

COMMENTS: Warts (verruca vulgaris) can occur anywhere on the body but are most common on the hands and feet. • Those occurring on the plantar surface of the foot can become highly painful. • Treatment options include cryotherapy, laser ablation, caustic

agents (salicylic acid), and electrodessication. • Surgical excision is associated with a high incidence of recurrence. • There are several types of **keratosis**, some considered premalignant, others not. • *Actinic* keratoses may be premalignant, although at least 25% spontaneously regress. • They occur in areas of sun-damaged skin. • Suspicious lesions should be examined by biopsy before treatment. • *Seborrheic* keratoses are not premalignant and develop mainly on the trunk in older persons. • They can be darkly pigmented and may be mistaken for melanomas. • Treatment consists of complete surgical excision, electrodessication, shave excision, or curettage. • A third type of keratosis, *arsenical* keratosis, is associated with dedifferentiation to squamous cell carcinoma. • **Keloids** are the result of exuberant scar formation outgrowing its original dimensions. • They can occur after trauma and have a predilection for the skin on the back, sternum, neck, face, ears, and feet. • They are more common in dark-skinned individuals. • Treatment includes excision with primary closure combined with pressure dressings, application of silicone gel sheets, intradermal steroids, or low-dose radiation therapy. • **Lipomas** are extremely common, often encapsulated, and cured by excision. • Malignant degeneration is uncommon. • **Neuromas** can be either neurilemmomas or neurofibromas. • The latter may be associated with von Recklinghausen's disease, which is actually two distinct heritable disorders of neuroectoderm (NF-1 and NF-2). • NF-1, the more common form, is an autosomal dominant disorder, affecting 1 in 5000 people and characterized by café-au-lait spots, axillary freckling, Lisch nodules of the iris, optic nerve gliomas, and cutaneous, subcutaneous, and visceral plexiform neurofibromas. • The NF-1 gene, located on 17q11.2, encodes a protein, neurofibromin, that is important in neuroectodermal differentiation and cardiac development. • Children with NF-1 have an increased risk for the development of central nervous system (CNS) tumors, Wilms' tumor, and lymphoma, and 10–30% develop malignant schwannomas. • NF-1–associated malignant schwannomas may be multiple and tend to occur at a younger age than do their sporadic counterparts. • There is also an increased incidence of other soft-tissue sarcomas among these patients.

A N S W E R :
A-b; B-a; C-c; D-d; E-e

---

10. With regard to keloids and hypertrophic scars, which of the following statements is/are true?

A. There are no histologic differences between the two.

B. The differences between hypertrophic scar and keloid are clinical, not pathologic.

C. Hypertrophic scars outgrow their original borders.

D. Hypertrophic scars and keloids have been treated successfully with intralesional injection of steroids.

E. Keloids are seen in dark-skinned individuals, whereas hypertrophic scars are seen in fair-skinned individuals.

Ref.: 1–3

COMMENTS: Histologically, keloids and hypertrophic scars appear the same. • Hypertrophic scars are thick, red, raised scars that do not outgrow their original borders, whereas keloids do. • Keloids are dense accumulations of fibrous tissue that form at the surface of the skin. • The defect appears to result from a failure in collagen breakdown rather than an increase in its production. • Keloids and hypertrophic scars have been successfully treated with intralesional steroid injection, radiation, pressure, and the use of silicone gel sheets.

A N S W E R :
A, B, D

11. Match each lesion in the left-hand column with the appropriate clinicopathologic feature in the right-hand column.

A. Atypical nevus	a. Precancerous melanosis of the face
B. Congenital nevus	b. Pigments located in the basal layer of the epidermis and upper dermis
C. Compound nevus	c. Often familial
D. Freckle	d. May contain hair
E. Hutchinson's freckle	e. Epidermal and intradermal melanocytes

Ref.: 1–3, 6

COMMENTS: Melanocytic nevi have been classified as congenital or acquired. • Congenital nevocellular nevi occur in 1% of newborns. • For small congenital nevi (<10 cm), the lifetime risk for the development of melanoma is about 5%. • Classification of acquired melanocytic nevi into intradermal, compound, and junctional nevi is based on the location of melanocytes within the skin. • Initially, most acquired nevi begin in the epidermis (junctional), extend partially into the dermis (compound), and then come to rest intradermally. • **Compound** nevi are smooth, usually slightly raised, and hairless. • **Atypical** (dysplastic) nevi are melanocytic nevi whose occurrence may be familial. • These nevi confer an increased risk for melanoma. • In some individuals, the nevi represent true precursors of malignant melanoma. • They are usually reddish to brown, have scalloped edges and variegated pigmentation, are usually larger than 6 mm in diameter, and often appear on areas not exposed to the sun. • **Hutchinson's freckle**, or lentigo maligna, occurs most often in the elderly and generally does not behave aggressively. • Most melanomas arise de novo or from preexisting "nondysplastic" nevi. • **Freckles** pose no threat and are found mostly in persons with light complexion. • The pigment is in the basal layer and upper dermis.

ANSWER:
A-c; B-d; C-e; D-b; E-a

12. With regard to basal cell and squamous cell carcinomas, which of the following statements is/are true?

A. Basal cell carcinomas grow more slowly than do squamous cell carcinomas. They can be darkly pigmented, resemble melanomas, and produce few signs of inflammation or induration.

B. Basal cell carcinomas grow more rapidly and metastasize to regional lymph nodes more readily than do squamous cell carcinomas, and they induce significant induration.

C. Ulceration without induration or inflammation is characteristic of the squamous cell carcinoma, which has been referred to as a "rodent ulcer."

D. Squamous cell carcinomas induce induration, may be surrounded by satellite nodules, can lead to ulceration with rolled edges, and metastasize more frequently than do basal cell carcinomas.

E. Squamous cell carcinomas can develop in postradiation dermatitis or in old burn-scar ulcers (Marjolin's ulcers).

Ref.: 1–3

COMMENTS: Basal cell carcinomas grow slowly and rarely metastasize, but they are capable of extensive local invasion. • Although most common in the head and neck, they can occur in any location. • They are often waxy or translucent, with underlying telangiectasia, but with time they can produce a flat ulcer with little induration or reaction that can become quite deep ("rodent ulcer"). • Superficial nonrecurrent basal cell carcinomas can be treated with topical 5-fluorouracil (5-FU), curettage, cryosurgery, or electrodessication,

but surgical excision is preferred (to confirm the diagnosis and because of higher cure rates). • **Squamous cell** carcinomas grow more rapidly and can metastasize. • They are common at the vermilion border, paranasal areas, and maxillary skin. • They tend to occur in persons with blond hair and light, thin, dry, irritated skin. • Central ulceration with marked induration is common. • These carcinomas arise often in patients with actinic keratosis, xeroderma pigmentosum, and atrophic epidermis and in persons exposed to arsenicals, nitrates, and hydrocarbons. • Excision of both types of lesion should be accompanied by a frozen section evaluation of the surgical margins. • Both lesions are radiosensitive, and in some cases radiotherapy offers better cosmetic results. • Operation is preferred in areas that have a burn scar or that have been irradiated. • Large lesions may require adjuvant radiotherapy after surgical excision. • Mohs' chemosurgery involves application of zinc chloride paste, followed by histologic examination of excised tissue. • This regimen is repeated until all tumor margins are clear. • Regional lymph node dissection for squamous cell carcinoma should be performed for clinically evident (palpable) disease.

ANSWER:
A, D, E

13. Which of the following statements regarding melanoma is/are true?

A. The most common histologic type is superficial spreading.

B. Depth of invasion (measured in millimeters), ulceration, and the patient's gender are important prognostic criteria.

C. Nodular melanomas carry a poorer prognosis than do superficial spreading melanomas of the same thickness.

D. Melanomas in dark-skinned people are frequently subungual or appear on the palms and soles.

Ref.: 1–3, 7

COMMENTS: The incidence of melanoma is increasing and may be related to increased exposure of fair-skinned people to solar radiation. • Melanomas are uncommon in dark-skinned people. • Superficial spreading melanoma accounts for about 70% of all melanomas. • Nodular and acral lentiginous melanomas tend to carry a poorer prognosis than do superficial spreading melanomas, but only because they are thicker. • Ulcerated melanomas and melanomas in men carry a poorer prognosis. • Two thirds of melanomas arise from a preexisting mole with junctional activity, and one third arise de novo.

ANSWER:
A, B, D

14. With regard to the classification of malignant melanoma, which of the following statements is/are true?

A. Stage I melanoma refers to melanoma in situ.

B. Clark's level IV denotes a melanoma extending as deep as the papillary dermis.

C. Clark's level I implies melanoma in situ.

D. A T4 melanoma is one with invasion of the subcutaneous tissue or that is more than 4.0 mm in thickness.

E. Stage III melanoma refers to those with involved lymph nodes or in-transit metastases.

Ref.: 1–3, 6

COMMENTS: Microstaging by level of invasion (Clark) or tumor thickness in millimeters (Breslow) is used to predict prognosis and the likelihood of regional and distant metastasis. • Breslow's measurements are considered more precise for predicting biologic behavior. • **Clark's** levels are defined as follows: I, above the basement membrane (i.e., melanoma in situ); II, into the papillary but not the reticular dermis; III, into an ill-defined interface between papillary and reticular dermis; IV, into reticular dermis; and V, into subcutaneous fat. • **Breslow's** method makes use of an oculomicrometer to determine maximal tumor thickness, as defined from the top of the granular layer of the epidermis to the deepest point of tumor invasion. • In ulcerated lesions, the base of the ulcer over the deepest point of penetration is used instead of the granular layer. • The American Joint Committee on Cancer staging system for melanoma has been revised. • T1 tumors = 1.0 mm, T2 = 1.01–2.0 mm, T3 = 2.01–4.0 mm, and T4 > 4.0 mm. • In addition, each T stage is subdivided into *a*, without ulceration, and *b*, with ulceration. • In addition, T1b also includes Clark's level IV or V. • See Tables 24-1 and 24-2.

A N S W E R :
C, D, E

Table 24-1. TNM Classification

Primary Tumor (T)

TX	Primary tumor cannot be assessed (e.g., shave biopsy or regressed melanoma)
T0	No evidence of primary tumor
Tis	Melanoma *in situ*
T1	Melanoma ≤ 1.0 mm in thickness with or without ulceration
T1a	Melanoma ≤ 1.0 mm in thickness and level II or III, no ulceration
T1b	Melanoma ≤ 1.0 mm in thickness and level IV or V or with ulceration
T2	Melanoma 1.01–2 mm in thickness with or without ulceration
T2a	Melanoma 1.01–2.0 mm in thickness, no ulceration
T2b	Melanoma 1.01–2.0 mm in thickness, with ulceration
T3	Melanoma 2.01–4 mm in thickness with or without ulceration
T3a	Melanoma 2.01–4.0 mm in thickness, no ulceration
T3b	Melanoma 2.01–4.0 mm in thickness, with ulceration
T4	Melanoma greater than 4.0 mm in thickness with or without ulceration
T4a	Melanoma > 4.0 mm in thickness, no ulceration
T4b	Melanoma > 4.0 mm in thickness, with ulceration

Regional Lymph Nodes (N)

NX	Regional lymph nodes cannot be assessed
N0	No regional lymph node metastasis
N1	Metastasis in one lymph node
N1a	Clinically occult (microscopic) metastasis
N1b	Clinically apparent (macroscopic) metastasis
N2	Metastasis in two to three regional nodes or intralymphatic regional metastasis without nodal metastases
N2a	Clinically occult (microscopic) metastasis
N2b	Clinically apparent (macroscopic) metastasis
N2c	Satellite or in-transit metastasis *without* nodal metastasis
N3	Metastasis in four or more regional nodes, or matted metastatic nodes, or in-transit metastasis or satellite(s) *with* metastasis in regional node(s)

Distant Metastasis (M)

MX	Distant metastasis cannot be assessed
M0	No distant metastasis
M1	Distant metastasis
M1a	Metastasis to skin, subcutaneous tissues or distant lymph nodes
M1b	Metastasis to lung
M1c	Metastasis to all other visceral sites or distant metastasis at any site associated with an elevated serum lactic dehydrogenase (LDH)

American Joint Committee on Cancer: *AJCC Staging Handbook*, 6th ed. Springer, New York, 2003.

Table 24-2. Pathologic Stage Grouping

Stage 0	Tis	N0	M0
Stage IA	T1a	N0	M0
Stage IB	T1b	N0	M0
	T2a	N0	M0
Stage IIA	T2b	N0	M0
	T3a	N0	M0
Stage IIB	T3b	N0	M0
	T4a	N0	M0
Stage IIC	T4b	N0	M0
Stage IIIA	T1-4a	N1a	M0
	T1-4a	N2a	M0
Stage IIIB	T1-4b	N1a	M0
	T1-4b	N2a	M0
	T1-4a	N1b	M0
	T1-4a	N2b	M0
	T1-4a/b	N2c	M0
Stage IIIC	T1-4b	N1b	M0
	T1-4b	N2b	M0
	Any T	N3	M0
Stage IV	Any T	Any N	M1

[a]Clinical staging includes microstaging of the primary melanoma and clinical/radiologic evaluation for metastases. By convention, it should be used after complete excision of the primary melanoma with clinical assessment for regional and distant metastases.
[b]Pathologic staging includes microstaging of the primary melanoma and pathologic information about the regional lymph nodes after partial or complete lymphadenectomy, except for *pathologic stage 0 or stage 1A patients who do not need pathologic evaluation of their lymph nodes.*
[c]There are no stage III subgroups for clinical staging.
From the American Joint Committee on Cancer Staging System for Cutaneous Melanoma.

15. Select the treatment option(s) in the right-hand column that is/are most appropriate for the melanoma case summaries outlined in the left-hand column.

A. Level III superficial spreading melanoma (0.4 mm thick) with clinically negative regional lymph nodes

B. Level IV nodular melanoma (2 mm thick) with satellitosis and clinically negative regional lymph nodes

C. Level IV superficial spreading melanoma (1.5 mm thick) with palpable regional lymph nodes

D. Level IV acral lentiginous melanoma (2 mm thick) with clinically negative regional lymph nodes

E. Level II lentigo maligna melanoma (0.3 mm)

a. Moh's micrographic surgery

b. Wide local excision with 0.5 cm margins

c. Wide local excision with 1.0 cm margins

d. Wide local excision with 2.0 cm margins

e. Wide local excision with 4.0 cm margins

f. Sentinel lymph node biopsy
g. Regional lymph node sampling
h. Radical regional lymphadenectomy

Ref.: 1–3, 6, 8

COMMENTS: Virtually all melanomas are best treated by wide excision. • The excision margin that minimizes the risk of local recurrence depends on the thickness of the tumor. • Melanoma in situ and thin lentigo maligna melanomas of the face are treated adequately by margins of 0.5 cm. • For melanomas less than 1.0 mm thick, 1-cm excision margins are appropriate. • For intermediate-thickness melanomas (1.0–4.0 mm) a 2-cm margin is sufficient. • Margins of 3–5 cm are generally employed for melanomas more than 4 mm in thickness and for those with associated satellitosis. • Moh's chemosurgery is not appropriate for the treatment of any melanomas. • The indications for elective lymph node dissection remain controversial. • Sentinel lymph node biopsy is indicated for patients with melanoma 1 mm or thicker with clinically negative nodes. • The indication is extended to patients with 0.75-mm thick melanomas if they are Clark's level IV or ulcerated. • Patients with clinically positive lymph nodes and no evidence of distant disease on metastatic workup (computed tomographic scan of the chest, abdomen, and pelvis; magnetic resonance imaging of the brain; or positron emission tomographic scan) should undergo radical regional lymphadenectomy. • The extent of operation may be modified to suit the individual situation (e.g., modified radical neck dissection for patients without bulky disease or gross involvement of the posterior triangle). • Random lymph node sampling, or "cherry-picking," is never indicated for treatment of melanoma. • Patients with primary tumors 4 mm or greater and clinically negative nodes should undergo metastatic workup before undergoing sentinel node biopsy and wide local excision.

ANSWER:
A-c; B-e,f; C-d,h; D-d,f; E-b

16. True or false: High-dose interferon (Intron, Schering Pharmaceuticals) has shown no biologic activity in patients with high-risk melanoma (T4N0 or any N1, N2, or N3).

Ref.: 1–3

COMMENTS: High-dose interferon was found to have biologic activity in patients with high-risk melanoma (who were in a disease-free state after resection of nodal disease) in the electrocorticography (ECOG) study. • In this study, high-dose interferon given intravenously for 1 month, followed by subcutaneous administration for the next 11 months, improved disease-free survival and overall survival for patients who had melanoma metastatic to lymph nodes. • Several subsequent studies that examined this effect confirmed the improvement in relapse-free survival but failed to confirm the improvement in disease-free survival seen in the original study. • Currently, patients who have melanomas greater than 4.0 mm thick or who are found to have positive lymph nodes should be offered the opportunity to undergo treatment with high-dose interferon or be enrolled in a clinical trial comparing a different adjuvant regime with high-dose interferon. • There are some exceptions to this recommendation, particularly for patients with advanced age or significant underlying medical disease.

ANSWER:
False

17. True or false: The use of preoperative lymphatic mapping before sentinel node biopsy is unnecessary for invasive melanomas of the distal extremities.

Ref.: 1–3

COMMENTS: Preoperative lymphatic mapping is indicated for all patients being injected for sentinel node biopsy because of the variability of the lymphatic drainage patterns among individuals, the presence of in-transit sentinel nodes in some individuals, and the possibility of drainage to more than one lymph node basin in some individuals.

ANSWER:
False

18. Match the lesion in the left-hand column with the appropriate characteristic in the right-hand column.

A. Cutaneous horn   a. Rapidly growing benign lesion that can mimic squamous cell carcinoma or basal cell carcinoma

B. Keratoacanthoma   b. Often seen after radiation exposure or extensive sun exposure

C. Squamous cell carcinoma   c. Premalignant lesion of skin

D. Bowen's disease   d. Squamous cell carcinoma in situ of the skin

E. Actinic keratosis

Ref.: 1–3

COMMENTS: Squamous cell carcinoma has been related to several premalignant conditions and environmental factors. • Chronic excessive sun exposure has been implicated as a cause. • Lesions appear on exposed ears, the lower lip, and the dorsum of the hands. • The potential for these cancers to metastasize is related to the cause, location, and size of the lesion. • Actinic (solar) keratosis and cutaneous horns are premalignant lesions found on the sun-exposed areas of skin in fair-skinned individuals, more commonly in those with prolonged exposure to the sun or to carcinogens. • These lesions can be treated topically (e.g., with cryotherapy or topical 5-FU). • Lesions resistant to this treatment should be excised. • Bowen's disease is squamous cell carcinoma in situ. • About 10% of these lesions progress to invasive squamous cell carcinoma. • They should be completely excised, with negative margins. • Keratoacanthoma, characterized by rapid growth, rolled edges, and a crater filled with keratin, can be confused with squamous and basal cell carcinoma. • Keratoacanthomas involute spontaneously over a period of several months. • A biopsy to include adjacent normal tissue is always necessary. • When the diagnosis is established, large lesions can be observed. • Small lesions can be excised in their entirety.

ANSWER:
A-b,c; B-a; C-b; D-d; E-b,c

19. With regard to UV radiation, which of the following statements is/are true?

A. Most of the UV radiation that reaches the earth is type B (290–320 nm).

B. Type A UV radiation (UVA) is responsible for most of the sun damage to human skin.

C. UVA radiation is within the photoabsorption spectrum of DNA, whereas type B UV radiation (UVB) is not.

D. Melanin content of skin is the single best intrinsic factor for protecting skin from the harmful effects of ultraviolet radiation.

E. Ultraviolet radiation is both a tumor initiator and tumor promoter.

Ref.: 1–3, 6

COMMENTS: UV radiation comprises the middle of the electromagnetic spectrum and is divided into UVA (320–380 nm), UVB (290–320 nm), and type C (240–290 nm). • Visible light is 700–400 nm. • UVC radiation is virtually eliminated by stratospheric ozone. • Only 5% of solar UV light is UVB, but it is responsible for much of the chronic sun damage and carcinogenic degeneration of the human skin. • UVB radiation is partially eliminated by stratospheric ozone, and a 1% decrease in stratospheric ozone increases UVB flux at the earth's surface by about 3%. • Whereas UVB and UVC radiation are within the photoabsorption spectrum of DNA, UVA radiation is not. • There is increasing evidence that UVA radiation contributes to the development of skin cancers via non-DNA targets. • Melanin is the most important factor in protecting the skin from the harmful effects of UV light. • Tightly woven clothing, sunscreen use, and sun avoidance also offer protection against the harmful effects of UV radiation. • UV light acts by both directly damaging DNA and other mechanisms, such as altering cellular immunity and DNA repair mechanisms.

ANSWER:
D, E

20. With regard to basal cell carcinoma, which of the following statements is/are true?

    A. It originates from the deep dermal appendages.

    B. It can be produced experimentally with UV light energy.

    C. The aggressive behavior of morpheaform basal cell carcinoma is related to collagenase production.

    D. The tumor metastasizes primarily through the hematogenous route.

Ref.: 1–3

COMMENTS: Basal cell cancer is the most common malignancy in the United States, accounting for about 70% of all skin cancers and one third of malignant tumors. • Basal cell carcinoma originates from the pluripotential basal epithelial cells of the epidermis and from hair follicles, not from the dermis. • The most common type of basal cell carcinoma is the nodular form, accounting for 70% of cases. • The morpheaform type is the most aggressive clinically. • This aggressive behavior may be related to the ability of this tumor to produce type IV collagenase, which facilitates local spread. • Other types of basal cell carcinoma include superficial and pigmented lesions. • Basal cell carcinomas rarely metastasize, but if they are unattended or are repeatedly recurrent, they can be locally destructive and problematic.

ANSWER:
C

21. Which of the following is/are appropriate treatment for in-transit metastasis from cutaneous malignant melanoma?

    A. Excision

    B. Injection

    C. Laser treatment

    D. Heated limb perfusion

    E. Amputation

Ref.: 1–3, 6, 8

COMMENTS: In-transit metastases are a specialized form of locoregional recurrence of cutaneous melanoma. • These lesions may be treated by local excision or ablation, although the recurrence rate is high. • Intralesional injection with immune modulators such as bacille Calmette-Guérin (BCG) has led to complete regression of both injected and neighboring lesions in some cases. • In patients with extensive in-transit metastases, limb perfusion with various cytotoxic agents (most commonly melphalan or tumor necrosis factor α [TNF-α]) results in complete response rates of 30–90% and a limb salvage rate of more than 80% in most series. • The overall 5-year survival rate after limb perfusion in these patients averages 50%, although it is lower (about 30%) for patients with concomitant regional lymph node metastases. • Major amputation may be performed for control of disease or palliation, although the indications for this have diminished since the advent of limb perfusion.

ANSWER:
A, B, C, D, E

22. Which of the following statements regarding genetic predisposition to skin cancer is/are true?

    A. About 10% of cases of malignant melanoma are familial.

    B. Familial melanoma is characterized by an earlier age of onset of disease, multiple primary tumors, and a frequent association with multiple dysplastic nevi.

    C. The p16/CDKN2A tumor suppressor gene, located on chromosome 9, has been implicated in 90% of cases of inherited melanoma.

    D. Mutations of PTC, a tumor suppressor gene, are responsible for most cases of basal cell nevus syndrome.

Ref.: 1–3, 6, 9–11

COMMENTS: About 1 in 10 cases of melanoma is familial. • Described initially as the familial mole and melanoma syndrome, the syndrome is characterized by patients who frequently present at a young age, have multiple primary tumors, and have multiple (>40) characteristic large dysplastic nevi. • Although linkage studies have implicated a number of candidate sites (including loci on chromosomes 1, 6, 7, and 9) in the etiology of familial melanoma, recent studies have shown that mutations of the MTS1 (p16/CDKN2A) gene on chromosome 9 are implicated in a number of kindreds. • Multiple mutations of this gene have been observed, and current data suggest that such mutations account for about one fourth of all familial cases of melanoma. • Mutations of the CDK4 gene have been identified in a few melanoma families. • Although commercial testing for p16 mutations is available, uncertainties regarding interpretation of the results of this genetic testing, as well as discrimination concerns, militate against the clinical use of the test at this time. • Mutations in PTC, the human homologue of the *Drosophila* patched gene, have been identified in most patients with the basal cell nevus (Gorlin's) syndrome. • Mutations have also been identified in a few sporadically occurring basal cell carcinomas. • The most common are frameshift mutations resulting in premature termination. • Determination of the functional significance of PTC may lead to innovative treatments (and prevention strategies) for basal cell carcinoma.

ANSWER:
A, B, D

REFERENCES

1. Schwartz SI, Shires GT, Spencer FC (eds): *Principles of Surgery*, 8th ed. McGraw-Hill, New York, 2004.
2. Townsend CM, Beauchamp RD, et al (eds): *Sabiston Textbook of Surgery: The Biological Basis of Modern Surgical Practice*, 17th ed. WB Saunders, Philadelphia, 2004.
3. Greenfield LJ, Mulholland MW, Oldham KT (eds): *Surgery: Scientific Principles and Practice*, 3rd ed. Lippincott, Williams & Wilkins, Philadelphia, 2001.
4. Williams PL, Warwick R, Dyson M, et al (eds): *Gray's Anatomy*, 37th ed. Churchill Livingstone, Edinburgh, 1989.
5. Das Gupta TK, Chaudhury P (eds): *Tumors of the Soft Tissues*, 2nd ed. Appleton-Century-Crofts, Norwalk, CT, 1998.
6. Lejeune FJ, Chaudhuri PK, Das Gupta TK (eds): *Malignant Melanoma: Medical and Surgical Management*. McGraw-Hill, New York, 1994.
7. Ridgeway CA, Hieken TJ, Ronan SG, et al: Acral lentiginous malignant melanoma. *Arch Surg* 130:88–92, 1995.
8. Coit D, Wallack M, Balch C: Melanoma surgical practice guidelines. *Oncology* 11:1317–1323, 1997.
9. Hahn H, Wicking C, Zaphiropoulous PG, et al: Mutations of the human homolog of *Drosophila* patched in the nevoid basal cell carcinoma syndrome. *Cell* 85:841–851, 1996.
10. Johnson RL, Rothman AL, Xie J, et al: Human homolog of patched, a candidate gene for the basal cell nevus syndrome. *Science* 272:1668–1671, 1996.
11. Huska FG, Hodi FS: Molecular genetics of familial cutaneous melanoma. *J Clin Oncol* 16:670–682, 1998.

C H A P T E R 25

Breast

Thomas R. Witt, M.D., and Mehra Golshan, M.D.

1. A 35-year-old woman with no personal history of breast disease and no family history of breast cancer visits a physician after her initial (normal) mammogram. Her menarche was at age 13, and her first child was born when she was 20. She has never taken contraceptives and drinks a glass of wine occasionally. She wants to know what the chance is that she will develop breast cancer in her lifetime. What should the physician tell her the approximate chance is?

   A. 1%

   B. 4%

   C. 9%

   D. 15%

   E. 20%

   Ref.: 1, 2

COMMENTS: The incidence of breast cancer has been steadily increasing worldwide in recent decades for reasons that are unclear. • Also poorly understood are the large geographic variations in its prevalence, with the United States, United Kingdom, and Scandinavian countries having high rates and Japan a low rate. • The American Cancer Society in 2002 estimated that there would be 203,500 new cases of breast cancer, with 39,600 deaths. • Approximately 11% of women in the United States can expect to develop breast cancer in their lifetime, but that figure assumes a longevity of more than age 80 years and includes those who are at high risk (in some cases >50%) because of multiple factors. • Using the Gail model, this patient would have a 0.2% 5-year risk and, if the patient lived to the age of 90, a 9.6% lifetime risk of developing breast cancer

ANSWER:
C

2. Which of the following are documented risk factors for breast cancer?

   A. Nulliparity

   B. Radiation exposure

   C. History of hormone replacement therapy

   D. Family history of breast cancer

   E. Cigarette smoke

   Ref.: 4

COMMENTS: Breast cancer risk has been shown to be elevated in nulliparous women and those who experience their first live birth after the age of 30. • With respect to radiation exposure, patients with multiple fluoroscopies and those who have received mantle radiation for treatment of Hodgkin's lymphoma have an elevated relative risk and incidence of breast carcinoma. • Prolonged use of birth control pills and hormone replacement therapy increase the risk of breast cancer. • The Women's Health Initiative study halted the estrogen-plus-progesterone arm of the study because of increased risk of stroke, coronary disease, and breast carcinoma. • An individual's risk of breast carcinoma is clearly related to the family history. • The greater the number of relatives affected, the closer the genetic relationship, the younger the age at diagnosis, and the presence of bilateral versus unilateral disease all increase the likelihood of the development of breast cancer in an individual. • Cigarette smoke has not been shown to be related to an increased incidence of breast carcinoma.

ANSWER:
A, B, C, D

3. With regard to the natural history of breast cancer, which of the following statements is/are true?

   A. On average, a 1-cm breast cancer has been subclinically present for approximately 1 year.

   B. Dimpling of the skin occurs as a result of glandular fibrosis and shortening of Cooper's ligaments.

   C. Skin edema in breast cancer results only from direct skin invasion by tumor.

   D. Lymph node metastasis usually presents in level 2 and 3 of the axilla.

   E. Ipsilateral lung involvement occurs most often as a result of direct chest wall invasion.

   Ref.: 2

COMMENTS: Most breast cancers are estimated to have volume-doubling times of 2–9 months, suggesting that the average 1-cm tumor has been present for at least 5 years before clinical detection. • Neither skin dimpling nor edema requires direct skin invasion. • These conditions can result from fibrosis (with shortening of Cooper's ligaments) and lymphatic blockage in the subdermal tissues, respectively. • The most common site of axillary lymph node metastasis is level 1, which is lateral to the pectoralis minor muscle. • All forms of distant metastases, including ipsilateral lung involvement, are due to <u>hematogenous</u> spread.

ANSWER:

B

4. With regard to the natural history of breast cancer, which of the following statements is/are true?

   A. Virtually all patients with untreated breast cancer die within 2 years of their diagnosis.

   B. The likelihood of distant metastasis is related to primary tumor size and involvement of axillary nodes.

   C. The most common initial site of distant metastasis is the liver.

   D. Stage for stage, the survival rate for breast cancer in males is lower than in females

   E. Mastectomy has been shown to improve survival when compared with breast conservation in patients with stage I and II breast carcinoma.

Ref.: 1, 2

COMMENTS: Breast cancer is a disease of wide biologic variability, and, although the median survival among untreated patients is 2.7 years, nearly 20% of patients survive 5 years and some as long as 15 years without treatment. • The 5-year survival rate for all stages of breast cancer is 86%. • For stage IV disease (distant metastasis), it is 21%. • The increased likelihood that distant metastases will occur in the presence of axillary nodal metastases and (to a lesser extent) large tumors has led, through the results of clinical trials, to the current recommendations of adjuvant systemic therapy in these high-risk patients. • Among patients dying of disseminated breast cancer, the <u>lung</u> is the most common site of distant disease. • However, as the initial site of distant metastasis, <u>bone</u> predominates, followed by lung, soft tissues, liver, and the central nervous system. • Appropriate local or regional therapy, including surgery and radiation therapy, has definitely improved both disease-free and overall survival. • Multiple large randomized trials have shown that <u>breast conservation achieves the same survival as that</u> of <u>mastectomy in patients with stage I and II breast cancer.</u>

ANSWER:

B

5. Each of the patients depicted in the accompanying figure has a breast cancer and a normal chest radiograph and blood chemistries. None has bone pain. What are the preoperative clinical TNM designation and the stage of each cancer?

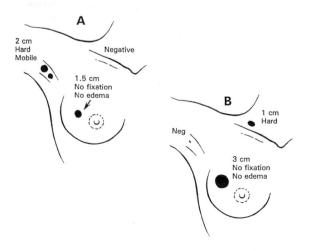

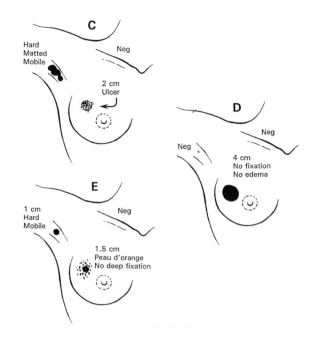

Ref.: 3

COMMENTS: The correct staging of breast cancer is important as a prognostic indicator. • The American Joint Committee on Cancer (AJCC) uses the TNM designation I in its staging system. • T denotes tumor size; N, lymph node involvement; and M metastases. • The sixth edition of the *Manual for Staging of Cancer*, published by the AJCC, includes the following. • T1 designates tumors less than 2 cm; T2, those between 2 and 5 cm; and T3, those larger than 5 cm. • Chest wall or direct skin involvement (T4) should also be assessed. • N1 designates suspicious mobile axillary nodes; N2, matted or fixed axillary nodes; and N3, ipsilateral internal mammary nodes. • M1 designates cases in which there is evidence of lung (chest radiograph) or liver or bone involvement (serum chemistries or scans). • Such evidence should be sought in each patient. • Supraclavicular nodes (formerly considered M1) are designated N3c and represent stage III disease, not stage IV, as formerly classified.

6. A 58-year-old woman presents with a chronic, erythematous, oozing, eczematoid rash involving the left nipple and areola. There are no breast masses palpable, and her mammogram is normal. Which of the following recommendations is appropriate?

   A. Referral to a dermatologist

   B. Oral vitamin E and topical aloe and lanolin

   C. Biopsy

   D. A nonallergenic brassiere

   E. Standard treatment that includes breast conservation

Ref.: 1, 2

COMMENTS: Paget's disease of the breast, unrelated to Paget's disease of the bone, is generally considered a <u>primary ductal carcinoma that secondarily invades the epithelium of the nipple and areola, although lobular carcinomas have been reported.</u> • The eczematoid rash described in this patient is a typical presentation. • Biopsy of any chronic nipple rash is mandatory and, in Paget's disease, shows distinctive pagetoid cells: large cells with pale cytoplasm and prominent nucleoli involving the epidermis of the nipple. • In 1874, Sir James Paget reported that this condition was invariably followed by cancer of the breast, usually within 1 year of diagnosis.

- Depending on the chronicity, Paget's disease may present with an intraductal carcinoma or an infiltrating carcinoma with or without a palpable mass. • The treatment is dictated by the extent of the underlying tumor. • Because of the rich network of lymphatics underneath the nipple-areolar complex and the proximity of the cancer to this plexus in Paget's disease of the breast, mastectomy is usually indicated. • However, breast-conserving therapies may be considered in selected cases. • Local treatment with ointments is not helpful and only delays diagnosis.

ANSWER:
C

7. Match each histologic type of breast cancer in the left-hand column with its associated features in the right-hand column.

A. Lobular carcinoma in situ	a. Lymphocytic infiltrate and a better-than-average prognosis
B. Ductal carcinoma in situ	b. Often large but quite mobile
C. Medullary carcinoma	c. Highest likelihood of multicentric ipsilateral disease
D. Inflammatory carcinoma	d. Highest likelihood of bilateral disease
E. Malignant cystosarcoma phylloides	e. Dermal lymphatic invasion
F. Infiltrating duct carcinoma	f. Most common carcinoma presenting as a breast mass

Ref.: 1, 2

COMMENTS: The clinical presentation, natural history, and biologic aggressiveness of breast cancer depend in large part on the histologic type. • **Lobular carcinoma in situ**, often called lobular neoplasia to emphasize that it is a risk marker rather than a true malignancy, usually presents as an incidental histologic finding at biopsy of another lesion in premenopausal women. • Its significance is that it portends an approximately 20–25% chance of developing an invasive carcinoma within 15 years of diagnosis, with both breasts being at essentially equal risk. • Owing to improved screening techniques, **ductal carcinoma in situ** (DCIS; intraductal carcinoma) is now most frequently seen as an area of clustered microcalcifications on the mammogram, whereas it previously tended to be manifested as a palpable mass. • The outlook for localized noncomedo DCIS treated with total excision alone is excellent. • Results from clinical trials, however, support radiation after total excision as the standard of treatment. • The comedo pattern, in contrast, is associated with a high incidence of multicentricity; and when it is treated conservatively, there is a correspondingly high recurrence rate, with half of the recurrences being invasive carcinoma. • **Medullary carcinoma** usually presents as a palpable mass with smooth mammographic borders that can mimic benign conditions. • Indeed, the appearance of this cancer on ultrasound can closely mimic the sonographic findings of a fibroadenoma, including smooth contour, homogeneous interior echogenicity, and posterior enhancement. • Grossly, the tumors are quite well circumscribed and may be mistaken for benign lesions. • These tumors are characterized by a lymphocytic infiltrate, are less likely to be associated with axillary nodal metastasis, and have a better-than-average prognosis. • **Inflammatory carcinoma**, a variant of infiltrating ductal carcinoma, is characterized by the clinical appearance of inflammation (peau d'orange, warmth, and erythema) secondary to dermal lymphatic invasion. • Although the overall prognosis is poor, it has recently improved with the addition of preoperative chemotherapy followed by mastectomy and irradiation. • Diagnosis is established histologically by skin biopsy revealing invasion of the dermal lymphatics. • **Cystosarcoma phylloides** resembles a giant fibroadenoma clinically and histologically, and it occurs in both benign and malignant forms. • The term *cystosarcoma phylloides* is now reserved for fully malignant lesions. • If the lesion is benign, adequate treatment consists of total excision with adequate (2- to 3-cm) margins. • Long-term follow-up is mandatory, since recurrences are not uncommon and can be malignant. • If the lesion is malignant, its primary mode of metastasis is vascular, and lymph node involvement is uncommon. • The malignant variety usually necessitates mastectomy to achieve local control, although, since the tumor is not multicentric, wide excision has been successfully performed. • Infiltrating ductal cancer is the most common carcinoma presenting as a breast mass.

ANSWER:
A-d; B-c; C-a; D-e; E-b; F-f

8. A 34-year-old woman underwent wide local excision, axillary dissection, and radiation therapy (5000 cGy over a 5-week period) to her left breast for a node-positive, estrogen receptor–negative, 2-cm infiltrating ductal carcinoma 3 years ago. She received four cycles of adjuvant chemotherapy with Cytoxan and Adriamycin at that time. The surgeon now performs a biopsy of a new 2-cm mass in the same breast, and it shows infiltrating ductal carcinoma. She has no other evidence of local, regional, or distant disease on imaging studies and clinical examination. Which of the following treatment plans is most appropriate?

A. Left total mastectomy without axillary exploration

B. Re-excision to free margins, sentinel lymph node biopsy, and a 5000-cGy "boost" to the breast

C. A 5000-cGy "boost" to the breast and combination 5-fluorouracil (5-FU)-based chemotherapy

D. Taxane-based chemotherapy alone

E. Bilateral total mastectomy

Ref.: 1, 2, 4

COMMENTS: Local recurrence of cancer in the breast occurs in approximately 10% of patients who are treated with wide local excision (lumpectomy), axillary dissection, and irradiation. • "Salvage" mastectomy is usually required and results in long-term survival approaching that seen when mastectomy is done for a first primary lesion. • In the absence of palpable nodes, a second surgical axillary evaluation is unnecessary and hazardous. • The effects of ionizing irradiation are cumulative and do not diminish with time. • Treatment with an additional 5000 cGy would therefore lead to serious normal-tissue toxicity in the irradiated area. • Treatment with chemotherapy alone would be inappropriate and would deny the patient the best chance for long-term survival and local control. • Given the patient's age, a detailed family history with genetic counseling would be appropriate. • A right total mastectomy would not be indicated, based on the information provided. • Tumor markers should be analyzed in the laboratory, and possible adjuvant therapy may be necessary, based on final pathologic findings.

ANSWER:
A

9. With regard to the management of patients with metastatic breast cancer that is estrogen receptor (ER)–positive, which of the following treatments is/are appropriate?

A. Bilateral oophorectomy

B. Antiestrogen drugs (tamoxifen)

C. Hypophysectomy

D. Adrenalectomy

E. Aromatase inhibitors

Ref.: 1, 2

COMMENTS: For reasons that are not completely understood, a variety of sometimes seemingly conflicting hormonal manipulations may cause a therapeutic response in patients with metastatic breast cancer, particularly in those who have significant amounts of ER and progesterone receptor (PR) protein on their cells (ER-positive and PR-positive). • Patients with high ER and PR levels, as determined by immunohistochemical techniques, also have a better prognosis than do those with low levels of or none of these proteins when other discriminants are comparable. • The most common hormonal manipulation is estrogen withdrawal, usually with the receptor-blocking agent tamoxifen (Nolvadex). • However, bilateral oophorectomy in premenopausal women is still a reasonable option, particularly since the advent of less invasive laparoscopic oophorectomy. • Surgical hypophysectomy and adrenalectomy were at one time common forms of hormonal manipulation, but they have been all but totally replaced by "medical adrenalectomy" with drugs such as anastrozole and letrozole, which inhibit the production of adrenal steroids and the conversion of androgens to estrogens in the adrenal gland and peripherally. • The aromatase inhibitors are beneficial only in postmenopausal women. • Recent studies suggest that they may be more beneficial than tamoxifen.

ANSWER:
A, B, E

10. A 39-year-old woman presents with an ill-defined 2-cm mass in the outer quadrant of her breast. Mammography shows very dense tissue but no discrete lesion. Ultrasound examination shows a solid lesion. An ultrasound-guided fine-needle aspiration (FNA) is performed, and the aspirate is plated, fixed, and sent to the laboratory for cytologic study. A highly cellular, monomorphic pattern is seen, with poorly cohesive intact cells, nuclear "crowding" with a variation in nuclear size, radial dispersion and clumping of the chromatin, and prominent nucleoli. Which of the following management choices is/are appropriate?

A. Modified radical mastectomy

B. Reassuring the patient that the process is benign

C. Lumpectomy, sentinel lymph node biopsy, and irradiation

D. Excision of a fibroadenoma with narrow margins

E. Lumpectomy and sentinel node biopsy without irradiation

Ref.: 1,2

COMMENTS: Aspiration biopsy with a 22-gauge needle is an effective and safe way of assessing palpable breast lesions. • Performing the aspiration under ultrasound guidance ensures that the lesion has been sampled thoroughly while under direct vision. • Although a smaller volume of tissue is obtained than with needle-core biopsy, FNA frequently yields results that may be equal to core biopsy if read by an experienced cytopathologist. • A fibroadenoma would show broad sheets of cohesive cells with nuclei that are uniform in size and shape. • The chromatin pattern would be finely granular, and large numbers of bare nuclei would be present. • The cytologic findings described in this question are diagnostic for carcinoma. • Appropriate management, therefore, includes either a modified radical mastectomy or lumpectomy, axillary evaluation by

either a sentinel lymph node biopsy or an axillary nodal dissection, and whole-breast irradiation.

ANSWER:
A, C

11. A 42-year-old woman underwent a lumpectomy and axillary dissection for a 2-cm, moderately differentiated, ER-negative infiltrating ductal carcinoma. Margins around the primary tumor were free, and 1 of 19 lymph nodes was positive for carcinoma. Which of the following treatment plans is most appropriate?

A. Radiation therapy alone

B. Radiation therapy and single-drug chemotherapy

C. Radiation therapy and multiple-drug chemotherapy

D. Radiation therapy, multiple-drug chemotherapy, and tamoxifen

E. Complete mastectomy and multiple-drug chemotherapy

Ref.: 1, 2, 4

COMMENTS: Multiple randomized prospective studies have shown both disease-free and overall survival benefit for adjuvant chemotherapy in node-positive premenopausal women, the greatest advantage being among those with one to three positive nodes. • Postmenopausal node-positive women have generally shown a more modest benefit. • Multiple-drug therapy has consistently been more effective than has single-drug therapy. • Adding tamoxifen to chemotherapy for node-positive premenopausal patients confers additional benefit when the cancer is ER positive but is not beneficial in ER-negative cancers. • Converting the local management of this tumor to mastectomy in the presence of free margins is not necessary and would not improve the survival rate.

ANSWER:
C

12. With regard to adjuvant radiotherapy following mastectomy, which of the following statements is/are true?

A. Local recurrence rate is reduced.

B. Disease-free survival is improved.

C. The side effects of cardiac toxicity and radiation pneumonitis are common after chest wall radiation.

D. It should be offered routinely to all patients whose primary tumors are larger than 2 cm.

Ref.: 1, 2, 4–6

COMMENTS: Adjuvant radiation therapy after mastectomy does decrease the local recurrence rates. • However, this has not been generally found to translate into longer overall or relapse-free survival, except in two recent reports involving node-positive patients. • Although relatively uncommon with modern radiation techniques, skin ulceration, arm edema, rib fracture, radiation pneumonitis, radiation-related chest wall sarcomas, and cardiac toxicity represent some of the potential side effects from chest wall irradiation. • Therefore, adjuvant radiotherapy after mastectomy should be reserved for patients who are at high risk for local recurrence (patients with large tumors, skin involvement, or more than four axillary lymph nodes involved).

ANSWER:
A

13. Which of the following 5-year survival rates by stage for treated breast cancer is/are correct?

A. Stage I: 90–95%

B. Stage II: 50–80%

C. Stage III: 30–50%

D. Stage IV: 1–5%   *20%*

Ref.: 1, 2, 4

COMMENTS: The wide range in rates of survival among patients with the same stages of breast cancer reflects the wide range of staging criteria used by various investigators as well as the variability in biologic behavior among the differing subtypes of breast cancer within a given stage. • Historically, there has been nonconformity among investigators in the criteria used to assign a cancer a particular stage, which has led to overlap in the staging designations. • The ability to detect and quantify the presence of certain tumor markers is providing investigators with the means to define these groups more precisely. • When reporting breast cancer follow-up data, one must differentiate between "survival" and "disease-free interval." Because of increasingly effective systemic therapies and the natural history of certain types of metastatic breast cancer, up to 20% of patients with stage IV disease are able to survive 5 years.

ANSWER:
A, B, C

14. With regard to chronic cystic mastitis, which of the following statements is/are true?

A. It is a well-defined abnormality of the breast with specific and consistent histologic features.

B. It is caused primarily by bacteria.

C. It is rarely seen in women younger than 45 years of age.

D. Cysts must measure at least 1 cm to warrant the diagnosis.

E. None of the above is true.

Ref.: 1, 2

COMMENTS: See Question 15.

15. Which of the following pathologic conditions of the breast does not belong to the chronic cystic mastitis group?

A. Papillomatosis

B. Blunt duct adenosis

C. Sclerosing adenosis

D. Apocrine metaplasia

E. Mondor's disease

Ref.: 1, 2

COMMENTS: Chronic cystic mastitis, commonly referred to as chronic cystic mastopathy, is a catchall phrase that refers to a poorly defined group of histopathologic processes in the breast of rather obscure etiology. • Indeed, many modern investigations now refer to this group of histologic findings as fibrocystic "change" rather than "disease" because of its widespread prevalence in the breast. • The various alterations in the stromal and epithelial architecture of the breast are unrelated to trauma or bacterial infection. • Pathologic changes commonly referred to by this name include fibrosis, mammary duct ectasia, apocrine metaplasia, blunt duct adenosis, sclerosing adenosis, epithelial hyperplasia, and papillomatosis. Mondor's disease, which does not belong in this group, is a superficial thrombophlebitis manifested as a characteristic painful, tender cord along the lateral aspect of the breast and inframammary chest wall.

ANSWERS:
Question 14: E
Question 15: E

16. A 42-year-old woman with no family history of breast cancer has an ill-defined thickening in the upper outer quadrant of her left breast. Her mammogram shows only minimal increase in the fibroglandular markings in that area. An ultrasound examination reveals no mass lesion. One month later, since the thickening seems slightly more prominent, the surgeon performs a biopsy of the area in question. The pathologic diagnosis is "stromal fibrosis," with the comments describing increased fibrosis, duct ectasia, periductal inflammation, and microcyst formation with no epithelial hyperplasia. What is the increase in likelihood that she will subsequently develop breast cancer?

A. Essentially none

B. Three times

C. Five times

D. Ten times

Ref.: 4

COMMENTS: Stromal fibrosis has not shown to increase the incidence of breast cancer. • The presence of proliferative lesions, such as papillomatosis (multiple tiny ductal papillomas) or hyperplasia of the usual variety, very slightly increases the risk of breast cancer. • Atypical hyperplasia increases the risk fourfold unless it accompanies a strong family history of breast cancer, in which case the risk is increased ninefold.

ANSWER:
A

17. With regard to breast infections, which of the following statements is/are true?

A. Acute bacterial infections occur most often as a result of preexisting chronic dermatitis.

B. Bacterial infections are usually indolent, taking up to several weeks to become clinically apparent.

C. Surgical drainage, once suppuration has occurred, is the treatment of choice for acute infections.

D. Tuberculosis is a rare cause of breast infection.

Ref.: 1, 2

COMMENTS: Acute bacterial breast infection most often occurs during lactation within the first several months following delivery. • Because the lactating breast is such an excellent culture medium, these infections usually develop rapidly, and their size is often underestimated on clinical examination. • If cellulitis without abscess formation is encountered, antibiotics may abort the infection. • Once suppuration has occurred, however, surgical drainage is required. • Ultrasound studies may be used diagnostically to identify the presence of one or more abscess cavities and in some instances can be used to guide catheters for closed drainage. • Depending on the extent of suppuration, local or general anesthesia may be used. • Chronic bacterial subareolar abscesses and fistulas occasionally occur and require surgical therapy. • Tuberculosis, once a common cause of breast infection, is now rare.

ANSWER:
C, D

18. With regard to breast development, which of the following statements is/are true?

   A. Breast enlargement in male neonates is indicative of an underlying estrogen-secreting adrenal tumor.

   B. Accessory nipples can be found anywhere from the axilla to the groin.

   C. Extramammary breast tissue is not under the influence of the hormonal status of the patient.

   D. Inverted nipples in children suggest underlying breast cancer.

Ref.: 1, 2

COMMENTS: If the embryologic mammary ridge extending from the axilla to the groin fails to involute fully, accessory nipples (polythelia) can appear along this route. • Accessory breast tissue (polymastia) is also seen frequently in the axilla and may enlarge during pregnancy and lactation as well as during the response to normal fluctuations in the patient's hormonal status during her menstrual cycle. • Accessory breast tissue can be detected on mammography and may present differential diagnostic difficulties for both the mammographer and the clinician. • Shortly after birth, both males and females may exhibit unilateral or bilateral breast enlargement, which is attributed to high levels of circulating maternal estrogens. • These changes regress spontaneously during the neonatal period. • In female infants, failure of one or both nipples to evert following birth and into adulthood leads to functional problems related to future breast-feeding but is unrelated to future breast cancer.

ANSWER:
B

19. With regard to mammography for evaluation of breast disease, which of the following statements is/are true?

   A. It can detect many cancers too small to be palpated.

   B. It accurately detects lesions in breasts regardless of the patient's age or glandular architecture.

   C. It delivers 2 cGy to the middle of the breast being studied.

   D. Although it occasionally misses small cancers, a highly suspicious reading (Birads V) for carcinoma on mammography is usually accurate.

Ref.: 1, 2, 4

COMMENTS: Mammography is an important aid in the overall evaluation of breast disease, frequently identifying carcinomas before they become palpable and, in many instances, before they become invasive. • The accuracy of mammography declines as breast density increases. • Accuracy increases as the breast parenchyma is replaced by adipose tissue as involution occurs with advancing age. • The overall false-negative and false-positive rates encountered in mammography screening are approximately 10%. • Current technology allows the delivery of as little as 0.1 cGy to the midbreast per study, making it safe for routine annual mammography in women older than 35 years of age. • Because the harmful effect of radiation is greatest in the breasts of younger women (i.e., those under age 35), because of the low incidence of breast cancer in younger women, and because of the inherent limitations of mammography in dense breasts often encountered within this age group, annual screening mammography is not performed routinely until age 40. • High-risk individuals are an exception to this rule. • Breast ultrasound studies, devoid of any harmful effect on the parenchyma of the breast, is an ideal imaging modality for younger patients with breast complaints regardless of the degree of breast density encountered. • It is also useful for breast evaluation of pregnant patients, in whom radiation exposure is avoided if possible.

ANSWER:
A, D

20. With regard to the current therapy for stage I and stage II breast cancer, which of the following statements is/are true?

   A. The Halsted radical mastectomy has resulted in a cure rate superior to that of other treatment options.

   B. The modified radical mastectomy involves preservation of the nipple to improve cosmesis following reconstruction.

   C. Wide local excision with axillary dissection and radiation therapy to the remainder of the breast is reserved for patients too debilitated to undergo the more radical mastectomy.

   D. Clinical trials have shown equivalent disease-free survival for selected patients randomized to receive either modified radical mastectomy or wide local excision, axillary dissection, and breast radiation therapy.

Ref.: 1, 2, 4

COMMENTS: The two most commonly employed modalities of definitive therapy for stage I and stage II breast cancer are (1) modified radical mastectomy, which preserves the pectoralis major muscle while excising all breast tissue, including the nipple, and the axillary nodal basin; and (2) a wide local excision of the breast tumor (lumpectomy) and axillary dissection in conjunction with postoperative whole-breast irradiation. • A number of large randomized trials have shown no significant disease-free survival advantage for the more radical (pectoralis-removing) Halsted mastectomy. • The National Surgical Adjuvant Breast Project (NSABP) has conducted a multi-institutional study (B-06) with more than 1800 patients with stage I or II breast cancer randomized to undergo modified radical mastectomy or wide local excision (lumpectomy) with axillary dissection with and without breast radiation therapy. • After 20 years of follow-up, there appear to be no statistically significant differences in disease-free survival between the mastectomy group and the breast preservation group. • Those undergoing wide local excision with axillary dissection but *without* radiotherapy had a higher local recurrence rate. • Patients too debilitated to undergo general anesthesia are not candidates for either a mastectomy or axillary dissection. • Elderly, high-risk patients are sometimes managed with lumpectomy or partial mastectomy under local anesthesia followed by tamoxifen, irradiation, or both. • Studies to date have shown that introduction of the sentinel node biopsy performed under local or intravenous sedation may well be an accurate, minimally invasive axillary staging procedure that can be used in even high-risk, clinically node-negative breast cancer patients, although results of large randomized trials are pending.

ANSWER:
D

21. Which of the following clinical characteristics of breast masses on physical examination are more suggestive of carcinoma than of benign disease?

    A. Indistinct borders blending into the surrounding breast tissue

    B. Hardness

    C. Excessive mobility within breast tissue

    D. Tethering to underlying muscular structures

    Ref.: 1, 2

COMMENTS: Although there are many exceptions to the classic physical findings of breast cancer, the typical breast carcinoma is hard and has fairly distinct borders. • Fixation to deeper structures is highly suggestive of malignancy. • A smooth, rubbery, mobile mass is more suggestive of fibroadenoma. • Fibrocystic disease may present as a disclike or polynodular thickening, with one or more of the borders blending indistinctly into the surrounding breast tissue.

A N S W E R :
B, D

22. With regard to subcutaneous mastectomy, which of the following statements is/are true?

    A. It involves removal of all breast tissue.

    B. It includes removal of the lower axillary lymph nodes.

    C. The best results are associated with this type of mastectomy.

    D. It is the treatment of choice for early (<1 cm) microinvasive cancers with clinically negative nodes.

    E. None of the above is true.

    Ref.: 1, 2

COMMENTS: Subcutaneous mastectomy is removal of the breast with preservation of the rim of the nipple. • When performing this operation, the incision line has been classically described as submammary. • In reality, the incisional line is within the breast compartment and by necessity must transect Cooper's ligaments as they attach to the anterior sheath of the superficial fascia. • Terminal ductal lobular units (TDLUs) are considered by many respected investigators as the site of development of both ductal and lobular carcinoma. • They are often in close proximity to the fascial sheaths (Cooper's ligaments) and are by necessity transected during operation. • Thus, remnants of TDLUs can be left attached to the dermis. • In addition, TDLUs are found sprouting from the ductal system at or near the nipple-areolar junction. • Axillary nodes are not removed as part of this operation. • In fact, exposure of the axilla to remove the entire tail of the breast is at times difficult. • Although incision location and nipple or areolar preservation can have cosmetic results that are superior to those following modified radical mastectomy, subcutaneous mastectomy is not an appropriate cancer operation.

A N S W E R :
E

23. With regard to cystosarcoma phylloides, which of the following statements is/are true?

    A. It bears a histologic relationship to fibroadenoma.

    B. Ten percent are malignant.

    C. As with ductal carcinoma, it has a high incidence of multicentricity within the breast.

    D. Axillary lymph nodal metastases are uncommon.

    E. Wide local excision or total (simple) mastectomy usually suffices for treatment.

    Ref.: 1, 2, 4

COMMENTS: Although only approximately 10% of all cystosarcomas are malignant, cystosarcoma is still the most common primary sarcoma of the breast. • The benign variant of cystosarcoma is considered by many to be a "giant fibroadenoma" and, as such, usually presents clinically as a solitary, discrete, mobile mass within the breast (usually quite a bit larger than the average fibroadenoma). • The diagnosis of malignancy in phylloides tumor is at times difficult because of the poor correlation between histologic features and clinical behavior. • The benign and malignant varieties may be differentiated by counting the number of mitoses seen per high power field, in addition to observing other features. • If the tumor is histologically benign, wide local excision is considered adequate treatment. • Even when benign, phylloides tumors have a high frequency of local recurrence, and therefore careful long-term follow-up is essential. • In the malignant variety, lymph node involvement is uncommon. • Therefore, total mastectomy without axillary dissection may be indicated, although, for small lesions, wide excision with 2-cm margins may be appropriate. • The malignant cystosarcoma has no significant incidence of multicentricity within the breast (unlike ductal or lobular carcinoma).

A N S W E R : *9% benign - WLE, close f/u*
A, B, D, E   *1% malig - WLE zm vs.*
total mastectomy

24. With regard to breast carcinoma in men, which of the following statements is/are true?

    A. It accounts for approximately 1% of all breast cancers.

    B. Stage for stage, the prognosis is poorer in affected men than it is in affected women.

    C. Modified radical mastectomy is usually the operation of choice.

    D. Unlike breast cancer in women, endocrine manipulation plays no significant role in its management.

    E. Gynecomastia is usually seen in association with male breast cancer.

    Ref.: 1, 4

COMMENTS: Breast cancer in men accounts for approximately 1% of all cases of breast cancer in the United States. • Its clinical presentation and natural history are similar to those in women. • A mass in the male breast must be differentiated from gynecomastia, which is clearly the more common cause of breast enlargement in men. • However, gynecomastia does not usually occur in association with male breast cancer. • Because of the relatively small amount of breast tissue present in men, pectoralis muscle involvement may be seen more frequently than in women. • However, a modified radical mastectomy is an appropriate operation for most male patients, and rarely will muscle have to be removed. • Stage for stage, the results of treatment are similar to those in women. • However, because men tend to present in later stages of the disease (partly owing to the lack of awareness that breast cancer can occur in men), the overall prognosis for male breast cancer is poorer. • Male breast cancer is similar to its female counterpart in that it may be affected by endocrine manipulation to a varying degree, and significant response rates in cases of advanced disease have been seen following orchiectomy and other hormonal manipulations.

ANSWER:
A, C

25. With regard to mammography as a screening tool, which of the following is/are current American Cancer Society recommendations?

  A. An initial screening mammogram should be obtained at age 40.

  B. Following initial screening, mammograms should be obtained between ages 40 and 50 only if there is clinical suspicion of a lesion present.

  C. Routine screening mammograms should be performed annually after the age of 40.

  D. Routine screening mammograms should be performed every 3 years after the age of 50.

Ref.: 2, 4, 7

COMMENTS: The principal determinant of recommendations for routine mammography are related to the risk-benefit ratio of tumor induction by unnecessary radiation versus detecting cancers at an earlier and therefore more curable stage. • Although unnecessary exposure to irradiation should always be avoided, especially in young persons, the benefits of appropriately prescribed and performed mammography probably outweigh the possible risks of oncogenesis. • Weighing all of these factors, the American Cancer Society has recommended an initial screening mammogram at age 40. • Annual mammograms should be obtained after the age of 40. • Large randomized screening trials have shown an overall risk reduction of mortality from breast cancer as high as 24% among women who underwent routine mammographic screening.

ANSWER:
A, C

26. ER-positive and PR-positive tumors are associated with which of the following?

  A. Better response to hormone manipulation

  B. Better response to chemotherapy

  C. Better prognosis following surgical therapy

  D. Better overall prognosis

  E. More well-differentiated tumors

Ref.: 2, 4

COMMENTS: Although ER and PR analysis is performed to predict the response of breast cancers to endocrine manipulation, tumors that are receptor-positive appear to have a generally better response to all forms of therapy. • Also, receptor-positive tumors tend to be well differentiated. • Hormone receptor status is a sufficiently reliable indicator of prognosis that it is now an integral part of the evaluation of breast cancer and is a major factor in determining appropriate adjuvant therapy. • Because of the importance of the results of hormone receptor analysis and the wide availability of this assay, it is considered inappropriate not to perform receptor analysis on all breast cancers.

ANSWER:
A, B, C, D, E

27. If wide local excision (lumpectomy), axillary dissection, and radiotherapy are being considered as definitive treatment for a given breast carcinoma, which one or more of the following factors bear favorably on that choice?

  A. T1 tumor

  B. Central (subareolar) location within the breast

  C. Extremely large breast

  D. Extremely small breast

  E. Multicentric disease

Ref.: 1, 4

COMMENTS: The choice of wide local incision (lumpectomy), axillary dissection, and radiotherapy versus modified radical mastectomy for stage I and II breast cancers depends on both subjective and objective factors. • Subjectively, the clinician must consider the patient's choice of operation after a fully informative preoperative consultation regarding the strengths and weaknesses of each operation. • Objectively, certain features of the tumor and breast itself may play a role in the appropriateness of the therapeutic choice. • Small lesions require a smaller resection and usually offer a better cosmetic result. • The size of the breast tumor, however, must be considered in relationship to the size of the breast. • Extremely small breasts do not lend themselves particularly well to a wide local incision, since a significant portion of the breast must be removed to achieve clear margins. • Large breasts present the radiotherapist with technical problems related to postoperative whole-breast radiotherapy, but technologic advances have diminished them. • Multicentric disease within the breast is considered a relative contraindication to breast preservation. • Because the nipple-areolar area of the breast is rich in lymphatic channels and because some studies have shown an increased likelihood of multicentric disease associated with subareolar cancers, the usual choice for a subareolar carcinoma is mastectomy.

ANSWER:
A

28. A 33-year-old woman underwent a modified radical mastectomy without reconstruction for a 3-cm, node-positive, ER-negative infiltrating ductal carcinoma. Two years later, she developed a 2-cm immobile nodule in her scar. Wide local resection showed infiltrating ductal carcinoma and clear margins. The chest film, bone scan, and computed tomographic (CT) scan of the liver were normal. After receiving appropriate irradiation to the involved chest wall, what is her chance of being alive with no evidence of recurrence at age 50?

  A. Less than 10%

  B. 20%

  C. 40%

  D. 60%

  E. More than 80%

Ref.: 4

COMMENTS: Local recurrence of breast cancer following mastectomy occurs in approximately 5% of patients. • Local excision plus irradiation is appropriate treatment. • Whether systemic therapy should be used in this situation remains controversial. • Chest wall recurrence in this setting is most often eventually accompanied by distant metastatic disease, even though evaluation may not detect it at the time. • The long-term prognosis is poor.

ANSWER:
A

29. A 10-week-pregnant, 28-year-old woman is referred to the clinician because her obstetrician felt a new breast mass. Mammography was not performed, and an ultrasound examination failed to show an abnormality. The clinician can feel a 1.5-cm, firm, nontender, discrete mass just lateral to the areola. Which of the following management options is appropriate?

 A. Perform a biopsy if the mass is still present 1 month after delivery.

 B. Perform a stereotactic core biopsy.

 C. Locally excise the mass, and, if cancer is found, recommend axillary dissection and irradiation.

 D. Perform a palpation-guided needle-core biopsy, and if, cancer is found, recommend mastectomy.

 E. Locally excise the mass and if cancer is found recommend termination of the pregnancy and mastectomy.

Ref.: 4

COMMENTS: Stage for stage, the prognosis of breast cancer is the same in pregnant as in nonpregnant women. • However, the overall prognosis for pregnant women is worse because they tend to present at a more advanced stage. • Reluctance to evaluate breast masses on the part of both the patient and her physician are contributing factors. • The evaluation and treatment of breast masses must not be delayed because of pregnancy. • Diagnostic mammograms can be safely performed in pregnant women. • However, radiation therapy, even with proper shielding, has a significant incidence of fetal injury and should be discouraged. • Mastectomy is usually appropriate during early and middle pregnancy. • During the third trimester, breast preservation may be considered if an early delivery after confirmation of fetal maturity would facilitate prompt commencement of whole-breast irradiation. • There is no evidence that the pregnancy itself is detrimental, and, for stage I or II disease, termination is not warranted.

ANSWER:
D

30. Which of the following treatments is best for a 40-year-old woman with extensive microcalcifications involving the entire upper aspect of the right breast and biopsy results that show a comedo pattern of ductal carcinoma in situ (DCIS)?

 A. Local excision alone

 B. Irradiation alone

 C. Local excision plus irradiation

 D. Right total mastectomy

 E. Right total mastectomy followed by irradiation

Ref.: 4

COMMENTS: The pendulum has swung toward more conservative management of DCIS. • For a small intraductal carcinoma of the solid, cribriform, or papillary variety, local excision with free margins with or without radiation is appropriate in many situations. • The calcifications described in this patient are too extensive to allow complete excision with a good cosmetic result. • In addition, a comedo pattern is more likely to be multifocal. • Multifocality is associated with a higher rate of recurrence after conservative surgical treatment because wide excision (lumpectomy) is less likely to remove all of the tumor. • Because the disease is noninvasive in this stage, axillary dissection is not necessary. • However, a sentinel lymph node biopsy would not be inappropriate because of the possibility that invasive cancer may be found in the mastectomy specimen at the time of mastectomy. • Postoperative irradiation offers no additional benefit, since total mastectomy is almost always curative.

ANSWER:
D

31. A 44-year-old woman comes to the clinician's office with a movable, nontender, palpable mass in the 12 o'clock position of the left breast. She says it was not present on self-examination 5 weeks earlier. Mammogram shows a 2.5-cm, well-circumscribed density in the area of the palpable abnormality. Ultrasound examination shows an anechoic, well-circumscribed mass with increased through transmission. There is no skin dimpling. Which of the following is the most appropriate first step in treatment?

 A. Schedule an excisional biopsy.

 B. Perform a palpation-guided needle-core biopsy in the office.

 C. Perform a palpation-guided fine-needle aspiration of the mass in the office.

 D. Recommend that she return in 1 month for follow-up.

 E. Obtain magnification compression mammogram views of the lesion.

Ref.: 4

COMMENTS: Fibrocystic disease is the most common cause of a mass in this age group, and the rapid onset in this patient suggests a cyst. • The mammographic findings support this impression. • Magnification compression views would add little information. • In this patient, the most direct and certain way of establishing the diagnosis would be immediate needle aspiration guided by palpation or ultrasound imaging. • When performing an ultrasound-guided aspiration in lieu of palpation-guided aspiration, certain advantages are realized. • It allows precise placement of the needle within the lesion and confirms compete resolution of the lesion. • Characteristics of benign solid lesions include sharp, smooth margins, a homogeneous (dark) interior, and posterior enhancement. • In contradistinction, malignant characteristics include irregular and jagged margins and heterogeneous interior and posterior shadowing. • Fine-needle aspiration (FNA) cytologic study or a core biopsy is the appropriate method of analysis for solid lesions. • A benign cyst is characterized by a sharp, smooth contour; a homogeneous, anechoic interior; and certain and strong posterior enhancement. • Needle aspiration is easily performed and can be seen to achieve complete evacuation. • If the fluid is not bloody and the mass completely disappears, cytologic evaluation rarely yields a diagnosis of carcinoma and is not cost effective.

ANSWER:
C

32. A 53-year-old woman with no family history of breast cancer is discovered on routine examination to have a firm, movable, well-defined, 2-cm mass in the upper outer quadrant of the

right breast. The mammogram shows only bilateral dense breast tissue, with no evidence of malignancy. No mass was seen on ultrasound examination. Which one or more of the following would be an appropriate next step?

A. Follow-up mammogram in 3–4 months

B. Fine-needle aspiration for cytologic studies

C. Bilateral breast magnetic resonance imaging (MRI)

D. Excisional biopsy

E. Clinical reevaluation of the mass in 3 months

F. Core biopsy

Ref.: 4

COMMENTS: Because most patients with breast cancer do not have a family history of breast cancer, any palpable mass requires investigation, regardless of history. • A cyst would be seen on ultrasound examination. • Either needle aspiration or needle-core biopsy of a solid mass would be acceptable as an initial diagnostic step. • Positive results for carcinoma would allow definitive local or regional treatment in a one-step operation. • Excisional biopsy is also an appropriate diagnostic procedure, especially if the lesion is suspicious, but has been largely supplanted by the less invasive needle technique. • Dense breast tissue decreases the diagnostic sensitivity of mammography and can easily obscure a carcinoma. • The absence of mammographic visualization in the presence of a palpable mass does not diminish the need for a tissue diagnosis. • In fact, up to 10% of breast cancers are found in the presence of a "negative" mammogram. • Delaying evaluation of a well-defined mass for 3 months is ill advised, and a follow-up mammogram at 3–4 months is of little value because this lesion is not mammographically detectable. • MRI is a very sensitive diagnostic tool but, at this point in the evaluation of this lesion, would not obviate the need for biopsy.

ANSWER:
B, D, F

33. A 33-year-old asymptomatic woman is referred to the clinician with an abnormal mammogram. No masses are palpable in either breast. The mammogram shows a tight cluster of microcalcifications at the 2 o'clock position of the left breast. Magnification compression views show at least 20 tiny, irregular calcifications in a 2-cm area, varying in shape and density, with no associated mass lesion. There are no other calcifications present in either breast. Which of the following is the most likely diagnosis?

A. Lobular carcinoma in situ

B. Fibroadenoma

C. Infiltrating ductal carcinoma

D. DCIS (intraductal carcinoma)

E. Fibrocystic changes

Ref.: 4, 8

COMMENTS: Mammographic calcifications are a hallmark of early breast cancer, particularly DCIS, but the common causes of calcifications identified on mammogram are varied. • Specific patterns, however, have been identified that are often associated with and predictive of these pathologic processes. • Parenchymal calcifications (i.e., those indicative of a pathologic breast process) occur in the lobar ductal system and in the terminal ductal lobular unit. • Certain patterns of ductal calcification are almost pathognomonic of DCIS, as is a specific bilateral pattern seen with plasma

cell mastitis. • One mammographic feature common to both high-grade DCIS and plasma cell mastitis is the appearance of calcium in a linear, branching pattern. • Evenly scattered calcifications, more often than not bilateral, are indicative of a lobular process. • This pattern is the one most commonly encountered and is indicative of either active or involutional fibrocystic change. • Clustered calcifications, whether single or multiple, present a diagnostic dilemma because of the varied pathologic processes that give rise to this pattern. • Close scrutiny of these areas by magnification views is required to delineate the finer characteristics of the calcifications. • Coarse, granular-appearing calcifications are seen with partially calcified fibroadenomas and papillomas, fibrocystic change, and low- to intermediate-grade DCIS. • Powdery calcifications are seen with sclerosing adenosis, with or without atypia, and low-grade DCIS. • Large, coarse calcifications (popcorn-like) are classically associated with a degenerating fibroadenoma and are readily discernible on mammogram. • Lobular carcinoma in situ and invasive lobular carcinoma are often mammographically featureless. • The clustered geographic distribution and characteristics of the calcifications described in this question make a diagnosis of DCIS more likely than that of an invasive carcinoma, which often has an associated mass lesion seen on mammogram.

ANSWER:
D

34. A 47-year-old woman with a history of breast pain presents with a recent onset of bilateral green nipple discharge. She has generalized bilateral tenderness and no palpable mass on breast examination. The discharge is Hemoccult negative. Mammogram shows diffuse fibroglandular tissue that is slightly more pronounced in the upper outer quadrants bilaterally but unchanged from a year earlier. Which of the following is the most appropriate first step in management?

A. Obtain an ultrasound scan.

B. Perform an ultrasound-guided core biopsy.

C. Reassure the patient.

D. Obtain a galactogram.

E. Excise the major retroareolar duct.

Ref.: 4

COMMENTS: Nipple discharge and breast tenderness are common complaints associated with mammary duct ectasia and fibrocystic change. • Surgery would be inappropriate in this case. • Reassurance is the appropriate management decision in this context, particularly in light of the clinical characteristics of the nipple discharge and the negative mammogram and physical examination findings. • If the drainage is bloody, serous, or watery, further diagnostic workup is indicated to determine the cause of the discharge. • Although such discharges demand evaluation, the cause is often benign (commonly an intraductal papilloma or papillomatosis). • Although some surgeons prefer a preoperative contrast radiograph of the involved duct (a galactogram) as a guide, the blood-distended duct is usually identifiable and can be removed through a circumareolar incision or a lacrimal probe-guided terminal duct excision. • If either preoperative or intraoperative ultrasound imaging is available, this modality can be used in real time to facilitate identification of the distended duct and to map precisely the area of operative excision. • More recently, ductoscopy has been added as a tool for the evaluation of clinically worrisome nipple discharge.

ANSWER:
C

35. A 35-year-old woman with no risk factors recently had her first mammogram. The breast tissue appeared fairly dense, but on the craniocaudad view, a 1.5-cm well-circumscribed, slightly lobulated, noncalcified density with smooth borders could be seen in the lateral aspect of the right breast. The lesion was not seen on the mediolateral view. Ultrasound examination showed no evidence of a cyst. No masses were palpable. Which of the following management choices is/are appropriate?

A. Follow-up mammogram in 4–6 months

B. Stereotactic core biopsy

C. Stereotactic localization and excisional biopsy

D. Reassurance of the patient that the lesion is benign and recommendation of routine follow-up

E. Radiofrequency ablation

Ref.: 4

COMMENTS: The probability is high that the lesion described above is benign, most likely a fibroadenoma or a lymph node. • If the patient is comfortable with accepting a small chance that the lesion represents a cancer, short-term mammographic follow-up is acceptable. • Stereotactic core biopsy is minimally invasive, is done on an outpatient basis, and provides a histologic diagnosis. • Excisional biopsy is more invasive and more traumatic but avoids the small risk of sampling error inherent in needle biopsies. • Localization of a lesion seen only on one view is best done stereotactically. • Reassurance without follow-up is inappropriate. • Percutaneous ablative techniques, including radiofrequency, cryoablation, and laser ablation, require tissue diagnosis of cancer and are considered experimental at this time.

ANSWER:
A, B, C

36. With regard to pure tubular carcinoma, which of the following is/are true?

A. Lymph node involvement is seen in less than 10% of cases.

B. It is a highly aggressive, frequently fatal carcinoma.

C. Lumpectomy with sentinel lymph node biopsy and irradiation is appropriate.

D. Halsted radical mastectomy with reconstruction is appropriate.

E. Neoadjuvant chemotherapy should be strongly considered.

Ref.: 4

COMMENTS: Tubular carcinoma represents a somewhat uncommon, well-differentiated variety of infiltrating ductal carcinoma that has a favorable prognosis. • Lymph node metastasis is encountered in less than 10% of patients with pure tubular carcinomas. • Lumpectomy with sentinel lymph node biopsy, followed by breast irradiation, would be appropriate for local control, as would modified radical mastectomy. • A radical mastectomy would not be indicated. • Neoadjuvant chemotherapy is appropriate for inflammatory or other locally advanced breast cancers but not for a tubular carcinoma.

ANSWER:
A, C

37. A 39-year-old woman with no family history of breast cancer underwent an excisional biopsy of a 2-cm breast mass.

Histologic sections show fibrosis, duct ectasia, atypical lobular hyperplasia, and several areas of lobular carcinoma in situ that involve the surgical margins. Which of the following statements is/are true?

A. At a minimum, she should undergo reexcision of the margins.

B. She has up to a ninefold increase in the chance of developing a subsequent breast cancer.

C. If she develops breast cancer, the area of the biopsy would be the most likely site.

D. If she develops breast cancer, it would most likely be lobular carcinoma.

E. Bilateral mastectomy is not an option at this point.

F. Tamoxifen can be recommended to reduce her future risk of breast cancer.

Ref.: 4

COMMENTS: Lobular carcinoma in situ (LCIS) is a histologic finding that is usually seen in tissue from a biopsy of some other lesion. • It represents a risk marker that predicts up to a ninefold increase in the chance of developing breast cancer. • Atypical lobular hyperplasia alone increases the risk fourfold. • In the face of a strong family history of breast cancer, atypical lobular hyperplasia also increases the risk ninefold. • Acquisition of free margins is not necessary, since it does not decrease the incidence of a subsequent cancer. • Either infiltrating lobular or, more commonly, infiltrating ductal carcinoma may develop. • Both breasts are at equal risk. • Bilateral mastectomy has been commonly performed in the past. • Recently, however, less aggressive management of this particular lesion has evolved, consisting of close follow-up with periodic physical examination and bilateral mammograms or the use of tamoxifen as chemoprevention, which has resulted in a nearly 50% reduction in the risk of developing breast cancer. • Bilateral total mastectomy remains an option that should be presented to the patient as part of the formal discussion of management.

ANSWER:
B, F

38. An otherwise healthy 55-year-old woman underwent excisional biopsy of a 2-cm mass in the upper outer quadrant of the right breast that showed a well-differentiated infiltrating ductal carcinoma with a minimal intraductal component and free margins. She has a palpable, firm, 2-cm right axillary node. Which of the following is/are considered appropriate local or regional therapy?

A. Right modified radical mastectomy with immediate reconstruction

B. Axillary dissection and breast irradiation

C. Sentinel lymph node biopsy and breast irradiation

D. Total mastectomy and axillary irradiation

E. Radical mastectomy with immediate reconstruction

Ref.: 4

COMMENTS: Because clinical examination of the axilla is unreliable (20–30% error rate), the presence of a palpable node should not automatically be considered a sign of metastatic involvement. • Similarly, the absence of clinically palpable nodes does not ensure that they are microscopically free of cancer. • The presence of positive axillary nodes, unless large and fixed, does not alter the local or regional management of breast cancer. • If invasive cancer is present, an axillary dissection or sentinel lymph node biopsy is indicated to determine overall prognosis and guide adjuvant therapy. • However, sentinel lymph node biopsy is not appropriate when, as in this case, there are clinically suspicious axillary nodes present. • Except in a small percentage of cases, the axillary dissection does not directly improve survival. • Modified radical mastectomy with or without reconstruction is always an option for the local or regional management of invasive breast cancer. • However, it confers no survival advantage. • A Halsted radical mastectomy would be inappropriate.

A N S W E R :
A, B

39. Mammograms show masses in two asymptomatic women in their mid-forties (see the figures). There are no previous mammograms available. On which of the patients would an excisional biopsy be the appropriate next step?

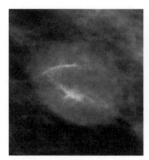 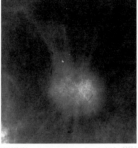

Patient 1   Patient 2

A: T1, N1, M0, stage IIA. B: T2, N3, M0, stage IIIC. C: T4, N2, M0, stage IIIB. D: T2, N0, M0, stage IIA. E: T4, N1, M0, stage IIIB.

A. Patient 1

B. Patient 2

C. Neither

Ref.: 4

COMMENTS: See Question 40.

40. With regard to asymptomatic, mammographically found breast masses, which of the following statements is/are true?

A. As a first step, biopsy of a single, dominant mass more than 1 cm in diameter in women older than 40 years must be performed.

B. Masses with a small, well-defined border and a "halo" sign around them are always benign.

C. The differential diagnosis of a small, dense stellate mass includes malignancy and postsurgical scar.

D. The presence of fat within a mass makes malignancy highly unlikely.

Ref.: 4

COMMENTS: Remember the ubiquitous cyst. • Before performing an open biopsy for a smooth-bordered or even a lobulated mass within the breast, an ultrasound examination should be performed. • Many such masses, even when they appear in postmenopausal women, are cysts (patient 1, Question 39), although solid focal lesions are also common. • Smooth, rounded masses cannot be assumed to be benign even if previous mammograms demonstrate a stable appearance over a long period of time. • Some malignant tumors, including mucinous and medullary carcinoma or cystosarcoma phylloides, can have a benign appearance on both ultrasound imaging and mammogram. • Stereotactic core biopsy and ultrasound-guided core biopsy offer good alternatives to open biopsy under these circumstances. • Dense stellate masses (patient 2, Question 39) should always be considered malignant until proved otherwise. • Although a surgical scar may have the same appearance as such a mass, the absence of a previous biopsy on history and physical examination excludes this possibility. • Most masses that contain fat are benign. • Typical examples are lymph nodes, with their fatty hilum; posttraumatic oil cysts; and hamartomas or fibrolipoadenomas of the breast.

A N S W E R S :
Question 39: B
Question 40: C, D

41. Five 38-year-old women with otherwise normal physical, laboratory, and radiographic findings underwent biopsies for small, nonpalpable mammographic abnormalities. Photomicrographs of each are shown in the figures. Assume that the disease extends to the edge of resection in each case and that it is difficult to be certain that the margins of excision are totally free.

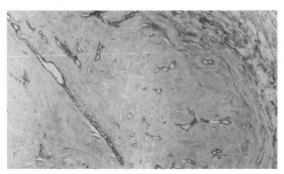 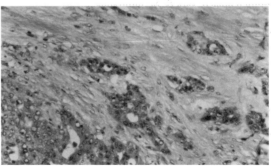

A   B

C

D

E

For each photomicrograph (A–E), select which one or more of the following treatment options would be appropriate.

A. Modified radical mastectomy

B. Routine follow-up with no further treatment

C. Re-excision with free margins and close follow-up

D. No further surgery and close follow-up

E. Total mastectomy without axillary dissection

F. Bilateral total mastectomy without axillary dissection

G. Re-excision with free margins, sentinel lymphatic biopsy or axillary dissection, and breast irradiation

H. Re-excision with free margins and breast irradiation

I. Tamoxifen for 5 years

Ref.: 1, 2, 4

COMMENTS: Prominent fibrous tissue compressing epithelial elements, as demonstrated in A, is typical of a **fibroadenoma**. • Involvement of margins is inconsequential, and re-excision is unwarranted. ∥ The nests of epithelial cells invading the stroma in random fashion, with a suggestion of tubule formation, as shown in B, are typical of **infiltrating ductal carcinoma**. • Either modified radical mastectomy or wide local excision with axillary dissection and breast irradiation is appropriate. ∥ The hyperchromatic nuclei in a fairly uniform population of neoplastic-appearing cells filling and distending the ducts, along with sharply defined punched-out (Swiss cheese) spaces, as seen in C, are typical of a **cribriform intraductal carcinoma**. • In contrast to a comedo pattern of intraductal carcinoma, this lesion can often be treated by excision to free margins and close follow-up. • If free margins are not obtained, the rate of recurrence is high. • Even if free margins are obtained, the lesion

occasionally recurs in an invasive form. • If the patient is unwilling to accept that small chance, total mastectomy or irradiation is appropriate, even though it may be overtreatment. • Axillary dissection is unnecessary, and long-term survival following mastectomy is essentially 100%. ∥ The uniform population of cells filling, expanding, and distorting the lobules, as seen in D, is typical of **lobular carcinoma in situ**. • This is a risk marker that indicates a ninefold increase in the likelihood that the patient will eventually develop invasive breast cancer. • There is no need to try to obtain free margins because it does not decrease the risk. • Even though the margins are involved, the cancer that may subsequently develop may be ductal or lobular and is no more likely to occur at the site of the biopsy than at any other location in either breast. • For this reason, if the surgeon recommends a prophylactic operation, bilateral total mastectomy should be considered. • This choice is rather aggressive, considering that it would be unnecessary in two thirds to three fourths of patients (only 25–30% of women with the lesion develop invasive cancer). • Many patients now choose close follow-up or chemopreventive treatment with tamoxifen instead of bilateral mastectomy. ∥ The ectatic duct with a single or double (epithelial and myoepithelial) cell layer, as shown in E, is typical of **fibrocystic disease**. • The condition is benign and requires only routine follow-up. • There is no need to try to achieve free margins.

ANSWER:
A-b; B-a,g; C-c,e,h; D-d,f,i; E-b

42. With regard to adjuvant tamoxifen therapy of invasive breast cancer, which of the following statements is/are true?

   A. It significantly reduces recurrence among women with negative nodes.

   B. It significantly reduces recurrence among women with positive nodes.

C. It significantly improves survival among women with negative nodes.

D. It significantly improves survival among women with positive nodes.

E. It is relatively more effective in postmenopausal than in premenopausal women.

F. The optimal duration of treatment is 2 years.

G. Patients with ER-positive tumors derive greater benefit.

Ref.: 9

COMMENTS: See Question 43.

43. With regard to adjuvant chemotherapy of invasive breast cancer, which of the following statements is/are true?

A. It significantly reduces recurrence among women with negative nodes.

B. It significantly reduces recurrence among women with positive nodes.

C. It significantly improves survival among women with negative nodes.

D. It significantly improves survival among women with positive nodes.

E. It is relatively more effective in postmenopausal than in premenopausal women.

F. Adriamycin cytoxan is associated with improved survival rates compared to CMF regimen.

Ref.: 10

COMMENTS: Adjuvant systemic therapy (both cytotoxic chemotherapy and hormonal therapy) plays a significant and growing role in the primary management of locally and regionally confined breast cancer. • In 1998, the Early Breast Cancer Trialists' Collaborative Group published updated results of their shared experiences with more than 130 randomized, prospective trials, involving more than 75,000 women, that investigated the role of adjuvant systemic therapy in breast cancer. • This meta-analysis has provided a number of generally accepted conclusions about the effectiveness of this therapy. • Both chemotherapy and tamoxifen resulted in a significantly reduced risk of recurrence and death from breast cancer among women with negative nodes or positive nodes, regardless of age or menopausal status. • Of note, however, was that tamoxifen resulted in greater risk reduction in postmenopausal women than in premenopausal women, and chemotherapy resulted in greater risk reduction in premenopausal women than in postmenopausal women. • In terms of duration of treatment, tamoxifen seems to be more effective the longer it is used, up to 5 years, with current recommendations being for a 5-year course. • More recently, adriamycin cytoxan has shown improved survival when compared with cmf with a shorter course of treatment. • Both tamoxifen and chemotherapy appear to be more effective in patients with ER-positive tumors. • Among all of the various groups and regimens, the reduction in "annual odds of death" or "annual odds of recurrence" ranged broadly, from approximately 10–40%. • Although it could be concluded from these data that all patients should receive adjuvant systemic therapy, it must be remembered that, for many populations of patients (e.g., a postmenopausal patient with a <1-cm, ER-positive, node-negative primary tumor), the likelihood of recurrence without adjuvant treatment may be only 5%. • A 30% reduction in this risk would reduce the

overall recurrence rate by only 1–2%. • However, because the 5% of patients who will experience recurrence cannot be identified at the outset, 98 or 99 of 100 patients would be receiving adjuvant therapy to benefit only 1 or 2. • This small benefit would have to be weighed against the cost and toxicity of the treatment itself.

ANSWERS:
Question 42: A, B, C, D, E, G
Question 43: A, B, C, D, F

44. Which one or more of the following factors could influence the choice of systemic adjuvant therapy for invasive breast cancer?

A. Tumor size

B. DNA ploidy

C. HER-2/neu

D. Axillary node status

E. ER status

F. Cathepsin D

G. Age or menopausal status

Ref.: 4

COMMENTS: Currently, the recommendation for adjuvant systemic therapy via cytotoxic chemotherapy or tamoxifen is based on consideration of tumor size, nodal status, ER status, and age or menopausal status. • In general, all node-positive tumors require chemotherapy, and tumors smaller than 1 cm that are node negative require no additional treatment. • The National Institutes of Health consensus panel and the international panel on the treatment of primary breast cancer recommend treating all node-negative tumors larger than 1 cm with adjuvant chemotherapy if they are ER negative or with tamoxifen if they are ER positive. • Current studies are evaluating the more liberal combining of tamoxifen with chemotherapy for all of these categories. • The other tumor characteristics mentioned above (DNA ploidy, HER-2/neu status, and cathepsin D status) have been variably reported to influence overall prognosis but are not yet considered factors that influence the choice of adjuvant therapy. • However, clinical trials are currently under way investigating the use of Herceptin (an anti-Her2/neu antibody) in the adjuvant and neoadjuvant setting among patients with positive Her2/neu expression.

ANSWER:
A, D, E, G

45. Germ-line mutations in which of the following genes is/are associated with a higher incidence of breast cancer.

A. APC

B. BRCA1

C. BRCA2

D. p53

E. hPMS1

Ref.: 11

COMMENTS: A germ-line mutation is a mutation that exists in every cell of the body and therefore is capable of being passed to the offspring via the sperm or egg. • The predominant genes responsible for hereditary breast cancer are BRCA1 (breast cancer 1) and BRCA2. • Women who carry a germ-line mutation in either of these genes have about an 85% likelihood of developing breast cancer by the age of 70, although most cancers occur before age 50. • Women with these mutations also have an increased risk (30–60%) of developing ovarian cancer. • Inherited mutations of the p53 gene result in Li-Fraumeni syndrome, which is associated with the development of a number of malignancies, including breast cancer, sarcomas, brain tumors, adrenocortical carcinomas, and leukemia. • The APC gene is involved in cell growth regulation and, when inherited in mutated form, leads to **familial adenomatous polyposis** and an increased incidence of colon cancer. • The hPMS1 gene is responsible for repair of DNA strands that become mismatched during cell division. • Mutations of this gene lead to **hereditary nonpolyposis colon cancer**. • The two genes do not increase the risk of breast cancer.

ANSWER:
B, C, D

---

46. A germ-line mutation in either BRCA1 or BRCA2 is associated with which of the following characteristics?

 A. Autosomal dominant transmission

 B. High incidence of breast and ovarian cancer in women

 C. Higher than average incidence of breast cancer in men

 D. Equal likelihood of a woman inheriting the mutation from her father or mother

 E. Incomplete penetrance

 F. Late-onset breast cancer

Ref.: 11

COMMENTS: Mutations in BRCA1 or BRCA2 result in a higher incidence of breast and ovarian cancer. • The risk of breast cancer is about 85% among individuals who carry the mutation and have a family history of breast cancer. • The risk of ovarian cancer is about 40% for BRCA1 mutations and 20% for BRCA2 mutations. • About 10% of males with BRCA2 mutations develop breast cancer. • Because the gene resides on an autosome (and is therefore not sex linked), men can pass the mutation to their children. • These genes are incompletely penetrant, that is, some mutation carriers can live to old age and not develop cancer. • The mutation is autosomal dominant, that is, a mutation in only one of the pair of chromosomes usually produces the disease. • Although women who carry germ-line mutations of these genes can develop post-menopausal breast cancer, most cancers arising in carriers occur premenopausally.

ANSWER:
A, B, C, D, E

---

47. A 32-year-old woman presents for evaluation of her breast cancer risk. She has five sisters, two of whom have developed premenopausal breast cancer. Her mother died of ovarian cancer at age 45. What should be the recommendation of the clinician?

 A. Discuss the availability of tests for a mutation in BRCA1 or BRCA2.

 B. Recommend bilateral mastectomy.

 C. Begin tamoxifen.

 D. Refer her for genetic counseling.

 E. Recommend mammography every 6 months after she has been treated for her breast cancer.

Ref.: 11

COMMENTS: There is a significant likelihood that the patient described above has a BRCA1 or BRCA2 mutation. • She could easily be tested for this with a simple but expensive blood test. • If she tests positive for a mutation in either of these genes, she has an approximately 85% lifetime risk of developing breast cancer and a 20–40% lifetime risk of developing ovarian cancer. • If such were the case, the patient might opt for aggressive prophylactic ablative surgery (mastectomy and oophorectomy). • Alternatively, she could opt for conservative management with careful surveillance to include clinical breast and pelvic examination, mammography, whole breast ultrasound, breast MRI, ovarian ultrasonography, and ovarian tumor marker assessment at appropriate intervals. • She could also opt for beginning tamoxifen, which has been shown in a recent chemoprevention trial to reduce the risk of developing breast cancer by close to 50% among patients considered to be at high risk. • Choosing among these options requires a firm understanding by the patient of the respective risks and benefits. • The patient should also understand that knowledge of one's status with regard to carrying a mutation of the BRCA1 or BRCA2 gene can result in discrimination by potential employers or insurance carriers unwilling to "take a chance" on such a high-risk individual. • Genetic testing has implications for the entire family, since the knowledge that one member carries a mutation alters the likelihood of other family members also being carriers. • For all these reasons, the current recommendation is for extremely high-risk individuals, as described above, to be referred for genetic counseling before actually undergoing testing for the presence of gene mutations.

ANSWER:
A, D

---

48. A 45-year-old woman had her first child at age 40. She began menstruating at age 9. She had a breast biopsy a year ago that showed atypical hyperplasia. Her mother had postmenopausal breast cancer. Reasonable options for this woman include which of the following?

 A. Bilateral prophylactic mastectomy

 B. Mammography every 6 months

 C. Tamoxifen for 5 years

 D. Raloxifene for 5 years

 E. Consuming a diet that is high in phytoestrogens

 F. Entering a clinical trial comparing tamoxifen with raloxifene

Ref.: 11

COMMENTS: The Breast Cancer Prevention Trial (BCPT), conducted by the National Surgical Adjuvant Breast Cancer Project (NSABP), compared tamoxifen with placebo in 13,000 women at high risk for breast cancer. • It showed that 5 years of tamoxifen reduced the short-term risk of breast cancer by 45%. • Complications included thromboembolic phenomena and postmenopausal endometrial cancer (each in the 1% or less range). • A randomized trial of postmenopausal women who received raloxifene versus placebo for osteoporosis revealed a reduction in breast cancer, although breast cancer was not the primary endpoint of the trial. • The NSABP will study 22,000 postmenopausal women at risk for breast cancer in the Study of Tamoxifen and Raloxifene (STAR) trial. • Participants will be randomized to tamoxifen versus raloxifene for 5 years. • Although there is tantalizing information from case-controlled and cohort studies that diets rich in phytoestrogens (e.g., soy or tofu) are associated with a reduced risk of breast cancer, there have as yet been no randomized trials addressing the issue. • Although this patient is at increased risk for developing breast cancer, she is not at a level of risk for which prophylactic mastectomy would be strongly considered, nor would she require screening mammography more often than once annually unless there were specific mammographic changes that required more frequent imaging.

A N S W E R :
C, F

49. Which of the following statements regarding of the human epidermal growth factor receptor-2 (HER-2) gene is/are true?

  A. It encodes a growth factor receptor.

  B. It controls normal cell growth.

  C. It is amplified in 25% of breast cancers.

  D. It is a target for biologic therapy.

  E. It is independently predictive of poor outcome in breast cancer.

Ref.: 11

COMMENTS: The HER-2 gene is responsible for encoding a transmembrane tyrosine kinase, a protein with potent growth-stimulating activity. • When the gene activity is amplified (i.e., the protein is present in abnormally increased amounts) in patients with breast cancer, more rapid growth and more aggressive behavior of the tumor can result. • This amplification can be measured and is known to occur in 25–30% of human breast cancers. • Such cancers are more likely to be associated with poor prognostic features, such as being ER negative, node positive, and poorly differentiated. • However, this overexpression of the gene is known to be an independent predictor of a worse prognosis, regardless of the status of the other variables. • The membrane receptor for the protein (not the gene itself) is a target for a new and promising monoclonal antibody therapy (Herceptin).

A N S W E R :
A, B, C, E

50. Select the true statement(s) regarding the use of tissue expanders for breast reconstruction.

  A. Tissue expansion works by stretching and thinning the overlying tissues. Diminished epidermal mitoses and dermal collagen synthesis are seen in areas of tissue expansion.

  B. Because tissue expansion frequently produces wound disruption when it is employed for immediate reconstruction, it is usually used for delayed reconstruction after mastectomy.

  C. Tissue expansion is contraindicated for patients who are smokers. A pedicled TRAM flap is a safer method of reconstruction for these patients.

  D. When a tissue expander is used for breast reconstruction, it is placed anterior to the pectoralis major muscle to produce an anatomically correct copy of the breast.

  E. Breasts reconstructed with tissue expanders do not usually feel as natural as those reconstructed with TRAM flaps.

Ref.: 1, 2, 12

COMMENTS: Tissue expansion is the most commonly employed method of breast reconstruction in the United States. • The device consists of a Silastic shell connected to an injection valve, through which saline solution can be added. • Tissue expansion is well suited for immediate reconstruction after mastectomy, since the operative time and blood loss are considerably less than for other methods of reconstruction. • The surgeon selects a tissue expander with a base dimension that matches the opposite breast and positions the device in the plane underneath the pectoralis major and serratus anterior muscles. • This submuscular location is critical because it prevents wound disruption and provides sufficient soft tissue camouflage for a reasonably natural breast shape to be created. • A small amount of saline solution is instilled at the time of reconstruction. • Weekly expansion is usually begun approximately 3 weeks after surgery. • The endpoint of tissue expansion is reached when sufficient saline solution has been added to produce a volumetric match of the opposite breast. • This process takes 2–3 months for an average-sized breast. • In most cases, the tissue expander is removed at the completion of the expansion process and replaced with a softer saline- or silicone gel-filled reconstructive implant. • Tissue expansion occurs by means of a combination of stretching overlying tissue, recruitment of adjacent tissue, and the production of new tissue. • Increased epidermal mitosis and increased dermal collagen synthesis have been demonstrated in expanded tissue. • The specific choice of reconstructive method is determined by a detailed analysis of the patient's medical history, goals, personal preferences, and body habitus. • In general, smoking is viewed as a contraindication to breast reconstruction with a pedicled TRAM flap because there is an unacceptably high incidence of flap necrosis in these patients. • Although smoking increases the risk of complications for any surgical procedure, tissue expander reconstruction can usually be carried out in smokers with acceptable morbidity. • One disadvantage of tissue expander and implant reconstruction is that the breast does not have as natural a feel as a breast reconstructed from the fat of the abdominal wall with a TRAM flap. • This advantage must be balanced against the longer recovery and abdominal donor site scar of the TRAM flap.

A N S W E R :
E

51. For which one or more of the following situations would postmastectomy radiation therapy be indicated?

  A. A primary breast tumor larger than 5 cm with positive axillary lymph nodes

  B. Four or more positive axillary lymph nodes

  C. A single positive axillary node with gross extracapsular extension

  D. Three of thirteen axillary nodes positive and matted together

  E. A node-negative, 4-cm cancer involving the deep margin of the mastectomy specimen

  F. Inflammatory breast cancer

Ref.: 5, 6, 16, 17

COMMENTS: In patients with T3 lesions (>5 cm) and positive axillary lymph nodes or in patients with four or more positive axillary lymph nodes (regardless of the primary tumor size), locoregional recurrence after mastectomy ranges from 25–30%. • This figure can be reduced to approximately 10% with postmastectomy irradiation. • Most commonly, the chest wall and regional nodal area (supraclavicular and axillary, with or without the internal mammary nodal regions) are treated to a dose of 50 Gy in 25–28 fractions.

• Additional fractions to a more limited field (a boost) may be given for close or positive margins. • Recently published trials from Denmark and British Columbia report that postmastectomy radiation therapy improves not only local control but also survival in node-positive patients. • Postmastectomy radiation therapy in patients with T3N0 disease or patients with T1 and T2 tumors with one to three positive axillary lymph nodes is more controversial. • Patients with T3N0 disease were included in the Danish study. • Furthermore, patients with one to three positive nodes were included in both the Danish and British Columbia trials and represented more than 50% of the patients in these trials. • Still, many argue that the risk of locoregional recurrence in these patients is less than 15%, and therefore postoperative radiation therapy may not be warranted. • Other indications for postmastectomy irradiation include N2 to N3 disease, gross extracapsular tumor extension, positive surgical margins, inflammatory breast cancer, or involvement of the skin, pectoral fascia, or skeletal muscle.

ANSWER:
A, B, C, D, E, F

52. Which of the following patients is considered an appropriate candidate for breast-preserving therapy with lumpectomy followed by radiation therapy?

A. A 40-year-old woman with a history of active scleroderma with a T1N0 infiltrating ductal carcinoma of the right breast

B. A 45-year-old woman with a T1N1 infiltrating ductal carcinoma of the left breast status postlumpectomy with negative surgical margins and axillary lymph node dissection with 2 of 12 positive lymph nodes

C. A 37-year-old woman with a T2N0 infiltrating ductal carcinoma of the right breast who has a history of Hodgkin's disease treated with 36 Gy to a mantle field 15 years ago

D. All of the above

E. None of the above

Ref.: 18, 19

COMMENTS: The National Surgical Adjuvant Breast and Bowel Project (NSABP) B-06 trial demonstrated that lumpectomy followed by radiation therapy to the breast is appropriate treatment for patients with primary tumors 4 cm or less in diameter with either positive or negative axillary lymph nodes. • Several other trials have confirmed these results for patients with stage I and II breast cancer. • The 20-year results from the NSABP B-06 trial show equal overall survival and disease-free survival for all patients whether they were treated with breast preservation or mastectomy. • However, the cohort of patients treated with lumpectomy alone without irradiation suffered a 35% recurrence rate in the ipsilateral breast. • This recurrence rate is considered unacceptably high when compared to the 10% risk of ipsilateral breast recurrences in patients who received radiation to the breast followed lumpectomy. • Several series have shown that patients with certain collagen vascular diseases may incur increased toxicity from radiation therapy. • Although excessive complications have not been consistently shown with all types of collagen vascular disorders, severe fibrosis and soft tissue necrosis have been associated with scleroderma, suggesting that patients with scleroderma may be better served with a mastectomy. • Patients with active systemic lupus erythematosus and rheumatoid arthritis may also be at increased risk for toxicity from radiation therapy. • Mastectomy is recommended for patients who have had prior radiation therapy to the chest or to a mantle field (which includes the neck, axilla, mediastinum, and

pulmonary hila) because radiation tolerance of the regional normal tissues may be exceeded, resulting in excessive toxicity.

ANSWER:
B

53. What recommendation regarding mammography should the clinician make to a woman whose mother was diagnosed with breast cancer at the age of 40 and whose sister was diagnosed with breast cancer at the age of 45?

A. First mammogram at age 25 and annually starting at age 40

B. First mammogram at age 30 and then annually thereafter

C. First mammogram at age 35 and then annually thereafter

D. First mammogram at age 40 and then annually thereafter

Ref.: 7

COMMENTS: The current recommendation is for the patient to have a baseline mammogram 10 years before the youngest age at diagnosis of breast cancer among first-degree relatives in the family. • This recommendation is often modified in cases where the first cancer is diagnosed earlier than age 35 because mammography in even high-risk women in their early twenties is rarely helpful.

ANSWER:
B

54. A 15-year-old girl is brought in by her mother because of asymmetric breast development. The physical examination reveals normal breast development on the left, a hypoplastic breast on the right, with noted hypoplasia of the pectoralis major muscle also on the right. What should the clinician explain to the mother?

A. This is a normal situation in this age group, since breast tissue often develops at different rates and is slightly asymmetric during adolescence

B. This is an example of Poland's syndrome.

C. This is an example of Li-Fraumeni syndrome.

D. This is an example of amazia.

Ref.: 7

COMMENTS: This patient is demonstrating Poland's syndrome, which is characterized by unilateral hypoplasia of the breast, pectoral muscles, and chest wall. • Li-Fraumeni syndrome is one of the inherited breast cancer syndromes in which there is an increased incidence of breast cancer, soft tissue and osteosarcomas, brain tumors, adrenocortical cancer, and leukemias in the same family. • Nearly 30% of the tumors in these families occur before the age of 15. • Amazia refers to a condition in which the nipple is present but the breast mound is absent.

ANSWER:
B

55. A 13-year-old girl is referred to a clinician for a palpable breast mass. Her breast development is normal for her age and is symmetric. Her mother was diagnosed with breast cancer at

the age of 29. The appropriate management of this lesion would include which of the following?

A. Excision of the nodule

B. Ultrasonography

C. Mammography

D. Fine-needle aspiration biopsy

E. Clinical follow-up in 3 months

Ref.: 7, 20

COMMENTS: Although there is a history of early-onset breast cancer in this girl's mother, the likelihood that this nodule is malignant is extremely low. • In young patients, mammography is difficult to interpret because the breast tissue is so dense, and radiation to the early developing breast should be avoided. • Ultrasound imaging would be the imaging technique of choice in this instance to delineate a solid lesion from a cystic lesion. • Even if it is a solid lesion, it is most likely a fibroadenoma and could be followed with a repeat examination in 3 months or repeat ultrasound scanning. • Excision of the nodule in a patient who is beginning breast development may result in abnormal breast development or amazia. • A fine-needle aspiration biopsy could be performed to confirm the benign nature of the lesion.

ANSWER:
B, D, E

56. Which of the following can mimic breast cancer on mammography or physical examination?

A. Radial scar

B. Fibromatosis

C. Granular cell tumor

D. Fat necrosis

Ref.: 7

COMMENTS: All of the lesions described can have an appearance similar to that of cancer on mammography or clinical examination. • **Radial scars** appear as a soft-tissue density with irregular edges and spiculation on the mammogram. • There is some controversy as to whether these lesions are premalignant. • **Fibromatosis** is characterized by locally invasive, nonencapsulated, proliferation of well-differentiated spindle cells. • Fibromatosis presents as a palpable mass and can entail skin retraction or fixation to underlying muscle. • Fibromatosis is indistinguishable from cancer on the mammogram. • **Granular cell tumors** also simulate cancer on both clinical examination and mammography. • These lesions present as palpable abnormalities with skin retraction and possible fixation to underlying structures. • They resemble scirrhous carcinoma on the mammogram. • **Fat necrosis** can appear similar to a cancer on mammography. • It can present as a palpable mass with poorly defined borders and may cause skin retraction. • Surgical excision is usually indicated for these lesions, owing to their mammographic resemblance to carcinoma and the small risk of sampling error associated with needle biopsy.

ANSWER:
A, B, C, D

57. An initial mammogram of a 45-year-old woman reveals a cluster of indeterminate microcalcifications in the upper outer quadrant

of the left breast. There is no family history of breast cancer, and the area in question is not palpable. Which of the following procedures would be appropriate?

A. Stereotactic-guided large core needle biopsy

B. Ultrasound-guided large core needle biopsy

C. Repeat mammogram of the involved breast in 6 months

D. Excisional biopsy with wire localization and specimen radiography

Ref.: 7

COMMENTS: See Question 60.

58. In which of the following situations would additional intervention be warranted?

A. Stereotactic 14-gauge core biopsy for indeterminate microcalcifications revealing "sclerosing adenosis with calcification in benign ductules"

B. Stereotactic 14-gauge core biopsy for a well-circumscribed mammographic density revealing "fibroadenoma"

C. Stereotactic 14-gauge core biopsy for a cluster of indeterminate microcalcifications revealing "atypical ductal hyperplasia"

D. Stereotactic 14-gauge core biopsy for a poorly defined 1-cm radiographic density revealing "apocrine metaplasia and fibrocystic changes"

Ref.: 7

COMMENTS: See Question 60.

59. A 38-year-old woman presents with a recently discovered 2-cm, tender mass in the 10 o'clock position of the upper outer right breast. Ultrasonography reveals a 2-cm, smooth-edged anechoic mass with bilateral edge shadowing and posterior acoustic enhancement as well as reverberation artifacts in the superficial portion of the mass. Which of the following interventional procedures would be appropriate at this point?

A. Stereotactic-guided large-core needle biopsy

B. Ultrasound-guided large-core needle biopsy

C. Ultrasound-guided needle aspiration

D. Excisional biopsy with wire localization and specimen radiography

E. Fine-needle aspiration by palpation

Ref.: 7

COMMENTS: See Question 60.

60. Routine screening mammography of a 57-year-old woman reveals a 1.5-cm, spiculated, centrally dense mass. An image-guided biopsy shows benign breast parenchyma. Which of the following is the most appropriate recommendation at this point?

A. Routine screening mammography in 1 year

B. Additional imaging with contrast-enhanced MRI

C. Short-term follow-up with diagnostic mammography in 4–6 months

D. Excisional biopsy with wire localization and specimen radiography

Ref.: 7

COMMENTS: One of the key advances in the diagnosis of pathologic conditions of the breast over the past 20 years has been the evolution of image-guided sampling of nonpalpable mammographically or sonographically detected lesions. • Several principles of management that have emerged from the growing experience with these techniques are brought out in the preceding four questions. • Indeterminate calcifications (Question 57) can be associated with a 10–30% chance of cancer accounting for the calcifications, and therefore some sort of tissue sampling would be indicated. • Stereo-guided core biopsy permits sampling with a low false-negative rate and allows the vast majority of persons whose condition is benign to avoid an open biopsy. • Ultrasound guidance for core biopsy is not appropriate when the target is a cluster of microcalcifications. • Excisional biopsy with wire localization is not inappropriate but would be better utilized as the initial biopsy technique for calcifications that are highly suspicious rather than indeterminate. • Although there is a small possibility of sampling error (false-negative results), it is generally thought that, when the mammographic target is not highly suspicious and the pathologic results are concordant with the radiographic features of the lesion, a clearly "benign" result without "atypia" would not require further intervention (Question 58). • The presence of "atypical hyperplasia" (ductal or lobular) generally suggests the need for additional tissue sampling, most often via a wire-localized excision. • When the mammographic changes are highly suspicious, as described in Question 60, however, a negative core biopsy result must be viewed with caution, since the possibility of sampling error must always be considered. • Definitive wide excision with wire localization in such circumstances would then be warranted. • The reasons for the initial core biopsy in such suspicious cases are multiple and include the value of having a tissue diagnosis (rather than just a "suspicion") when discussing diagnosis and management options with the patient and the ability to more accurately inject the radionuclide or blue dye into the area of the relatively undisturbed primary tumor when sentinel node biopsy is chosen as the method of axillary assessment. • In Question 59, the ultrasound findings are those of a simple or slightly complex cyst. • Such cysts carry essentially no risk of harboring cancer and therefore do not normally require any intervention unless they are symptomatic, as in this case. • Aspiration is then appropriate and can be done either by palpation or with ultrasound guidance.

ANSWERS:
Question 57: A, D
Question 58: C
Question 59: C, E
Question 60: D

61. In a patient who has undergone an axillary dissection for breast cancer, match the postoperative affliction in the left-hand column with the most likely cause in the right-hand column.

A. Hypesthesia of the upper inner aspect of the ipsilateral arm
a. Lymphatic fibrosis

B. Progressive atrophy of the pectoralis major muscle
b. Medial pectoral pedicle injury

C. Sudden, painful, early postoperative swelling of the involved arm
c. Thoracodorsal pedicle injury

D. Painless, slow, progressive swelling of the involved arm
d. Long thoracic nerve injury beginning 18 months after surgery

E. Asymmetric protrusion of the ipsilateral scapula, especially during "pushing" maneuvers of the arm
e. Second intercostal brachiocutaneous nerve injury

F. Ischemic loss of the entire latissimus dorsi flap utilized for reconstruction
f. Axillary vein thrombosis

Ref.: 7

COMMENTS: A number of neurovascular structures are identified and dissected during an axillary dissection and are at risk of injury. • The axillary vein can be narrowed or ligated, owing to surgical error during the procedure, or can undergo acute spontaneous thrombosis during the immediate postoperative period. • Because collateral channels have not had a chance to develop, the resulting swelling of the ipsilateral arm is usually acute and painful. • The long thoracic nerve is the motor nerve to the serratus anterior muscle, which functions to stabilize the scapula against the posterior chest wall, especially during pushing maneuvers. • Injury to this structure leads to "winging" of the scapula. • The thoracodorsal pedicle contains the motor nerve and the principal artery and vein serving the latissimus dorsi muscle. • Injury to the nerve leads to atrophy, but this is rarely clinically significant, except in athletes. • Loss of the vascular pedicle distal to its branch to the serratus muscle, however, would lead to ischemic loss of the latissimus dorsi myocutaneous rotation flap, one of the principal sources of autologous tissue for breast reconstruction and for closure of soft tissue deficits of the chest wall. • The medial pectoral pedicle contains the principal motor nerve and partial blood supply to the pectoralis major muscle. • Injury leads to atrophy but not ischemia, as the blood supply to this muscle is from many sources. • The second intercostal brachiocutaneous nerve is sensory to the upper lateral chest wall and medial and posterior upper arm. • It passes transversely across the axilla about 1–2 cm caudal to the axillary vein. • In the past, it was routinely sectioned to allow cleaner en bloc removal of the axillary contents, but many surgeons now choose to preserve it in cases where it is not in close proximity to clinically suspicious lymph nodes. • The axilla is rich in lymphatic vessels draining the ipsilateral arm. • Some of these lymphatics are disrupted during axillary dissection, but continued fibrosis of the remaining lymphatics, especially in cases where the dissected axilla has been irradiated, may lead to progressive lymphedema of the arm, which can begin years after therapy. • The possibility of developing occasionally unsightly and disabling lymphedema has led to a generally more conservative surgical approach toward axillary dissection for breast cancer in recent years.

ANSWER:
A-e; B-b; C-f; D-a; E-d; F-c

62. A 48-year-old woman has undergone a lumpectomy for a 4-mm infiltrating ductal carcinoma of the lower outer quadrant of the right breast. The margins of resection are free of tumor. Which one of the following options for further local therapy would be the most appropriate?

A. Right modified radical mastectomy

B. Right axillary sentinel lymph node biopsy followed by radiation therapy to the right breast

C. Right axillary sentinel lymph node biopsy followed by radiation therapy only if the lymph node is positive for cancer

D. A right level I and II axillary dissection followed by radiation therapy to the right breast.

E. A right level I axillary dissection followed by radiation therapy only if one or more of the axillary lymph nodes are positive for cancer

Ref.: 21

COMMENTS: See Question 63.

63. Which of the following statements regarding axillary sentinel lymph node biopsy for breast cancer is/are true?

A. Axillary sentinel lymph nodes are successfully identified over 90% of the time in experienced hands.

B. If there is concordance of identification of the sentinel lymph node by both radionuclide and blue dye techniques, the false-negative rate for diagnosing positive axillary lymph nodes is essentially zero.

C. The risk of arm swelling, sensory deficits, and shoulder stiffness is much lower following sentinel lymph node biopsy than following standard axillary dissection.

D. If the sentinel lymph node is positive for cancer, a more complete axillary dissection (level I or level I and II) should usually be performed.

Ref.: 21

COMMENTS: All invasive breast cancers have the potential to metastasize to axillary lymph nodes. • The accurate pathologic assessment of these nodes affects the prognosis and may affect the recommendation for adjuvant systemic therapy, depending on features of the primary tumor. • This is especially true for small cancers (<1 cm), for which systemic therapy would not generally be recommended if the nodes are negative. • The increasing use of sentinel lymph node biopsy for axillary assessment for breast cancer has come from a desire to assess the axillary status accurately, with lower risks of lymphedema, numbness, and shoulder stiffness, which are attendant to the more aggressive standard axillary dissection techniques. • The sentinel lymph node biopsy procedure is especially well suited for small primary tumors where the likelihood of axillary metastasis is low (Question 62). • In such cases, whether the axilla is assessed by sentinel lymph node biopsy or standard axillary dissection, radiation therapy is still indicated to reduce the incidence of in-breast tumor recurrence, regardless of the nodal status. • Mastectomy would not be required for such a patient, since the cure rate would not be improved.

The sentinel lymph node biopsy technique is accomplished by injecting a small amount of radioactive material (technetium sulfur colloid) and/or blue dye (usually isosulfan blue dye) into the area of the tumor, subdermally around the tumor site or in the periareolar area. • The periareolar injection is especially well suited for cases in which the primary tumor has already been excised or when it is located in close proximity to the axillary nodes. • These materials are transported through the same lymph vessels to the same lymph node as cancer cells from the primary tumor would be if lymph node metastases were to have occurred. • By scanning the axilla with a gamma probe for a "hot" area or by visually searching for a "blue" node, a much more limited incision and exploration of the axilla can be performed, reducing the risk of lymphedema, sensory deficits, and shoulder stiffness to negligible levels. • One or more lymph nodes (rarely more than three) are usually identified and can be carefully assessed pathologically by both standard histologic and immunohistochemical staining techniques. • Using one or both of these localizing techniques results in identifying at least one sentinel lymph node in approximately 95% of cases. • Unfortunately, the sentinel lymph node technique is not 100% accurate. • Among patients with histologically positive nodes, the sentinel lymph node technique failed to identify the positive node in up to 10% of cases, even if the node was identified by both radioactive and blue dye techniques. • When the sentinel lymph node is shown to contain tumor, it is generally thought that the axillary assessment should be completed with a level I and II dissection to look for other nodal involvement, which could bear on the prognosis and postoperative therapy recommendations. • This is somewhat controversial, however, because in most cases the recommendation for subsequent therapy may not change. • Sentinel lymph node biopsy has become an appropriate alternative to standard axillary dissection for clinically node-negative breast cancers, although results of large randomized trials are still pending. • Sentinel lymph node biopsy is not appropriate for evaluation of the clinically positive axilla.

ANSWERS:
Question 62: B
Question 63: A, C, D

64. What is the incidence of lymphedema after axillary node dissection (levels I and II)?

A. 5%

B. 10%

C. 20%

D. 40%

E. 50%

Ref.: 4

COMMENTS: The incidence of lymphedema after axillary node dissection ranges from 15–30% depending on the definition used. • The probability of lymphedema increases with greater dissection and level of nodes removed, the tumor burden in the axilla, the presence of lymphedema before surgery, and if radiation is applied to the field after surgery. • With the advent of sentinel node biopsy, the rate of lymphedema has been shown to be much lower, in the range of 2–4%.

ANSWER:
C

65. Radiation delivered to the breast after lumpectomy and sentinel node biopsy for a 1.2-cm node-negative infiltrating ductal carcinoma is likely to be associated with which of the following?

A. Decreased risk of systemic relapse

B. Increased risk of lymphoma

C. Cardiac toxicity

D. Radiation pneumonitis

E. Decreased risk of local relapse

Ref.: 4

COMMENTS: The addition of breast irradiation after breast conservation has been shown in multiple randomized trials to decrease the incidence of breast tumor recurrence. • Some studies have shown a survival benefit although this is not a uniformly accepted result. • Lymphoma is not associated with breast irradiation.

- The incidence of cardiac toxicity and radiation pneumonitis with modern techniques of radiation therapy planning and dosimetry is very low.

ANSWER:

E

66. For which patients are aromotase inhibitors, such as Arimidex or Femara, useful?

    A. Premenopausal women

    B. Perimenopausal women

    C. Postmenopausal women

    D. High-risk 35-year-old woman with LCIS

Ref.: 4,7

COMMENTS: Aromotase inhibitors are useful only in the postmenopausal setting. • In postmenopausal women, the ovaries stop producing estrogen, but low levels of estrogen remain because aromatase converts other steroid hormones into estrogen. • Aromatase inhibitors block production of estrogen by aromatase in postmenopausal women. • The ATAC trial results showed that, in postmenopausal women taking Arimedex, there was a lower recurrence rate, a lower chance of developing a new primary, and less toxicity than in women taking tamoxifen.

ANSWER:

C

67. What additional treatment should a patient with a 2-cm focus of ER-positive DCIS transected at a surgical margin by lumpectomy receive?

    A. Radiation only

    B. Tamoxifen only

    C. Surgical re-excision, radiation, and tamoxifen

    D. Surgical re-excision only

Ref.: 4,7

COMMENTS: If ductal carcinoma has been transected at the margin of resection, its rate of recurrence is unacceptably high in both the noninvasive and invasive forms. • Re-excision to clear margins is the standard of care. • Subsequent radiation therapy significantly reduces local recurrence and is recommended for all but the smallest of tumors. • The addition of tamoxifen has been shown to further decrease the incidence of recurrent DCIS and new invasive breast cancer. • Recent studies have shown that this benefit is best seen in ER-positive DCIS.

ANSWER:

C

68. For a 44-year-old woman with a core-biopsy-proven 7-cm infiltrating ductal carcinoma in her right breast with a clinically negative axilla, which of the following treatment plans would be appropriate?

    A. Modified radical mastectomy followed by chemotherapy and radiation

    B. Lumpectomy with clear margins, sentinel node biopsy, and radiation therapy

    C. Preoperative radiation followed by modified radical mastectomy

    D. Preoperative chemotherapy followed by modified radical mastectomy

    E. Preoperative tamoxifen followed by modified radical mastectomy

Ref.: 1, 2

COMMENTS: Large breast cancers (>5 cm) are usually not amenable to breast conservation. • Neoadjuvant chemotherapy results in survival rates that are equivalent to those achieved with postoperative adjuvant therapy and in some instances has reduced the primary tumor size to that which would permit an attempt at lumpectomy. • Neoadjuvant therapy can result in pathologic downstaging of the axilla, which has led some to recommend sentinel node biopsy of the clinically negative axilla before commencing the neoadjuvant treatment.

ANSWER:

A, D

69. Which of the following is/are associated with the appearance of invasive lobular carcinomas on mammograms and ultrasound images?

    A. Discrete masses

    B. Multicentric appearance

    C. Partially cystic appearance

    D. Indistinct masses with poorly defined borders

    E. Calcifications

Ref.: 8

COMMENTS: Compared with invasive ductal carcinomas, invasive lobular carcinomas tend to be more indistinct and difficult to visualize on mammograms. • The extent of the tumor is often underestimated on the mammogram and may be more accurately appreciated by ultrasound imaging or MRI. • Nonetheless, recurrence and survival rates for invasive lobular carcinoma are equivalent to those for ductal carcinoma, stage for stage.

ANSWER:

D

70. In which population is the incidence of BRCA mutations highest?

    A. Pima Indians

    B. Inhabitants of southern China

    C. Ashkenazi Jews

    D. Patients with a first-degree relative age 55 with breast cancer

    E. Patients with a history of radiation therapy for Hodgkin's disease

Ref.: 11

COMMENTS: The BRCA mutation rate is highest among Ashkenazi Jews, ranging from 1–3%. • The incidence of breast cancer in those who have received mantel radiation for Hodgkin's disease is five times that of the general population. • A person with a first-degree relative with postmenopausal breast cancer has a relative risk of 1.8 times that of the general population.

ANSWER:
C

71. What is the increased relative risk of breast cancer associated with hormone replacement therapy of more than 5 years' duration?

    A. 1.0

    B. 1.3

    C. 2.0

    D. 5.5

    E. 10.2

Ref.: 7, 9

COMMENTS: Results of the Women's Health Initiative (WHI) study of postmenopausal women receiving hormone replacement therapy has shown that the relative risk of developing breast cancer after 5 years of use is 1.35, or a 26% increase in risk. • In addition, there was an increased risk of stroke and an unexpected increase in the risk of coronary artery disease in long-term hormone replacement therapy users.

ANSWER:
B

72. A patient has an excisional biopsy of a well-defined, palpable mass. The final pathologic studies revealed a 2-cm fibradenoma containing a small focus of LCIS. What should the clinician do next?

    A. Recommend wide local re-excision of the LCIS

    B. Recommend radiation therapy

    C. Recommend a modified radical mastectomy

    D. Inform the patient that she has an increased incidence of invasive carcinoma in the ipsilateral breast only

    E. Inform the patient that she has an increased risk of invasive cancer in either breast

Ref.: 4, 7

COMMENTS: The diagnosis of LCIS is a risk factor for the development of invasive carcinoma, although LCIS is not itself necessarily a preinvasive condition. • The increased risk applies to both breasts equally for both invasive ductal and lobular carcinoma. • Surgical excision will have no therapeutic value. • Appropriate management options include careful surveillance, tamoxifen chemoprevention, or bilateral total mastectomies. • The relative risk is 16.4, or an annual incidence of 1.8%.

ANSWER:
E

73. What is the approximate false-negative rate for a sentinel node biopsy?

    A. 1%

    B. 8%

    C. 15%

    D. 20%

    E. 25%

Ref.: 4, 7

COMMENTS: The sentinel node biopsy technique has a learning curve of approximately 30 cases before proficiency is attained. • In experienced hands, the false-negative rate ranges from 4–12%. • The use of tracer blue dye versus technetium-labeled sulfur colloid or both has not been shown to affect the detection rate or false-negative rate if the surgeon is proficient. • Isosulfan blue dye, however, is associated with a small incidence of anaphylactoid reactions.

ANSWER:
B

74. What is the relative risk of developing breast carcinoma that is associated with a finding of atypical duct hyperplasia on the cytologic evaluation of nipple fluid aspirate?

    A. 1

    B. 2.5

    C. 4.9

    D. 18

    E. 20

Ref.: 4, 7

COMMENTS: The evaluation of nipple fluid aspirate for the presence of atypia has been gaining more interest recently with the advent of ductal lavage, which helps in obtaining larger cell samples. The technique currently raises as many questions as answers and should be utilized only in the setting of a clinical research protocol. Studies of patients having nipple fluid aspirate with atypia have shown an increased risk of breast cancer that is even greater with a first-degree relative with breast cancer.

ANSWER:
C

75. Which of the following statements regarding skin-sparing mastectomy is/are true?

    A. It leaves additional breast tissue to form a better mound for reconstruction.

    B. It improves the cosmetic result, with a more symmetrical and natural breast envelope.

    C. It has been associated with a higher risk of skin recurrence.

    D. It includes preserving the nipple-areolar complex.

Ref.: 7, 12

COMMENTS: The use of skin-sparing mastectomy has been shown to improve the cosmetic result by leaving a more symmetrical and natural breast mound. • Skin-sparing mastectomy should not be used if breast reconstruction is to be delayed or not performed at all, since excess skin negatively affects the cosmetic result. • The oncologic safety of skin-sparing mastectomy has been demonstrated with T1 and T2 tumors. • The nipple-areolar complex should not be preserved because it contains ductal tissue.

ANSWER:
B

76. Which of the following is/are typically associated with breast pain?

A. Breast cancer

B. Excessive caffeine intake

C. DCIS

D. LCIS

E. Cyclical hormonal changes

Ref.: 4

COMMENTS: Although breast pain may be the most common presenting breast symptom, it is rarely associated with carcinoma. • Often, lifestyle and dietary changes result in improvement of mastalgia. • Decreasing caffeine intake and use of better support bras are the first steps in management of breast pain. • Medications such as danazol, primrose oil, and nonsteroidal anti-inflammatory drugs have been shown to be occasionally effective in refractory cases. • In many cases, patients report a lessening of the pain after being reassured that the pain is not associated with cancer.

ANSWER:
B, E

77. An ultrasound image of a patient's breast reveals a 2-cm simple cyst. Aspiration yields straw-colored, clear fluid, and there is complete resolution on postprocedure ultrasound imaging. What should the clinician's next step be?

A. Order repeat ultrasound imaging in 3 months.

B. Have the fluid sent to the laboratory for Hemoccult testing, cytologic studies, and assessment for tumor markers.

C. Perform wire-localized excision of the cavity.

D. Place the patient on antibiotics.

E. Advise the patient to continue with routine clinical breast examinations and mammograms.

Ref.: 7

COMMENTS: A simple cyst that completely resolves after aspiration of straw-colored fluid needs no further diagnostic or surgical evaluation. • Routine follow-up with clinical examination and scheduled mammograms is indicated. • If the cyst recurs, especially in the postmenopausal setting, surgical excision should be considered.

ANSWER:
E

78. Contraindications to breast-conserving therapy include which of the following?

A. Pregnancy in the first or second trimester

B. Two or more tumors in separate quadrants of the breast

C. Diffuse malignant-appearing calcifications

D. History of therapeutic irradiation to the breast or chest region

E. Inability to achieve a free margin of excision

Ref.: 4, 7

COMMENTS: Contraindications to breast-conserving therapy include early pregnancy, since the required radiation being delivered to the pregnant patient would harm the fetus. • However, breast-conserving therapy may be performed in the third trimester, with irradiation given after delivery. • Patients with multicentric disease and diffuse malignant-appearing calcification are not considered candidates for breast-conserving therapy. • The normal therapeutic dose of radiation combined with previous breast irradiation would result in excessive normal-tissue toxicity. • Persistent unsuccessful attempts at clearing a positive margin is another contraindication.

ANSWER:
A, B, C, D, E

79. Regarding lumpectomy skin incision placement, which of the following yield(s) the best cosmetic results?

A. Curvilinear incisions along Langer's line

B. Radial incisions at the 3 o'clock and 9 o'clock positions

C. Excision of a segment of skin overlying the tumor

D. Periareolar incisions for peripheral tumors

Ref.: 4, 12

COMMENTS: Placement of the skin incision is of critical importance to the quality of cosmesis. • Often, using curvilinear skin incisions in Langer's lines in the superior breast above the 3 o'clock position achieves the best cosmetic results. • However, certain areas, such as the inferior breast between the 3 o'clock to 9 o'clock positions, are best served with radial incisions. • The incision should be close to the lesion. • When possible, preservation of the subcutaneous tissue improves the cosmetic result.

ANSWER:
A, B

80. What is the typical local recurrence rate after mastectomy?

A. 1%

B. 6%

C. 15%

D. 20%

E. 30%

Ref.: 7, 16

COMMENTS: Results of prospective randomized trials comparing breast conserving to mastectomy revealed a local recurrence rate for mastectomy ranging from 4–8%. • Local recurrence in the breast after lumpectomy and radiation is about 10%, while that following lumpectomy without radiation is as high as 40%. • Local control, however, does not necessarily translate to improved survival.

ANSWER:
B

81. What is the percentage of patients who have DCIS detected by mammography as opposed to a palpable finding?

A. 60%

B. 70%

C. 80%

D. 90%

Ref.: 1, 2

COMMENTS: Over the last 10 years, there has been an increase in the detection of DCIS by mammography, most often manifested by the presence of microcalcifications. • This has led to an increase in the use of breast conservation and radiotherapy as treatment for this condition.

ANSWER:
D

REFERENCES

1. Townsend CM, Beauchamp RD, Evers BM, et al (eds): *Sabiston Textbook of Surgery: The Biological Basis of Modern Surgical Practice,* 16th ed. WB Saunders, Philadelphia, 2001.
2. Schwartz SI, Shires GT, Spencer FC: *Principles of Surgery,* 7th ed. McGraw-Hill, New York, 1999.
3. American Joint Committee on Cancer: *Manual for Staging of Cancer,* 6th ed. Springer-Verlag, 2002.
4. Bland KI, Copeland EM: *The Breast: Comprehensive Management of Benign and Malignant Diseases.* WB Saunders, Philadelphia, 1998.
5. Overgaard M, Hanson P, Overgaard J, et al: Postoperative radiotherapy in high-risk premenopausal women with breast cancer who receive adjuvant chemotherapy. *N Engl J Med* 337:949–955, 1997.
6. Ragaz J, Jackson S, Le N, et al: Adjuvant radiotherapy and chemotherapy in node-positive premenopausal women with breast cancer. *N Engl J Med* 337:956–962, 1997.
7. Harris J, Lippman M, Morrow M, et al: *Diseases of the Breast.* Lippincott-Raven, Philadelphia, 2000.
8. Tabar L, Dean PB: *Teaching Atlas of Mammography.* Thieme, New York, 2001.
9. Early Breast Cancer Trialists' Collaborative Group: Tamoxifen for early breast cancer: an overview of the randomised trials. *Lancet* 351:1451–1467, 1998.
10. Early Breast Cancer Trialists' Collaborative Group: Polychemotherapy for early breast cancer: an overview of the randomised trials. *Lancet* 352:930–941, 1998.
11. Olopade O, Weber B: Breast cancer genetics: toward molecular characterization of individuals at increased risk for breast cancer. In: *PPO Updates: Principles and Practice of Oncology,* vol 12, nos 10, 11, 1998.
12. Hartrampf C (ed): *Breast Reconstruction with Living Tissue.* Hampton Press, Norfolk, VA, 1991.
13. Goldwyn R (ed): *Reduction Mammoplasty.* Little, Brown, Boston, 1990.
14. Hunt KK, Baldwin BJ, Strom EA, et al: Feasibility of postmastectomy radiation therapy after TRAM flap breast reconstruction. *Ann Surg Oncol* 4:377–384, 1997.
15. Deapen DM, Bernsteri L, Brody GS: Are breast implants anticarcinogenic: a 14-year follow-up of the Los Angeles study. *Plast Reconstr Surg* 99:1346–1353, 1997.
16. Taylor ME: Breast: locally advanced (T3 and T4), inflammatory, and recurrent tumors. In: Perez CA, Brady LW (eds) *Principles and Practice of Radiation Oncology,* 3rd ed. Lippincott-Raven, Philadelphia, 1998.
17. Fowble B: Postmastectomy radiation: then and now. *Oncology* 11:213–239, 1997.
18. Fisher B, Anderson S, Redmond C, et al: Re-analysis and results after 12 years of follow-up in a randomized clinical trial comparing total mastectomy with lumpectomy with or without irradiation in the treatment of breast cancer. *N Engl J Med* 333:1456–1461, 1995.
19. Perez CA, Taylor ME: Breast: stage Tis, T1 and T2 tumors. In: Perez CA, Brady LW (eds) *Principles and Practice of Radiation Oncology,* 3rd ed. Lippincott-Raven, Philadelphia, 1998.
20. Cameron J: *Current Surgical Therapy.* Mosby, St. Louis, 1998.
21. Krag D, Weaver D, Ashikaga T, et al: The sentinel node in breast cancer: a multicenter validation study. *N Engl J Med* 339:941–946, 1998.

Head and Neck

José M. Velasco, M.D., and Tina J. Hieken, M.D.

1. Match the lettered parts (A–F) of the illustrated pharynx and larynx with the anatomic structures listed below.

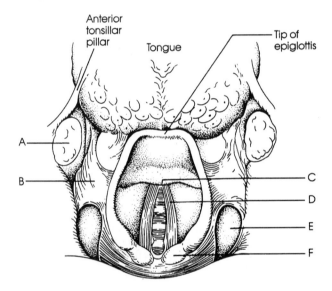

Anterior tonsillar pillar
Tongue
Tip of epiglottis

a. Arytenoid process
b. Vocal cord
c. Pharyngoepiglottic fold
d. Anterior commissure
e. Palatine tonsil
f. Piriform sinus

A. Arytenoid process
B. Vocal cord
C. Pharyngoepiglottic fold
D. Anterior commissure
E. Palatine tonsil
F. Piriform sinus

Ref.: 1

COMMENTS: The larynx extends from the tip of the epiglottis superiorly to the cricoid cartilage inferiorly and from the posterior commissure and mucoperichondrium of the cricoid posteriorly to the lingual surface of the epiglottis, thyrohyoid membrane, and thyroid and cricoid cartilages anteriorly. • The larynx may be divided into three regions: the supraglottic, glottic, and subglottic larynx. • The **supraglottic larynx** consists of structures superior to the true vocal cords and includes the laryngeal ventricle, false vocal cords (ventricular bands), arytenoids, aryepiglottic folds, and epiglottis. • The **glottic larynx** consists of the true vocal cords only. • The **subglottic larynx** extends from the undersurface of the true cords to the inferior border of the cricoid cartilage. • The **hypopharynx** is made up of the piriform sinuses, the postcricoid mucosa, and the lateral and posterior pharyngeal walls. • Knowledge of these anatomic sites is required for proper staging and treatment of tumors in this area.

ANSWER:
A-e; B-c; C-d; D-b; E-f; F-a

2. Which one of the following anatomic sites is considered to be part of the oral cavity?

A. Retromolar trigone

B. Palatine tonsil

C. Soft palate

D. Posterior third of tongue

Ref.: 1, 2

COMMENTS: The **oral cavity** is bounded *anteriorly* by the skin-vermilion border of the lips and includes the buccal mucosa, upper and lower alveolar ridges, retromolar trigone, floor of the mouth, anterior two thirds of the tongue, and hard palate. • *Posteriorly*, the oral cavity is bounded by the junction between the hard and soft palates and the junction between the anterior two thirds and the posterior one third of the tongue. • The *lateral* borders are defined by the anterior tonsillar pillars.

The **oropharynx**, which is not considered part of the oral cavity, is bounded by the palatine tonsils, soft palate, posterior third of the tongue, and posterior pharyngeal wall. • The more posterior oropharyngeal tumors have a higher likelihood of regional lymph node metastases than do those in a more anterior location because of the rich lymphatic network in the pharyngeal submucosa. • Among tumors within the oral cavity, there are also differences in the likelihood of regional nodal disease (e.g., tumors of the gingiva are less likely to have nodal metastases than are tumors of the floor of the mouth).

ANSWER:
A

3. Regarding the anatomy of the parotid gland, which one of the following statements is true?

   A. The parotid gland is bilobar, divided into two well-defined lobes (superficial and deep) based on the neurovascular supply of the gland and embryologic lobar encapsulation.

   B. The facial nerve and its branches course superficially to the external parotid fascia and therefore may be injured during parotid surgery.

   C. Injury to one or more branches of the facial nerve may occur during operations on the submandibular salivary gland as well as on the parotid gland.

   D. The main trunk of the facial nerve and its divisions are more craniad (superior) and deep in infants than in adults.

Ref.: 1, 3, 4

COMMENTS: The parotid gland is a unilobar structure embryologically and is considered clinically to be divided into a superficial (or lateral) and a deep lobe, as defined by the portions of the gland that lie, respectively, superficial and deep to the facial nerve, which ramifies through the gland. • Superficial lobe tumors necessitate identification of the trunk and branches of the facial nerve, with dissection of the tumor and superficial lobe off the underlying nerve. • Deep lobe tumors are usually approached by an initial superficial lobectomy, followed by removal of the deep lobe from between or underneath the branches of the facial nerve. • Swinging around the tail of the gland, without following the marginal mandibular branch proximally to distally, the so-called "flanking maneuver," is the most common cause of a facial nerve injury. • Injury to the marginal mandibular branch of the facial nerve may also occur during submandibular salivary gland surgery, since this nerve courses deep to the platysma over the external facial vessels, which are in close approximation to the lateral capsule of the gland. • The lingual and hypoglossal nerves are also at risk during submandibular gland surgery and should be identified to avoid inadvertent injury. • In infants and young children, the facial nerve trunk is located more caudad (inferiorly) and superficially than in adults. • Transection of the nerve trunk has been reported after excision of upper cervical as well as parotid lesions in these young patients.

ANSWER:
C

4. Match the description in the left-hand column with the correct anatomic triangle in the right-hand column.

   A. Formed by the anterior margin of the sternocleidomastoid muscle, the midline of the neck, and the inferior margin of the mandible — a. Anterior triangle

   B. Formed by the posterior margin of the sternocleidomastoid muscle, the trapezius muscle, and the middle third of the clavicle — b. Posterior triangle

   C. Formed by the anterior and posterior bellies of the digastric muscle and the inferior border of the mandible — c. Submandibular triangle

   D. Formed by the midline of the neck, the superior belly of the omohyoid muscle, and the anterior border of the sternocleidomastoid muscle — d. Muscular triangle

Ref.: 5

COMMENTS: The bones and muscles of the neck divide it into anatomic triangles. • The **anterior triangle** is bounded by the anterior margin of the sternocleidomastoid muscle, the midline of the neck, and the inferior margin of the mandible. • It is further subdivided into the submental, submandibular, carotid, and muscular triangles by the digastric muscle, the hyoid bone, and the superior belly of the omohyoid muscle. • The **posterior triangle** of the neck is bounded by the sternocleidomastoid and trapezius muscles (which attach on the superior nuchal line, forming the apex of this triangle) and the middle third of the clavicle (which forms its base). • The posterior triangle is further subdivided into the occipital and subclavian triangles by the posterior belly of the omohyoid muscle.

ANSWER:
A-a; B-b; C-c; D-d

5. Match the cervical lymph node level in the left-hand column with the corresponding anatomic description in the right-hand column.

   A. Level I   a. Prelaryngeal, pretracheal, and paratracheal
   B. Level II   b. Upper jugulodigastric
   C. Level III   c. Posterior triangle
   D. Level IV   d. Submental and submandibular
   E. Level V   e. Middle jugulodigastric
   F. Level VI   f. Upper mediastinal
   G. Level VII   g. Lower jugulodigastric

Ref.: 1, 5, 6

COMMENTS: The cervical lymphatics have been grouped into seven basins. • Knowledge of the anatomy of each nodal group is critical to proper identification and staging of head and neck tumors. • **Level I** contains the submental and submandibular nodes and is bounded by the anterior and posterior bellies of the digastric muscle, the mandible superiorly, and the hyoid bone inferiorly. • **Level II** is the upper jugular nodal group, extending from the posterior belly of the digastric muscle medially to the posterior border of the sternocleidomastoid muscle laterally and from the skull base superiorly to the hyoid bone inferiorly. • **Level III** is the middle jugular nodal group, extending from the hyoid bone superiorly to the cricoid cartilage inferiorly. • **Level IV** is the lower jugular nodal group, extending from the level of the cricoid cartilage superiorly to the clavicle inferiorly. • Levels III and IV share the same lateral border: the posterior margin of the sternocleidomastoid muscle. • Posterior and lateral to levels II, III, and IV is **Level V**, consisting of the lymph nodes of the posterior triangle. • **Level VI** is the anterior compartment nodal group, including the prelaryngeal, pretracheal, and paratracheal nodes from the hyoid superiorly to the sternal notch inferiorly and laterally to the medial borders of the carotid sheaths. • **Level VII** contains the upper mediastinal lymph nodes inferior to the suprasternal notch. • Other lymph node groups that may be involved in metastases from head and neck cancers include the suboccipital, retropharyngeal, parapharyngeal, preauricular, and parotid lymph nodes.

ANSWER:
A-d; B-b; C-e; D-g; E-c; F-a; G-f

6. Match each of the clinical characteristics of cleft lip and palate in the left-hand column with the appropriate anatomic defect in the right-hand column.

   A. Involves the lip, alveolus, or both — a. Cleft of primary palate

   B. Involves the hard and soft palates — b. Cleft of secondary palate

C. Should be closed between 10 and 14 weeks of age

D. Should be closed between 10 and 14 months of age

c. Both cleft of primary palate and cleft of secondary palate

d. Neither cleft of primary palate nor cleft of secondary palate

Ref.: 1, 2, 7

COMMENTS: Vertical paramedian clefts of the lip and palate are considered in two principal categories: clefts of the primary palate (the lip and alveolar ridge) and clefts of the secondary palate (hard and soft palate). • These clefts may occur alone or in association with each other, but the most common anomaly is a combined cleft lip and palate. • The timing of surgical correction varies with the specific type of defect. • Clefts of the lip are best repaired at 10 to 14 weeks of age, enabling the infant to achieve more normal patterns of feeding. • Repair of a cleft palate is usually delayed until sometime between 10 and 14 months of age to facilitate the technical closure. • Lip coaptation may be performed earlier to decrease the gap at the time of definitive surgery. • Delay beyond the age of 2 years, when the child is beginning to develop skills of speech, may result in permanent speech disability. • These closures are usually performed by means of local rotation flaps and are technically challenging. • Patients benefit from multidisciplinary care from a cleft and craniofacial team that includes audiologists, facial plastic surgeons, geneticists, orthodontists, oral surgeons, otolaryngologists, and speech pathologists.

ANSWER:
A-a; B-b; C-a; D-b

7. Regarding obstructive sleep apnea (OSA), which one of the following statements is true?

A. It is a rare disorder.

B. It is seen only in morbidly obese patients who are more than 100% over their expected body weight.

C. Initial surgical treatment usually involves tracheostomy.

D. It may be associated with cardiac arrhythmias, myocardial infarction, and death.

E. It is a contraindication for weight reduction surgery.

Ref.: 2, 7, 8

COMMENTS: OSA is a common disorder that affects at least 10% of the population. • It is more common and more severe in morbidly obese patients but occurs in patients who are not obese. • It is more common in patients with relative micrognathia or retrognathia. • It is often associated with difficult anesthetic intubation. • Symptoms include snoring and excessive daytime somnolence. • There are many surgical and nonsurgical treatments available to treat OSA. • Nasal continuous positive airway pressure (CPAP) used by the patient during sleep is the mainstay of treatment. • Surgical options include uvulopalatopharyngoplasty and hyoid suspension procedures. • Occasionally, patients require permanent tracheostomy. • Eligible morbidly obese patients with sleep apnea will benefit from weight reduction operations. • Other surgical procedures that are more specific and less common include orthognathic surgery to correct retrognathia and procedures to reduce the volume of tissue at the tongue base. • Patients with OSA desaturate during periods of apnea. • This is usually worse if a patient has been sedated or received narcotics. • Desaturation may be a cause of arrhythmias, myocardial infarction, and death in the postoperative patient.

ANSWER:
D

8. Regarding sinusitis in the critically ill patient, which of the following statements is true?

A. The diagnosis is based on plain radiographs.

B. The diagnosis is based on computed tomographic (CT) scan evidence of sinusitis.

C. The predominant organisms are gram-positive bacteria.

D. The correlation between clinical infectious sinusitis and radiographic signs is poor.

E. Treatment includes high-dose corticosteroids.

Ref.: 10

COMMENTS: Acute sinusitis is a nosocomial infection. • Diagnosis should be entertained in intubated patients with fever of unknown origin. • The incidence is higher among neurosurgical patients. • Diagnosis requires identification of an organism, usually gram-negative organisms *(Pseudomonas)*, and radiographic evidence of sinusitis. • Plain radiographs were formerly used to establish the diagnosis in patients with and without nasal discharge, but the maxillary, ethmoid, and sphenoid sinuses are best evaluated by CT scan. • The classic findings of sinusitis—mucosal thickening, opacification, and air-fluid levels—alone do not predict infection. • The diagnosis requires the presence of purulent discharge and positive bacteriologic study results. • Treatment is based on removal of nasogastric and/or nasotracheal tubes and administration of antibiotics, antihistamines, and decongestants, including α-agonists. • Operative drainage is reserved for refractory cases.

ANSWER:
D

9. Which one of the following statements accurately pertains to the management of full-thickness lacerations of the lip?

A. Layered closure is unnecessary except when required for hemostasis.

B. A frequent cause of wound breakdown is ischemic necrosis secondary to the relatively poor labial blood supply.

C. The extent of soft-tissue loss in labial lacerations is frequently underestimated.

D. Proper apposition of the vermilion border is the principal determinant of cosmetic outcome.

Ref.: 1

COMMENTS: The proper management of full-thickness labial lacerations involves débridement of devitalized tissue and a layered closure of the mucosa, labial musculature, and skin with fine absorbable and nonabsorbable sutures, with particular attention paid to the accurate apposition of the vermilion border. • Because of the circular and radial orientation of the labial musculature, labial lacerations frequently open widely, leading to the erroneous assumption that there has been significant soft-tissue loss. • The blood supply of the perioral area is excellent and is rarely of concern when repairing these wounds. • Pathogenic oral anaerobes have occasionally been implicated as the cause of wound breakdown and local infection. • For this reason, some clinicians recommend prophylactic antibiotic therapy.

A N S W E R :
D

10. Regarding disorders of the external ear, which one of the following statements is true?

   A. The "cauliflower ear," as seen in wrestlers and boxers, is caused by repeated soft-tissue infection of the pinna.

   B. Full-thickness lacerations of the pinna should be managed with sutures placed both on cutaneous surfaces and through the perichondrium or disrupted cartilage.

   C. Infections of the pinna superficial to the perichondrium should not be surgically drained, since they may be the cause of perichondritis.

   D. A foreign body in the ear canal should be removed immediately.

Ref.: 2, 7

COMMENTS: The presence of cartilage and its relationship to the perichondrium are important anatomic considerations when determining management of disorders of the pinna. • **Hematomas** usually occur between the perichondrium and underlying cartilage and should be drained by aspiration, if possible, or by incision. • Suturing a bolster to the site of drainage avoids reaccumulation. • Untreated hematomas can organize and calcify, resulting in a cauliflower ear.

For **full-thickness lacerations** of the pinna, a few sutures placed through cartilage help with alignment. • These lacerations should be repaired by reapproximating cartilage, perichondrium, and both skin surfaces.

Infections deep to the perichondrium should be promptly drained because, if untreated, they can lead to cartilage necrosis. • Superficial furuncles also may need to be drained if they do not resolve with warm soaks and antibiotics.

A **foreign body** in the ear canal is a problem particularly common in children. • A microscope is usually essential. • A foreign body is never an emergency, and removal should not be attempted by one not trained to do so. • The use of forceps may push a foreign body farther into the ear canal, injuring the tympanic membrane and ossicles. • With an uncooperative child, general anesthesia may be warranted for removing foreign bodies from the ear canal. • Animal or vegetable matter should not be irrigated in an attempt at removal, since this may cause the material to swell and make removal more difficult. • Removal of inanimate objects may be delayed if the canal is already irritated from previous attempts. • Irregularly shaped objects may be removed with fine forceps under the operating microscope. • Round objects, such as beads, can be removed only with strong suction or by passing a right-angle hook deep to them, turning them, and teasing them out. • After removal, the canal should be inspected for a second foreign body and to assess the status of the canal wall and tympanic membrane.

A N S W E R :
B

11. Regarding nasal trauma, which one of the following statements is true?

   A. Undisplaced nasal fractures require wire fixation to prevent subsequent displacement during the healing process.

   B. Septal hematomas rarely require surgical intervention.

   C. Cerebrospinal fluid (CSF) rhinorrhea requires urgent surgical intervention in order to prevent meningitis.

   D. Complications of retained nasal foreign bodies may include nasal septal abscess, sinusitis, orbital cellulitis, brain abscess, and cavernous sinus thrombosis.

   E. Nasal defects with exposed cartilage are best managed by a full-thickness skin graft.

Ref.: 1, 2, 7, 8

COMMENTS: Nasal fractures are the most common fractures of the facial skeleton and are nearly always associated with tearing of the overlying mucosa, thereby making them open fractures. • Clinical examination revealing displacement of nasal bones, localized bone tenderness, or crepitance on light palpation suggests the diagnosis. • Facial radiographs should be obtained to confirm the fracture as well as to look for fractures of other facial bones. • Undisplaced fractures require no specific therapy except external splinting for protection. • Radiographs of the nasal bones show them in lateral view and therefore can detect only anteroposterior displacement. • Lateral displacement can be assessed clinically and by CT scanning. • Many noncomminuted, displaced fractures can be treated by simple closed reduction.

Septal hematomas develop between the perichondrium and the underlying cartilage of the nasal septum. • Such hematomas frequently become infected and may produce avascular necrosis of the underlying cartilage because of separation from the perichondrium, resulting in a "saddle nose" deformity. • To prevent this problem, early diagnosis, prompt incision and drainage, septal splinting, and antibiotics to cover *Staphylococcus aureus* are indicated.

Severe nasal injury may be associated with **CSF rhinorrhea**, which may be suspected if clear fluid drains from the nose after injury. • It is strongly suggested if there is a high glucose content in the fluid. • The presence of β_2-transferrin in the fluid confirms that it is CSF. • Thin-cut CT scans should be used in all cases of traumatic CSF rhinorrhea to determine the site of the skull base injury. • Usually, a cribriform plate fracture is identifiable. • Most traumatic leaks seal without treatment. • The initial management is observation, head elevation, avoidance of nose blowing and straining, and possibly administration of antibiotics. • If the leak persists for more than 4–6 weeks or meningitis develops, the leak should be repaired surgically. • In most cases, the leak can be repaired via an endoscopic or traditional extracranial approach. • A frontal craniotomy may be used for more recalcitrant or cryptically located leaks. • Repair of facial fractures should not be delayed during a trial of conservative management for a CSF fistula because realignment of the bony fragments helps speed healing of the dural tear. • If leaking fluid cannot be collected or if the site of the leak cannot be determined, radiologic contrast studies are indicated. • As an adjunct to both surgical and conservative management, lumbar puncture and the use of a closed drainage system helps decrease the intracranial pressure, thus giving the dura a better chance to heal.

Nasal foreign bodies are quite common in children. • They are best managed either by placing a blunt hook deep to the foreign body and teasing it out or by using a Frazier suction tip. • Topical vasoconstrictors may decrease bleeding, which may be significant after removal of the object, especially if it has been present for some time. • Life-threatening aspiration may occur during attempts at foreign-body removal in an awake, uncooperative patient. • Therefore, general anesthesia should be considered. • Nasal foreign bodies should be removed promptly, since overlooked or retained nasal foreign bodies may lead to significant complications.

Nasal defects with exposed cartilage require coverage with a local nasal flap if the defect is small. • Larger defects may require a forehead flap or microvascular free flap for coverage.

ANSWER:
D

12. Match each of the benign conditions involving the tongue in the left-hand column with its appropriate characteristic in the right-hand column.

A. Lingual thyroid
B. Thyroglossal duct cyst
C. Median rhomboid glossitis
D. Granular cell myoblastoma

a. It requires no treatment.
b. It arises from nerve cells.
c. Resection may necessitate lifelong medication.
d. Surgical treatment involves resection of bone.

Ref.: 1, 3

COMMENTS: The four entities listed are among the many benign conditions that may involve the tongue. • **Lingual thyroid** results from failure of descent of the thyroid gland into the lower anterior neck. • This results in the clinical appearance of a reddish-brown mass emanating from the base of the tongue. • Resection of a lingual thyroid may be necessary because of pharyngeal obstruction from the mass. • Since this structure may represent the patient's only thyroid tissue, resection may render the patient hypothyroid and necessitate thyroid replacement therapy. • Thyroid scanning can establish the existence of other thyroid tissue.

Thyroglossal duct cysts also represent an anomaly of thyroid embryology in which there is failure of obliteration of the midline pharyngeal diverticulum during thyroid descent. • The clinical presentation is that of a midline cystic mass, usually appearing during childhood or adolescence. • A thyroglossal duct cyst may be distinguished from other midline neck masses by watching it elevate with protrusion of the tongue. • Proper surgical treatment involves excision of the entire tract, including the midportion of the hyoid bone.

Median rhomboid glossitis results from the failure of fusion of the lateral halves of the tongue. • It is a clinically innocuous anomaly and requires no treatment.

Granular cell myoblastoma is a benign proliferation of Schwann cells that occurs in the tongue as well as in other sites of the aerodigestive tract, especially the larynx. • It may appear clinically similar to carcinoma of the tongue but has no malignant potential and is properly treated by local surgical (wedge) excision.

ANSWER:
A-c; B-d; C-a; D-b

13. Regarding oropharyngeal abscesses, which one of the following statements is true?

A. Peritonsillar, parapharyngeal, and retropharyngeal abscesses occur with approximately equal frequency among children younger than 10 years of age.

B. Parapharyngeal and retropharyngeal abscesses can progress rapidly to cause airway obstruction.

C. Drainage of peritonsillar, parapharyngeal, and retropharyngeal abscesses is best accomplished through the pharyngeal wall.

D. As with abscesses in other locations in the body, small drains should be placed into transpharyngeally drained abscesses to promote continued evacuation of the abscess cavity.

Ref.: 1, 2, 7, 9

COMMENTS: Oropharyngeal abscesses have distinct epidemiologic characteristics and management protocols, depending on their location. • **Peritonsillar** abscesses are rare in children younger than age 10, even though they represent complications of acute tonsillitis. • The patient may be quite ill and present with trismus and severe odynophagia. • An initial trial of antibiotics and needle aspiration of the abscess are warranted. • If there is no response within 24 hr, aspiration should be repeated or incision and drainage performed. • Unlike a parapharyngeal or retropharyngeal abscess, which may progress rapidly and cause airway obstruction, the peritonsillar abscess is more limited and rarely causes airway obstruction.

Retropharyngeal abscesses occur in infants, young children, and elderly adults. • They are rare after the age of 10 years. • In children, these infections are due to the lymphadenitis associated with pharyngitis. • In elderly individuals, they are caused by foreign bodies or Pott's disease. • The infant may present in opisthotonus, and the clinical picture is often confused with that of meningitis. • The fever is often high, and the patient may drool as a result of odynophagia. • Physical examination reveals a boggy, fluctuant texture of the retropharyngeal tissues and inability to palpate the normally palpable vertebral bodies. • The swelling is unilateral because of the midline laryngeal raphe. • Radiologic evaluation may show gas in the retropharyngeal soft tissue or widening of this space. • Loss of the airway is a potential hazard. • Antibiotics and surgical drainage through the posterior pharyngeal wall or the neck are the treatments of choice. • With both peritonsillar and retropharyngeal abscesses, aspiration of pus into the tracheobronchial tree is a distinct hazard and can be prevented by careful endotracheal intubation and placing the patient in the Trendelenburg position before drainage. • Drains are not required, since these abscess cavities tend to empty themselves during each swallowing motion.

Parapharyngeal abscesses occur in all age groups and may be secondary to dental infection, pharyngitis, or tonsillitis. • Because these abscesses occur more laterally, drainage through the oropharynx is hazardous, owing to the proximity to the internal carotid artery and jugular vein. • Parapharyngeal abscesses should be drained through the lateral neck, with a drain left in place to permit continued evacuation of the cavity. • An important concern is the ability of infection to spread from one space to another. • The greatest morbidity associated with these abscesses is from internal jugular vein thrombosis, vascular erosion, or spread into the mediastinum or abdomen via the prevertebral or retropharyngeal spaces.

ANSWER:
B

14. Regarding tracheotomy, which one of the following statements is not true?

A. Indications for tracheotomy include the inability to handle upper and lower respiratory secretions, respiratory obstruction, and prolonged intubation of greater than 5 days.

B. Elective temporary tracheotomy is often performed at the time of major resections of oral-cavity and oropharyngeal cancers to avoid airway compromise secondary to bleeding or edema in the postoperative period.

C. Alternatives to tracheotomy include percutaneous tracheotomy and tracheostomy.

D. Cricothyroidotomy has been associated with a higher incidence of vocal cord dysfunction and subglottic stenosis than has standard tracheotomy.

E. Percutaneous tracheotomy has a lower incidence of tracheal stenosis than does standard tracheotomy.

Ref.: 1, 2, 7, 8, 11

COMMENTS: The principal indications for tracheotomy include respiratory obstruction that cannot properly be managed with endotracheal intubation and the inability to evacuate secretions from the upper or lower respiratory tree. • Prolonged endotracheal intubation may lead to interarytenoid scarring or subglottic stenosis and necessitate tracheotomy. • However, the currently available low-pressure soft cuffs allow safe endotracheal intubation for up to 14 days. • Elective temporary tracheostomy is indicated to prevent loss of the airway after many major head and neck cancer resections that may be associated with bleeding into or edema of the surrounding soft tissues.

Advantages of tracheotomy include decreased tracheo-bronchial dead space and improved tracheobronchial toilet, oral hygiene, and comfort for the patient. • Patients with tracheotomy tubes can eat and speak, unlike patients with endotracheal tubes. • Disadvantages of tracheotomy include an inability of the patient to cough (because of bypass of the glottic closure mechanism), bypassing of the normal warming and humidification of inspired air in the upper respiratory tract, and direct exposure of the lower respiratory tract to environmental pathogens. • Postoperative complications of tracheotomy include pneumothorax, pneumome-diastinum, recurrent laryngeal nerve damage, airway stenosis, wound infection, and aspiration.

Percutaneous dilatational tracheotomy (PDT), with or without bronchoscopic guidance, has been proven to be a safe and reasonable alternative to standard tracheotomy. • Standard systems include a needle that pierces the soft tissue and trachea. • A guide wire is then used to guide dilators through the perforation until a tracheotomy tube is placed. • Bronchoscopy should be used to guide the PDT.

Tracheostomy involves suturing skin flaps directly to the trachea so that the stoma is epithelium lined and remains open without a tube. • Patients who require permanent tracheotomy for severe sleep apnea or laryngeal scarring not amenable to correction should have a tracheostomy instead of a tracheotomy.

Cricothyrotomy is a procedure to establish an immediate airway when airway obstruction is imminent or present and endotracheal intubation is not possible. • Packaged cricothyrotomy kits are easy to use, but any incision through the skin and directly through the cricothyroid membrane can establish an airway. • An endotracheal tube should be pushed through the incision if possible. • It should be converted to a standard tracheotomy within a few days, since prolonged cricothyrodotomy use has been associated with a higher incidence of long-term sequelae than has tracheotomy.

Tracheal stenosis is the most common long-term complication of tracheotomy. • It occurs distal to the stoma where the balloon is. • PDT has a lower incidence of stenosis than does conventional tracheotomy. • The use of high-volume, low-pressure balloons has significantly lowered the incidence of clinically significant stenosis.

ANSWER:
A

15. Regarding epistaxis, which one of the following statements is not true?

    A. In most cases, epistaxis occurs from the anteroinferior part of the nasal septum.

    B. Properly applied anteroposterior packing controls bleeding in 95% of cases.

    C. Hypoxemia is a potential complication of nasal packing.

    D. Ligation of the internal maxillary artery is ineffective for controlling epistaxis and should be avoided.

    Ref.: 1, 2, 7, 8, 11

COMMENTS: Approximately 90% of cases of epistaxis arise from a plexus of vessels (Kiesselbach's plexus) in the anteroinferior part of the nasal septum. • In most cases, it is easily controlled with simple digital pressure. • If this fails and if the bleeding site can be visualized, it can be cauterized chemically or electrically, although occasionally anterior nasal packing is required. • Absorbable packing is recommended for patients with coagulopathies.

In 10% of cases of epistaxis, the source is posterior, in the area of Woodruff's plexus. • This situation poses a potentially serious problem, since posterior epistaxis frequently occurs in patients with arteriosclerosis and hypertension and may be difficult to control. • It has significant associated morbidity, including hypoxia, sepsis, respiratory obstruction, cardiac arrhythmia or ischemia (or both), aspiration pneumonia, nasal necrosis, and sinusitis. • The initial attempt at controlling the bleeding should be with readily available anterior or combined anterior and posterior packs, which is successful in up to 95% of cases. • When such packing is utilized, antibiotics should be given prophylactically in an effort to prevent sinusitis and otitis media. • Air exchange is frequently hindered by the packing. • Since many of these patients have associated systemic and cardiopulmonary disease, supplemental oxygen (28% O_2 or less) should be administered. • Patients with cardiac or severe pulmonary disease should be placed on a monitor. • Posterior epistaxis that cannot be controlled with packing may be treated by transantral or transnasal endoscopic ligation of the internal maxillary artery. • The anterior ethmoid artery should be ligated if the bleeding site can be identified high in the lateral nasal walls. • Alcoholics or patients with chronic obstructive pulmonary disease should be considered for early internal maxillary or ethmoid artery ligation (or both). • This maneuver avoids nasal packing in this high-risk group. • Transfemoral carotid angiography and embolization with absorbable Gelfoam or polyvinyl alcohol particles is an option that may be utilized for recurrent epistaxis after unsuccessful surgical intervention in patients with nonoperable nasal tumors or who are poor anesthetic risks.

ANSWER:
D

16. Regarding laryngeal injury, which one of the following statements is true?

    A. Trauma is the second most common cause of laryngeal stenosis.

    B. Iatrogenic laryngeal stenosis occurs most often in the supraglottic location as a result of traumatic intubation attempts.

    C. Laryngeal trauma with associated respiratory difficulty should initially be managed with urgent tracheostomy rather than endotracheal intubation.

    D. Because the rigid component of the larynx is cartilage and not bone, fractures of the larynx do not occur.

    Ref.: 1, 2

COMMENTS: Because of high rates of compliance with vaccination programs and improved antibiotic therapy, trauma has replaced infectious diseases as the most common cause of laryngeal stenosis. • A significant proportion of laryngeal injuries are iatrogenic, related primarily to subglottic injury caused by prolonged intubation with a cuffed endotracheal tube. • The incidence of this complication has been reduced significantly by the use of endotracheal tubes with soft, low-pressure cuffs. • Posttraumatic stenoses may be managed by dilatation, laser therapy, or local excision with reconstruction of the stenotic segment. • Direct blows to the neck may result in fracture of the laryngeal cartilage or laryngotracheal disruption. • When such an injury is suspected and the patient is having difficulty breathing, urgent tracheotomy, under local anesthesia, should be performed. • Attempts at endotracheal intubation may be unsuccessful, compound the injury, or result in loss of the airway. • In the stable patient, preliminary evaluation should include fiberoptic nasolaryngoscopy and CT scanning. • Some patients, such as those with edema, small hematomas, small lacerations, or nondisplaced thyroid cartilage fractures, may be observed. • Those with more significant injuries require neck exploration (with or without laryngeal thyrotomy), open reduction and internal fixation of fractures (with wires or miniplates), and repair of mucosal lacerations to facilitate anatomic restoration of the larynx. • Exposed cartilage must be covered meticulously to prevent granulation and subsequent fibrosis. • Mucosal advancement flaps may be needed. • Early repair leads to the best outcome. • Stents may be needed in cases of severe injury.

ANSWER:
C

17. Regarding foreign bodies of the larynx and tracheobronchial tree, which of the following statements is/are true?

    A. The ability to speak is an important differentiating sign for diagnosing the cause of cyanosis and respiratory difficulty that occurs while eating.

    B. Complete occlusion of the larynx with a food bolus should be managed immediately by tracheostomy.

    C. Radiographs are not beneficial in localizing the site of bronchial obstruction by radiolucent foreign bodies.

    D. The cessation of coughing 30 minutes after inhalation of a foreign body indicates that the foreign body has been coughed out.

    E. Infectious complications are the rare long-term sequelae of retained tracheobronchial foreign bodies.

Ref.: 1, 2, 7

COMMENTS: The "café coronary," in which a patient becomes dyspneic and cyanotic while eating, may be due to myocardial infarction, arrhythmia, or airway obstruction from a food bolus. • The inability to exchange air and to speak suggests aspiration as the cause of the difficulty. • If the choking person is able to exchange adequate amounts of air, he or she should be left alone but observed closely. • If there is complete obstruction of air exchange, initial treatment includes an attempt to dislodge the foreign body with the Heimlich (abdominal thrust) maneuver. • Emergency tracheostomy is hazardous and should be employed only as a last-resort, lifesaving measure. • Inhalation of foreign bodies into the tracheobronchial tree where air exchange is still ongoing usually produces severe coughing that lasts up to 30 minutes. • After this time, the coughing may stop due to sensory neural adaptation. • This may be erroneously interpreted as a sign that the foreign body has been expelled and lead to a delay in diagnosis. • In most cases of a retained foreign body, this relatively asymptomatic latent period is followed by a cough productive of purulent sputum. • Infectious complications, including bronchiectasis, recurrent pneumonitis, lung abscess, and empyema, can follow. • Even when radiolucent objects have been inhaled, standard chest radiographs may assist in localizing the site of bronchiolar obstruction, as in cases in which a ball-valve type of expiratory obstruction produces a localized pulmonary emphysema or air trapping with mediastinal shift.

• The proper initial management of aspirated foreign bodies is retrieval via tracheobronchial endoscopy.

ANSWER:
A

18. Regarding foreign bodies of the esophagus, which of the following statements is/are true?

    A. Most esophageal foreign bodies are found just above the gastroesophageal junction.

    B. Fever during the first 12 hr after esophagoscopy is usually a sign of atelectasis.

    C. Dysphagia without pain is the clinical hallmark of the presence of a foreign body in the esophagus.

    D. Retrieval of esophageal foreign bodies through a rigid esophagoscope with the patient under general anesthesia is the treatment of choice.

    E. Follow-up esophagoscopy should be performed to diagnose possible underlying pathologic conditions.

Ref.: 1, 2, 7

COMMENTS: Esophageal foreign bodies lodge at points of natural narrowing: below the cricopharyngeus muscle, near the arch of the aorta, behind the right main stem bronchus, and at the gastroesophageal junction. • Approximately 95% of all esophageal foreign bodies are found immediately below the cricopharyngeus muscle. • Large foreign bodies in this area can produce partial airway obstruction as a result of extrinsic pressure on the membranous trachea. • In most instances, the clinical presentation is that of dysphagia and associated suprasternal pain. • Perforation may occur immediately, or it may be delayed. • The risk of perforation increases with the length of time the foreign body remains in the esophagus. • Perforation is diagnosed by the presence of tachycardia, fever, pain radiating to the back, soft-tissue crepitance, or radiographic demonstration of air in soft tissues. • The presence of a foreign body may be documented by standard and contrast x-rays. • Appropriate treatment involves rigid endoscopic retrieval of the foreign body with the patient under general anesthesia. • Fever or pain after esophagoscopy must be considered a sign of perforation until proved otherwise. • A chest x-ray (to rule out air in the mediastinum) and a thin barium swallow should be performed immediately. • Urgent drainage of the mediastinum and, if possible, closure of the perforation are essential and minimize the mortality associated with esophageal perforation. • Adult patients should be followed up to exclude underlying pathologic conditions, such as a neoplasm or reflux esophagitis.

ANSWER:
D, E

19. Regarding mandibular trauma, which one of the following statements is true?

    A. Most mandibular fractures are open fractures.

    B. Open reduction has fallen out of favor.

    C. Teeth lying within the fracture line of the mandible should be removed to prevent root abscesses.

    D. Malocclusion is the most common long-term complication of mandibular fractures.

E. Dislocations of the temporomandibular joint usually require open reduction and repair of the anterior capsule with the patient under general anesthesia.

Ref.: 1, 3, 7

COMMENTS: The diagnosis of mandibular fracture is usually easily made on careful clinical examination. • Signs of mandibular fracture are point tenderness, malocclusion, intraoral mucosal ecchymosis and laceration, instability on bimanual manipulation, and numbness of the lower lip due to inferior alveolar nerve damage. • Radiographs should be obtained to confirm the clinical impression and to search for associated occult facial bone fractures. • Most mandibular fractures are open fractures because they communicate with the oral cavity or skin. • Prophylactic antibiotics should be given in these cases. • The majority of mandibular fractures are adequately treated by intermaxillary wiring or with arch bars and elastic band stabilization. • Open reduction with internal fixation of mandibular fractures results in faster healing and greater comfort for the patient than after intermaxillary fixation and is gaining popularity. • Disadvantages of this technique include foreign-body implantation and decreased periosteal coverage of the fracture site. • It was formerly recommended that teeth lying within the fracture line be removed. • More recently, however, it has been recognized that many of these teeth are salvageable if the fracture is managed conservatively. • Malocclusion is the most common complication of mandibular fracture. • It results from failure to restore preinjury occlusion or from fragment destabilization. • If significant malocclusion occurs, a corrective operation is indicated. • Temporomandibular joint dislocations usually occur when the head of the mandibular condyle moves forward through a tear in the anterior joint capsule. • This problem can usually be managed with injection of anesthetic into the joint capsule and downward traction on the posterior molar teeth. • Cases of recurrent dislocation may require operative intervention.

ANSWER:
A, D

20. Match each type of maxillary fracture in the left-hand column with its appropriate anatomic description in the right-hand column.

A. Le Fort I	a. Transverse maxillary fracture
B. Le Fort II	b. Craniofacial dissociation
C. Le Fort III	c. Pyramidal fractures

Ref.: 1, 3, 7

COMMENTS: In 1900, Rene Le Fort classified midface fractures. • With **Le Fort I** fractures (transverse), fracture segments include the upper teeth, palate, lower portions of the pterygoid processes, and a portion of the wall of the maxillary sinus. • **Le Fort II** fractures (pyramidal) also contain the nasal bones and frontal processes of the maxilla. • Clinically, the malar eminences are usually not displaced, but there may be significant widening of the inner canthi of the eyes and bridge of the nose. • **Le Fort III** fractures (craniofacial dissociation) involve separation of the maxillae, nasal bones, and zygomas from their usual cranial attachments. • Treatment of these fractures is best carried out with direct operative exposure, manipulation of the fracture segments, and internal fixation with miniplates and microplates. • The incidence of these injuries has decreased significantly with the increased use of air bags, shoulder-lap seatbelts, padded dashboards, collapsible steering wheels, and the 55-mph speed limit.

• Multiple Le Fort fractures are common (e.g., a Le Fort I on one side with a Le Fort II on the other).

ANSWER:
A-a; B-c; C-b

21. Regarding acute suppurative parotitis, which one of the following statements is not true?

A. It usually occurs in elderly or debilitated patients.

B. Dehydration is a major contributing factor.

C. Immediate surgical drainage is mandatory.

D. The numerous vertically oriented fascial septa of the parotid space lead to multiloculated abscesses when infection progresses.

E. *S. aureus* is the most frequent causative organism.

Ref.: 1–3, 7

COMMENTS: Acute suppurative parotitis is a severe, life-threatening infection most often seen in dehydrated elderly or debilitated patients with poor oral hygiene. • Its pathogenesis is thought to be related to stasis within the salivary ducts as a result of increased viscosity. • *S. aureus* is the usual causative organism, but other organisms can be responsible in immunocompromised patients. • Initial treatment with appropriate intravenous hydration, warm packs, sialagogues, and antibiotics may be successful. • If improvement is not seen within 12 hr of initiating this treatment, surgical treatment is warranted. • Drainage is performed through a preauricular incision, with elevation of the skin to expose the parotid capsule and vertical incisions through the gland in a direction parallel to the branches of the facial nerve.

ANSWER:
C

22. Regarding nonneoplastic parotid disease, which one of the following statements is true?

A. A lacerated Stensen's duct should be ligated.

B. Recurrent acute sialoadenitis is thought to be an ascending infection from the oral cavity.

C. Most cases of chronic recurrent Sialodenitis are bilateral.

D. Parotidectomy, with its inherent risk of facial nerve injury, is considered too morbid a procedure for treatment of nonneoplastic conditions of the parotid gland.

Ref.: 1, 2, 11

COMMENTS: A transection of Stensen's duct should be repaired, if possible, by direct suture approximation over a small-catheter stent. • Ligation of the duct is sometimes required but may result in painful atrophy of the parotid gland, producing a contour deformity of the face. • Inflammatory conditions of the parotid gland include calculous disease and sialectasis, both of which may result in recurrent sialoadenitis. • Infection is thought to result from ascending involvement of the parenchyma from the oral cavity by way of the major duct. • Usually, only one gland is affected. • In the case of calculous disease, improper diet and abnormal salivary pH may predispose to the formation of stones in the major ducts. • These stones are usually present near the duct orifice and may be successfully treated by incising the duct orifice and removing the stone transorally. • Occasionally, infections continue to occur despite stone extraction, alteration of diet and oral hygiene, stimulation of salivary secretions, adequate hydration, and antibiotics. • In such circumstances, parotidectomy may be indicated. • Observing the principles of facial nerve identification and dissection reduces the risk of the operation.

ANSWER:
B

23. Regarding the technical aspects of parotid surgery, which one of the following statements is true?

   A. The facial nerve is best identified by locating its trunk after it has exited the stylomastoid foramen and before it enters the posterior aspect of the parotid gland as it runs deep to the posterior facial vein.

   B. Complete postoperative paralysis of the muscles supplied by one or more divisions of the facial nerve suggests that there has been disruption of or permanent injury to that division during surgery.

   C. The auriculotemporal nerve, although not specifically sought during parotid surgery, may be involved in postoperative morbidity.

   D. Sectioning the facial nerve during parotid surgery results in permanent degeneration of the nerve distal to the cut, making attempts at nerve reconstruction futile.

   E. The greater auricular nerve is rarely injured during parotid surgery, since it lies outside the usual anatomic borders of parotid dissection.

Ref.: 1, 2, 11

COMMENTS: Proper identification and preservation of the facial nerve and its branches are the keys to successful parotid surgery. • Formerly, it was believed that most parotid malignancies should be treated by radical parotidectomy, with deliberate sacrifice of the facial nerve. • Currently, it is thought that deliberate sacrifice of the nerve or its branches may be required only in instances of direct nerve invasion by tumor. • Nerve preservation and adjuvant postoperative radiation therapy have yielded local control rates equivalent to those seen with more radical surgery but without the inherent morbidity of facial nerve sacrifice. • Identifying its trunk as it exits the stylomastoid foramen best protects the facial nerve. • The trunk crosses superficial to the external carotid artery and posterior facial vein to enter the posterior aspect of the parotid gland approximately 1.5 cm deep to the gland surface. • Meticulous attention to technique and knowledge of surgical landmarks make identification safer. • Some surgeons advocate the use of a facial nerve monitor. • When scarring or tumor prevents initial dissection of the main trunk, the nerve may be found in a retrograde fashion by dissecting out its more peripheral branches first.

   Paresis or even complete paralysis of the muscles supplied by the facial nerve may occur in the absence of obvious nerve injury. • This is almost always a temporary phenomenon, and function usually returns within several months. • If the facial nerve or one of its major branches is deliberately or inadvertently cut during parotid surgery, immediate nerve repair or interposition nerve graft should be attempted, since there is at least some expectation of partial recovery in such circumstances. • When this fails, there are numerous techniques of neuromusculofascial transfers that may be employed in an effort to restore facial symmetry and animation. • Although the auriculotemporal nerve is not specifically sought during parotid surgery, disruption of these parasympathetic fibers and subsequent possible cross-reinnervation with branches of the

sympathetic supply to the skin may result in postoperative gustatory sweating (Frey's syndrome). • The most frequently injured nerve during parotid surgery is not the facial nerve but the greater auricular nerve, which usually ramifies through the posteroinferior portion of the gland. • Sectioning the nerve produces numbness of the lower portion of the auricle and periauricular skin.

ANSWER:
C

24. Match the grouped primary tumor sites in the left-hand column with the corresponding shared characteristic location of cervical lymph node metastases in the right-hand column. More than one answer may be appropriate.

   A. Oral cavity and facial skin
   B. Thyroid, oropharynx, hypopharynx, larynx, and cervical esophagus
   C. Posterior scalp, nasopharynx, breast, and gastrointestinal (GI) tract
   D. GI tract and breast
   E. Thyroid

   a. Level I
   b. Level II
   c. Level III
   d. Level IV
   e. Level V
   f. Level VI

Ref.: 1, 6, 9

COMMENTS: See Question 5. • Examination of the neck is a critical component of the staging evaluation of patients with a head and neck cancer. • An understanding of the usual paths of regional cervical lymph node drainage is critical. • Such knowledge may prompt the search for a second primary tumor when disease metastasizes to an unexpected site and is crucial for determining the proper evaluation of a patient with an enlarged cervical lymph node. • While characteristic nodal drainage patterns exist, drainage to various or multiple sites may occur, as the primary site groupings illustrate.

   Primary tumors from the facial skin and oral cavity, including the lip, often drain first to the submental and submandibular (level I) lymph nodes and then to levels II and III (upper and middle jugular groups). • Skip metastases can occur, however, with involvement of lower-echelon nodes occurring before upper-echelon nodes are involved. • Tumors arising in the oropharynx, hypopharynx, and larynx usually spread first to the upper, middle, and lower jugular nodes (levels II, III, and IV). • Tumors of the nasopharynx and the skin of the posterior scalp often metastasize to posterior triangle (level V) nodes. • Nasopharyngeal tumors may also metastasize to the jugular nodes (II, III, and IV). • Metastatic nodes in the posterior triangle also may be from a GI tract or breast primary tumor. • Thyroid tumors often spread to the middle and lower jugular nodes and/or involve the anterior compartment (level VI) nodes.

ANSWER:
A-a; B-e; C-d; D-c; E-b

25. Regarding neoplasms of the ear, which one of the following statements is not true?

   A. Most carcinomas of the pinna are related to excessive exposure to ultraviolet irradiation.

   B. Cancers of the external ear are more common in men than in women.

   C. Treatment of squamous cell carcinoma of the ear may involve surgical excision, Mohs micrographic resection, or radiotherapy.

D. Surgical excision of a high-grade, 1-cm squamous cell carcinoma of the ear should include 1-cm margins.

E. Rhabdomyosarcoma is the most common childhood aural malignancy.

Ref.: 1, 6, 12

COMMENTS: The most common tumors of the external ear—squamous cell carcinoma and basal cell carcinoma—are related to ultraviolet light exposure. • The majority (90%) occur in males. • Poor prognostic features of squamous cell carcinoma of the ear include deep dermal (or deeper) invasion, size greater than 2 cm, and perineural extension. • When the latter is present, the tumor often extends beyond the clinically apparent margins of disease.

Treatment of squamous cell carcinoma of the ear may include surgical excision with frozen-section evaluation of the margins, Mohs surgery, and/or radiation. • Radiotherapy, which is associated with excellent local control rates, may be used as primary treatment for small, superficial lesions or as an adjunct to definitive surgical treatment for advanced or poor prognosis lesions. • Generally, surgical margins of 0.5 cm are advocated for most cutaneous squamous cell carcinomas, although slightly larger margins, of 0.6–0.9 cm, have been recommended for very large or deep tumors or those exhibiting perineural invasion.

The incidence of lymph node metastases from squamous cell carcinoma of the ear is reported to be 6–20%. • Lymph node dissection should be performed in the presence of clinically evident lymph node metastases. • The lymphatic drainage of the external ear may include the parotid nodes as well as the jugular chain.

Rhabdomyosarcoma is the most common childhood aural malignancy.

ANSWER:
D

26. Regarding neoplasms of the nasopharynx, which one of the following statements is true?

A. Lymphoma is the most common nasopharyngeal neoplasm in adults.

B. There is an unusually high incidence of nasopharyngeal carcinoma among the Chinese.

C. Elevated titers of anti–viral Epstein-Barr antibodies are present in 20% of patients.

D. The most common presentation of nasopharyngeal carcinoma is bleeding or nasopharyngeal obstruction.

E. Surgery is the treatment of choice for small, well-localized nasopharyngeal carcinomas.

Ref.: 1, 2, 6, 9, 11

COMMENTS: Malignant neoplasms of the nasopharynx include squamous carcinoma, adenocarcinoma (usually of minor salivary gland origin), sarcoma, lymphoma, and melanoma. • Among children, lymphoma is the most common malignancy in the nasopharynx. • In adults, squamous carcinoma and its variants with or without lymphoid stroma (formerly called lymphoepithelial carcinoma) are the most common types. • There is an unusually high incidence of nasopharyngeal carcinoma among the Chinese, comprising almost 20% of cancers in this population, and it appears at an earlier age than do other squamous carcinomas of the upper aerodigestive tract. • Elevated titers of anti–Epstein-Barr virus antibodies are seen in up to 70% of patients with nasopharyngeal carcinoma, suggesting a possible viral cause.

The most common clinical presentation of nasopharyngeal carcinoma is painless cervical lymphadenopathy, usually involving the posterior triangle of the neck. • Other symptoms may include bleeding, nasopharyngeal obstruction, and the sequelae of invasion of the skull base, such as cranial nerve palsy. • Imaging with CT and magnetic resonance imaging (MRI) delineates the extent of disease in the nasopharynx and neck.

Carcinoma of the nasopharynx is best treated with irradiation alone for stage I and II disease and with chemotherapy for more advanced disease. • Difficult access and the inability to obtain a wide surgical margin because of the proximity of the nasopharynx to the base of the skull and vertebral column make surgical excision of even the earliest lesions inappropriate. • The role of surgery is usually limited to nasopharyngoscopy and biopsy.

The tumor has a high propensity to metastasize to cervical lymph nodes. • More than 80% of patients are stage III or IV at the time of diagnosis, including approximately 20% with bilateral neck disease at presentation. • Distant metastatic disease at presentation is uncommon (3%). • The overall 5-year survival rate for squamous cell carcinoma of the nasopharynx is approximately 35%.

ANSWER:
B

27. Regarding carcinoma of the tonsil, which one of the following statements is true?

A. Lymphomas are the most common tumor in this area, arising from Waldeyer's ring.

B. Early tumors may present with dysphagia and ear pain.

C. Biopsy of a suspected tonsillar carcinoma may be done in the office setting with topical anesthesia.

D. Clinically evident lymph node metastases, usually level II jugulodigastric lymph nodes, are found in approximately 25% of patients at presentation.

E. Advanced tumors, T3 and T4, initially should be treated with combination chemotherapy and radiation.

Ref.: 1–3, 6, 9, 11

COMMENTS: The most frequent malignant tumor of the oropharynx, the tonsil, and the tonsillar fossa is squamous cell carcinomas (95%). • As with other squamous cell carcinomas of the upper aerodigestive tract, there is a distinct male predominance and an association with excessive use of tobacco and alcohol. • An association with human papillomavirus, human immunodeficiency virus (HIV), and vitamin A deficiency also has been described. • Mild sore throat or a tonsillar ulceration may be seen with early lesions, although most tumors are asymptomatic until reaching considerable size. • Dysphagia, odynophagia, slurred speech, ear pain, and trismus are symptoms of advanced disease. • Tonsillar carcinomas may extend to the soft palate, nasopharynx, base of tongue, or the lateral pharyngeal wall. • This area is easily visualized. • Biopsy of a suspected tonsillar carcinoma may be done in the office with topical anesthetic. • Patients with advanced lesions involving the base of tongue or pharyngeal wall may benefit from further endoscopic examination in the operating room to delineate the precise extent of disease. • This is important in planning appropriate therapy.

Extensive local growth and the abundant lymphatics of the tonsillar fossa lead to a high frequency of cervical lymph node metastases, usually first to the level II jugulodigastric nodes, clinically evident in two thirds to three quarters of patients at presentation. • Among patients with clinically negative nodes at presentation, approximately 10% will have occult cervical metastases. • T1 and

T2 lesions are usually treated with irradiation (either external beam or interstitial or both), and results are comparable to those achieved with surgery and there is less cosmetic and functional disturbance. • T3 lesions that do not invade the mandible also may be treated by primary radiotherapy, but the mainstay of treatment for T3 and T4 lesions is surgery followed by irradiation. • The role of adjuvant or neoadjuvant chemotherapy for tonsillar carcinoma is not established. • Surgical treatment of oropharyngeal tumors is apt to leave the patient with impaired swallowing and an inability to protect the airway unless meticulous reconstruction is planned. • The ipsilateral neck should be treated, usually with radiation for N0 disease and with neck dissection for clinically positive disease, followed by adjuvant radiotherapy when there is extracapsular spread of disease or when there are multiple involved lymph nodes. • Tonsillar carcinoma has the most favorable survival rates among oropharyngeal carcinomas, with a 5-year survival of approximately 80% for stage I and II disease and 50% for stage III disease.

ANSWER:
C

28. Match each of the clinical characteristics of laryngeal carcinoma in the left-hand column with the appropriate anatomic site or sites of origin in the right-hand column. Items in the right-hand column may be used more than once.

    A. Symptoms occur early.   a. Supraglottic larynx
    B. Regional lymph node   b. Glottic larynx
       metastases are common.
    C. It may be managed with   c. Subglottic larynx
       voice preservation.
    D. Primary radiotherapy may be
       the treatment of choice.

Ref.: 1, 2, 6, 9, 11

COMMENTS: The larynx is divided into three areas: the *supraglottic larynx* extends from the valleculae to the laryngeal ventricles, the *glottis* includes the true vocal cords and vocal process of arytenoids, and the *subglottic larynx* extends from 5 mm below the vocal cords to the inferior margin of the cricoid cartilage. • Glottic carcinomas, in contradistinction to other laryngeal tumors, produce symptoms early because of the small degree of anatomic change required to produce hoarseness. • They therefore tend to be diagnosed at an early stage. • In addition, because true glottic cancers have limited lymphatic access, the likelihood of regional nodal metastases is low. • For T1 and early T2 lesions, surgery and irradiation are equally effective. • For T2b lesions with impaired cord mobility, functional outcome after surgical treatment is usually superior. • Lasers have added a new dimension to the treatment of glottic cancer, with high cure rates and low morbidity.

Carcinomas of the supraglottic and subglottic larynx usually grow to a considerable size before producing symptoms (hoarseness, sore throat, dysphagia, and dyspnea). • Because of their relatively large size and the abundant lymphatics in the area, regional lymph node metastases are relatively common (30–50%) at the time of diagnosis. • For these reasons, symptomatic tumors in these areas rarely are managed successfully by radiotherapy alone. • Surgery, with or without irradiation, is the preferred treatment. • Direct involvement of the glottic larynx or paralysis of the vocal cords by supraglottic or subglottic lesions may require total laryngectomy. • In selected patients, conservative surgery, including vertical hemilaryngectomy, allows preservation of the voice and swallowing. • For patients with more advanced tumors, neoadjuvant chemoradiation may permit organ preservation in up to two thirds of eligible patients. • Salvage laryngectomy for persistent or recurrent disease is successful in 50% of cases. • After total laryngectomy,

rehabilitation includes esophageal speech, use of the electrolarynx, and the surgically created tracheoesophageal fistula with a one-way valve. • Patients with T3 and T4 tumors should have the ipsilateral neck treated (with either irradiation or surgery), even in N0 cases, because subsequent failure in the neck occurs in 10–30% of these patients.

ANSWER:
A-b; B-a,c; C-a,b,c; D-b

29. Which one of the following statements accurately describes carcinoma of the lip?

    A. The primary risk factor is tobacco use.

    B. It is approximately equally distributed between the upper and the lower lip.

    C. More than 75% are basal cell carcinomas.

    D. Surgery and radiotherapy are equally effective treatments for T1 and T2 tumors.

    E. Carcinomas that recur locally after surgical treatment should be treated with chemotherapy and radiation.

Ref.: 1, 6, 9

COMMENTS: Carcinoma of the lip occurs almost exclusively in males (95%), and actinic damage from ultraviolet radiation exposure is the major risk factor. • Other risk factors include tobacco use of all types, alcohol abuse, and immunosuppression. • About 90% of lip cancers occur on the lower lip, and most are squamous cell carcinomas, with basal cell carcinoma, melanoma, and minor salivary gland carcinoma seen less commonly in this location. • T1 and T2 lesions (≤ 4 cm) may be treated with either surgery or radiation with comparably excellent results. • Since 30% or more of the lip width can be resected and closed primarily after simple V-shaped excision with good cosmesis and function, this method is used most frequently. • Larger lesions require flap reconstruction. • T3 and T4 tumors should be treated surgically, followed by postoperative adjuvant radiation. • Prophylactic supraomohyoid neck dissection should be considered for patients with tumors greater than 4 cm, desmoplastic tumors, and those exhibiting perineural invasion, although, overall, only 10% of patients have lymph node metastases at the time of initial presentation.

Cervical node involvement usually appears first in the submental and submandibular regions, although tumors of the upper lip or commissure may spread to preauricular nodes. • When lymph node involvement is found after prophylactic node dissection, a modified radical neck dissection should be performed. • Patients with a local recurrence should undergo resection, radiotherapy (if not performed as the initial therapy), and selective neck dissection. • Prognosis for patients with lip carcinoma is the most favorable among head and neck cancers, with a 90% overall 5-year survival rate. • When there is lymph node involvement, the 5-year overall survival rate drops to 50%.

ANSWER:
D

30. Match the characteristics in the left-hand column with the appropriate tumor site in the right-hand column.

    A. Patients are predominantly male.   a. Cancer of the oral
                                                 cavity
    B. Tobacco abuse and alcohol abuse   b. Cancer of the
       are major risk factors.   oropharynx

C. Lymphoma occurs most commonly here.

D. Minor salivary gland carcinomas are the second most common histologic subtype.

E. Bilateral cervical node metastases are not uncommon.

F. It includes carcinoma of the tongue

c. Both cancer of the oral cavity and cancer of the oropharynx

d. Neither cancer of the oral cavity nor cancer of the oropharynx

Ref.: 1, 2, 6, 9, 11

COMMENTS: Cancers of both the oral cavity and oropharynx exhibit a male predominance and are related to tobacco and ethanol abuse. • While the majority of lesions from both sites are squamous cell carcinomas, there is much higher incidence of lymphoma in the oropharynx (occurring primarily in the lymphoid-rich Waldeyer's ring). • Minor salivary gland carcinomas are the second most common type of oral-cavity cancer. • Overall, the prognosis of patients with oropharyngeal carcinoma is worse than that of patients with cancer of the oral cavity. • This is due to a number of factors, including the larger size that primary oropharyngeal tumors usually achieve before producing symptoms or resulting in clinical detection and the greater propensity for lymph node metastases. • Oropharyngeal tumors are also more likely than are oral cavity tumors to metastasize to bilateral cervical lymph nodes. • Tumors of the mobile (anterior) tongue are classified as oral-cavity tumors, while those of the base of the tongue are classified as oropharyngeal tumors.

ANSWER:
A-c; B-c; C-d; D-a; E-b; F-c

31. Regarding carcinoma of the tongue, which of one of the following statements is not true?

A. Iron-deficiency anemia and submucosal fibrosis may be risk factors.

B. The most common location of tongue carcinoma is at the midportion of the lateral tongue.

C. Tumors arising behind the circumvallate papillae generally have a better prognosis because they are detected at an early stage.

D. Primary radiotherapy is effective for T1 tongue carcinomas, with local control and survival rates equivalent to those after primary surgical therapy.

E. Because the incidence of cervical lymph node metastases is high, even for early-stage tumors, treatment of the ipsilateral neck is almost always indicated.

Ref.: 1, 3, 6, 7, 9

COMMENTS: Carcinoma of the tongue includes tumors of the oral (anterior, mobile) tongue and tumors of the base of tongue. • The epidemiologic features of carcinoma of the tongue are similar to those of other head and neck cancers (i.e., male predominance, history of tobacco and alcohol abuse, and epidermoid carcinoma prevalence). • There is a high incidence of tongue carcinoma in India, where submucosal fibrosis is believed to be an etiologic factor. • There is also an increased incidence of tongue carcinoma in patients with Plummer-Vinson syndrome (i.e., cervical dysphagia, iron-deficiency anemia, atrophic oral mucosa, brittle spoon-shaped

fingernails, and Scandinavian predominance). • Most tumors are squamous cell carcinoma, but minor salivary gland tumors, sarcomas, and lymphomas also occur in this location.

The most common site is at the midportion of the lateral tongue. • These tumors may grow in an exophytic or infiltrative fashion. • Tumors of the base of tongue (those arising behind the circumvallate papillae) frequently present at an advanced stage because of their silent location and generally have a poor prognosis. • Radiotherapy (either brachytherapy and/or external beam) and surgery yield equivalent results for early lesions. • However, carcinoma of the oral tongue frequently presents with extension to the floor of mouth and invasion of the inner table of the mandible. • In such circumstances, a composite resection including partial mandibulectomy should be performed. • Carcinoma of the base of tongue may extend to the oral tongue, surrounding oropharynx, and/or larynx. • Radiation therapy alone is unlikely to be successful with large, locally advanced lesions, and most are treated with surgery followed by radiation with or without chemotherapy. • The morbidity of hemiglossectomy or total glossectomy with or without laryngectomy is related to the critical functions of the tongue regarding speech, deglutition, and airway protection. • Reconstruction is critical. • Partial glossectomy may require the use of free lateral arm or radial forearm flaps, which provide better restoration of function (mobility and sensation) than do the bulkier, insensate myocutaneous flaps used in the past. • After a total glossectomy, a pectoralis major myocutaneous or jejunal free flap may be needed to restore the entire floor of mouth and pharynx.

The incidence of cervical lymph node metastases at the time of diagnosis is approximately 50% for tumors of the oral tongue and 70% or more for tumors of the base of tongue. • The latter are bilateral in 25% of cases. • Level II nodes are most frequently affected, but level I, III, and IV nodes are also often involved. • Therefore, the ipsilateral cervical lymph nodes should be treated in most cases. • Modified or radical neck dissection is performed for clinically evident disease. • Selective (levels I–IV) or supraomohyoid (levels I–III) neck dissection or radiotherapy may be used for the clinically N_0 neck, otherwise, more than one third of these patients with cervical lymph node metastases will experience recurrence in the neck.

ANSWER:
C

32. Match each of the tumors of the jaw in the left-hand column with its appropriate characteristic in the right-hand column.

A. Radicular cyst

B. Ameloblastoma

C. Osteogenic sarcoma

D. Carcinoma

a. It usually requires multimodality therapy.

b. Local excision or curettage is appropriate.

c. It is a slow-growing malignancy with "soap-bubble" radiographic appearance.

d. It may be metastatic from another primary site.

Ref.: 1, 3

COMMENTS: Although the mandible and maxilla are most often involved in head and neck cancer by virtue of direct extension of contiguous epithelial tumors, a number of benign and malignant primary tumors of the jaws exist. • **Radicular cysts** (dental cysts or root cysts) are usually easily diagnosed by their appropriate lucent appearance on radiographs. • Local resection or enucleation, with curettage of the cyst cavity, is usually all that is required for treatment. • Many other benign jaw cysts exist, and they require preoperative radiologic assessment and a histologic diagnosis before appropriate treatment can be instituted. • These steps are necessary to avoid under- or overtreatment.

Ameloblastoma (adamantinoma) is a slow-growing, low-grade malignancy that has the capability to metastasize to distant sites. • The characteristic radiographic appearance is that of soap bubbles. • Wide excision with appropriate bone reconstruction is the treatment of choice.

Osteogenic sarcoma may occur in either the mandible or the maxilla and usually carries a grave prognosis. • Wide surgical excision alone may be curative, but improved results are possible with multimodality therapy, including preoperative chemotherapy and possible adjuvant radiotherapy.

Carcinoma, most often breast, thyroid, or prostate, can metastasize to the mandible and present clinically as a primary tumor.

A N S W E R :
A-b; B-c; C-a; D-d

33. Regarding salivary gland tumors, which one of the following statements is true?

   A. The majority of malignant salivary gland tumors arise in the parotid gland.

   B. Most parotid neoplasms are malignant.

   C. Fine-needle aspiration biopsy is recommended for all suspected salivary gland malignancies.

   D. Minor salivary gland tumors occur most commonly in the floor of the mouth.

Ref.: 1, 3, 6

COMMENTS: The likelihood of a given tumor's being malignant is lowest in the parotid gland (approximately 20%), followed by the submandibular salivary gland (approximately 50%), minor salivary glands (approximately 80%), and sublingual glands (nearly 100%). • However, because more than 75% of all salivary gland tumors occur in the parotid gland, the parotid gland accounts for the majority of malignant salivary gland tumors. • The diagnostic evaluation of a salivary gland mass depends on the location and clinical scenario. • Fine-needle aspiration biopsy (FNAB) is not indicated for all parotid tumors, since a tissue diagnosis does not change the treatment plan for a patient with a small, mobile mass clearly within the gland. • When the location is uncertain, the history suggests the possibility of metastatic disease, or the tumor size or location indicates a difficult facial nerve dissection, FNAB may be helpful. • FNAB should be employed for submandibular masses, since the majority are lymph nodes, not true glandular lesions. • Nonetheless, FNAB gives an accurate preoperative diagnosis only about 80% of the time. • Biopsy, usually a punch or excisional biopsy, should be performed for suspected minor salivary gland tumors, the most common site of which is the palate, usually at the junction of the hard and soft palate. • Like FNAB, imaging studies (CT or MRI) should be used when they are likely to augment the clinical assessment of staging and affect treatment planning.

A N S W E R :
A

34. Match each histologic type of salivary gland tumor in the left-hand column with its appropriate characteristic in the right-hand column.

   A. Pleomorphic adenoma   a. It accounts for 20% of malignant salivary tumors.

   B. Warthin's tumor   b. Parotidectomy may be indicated, even when distant metastatic disease is present.

   C. Mucoepidermoid carcinoma   c. It is the most common salivary gland tumor.

   D. Adenoid cystic carcinoma   d. Biologic aggressiveness varies widely according to tumor grade.

   E. Adenocarcinoma   e. It may represent malignant degeneration of a benign tumor.

   F. Malignant mixed tumor   f. It exhibits marked male predominance.

Ref.: 1–3, 6, 9, 11

COMMENTS: The histologic and biologic spectrum of major and minor salivary gland tumors is broad, since the glands are composed of diverse cell types, any of which may give rise to neoplasia. • Most salivary gland tumors grow slowly and are asymptomatic. • On occasion, malignant tumors present with signs of rapid growth, pain, paresthesias, and nerve deficits. • Among the benign tumors, **pleomorphic adenoma** (benign mixed tumor) is the most common. • It is found most often in the parotid gland and is best managed by superficial lobectomy (or wide excision) with preservation of the facial nerve. • Although grossly these lesions appear encapsulated, microscopically they extend beyond the apparent borders, a feature that leads to high recurrence rates after enucleation.

The second most common benign tumor is **Warthin's tumor** (papillary cystadenoma lymphomatosum). • These tumors are typically cystic lesions in the tail of the parotid, mainly in men, often multicentric, and bilateral in 10% of cases.

Mucoepidermoid carcinoma is the most common malignant salivary gland tumor. • Low-grade mucoepidermoid carcinoma (of predominantly mucin-secreting cells) has an excellent prognosis, whereas high-grade mucoepidermoid carcinoma (of predominantly epidermoid cells) has a poor prognosis. • Even after aggressive treatment, consisting of total parotidectomy, neck dissection, and postoperative radiotherapy, the 5-year survival rate for high-grade tumors is only 50%. • **Adenoid cystic carcinoma** is the most common malignant tumor of the submandibular gland and second most common malignant tumor of the parotid. • These tumors have a propensity for perineural spread and regional or distant recurrence after a prolonged disease-free interval of 10 or even 20 years. • Even with disseminated disease, patients may experience prolonged survival. • Therefore, patients with metastatic disease, such as a solitary lung nodule, at presentation may benefit from resection of the primary tumor. • **Adenocarcinoma** accounts for 20% of malignant salivary gland tumors. • Malignant **mixed tumors** probably represent malignant transformation of a benign mixed tumor. • This possibility has been suggested by findings of malignant elements in tumors that otherwise appear to be pleomorphic adenomas. • These findings support the rationale for resection of major salivary gland tumors, even if they have been present and unchanged for many years. • Nodal metastases occur in only about 20% of patients with malignant salivary gland tumors, most often in those with high-grade tumors and rarely in those with low-grade or adenoid cystic carcinoma.

A N S W E R :
A-c; B-f; C-d; D-b; E-a; F-e

35. Regarding neck dissections, which one of the following statements is true?

   A. In a classical radical neck dissection, the internal jugular vein, spinal accessory nerve, phrenic nerve, and sternocleidomastoid muscle are routinely resected en bloc with the specimen.

B. Bilateral simultaneous radical neck dissections are well tolerated and should be performed in cases of midline lesions that have or may have metastasized to both sides of the neck.

C. The term *modified radical neck dissection* refers to the dissection of all but the posterior triangle portion of the classic radical neck dissection.

D. Sentinel lymph node biopsy with selective neck dissection is now the standard of care for clinically N0 squamous cell carcinomas of the oral cavity.

E. Preservation of the spinal accessory nerve significantly reduces the morbidity of neck dissection.

Ref.: 1–5,11,13

COMMENTS: The **classical radical neck dissection**, as described by George Crile in 1906, is designed to remove the lymph node–bearing tissue that accompanies the great vessels within the carotid sheath as well as that found in the submandibular and posterior cervical triangles. • The dissection involves removal of the sternocleidomastoid muscle, internal jugular vein, spinal accessory nerve, submandibular gland, and associated lymph node–bearing tissue. • Although branches of the external carotid artery may be sacrificed, the external, internal, and common carotid arteries are left intact. • The cervical branch of the facial nerve is, of necessity, sacrificed, but the marginal mandibular branch is preserved. • The sensory branches of the anterior roots of C-2, C-3, and C-4 are sacrificed during the procedure, accounting for the relatively low level of pain during the postoperative period. • The lingual, hypoglossal, and phrenic nerves are preserved, as are the branches of the brachial plexus and the intrinsic deep musculature of the neck.

Occasionally, clinical bilateral cervical nodal disease necessitates **bilateral radical neck dissection**. • Such an operation significantly increases surgical morbidity in terms of risk for facial, pharyngeal and orbital edema, and changes in mental status due to increased central nervous system venous pressure, although the published complication rate is not very high. • Temporally staging the neck dissections (to allow collaterals to develop) and preserving one of the internal jugular veins, if technically feasible, may reduce these postoperative risks. • Prophylactic or elective bilateral simultaneous neck dissections should be avoided.

The **modified radical neck dissection** involves removal of the lymph node–bearing areas in the classical radical neck dissection but with preservation of the nonlymphatic structures, including one or more of the following: the sternocleidomastoid muscle, internal jugular vein, and/or spinal accessory nerve. • This technique is widely accepted for treatment of the clinically negative neck at high risk for occult nodal metastases. • Its use is also gaining acceptance for the treatment of the clinically positive neck, but this remains controversial. • **Selective neck dissection** entails preservation of one or more lymph node groups. • With these dissections, the internal jugular vein, sternocleidomastoid muscle, and spinal accessory nerve are routinely spared. • **Supraomohyoid neck dissection** is the removal of level I, II, and III nodes; **lateral neck dissection** entails removal of level II, III, and IV nodes; and **posterolateral neck dissection** is lateral dissection plus removal of the posterior triangle (level V), retroauricular, and suboccipital lymph nodes. • While sentinel lymph node biopsy with selective lymph node dissection is now accepted for the treatment of appropriately selected melanomas of the head and neck, its application to squamous cell carcinomas of the head and neck is still investigational. • The syndrome of shoulder droop, scapular displacement, discomfort, and

weakness that accompanies loss of the spinal accessory nerve is the major source of morbidity following radical neck dissection. • In patients who are candidates for modified neck dissection, preservation of this nerve significantly reduces the likelihood of this aspect of postoperative morbidity.

ANSWER:
E

36. Which one of the following statements regarding recent advances in head and neck reconstruction is most accurate?

A. Esophageal speech following laryngectomy is one of the most significant advances in the rehabilitation of head and neck cancer patients in recent years.

B. Unlike the fasciocutaneous forearm flap, the pectoralis major myocutaneous flap usually provides thin, sensate tissue for intraoral reconstruction.

C. Refinements in microvascular techniques have contributed significantly to reconstruction of composite defects of the oral cavity, oropharynx, pharynx, and esophagus.

D. Increasingly complicated extirpative procedures used for the treatment of head and neck cases have resulted in an increased need for multiple, staged reconstructive procedures.

E. Use of microvascular flaps increases hospital stay and prolong rehabilitation of patients.

Ref.: 1, 2, 11

COMMENTS: Advances in the extirpative portion of the surgical management of head and neck cancer include improvements in anesthetic techniques, the development of larynx-conservation techniques, and the introduction of lasers and microscopically controlled stepwise excision of neoplasms. • Advances in head and neck reconstruction include refinements in microvascular surgery. • This has led to decreased length of stay and improved functional restoration. • Advantages of free flaps include the ability to provide thin, sensate tissue with an improved ability to shape and inset the flap. • Before these developments, reconstruction was either deferred, leaving the patient an oral cripple, or required multiple, staged procedures. • Although the pectoralis major myocutaneous flap is often regarded as the workhorse of head and neck reconstruction, the radial forearm free flap and the vascularized fibula flap have the ability to provide virtually unlimited bone and soft tissue for head and neck reconstruction. • In addition, the free jejunal flap is an excellent option for esophageal reconstruction. • Free tissue transfers have resulted in improved restoration of functional swallowing and airway protection and decreased the need for permanent tracheostomy and gastrostomy in selected patients. • Furthermore, immediate reconstruction has reduced costs, allowed patients to begin oral rehabilitation and adjuvant therapy more expeditiously, and avoided the disfigurement and social ostracism patients may otherwise suffer. • Composite free-tissue transfers, especially in cases involving mandibulectomy, are invaluable in head and neck reconstruction.

ANSWER:
C

37. Regarding the use of chemotherapy for head and neck cancer, which one of the following statements is true?

A. Induction chemotherapy for locally advanced squamous cell carcinoma of the head and neck is associated with a complete response rate of up to 50%.

B. Induction chemotherapy increases the morbidity of subsequent surgery or radiotherapy.

C. Postoperative adjuvant chemotherapy decreases the rate of development of distant metastatic disease and improves survival in high-risk patients.

D. Concurrent chemoradiotherapy has been shown to improve locoregional disease control and overall survival in patients with advanced oropharyngeal carcinomas, but significant (grade 3 or 4) toxicity occurs in up to 25% of treated patients.

Ref.: 2, 14

COMMENTS: Data from numerous randomized trials over the past two decades demonstrate that **induction chemotherapy** (given before any local therapy) for locally advanced squamous cell carcinomas of the head and neck results in a 60–90% major response rate and a complete clinical response rate of 20–50%. • While overall there is no survival advantage to induction chemotherapy, among the clinically complete responders, two thirds have a pathologically complete response, and these patients do appear to have a survival advantage. • Induction chemotherapy does not increase the morbidity of subsequent locoregional therapy. • Induction chemotherapy may permit organ preservation and improved quality of life.

Postoperative adjuvant chemotherapy alone has been poorly accepted by patients, with more than half not completing treatment. • While some studies have shown a decreased incidence of distant metastases, this has not translated into an effect on overall survival. • To date, only one of four published trials of **postoperative adjuvant chemoradiation** has shown a survival benefit. • In this small trial of patients with extracapsular extension of nodal metastatic disease, both locoregional control and overall survival were improved compared with adjuvant radiotherapy alone. • Recent meta-analyses have demonstrated a small (2–8%) but significant absolute survival benefit to various regimens of chemotherapy plus radiotherapy compared to radiotherapy alone. • The most striking benefits have been seen in more recent large, multicenter, randomized trials employing concurrent cisplatin-based chemotherapy and standard or altered fraction radiotherapy. • Several studies have demonstrated improved locoregional control and disease-free and overall survival compared to radiotherapy alone. • In these study populations, the group that appears to benefit is patients with stage III or IV unresectable oropharyngeal carcinomas. • Toxicity with these regimens is significant, with up to 75% of patients experiencing grade 3 or 4 side effects. • Patients can expect to require vigorous supportive care during treatment, including a gastrostomy for nutritional support.

ANSWER:
A

38. Regarding the diagnosis and management of a solitary neck mass, which one of the following statements is true?

A. About 20% of metastatic cervical lymph nodes are from primary tumors in the chest and abdomen.

B. Midline nonthyroidal neck masses are usually neoplastic.

C. The first step in management is an incisional or excisional biopsy to establish the diagnosis, avoiding other unnecessary testing.

D. Fine-needle aspiration biopsy is particularly helpful in diagnosing lymphomas, sarcomas, and poorly differentiated adenocarcinomas.

E. Radical neck dissection should not be performed for metastatic cervical disease if the primary tumor is not identified.

Ref.: 2, 6, 9, 11

COMMENTS: Solitary neck masses may represent congenital abnormalities, inflammatory or infectious lymph nodes, metastatic carcinoma from sites in the upper aerodigestive tract, metastases from other sites (e.g., lung, breast, GI tract, or kidney), lymphoma, or rare primary tumors (e.g., a carotid body tumor). • The age of the patient, past medical history (especially of cancer), clinical presentation, and physical characteristics of the mass frequently give some indication as to the nature of the pathologic condition. • Metastatic cancer is the most common nonthyroidal neck mass in patients over age 40. • About 80% of metastatic cervical lymph nodes are from primary tumors above the clavicles, while 20% are from tumors elsewhere. • Most extrathyroidal midline neck masses are congenital lesions (e.g., thyroglossal duct cysts).

The first step in the evaluation should be thorough inspection and palpation of the head and neck area, including indirect laryngoscopy and nasopharyngoscopy. • The chest, abdomen, and other major lymph node groups should also be examined. • Any mass that is hard should be considered neoplastic until proven otherwise. • When a neoplasm is suspected, fine-needle aspiration biology (FNAB) should be performed. • FNAB is a safe procedure, but it is nondiagnostic in approximately 10% of cases (usually due to inadequate specimen or histologic features not amenable to cytologic diagnosis) and falsely negative in another 5–10% of cases. • Therefore, a negative FNAB should not preclude further evaluation when malignancy is suspected. • While squamous cell carcinoma, thyroid cancer, melanoma, and well-differentiated adenocarcinoma usually are easily diagnosed by FNAB, sarcomas, lymphomas, and poorly differentiated tumors are not. • Core-needle biopsies may be more helpful in some settings, but, not infrequently, an open biopsy is required to establish a diagnosis.

If open biopsy is needed, it should be excisional, if possible, since incisional biopsies are associated with greater risk of tumor seeding and infectious complications. • The incision should be placed in a manner that will accommodate future neck dissection, if required. • If no primary tumor is identified by physical examination and indirect laryngoscopy, CT scans (or MRI) of the head, neck, and chest are indicated for metastatic squamous cell carcinoma and scans of the neck, chest, abdomen, and pelvis for metastatic adenocarcinoma. • If there is still no evidence of a primary tumor, triple endoscopy (direct laryngoscopy, bronchoscopy, and esophagoscopy) under general anesthesia should be done. • If no primary tumor is visualized, random biopsies of the statistically most likely sites of disease (nasopharynx, tonsillar fossa, base of tongue, and piriform sinus) are performed. • Neck dissection for an unknown primary tumor should be followed by irradiation to the pharynx and the neck. • Up to one half of the patients so managed survive 5 years free of disease, despite the fact that the primary tumor may never be found.

ANSWER:
A

39. Which one of the following statements regarding Kaposi's sarcoma (KS) associated with HIV infection is true?

A. As in non–HIV-associated KS, the oral and pharyngeal mucosa are common sites of disease.

B. A sexual mode of transmission of KS is likely.

C. While bleeding is common, severe odynophagia and dysphagia are infrequently seen with oral KS.

D. The primary goal of treating KS is prevention of malignant degeneration.

E. Surgery is the mainstay of treatment.

Ref.: 3

COMMENTS: HIV and autoimmune deficiency syndrome (AIDS) patients experience a variety of nonneoplastic and neoplastic head and neck problems. • KS, once a rare cutaneous malignancy of the lower extremities of elderly males, is now the most common neoplasm associated with AIDS, arising in 15% of patients. • The most common site is the oral or perioral mucosa (55% of cases), with the palate the most frequent location of disease. • It is interesting to note that, while KS is rare in hemophiliacs and intravenous drug abusers with AIDS, it is common among homosexual or bisexual AIDS patients, suggesting a sexual mode of transmission, possibly linked to cytolomegalovirus infection or virally induced angiogenic factors. • Symptoms are minor until the lesion undergoes ulceration or secondary infection. • Then, severe odynophagia and dysphagia often occur. • Pharyngeal or laryngeal KS may cause airway obstruction. • The treatment of HIV-associated KS is primarily palliative. • Although low-dose radiotherapy is effective for cutaneous KS, mucosal lesions do not respond as well. • Laser ablation, photodynamic therapy, and systemic or intralesional vinblastine, etoposide, and interferon-α have been tried, with response rates of up to 30%. • Ultimate survival is probably determined by the infectious complications of AIDS, not by the neoplasm. • The median survival after diagnosis is 2 years, with a 5-year survival rate of only 10%.

ANSWER:
B

REFERENCES

1. Townsend CM, Beauchamp RD, Evers BM, et al (eds): *Sabiston Textbook of Surgery: The Biological Basis of Modern Surgical Practice*, 16th ed. Saunders, Philadelphia, 2001.
2. Cummings CW, Frederickson JM, Harker LA, et al: *Otolaryngology: Head and Neck Surgery*, 3rd ed. CV Mosby, St. Louis, 1998.
3. Schwartz SI, Shires GT, Spencer FC, et al: *Schwartz's Principles of Surgery*, 7th ed. McGraw-Hill, New York, 1999.
4. Loré JM Jr: *An Atlas of Head and Neck Surgery*, 3rd ed. Saunders, Philadelphia, 1988.
5. Wood WC, Skandalakis JE: *Anatomic Basis of Tumor Surgery*. Quality Medical Publishing, St. Louis, 1999.
6. Saclarides TJ, Millikan KW, Godellas CV: *Surgical Oncology: An Algorithmic Approach*. Springer-Verlag, New York, 2003.
7. Gates GA: *Current Therapy in Otolaryngology: Head and Neck Surgery*, 6th ed. CV Mosby, St. Louis, 1998.
8. Bailey BJ, Calhoun KH, Derkay CS, et al: *Head and Neck Surgery: Otolaryngology*, 3rd ed. JB Lippincott, Philadelphia, 2001.
9. Greenfield L, Mullholland MW, Oldham KT, et al: *Greenfield's Surgery: Scientific Principles and Practice*, 3rd ed. Lippincott, Williams & Wilkins, Philadelphia, 2001.
10. Talmor M, Li P, Barie PS: Acute paranasal sinusitis in critically ill patients: guidelines for prevention, diagnosis, and treatment. *Clin Infect Dis* 25:1441–1446, 1997.
11. Thawley SE, Panje WR, Batsa JG, et al: *Comprehensive Management of Head and Neck Tumors*, 2nd ed. Saunders, Philadelphia, 1999.
12. Estrem SA, Renner GJ: Special problems associated with cutaneous carcinoma of the ear. *Otolaryngol Clin North Am* 26(2):231–245, 1993.
13. Pitman KT, Ferlito A, Devaney KO, et al: Sentinel lymph node biopsy in head and neck cancer. *Oral Oncol* 39(4):343–349, 2003.
14. DeVita VT, Hellman S, Rosenberg SA: *Cancer: Principles and Practice of Oncology*, 6th ed. Lippincott, Williams & Wilkins, Philadelphia, 2001.

C H A P T E R 27

Thyroid

Roderick Quiros, M.D., and Richard A. Prinz, M.D.

1. With regard to the vascular structures and their relationships to the thyroid gland, which of the following is/are true?

   A. Thyroidea ima arteries can arise from the aorta.

   B. The superior thyroid artery originates from the external carotid, and the inferior thyroid originates from the subclavian artery.

   C. The inferior thyroid artery is in close proximity to the recurrent laryngeal nerve, which generally runs posterior to the artery.

   D. The superior thyroid artery supplies the parathyroid glands.

   E. Venous vessels parallel the arterial circulation.

   F. The superior laryngeal nerve can be injured when ligating the superior thyroid artery.

   Ref.: 1–4

COMMENTS: The thyroid gland is a highly vascular organ that is second only to the carotid body in this respect. • It is supplied by two superior and two inferior arteries. • The superior thyroid arteries branch from the external carotid artery just above the carotid bifurcation. • The inferior thyroid arteries arise from the thyrocervical trunk and course posterior to the carotid sheath and then downward and medial to enter the middle of the thyroid gland. • The inferior thyroid arteries also provide blood supply to the superior and inferior parathyroid glands. • The relationship with the recurrent laryngeal nerve has important surgical implications. • In 1–4% of individuals, thyroidea ima arteries arise from either the innominate artery or aorta. • They generally course along the trachea and then enter the lower surface of the isthmus. • Venous drainage of the thyroid gland consists of three pairs of principal veins. • The superior thyroid veins course along with the superior thyroid artery and then empty into the internal jugular vein. • The middle thyroid vein, present in only 50% of individuals, drains directly into the internal jugular vein. • This vein is ligated during thyroid surgery to provide adequate mobilization of the thyroid lobe. • Inferior thyroid veins follow the course of the thyrothymic ligament before draining into the innominate or brachiocephalic veins.

ANSWER:
A, C, F

2. With regard to the anatomic relationship of the thyroid gland to nearby nerves, which of the following statements is/are true?

   A. Both superior and inferior thyroid arteries bear a fairly constant relationship to the recurrent laryngeal nerves.

   B. The superior laryngeal nerves provide both sensory and motor function to the larynx.

   C. Injury to the external branch of the superior laryngeal nerve may go unnoticed in most individuals.

   D. The "recurrent" nature of the recurrent laryngeal nerves is one of the few anatomic relationships for which anomalies or variations have not been reported.

   E. Unilateral recurrent laryngeal nerve injury results in airway compromise that may necessitate tracheostomy.

   Ref.: 1–4

COMMENTS: The thyroid gland is innervated via sympathetic fibers from the cervical ganglion and parasympathetic fibers from the vagus that reach the gland through the laryngeal nerves. • Because of their proximity to the gland, the laryngeal nerves are at risk of injury during thyroidectomy.

The **superior laryngeal** nerve provides both sensory and motor function to the larynx. • Its external branch provides motor innervation to the cricothyroid muscle and is at risk during thyroid surgery because of its close relationship to the superior thyroid vessels. • Injury to this nerve branch results in bowing of the vocal cord during phonation. • This effect may go unnoticed except in individuals, such as singers, who find themselves unable to reach high-pitched notes or professional speakers, who notice an increased fatigability of their voice.

The **recurrent laryngeal** nerve is so named because of its oblique course around the subclavian artery on the right and the aorta near the ductus arteriosus on the left. • The nerve then ascends on either side in the tracheoesophageal sulcus to the thyroid gland. • The relationship of the recurrent nerve to the inferior thyroid artery is variable. • In 75% of persons, the nerve traverses posterior to the inferior thyroid artery, whereas in 25% it courses anterior to the artery, and in as many as 10% it courses over the thyroid gland before entering the larynx.

In rare instances (<0.5% of persons) and almost exclusively on the right side, a **nonrecurrent** nerve exists, usually in association with vascular anomalies of the aortic arch. • In such circumstances, the nerve approaches the cricothyroid membrane obliquely from above, and during thyroid surgery it may be inadvertently divided if not recognized.

The recurrent laryngeal nerve provides motor function to most of the intrinsic laryngeal muscles, and its unilateral injury results in paralysis of the vocal cord, which changes the quality of the voice but rarely compromises the airway. • Bilateral recurrent laryngeal nerve injury, in contrast, may severely compromise airflow, necessitating tracheostomy.

ANSWER:
B, C

3. With regard to thyroid anatomy and associated structures, which of the following is/are true?

   A. Delphian lymph nodes are located along the internal jugular vein.

   B. The ligament of Berry is a posteromedial suspensory ligament that is in close relationship to the recurrent laryngeal nerve.

   C. The tubercle of Zuckerkandl is the most lateral posterior extension of thyroid tissue and is closely associated with the recurrent laryngeal nerve.

   D. The tubercle of Zuckerkandl is removed during a subtotal thyroidectomy.

   E. Injury to the loop of Galen is associated with ligation of the superior thyroid artery.

Ref.: 1–4

COMMENTS: The thyroid gland lies in the visceral compartment, covered with a thin layer of connective tissue derived from pretracheal fascia. • **Delphian lymph nodes** are closely associated with the pyramidal process and are enveloped by pretracheal fascia. • Another name for the **ligament of Berry** is the posteromedial suspensory ligament. • The location of this ligament is surgically important, owing to its close proximity to the recurrent laryngeal nerve. • In most patients, the nerve lies lateral to the ligament of Berry, but, in 25% of patients, the ligament surrounds the nerve. • The most lateral posterior extension of thyroid tissue is referred to as the **tubercle of Zuckerkandl**. • To identify the location of the recurrent laryngeal nerve, this portion of thyroid tissue must be rotated medially. • Because of the posterior location and close approximation to the recurrent laryngeal nerve, this portion of tissue is left behind during subtotal thyroidectomy. • The superior laryngeal nerve branch of the vagus arises high in the neck and descends medially and deep to the internal carotid artery along the pharynx toward the superior cornu of the hyoid bone. • It lies on the middle constrictor muscle and divides into internal and external branches. • The **loop of Galen** is where the pharyngeal branches of the recurrent laryngeal nerve communicate with the branches of the superior laryngeal nerve. • This structure may be injured when dissecting or ligating the superior thyroid artery.

ANSWER:
B, C, E

4. With regard to anomalous variations in thyroid embryologic development, which of the following statements is/are true?

   A. Lingual thyroid tissue should always be removed because it carries a high risk of malignancy.

   B. Removal of a thyroglossal duct cyst generally requires resection of the midportion of the hyoid bone to prevent cyst recurrence.

   C. In 70% of patients with lingual thyroid, it is the only thyroid tissue.

   D. Most mediastinal thyroid glands result from an abnormally caudad embryologic descent.

   E. So-called lateral aberrant thyroid rests may in fact be metastases of well-differentiated thyroid cancer.

Ref.: 1–4

COMMENTS: Embryologically, the thyroid gland is derived from the endoderm of the primitive foregut. • It results from a median endodermal down growth from the first and second pharyngeal pouches in the area of the foramen cecum. • These cells separate from the pharyngeal connections by the fifth gestational week and migrate caudally. • During their descent, the follicular cells fuse with parafollicular cells, which are derived from the ultimobranchial bodies of the fourth and fifth branchial pouches. • Abnormalities in descent of the thyroid tissue from the pharyngeal floor may result in a lingual thyroid or persistence of solid or cystic structures along the course of the midline descent, which results, respectively, in a persistent **pyramidal lobe** or a **thyroglossal duct cyst**.

In about 70% of patients with **lingual thyroids**, it represents the only thyroid tissue. • It is rarely symptomatic unless it enlarges and produces pharyngeal obstruction. • It carries a 3% risk of becoming malignant. • Treatment by radioiodine ablation or surgical excision is required only for symptoms or suspicion of malignancy.

A **thyroglossal duct cyst** may occur anywhere in the midline from the base of the tongue to the thyroid gland, but it is generally found just inferior to the hyoid bone. • The cyst classically moves upward with swallowing. • These lesions should be removed because they are susceptible to infections and, in rare instances, may be premalignant. • Removal of the cyst generally requires resection of the midportion of the hyoid bone to prevent recurrence.

Although the initial embryologic descent of the thyroid may proceed into an abnormally caudad position, resulting in a mediastinal or substernal thyroid, most intrathoracic goiters represent inferior extensions of acquired pathologic processes in a normally located gland.

Most benign "**lateral aberrant thyroid rests**, in fact, represent metastases of well-differentiated thyroid cancers. • This is certainly true when papillary features or severely atypical follicular features are found. • However, failure of lateral thyroid elements to be incorporated into the thyroid capsule occasionally results in embryologic thyroid rests in the lateral neck.

ANSWER:
B, C, E

5. Which of the following is/are true about iodine metabolism?

   A. The thyroid gland has 90% of the body's iodine stores.

   B. Iodide transport into follicular cells takes place via passive diffusion.

   C. TSH stimulates iodide movement into the follicular cells.

   D. Iodide excess may lead to multinodular goiter.

   E. Iodide transport is linked to a sodium-potassium adenosine triphosphatase system.

Ref.: 1–4

COMMENTS: Iodide is absorbed from the gastrointestinal (GI) tract in inorganic form before being taken up into the thyroid. • Up to 90% of total body iodine is stored by the thyroid gland. • Iodide entry into the follicular cells from the extracellular space involves an active transport mechanism, specifically the sodium-potassium adenosine triphosphatase system. • Iodide transport is regulated by thyroid-stimulating hormone (TSH) as well as the iodide content of the follicular cells, and its entry into the follicular cell creates a large gradient across the cell. • Iodide deficiency leads to multinodular goiter, hypothyroidism, mental retardation, and (possibly) follicular cancer. • Iodide excess has been linked to Graves' disease and Hashimoto's thyroiditis.

A N S W E R :
A, C, E

---

6. With regard to thyroid hormone synthesis and physiology, which of the following statements is/are true?

   A. The iodide used in thyroid hormone synthesis is derived primarily from dietary sources.

   B. The amino acid threonine binds to iodine to form active thyroid hormone.

   C. When the active thyroid hormones triiodothyronine (T_3) and thyroxine (T_4) are released into the plasma, they bind to thyroglobulin for transport.

   D. In the periphery, T_3 is converted to the metabolically more active T_4.

   E. TSH regulates most aspects of iodine uptake and oxidation.

Ref.: 1–4

COMMENTS: Thyroid hormones play an active regulatory role in many aspects of energy substrate metabolism, including increased oxygen consumption and calorigenesis, stimulation of protein synthesis, regulation of most aspects of carbohydrate metabolism, and metabolism of cholesterol and phospholipids.

   Thyroid hormone synthesis begins with the active transport of iodide (a process referred to as iodide trapping) from dietary sources into the thyroid gland, in which iodide is oxidized by thyroid peroxidase to iodine. • Successive organic iodinization of tyrosine to monoiodotyrosine (MIT) and diiodotyrosine (DIT) results in the eventual production of triiodthyronine (T_3) and tetraiodothyronine (T_4). • Through a process of coupling, two molecules of DIT form T_4, and one of DIT and one of MIT form T_3. • There is evidence that T_3 may be formed from T_4 within the thyroid and in the peripheral circulation. • T_3 and T_4 are stored in the thyroid bound to the protein thyroglobulin. • When cleaved from thyroglobulin, T_3 and T_4 are released into the plasma and become bound to thyronine-binding globulin (TBG) for transport. • In plasma, the T_4/T_3 ratio is between 10:1 and 20:1. • Most T_4 is converted to T_3, which is several times more active than T_4 and accounts for approximately half the metabolic effect of the thyroid hormone. • Most of the aspects of iodide uptake, oxidation, organic iodine binding, and thyroid hormone release are regulated by TSH, which is synthesized and released from the anterior pituitary gland. • Thyrotropin-releasing hormone (TRH), which is produced in the hypothalamus, and both thyroid hormones modulate TSH secretion. • Thyroid hormones inhibit TSH release, whereas TRH stimulates TSH production.

[handwritten: TRH (hypothalamus)]
[handwritten: TSH (ant pit)]
[handwritten: $T_3 T_4$ (thyroid)]

A N S W E R :
A, E

---

7. With regard to thyroid scanning, which of the following statements is/are true?

   A. The dose of radiation delivered to the thyroid is the same regardless of whether iodine 131 (^{131}I), iodine 123 (^{123}I), or technetium 99m (^{99m}Tc) is used.

   B. Thyroid scanning is useful for assessing the thyroid gland when it is normally located, but it does not evaluate ectopic thyroid tissue.

   C. Thyroid scintigraphy is highly accurate, even for detecting lesions as small as 1 cm in diameter.

   D. Metastases from well-differentiated thyroid carcinoma are unlikely to be detected by ^{131}I imaging if substantial normal thyroid tissue is present.

Ref.: 1–4

COMMENTS: See Question 8.

---

8. Match each thyroid test in the left-hand column with one or more appropriate test characteristics in the right-hand column.

A. ^{99m}Tc	a. May be used in conjunction with TSH level to determine thyroid function and status of the thyroid-pituitary feedback mechanism
B. ^{131}I	b. Useful for identifying metastatic deposits of differentiated thyroid cancer
C. Ultrasound imaging (US)	c. May be used to treat cystic thyroid nodules and determine the need for operating on solid thyroid nodules
D. T_3 and T_4 assays	d. Low-radiation nuclide used to provide information about the function of a thyroid nodule
E. Fine-needle aspiration (FNA) biopsy	e. May provide information on thyroid anatomy and the solid or cystic nature of thyroid nodules
F. Thyroid autoantibodies	f. Useful for diagnosing Graves' disease and Hashimoto's thyroiditis

Ref.: 1–4

COMMENTS: Thyroid scanning involves measuring the emitted radioactivity of a radionuclide that is taken up by the thyroid gland. • The nuclides technetium 99m pertechnetate (^{99m}Tc) and iodine (both ^{123}I and ^{131}I) are used primarily to assess the function of nodules (generally those >1.5 cm in diameter) within the thyroid gland but also to identify ectopic thyroid tissue, such as a lingual thyroid. • ^{99m}Tc and ^{123}I are the standard agents used because the radiation exposure to the patient is relatively small (10 and 30 mrad, respectively). • ^{131}I (500 mrad) remains useful for detecting distant metastases of differentiated thyroid cancer and for detecting retrosternal thyroid masses. • The use of ^{131}I for detecting thyroid metastases is limited by the presence of normally functioning thyroid tissue, which preferentially takes up the iodine. • The amount of radioactivity detected during the scan is a measure of the thyroid uptake of the nuclide and thus indirectly indicates the metabolic activity of the gland. • **US imaging** of the thyroid is useful for determining the number and distribution of thyroid nodules and whether they are cystic or solid, but it does not assess thyroid function. • **Thyroid hormone** (T_3 or T_4) and **TSH assays** of peripheral blood are useful for determining the presence of hyper- or hypofunction of the gland and the status of the thyroid-pituitary feedback mechanism. • The TSH level is more sensitive to subclinical hypothyroidism than are the thyroid hormone levels. • **Fine-needle aspiration (FNA)** biopsy is the prime method of evaluating thyroid nodules. • Cystic lesions with a negative result on cytologic evaluation can be entirely treated by aspiration. • If the lesion is solid, cytologic studies can be performed to estimate the likelihood of underlying malignancy and to determine reliably the need for resection. • To decrease the already low rate of false-negative diagnoses, current recommendations are for repeat aspiration of cytologically benign nodules at a later time. • Atypical, suspicious, or malignant cytologic findings mandate resection. • High titers of **thyroid autoantibodies** may be useful for identifying Graves' disease (hyperfunction) or Hashimoto's disease (hyper- or hypofunction).

ANSWERS:
Question 7: D
Question 8: A-d; B-b; C-e; D-a; E-c; F-f

9. With regard to thyroid function tests, which of the following statements is/are true?

    A. Estrogens increase the amount of TBG and therefore may falsely suggest hyperthyroidism.

    B. Administration of exogenous thyroid may lead to an increase in the radioactive iodine uptake (RAIU).

    C. Both barium enema and intravenous pyelography can affect the RAIU.

    D. Failure of exogenous T_3 to suppress TSH secretion may be seen in Graves' disease and in toxic adenomas.

Ref.: 1–4

COMMENTS: Most plasma T_4 assays measure total T_4, which reflects the amount bound to TBG as well as T_4. • Estrogen administration or pregnancy usually results in elevated TBG values, which elevates the total T_4 level even though the patient has a normal free T_4 level and is not hyperthyroid. • Androgens have the opposite effect. • Administration of exogenous thyroid hormone or of dietary or intravenous iodine usually results in a reduction of RAIU even though the patient is clinically not hypothyroid. • Contrast studies that do not involve iodine use do not affect the iodine uptake assay. • Normally, plasma TSH levels should fall to 50% of control values when T_3 is administered for 7–10 days. • In conditions exhibiting autonomous function of the thyroid (as may be seen in Graves' disease and toxic adenomas), TSH may already be suppressed, and further depression cannot be obtained by administration of exogenous thyroid hormone.

ANSWER:
A, D

10. With regard to thyroid function tests, which of the following is/are true?

    A. TSH levels are decreased in hyperthyroidism.

    B. Suppression of iodine uptake in patients with increased T_3 and T_4 levels is pathognomonic for subacute thyroiditis.

    C. Serum antibodies (antimicrosomal and antithyroglobulin) are present in both Graves' disease and Hashimoto's thyroiditis.

    D. The TRH assay can evaluate the pituitary TSH-secreting mechanism.

    E. The RAIU is elevated in patients receiving L-thyroxine or iodine.

Ref.: 1–4

COMMENTS: Many consider the measurement of **circulating TSH** concentrations to be the single best test of thyroid function in most patients. • Normal levels are between 0.4 and 4.2 µU/ml. • Hypothyroid patients have a TSH level of more than 4.0, whereas hyperthyroid patients have a level less than 0.5.

Serum T_4 assay is completed by measuring the total T_4 by radioimmunoassay (RIA). • Both bound and free T_4 levels are measured. • Total T_4 levels are elevated in most patients with hyperthyroidism but are also elevated in normal patients who have elevated TBG levels from estrogen use, pregnancy, and congenital TBG excess. • Total T_4 levels are reduced in patients with hypothyroidism, with nephrotic syndrome, or who are taking anabolic steroids. • The increase in serum T_3 and T_4 levels with thyroiditis and consequent hyperthyroidism result from leakage of colloid and thyroid hormone into the interstitial tissue and blood from disrupted follicles. • Suppression of iodine uptake in patients with increased T_3 and T_4 levels is pathognomonic for subacute thyroiditis.

The **TRH** stimulation test determines the functional status of the pituitary TSH secretory mechanism. • It has currently been replaced by the more sensitive serum TSH assay. • Its use is confined to evaluating pituitary gland function. • Serum thyroid antibodies, such as antimicrosomal and antithyroglobulin, may be present in autoimmune diseases such as Hashimoto's thyroiditis and Graves' disease. • About 80% of patients with Hashimoto's thyroiditis have detectable autoantibodies.

RAIU is also an effective measure of thyroid function but is less frequently used. • This study works on the premise that more iodine is trapped by the thyroid in those with hyperthyroidism, resulting in an elevated value. • The opposite is true for hypothyroidism. • It is important to note that both L-thyroxine and iodine administration during radiologic studies, such as angiography, computed tomography (CT), and cystography, can give falsely low results.

ANSWER:
A, B, C, D

11. Which of the following is/are accurate regarding cervical US imaging?

    A. Can differentiate between solid and cystic lesions

    B. May detect lesions as small as 2 mm

    C. Differentiates benign from malignant lesions

    D. Allows follow-up of thyroid nodules in response to therapy

    E. Useful in evaluating other structures, including lymph nodes and parathyroid glands

Ref.: 1–4

COMMENT: US imaging is a fast, sensitive, and noninvasive means of evaluating the thyroid gland. • It can also be used to detect pathologic conditions of the parathyroid and cervical lymph nodes. • It easily differentiates solid and cystic lesions and may be used to help guide an FNA biopsy of a suspicious lesion. • High-resolution US can detect nodules as small as 2 mm. • Because there is no pathomnemonic feature distinguishing malignant from benign lesions, it cannot be used to exclude malignancy. • US findings suggestive of malignancy include hypoechoic lesions, punctuate calcifications (papillary carcinoma), and nodularity or intramural projections within a thyroid cyst. • US findings suggestive of benign disease include simple cysts or solid, hyperechoic lesions. • If a patient with a benign-appearing nodule is observed or treated with TSH-suppressive doses of exogenous thyroid hormone or if a simple cyst is aspirated, US is useful in following any changes in the lesion in response to these interventions. • In addition, US can evaluate other cervical structures, including lymph nodes, major vessels, and the parathyroid glands.

ANSWER:
A, B, D, E

12. Match the imaging modality on the left with the statement on the right.

A. MRI	a. May be used for imaging as well as treatment
B. Radioiodine	b. Most useful as an imaging agent for lymphoma or anaplastic cancer
C. Gallium	c. Optimal for imaging the mediastinum
D. US	d. Assesses adenopathy and assists in node biopsy
E. Computed tomography (CT)	e. May be promising for differentiating follicular cancer from follicular adenoma

Ref.: 1–4

COMMENTS: No current imaging method is capable of reliably differentiating a benign nodule from a malignant one. • **Radioactive iodine** is most specific and predicts the subsequent ability to treat with a larger iodine dose. • It is useful only for well-differentiated thyroid cancer. • Even so, some papillary tumors and approximately 50% of metastases from both papillary and follicular carcinomas cannot be detected. • ^{123}I is the best isotope for diagnosis, and ^{131}I is best for treatment.

Gallium is most useful as an imaging agent for patients with anaplastic carcinoma or thyroid lymphoma. • Imaging with gallium frequently is positive in these iodine-negative tumors. • Although a negative scan essentially excludes thyroid lymphoma, interpretation of a positive scan is complicated by the frequency of uptake in Hashimoto's thyroiditis, a common underlying disorder.

Positron emission tomography (PET), although not widely available, is useful for measuring nodule volume. • Its combination with **fluorine-18-fluorodeoxyglucose (FDG) imaging** is intriguing and requires further study. • Nonisotopic imaging is useful as an adjunct to the methods described previously.

US imaging is useful for evaluating the neck for adenopathy or recurrence. • It has the additional benefit of allowing directed biopsy of the nodule or area in question.

CT scanning may be optimal for imaging the mediastinum. • Its use in thyroid cancer should be limited to noncontrast studies, if possible, to avoid interference with iodine imaging or treatment.

MRI, although more expensive than CT, introduces no radiation exposure, does not use iodinated contrast, and can produce images in three planes. • It permits differentiation of fibrosis from residual or recurrent disease and identification of muscle invasion.

The recent demonstration of the use of proton magnetic imaging to distinguish between follicular cancer and follicular adenoma is encouraging.

A N S W E R :
A-e; B-a; C-b; D-d; E-c

13. With regard to the recurrent laryngeal nerve (RLN), which of the following statements is/are true?

A. Following a month without clinical improvement, unilateral injured vocal cords should be assessed and treated with injection of collagen or Teflon.

B. Bilateral injury may result in tracheostomy.

C. Anatomically, the most common location of the RLN is along the tracheoesophageal groove.

D. Re-exploration is associated with an increased risk of injury.

E. If tumor has encompassed the RLN, the nerve should always be divided to obtain adequate margins.

Ref.: 1–4

COMMENTS: The anatomic relationships of greatest importance to the thyroid are those related to the RLN. • Injury to the RLN results in paralysis of the vocal cords on the ipsilateral side. • The cord may remain in a paramedial position or be adducted toward the midline. • Clinically, patients present with hoarseness, a weakened voice, and occasionally shortness of breath. • It is important to assess cord function preoperatively as well as postoperatively. • The RLN generally courses in the tracheoesophageal groove posterior to the inferior thyroid artery, although in approximately 20% of patients it travels anteriorly to the inferior thyroid artery. • Permanent RLN injuries occur during 1–2% of thyroid operations performed by experienced surgeons. • Re-explorations increase the risk to 5%. • Temporary RLN injuries occur more commonly. • Therefore, one should follow the patient for a period of 6–9 months to see whether vocal cord function returns. • If no function returns by then, injection of the paralyzed vocal cord with collagen or Teflon helps tighten it, thereby improving function. • Bilateral injury is much more serious because both cords assume a median or paramedian position, resulting in airway obstruction. • If this occurs, the patient often requires an emergent tracheostomy. • Sometimes the RLN must be sacrificed because of tumor involvement, although generally it can be preserved and dissected free from the tumor when it is functioning preoperatively. • When it is encompassed by tumor, the nerve should be identified where it enters the tumor and then dissected free from the tumor. • This is not possible in some patients.

A N S W E R :
B, C, D

14. Match each cause of hyperthyroidism in the left-hand column with one or more appropriate descriptions in the right-hand column.

A. Graves' disease	a. Autonomous function independent of TSH, long-acting thyroid stimulator (LATS), and thyroid-stimulating immunoglobulins (TSI)
B. Toxic multinodular goiter	b. Diffuse glandular involvement, with increased vascularity and lymphoid aggregates
C. Toxic adenoma	c. Extrathyroidal manifestations
	d. Possible presence of cervical compression symptoms

Ref.: 1–4

COMMENTS: Overactivity of the thyroid gland may be manifested only as an elevation in the amount of circulating thyroid hormone, or it may be clinically evident from a number of signs and symptoms, many of which mimic catecholamine excess (e.g., hypertension, tachycardia, flushing, and sweating). • Overproduction of thyroid hormone may occur with diffuse involvement of the gland (diffuse toxic goiter or Graves' disease). • Alternatively, it may occur in the setting of a single "hot" nodule (toxic adenoma) or in a multinodular gland (Plummer's disease). • Each of these causes of hyperthyroidism is several times more common in women than in men. • Graves' disease occurs most commonly during the third and fourth decades, whereas toxic thyroid nodules are found most commonly in patients over 50 years of age. • Other rare causes of hyperthyroidism include trophoblastic tumors and TSH-secreting pituitary tumors. • With toxic adenoma or toxic multinodular goiter, the hyperfunctioning nodules are thought to represent adenomas that are functioning autonomously. • In contradistinction, Graves' disease is thought to be an autoimmune phenomenon in which TSH receptors within the thyroid gland are stimulated by binding with immunoglobulins (LATS and TSI). • Increased vascularity (a bruit) and lymphoid tissue may be present. • Among the entities producing hyperthyroidism, Graves' disease is unique in its association with extrathyroidal manifestations (e.g., exophthalmos and pretibial myxedema), which may bear no relationship to the presence or severity of thyroid overactivity. • Enlargement of the thyroid gland associated with any of the aforementioned causes of thyrotoxicosis may produce tracheal or pharyngoesophageal compression symptoms.

ANSWER:
A-b,c,d; B-a,d; C-a,d

15. With regard to the use of radioiodine to treat hyperthyroidism, which of the following statements is/are true?

   A. Hypothyroidism occurs in essentially all cases.

   B. There is a marked increased risk of future thyroid cancers after radioiodine therapy.

   C. Radioiodine ablation is generally accomplished through the use of ^{123}I.

   D. Radioiodine may pass through the placenta and lactating breasts to produce hypothyroidism in fetuses and infants.

Ref.: 1–4

COMMENTS: See Question 16.

16. Match each clinical situation in the left-hand column with the most appropriate treatment in the right-hand column.

   A. A 25-year-old with Graves' disease and a markedly enlarged gland with compressive symptoms

   B. An 8-year-old with Graves' disease and a small gland

   C. A 38-year-old with a toxic adenoma

   D. A 35-year-old with a toxic, diffuse goiter, and keloid formation

   E. A 40-year-old with Graves' disease and a nodule in one lobe

   a. Surgery
   b. Radioiodine
   c. Antithyroid drugs

Ref.: 1–4

COMMENTS: The treatment of Graves' disease is controversial and may be accomplished effectively with a subtotal or total thyroidectomy, radioiodine therapy, or antithyroid drugs. • All of these forms of treatment have particular advantages and shortcomings. • **Antithyroid drugs** exert their effect by interfering with the conversion of iodine to organic compounds (iodine binding) and by preventing the coupling of iodotyrosine. • Treatment with these drugs is long term—up to 2 years—and may be associated with drug fever, rash, and granulocytopenia. • Agranulocytosis occurs in fewer than 0.4% of treated patients, but it can be fatal. • Furthermore, recurrence of hyperthyroidism after cessation of the drugs occurs in as many as 60% of patients. • **Radioiodine ablation** of the thyroid with ^{131}I may take several weeks to months to exert its effect and is associated with the almost certain occurrence of future hypothyroidism. • Radioiodine may pass through the placenta and lactating breasts, thereby producing hypothyroidism in fetuses and infants. • Radioiodine should be avoided in children. • Although the carcinogenic effects of radioiodine are theoretically possible, clinical experience has not supported this concern. • Such therapy is safe and effective and, in comparison with surgery, relatively inexpensive. • **Thyroidectomy** confers the risk of anesthesia and trauma to the recurrent laryngeal nerves and parathyroids. • Thyroidectomy has the advantage of an

immediate response and the reversal of compression symptoms. • Hypothyroidism after subtotal thyroidectomy also is common.

Each of these three forms of treatment may be appropriate for a particular patient with Graves' disease. • Specific circumstances occasionally influence the therapeutic choice. • Antithyroid medications are used initially in most patients to render them euthyroid. • Antithyroid medications are also used for young patients and for patients with relatively small goiters and only mild elevation of serum thyroid hormone levels. • Patients with extremely large glands, particularly those causing compressive symptoms, are most readily treated by thyroidectomy. • Surgery is indicated in patients with "cold" nodules within toxic glands because these nodules carry the same risk of malignancy as those found in a euthyroid gland. • Toxic multinodular goiters probably are most effectively treated by surgical excision. • Radioiodine may be less effective for this condition than it is for Graves' disease because of the inhomogeneous uptake of the nuclide by the multinodular gland. • Toxic adenomas are best treated by surgery involving lobectomy on the involved side, which provides an immediately effective treatment, frequently with preservation of enough thyroid tissue that there is no need for thyroid replacement therapy. • Pregnant patients whose condition is not readily controlled with antithyroid medications should undergo surgical resection of the thyroid.

ANSWERS:
Question 15: A, D
Question 16: A-a,c; B-c; C-a,c; D-b,c; E-a,c

17. Which of the following is/are true about the treatment and management of Graves' disease?

   A. Treatment of choice is subtotal thyroidectomy.

   B. Subtotal thyroidectomy and irradiation have similar recurrence rates.

   C. Radioactive iodine is the treatment of choice other than in children and women of childbearing age.

   D. Recurrence rates for antithyroid drugs are comparable to that for subtotal thyroidectomy.

   E. Subtotal thyroidectomy results in an improvement in exophthalmos.

Ref.: 1–4

COMMENTS: Graves' disease is an autoimmune disorder that targets the thyroid, extraocular muscles, and skin. • Patients with this disorder complain of fatigue, palpitations, tremors, shortening of menstrual cycles, anxiety, weight loss, and heat intolerance. • The diagnosis of thyrotoxicosis can be established by demonstrating elevation of the free thyroxine (T_4) index and suppression of the serum concentration of TSH. • The diagnosis of Graves' disease is established by high thyroid RAIU in a thyrotoxic patient who has a diffuse goiter. • Therapy may consist of treatment with ^{131}I, antithyroid drugs, and subtotal thyroidectomy. • Radioactive iodine therapy is most commonly used, rendering 90% of patients euthyroid or hypothyroid. • The relapse rate is 10–25%. • This form of therapy is contraindicated during pregnancy. • Antithyroid drugs, propylthiouracil or methimazole, are used with the intent of inducing remission of Graves' disease. • Remission rates approach 40% at 1 year and 65% at 2 years, but recurrence rates can be as high as 72%. • Subtotal thyroidectomy removes most of the thyroid tissue, leaving behind a thyroid remnant of 2–7 g, which may cause the patient to become euthyroid. • The recurrence rates are equal to that of irradiation (up to 10%). • Subtotal thyroidectomy can be associated with recurrent laryngeal nerve injury and transient or permanent hypocalcemia. • It is imperative that the patient be made pharmacologically euthyroid preoperatively to avoid thyroid storm. • Surgery does not reliably result in an alleviation of exophthalmos, but there are reports that total thyroidectomy may be beneficial.

ANSWER:
B, C

18. Which of the following statements about drug therapy for thyroid disease is/are true?

A. Both propylthiouracil (PTU) and methimazole inhibit linking of iodotyrosine molecules MIT and DIT.

B. Methimazole can inhibit peripheral conversion of T4 to T3.

C. Methimazole can cross the placenta and affect fetal development.

D. Steroids can be used to inhibit T3 formation in acute conditions.

E. β-Blockers effectively inhibit T3 formation, but are slower in doing so compared to PTU.

Ref.: 1–4

COMMENTS: Both PTU and methimazole inhibit the organification and oxidation of inorganic iodine and the linking of MIT and DIT. • In addition, PTU inhibits peripheral conversion of T4 to T3. • Methimazole has a longer half-life and can cross the placenta in pregnant women, with a possible adverse effect on fetal development. • Both drugs can cause agranulocytosis in 1% of patients. • Steroids can actually suppress the pituitary-thyroid axis. • Steroids can inhibit peripheral conversion of T4 to T3 and can lower serum TSH as well. • Because they act quickly, steroids may be used as a rapid inhibitory agent in severe or acute hyperthyroid conditions. • β-Blockers do not inhibit thyroid hormone synthesis but are used to control peripheral sensitivity to catecholamines. • In short, β-blockers control the symptoms of hyperthyroidism.

ANSWER:
A, C, D

19. Which of the following is true regarding thyroid storm?

A. It results from the inability of the thyroid to produce enough T3 or T4 in response to stress.

B. It may be seen in a patient with untreated Graves' disease who undergoes physiologic stress, such as an operation.

C. The treatment of choice is immediate resuscitation and resection of the thyroid nodule causing the symptoms.

D. Treatment consists of β-blockers, cooling blankets, and PTU.

Ref.: 1–5

COMMENT: Thyroid storm is a life-threatening emergency caused by severe thyrotoxicosis. • Stress, including trauma, sepsis, or surgery, may precipitate this condition, particularly in hyperthyroid patients who are untreated. • Treatment consists of correcting the precipitating event and controlling the thyrotoxicosis and its attendant symptoms. • Thyrotoxicosis is managed with PTU and inorganic iodide, which block T3 and T4 synthesis and slow the release of existing hormone. • β-Blockers do not control hormone release per se but help attenuate the symptoms of hyperthyroidism, including fever, diaphoresis, tachycardia, restlessness, and agitation.

• Supportive measures, including fever reduction and fluid administration, should also be initiated.

ANSWER:
B, D

20. A 50-year-old woman presents with a 2-year history of mild, diffuse, tender thyroid enlargement; a 10-pound weight gain; and fatigue. Of the following diagnoses, which is the most likely?

A. Riedel's thyroiditis

B. Hashimoto's thyroiditis

C. Subacute thyroiditis

D. Acute suppurative thyroiditis

E. Papillary thyroid carcinoma

Ref.: 1–4

COMMENTS: See Question 21.

21. Match each form of thyroiditis in the left-hand column with the proper clinical description in the right-hand column.

A. Acute suppurative thyroiditis

B. Subacute (de Quervain's) thyroiditis

C. Hashimoto's disease

D. Riedel's thyroiditis

a. May be associated with retroperitoneal fibrosis

b. Acute illness of bacterial origin

c. Most common form of thyroiditis

d. Probably of viral origin

Ref.: 1–4

COMMENTS: Hashimoto's disease is the most common form of chronic thyroiditis. • It most often occurs in middle-aged women, who present with complaints of fatigue and a diffusely enlarged thyroid that may be tender. • Although hyperthyroidism may be present in patients with Hashimoto's disease, most are either euthyroid or hypothyroid. • The disease is thought to be an autoimmune process, and one of the confirming diagnostic findings is the presence of antithyroid antibodies. • Frequently, no treatment is needed. • However, thyroid replacement therapy is used if the patient is hypothyroid. • The incidence of papillary thyroid carcinoma among patients with Hashimoto's disease is not higher than that among the general population. • Therefore, prophylactic thyroidectomy is not warranted. • Operation generally is reserved for symptoms of compression or for removal of nodules within the diseased gland that are potentially malignant. • **Acute suppurative thyroiditis** is rare. • It manifests as a sudden onset of severe pain associated with fever, chills, and dysphagia. • It almost always follows an acute upper respiratory infection and is of bacterial origin. • Treatment is with antibiotics and occasionally drainage. • **Subacute (de Quervain's) thyroiditis** also frequently follows an upper respiratory infection. • Although association with a viral cause is considered most likely, an autoimmune mechanism has been suggested because of the presence of thyroid antibodies. • Although the onset is fairly abrupt, the clinical course is less fulminant than that of acute suppurative thyroiditis. • It is characterized by moderate swelling and tenderness of the thyroid gland with repeated exacerbations and remissions over several months. • Recovery is frequently spontaneous but may be facilitated by a course of salicylate or corticosteroid therapy. • **Riedel's struma** is a rare, chronic inflammatory condition characterized by dense fibrosis throughout the thyroid and periglandular tissues. • It frequently results in hypothyroidism and symptoms of tracheal and esophageal compression. • It has been associated with other fibrotic reactions, including retroperitoneal fibrosis and sclerosing mediastinitis. • When unilateral, it is difficult to distinguish from carcinoma. • Treatment usually includes thyroid hormone therapy, and operation may be necessary for relief of tracheoesophageal obstruction.

ANSWERS:
Question 20: B
Question 21: A-b; B-d; C-c; D-a

22. With regard to goiter, which of the following statements is/are correct?

A. The term *goiter* can refer to any abnormal enlargement of the thyroid gland.

B. The term *familial goiter* implies that a genetic defect may play a role in the etiology.

C. The most identifiable cause of endemic goiter is iodine deficiency.

D. Immediate operation is indicated for patients with extremely large iodine-deficiency goiters because of the increased risk of cancer in the larger glands.

Ref.: 1–4

COMMENTS: The term *goiter* refers broadly to any abnormal enlargement of the thyroid gland, whether diffuse or nodular. • Diffuse enlargement of the thyroid without evidence of a functional abnormality is usually the result of a colloid goiter (simple or nontoxic goiter). • On occasion, there is a familial tendency toward diffuse thyroid enlargement (*familial goiter*), in some circumstances caused by an inherited enzymatic defect that results in impaired iodine metabolism. • Affected patients are often hypothyroid. • Diffuse thyroid enlargement is often caused by environmental effects, including the ingestion of goitrogenic foods or drugs (e.g., paraaminosalicylic acid), but the most common is dietary iodine deficiency. • Many countries have so-called goiter belts (endemic goiter), the result of environmental iodine deficiencies that occur in specific geographic locations. • In the United States this is primarily of historical interest today because the use of iodized table salt has become nearly routine. • Diffuse goiters may cause problems by virtue of their cosmetic effect or compression symptoms. • They can occasionally be made smaller with iodine or thyroid hormone administration, but operation may be required. • The risk of cancer is not increased in these glands and is not an indication for operation.

ANSWER:
A, B, C

23. Which of the following statements about a substernal goiter is/are true?

A. It may be associated with subclinical hypothyroidism.

B. CT scan is the best modality for its imaging.

C. Airway compression is an unusual presentation clinically.

D. It can involve the posterior mediastinum as well as the anterior mediastinum.

E. Primary substernal goiter vessels originate from the innominate artery, whereas secondary substernal goiter vessels originate from the superior and inferior thyroid arteries.

F. Treatment is total thyroidectomy.

Ref.: 1–4

COMMENTS: Endemic goiter is primarily the result of dietary iodine deficiency. • It results in primary hypothyroidism, which is associated with an elevated TSH level. • A plain radiograph may demonstrate tracheal deviation, but CT scanning of the neck demonstrates continuity of the mediastinal mass with a cervical goiter and permits identification of tissue planes of intrathoracic goitrous components. • Airway compression is the most common symptom of substernal goiter. • Other symptoms include dysphagia, wheezing, vocal cord paralysis, and rarely superior vena cava (SVC) compression syndrome. • Anatomically, substernal goiters are classified into two types: primary, in which the origin of the blood supply is intrathoracic; and secondary, in which the blood supply is cervical in origin. • Both can be present in either the anterior or the posterior mediastinum. • The surgical procedure of choice is total lobectomy on the side of the substernal goiter. • Most substernal goiters can be removed through a cervical incision. • Rarely, a median sternotomy must be performed. • If patients are kept on thyroid hormone substitution therapy, the recurrence rate is low (2.5%). • Total thyroidectomy is not recommended as an approach to this benign disease unless both lobes are clearly involved.

ANSWER:
A, B, D, E

24. Which of the following is/are associated with an increased risk for developing thyroid cancer.

A. Smoking

B. Dental radiography

C. Medical treatment with [131]I

D. Child undergoing radiation therapy for a Wilms' tumor

E. Individual who lived near Chernobyl

Ref.: 1–4

COMMENTS: A family history of thyroid neoplasms, benign or malignant, of follicular cell origin does not appear to increase the risk of thyroid cancer significantly. • However, a family history of medullary carcinoma of the thyroid (parafollicular cell origin) does increase the risk of developing the same type of thyroid cancer. • Risk is also increased in patients exposed to external radiation (e.g., those receiving upper mantle radiation therapy for Hodgkin's disease up to 5000 rad). • Patients with Wilms' tumor and associated childhood tumors such as neuroblastoma and leukemias have an increased risk for developing thyroid cancer secondary to their radiation exposure. • Therapeutic radioiodine administration, as used for treatment of hyperthyroidism, has not been associated with an increased subsequent risk of thyroid cancer; it is presumed that this is because of the nearly total destruction of the follicular cells. • Smoking is not a risk factor for the development of thyroid carcinoma. • Medical treatment with ^{131}I at low doses for diagnostic imaging or high doses for thyroid ablation does not appear to increase the incidence of thyroid cancer. • On the other hand, the nuclear fallout present at Chernobyl released multiple short-lived isotopes ^{131}I, [133]I, and [135]I, and there has been an increase in the incidence of papillary carcinoma with a high incidence of lymph node metastases in patients living in the Chernobyl region. • Papillary cancer is the most common thyroid cancer associated with radiation exposure. • Patients with a history of radiation exposure and who have papillary cancer require total thyroidectomy. • It is of note that patients are at increased risk for developing thyroid cancer for periods as long as 50 years after exposure. • Dental radiographs are usually not associated with an increased risk.

ANSWER:
D, E

25. Which of the following thyroid adenomas in rare instances behaves in a malignant manner?

    A. Colloid adenoma

    B. Embryonal adenoma

    C. Fetal adenoma

    D. Hürthle cell adenoma

Ref.: 1–4

COMMENTS: The clinical significance of thyroid adenomas is related to the need to differentiate them from thyroid carcinoma. • Such differentiation frequently requires thyroid lobectomy for tissue diagnosis. • Once the histologic diagnosis is known, no further treatment is necessary. • Some clinicians believe that thyroid suppression should be used to reduce the risk of development of future adenomas. • The **colloid**, **embryonal**, and **fetal** adenomas are all considered subcategories of follicular adenoma and are differentiated from each other by the relative amount of colloid present and the architectural arrangement of the epithelial cells. • Cytologically, all these cells appear to be similar to the normal thyroid follicular cell. • These follicular adenomas are entirely benign and do not increase the risk of carcinoma. • **Hürthle cell adenoma** is characterized by Hürthle cells (variable enlargement, hyperchromatic nuclei, and granular cytoplasm) and is considered by some pathologists to be, in fact, a low-grade follicular carcinoma. • Although it is rare for a benign-appearing Hürthle cell adenoma to behave in a malignant manner, the noncommittal term *Hürthle cell tumor* has been used to describe these neoplasms. • The term *Hürthle cell carcinoma* is reserved for the clearly malignant variant. • Some clinicians believe that a more aggressive surgical approach (total thyroidectomy) is indicated for routine management of Hürthle cell tumors because of their potentially (albeit rare) malignant behavior.

ANSWER:
D

26. From each of the following pairs of features of thyroid nodules, select the one that is associated with the greater likelihood of malignancy.

    A. Solid versus cystic

    B. Solitary versus multiple.

    C. "Hot" versus "cold"

    D. Rapid enlargement overnight versus slow enlargement over many months

    E. Hard versus soft

    F. Male versus female patient

    G. Child versus adult patient

Ref.: 1–4

COMMENTS: The management of thyroid nodules, particularly the decision as to whether surgical intervention is required, depends on the clinical index of suspicion that the nodule is malignant.

• Numerous factors in the history, physical examination, and laboratory examination of the patient raise or lower one's index of suspicion. • Epidemiologically, thyroid cancers are more common in adults than in children and in women than in men because thyroid nodules themselves are more common in those populations. • The likelihood that a given nodule is malignant, however, is greater in males than in females and in children than in adults. • Most thyroid cancers grow slowly and indolently. • Extremely rapid growth (e.g., described as sudden enlargement overnight) usually is caused by hemorrhage into a previously undetected nodule. • A history of recent voice change or difficulty swallowing, particularly when the lesion is small, should raise the index of suspicion of malignancy. • On physical examination, soft or fleshy lesions suggest benign disease, whereas hardness is more often associated with malignancy. • Indirect laryngoscopy should be performed to search for ipsilateral vocal cord paresis or paralysis, which suggests that the thyroid nodule may be invading or compressing the recurrent laryngeal nerve. • Radionuclide scans can provide information about the metabolic activity of the nodule and the number of nodules present. • US imaging can provide information about the number of nodules and their solid or cystic nature. • A single nodule, decreased or absent function ("cold"), and solid consistency increase the likelihood of malignancy compared to multiple nodules, hyperfunction ("hot"), and cystic consistency. • A solitary, solid, cold thyroid nodule carries a 10–20% risk of malignancy; whereas cystic structure, multinodularity, and normal or hyperfunctioning status carry risks in the range of 5% or less.

ANSWER:
A-solid; B-solitary; C-cold; D-slow; E-hard; F-male; G-child

27. With regard to the technique of FNA biopsy of the thyroid, which one of the following statements is/are true?

    A. It is generally contraindicated because of the extremely vascular nature of the thyroid gland.

    B. False-positive results are rare.

    C. False-negative results occur less often than false-positive results.

    D. There is a 3% risk that cancer cells will implant along the needle tract.

    E. Benign versus malignant follicular neoplasms can be easily differentiated.

Ref.: 1–4

COMMENTS: FNA biopsy is a standard technique for evaluating thyroid nodules. • Using 18- to 25-gauge needles, in the absence of coagulopathy, hemorrhagic complications are rare. • The theoretic complication of cancer cell implantation along the needle tract has not been observed. • Although false-negative results are rare (<5%), when the clinical suspicion of malignancy is high a negative needle biopsy should not deter surgery. • Because of the possibility of a false-negative result, patients should undergo repeated needle aspirations and follow-up observation. • Changes in examination or cytologic findings to those of a more suspicious nature dictate surgical resection of the nodule. • False-positive results are rare (<1%) when the specimens are of good quality and examined by an experienced cytologist. • Therefore, such nodules should be resected. • It has a reported sensitivity of 68–98% and a specificity of 56–100% for malignancy. • An adequate FNA specimen is categorized as benign, suspicious, indeterminate, or malignant. • Up to 75% of lesions are diagnosed as benign, while 5% of FNA specimens confirm malignancy. • The remainder are suspicious lesions. • With regard to malignancy, FNA can diagnose papillary, medullary, and anaplastic thyroid cancer. • FNA can also be used to diagnose and treat cystic thyroid lesions. • The area of greatest difficulty during interpretation is with follicular neoplasms, for which differentiation of benign from malignant depends more on gross and histologic tumor architecture than on cytologic findings. • Nodules whose cytologic features are reportedly atypical, suspicious, possibly malignant, or consistent with a follicular neoplasm should be resected because approximately 20% of them are carcinomas.

ANSWER:
B

28. Which of these are prognostic factors in patients with papillary thyroid cancer?

A. Age

B. Metastases (distant)

C. Grade of the tumor

D. Extent of the primary tumor

E. Size of the primary tumor

Ref.: 1–4

COMMENTS: Clinical scoring systems have been constructed to help predict prognosis in patients with thyroid cancer. • The AMES system is based on age, distant metastasis, extent of primary tumor, and tumor size, while the AGES system is based on age, grade of the tumor, extent of the tumor, as well as its size. • In both systems, age (<40 years of age in men and <50 years of age in women) is the most important prognostic factor in determining long-term survival.

ANSWER:
A, B, C, D, E

29. Match each type of thyroid cancer in the left-hand column with the appropriate response in the right-hand column.

A. Papillary	a. Worst prognosis
B. Follicular	b. Most commonly associated with radiation exposure
C. Medullary	c. Associated with hyperparathyroidism
D. Anaplastic	d. Hematogenous metastatic spread to bone
E. Lymphoma	e. Usually requires systemic chemo- or radiation therapy

Ref.: 1–4

COMMENTS: Papillary cancer is the most common thyroid cancer (80% of cases) and has the best prognosis. • It is associated with a history of prior irradiation, as in treatments for tonsillitis in the 1950s or exposure to areas of nuclear fallout (e.g., at Chernobyl). • Follicular cancer is the next most common thyroid cancer (10% of cases). • Unlike papillary thyroid cancer, which tends to spread through the lymphatic system, follicular cancer spreads hematogenously, with bone and liver most commonly involved as distant metastatic sites. • Medullary cancer (3–5% of cases) occurs sporadically or in the setting of the MEN II syndromes. • Those cancers in patients with MEN IIa are associated with hyperparathyroidism as well as pheochromocytomas. • Patients with medullary cancers should be screened for these other cancers, particularly if there is a family history to suggest the MEN syndrome.

• Anaplastic cancer is the least common (1–2% of cases), yet most aggressive thyroid cancer. • It progresses rapidly, often causing symptoms of airway obstruction, cervical pain, or even superior vena cava syndrome. • Overall survival of patients with anaplastic cancer is dismal, and surgery is most often palliative. • Thyroid lymphoma (1% of cases) should be considered in patients with rapidly growing goiter. • Diagnosis is made by FNA. • Treatment consists primarily of chemotherapy (CHOP regimen: cyclophosphamide, doxorubicin/adriamycin, vincristine, prednisolone), though surgical debulking may help increase patient survival.

ANSWER:
A-b; B-d; C-c; D-a; E-e

30. With regard to papillary carcinoma, which of the following is/are true?

A. It is the most common thyroid malignancy.

B. It has the best prognosis.

C. Children are more likely to have lymph node metastases on presentation.

D. It often metastasizes to bone and lung.

E. It is the most common thyroid malignancy associated with previous radiation exposure.

F. Gardner syndrome is a risk factor for the development of papillary cancer.

G. Most tumors are unilateral.

Ref.: 1–4

COMMENTS: Papillary thyroid carcinoma is the most common form of thyroid cancer and carries the best prognosis. • It manifests primarily as local and regional involvement. • Distant metastases are present in fewer than 1% of patients at initial presentation. • It accounts for most thyroid cancers seen in patients with prior exposure to radiation. • There is a high likelihood (up to 80%) of occult multicentric disease when the gland is examined pathologically with special care. • These pathologic findings and autopsy data reveal a much higher incidence of occult disease than clinical disease indicates and raise the question as to the biologic importance of these occult papillary cancers. • In contrast to most other epithelial cancers, the presence of regional lymph node metastases in patients does not appear to affect prognosis adversely so long as the disease is resectable. • The incidence of local metastases is high with papillary carcinoma, ranging from 37% to 65% in adults, but the incidence is higher for children, ranging from 50–80%. • Evaluations of large numbers of patients with papillary carcinoma in several series have failed to demonstrate any significant adverse mortality effects of local metastases of papillary carcinoma. • The overall mortality rate from papillary thyroid cancer ranges from 1–10%, generally occurring only in older patients with large primary tumors. • Death from papillary thyroid cancer is usually caused by aggressive local and regional behavior with tracheoesophageal and mediastinal involvement or by differentiation to a more anaplastic form. • It is of note that familial adenomatous polyposis (Gardner syndrome) is associated with excessive rates of differentiated thyroid carcinoma: 89% papillary with a high 17:1 female/male ratio.

ANSWER:
A, B, C, E, F

31. Fine-needle aspiration of a 3-cm thyroid nodule reveals papillary cancer. Which of the following is/are true?

    A. Orphan Annie-eye nuclei can be present histologically.

    B. The patient should undergo further radiologic evaluation of the neck with CT scans to assess lymph nodes and tumor extension due to the large size of the nodule.

    C. Psammoma bodies can be present histologically.

    D. Multiple histologic subtypes of papillary carcinoma exist.

    E. The tall cell variant of papillary cancer carries a poor prognosis.

    Ref.: 1–4

COMMENTS: FNA is considered the gold standard for evaluation of a thyroid nodule. • The false-negative rate is less than 5% and the false-positive rate less than 1–2% when an experienced cytologist evaluates the specimen. • Distinctive features of papillary carcinoma include large nuclei with a pale-staining, "ground glass appearance." These optically clear nuclei are referred to as **Orphan Annie-eye nuclei**. • Also present are **psammoma bodies**, which represent degenerative changes in the papillae of papillary carcinoma that appear as laminated, basophilic structures. • They appear in 40–50% of papillary carcinomas and are virtually pathognomonic. • Further radiologic evaluation of the neck with CT does not change the treatment of this patient, which is total thyroidectomy. • A more cost-effective means of identifying suspicious but not palpable lymph nodes is US imaging of the neck. • There are multiple histologic subtypes of papillary carcinoma: encapsulated, follicular, tall cell, diffuse sclerosing, oxyphilic, and others, including columnar cell, clear cell, insular, lipomatous, and trabecular. • Tall-cell carcinoma of the thyroid is a histologic variant that is more invasive, highly aggressive, and more common in elderly patients. • Tall-cell variants carry a poor prognosis. • It is of note that according to the World Health Organization classification, all carcinomas displaying any papillary features, either pure or in mixed form (with follicular elements), are classified as papillary carcinomas.

ANSWER:
A, C, D, E

32. A 29-year-old man presents with a firm 2-cm mass in the right thyroid lobe and an ipsilateral lower deep jugular lymph node 1.5 cm in diameter. Both are examined cytologically by FNA biopsy and are found to contain papillary cancer. Which of the following therapies is/are most appropriate?

    A. Thyroid lobectomy with external beam radiotherapy to the involved part of the neck

    B. Total thyroidectomy and ipsilateral radical neck dissection

    C. Total thyroidectomy with ipsilateral modified radical neck dissection

    D. Total thyroidectomy and bilateral modified radical neck dissection

    E. Excision of thyroid lobe and isthmus with ipsilateral modified radical neck dissection

    F. Enucleation of the primary tumor from the thyroid gland

    G. Excision of thyroid lobe and isthmus and paratracheal node dissection

    Ref.: 1–4

COMMENTS: Papillary thyroid cancer is primarily a surgically treated disease. • External beam radiation therapy is indicated only for unresectable disease. • Radioiodine ablation is appropriate in high-risk patients (i.e., those who are older, have large primary tumors, and whose tumors have extrathyroidal extension or lateral cervical metastases). • The extent of the surgical management of the primary tumor is also controversial.

Enucleation of the tumor without anatomic dissection of the involved lobe is not appropriate. • It carries the risk of hemorrhage, injury to the nonvisualized recurrent laryngeal nerve, and implantation of the wound with cancer.

Excision of the involved thyroid lobe and isthmus is an acceptable approach for small (<1.5 cm in diameter) papillary carcinomas that are contained within that lobe. • Clinicians who prefer this approach do so because of the risk of hypoparathyroidism and nerve injury and the lack of evidence of a survival benefit when the clinically uninvolved contralateral lobe is resected.

Other clinicians believe that a near-total or total thyroidectomy is warranted. • The rationale for this more aggressive approach is based on the recognized incidence of multicentric disease (albeit with an unclear clinical significance), facilitation of possible postoperative radioiodine therapy by surgical ablation of the remaining thyroid parenchyma, and a decreased incidence of recurrence in the contralateral lobe. • Some authors have advocated subtotal resection of the contralateral lobe (particularly in high-risk patients) to obtain the potential benefits of the more extensive resections without the added risks of nerve or parathyroid injury.

The management of cervical lymph node metastases has become more conservative. • It is now generally accepted that a modified radical neck dissection (sparing the sternocleidomastoid muscle, internal jugular vein, and spinal accessory nerve) is appropriate management of clinically evident cervical node metastases.

Some clinicians believe that even less radical surgery that removes only the grossly positive nodes (the so-called berry-picking procedure) may also be appropriate.

Prophylactic dissection of the clinically uninvolved part of the neck for papillary thyroid carcinoma (ipsilateral or contralateral) has not been shown to be beneficial. • For patients in whom the neck is clinically uninvolved with a proven papillary carcinoma, prophylactic paratracheal lymph node dissection may be appropriate because it can easily be performed without extending the incision and without functional or cosmetic compromise. • Furthermore, it involves removal of the stage I lymph nodes that are most likely to be involved by papillary carcinoma.

ANSWER:
C

33. A 23-year-old male patient is found to have a 1.5-cm papillary carcinoma completely contained in his right thyroid lobe. True or false: central compartment lymph nodes portend a poorer prognosis for this patient compared to a similar tumor without cervical metastasis.

    Ref.: 1–4

COMMENTS: Younger patients have a higher incidence of lymph node metastasis with papillary thyroid cancer compared to older patients. • However, this does not appear to worsen prognosis or mortality considerably when the primary tumor is completely intrathyroidal. • Extension of the primary tumor through the capsule portends a poorer prognosis, particularly in the presence of lymph node metastasis.

ANSWER:
False

34. In regard to follicular thyroid cancer, which of the following is/are true?

  A. It is more common in geographic regions that are iodine deficient.

  B. It occurs predominantly in females, and estrogens have been recently found to be a risk factor.

  C. The major histologic criterion for diagnosis is unequivocal capsular and vascular invasion.

  D. Both minimally invasive and widely invasive follicular cancers are likely to have regional lymph node involvement on presentation.

  E. Cytologically, it can be easily differentiated from a benign adenoma.

Ref.: 1–4

COMMENTS: Follicular carcinoma constitutes approximately 15% of all thyroid cancers. • Patients with follicular thyroid cancer (FTC) tend to be older than those with papillary thyroid cancer. • Due to the preponderance of FTC in female patients, it has been suggested that estrogens may be associated with thyroid cancer. • Experiments have shown that thyrocytes express estrogen receptors, and estrogen stimulates the growth of thyrocytes. • However, pregnancy has not been shown to increase the risk for thyroid cancer, and the role of estrogen in thyroid cancer currently remains unresolved. • FTC is common in regions that are iodine deficient, and rates of FTC have decreased in regions that have received iodine supplementation. • Characteristics of both papillary and follicular tumors are frequently found within the same neoplasm, and these so-called mixed cancers tend to behave like a pure papillary thyroid cancer. • Pure follicular carcinoma is difficult to diagnose on the basis of cytologic characteristics alone because its cells appear similar to those of its benign counterpart, the follicular adenoma. • The diagnosis is more reliably obtained by the identification of vascular or capsular invasion of the tumor. • Such invasive characteristics may be present, even though the capsule appears to be discrete and intact grossly. • This is why one must do a thyroid lobectomy on a patient with an FNA diagnosis of a follicular neoplasm. • These patients have a 20% risk of malignancy. • If the thyroid lobectomy reveals follicular cancer, the patient undergoes total thyroidectomy. • Unlike papillary carcinomas of the thyroid, follicular carcinomas usually spread hematogenously, and their metastatic potential is more likely distant than regional. • Both minimally invasive and widely invasive follicular carcinomas involve the regional lymph nodes in only 10% of patients on presentation. • The most common sites of distant metastases are lung and bone.

ANSWER:
A, C

35. A 40-year-old woman comes to the clinician's office with a thyroid mass, which is confirmed on FNA and US to be a unilateral, 3.2-cm follicular neoplasm. She has been completely asymptomatic. What will the next intervention be?

  A. Total thyroidectomy

  B. Hemithyroidectomy or isthmusectomy

  C. Excisional biopsy

  D. Core-needle biopsy

  E. Thyroid suppression via T3 or T4 analogues

Ref.: 1–4

COMMENTS: The presence of a follicular neoplasm as confirmed by FNA mandates further evaluation, since FNA does not provide enough information about tissue architecture to differentiate between a benign follicular adenoma and a follicular carcinoma. • Vascular or capsular invasion confirms the presence of carcinoma. • The management of small, unilateral follicular lesions is controversial (total versus hemi-thyroidectomy with frozen section). • However, lesions larger than 4 cm should be treated by a total thyroidectomy, since multicentricity becomes more common as tumor size increases. • Total thyroidectomy also facilitates the effectiveness of postoperative radioactive iodine, since no residual thyroid tissue remains to serve as a sink for the radioisotope.

ANSWER:
A, B

36. A 45-year-old woman with a firm 3-cm nodule in the left thyroid lobe undergoes left thyroid lobectomy. Frozen section reveals a follicular carcinoma with capsular invasion. Which of the following additional therapeutic modalities is/are appropriate in this situation?

  A. Near-total or total thyroidectomy

  B. Radical neck dissection on the involved side

  C. Exogenous thyroid administration to suppress TSH

  D. Radioiodine scan to detect pulmonary metastases with appropriate surgical resection if found

  E. Ablation of residual thyroid tissue and any demonstrated metastases with radioiodine

Ref.: 1–4

COMMENTS: Near-total or total thyroidectomy is favored for follicular carcinoma because it allows detection of metastases by radioiodine postoperatively. • Because regional lymph node metastases from pure follicular thyroid carcinomas are relatively uncommon, prophylactic neck dissection is inappropriate. • Involved cervical lymph nodes are best managed by a modified neck dissection, with preservation of the sternocleidomastoid muscle, internal jugular vein, and spinal accessory nerve. • Radioiodine scanning for the presence of metastases is useful for diagnosing follicular thyroid carcinoma, but its accuracy increases when the residual normal thyroid tissue has been ablated either by surgery or by a prior ablative dose of radioiodine. • If metastases are subsequently found by radioiodine scanning, they are best treated by ablative doses of radioiodine. • In rare instances, resection of isolated metastases is appropriate if they do not have an affinity for iodine. • The growth of well-differentiated (papillary and follicular, nonmedullary) thyroid carcinomas may to some extent be under the influence of TSH, and many such cancers have cell-surface TSH receptors. • The recurrence and survival rates appear to be improved with thyroid hormone administration to obtain TSH suppression. • In fact, regression of known metastatic follicular carcinoma with exogenous thyroid therapy alone has been reported.

ANSWER:
A, C, E

37. With regard to thyroid cancer, which of the following is/are indications for the use of radioiodine therapy (^{131}I)?

  A. Inoperable primary tumor

  B. Postoperative residual disease in neck

  C. Distant metastases

D. Invasion of thyroid capsule

E. Cervical or mediastinal node metastases

F. Recurrent thyroid cancer

Ref.: 1–4

COMMENTS: All of the above are indications of the use of ^{131}I for thyroid cancer. • Patients who undergo near-total or total thyroidectomy improve the ability of ^{131}I to ablate the remaining gland and treat distant metastases. • Patients with treated well-differentiated thyroid cancer are maintained on suppressive doses of thyroid hormone. • Before body imaging with ^{131}I, thyroid hormone must be discontinued to allow the TSH level to rise. • The TSH level usually reaches a maximum 4–6 weeks following total thyroidectomy. • Elevated TSH levels are needed to optimize the ^{131}I scan. • A suggested protocol is as follows. • During the fourth to sixth week after discontinuing thyroid hormone, patients are given a diagnostic dose of 5 or 10 mCi ^{131}I and are scanned 3–4 days later. • If there is any meaningful uptake, patients undergo radioiodine ablation or therapy. • Patients undergo post-therapy scanning 3–7 days later to evaluate the responsiveness of the tumor. • Side effects consist of sialadenitis, gastrointestinal symptoms, male and female infertility, bone marrow suppression, parathyroid dysfunction, and leukemia.

ANSWER:
A, B, C, D, E, F

---

38. All but which of the following statements is/are true about Hürthle cell carcinoma?

A. It is a subtype of follicular cancer.

B. It is composed of oxyphilic cells.

C. It carries a worse prognosis than does follicular cancer.

D. It has a higher rate of recurrence than does follicular cancer.

Ref.: 1–4

COMMENTS: Hürthle cell carcinoma is a subtype of follicular thyroid cancer. • Histologically, it contains oxyphilic cells derived from follicular cells. • Hürthle cell cancer does not necessarily have a worse prognosis than does follicular cancer, but it does have a higher recurrence rate, with regional lymph nodes most commonly affected.

ANSWER:
C

---

39. With regard to medullary thyroid carcinoma, which of the following statements is/are correct?

A. It is derived from a dedifferentiated variant of the same cell that produces papillary and follicular carcinomas.

B. Its pattern of metastatic spread is almost exclusively to distant sites.

C. The serum calcitonin level is useful for diagnosis and management.

D. The prognosis is approximately the same as that of papillary carcinoma.

Ref.: 1–4

COMMENTS: Medullary carcinoma accounts for less than 10% of all thyroid carcinomas. • Its cell of origin is the C-cell, or parafollicular cell, which originates in the neural crest. • It bears no embryologic association with the epithelial cell origin of papillary and follicular tumors. • This cell produces calcitonin, which is involved in calcium homeostasis. • Elevations of serum calcitonin levels occur with C-cell hyperplasia (considered to be a premalignant condition) and frank medullary carcinoma. • Changes in the serum calcitonin level may be useful for monitoring the success of treatment and the presence of recurrent disease. • Medullary thyroid carcinoma has the propensity to spread to both regional lymph nodes and distant metastatic sites, and its prognosis depends on the presence or absence of regional and distant metastases. • The overall 5-year survival rate is approximately 50%, which is considerably less than that for papillary or follicular thyroid carcinoma.

ANSWER:
C

---

40. Match the following characteristics of medullary thyroid carcinoma (MTC) in the left-hand column with either its sporadic form, or its hereditary form, or both in the right-hand column.

A. Contains parafollicular cells that secrete calcitonin

B. Multifocal and bilateral

C. Associated with MEN-IIA and MEN-IIB

D. Worse prognosis

E. Treatment consists of total thyroidectomy with central node dissection

a. Sporadic MTC

b. Hereditary MTC

c. Both

Ref.: 1–4

COMMENTS: MTC, first described in 1959, is a tumor of the C cells, or parafollicular cells. • These cells secrete calcitonin, which is involved in calcium homeostasis. • Calcitonin is used as a tumor marker used to screen patients with multiple endocrine neoplasia types IIA and IIB (MEN-IIA and MEN-IIB) and is useful for following these patients for recurrence and response to treatment. • Medullary cancer can occur in a sporadic form (75% of cases) and a familial form (25% of cases). • In its sporadic form, the tumor is often single and unilateral and occurs without a pattern of familial predisposition. • The tumor generally presents as a solitary thyroid nodule with lymph node metastases at the time of exploration. • In the hereditary form, the tumor occurs as multifocal, bilateral disease with an autosomal dominant pattern of inheritance. • These tumors also occur at an earlier age. • The familial form can be associated with pheochromocytoma and parathyroid hyperplasia (MEN-IIA) or with pheochromocytoma, multiple mucosal neuromas, intestinal ganglioneuromas, and megacolon (MEN-IIB). • MTC tends to be more aggressive in MEN-IIB. • The overall 5-year survival rate is 50%, with a better prognosis for the sporadic than for the hereditary, or familial, form.

ANSWER:
A-c; B-b; C-b; D-b; E-c

---

41. With regard to the management of a patient with MTC, which of the following statements is/are correct?

A. The patient should be screened for hyperparathyroidism and pheochromocytoma.

B. Total thyroidectomy is the procedure of choice.

C. If cervical lymph node metastases are present and no distant metastases are evident, neck dissection results in little benefit with regard to long-term survival.

D. If pheochromocytoma is found, adrenal surgery should precede the thyroid surgery.

E. If hyperparathyroidism is found, it may be surgically managed at the time of thyroidectomy by removing the two largest parathyroid glands.

Ref.: 1–4

COMMENTS: The incidence of familial MTC is probably underestimated, inasmuch as the disease may go unrecognized (or unreported) in other family members. • It is also possible that any patient with an MTC may be the index case for a familial type. • It is reasonable, therefore, to screen for hyperparathyroidism (parathyroid hormone and calcium levels) and pheochromocytoma (urinary catecholamine, metanephrine, and vanillylmandelic acid levels) in all patients with MTC. • The best current method of screening for familial MTC is genetic analysis for abnormality of the *ret* proto-oncogene or chromosome X. • It predicts the potential need for total thyroidectomy. • If MTC is detected in children, then total thyroidectomy should be performed when the child is 5–6 years old, before clinical disease is evident.

If evidence of pheochromocytoma exists, this problem must be dealt with first because there is a significant risk of catastrophic blood pressure fluctuations during other (thyroid) surgery.

Hyperparathyroidism, if present, is almost always caused by four-gland hyperplasia and is best treated by excision of three and one-half glands (subtotal parathyroidectomy) or by a total parathyroidectomy, with implantation of a small amount of parathyroid tissue in the forearm musculature. • The parathyroid surgery should be carried out at the same time as the thyroid surgery.

Truly sporadic cases of MTC can be managed by excision of the involved thyroid lobe and isthmus alone because multicentricity is rare in the sporadic form. • Total thyroidectomy, however, is considered the treatment of choice because the patient may have an unrecognized familial form in which multicentricity is common. • MTC tends to spread first to the regional lymph nodes and then to distant sites. • Therefore, thyroidectomy with neck dissection in the presence of clinically evident cervical lymph nodes is appropriate therapy and is associated with 10-year survival rates approaching 50%.

ANSWER:
A, B, D

42. With regard to genetic analysis in patients with thyroid cancer, which of the following is/are true about the *ret* proto-oncogene?

A. Is associated with anaplastic thyroid cancer

B. Is located on chromosome 10

C. Is associated with familial MTC

D. Is associated with MEN-IIA and MEN-IIB

E. Is associated with follicular cancer of the thyroid

Ref.: 1–4

COMMENTS: The *ret* proto-oncogene was first cloned by M. Takahashi et al. in 1985. • It codes for two isoforms of a tyrosine-kinase receptor in the cell membrane. • The gene was translocated and rearranged on the same chromosome 10 to an unknown 5′ sequence. • A relationship has been described between the *ret* proto-oncogene and papillary thyroid cancer. • In Italy, approximately 30% of patients with thyroid cancer have *ret* rearrangements. • Recently, studies of the tyrosine kinase domain of the *ret* proto-oncogene revealed that specific germline mutations of *ret* led to MEN-IIA, MEN-IIB, and familial MTC. • The oncogene

was mapped on chromosome 10q11–12. • In 1994, CJM Lips et al. documented that patients who have the *ret* proto-oncogene mutation develop MTC and that *ret*-negative patients are not at risk. • In fact, the presence of the *ret* proto-oncogene on chromosome 10 more accurately detected MTC than calcitonin. • Continuing research in the field of genetics will provide further information about familial disease processes and help physicians manage these ailments clinically.

ANSWER:
B, C, D

43. Thyroid lymphoma is characterized by which of the following?

A. Should be suspected in patients presenting with a rapidly enlarging goiter

B. May be associated with Hashimoto's thyroiditis

C. May be associated with prior neck irradiation

D. May be associated with HIV infection

Ref.: 1–4

COMMENTS: Thyroid lymphoma is relatively uncommon but should be suspected in the patient with a rapidly enlarging goiter. • It may progress quickly, often causing hoarseness, dysphagia, and airway compromise in some cases. • There appears to be an association between thyroid lymphoma and Hashimoto's thyroiditis but not between a history of neck irradiation or HIV infection.

ANSWER:
A, B

44. Match the terms in the left-hand column with the definitions in the right-hand column.

A. Total thyroidectomy	a. Removes all of the thyroid tissue except for a rim of thyroid tissue bilaterally to ensure parathyroid viability and avoid damage to the recurrent laryngeal nerves
B. Near-total thyroidectomy	b. Removes a complete lobe while leaving a small remnant of thyroid tissue laterally on the contralateral side to avoid damage to the parathyroid glands and recurrent laryngeal nerve
C. Subtotal thyroidectomy	c. Involves division and removal of all thyroid tissue between the entrance of the recurrent laryngeal nerves bilaterally by the ligament of Berry

Ref.: 1–4

COMMENTS: A total thyroidectomy involves dissection and removal of all visible thyroid tissue bilaterally, which usually reveals the entrance of the recurrent laryngeal nerves as they enter the ligament of Berry. • A near-total thyroidectomy is a complete hemithyroidectomy and isthmusectomy. • In addition, most of the contralateral side is also removed, but a remnant of thyroid tissue is left to prevent damage to the parathyroid glands. • A subtotal thyroidectomy involves removal of all visible thyroid tissue except for a rim of thyroid issue bilaterally. • This reduces risk of injury to parathyroid glands and recurrent laryngeal nerves on both sides.

ANSWER:
A-c, B-b, C-a

---

45. During a total thyroidectomy for papillary cancer, the clinician observes an intact recurrent laryngeal nerve on the right side and a completely transected nerve on the left, with both ends in view. What should management of this patient at this point entail?

A. Complete the operation and evaluate the vocal cords postoperatively via flexible bronchoscopy.

B. Perform intraoperative flexible bronchoscopy to evaluate the vocal cords.

C. Repair the nerve using 8-0 monofilament sutures.

D. None of the above

Ref.: 1–4

COMMENTS: If the recurrent laryngeal nerve is injured or transected during an otherwise uncomplicated operation, it should be repaired using loupes or an operating microscope to visualize the field, and 8-0 or 9-0 monofilament sutures to anastomose the cut ends of the nerve. • There is no role for flexible bronchoscopy either intraoperatively or postoperatively unless there is uncertainty about the injury or the function of the contralateral nerve.

ANSWER:
C

---

46. What is the incidence of permanent recurrent laryngeal nerve after thyroid surgery?

A. 0–4%

B. 8–12%

C. 15–20%

D. 20–25%

Ref.: 1–4

COMMENTS: Recurrent laryngeal nerve injury is an uncommon and preventable injury in thyroid surgery. • Injury results from ligation, traction, suture entrapment, electrocautery injury, or hematoma. • Some injuries are transient, with function returning within 6–12 months of surgery, while others may be permanent. • The incidence of permanent injury after thyroid surgery is 0–4%.

ANSWER:
A

REFERENCES

1. Clark O, Duh Q, Kebebew E: *Textbook of Endocrine Surgery,* 2nd ed. Saunders, Philadelphia, 2005.
2. Greenfield LJ, Mulholland MW, Oldham KT, et al (eds): *Surgery: Scientific Principles and Practice*, 3rd ed. Lippincott, Williams & Wilkins, Philadelphia, 2001.
3. Townsend CM, Beauchamp RD, Evers BM, et al (eds): *Sabiston Textbook of Surgery: The Biological Basis of Modern Surgical Practice*, 17th ed. WB Saunders, Philadelphia, 2004.
4. Brunicardi FC, Andersen DK, Billiar TR, et al: *Schwartz's Principles of Surgery*, 8th ed. McGraw-Hill, New York, 2004.
5. Prinz RA, Rossi HL, Kim AW: Difficult problems in thyroid surgery. *Curr Probl Surg* 39:5-91, 2002.

C H A P T E R **28**

Parathyroid

Edie Chan, M.D., and Richard A. Prinz, M.D.

1. With regard to the embryology of the inferior parathyroid glands, which of the following statements is false?

   A. They arise from the third branchial pouch.

   B. They are more likely to be found in an ectopic location than are the superior parathyroid glands.

   C. They are embryologically associated with the thyroid gland.

   D. They are embryologically associated with the thymus gland.

   Ref.: 1, 2

COMMENTS: The superior parathyroid glands arise from the fourth branchial pouch in association with the lateral thyroid complex. • Paradoxically, the inferior parathyroid glands arise from a higher branchial pouch (the third) in association with the thymus (hence the name *parathymus*). • They achieve their characteristically lower position in adults because of the more caudal descent of the thymus gland into the mediastinum. • Because of this long descent by elements of the third branchial pouch, the inferior parathyroids are found over a wider anatomic range (from the pharynx to the pericardium) than are the superior parathyroids, which bear a fairly constant relationship to the posterolateral aspect of the thyroid gland.

ANSWER:
C

2. With regard to parathyroid anatomy, which of the following statements is correct?

   A. The superior parathyroids usually receive their blood supply from the superior thyroid artery.

   B. The inferior parathyroids usually receive their blood supply from the inferior thyroid artery.

   C. Either the superior or the inferior parathyroids may be located in the mediastinum.

   D. Supernumerary glands are found in one third of patients.

   Ref.: 1, 2

COMMENTS: Normal parathyroid glands in adults are flat, ovoid structures measuring approximately 3×6 mm and weighing approximately 25–40 mg each. • In most cases, both the superior and inferior parathyroids derive their blood supply from the inferior thyroid artery. • On occasion, the superior parathyroids are supplied by branches of the superior thyroid artery. • The superior parathyroids are almost always located on the dorsal aspect of the thyroid at the level of the cricoid cartilage. • The inferior parathyroids are more variable in their location. • In 50% of patients, they are found on the lateral surface of the lower thyroid pole, whereas in the remaining 50% they are associated with the thymus (mostly in the neck and occasionally in the superior mediastinum). • About 90% of patients have four parathyroid glands. • The other 10% have supernumerary glands (usually totaling five or six), which may be a result of fragmentation of the original four glands during embryologic descent. • The presence of fewer than the usual four glands has been reported, but such reports must be viewed with caution because the inability to find a gland is not proof of its absence.

ANSWER:
B

3. With regard to the physiology of parathyroid hormone (PTH), which of the following statements is false?

   A. Normally, PTH secretion is inversely related to the serum calcium level.

   B. PTH secretion is under partial control of the pituitary via the parathyroid-stimulating hormone (PSH).

   C. PTH has a direct action on bone, stimulating osteoclastic activity.

   D. PTH has a direct effect on the increased renal tubular reabsorption of calcium and the decreased reabsorption of phosphate.

   E. Assays specific for the intact PTH molecule are the most accurate for evaluating the serum PTH level.

   Ref.: 1, 2

COMMENTS: PTH, the principal mediator of calcium homeostasis, is secreted by the parathyroid gland in response to fluctuations in the serum calcium concentration. • This is a direct feedback system in which PTH secretion is inversely related to the serum level of ionized calcium. • There is no pituitary control over PTH secretion. • PTH has direct effects on the bone and kidneys and an indirect effect on the gut, all of which result in an increased serum calcium concentration. • In bone, PTH stimulates calcium release by enhancing resorption of bone matrix by osteoclasts. • In the kidneys, PTH increases tubular reabsorption of filtered calcium and decreases tubular reabsorption of filtered phosphate (phosphaturic effect). • Increased intestinal absorption of dietary calcium occurs indirectly through PTH stimulation of renal vitamin D complex synthesis. • The PTH molecule is made up of a fully active amino (N)-terminal fragment and a carboxyl (C)-terminal fragment with no known biologic activity. • The ability to measure the intact PTH molecule is the most sensitive and specific means of diagnosing hyperparathyroidism. • The intact PTH level is elevated in more than 95% of patients with primary hyperparathyroidism.

ANSWER:
B

4. With regard to vitamin D physiology, which of the following statements is false?

 A. The major source of vitamin D is dietary.

 B. Vitamin D increases intestinal absorption of dietary calcium.

 C. Vitamin D has a direct effect on bone, resulting in its ossification.

 D. Decreased levels of serum phosphate stimulate the hydroxylation of 25-hydroxycholecalciferol in the kidneys.

Ref.: 1, 2

COMMENTS: Vitamin D (in the form of vitamin D_3 or cholecalciferol) is produced primarily by ultraviolet activation of 7-dehydrocholesterol in the skin. • Vitamin D_3 undergoes initial hydroxylation in the liver to 25-hydroxycholecalciferol and a second hydroxylation in the kidneys to its most active form, 1,25-dihydroxycholecalciferol. • This dihydroxy vitamin D_3 is the form that is primarily responsible for the physiologic functions: facilitation of intestinal absorption of dietary calcium and ossification of the bone. • Low serum phosphate and increased serum PTH levels stimulate the renal conversion of 25- hydroxycholecalciferol to 1,25-dihydroxycholecalciferol.

ANSWER:
A

5. Which of the following is false regarding calcitonin?

 A. It is secreted by thyroid parafollicular cells.

 B. It induces urinary excretion of both phosphate and calcium.

 C. It is an effective tumor marker.

 D. The most potent secretagogues for calcitonin are calcium and pentagastrin.

 E. Its abundance with medullary carcinoma of the thyroid causes hypocalcemia.

Ref.: 1–5

COMMENTS: Calcitonin is a hormone secreted by the **parafollicular cells** (C cells) of the thyroid. • Its physiologic effects relate to lowering of serum calcium levels by promoting urinary excretion of calcium and phosphate. • In rats, calcitonin has also been demonstrated to inhibit bone resorption. • As a matter of fact, the physiologic effects of calcitonin appear to be more important for calcium homeostasis in certain animals than in humans. • The fact that calcitonin does not play a central role in the control of serum calcium in humans is exemplified by the relatively normal serum calcium levels found in patients who have low levels of calcitonin

after total thyroidectomy and in those with high levels of calcitonin from advanced medullary carcinoma of the thyroid. • Synthetic salmon calcitonin in large doses (200–800 U/day) reduces the serum calcium level rapidly and is a useful adjunct to pamidronate, whose action has a delayed onset. • Its most potent secretagogues are calcium and pentagastrin, which have been used for diagnosis and for monitoring tumor persistence and recurrence. • Others include β-adrenergic catecholamines, glucagon, and cholecystokinin. • PTH and calcitonin activity is mediated by cyclic adenosine monophosphate (cAMP) through a number of specific enzyme activations that occur in the kidney and bone. • Calcitonin is a tumor marker for medullary thyroid carcinoma and provides a mechanism to diagnose and monitor patients for the presence and recurrence of disease.

ANSWER:
E

6. True or false:

 A. PTH stimulates the reabsorption of calcium in the kidney and has no direct effect on the intestine.

 B. Vitamin D stimulates reabsorption of calcium in the kidney and stimulates absorption of calcium in the intestine.

 C. Calcitonin inhibits resorption of calcium and phosphate from bone.

 D. Calcitonin stimulates reabsorption of phosphate in the kidney.

Ref.: 1–3

COMMENTS: Parathyroid hormone is composed of 84 amino acids with a hormonally active N-terminal and an inactive C-terminal. • In the skeleton, PTH inhibits osteoblasts and stimulates osteoclasts, resulting in a decrease in bone density. • In the kidney, PTH causes a decrease in calcium clearance by stimulating the reabsorption of calcium and the conversion of 25-hydroxy vitamin D_3 (25[OH]D_3) to 1,25(OH)2D_3. • This metabolite then goes on to stimulate absorption of calcium and phosphate in the intestine. • In contrast, PTH does not have a direct effect on calcium absorption in the intestine. • Vitamin D_3 is derived from the ultraviolet activation of 7-dehydrocholesterol in the skin. • Vitamin D is then hydroxylated in both the liver (25[OH]D_3) and the kidney (1,25[OH]2D_3). • Vitamin D increases the intestinal absorption of calcium and phosphate and the mobilization of calcium and phosphate from bone to blood. • Calcitonin inhibits resorption of calcium and phosphate from bone and inhibits reabsorption of calcium and phosphate in the kidneys of some animals. • Calcitonin does not have any direct effect on the intestine.

ANSWER:
A-True; B-False; C-True; D-False

7. Match each laboratory or physiologic finding in the left-hand column with the appropriate categorization of hyperparathyroidism in the right-hand column.

 A. High-normal to elevated serum calcium levels, high serum PTH levels

 a. Primary hyperparathyroidism

 B. Low-normal to low serum calcium levels, high serum PTH levels

 b. Secondary hyperparathyroidism

C. Compensatory hyperfunction

D. Autonomous hyperfunction

E. When surgery is indicated, treatment is always by subtotal parathyroidectomy or total parathyroidectomy with autotransplantation.

c. Tertiary hyperparathyroidism

Ref.: 1, 2

COMMENTS: Hyperparathyroidism is the production of abnormally large amounts of PTH. • This condition may be associated with high, normal, or low serum calcium levels, depending on the underlying mechanism. • In **primary** hyperparathyroidism, one or more parathyroid glands are autonomously functioning without the normal negative feedback response to the serum calcium level, which usually results in elevations of serum calcium and PTH levels. • **Secondary** hyperparathyroidism is considered a compensatory response by the parathyroid glands to hypocalcemia. • Most often the hypocalcemia is secondary to underlying renal disease (causing hyperphosphatemia and a reduction of 1,25-dihydroxy vitamin D_3) or to intestinal malabsorption syndromes. • In secondary hyperparathyroidism the PTH level is elevated, but, because of abnormal calcium losses, the serum calcium level may not rise above the low-normal range. • Most patients (approximately 90%) with secondary hyperparathyroidism from renal failure can be managed by diet, calcium, or vitamin D and phosphate-binding agents (or some combination). • However, patients in whom severe renal osteodystrophy develops require subtotal parathyroidectomy or total parathyroidectomy with autotransplantation. • **Tertiary** hyperparathyroidism occurs in long-standing secondary hyperparathyroidism when stimulation of the parathyroid glands by hypocalcemia results in autonomous hyperfunction of those glands. • These glands remain overactive when renal failure is corrected by renal transplantation. The parathyroid hormone level remains high, and the serum calcium level becomes high-normal to elevated. • Patients with tertiary hyperparathyroidism generally are asymptomatic. • Surgery is required for only about 10% of those patients. • Indications for surgery are persistent hypercalcemia and elevated PTH levels with normal renal function. • As with secondary hyperparathyroidism, surgery involves either subtotal parathyroidectomy or total parathyroidectomy with autotransplantation.

ANSWER:
A-a,c; B-b; C-b; D-a,c; E-b,c

8. Which of the following is/are not a risk factor(s) for primary hyperparathyroidism?

A. Postmenopausal female

B. Previous exposure to ionizing radiation

C. Family history of multiple endocrine neoplasia type I (MEN-I) syndrome

D. Renal failure

Ref.: 1–5

COMMENTS: The incidence of hyperparathyroidism is approximately 25 per 100,000 (0.025%) general population. • The incidence of the disease markedly increases with age, especially in postmenopausal women. • In women older than 65, the incidence is 2.5%. • Although the cause of primary hyperparathyroidism is unknown, some studies have identified associated risk factors. • Exposure to low-dose ionizing radiation during childhood increases the risk for development of hyperparathyroidism, analogous to the increased incidence of well-differentiated thyroid cancer and salivary gland tumors in similarly exposed patients. • Some reports suggest that exposure to radioactive iodine, as used for treatment of Graves' disease, may increase the risk of developing hyperparathyroidism, but this is not conclusive. • Members of a family with MEN-I or MEN-IIA syndrome are at risk for developing hyperparathyroidism. • Genetic studies have identified a proto-oncogene, *PRAD1*, that has been associated with overexpression in parathyroid adenomas. • Male gender and renal failure are not risk factors for primary hyperparathyroidism.

ANSWER:
D

9. Most patients with primary hyperparathyroidism have elevations of all but which of the following?

A. Total serum calcium

B. Ionized serum calcium

C. Serum alkaline phosphatase

D. Urinary cAMP

E. Urinary calcium

Ref.: 1–3

COMMENTS: The diagnosis of hyperparathyroidism is usually based on the presence of elevated serum levels of calcium and intact PTH. • Measurement of ionized calcium is superior to determination of the total calcium level for evaluating patients with hyperparathyroidism. • Since only a few patients (10–40%) with hyperparathyroidism have an elevated serum alkaline phosphatase level, this assay is not helpful for diagnosis. • PTH interacts with cells lining the renal tubule, resulting in activation of cAMP. • This results in the leakage of cAMP into tubular fluid, leading to an elevated urinary cAMP level. • This finding has been demonstrated in up to 95% of patients with hyperparathyroidism. • Hyperparathyroidism is associated with elevated urinary calcium levels, whereas benign familial hypocalciuric hypercalcemia (BFHH), which also causes hypercalcemia, is not. • This distinction is critical because patients with BFHH do not benefit from an operation. • Other typical biochemical features of primary hyperparathyroidism include elevated serum chloride and decreased serum phosphate levels. • A chloride/phosphate ratio exceeding 33 is highly suggestive of the condition.

ANSWER:
C

10. With regard to the pathologic features of primary hyperparathyroidism, which of the following statements is false?

A. The presence of hyperplastic tissue surrounded by a rim of normal-appearing parathyroid tissue essentially confirms the diagnosis of adenoma.

B. Chief-cell hyperplasia is the most common form of parathyroid hyperplasia.

C. Clear-cell hyperplasia of the parathyroid gland is a rare cause of primary hyperparathyroidism.

D. When more than one gland is pathologically enlarged, the diagnosis of hyperplasia must be made.

Ref.: 1, 2

COMMENTS: The differentiation of **adenoma** from **hyperplasia** as the cause of primary hyperparathyroidism is difficult at times. • The classic gross findings diagnostic of adenoma are a single enlarged gland with three normal or small remaining glands associated with the histologic finding of hyperplastic tissue surrounded by a rim of normal-appearing parathyroid tissue. • This adenoma is the cause of primary hyperparathyroidism in approximately 80–85% of patients. • When two glands are found to be enlarged and one or more glands are normal, the diagnosis is **multiple adenomas**, rather than hyperplasia. • This condition is uncommon, accounting for fewer than 2–8% of cases. When three (or more) glands are abnormally enlarged, the likely diagnosis is hyperplasia. • **Chief-cell hyperplasia** is the most common subtype of parathyroid hyperplasia. **Clear-cell hyperplasia** and **carcinoma** are rare causes of primary hyperparathyroidism. It is often difficult to differentiate hyperplasia from adenoma on the basis of frozen sections. • Unless the characteristic rim of normal tissue is seen, the hyperplastic nature of adenomas is similar to that of true hyperplasia. • Most commonly, the decision as to whether the entity is an adenoma or hyperplasia depends on the gross characteristics of the glands identified at exploration.

ANSWER:
D

11. Which of the following is not associated with hyperparathyroidism?

    A. Muscle weakness

    B. Myalgia and arthralgia

    C. Nephrolithiasis

    D. Pancreatitis

    E. Peptic ulcer disease

    F. Depression

    G. Carpopedal spasm

    Ref.: 1–3

COMMENTS: Most patients with primary hyperparathyroidism are not overtly symptomatic, and the condition is diagnosed most frequently after routine serum chemistry testing. • The most common complaints consist of myalgias, arthralgias, constipation, muscle weakness, and polyuria. • These symptoms are nonspecific and often do not cause the examining physician to suspect hyperparathyroidism. • Nephrolithiasis is present in approximately 10–25% of patients, whereas nephrocalcinosis (calcification within the parenchyma) is present in 5%. • Renal function can be impaired with time, which may be a reason why 70% of patients with hyperparathyroidism have hypertension. • Patients with MEN-I syndrome and hyperparathyroidism have an increased risk for peptic ulcer disease. • In these patients, an elevated PTH level augments the hypergastrinemia caused by gastrinoma, leading to further increased gastric acid secretion. • Of 1000 patients with hyperparathyroidism at 26 hospitals in Great Britain, only 1% were found to have a history of pancreatitis. • Although pancreatitis can occur with other disease processes associated with hypercalcemia, the relationship between hyperparathyroidism and pancreatitis remains unconfirmed. • Patients with hypercalcemia can develop neurologic or psychiatric disturbances ranging from depression or anxiety to psychosis or coma. • Carpopedal spasm is associated with hypocalcemia, not hypercalcemia.

ANSWER:
G

12. Which of the following is/are not indication(s) for operative treatment of asymptomatic **patients with primary hyperparathyroidism?**

    A. Serum calcium of 10 mg/dl

    B. Reduced creatinine clearance

    C. Presence of kidney stones detected by abdominal radiogram

    D. Markedly elevated 24-hr urinary calcium excretion

    E. Substantially reduced bone mass, as determined by direct measurement

    Ref.: 1–3

COMMENTS: In 1990, the National Institutes of Health Consensus Development Conference reviewed available data on the subject of managing patients with asymptomatic primary hyperparathyroidism. • The panel agreed that a patient who is symptomatic requires operative therapy. • The indications for operating on asymptomatic patients are as follows: history of an episode of life-threatening hypercalcemia, reduced creatinine clearance, presence of kidney stones detected by abdominal imaging, markedly elevated 24-hr urinary calcium excretion, and substantially reduced bone mass, as determined by direct measurement. • Patients who do not fall into one of these categories may be followed with semiannual examinations. • Operative treatment was recommended if one of the following developed: typical symptoms of the skeletal, renal, or gastrointestinal systems; sustained serum calcium levels of more than 1.0–1.6 mg/dl above normal; substantial decline in renal function; nephrolithiasis or worsening calciuria; substantial decline in bone mass; onset of neuromuscular or psychological symptoms; or inability or unwillingness of a patient to continue medical surveillance. • Some studies have demonstrated an increased death rate from cardiovascular disease among patients with asymptomatic hyperparathyroidism followed nonoperatively.

ANSWER:
A

13. A pregnant mother in her first trimester arrives at the clinician's office with the diagnosis of primary hyperparathyroidism. What is the correct management?

    A. Parathyroidectomy during the first trimester

    B. Parathyroidectomy during the second trimester

    C. Cesarean section and parathyroidectomy at term

    D. Close observation and parathyroidectomy following delivery

    Ref.: 1–3

COMMENTS: Primary hyperparathyroidism during pregnancy, although rare, is associated with complications of fetal tetany, stillbirth, and abortion. • The risk of fetal complications is higher if the hyperparathyroidism remains untreated. • Therefore, such a patient should undergo parathyroidectomy during the second trimester. • The procedure is not done during the first trimester because of the risk of miscarriage and the teratogenic effects of anesthesia on the fetus. • Operations during the third trimester have an increased risk of inducing labor. • Overall, for operations that must be done during pregnancy, the second trimester offers the lowest morbidity and mortality for both mother and fetus.

ANSWER:
B

14. In regard to secondary hyperparathyroidism, which of the following is false?

A. Bone pain is the most common indication for operation.

B. Intractable pruritus is alleviated in 85% of patients following parathyroidectomy.

C. Total parathyroidectomy with autotransplantation is superior to subtotal parathyroidectomy.

D. Transcervical thymectomy should be performed routinely in operated patients.

Ref.: 1–3, 5

COMMENTS: Only 5–10% of patients with secondary hyperparathyroidism require operative management. • Most respond well to medical treatment with phosphate binders, supplemental calcium and vitamin D$_3$, and diet. • Bone pain is the most common indication for operation, and the symptoms are relieved in 85% of patients following parathyroidectomy. • Intractable pruritus is the second most frequent indication for parathyroidectomy and is also alleviated in 85% of patients. • Malaise is another frequent symptom that diminishes in most patients undergoing parathyroidectomy. • **Subtotal parathyroidectomy** was first introduced by S.W. Stanbury and colleagues in 1960. • The procedure typically involves resection of three and a half of the four glands. • **Total parathyroidectomy**, popularized by S.A. Wells in 1975, consists of removing all four enlarged parathyroidectomy glands and **autotransplanting** part of one parathyroid gland into the forearm. • Roughly equivalent results have been obtained with the two procedures, and debate continues as to which is better. • A **transcervical thymectomy** is performed routinely to remove supernumerary parathyroid glands or embryologic nests of parathyroid tissue. • The most common cause of persistent hyperparathyroidism after subtotal or total parathyroidectomy plus autotransplantation is an undiscovered or supernumerary parathyroid gland in the neck or anterior mediastinum.

ANSWER:
C

15. A patient with a previous diagnosis of primary hyperparathyroidism presents with rapidly developing muscular weakness, nausea, vomiting, and confusion. Which of the following is the best initial step in management?

A. Vigorous hydration with intravenous saline solution

B. Intravenous furosemide

C. Intravenous mithramycin

D. Intravenous calcitonin

E. Immediate parathyroid exploration

Ref.: 1, 2, 4

COMMENTS: For reasons that are unclear, patients with mild-to-moderate hypercalcemia from primary hyperparathyroidism may suddenly develop **hypercalcemic crisis** in which the serum calcium level rises to 14.5 mg/dl or higher. • Symptoms may include weakness, nausea, vomiting, confusion, and even coma. • Such a crisis is considered a medical emergency, and the initial management should be designed to lower the serum calcium level acutely. • This is best accomplished by vigorous saline intravenous infusion to expand the intravascular volume, followed by administration of loop diuretics, such as furosemide, to increase urinary calcium excretion. • Furosemide should not be used until the patient is well hydrated, as indicated by adequate urine output. • Cardiac monitoring is required, particularly when the calcium level is higher than 16 mg/dl. • When calcium levels remain elevated, other hypercalcemia agents are administered. • **Calcitonin** given intravenously or subcutaneously has a rapid effect. • Intravenous **mithramycin,** which inhibits bone resorption, can effectively lower the serum calcium concentration within 24 hr of administration. • Its potential hematologic, renal, and hepatic toxicity limits its use to (1) palliation of malignancy and (2) cases in which conventional therapy for hypercalcemia is ineffective or contraindicated. • **Parathyroid exploration,** with resection of the offending gland or glands, represents the definitive treatment of this entity but should be delayed until the serum calcium level is reduced to a safer level.

ANSWER:
A

16. A patient requires parathyroid exploration for primary hyperparathyroidism. During the exploration, an abnormally large parathyroid gland is found posterior to the lower pole of the right thyroid lobe. Which of the following choices is/are appropriate at this point?

A. Excise the enlarged gland without identifying the other parathyroid glands.

B. Excise the enlarged gland and then identify the three remaining glands. If they appear normal, perform biopsies of all three to confirm normal histologic features.

C. Identify the remaining glands, and if they appear normal in size, excise the largest one only.

D. Identify the remaining glands and excise the largest one or two of the three remaining ones.

Ref.: 1–4

COMMENTS: See Question 17.

17. On further exploration of the patient described in Question 16, the three remaining glands are encountered, and all appear to be abnormally enlarged, as was the first gland found. Which of the following options is/are appropriate at this point?

A. Resect all four glands.

B. Resect only the two largest glands.

C. Resect three glands and a portion of the fourth.

D. Resect the largest gland and half of each of the three remaining glands.

Ref.: 1–4

COMMENTS: The differentiation between an adenoma and four-gland hyperplasia as the cause of hyperparathyroidism frequently is most easily made by the gross findings at operation rather than by the histologic findings. • When a large gland is found during exploration, the surgeon must identify at least one normal-sized gland to confirm the diagnosis of an adenoma. • Nevertheless, because multiple adenomas are encountered in 2–8% of patients, the surgeon must attempt to identify the remaining three glands. • Ideally, all three remaining glands are found. • If they are normal in size, only the enlarged gland need be removed. • A shave biopsy of one of the three normal-appearing glands may be useful for confirming its normal histologic features. • A biopsy of all three remaining glands carries the risk of injuring or devascularizing all three and causing permanent hypoparathyroidism. • If one large and one normal-sized gland are found but the other two glands are not easily identified, many surgeons would not pursue a more intense search for the remaining glands on the grounds that the risk of injuring those glands and causing hypoparathyroidism may outweigh the small possibility of multiple adenomas. • If more than one enlarged gland is found, four-gland hyperplasia must be suspected as the cause of the hyperparathyroidism. • In such cases, it is even more important that all four glands be identified. • If all four are enlarged, the generally accepted options for management include either subtotal parathyroidectomy, resecting three glands and a portion of the fourth (leaving approximately 40–60 mg of a single gland in place), or a total parathyroidectomy, resecting all four glands and implanting a morcellated portion of one of the glands into a readily accessible muscle. • Implantation into the forearm musculature permits re-exploration of that area if hyperparathyroidism persists, without the inherent dangers of a cervical re-exploration. • The goal of managing four-gland hyperplasia is to leave enough parathyroid tissue to prevent permanent hypoparathyroidism.

ANSWERS:
Question 16: C
Question 17: C

18. During exploration for primary hyperparathyroidism, two normal-appearing glands on the left and one normal-appearing gland on the right are found after the paratracheal areas are explored bilaterally. The fourth gland is not found. Which of the following course(s) of action is/are the most appropriate?

   A. Terminate the operation with no further dissection.

   B. Extend the exploration through the existing cervical incision to include the central compartment of the neck between carotid arteries, posteriorly to the vertebral body, superiorly to the level of the pharynx and carotid bulb, and inferiorly into the mediastinum. Terminate the operation if the fourth gland is not found.

   C. Resect the three glands found, leaving the fourth to maintain normal PTH levels.

   D. Extend the incision into the right side of the neck laterally to explore the entire neck, including the posterior triangle.

   E. Close the cervical incision and perform a median sternotomy to explore the mediastinum for an ectopic parathyroid.

Ref.: 1, 2, 4

COMMENTS: One of the more frustrating aspects of parathyroid surgery is the inability to find one of the parathyroid glands that is suspected to be the cause of hyperparathyroidism. • In the clinical situation described, three normal-appearing glands are found, raising the likelihood that an adenoma of the fourth gland exists in an ectopic location. • An understanding of the embryology of the parathyroids enables the surgeon to select the areas in which the gland is most likely to be found, which include the central compartment of the neck between the carotid arteries, moving posteriorly to the vertebral body, superiorly to the level of the pharynx and carotid bulb, and inferiorly into the mediastinum. • All of these areas, including the upper portion of the mediastinum, can be explored through the existing cervical collar incision, and this exploration should be conducted at the time of the initial operation. • If the adenoma is not found after this extensive search, it is likely that the adenoma is in the mediastinum in an area not accessible through the collar incision. • There is a small possibility that the adenoma is truly subcapsular within the ipsilateral thyroid lobe, and some surgeons would perform a thyroid lobectomy on the side of the missing gland. • Extending the cervical exploration to include the posterior triangle would not be fruitful because the parathyroid gland would not be found in that location. • Although sternotomy may be required to identify the missing gland, most surgeons delay this procedure until after the performance of sophisticated localization studies. • Before closing, normal histologic features (i.e., nonhyperplastic tissue) should be confirmed by biopsy of one or two of the three normal-appearing glands that were found. • Most surgeons mark the normal glands with surgical clips or nonabsorbable suture {the latter is preferred, to avoid computed tomography [CT] scan interference} to facilitate their identification if re-exploration becomes necessary. • It is inappropriate to resect all three glands because hypoparathyroidism would result once the adenoma is found and resected.

ANSWER:
B

19. Signs or symptoms of hypocalcemia include which of the following?

   A. Electrocardiogram (ECG) with a shortened QT interval

   B. ECG with inverted T waves

   C. Bone pain due to "bone hunger"

   D. Muscular paralysis

   E. Muscular tetany

Ref.: 1–3

COMMENTS: Hypocalcemia can occur in as many as 30% of patients following parathyroidectomy, but only 1% develop permanent hypocalcemia. • The major clinical manifestations result from reduced plasma ionized calcium levels and consequent neuromuscular excitability. • The earliest manifestations are numbness and tingling in the circumoral area, fingers, and toes. • Tetany may develop, characterized by carpopedal spasm. • In severe cases, patients have mental status changes eventually leading to coma. • On physical examination, contraction of the facial muscles is elicited by tapping on the facial nerve anterior to the ear (Chvostek's sign). • Trousseau's sign (development of carpopedal spasm) can be elicited by occluding blood flow to the forearm for 3 minutes using a blood pressure cuff. • The ECG may reveal a prolonged QT interval and peaked T waves. • Mild symptoms can be treated with oral calcium. • Up to 6 g of oral calcium may be given daily. • One must be careful when giving intravenous calcium peripherally, since calcium carbonate can damage the skin and surrounding tissue, resulting in full-thickness skin burns and, in severe cases, loss of the distal extremity. • If possible, intravenous calcium is administered centrally. • Three causes of postoperative hypocalcemia are hungry bone syndrome, hypomagnesemia, and failure of the parathyroid remnant or autograft. • In patients with long-standing hyperparathyroidism and bone disease, there may be substantial skeletal calcium deposition, so-called bone hunger. • Postoperatively, these patients have decreasing calcium levels for 2–3 days, which returns to normal over the next couple of days.

ANSWER:
E

20. A 50-year-old woman presents to the clinician's office with a history of renal stones, peptic ulcer disease refractory to H$_2$-blockers, and nipple discharge. Which of the multiple endocrine neoplasia (MEN) syndromes does this suggest?

A. MEN-I

B. MEN-IIA

C. MEN-IIB

D. Any of the above

Ref.: 1–4

COMMENTS: See Question 22.

21. For each MEN syndrome in the left-hand column, choose the appropriate biochemical screening test(s) from the right-hand column.

A. MEN-I
B. MEN-IIA
C. MEN-IIB

a. serum PTH
b. Serum somatomedin C
c. Serum gastrin
d. Serum calcitonin
e. Urinary catecholamines

Ref.: 1–3

COMMENTS: See Question 22.

22. Which of the following is/are appropriate treatment of the patient in Question 20?

A. Adrenalectomy

B. Unilateral parathyroidectomy

C. Total parathyroidectomy with heterotopic transplantation

D. Total thyroidectomy

Ref.: 1–3

COMMENTS: Most cases of primary hyperparathyroidism occur in sporadic distribution in the general population. • There is a small subset of patients, however, who manifest a familial tendency to develop hyperparathyroidism. • It may occur alone as the only endocrine abnormality, or it may occur in association with other endocrine abnormalities (MEN syndromes). • The **MEN-I syndrome** in its fully expressed state consists of pituitary adenomas (prolactin-secreting adenomas are the most common), parathyroid hyperplasia, and pancreatic islet cell neoplasia (e.g., gastrinoma and insulinoma). • The **MEN-II syndrome** consists of medullary

carcinoma of the thyroid variably associated with hyperparathyroidism and pheochromocytoma. • The hyperparathyroidism may be due to hyperplasia or adenomas. • In the fully expressed form of the subtype **MEN-IIA**, all three of these entities are present. • **MEN-IIB syndrome** consists of medullary carcinoma of the thyroid and pheochromocytoma in association with ganglioneuromas, soft-tissue nodules, and a marfanoid habitus but without hyperparathyroidism.

Screening for MEN-I consists of (1) measurement of intact serum PTH and albumin-corrected total serum calcium levels to detect hyperparathyroidism; (2) prolactin and somatomedin C assays to detect pituitary adenoma; and (3) measurements of fasting glucose and insulin, pancreatic polypeptide, and serum gastrin levels to detect pancreatic islet cell neoplasia. • The calcitonin assay is used for diagnosing and following patients with medullary thyroid cancer, which can be present in MEN-IIA and MEN-IIB patients. • A 24-hr urine collection to measure catecholamines and their metabolites is used as a screening test for pheochromocytoma, which can be present with MEN-IIA and MEN-IIB.

The **management** of patients with MEN-I depends on the severity of symptoms associated with the individual components. • Resection of the pituitary adenoma, parathyroidectomy, and pharmacologic or surgical management of the pancreatic tumor may be appropriate. • In MEN-I patients, hyperparathyroidism is associated with hyperplasia of all four glands, rather than a single adenoma. • Patients with evidence of hyperparathyroidism with an elevated gastrin level are advised strongly to first undergo parathyroidectomy. • Hypercalcemia is associated with increased gastrin levels, which may result in peptic ulcer disease. • Peptic ulcer disease is the number-one cause of death among families with MEN-I syndrome. • Elevated gastrin levels in patients with MEN-I indicate the presence of gastrinoma, resulting in Zollinger-Ellison syndrome. • Identification and resection constitute the preferred treatment. • Small duodenal gastrinomas must be directly searched for. • Antisecretory drugs or parietal cell vagotomy may reduce medication requirements. • Insulinoma is treated operatively. • Pharmacologic agents such as diazoxide and octreotide may be useful, as may streptozocin for patients with metastases. • The prevalence of pituitary adenomas in patients with MEN-I varies from 10 to 65%. • Prolactin-secreting adenomas are the most common, followed by growth hormone–secreting adenomas. • Surgery has been supplanted by medical treatment with dopamine analogues because of their ability to inhibit prolactin release. • Approximately 70–90% of patients respond to the dopamine agonist bromocriptine. • Somatostatin analogues and surgery are the preferred treatment for pituitary acromegaly. • Patients with MEN-II and medullary thyroid cancer must be evaluated for pheochromocytoma. • If present, the pheochromocytoma is resected first, followed by staged neck exploration. • Total parathyroidectomy with heterotopic transplantation is performed for patients with MEN-IIA and hyperparathyroidism and for those undergoing thyroidectomy even if normocalcemic.

ANSWERS:
Question 20: A
Question 21: A-a,b,c; B-a,d,e; C-d,e
Question 22: C

23. With regard to parathyroid carcinoma, which of the following statements is/are correct?

A. It is a rare cause of hyperparathyroidism.

B. Only 5–10% of patients with parathyroid carcinoma manifest hypercalcemia.

C. The cytologic criteria differentiating parathyroid carcinoma from adenoma are well established.

D. Parathyroidectomy is usually curative.

Ref.: 1, 2, 5

COMMENTS: Parathyroid carcinoma is a rare cause of hyperparathyroidism, accounting for fewer than 1% of cases. • Like many other neuroendocrine tumors, carcinoma of the parathyroid may not prevent the gland from carrying out its normal endocrine function (i.e., PTH production). • However, regulation of PTH production is usually impaired, and as many as 85% of patients with parathyroid carcinoma present with hypercalcemia. • It is of note that the hypercalcemia is usually severe, frequently manifesting serum calcium concentrations in excess of 14 mg/dl. • Approximately 50% of patients with parathyroid cancer have a palpable tumor, in contrast to its rarity in patients with benign hyperparathyroidism. • The cytologic criteria for malignancy are poorly defined, and it may be difficult to differentiate a parathyroid carcinoma from adenoma on histologic basis alone. • Evidence of local invasion or regional or distant metastases may be needed to confirm the diagnosis of carcinoma. • The surgeon must therefore be suspicious of carcinoma when the tumor is firmly attached to adjacent structures. • The likelihood of cure is greatest when all known disease can be surgically resected, which involves en bloc resection of the parathyroid and ipsilateral thyroid lobe with adjacent muscle and fibrofatty tissue. • Surgical debulking of known disease may be beneficial in reducing the PTH levels and thereby palliating the symptoms of severe hypercalcemia. • The long-term prognosis is usually poor.

ANSWER:
A

24. Which of the following is the most common cause of hypoparathyroidism?

A. Previous thyroid surgery

B. Previous parathyroid surgery

C. Previous viral infection involving the parathyroid glands

D. Genetic disorder of PTH metabolism

Ref.: 1, 2

COMMENTS: The most common cause of hypoparathyroidism is surgical trauma to the parathyroid glands during thyroid or parathyroid exploration. • Because thyroid operations are much more common than parathyroid operations, previous thyroid surgery accounts for most cases of hypoparathyroidism. • There is no known association between viral infections and the development of hypoparathyroidism. • There is a rare genetic disorder (pseudohypoparathyroidism) in which the serum PTH level is normal to elevated but the end-organ response of the kidney to circulating PTH is abnormal, resulting in hyperphosphatemia and hypocalcemia. • Most postoperative hypocalcemia is temporary. • If viable parathyroid tissue does remain, the PTH and serum calcium levels return to normal. • These patients may need to be supported temporarily with exogenous calcium and, on occasion, vitamin D. • If the patient remains asymptomatic, it is usually wise to avoid calcium administration alone because a low serum calcium level serves as the stimulus for the compensatory growth and function of the remaining parathyroid tissue. • If clinical signs of hypocalcemia develop (e.g., carpopedal spasm, tetany, Chvostek's sign, Trousseau's sign, and ECG changes) or if the

hypoparathyroidism appears to be permanent, treatment with exogenous calcium (up to 2 g of elemental calcium per day) and vitamin D₃ (up to 100,000 units/day) is needed.

ANSWER:
A

25. True or false: Technetium sestamibi scanning for preoperative localization has become a standard localization test in the setting of reoperation.

Ref.: 4

COMMENTS: Sestamibi was originally developed for cardiac imaging but was discovered to concentrate in parathyroid tissue, allowing localization on delayed scans. • Its short half-life and high energy profile made it more advantageous then thallium-technetium subtraction scanning. • It is now standard in the reoperative setting and in patients undergoing focused, minimally invasive parathyroidectomy. • Cervical ultrasound is also commonly used for parathyroid localization.

ANSWER:
True

26. Indications of parathyroidectomy in patients with secondary hyperparathyroidism include all but which of the following?

A. Development of open ulcerative skin lesions from calcinosis

B. Bone pain or pathologic fractures

C. Ectopic calcifications

D. Intractable pruritus

E. Renal failure

Ref.: 4

COMMENTS: Most renal patients will have some degree of hyperparathyroidism, but only 5–10% require surgical intervention. • Parathyroidectomy is recommended when complications that carry a substantial morbidity occur or when medical management has failed. • Complications include the development of open ulcerative skin lesions from calcinosis or calciphylaxis, which can carry a high mortality rate without surgical intervention; persistent bone pain or pathologic fractures; ectopic calcifications; and intractable pruritus. • Renal failure is not an indication for parathyroidectomy.

ANSWER:
E

27. True or false: Hungry bone syndrome usually occurs in patients with an increased serum alkaline phosphatase levels.

Ref.: 4

COMMENTS: The serum concentration of alkaline phosphatase is normally less than 110 IU/100 ml. • Ten to 40% of patients with hyperparathyroidism have increased levels. • After surgery, systemic hypocalcemia may occur, especially in patients with large adenomas. • It also occurs in patients with total parathyroidectomy and autotransplantation. • The serum calcium level falls rapidly to lower levels in these patients than in patients with normal alkaline phosphatase levels, because of their underlying bone disease. • This is known as hungry bone syndrome.

ANSWER:
True

28. Which of the following regarding minimally invasive parathyroidectomy is false?

A. Minimally invasive parathyroidectomy involves localizing a parathyroid adenoma with a preoperative sestamibi scan.

B. A baseline PTH level is compared with a 5-minute postexcision PTH level.

C. Because circulating PTH has a half-life of 30 minutes, a 10% reduction is expected 5 minutes after excision.

D. Ninety-five percent of patients demonstrate a fall in PTH levels, and approximately 5% have additional hyperfunctioning glands.

Ref.: 4

COMMENTS: Minimally invasive parathyroidectomy is an emerging technique, in which the parathyroid adenoma is first localized preoperatively by a sestamibi scan. • An abbreviated Kocher incision is made on the side of the localized adenoma. • Often, general anesthesia can be replaced with cervical block anesthesia and sedation. • A baseline PTH level is obtained before the start of the operation. • After the adenoma is removed, postexcision PTH levels are measured at 5 and 10 minutes. • Since circulating PTH has a half-life of 3–4 minutes, a 50% reduction is expected after adenoma excision. • Although 95% of patients exhibit a fall in PTH level, about 5% have a sustained PTH level because of additional hyperfunctioning glands. • If an adequate parathyroidectomy is performed, there will be a greater than 50% drop in baseline PTH levels.

ANSWER:
C, D

29. True or false:

A. Persistent hyperparathyroidism is defined as biochemical evidence of primary hyperparathyroidism immediately after an operation or within 6 months.

B. Recurrent hyperparathyroidism is defined by chemical evidence of primary hyperparathyroidism occurring after the sixth postoperative month.

Ref.: 4

COMMENTS: Causes of persistent hyperparathyroidism include failure to locate a causative adenoma or an unrecognized second adenoma. • It can also be caused by failure to recognize parathyroid hyperplasia or adequately resect parathyroid hyperplasia. • Other causes include residual or metastatic disease from parathyroid carcinoma or, rarely, the secretion of PTHrP by a lung, pancreatic, or ovarian cancer. • Recurrent hyperparathyroidism can

occur from hyperplastic parathyroid tissue left behind in a first operation, autotransplanted parathyroid tissue, or rupture of a tumor or rough handling at initial operation, leading to implantation of hyperplastic parathyroid cells (parathyromatosis). • The most common cause is missed adenocarcinoma.

ANSWER:
A-True; B-True

30. Which of the following would not be elevated in patients with hypercalcemia due to malignancy?

A. Urinary cAMP

B. Intact PTH

C. C-Terminal PTH

D. PTH-related peptide

Ref.: 1–3

COMMENTS: In hospitalized patients, malignancy rather than hyperparathyroidism is the most common cause of hypercalcemia. • Most patients with hypercalcemia and malignancy have suppressed PTH levels. • Generally, hypercalcemia from malignancy can be divided into two groups: (1) those with hematologic malignancies and (2) those with solid tumors. • Hematologic diseases associated with hypercalcemia include multiple myeloma, lymphoma, and leukemia. • These patients typically have lytic bone lesions radiographically and demonstrate increased osteoclast activity histologically. • At the cellular level, the cause of hypercalcemia is stimulation of osteoclast activity by interleukin-1B and tumor necrosis factor-β. • Unlike patients with hyperparathyroidism, these patients have low urine levels of cAMP. • The solid tumors generally associated with hypercalcemia are in the breast, lung, and kidney or are neuroendocrine tumors of the pancreas. • These patients have a normal serum PTH level, but their urinary cAMP levels are elevated. • The cause of hypercalcemia in these solid tumors has been linked to tumor production of a PTH-related peptide, which may be elevated in 85–90% of patients.

ANSWER:
B, C

REFERENCES

1. Townsend CM, Beauchamp RD, Evers BM, et al (eds): *Sabiston Textbook of Surgery: The Biological Basis of Modern Surgical Practice*, 17th ed. Saunders, Philadelphia, 2004.
2. Schwartz SI, Shires GT, Spencer FC (eds): *Principles of Surgery*, 8th ed. McGraw-Hill, New York, 2004.
3. Greenfield LJ, Mulholland MW, Oldham KT (eds): *Surgery: Scientific Principles and Practice*, 3rd ed. Lippincott, Williams & Wilkins, Philadelphia, 2001.
4. Clark OH, Duh QY (eds): *Textbook of Endocrine Surgery*, 2nd ed. Saunders, Philadelphia, 2005.
5. Packman KS, Demeure MJ: Indications for parathyroidectomy and extent of treatment for patients with secondary hyperparathyroidism. *Surg Clin North Am* 75:465–428, 1995.

CHAPTER 29

Pituitary

Scott Wilhelm, M.D., and Richard A. Prinz, M.D.

1. The pituitary gland is bordered by which of the following sinuses?

A. Frontal sinus

B. Sphenoid sinus

C. Maxillary sinus

D. Cavernous sinus

E. Ethmoid sinuses

Ref.: 2, 3

COMMENTS: The pituitary gland sits within the sella turcica, or "Turkish saddle," which is a portion of the sphenoid bone. • The floor of the sella forms the roof of the sphenoid sinus. • This unique anatomic border allows for a relatively straightforward surgical approach to tumors of the pituitary gland. • Approximately 95% of all pituitary tumors can be removed through a transnasal, transsphenoidal approach. • The pituitary is laterally bordered by the paired cavernous sinuses. • Macroadenomas of the pituitary can exert external compression on the cavernous sinus and its contents, including the internal carotid artery and cranial nerves III, IV, V (roots 1 and 2), and VI. • The frontal, maxillary, and ethmoid sinuses do not directly border the pituitary gland.

ANSWER:
B, D

2. Compression of surrounding cranial nerves by a pituitary macroadenoma can cause various symptoms. Match the pathologic symptoms in the left-hand column with the cranial nerve (CN) involved in the right-hand column.

A. Bitemporal hemianopsia	a. CN II
B. Abducted, downward gaze, ptosis, and dilated pupil	b. CN III
C. Abducted gaze with compensatory head tilt	c. CN IV
D. Absent corneal reflex	d. CN V
E. Adducted eye (medial strabismus) and diplopia	e. CN VI

Ref.: 2, 3

COMMENTS: As pituitary adenomas increase in size, they can begin to exert external compression superiorly into the optic chiasm of CN II. • This results in the classic symptom associated with macroadenomas: bilateral temporal hemianopsia. • However, because this field deficit is variable, formal visual field testing of all of these patients is mandatory. • Lateral growth of these tumors can compress the cavernous sinuses, which contain cranial nerves III–VI. • Nerves III (oculomotor), IV (trochlear), and VI (abducens) control the various extraocular muscles. • CN III innervates four of the six extraocular muscles as well as the levator palpebrae. • Palsy results in abducted downward lateral gaze and lid lag, or ptosis. • CN III also supplies parasympathetic innervation to the pupillary constrictor muscles. • Thus, palsy results in a dilated pupil. • CN IV innervates only the superior oblique muscle of the eye. • Palsy results in an outward rotation of the eye, or abducted gaze. • The patient often compensates for this deficit by tilting the head away from the side of the lesion. • CN V supplies sensory innervation to the ipsilateral face and cornea as well as motor activity to the muscles of mastication. • CN VI innervates only the lateral rectus muscle. • Thus, palsy results in a medial strabismus, or adduction of the eye. • Approximately 80% of all CN palsies will improve or resolve completely with pituitary decompression.

ANSWER:
A-a, B-b, C-c, D-d, E-e

3. With regard to the anatomy of the pituitary gland, which of the following statements is/are true?

A. As with other portions of the central nervous system (CNS), there is an anatomic and physiologic blood-brain barrier within the neurohypophysis.

B. The adenohypophysis does not have its own direct arterial blood supply.

C. The neurohypophysis contains both neuronal cell bodies and axons.

D. The adenohypophysis contains axons only.

E. No nerves terminate within the adenohypophysis.

Ref.: 1, 2

COMMENTS: The special neuroendocrine function of the pituitary gland and its interrelationship with the hypothalamus are facilitated by several distinct anatomic features. • For example, the hormonal mediators released within the neurohypophysis gain access to the vascular system through fenestrated epithelium, and thus the neurohypophysis does not have a "blood-brain barrier," unlike most of the rest of the CNS. • The vascular anatomy of the adenohypophysis is unusual in that it does not derive its blood supply from a direct arterial source but, rather, from a system of portal vessels that first pass through the capillary bed of the neuro-hypophysis. • Because no nerves terminate directly within the adenohypophysis, it is dependent on this portal capillary system for receiving the hormones that influence its function. • The neurohy-pophysis, on the other hand, is regulated in part by hormonal influ-ences from the periphery (and possibly feedback directly from the adenohypophysis) and by direct neural input from the hypothala-mus. • The latter occurs by means of axons, the cell bodies of which lie within the hypothalamus. • The neurohypophysis itself contains no neuronal cell bodies. • Such an anatomic arrangement allows complicated interplay of neural and hormonal factors among the hypothalamus, neurohypophysis, adenohypophysis, and peripheral endocrine function.

ANSWER:
B, E

4. A 33-year-old woman develops a visual field loss. Computed tomography (CT) scanning of the brain demonstrates a cystic sellar mass with calcification. Which of the following state-ments about this patient is/are true?

   A. The most common masses involving the sellar and parasel-lar region include pituitary adenomas, hypothalamic or optic nerve gliomas, craniopharyngiomas, aneurysms, menin-giomas, germinomas, and inflammatory lesions.

   B. Calcification is typical of pituitary adenomas.

   C. Craniopharyngiomas are usually cystic.

   D. Suprasellar extension of the tumor can lead to obstructive hydrocephalus.

Ref.: 2

COMMENTS: Certain lesions are commonly found in the sella and parasellar region. • They include pituitary adenomas, gliomas of the optic nerve or chiasm and of the hypothalamus, cranio-pharyngiomas, aneurysms, meningiomas, germinomas, and inflammatory lesions, such as a sarcoid. • Although most of these abnormalities can cause visual symptoms, the presence of calcification in a cyst on a CT scan makes craniopharyngioma the most likely diagnosis. • These tumors account for 2–4% of brain tumors and originate from remnants of Rathke's pouch. • Pathologically, most craniopharyngiomas contain a solid and a cystic component containing calcifications. • They are com-posed of columnar epithelium, with squamous cells forming the interior. • These tumors can cause visual symptoms, headache, or hydrocephalus. • Treatment consists of surgical resection followed by radiation therapy. • As with any tumor of the sellar region, suprasellar extension of sellar tumors commonly leads to compres-sion of the third ventricle and the foramen of Monro, with result-ant obstructive hydrocephalus.

ANSWER:
A, C, D

5. Match the hormones in the left-hand column with their place of origin in the right-hand column.

   A. Adrenocorticotropic hormone (ACTH)

   a. Adenohypophysis (anterior pituitary)

   B. Dopamine

   b. Neurohypophhsis (posterior pituitary)

   C. Oxytocin

   c. Hypothalamus

   D. Thyroid-stimulating hormone (TSH)

   E. Vasopressin

Ref.: 2, 3

COMMENTS: The anterior pituitary, or adenohypophysis, repre-sents 80% of the total gland weight. • It contains various cell types, which secrete prolactin, growth hormone (GH), ACTH, TSH, and the gonadotropins, follicle-stimulating hormone (FSH), and luteinizing hormone (LH). • The posterior pituitary receives neural stimuli from the supraoptic and paraventricular nuclei in the hypothalamus, which lead to the release of oxytocin and antidiuretic hormone (ADH), also known as vasopressin. • The hypothalamus is also responsible for production of corticotropin-releasing hormone (CRH), which stimulates release of ACTH; thyrotropin-releasing hormone (TRH), which stimulates TSH secretion; dopamine, which inhibits prolactin release; growth hormone–releasing hormone, which stimulates release of GH; gonadotropin-releasing hormone (GnRH), which stimulates FSH and LH release; and somatostatin, which inhibits the release of GH. • There are many complex inter-actions among the hypothalamic-pituitary axis and its end organs—thyroid, adrenal, kidneys, and gonads, among other organs—that are beyond the scope of this review.

ANSWER:
A-a; B-c; C-b; D-a; E-b

6. A patient is involved in a motor vehicle accident and sustains a severe head injury with a Glasgow Coma Scale (GCS) classifi-cation of 7. After 24 hr in the intensive care unit, the patient's urine output increases to 300–500 ml/hr and has a specific gravity of 1.000. Which of the following statements with regard to this patient is/are true?

   A. Electrolyte analysis would show hypernatremia.

   B. Vasopressin excess causes diabetes insipidus (DI).

   C. Serum osmolarity is typically less than 285 mOsm.

   D. Treatment of this patient includes immediate administration of deamino-D-arginine-vasopressin (DDAVP).

   E. The head CT scan of this patient would likely demonstrate a posterior fossa contusion.

Ref.: 1–3

COMMENTS: This history of excessive dilute urine after severe head trauma is highly suggestive of DI, which is the result of defi-cient vasopressin release. • This can result from traumatic injury of either the hypothalamus or the pituitary itself. • DI can also occur as a result of pituitary or other sellar or suprasellar tumors (see Question 4). • Vasopressin, or ADH, binds to receptors on the distal renal tubules and collecting ducts, where it activates the gen-eration of cyclic adenosine monophosphate (cAMP), which increases the reabsorption of water. • DI results in an excessive volume of dilute urine, hypovolemia, and hypernatremia, with resultant polydipsia as a prominent clinical feature. • Serum osmolarity is typically increased to a level greater than 285 mOsm as a result of the increased urinary volume. • Serum osmolarity can roughly be estimated by the following formula if one knows the serum electrolyte levels:

$$2 \times \text{serum sodium} + \text{blood glucose}/18 + \text{blood urea nitrogen}/3$$

When treating a patient who develops a mild case of DI and who is alert and able to tolerate oral rehydration, increased fluid intake prompted by the patient's normal thirst mechanism can often compensate for the decreased vasopressin production. • As in the case described in this question, exogenous vasopressin is often necessary.

ANSWER:
A, D

7. With regard to the physiologic aspects of prolactin secretion, which of the following statements is/are true?

   A. Prolactin is secreted from the neurohypophysis in response to suckling.

   B. Males and nonpregnant females have similar blood levels of prolactin.

   C. Prolactin has physiologic effects on the breast, ovary, and testis.

   D. The principal hypothalamic effect on prolactin secretion is inhibitory.

   E. Prolactin secretion may be stimulated by pregnancy, stress, exercise, and breast stimulation.

Ref.: 1, 2

COMMENTS: Prolactin is a peptide secreted from the adenohypophysis in response to numerous peripheral factors, including pregnancy, stress, exercise, and direct breast stimulation. • Hypothalamic control of prolactin secretion is primarily inhibitory via prolactin-inhibiting factor, which evidence suggests may be dopamine. • In the nonstimulated state, men and women have similar blood levels of prolactin. • Its most important physiologic effect is mammotropic, stimulating duct development and lactation. • It also has gonadal effects and is thought to partly modulate ovarian progesterone synthesis and testicular testosterone synthesis.

ANSWER:
B, C, D, E

8. Which of the following are causes of hyperprolactinemia?

   A. Intravenous dopamine

   B. Pregnancy

   C. Sheenan's syndrome

   D. Hyperthyroidism

   E. Chronic renal failure

Ref.: 3

COMMENTS: Prolactinomas are the most common pituitary tumor. • They are the cause of hyperprolactinemia in approximately 60–70% of patients. • There are, however, several other important causes. • Pregnant females have a normal increase in prolactin levels, which remain elevated in breast-feeding mothers. • In females with a known prolactinoma, increased estrogen levels can lead to growth of the existing prolactinoma. • Thus, all females who have a known prolactinoma should have baseline visual field testing performed if they intend to become pregnant. • Two other important causes are hypothyroidism and chronic

renal failure. • Sarcoidosis and various drugs are also known causes. • Dopamine is the presumed prolactin-inhibitory factor that is released from the hypothalamus and suppresses prolactin release. • Intravenous dopamine infusion leads to low prolactin levels. • Sheenan's syndrome occurs as a result of pituitary necrosis after postpartum hemorrhage and hypovolemia. • The extent of necrosis determines the degree of hypopituitarism. • Thus, secretion of any pituitary hormone, including prolactin, would be decreased.

ANSWER:
B, E

9. With regard to ACTH, which of the following statements is/are true?

   A. ACTH release is presumed to be under partial hypothalamic control.

   B. ACTH release may be affected by direct feedback inhibition of circulating cortisol levels on the adenohypophysis.

   C. ACTH levels are fairly constant during any given 24-hr period but may rise abruptly in response to stress.

   D. There is a circadian rhythm of ACTH release that cannot usually be overcome by peripheral stimulatory influences.

Ref.: 1–3

COMMENTS: ACTH is secreted by the adenohypophysis under the influence of both CRF from the hypothalamus and the negative feedback of circulating cortisol levels. • Although there are several surges of ACTH release during a given 24-hr period, the largest characteristically occurs at night and during the early morning hours, accounting for the typical diurnal variation of blood cortisol levels. • These central and negative feedback regulatory mechanisms are easily overridden during periods of stress, such as acute illness, fever, hypoglycemia, and emotional upset. • An abrupt increase in ACTH secretion in response to these factors can lead to as much as a tenfold increase in cortisol production within a short period of time.

ANSWER:
A, B

10. Match each of the physiologic effects in the left-hand column with its respective gonadotropic hormone in the right-hand column.

A. Promotes spermatogenesis	a. FSH
B. Stimulates testicular testosterone production	b. LH
C. Facilitates development of corpus luteum	c. Both FSH and LH
D. Promotes ovarian follicle maturation	d. Neither FSH nor LH
E. Production stimulated by GnRH	

Ref.: 1, 2

COMMENTS: Sexual and reproductive physiology involves a complex interaction of hypothalamic, pituitary, gonadal, adrenal, and circulating hormonal factors. • The role of the pituitary in this complex scheme involves the production of FSH and LH.

• These two hormones are produced by the same adenohypophyseal cell under the influence of a single GnRH from the hypothalamus. • This hypothalamic-pituitary interaction is modulated by feedback from adrenal and gonadal hormone production.

ANSWER:
A-a; B-b; C-d; D-a; E-c

---

11. With regard to TSH, which of the following statements is/are true?

   A. TSH release is under hypothalamic influence by means of TRH.

   B. TSH release is directly influenced by circulating thyroid hormones.

   C. As with other adenohypophyseal hormones, TSH has numerous effects in addition to its stimulatory effect on the thyroid gland.

   D. TSH levels can be pharmacologically manipulated to affect the growth of thyroid neoplasms.

Ref.: 1, 2

COMMENTS: Unlike prolactin and GH, which have numerous metabolic effects, TSH appears to exert influence only on the thyroid gland. • It stimulates both growth of the gland and secretion of thyroid hormones. • Circulating thyroid hormones exert a well-defined feedback inhibition on TSH-producing cells in the adenohypophysis, both directly and by the inhibiting effect on hypothalamically derived TRH. • The growth of thyroid neoplasms, similar to the growth of the normal thyroid gland, may be stimulated by high TSH levels. • For this reason, pharmacologic reduction of TSH levels by administration of exogenous thyroid hormone may shrink both benign and malignant thyroid tumors.

ANSWER:
A, B, D

---

12. With regard to excess ACTH production by the pituitary, which of the following statements is/are true?

   A. Cushing's syndrome and Cushing's disease are synonymous terms.

   B. ACTH-producing pituitary adenomas are the most common cause of excess adrenal cortisol production.

   C. Most hypothalamic or pituitary causes of excess ACTH production are due to pituitary microadenomas.

   D. The sella is enlarged in most patients with ACTH-producing pituitary adenomas.

   E. Bilateral adrenalectomy is preferable to hypophysectomy for the management of Cushing's disease.

Ref.: 1, 2

COMMENTS: Cushing's syndrome refers to the clinical sequelae of excess adrenal cortisol production. • It may be due to an adrenal carcinoma, an adrenal adenoma, nodular dysplasia of the adrenal, or diffuse adrenal hyperplasia in response to excess ACTH production from a pituitary adenoma, ectopic ACTH production by a benign or malignant nonpituitary and nonadrenal tumor, or excess CRF production from the hypothalamus. • When Cushing's syndrome is due to a pituitary adenoma, it is known as

Cushing's disease, in honor of Harvey Cushing, a pioneering American neurosurgeon. • Cushing's disease accounts for 60–80% of naturally occurring Cushing's syndrome. • Of the hypothalamic or pituitary causes of Cushing's syndrome, pathologic studies have demonstrated that up to 80% are due to a pituitary microadenoma that produces ACTH. • In most of these cases, the adenoma is too small to cause any changes in the radiographic appearance of the sella. • When appropriate studies have revealed that a pituitary adenoma is the cause of bilateral adrenal hyperplasia, the preferred method of treatment is transsphenoidal excision of the adenoma, rather than bilateral adrenalectomy.

ANSWER:
B, C

---

13. Which one or more of the following statements characterize pituitary endorphins?

   A. They are opiate-like peptides.

   B. They share a common amino acid sequence with other adenohypophyseal hormones.

   C. They are also found in the brain and gut.

   D. Despite their biochemical identification, physiologic or behavioral effects of these substances have not yet been demonstrated.

Ref.: 1, 2

COMMENTS: Pituitary endorphins are opiate-like peptides that represent fragments of a larger prohormone called pro-opiocortin. • Melanocyte-stimulating hormone and ACTH possess amino acid sequences that are identical to portions of the pro-opiocortin and β-lipotropin structures. • These endorphins, which are also found throughout the brain and gut, are capable of exerting potent analgesic effects and may be key factors in an individual's behavioral and physiologic response to pain.

ANSWER:
A, B, C

---

14. Amenorrhea and progressive hypothyroidism occurring after recovery from shock due to placental hemorrhage may be known as which of the following?

   A. Sheehan's syndrome

   B. Postpartum pituitary ischemia

   C. Thyrogenital syndrome

   D. A form of pituitary apoplexy

Ref.: 1–3

COMMENTS: During pregnancy, the size of the pituitary may increase as much as 50%, with a proportionate increase in its blood flow. • If a state of hypoperfusion occurs during late pregnancy or delivery, the pituitary may become ischemic and subsequently necrotic, resulting in panhypopituitarism. • The most obvious subsequent clinical manifestations of this condition are amenorrhea and hypothyroidism. • Once the diagnosis is made, treatment involves appropriate hormone replacement therapy.

ANSWER:
A, B, D

15. With regard to growth hormone hypersecretion, which of the following statements is/are true?

   A. Acromegaly may occur in both adults and children.

   B. GH-secreting tumors may produce symptoms that are not related to GH excess.

   C. Acromegalics frequently die of cardiac complications.

   D. Surgery has been supplanted by radiation therapy as the treatment of choice for excessive GH secretion.

   E. Somatostatin analogues are a useful medical adjunctive therapy.

Ref.: 1–3

COMMENTS: Excessive production of GH by pituitary adenomas leads to morphologic changes that differ according to the age and skeletal maturity of the patient. • In children (before epiphyseal closure), there is generalized overgrowth of most of the somatic structures, resulting in gigantism. • In adults (after epiphyseal closure), the somatic enlargement is most evident in the face, hands, and feet and is termed acromegaly. • In patients with acromegaly, enlargement of the heart, with subsequent valvular dysfunction and cardiomyopathy, may also occur and is a common cause of death. • Although the characteristic physical appearance of patients with GH excess dominates the clinical presentation, the adenoma itself occasionally grows to such a size as to produce symptoms due to an expanding pituitary mass (e.g., visual disturbances, headaches, or pituitary hypofunction). • Surgical excision of the adenoma is the treatment in most circumstances, although radiation therapy is finding increasing applicability. • Octreotide decreases serum levels of GH as well as somatomedian C, a downstream growth factor. • It may be useful in the preoperative setting or after surgical failure. • Octreotide has also been used as primary therapy in patients who are not operative candidates

ANSWER:
B, C, E

16. With regard to GH, which of the following statements is/are true?

   A. GH is a peptide that affects the growth of somatic structures, such as bone and muscle, but does not affect the growth of visceral organs or physiologic homeostasis.

   B. GH secretion is stimulated by a hypothalamic-releasing factor, but no hypothalamic inhibitory factor has yet been identified.

   C. Under normal circumstances, the largest surge of GH in the peripheral blood occurs during the evening.

   D. GH secretion may be stimulated by exercise, stress, or hypoglycemia.

Ref.: 1, 2

COMMENTS: GH is a large peptide secreted from the lateral aspect of the adenohypophysis. • Its secretion is regulated by releasing factors and inhibitory factors (somatostatin) from the hypothalamus. • Furthermore, its release is stimulated directly or indirectly by exercise, physiologic stress, and hypoglycemia. • In addition to its positive effect on the growth of somatic structures, GH also stimulates the growth of visceral organs. • In addition, it has numerous anabolic effects, including the elevation of blood glucose and free fatty acid levels and the incorporation of amino acids into protein. • GH is released into the peripheral blood as

a result of secretory surges occurring six to eight times daily. • The largest surge occurs during the early morning hours. • During adolescence, the total amount of GH secreted daily increases, owing to an increase in the number of surges.

ANSWER:
D

17. With regard to pituitary-releasing factors, which of the following statements is/are true?

   A. Releasing factors are formed in the hypothalamus and proceed directly to the adenohypophysis, bypassing the neurohypophysis.

   B. Releasing factors are derivatives of steroids similar to those seen in the adrenal cortex.

   C. Release of TSH is under partial control of TRH and partial control of peripheral triiodothyronine (T_3) and thyroxine (T_4) levels.

   D. The concept of feedback inhibition of pituitary function is outdated.

Ref.: 1, 2

COMMENTS: The concept of feedback inhibition is fundamental to the understanding of the hypothalamic-pituitary-peripheral endocrine axis. • In its most simplified form, the hypothalamus, sensing and reacting to peripheral blood hormone levels, synthesizes releasing factors (small peptides), which are released as neurosecretory granules from the axons within the neurohypophysis. • These are then transported through the portal vascular system to the adenohypophysis to influence adenohypophyseal hormone output. • These hormones in turn influence endocrine function of the peripheral end organ, which alters the circulating blood levels of the hormone it produces, completing the cycle. • The adenohypophysis may be directly sensitive to blood levels of circulating hormones, as in the case of TSH production, which may be altered not only by TRH but also by peripheral T_3 and T_4 levels.

ANSWER:
C

18. With regard to pituitary tumors, which of the following statements is/are true?

   A. The classification of pituitary tumors depends solely on their aniline dye affinity.

   B. The most common pituitary tumor is endocrine inactive.

   C. Common parasellar symptoms include cerebrospinal fluid obstruction.

   D. Prolactin excess in males causes decreased potency and infertility.

   E. Surgery and radiation therapy are the mainstays of treatment.

Ref.: 1, 2

COMMENTS: Pituitary tumors were formerly classified according to their affinity for aniline dyes (chromophobe, eosinophils, or basophilic adenomas). • The more recent classification divides them into endocrine-active and endocrine-inactive tumors. • A great deal of additional classification has been performed based on more specific immunohistochemical techniques and more recently by polymerase chain reaction techniques. • The most common pituitary adenoma is the prolactin-producing adenoma, followed (in decreasing order of frequency) by endocrine-inactive tumors, GH-producing tumors, ACTH-producing tumors, TSH-producing tumors, and LH- or FSH-producing tumors. • Tumors less than 1 cm in diameter are termed microadenomas, whereas those larger than 1 cm in diameter are called macroadenomas. • Symptoms depend on the type of hormone produced, the degree of compromise of the surrounding anterior pituitary (symptoms of hormone insufficiency), and the mass effect of the tumor itself, producing parasellar neurologic deficits. • In females, prolactin excess causes menstrual irregularities, infertility, and galactorrhea. • In males, it leads to decreased potency and infertility. • GH excess causes gigantism in young patients and acromegaly in patients whose epiphyses are closed. • ACTH-producing adenomas cause Cushing's disease. • TSH-producing adenomas are associated with hyperthyroidism, whereas LH- and FSH-producing adenomas lead to gonadal insufficiency. • Parasellar deficits include optic nerve dysfunction, extraocular motor loss, hypothalamic dysfunction, or frontal and medial temporal lobe signs and symptoms. • The most effective therapies for symptomatic pituitary adenomas remain surgery and radiation therapy, although TSH-producing and FSH- and LH-producing adenomas may shrink in response to bromocriptine therapy.

A N S W E R :
D, E

19. In regard to imaging modalities of the pituitary gland, which of the following is/are correct?

   A. Lateral skull x-rays can demonstrate the presence of a pituitary macroadenoma.

   B. CT scanning with intravenous contrast is the preferred imaging modality for pituitary lesions.

   C. Magnetic resonance imaging (MRI) with gadolinium can distinguish a pituitary tumor from an aneurysm.

   D. Angiography has no role in evaluating pituitary disease.

Ref.: 3

COMMENTS: Plain skull x-rays can detect pituitary macroadenomas, since these lesions typically lead to a characteristic widening of the sella turcica. • However, neither skull x-rays nor CT scans are the preferred imaging modality for pituitary lesions. • MRI with gadolinium has become the gold standard for evaluating these lesions and can detect pituitary microadenomas as small as 3–5 mm. • MRI can also be used to distinguish vascular anomalies such as aneurysms from pituitary tumors. • Angiography is no longer frequently used in the evaluation of pituitary lesions. • However, in cases where large sellar masses cause compression of the neighboring cavernous sinus, the internal carotid artery can be compressed, leading to a cerebrovascular aneurysm. • Angiography is still useful in this situation or to further evaluate aneurysms mimicking sellar lesions.

A N S W E R :
A, C

20. Match the sellar lesion in the left-hand column with the common presenting symptom(s) in the right-hand column.

   A. Macroadenoma   a. Gigantism in children and acromegaly in adults

   B. Craniopharyngioma   b. Bitemporal hemianopsia

   C. GH microadenoma   c. Galactorrhea, amenorrhea, and impotence

   D. ACTH microadenoma   d. Cushing's disease

   E. Prolactin adenoma   e. DI

Ref.: 1, 2

COMMENTS: The pituitary gland acts as the master gland of the endocrine system. • Its most common tumors are pituitary adenomas. • Frequently, these adenomas are not hormonally active but, instead, cause symptoms by local mass effect. • Because they present by pressing on local structures, such as the optic chiasm or other cranial nerves, they are usually more than 1 cm in diameter and are referred to as macroadenomas. • Microadenomas, pituitary tumors less than 1 cm in diameter, present because of the hormone-stimulating factors they secrete. • ACTH-secreting tumors cause Cushing's disease. • They can be differentiated from adrenal tumors that produce cortisol and ectopic tumors that secrete ACTH by the dexamethasone suppression test. • GH-secreting tumors cause gigantism in children and acromegaly in adults. • They are best treated surgically if no contraindications exist. • Prolactinomas cause amenorrhea, galactorrhea, impotence, and symptoms of mass effect. • These symptoms can be controlled in some patients with bromocriptine, a dopamine agonist. • Craniopharyngioma, an epithelium-lined tumor, usually involves the sella. • It is more common during childhood and can present with mass effect or hypopituitary symptoms, such as DI.

A N S W E R :
A-b; B-e; C-a; D-d; E-c

21. Decreased secretion of the hormones in the right-hand column results in which of the syndromes or symptoms in the left-hand column?

   A. Amenorrhea   a. ACTH

   B. Addison's disease   b. LH

   C. DI   c. TSH

   D. Weight gain and constipation   d. Vasopressin

Ref.: 3

COMMENTS: Depressed secretion of either of the gonadotropins (FSH or LH) can lead to amenorrhea, which also can result from excess prolactin secretion. • Addison's disease results from low cortisol production, which may be caused by depressed ACTH levels. • This is a life-threatening situation that requires immediate administration of exogenous steroids. • As previously mentioned, a lack of vasopressin from traumatic injury, tumor, pituitary irradiation, or pituitary resection can result in diabetes insipidus. • Low TSH levels can lead to hypothyroidism, with a well known constellation of symptoms.

A N S W E R :
A-b; B-a; C-d; D-c

22. In regard to Nelson's syndrome, which of the following is/are true?

   A. It is treated with bilateral adrenalectomy.

   B. It is characterized by elevated ACTH levels.

   C. It results in pituitary atrophy.

D. It is also known as empty sella syndrome.

E. It can result in increased skin pigmentation.

Ref.: 3

COMMENTS: In 1958, D.H. Nelson and coworkers identified a syndrome of progressive hyperpigmentation, visual field loss, and amenorrhea associated with elevated ACTH levels. • This syndrome was discovered in a patient who had undergone bilateral adrenalectomy as treatment for bilateral adrenal hyperplasia causing Cushing's syndrome. • Lack of cortisol feedback typically leads to pituitary hypertrophy and ACTH hypersecretion. • The hyperpigmentation is due to the cosecretion of melanocyte-stimulating hormone along with ACTH. • Empty sella syndrome results from arachnoid herniation due to a congenital defect in the diaphragma sella. • Pituitary function in patients with empty sella syndrome is typically normal, but occasionally hyperprolactinemia is observed. • No treatment is necessary.

ANSWER:
B, E

REFERENCES

1. Brunicardi FC, Andersen DK, Billiar TR, et al: *Schwartz's Principles of Surgery*, 8th ed. McGraw-Hill, New York, 2004.
2. Townsend CM, Beauchamp RD, Evers BM, et al: *Sabiston Textbook of Surgery*: *The Biological Basis of Modern Surgical Practice*, 17th ed. Saunders, Philadelphia, 2004.
3. Mullholland MW, Lillemoe KD, Doherty GM, et al: *Greenfield's Surgery: Scientific Principles and Practice*, 4th ed. Lippincott, Williams & Wilkins, Philadelphia, 2006.

C H A P T E R 30

Adrenal

Theresa W. Ruddy, M.D., and Richard A. Prinz, M.D.

1. Which of the following statements about the embryologic development of the adrenal gland is/are true?

   A. Adrenal cortex is derived from ectodermal tissue.

   B. Adrenal medulla is derived from ectodermal tissue.

   C. Extra-adrenal medullary tissue is most commonly found adjacent to the aorta.

   D. Extra-adrenal cortical tissue is most commonly found along the sympathetic nerve chain.

   Ref.: 1–3

COMMENTS: The adrenal gland is composed of a cortex and a medulla, which have different embryologic origins and different physiologic functions. • The cortex is derived from mesoderm between the dorsal mesentery and the primitive gonad located along the urogenital ridge. • This development occurs between the fourth and sixth weeks of fetal life. • The medulla is derived from ectodermal cells and the neural crest during the seventh week of fetal development. • These ectodermal cells migrate from the neural crest of the periaortic area, resulting in the development of the sympathetic ganglia and the adrenal medulla. • In lower vertebrates, the cortical and medullary tissues remain separate. • In humans, the cortex envelops the medulla to form a single gland. • The adrenal is larger than the kidney during fetal development but gradually decreases in size during the first postpartum year. • During the course of fetal development, both adrenal cortical and adrenal medullary rests may persist along the paths of cellular migration. • Extra-adrenal medullary (chromaffin) tissue is found more commonly and over a wider anatomic range than is extra-adrenal cortical tissue. • This aberrant medullary tissue is responsible for extra-adrenal pheochromocytomas. • The most common extra-adrenal site of medullary tissue is the organ of Zuckerkandl, located near the origin of the inferior mesenteric artery to the left of the aortic bifurcation.

ANSWER:
B, C

2. Which of the following statements describe(s) the typical venous drainage of the adrenal glands?

   A. Plexuses of small veins provide the major drainage of each gland.

   B. A primary central vein provides the major drainage of each gland.

   C. Both glands drain into the inferior vena cava.

   D. The right gland drains into the inferior vena cava.

   E. The left gland drains into the inferior vena cava.

   Ref.: 1–3

COMMENTS: Each adrenal gland is usually drained by one main central vein. • On the right side, the adrenal vein leaves the gland medially and goes directly into the inferior vena cava. • This vein is typically short and can be the source of hazardous bleeding if not handled correctly. • On the left side, the adrenal vein leaves the gland anteriorly and joins the left renal vein. • The left adrenal anatomy makes selective catheterization of the adrenal vein simpler on the left. • Occasionally, the left adrenal vein enters the inferior vena cava directly. • Small accessory adrenal veins may also be present.

ANSWER:
B, D

3. The arterial blood supply of both the right and left adrenal glands comes from which of the following?

   A. Branch of the inferior phrenic artery

   B. Direct aortic branch

   C. Branch of the renal artery

   D. None of the above; each gland is supplied by a different pattern.

   Ref.: 1–3

COMMENTS: The arterial blood supply to both the adrenal glands is similar and typically from three sources. • The **superior adrenal artery** originates from a branch of the inferior phrenic artery, which comes off the aorta. • The **middle adrenal artery** comes directly from the aorta. • The **inferior adrenal artery** arises from the renal artery on each side.

ANSWER:
A, B, C

4. Match each of the hormones in the left-hand column with one or more of the parts of the adrenal gland where it is primarily manufactured in the right-hand column.

A. Cortisol	a. Zona glomerulosa
B. Aldosterone	b. Zona fasciculata
C. Sex steroids	c. Zona reticularis

D. Epinephrine

E. Norepinephrine

F. 17-Hydroxylase

G. 11-Hydroxylase

H. 21-Hydroxylase

I. Corticosterone methyloxidase

d. Adrenal medulla

Ref.: 1–3

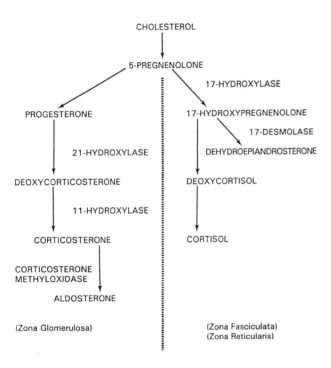

CHOLESTEROL

5-PREGNENOLONE

17-HYDROXYLASE

PROGESTERONE   17-HYDROXYPREGNENOLONE

17-DESMOLASE

21-HYDROXYLASE   DEHYDROEPIANDROSTERONE

DEOXYCORTICOSTERONE   DEOXYCORTISOL

11-HYDROXYLASE

CORTICOSTERONE   CORTISOL

CORTICOSTERONE
METHYLOXIDASE

ALDOSTERONE

(Zona Glomerulosa)   (Zona Fasciculata)
                        (Zona Reticularis)

COMMENTS: Adrenal cortical hormones are manufactured as a result of hydroxylation and oxidation of certain sites on the cholesterol molecule. • These processes occur in various areas of the adrenal cortex, depending on the enzymes present or absent in each anatomic zone. • The three anatomic zones of the adrenal cortex are arranged concentrically from the capsule inward to the medulla: zona glomerulosa, zona fasciculata, and zona reticularis. • Adrenal cortical hormones are synthesized from cholesterol, which is converted to 5-pregnenolone. • In the presence of 17-hydroxylase (contained in the zona fasciculata and zona reticularis but *not* in the zona glomerulosa), 5-pregnenolone is converted to 17-hydroxypregnenolone, which is the precursor of both cortisol and the androgens. • In the absence of 17-hydroxylase, 5-pregnenolone is converted to progesterone, which is the precursor of aldosterone. • Each of the three zones in the adrenal cortex contains 11- and 21-hydroxylating enzymes. • Aldosterone is produced exclusively by the zona glomerulosa because of the presence of corticosterone methyloxidase. • Cortisol is produced in both the zona fasciculata and the zona reticularis. • The sex steroids are produced primarily in the zona reticularis but can also be manufactured in the zona fasciculata. • The catecholamines are not cholesterol derivatives. • They are synthesized from phenylalanine and tyrosine. • The conversion of norepinephrine to epinephrine requires methylation by the enzyme phenylethanolamine-*N*-methyltransferase, which is present almost exclusively in the

adrenal medulla and organ of Zuckerkandl. • Therefore, nearly all epinephrine is synthesized in the adrenal medulla.

ANSWER:
A-b,c; B-a; C-b,c; D-d; E-d; F-b,c; G-a,b,c; H-a,b,c; I-a

5. Physiologic results of normal cortisol production include which of the following?

A. Gluconeogenesis

B. Protein catabolism

C. Fat storage

D. Decreased serum triglyceride and free fatty acid levels

E. Decreased urinary sodium levels

Ref.: 1–3

COMMENTS: Cortisol is produced in the zona fasciculata and zona reticularis. • Cortisol binds to cell receptors. • The steroid-receptor complex directly binds DNA, leading to gene transcription, ultimately producing the metabolic effects of cortisol. • Glucocorticoids are necessary to maintain hepatic glycogen stores by stimulating gluconeogenesis. • Cortisol also stimulates glucagon release, protein catabolism, and lipolysis. • The lipolysis leads to **increased** serum triglyceride and free fatty acids levels. • Glucocorticoids act at the distal renal tubule by inducing resorption of sodium.

ANSWER:
A, B, E

6. Cushing's disease is caused by which of the following?

A. Adrenal adenoma

B. Adrenal carcinoma

C. Pituitary adenoma

D. Ectopic ACTH production

Ref.: 1–3

COMMENTS: Cushing's syndrome refers to the clinical manifestations of excess glucocorticoids. • The most common cause of Cushing's syndrome is iatrogenic, from exogenous administration of corticosteroids. • Endogenous overproduction of cortisol is either **ACTH dependent** (80% of cases) or **ACTH independent**. • The most common cause of ACTH-dependent hypercortisolism is a pituitary adenoma. • Cortisol excess from a pituitary tumor is known as **Cushing's disease.** • Other ACTH-dependent causes of cortisol excess include ectopic ACTH produced by tumors, such as small-cell lung cancers or bronchial carcinoids. • Bilateral adrenal hyperplasia is seen with ACTH-dependent hypercortisolism. • ACTH-independent Cushing's syndrome is caused directly by pathologic conditions of the adrenal gland, including adrenal adenoma, adrenal carcinoma, and the rare adrenocortical hyperplasia.

ANSWER:
C

7. Clinical features of Cushing's syndrome include which of the following?

A. Hypoglycemia

B. Hyperkalemia

C. Hypertension

D. Truncal obesity

Ref.: 1–3

COMMENTS: Cushing's syndrome produces clinical features consistent with excess glucocorticoids. • These features include truncal obesity, hypertension, and glucose intolerance. • Abnormal patterns of fat deposition produce the characteristic "buffalo hump" and "moon facies." Females manifest hirsutism and menstrual disorders. • Sexual dysfunction is common in both sexes. • Purple striae over the abdomen and extremities; proximal muscle atrophy with weakness, peripheral edema, acne, and easy bruisability; and osteoporosis are seen. • Patients may also suffer from fungal skin infections. • Other features may include back pain; poor wound healing; neurologic symptoms, such as headaches; and psychiatric disturbances. • Hypokalemia may occur, owing to the weak mineralocorticoid effect of cortisol. • Osteopenia, diabetes mellitus, and nephrolithiasis may be part of the syndrome. • Patients often have a persistent leukocytosis.

ANSWER:
C, D

8. An obese 45-year-old man complains of impotence. Examination demonstrates a blood pressure of 180/90, proximal muscle wasting, and purple abdominal striae. Which of the following is the most sensitive screening test for hypercortisolism?

A. Plasma cortisol level at 8 PM

B. Plasma cortisol level at 4 AM

C. Random plasma cortisol level

D. 24-hr urinary free cortisol level

E. 24-hr urinary 17-OH corticosteroid level

Ref.: 1–3

COMMENTS: Patients suspected of having Cushing's syndrome should first have excess cortisol production confirmed and then its source determined. • Cortisol is normally secreted intermittently, with a diurnal variation such that evening levels are lower (by about one half) than are morning levels. • Therefore, a random sample is not useful. • Although patients with Cushing's syndrome typically have elevated evening levels, there is sufficient overlap with normal levels to limit the accuracy of evening testing. • The most sensitive screening test is a 24-hr determination of urinary free cortisol levels. • Normally, little free cortisol is excreted in the urine. • Excess cortisol is present in the urine when cortisol-binding sites are saturated during hypercortisolism. • Two or three consecutive urine samples should be obtained. • The urinary creatinine level should be measured concomitantly to ensure that the sample is adequate. • 17-Hydroxy (OH) corticosteroids and 17-OH ketosteroids are metabolites of cortisol and androgens that can be measured in the urine, but these determinations are less accurate than is the free cortisol assay.

ANSWER:
D

9. The patient described in Question 8 is found to have mild elevation of the urinary free cortisol level. Which test should be performed next to confirm a diagnosis of Cushing's syndrome?

A. Plasma ACTH level

B. Corticotropin-releasing hormone (CRH) stimulation

C. Metyrapone stimulation

D. High-dose dexamethasone suppression

E. Low-dose dexamethasone suppression

Ref.: 1–3

COMMENTS: The low-dose dexamethasone suppression test can confirm hypercortisolism. • The other tests listed are used to determine the cause of Cushing's syndrome once a diagnosis has been made. • Dexamethasone is a synthetic corticosteroid that suppresses pituitary secretion of ACTH and consequent adrenal corticosteroid production. • Plasma cortisol is sampled in the morning after oral administration of 1 mg dexamethasone the night before. • Plasma cortisol levels are low (<3 mg/dl) in normal individuals but elevated in patients with Cushing's syndrome. • False-positive test results may be obtained in patients who are obese, chronically ill, alcoholic, or taking certain medications (e.g., Dilantin, rifampin, estrogens, or tamoxifen). • Plasma ACTH levels are measured to determine whether the cause is excessive ACTH production from a pituitary or ectopic source. • CRH stimulation can differentiate Cushing's disease from an ectopic source of ACTH. • CRH stimulation leads to increased ACTH levels in Cushing's disease but usually no change when ACTH is from an ectopic source. • Metyrapone stimulates ACTH in patients with Cushing's disease. • The high-dose dexamethasone-suppression test is used to differentiate a pituitary from an ectopic source of ACTH. • The high dose of dexamethasone will usually suppress a pituitary adenoma but will have little or no effect on ectopic sources or adrenal tumors.

ANSWER:
E

10. In which of the following ways is inferior petrosal sinus sampling helpful in the evaluation of a patient with hypercortisolism (Cushing's syndrome)?

A. It lacks sensitivity for pituitary adenoma.

B. Procedural complications limit its clinical availability.

C. It differentiates pituitary from nonpituitary ACTH-dependent Cushing's syndrome.

D. It differentiates ACTH-independent from ACTH-dependent Cushing's syndrome.

E. It can precisely determine the location of a pituitary adenoma.

Ref.: 1–3

COMMENTS: Bilateral simultaneous inferior petrosal sinus sampling is the most accurate method of distinguishing between ACTH excess from pituitary sources and that from ectopic sources. • It is 100% sensitive and specific for pituitary adenoma. • Comparisons are made between the ACTH levels in peripheral blood and blood from the inferior petrosal sinus draining the pituitary gland both before and after stimulation with CRH. • This test is appropriate when other biochemical and imaging studies have not succeeded in differentiating the source of ACTH-dependent Cushing's syndrome. • Comparison between the right and left sides may also be useful for lateralizing a pituitary adenoma. • Inferior petrosal sinus sampling is an invasive test that requires skilled intervention to catheterize the sinuses via the internal jugular vein. • In experienced hands, it has proved safe and reliable.

ANSWER:
B, C

11. A 29-year-old man presents with truncal obesity, hypertension, and muscular weakness. He is found to have increased serum cortisol levels, elevated plasma ACTH levels, and suppression of urinary free cortisol after administration of high-dose but not low-dose dexamethasone. A computed tomographic (CT) brain scan reveals a small mass in the pituitary. Which of the following is the preferred treatment?

A. Bilateral adrenalectomy

B. Transsphenoidal resection of the microadenoma

C. Chemotherapy

D. Aminoglutethimide administration

E. Pituitary irradiation

Ref.: 1–3

COMMENTS: The patient described has a pituitary adenoma. • The primary treatment is transsphenoidal resection of the tumor. • This procedure is successful in 90–95% of patients treated by experienced neurosurgeons. • Irradiation can be used as an adjunct. • Aminoglutethimide blocks production and secretion of adrenocortical steroids. • It is not appropriate initial treatment and is reserved for those who are not surgical candidates. • Bilateral adrenalectomy is not indicated for Cushing's disease. • The pituitary adenoma is not malignant, and therefore chemotherapy has no role.

ANSWER:
B

12. A 35-year-old woman presents with clinical and laboratory evidence of Cushing's syndrome and is found to have a depressed plasma ACTH level and a well-defined 3-cm left adrenal mass. Which of the following is the preferred treatment?

A. Bilateral adrenalectomy

B. Left adrenalectomy

C. Mitotane administration

D. Left adrenal irradiation

Ref.: 1–3

COMMENTS: Unilateral adrenalectomy of the affected gland is indicated for the treatment of an adrenal adenoma. • A laparoscopic approach is preferred unless the lesion is greater than 6 cm in size. • In that case, an open approach should be considered because of a higher likelihood of malignancy. • Bilateral adrenalectomy is not necessary for a unilateral adenoma. • The remaining gland has been suppressed by the hypercortisolism from the adrenal adenoma. • The patient will require exogenous glucocorticoids until the remaining gland regains function. • Mitotane is an adrenal cytotoxic agent. • It is used with limited effectiveness for adrenocortical carcinoma. • It and irradiation are not indicated for the treatment of adrenal adenoma.

ANSWER:
B

13. Which one of the following findings is most consistent with the diagnosis of primary hyperaldosteronism (Conn's syndrome)?

A. Sodium 145 mEq/L, potassium 4.8 mEq/L, blood pressure 90/60, and expanded blood volume

B. Sodium 132 mEq/L, potassium 5.4 mEq/L, blood pressure 160/100, and expanded blood volume

C. Sodium 149 mEq/L, potassium 3.0 mEq/L, blood pressure 160/100, and contracted blood volume

D. Sodium 149 mEq/L, potassium 3.0 mEq/L, blood pressure 160/100, and expanded blood volume

Ref.: 1–3

COMMENTS: The clinical and laboratory findings characteristic of primary hyperaldosteronism are hypernatremia, hypokalemia, elevated plasma aldosterone levels, normal cortisol levels, expanded blood volume, and sustained hypertension. • These findings are all attributable to physiologic of aldosterone effect on the distal convoluted tubule, causing sodium retention in exchange for potassium and hydrogen ion excretion. • Alkalosis, polydipsia, nocturnal polyuria, and paresthesias also are common.

ANSWER:
D

14. Which one of the following is the most common cause of primary hyperaldosteronism?

A. Adrenocortical carcinoma

B. Solitary adrenal adenoma

C. Bilateral adrenocortical hyperplasia

D. Pituitary neoplasm

E. Ovarian or testicular neoplasm

Ref.: 1–3

COMMENTS: Primary hyperaldosteronism is an uncommon disease, first described by J.W. Conn in 1955, characterized by autonomous excess secretion of aldosterone from the adrenal cortex. • In 60–70% of cases, primary hyperaldosteronism is due to a solitary adrenal adenoma. • Most of the remaining cases are due to bilateral adrenocortical hyperplasia, the cause of which is not precisely known. • Occasionally, adrenocortical carcinoma is associated with excess aldosterone secretion. • There have been a few reports of ectopic production of aldosterone from ovarian neoplasms. • Autosomal-dominant glucocorticoid-suppressible hyperaldosteronism is another rare cause of primary hyperaldosteronism. • **Secondary** hyperaldosteronism is a relatively common clinical condition in which a relative deficit of circulating volume or sodium content stimulates renin synthesis, leading to aldosterone production. • Secondary hyperaldosteronism can occur in patients with renal artery stenosis, congestive heart failure, or hepatic cirrhosis and during pregnancy.

ANSWER:
B

15. Match each anatomic location in the left-hand column with its physiologic function in the right-hand column.

A. Macula densa   a. Synthesizes renin

B. Juxtaglomerular cells   b. Produces aldosterone

C. Zona glomerulosa   c. Produces angiotensinogen

D. Liver   d. Converts angiotensin I to angiotensin II

E. Lung

e. Sensitive to decreases in renal arterial blood pressure

f. Sensitive to changes in sodium concentration in the distal tubule

Ref.: 1–3

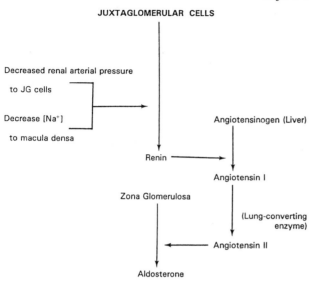

JUXTAGLOMERULAR CELLS

Decreased renal arterial pressure to JG cells

Decrease [Na⁺] to macula densa

Angiotensinogen (Liver)

Renin →

Angiotensin I

Zona Glomerulosa

(Lung-converting enzyme)

← Angiotensin II

Aldosterone

COMMENTS: Aldosterone is the only clinically important mineralocorticoid in humans. • It is secreted by the zona glomerulosa of the adrenal cortex under the influence of the renin-angiotensin system, serum potassium levels, and plasma ACTH levels. • Stimulation by ACTH is the weakest and only occurs when pathologic levels of ACTH are present. • Elevated serum potassium levels directly stimulate adrenal secretion of aldosterone. • The major regulator of aldosterone secretion is the renin-angiotensin system, where decreases in renal arterial blood pressure stimulate renin secretion from the juxtaglomerular cells of the kidney. • Renin converts angiotensinogen, which is synthesized in the liver, to inactive angiotensin I. • Angiotensin-converting enzyme in the lung converts angiotensin I to active angiotensin II. • Angiotensin II is a potent vasoconstrictor and stimulant of aldosterone secretion. • Aldosterone acts on the distal tubule, resulting in sodium and chloride retention in exchange for potassium and hydrogen ions. • Primary hyperaldosteronism is a condition in which autonomous production of aldosterone (e.g., an aldosterone-producing adenoma) functions outside the normal influence of the negative feedback loop. • Classic findings include hypertension, hypokalemia, and metaboli alkalosis. • Secondary hyperaldosteronism is a physiologic compensatory mechanism in which elevated serum aldosterone levels are found in response to increased renin secretion. • The macula densa is a specialized area of the thick ascending limb adjacent to the glomerulus. • The cells of the macula densa are sensitive to change in the intraluminal concentration of sodium and chloride in the distal tubule. • Signals from the macula densa regulate the renin-secreting cells and glomerular infiltration rate.

ANSWER:
A-f; B-e,a; C-b; D-c; E-d

16. Primary hyperaldosteronism can be differentiated from secondary by which of the following tests?

A. Plasma aldosterone level

B. Plasma renin level

C. Plasma cortisol level

D. CT scan

E. Adrenal vein sampling

Ref.: 1–3

COMMENTS: In primary hyperaldosteronism, plasma renin levels are suppressed, whereas in secondary hyperaldosteronism they are not. • Various tests to confirm the overproduction of aldosterone, seen in primary disease, include saline loading and the administration of captopril. • These tests would normally suppress aldosterone levels unless the elevated levels are caused by primary disease. • The plasma aldosterone/plasma renin activity ratio is greater than 20 with primary hyperaldosteronism. • Measurements of 24-hr urinary aldosterone levels are more accurate than are measurements of plasma levels. • Medications such as spironolactone, angiotensin-converting enzyme (ACE) inhibitors, and diuretics can affect renin-aldosterone regulation and need to be withheld when performing these tests.

ANSWER:
B

17. Which of the following is true regarding hyperaldosteronism due to adrenal adenoma versus that due to adrenal hyperplasia?

A. Operation can be performed based on postural aldosterone levels, renin levels, and measurement of 18-hydroxycorticosterone.

B. Preoperative distinction is critical because unilateral adrenalectomy is indicated for adenoma, and bilateral adrenalectomy is usually not performed for hyperplasia.

C. Initial distinction is not critical because both are treated with potassium-sparing diuretics.

D. Adrenal venous sampling may be necessary to diagnose and identify the hyperfunctioning glands.

Ref.: 1–3

COMMENTS: The distinction between adrenal adenoma and bilateral adrenal hyperplasia is critical for proper treatment. • Adenoma is treated with unilateral adrenalectomy, and bilateral hyperplasia is treated with spironolactone and calcium-channel blockers. • Postural levels of aldosterone and renin are persistently elevated in patients with adenoma. • For patients with hyperplasia, variation is observed. • 18-Hydroxy-corticosterone is an aldosterone precursor, and levels are usually elevated in patients with adenomas but not those with hyperplasia. • CT scanning is the first study used to localize an adenoma. • Adrenal scintigraphy with iodocholesterol identifies hyperfunctioning cortical activity with 90% accuracy. • Adrenal venous sampling is done when bilateral adenomas are apparent on CT scan. • An adrenal vein aldosterone/cortisol ratio that is four to five times higher on one side is 90% predictive.

ANSWER:
B, D

18. The rate-limiting step of catecholamine synthesis involves which enzyme?

A. Catechol-*O*-methyltransferase (COMT)

B. Dihydroxyphenylalanine (DOPA) decarboxylase

C. Monoamine oxidase (MAO)

D. Tyrosine hydroxylase

E. Phenylethanolamine-*N*-methyltransferase (PNMT)

Ref.: 1–3

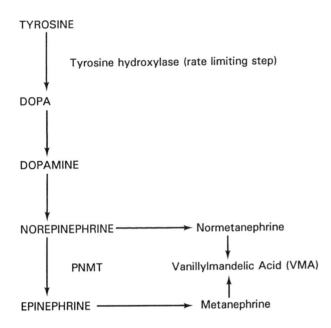

COMMENTS: Catecholamine synthesis, which occurs in the adrenal medulla, begins with tyrosine, which is acquired in the diet or converted from phenylalanine. • Tyrosine is hydroxylated by tyrosine hydroxylase to DOPA, which is decarboxylated to form dopamine. • Dopamine is carboxylated to form norepinephrine. • PNMT converts norepinephrine to epinephrine. • Epinephrine accounts for 80% of the catecholamines produced by the adrenal medulla. • The catecholamines, particularly norepinephrine, exert a negative feedback inhibition on tyrosine hydroxylase. • Therefore, tyrosine hydroxylase inhibits the rate-limiting step of catecholamine synthesis, specifically converting tyrosine to DOPA. • Inactivation of catecholamines may occur by uptake and retention in postganglionic neurons and sympathetic nerves. • In addition, the catecholamines can be inactivated by enzymes, specifically COMT or MAO. • The metabolites of catecholamine degradation are normetanephrine, metanephrine, and vanillylmandelic acid (VMA). • Measurement of these products in urine may be helpful in diagnosis of pheochromocytoma.

ANSWER:
D

19. What signs and symptoms are seen in patients with pheochromocytoma?

A. Headache

B. Paroxysmal hypertension

C. Palpitations

D. Sweating

E. All of the above

Ref.: 1–3

COMMENTS: The clinical signs and symptoms of a pheochromocytoma are the result of catecholamine excess. • One would expect to see hypertension, tachycardia, palpitations, excessive sweating, anxiety, tremulousness, nausea, and vomiting. • Headache occurs in 80% of patients with a pheochromocytoma. • The hypertension can be episodic or persistent, depending on whether the catecholamine secretion from the tumor is intermittent or continuous. • Severe hypertension can be precipitated with anesthesia induction.

ANSWER:
E

20. Pheochromocytoma may be associated with which of the following syndromes?

A. von Hippel-Lindau disease

B. von Recklinghausen's disease

C. Multiple endocrine neoplasia type I (MEN-I)

D. MEN-IIA

E. MEN-IIB

Ref.: 1–3

COMMENTS: Pheochromocytomas most commonly occur in an isolated sporadic form. • They are found in MEN-IIA (pheochromocytoma, medullary carcinoma of the thyroid, and multiple mucosal neuromas). • It is also seen in other neurocutaneous syndromes, including von Recklinghausen's disease (neurofibromatosis), Bourneville's disease (tuberous sclerosis), and Sturge-Weber syndrome (meningofacial angiomatosis). • It is recommended that patients diagnosed with these syndromes be screened for the presence of a pheochromocytoma, to avoid a potential catastrophic hypertensive event.

ANSWER:
A, B, C

21. Which of the following is/are true regarding pheochromocytoma?

A. Fifty percent are malignant.

B. Thirty percent are extra-adrenal.

C. One fourth are bilateral.

D. Ten percent occur in children.

Ref.: 1–3

COMMENTS: The "rule of tens," meaning 10% of those affected, applies to patients with pheochromocytomas. • In particular, 10% of pheochromocytomas are malignant, 10% are extra-adrenal, 10% are bilateral, and 10% occur in children. • These pecentages increase within certain subsets of patients. • Specifically, in familial cases, there is increased risk of malignancy, bilateral tumors, extra-adrenal tumors, and tumors appearing at an earlier age. • The organ of Zuckerkandl is the most common extra-adrenal site. • It is located generally left of the aorta near the origin of the inferior mesenteric artery.

ANSWER:
D

22. Which of the following studies are useful for the diagnosis of a pheochromocytoma?

A. Clonidine suppression test

B. 24-hr urine metanephrine levels

C. 24-hr urine vanillylmandelic acid levels

D. Plasma catecholamine levels

Ref.: 1–3

COMMENTS: A pheochromocytoma is diagnosed by the presence of increased urine catecholamine and metabolite levels. • Plasma levels of catecholamines are not helpful for diagnosis because they are also elevated in essential hypertension. • Testing for pheochromocytoma is indicated for patients with paroxysmal hypertension, pregnant patients with new-onset hypertension, patients with a history of pheochromocytoma, and patients with conditions associated with pheochromocytomas. • In addition, patients with an incidental adrenal mass revealed on CT scanning or magnetic resonance imaging (MRI) should be evaluated. • Less than 2% of pheochromocytomas are missed when 24-hr urine metanephrine and VMA levels are measured. • However, the presence of iodine contrast and α- or β-blockers can render these tests inaccurate. • The clonidine suppression test is also useful. • Failure to suppress catecholamines with administration of clonidine is a positive indication of the presence of a pheochromocytoma.

ANSWER:
A, B, C

23. Which studies are appropriate for localizing a pheochromocytoma?

A. CT scan

B. MRI

C. I-meta-iodobenzylguanidine (MIBG) scan

D. Iodocholesterol (NP-59) scan

E. Venography

Ref.: 1–3

COMMENTS: CT scanning can detect tumors larger than 1 cm and is 87–100% sensitive. • MRI is also very sensitive, and T2-weighted image brightness that is three times greater than that of the liver is highly specific for pheochromocytoma. • I-MIBG scanning is most useful for localizing extra-adrenal tumors and following patients diagnosed with malignant pheochromocytomas. • Venography is no longer performed because it can induce a lethal hypertensive crisis. • Iodocholesterol scintigraphy identifies adrenocortical tissue.

ANSWER:
A, B, C

24. Which of the following is/are used in preoperative preparation of patients with pheochromocytomas?

A. Fluids, blood, or both

B. Diuretics

C. α-Antagonists

D. β-Antagonists

E. β-Agonists

Ref.: 1–3

COMMENTS: The pathologic conditions associated with pheochromocytoma are due to increased α- and β-catecholamine synthesis. • The elevation of catecholamine levels leads to increased peripheral vascular resistance, hypertension, tachycardia, and contracted blood volume. • When the pheochromocytoma is removed during adrenalectomy, there is an abrupt drop in catecholamine release, which can lead to profound hypotension and hypovolemia. • To avoid this situation, α- and often β-blockade (with the latter added only after α-blockade is well established) are provided before surgery. • α-Blockade is achieved with phenoxybenzamine, prazosin, or phentolamine 1–3 weeks before surgery. • β-Blockade is indicated for patients with significant tachycardia, arrhythmias, or tumors that secrete predominantly epinephrine. • Administration of β-blockade before establishment of α-blockade can result in cardiomyopathy and unrelieved afterload. • Fluids, blood, and diuretics are not indicated before adrenalectomy for pheochromocytoma.

ANSWER:
C, D

25. Which of the following are typical characteristics of acute adrenal insufficiency?

A. Fever, hypertension, high cardiac output, and low systemic vascular resistance

B. Hypothermia, hypotension, low cardiac output, and high systemic vascular resistance

C. Fever, hypotension, high cardiac output, and low systemic vascular resistance

D. Hyperkalemia, hyponatremia, and hypoglycemia

E. Hypokalemia, hypernatremia, and hyperglycemia

Ref.: 1–3

COMMENTS: See Question 26.

26. Treatment of acute adrenal insufficiency involves administration of which of the following?

A. Normal saline solution and glucose

B. Normal saline solution, potassium, and glucose

C. Hypertonic saline solution and potassium

D. Intravenous glucocorticoids

E. Intravenous mineralocorticoids

Ref.: 1–3

COMMENTS: Acute adrenal insufficiency or adrenal crisis results in cardiovascular collapse. • Clinical features include fever, hypotension due to high-output circulatory failure and low systemic vascular resistance, nausea, vomiting, abdominal pain and distention, and mental lethargy or obtundation. • This presentation obviously overlaps with a large number of other surgical and medical catastrophes, and diagnosis requires a high index of suspicion. • Laboratory features of adrenal crisis include hyponatremia, hyperkalemia, hypoglycemia, and azotemia. • Treatment must be prompt and intensive. • Volume resuscitation is achieved with normal saline solution, glucose is administered, and intravenous glucocorticoids in the form of dexamethasone and hydrocortisone must be given. • After the patient has been stabilized, the cause of the crisis and the underlying adrenal deficit are investigated. • Mineralocorticoids are not necessary for the management of acute adrenal crisis, but fluorocortisone may be administered later, when infusion of saline solution has been discontinued.

• Mineralocorticoids are important for the maintenance of patients with chronic adrenal insufficiency.

ANSWERS:
Question 25: C, D
Question 26: A, D

27. Which of the following is the most common cause of adrenal insufficiency?

    A. Tuberculosis

    B. Autoimmune disease

    C. Adrenal hemorrhage

    D. Metastases to the adrenal gland

    E. Exogenous steroid administration

    Ref.: 1–3

COMMENTS: Exogenous steroid administration is overall the most common cause of adrenal insufficiency. • Among the *primary* disorders that result in adrenal insufficiency, autoimmune disease is the most common, accounting for two thirds or more of spontaneous cases. • Tuberculosis remains an important cause as well, although it is less commonly so than in the past. • Acquired immunodeficiency syndrome (AIDS)-related infections have been increasingly important. • Adrenal hemorrhage may occur as a result of trauma, coagulopathy, or fulminant bacterial sepsis (Waterhouse-Friderichsen syndrome). • Metastases to the adrenal glands are common in a number of malignancies (e.g., breast, lung, and melanoma) and may also produce insidious adrenal insufficiency.

ANSWER:
E

28. A 46-year-old woman who has been on long-term prednisone therapy for rheumatoid arthritis needs an abdominal hysterectomy for fibroid tumors. Which of the following complications may be expected to occur in this patient with greater-than-average frequency?

    A. Poor wound healing

    B. Pulmonary embolus

    C. Myocardial infarction

    D. Ileus

    E. Renal failure

    Ref.: 1–3

COMMENTS: See Question 29.

29. Appropriate perioperative steroid support for the patient described in Question 28 includes which one of the following?

    A. Cortisone (10 mg) 8 hr before and after operation

    B. Prednisone (10 mg) 8 hr before and after operation

    C. Hydrocortisone (300 mg) in a single dose immediately after operation

    D. Cortisone (200 mg) in divided doses before operation, 100 mg hydrocortisone during the procedure, and in doses tapered over several days to baseline after operation

    E. Cortisone (10 mg) 8 hr before operation and 1 g methylprednisolone 8 hr after operation

    Ref.: 1–3

COMMENTS: Poor wound healing and increased frequency and severity of a variety of postoperative infections occur more commonly in patients on long-term steroid therapy. • Poor wound healing is primarily due to the protein catabolic effect and inhibition of normal fibroblast function. • The increased incidence of infection is related to the broad immunosuppressive activity of steroids. • Although the association is somewhat controversial, chronic steroid therapy is also frequently linked to an increased incidence of several other complications, including gastric and duodenal ulcers and pancreatitis. • Pulmonary embolus, myocardial infarction, ileus, and renal failure do not occur with greater frequency in a patient on long-term steroids.

Adrenocortical insufficiency may occur in patients on chronic corticosteroid therapy because of inhibition of the normal adrenal response to stress. • Both pituitary ACTH and endogenous adrenal steroid production are suppressed by exogenous steroid administration and cannot, therefore, respond to physiologic or surgical stress in a normal manner. • The adrenal cortex normally produces 10–30 mg cortisol per day, but in times of stress, many times this amount may be required. • To protect the patient against acute adrenal insufficiency, a "steroid prep" should be administered before surgery. • One of the acceptable regimens includes administration of 100 mg hydrocortisone the evening before and the morning of a major operation, with 100 mg of hydrocortisone administered every 8 hr for the next 24 hr. • Cortisone (or other corticosteroids in doses with comparable potency, as shown in the table) 300 mg/day perioperatively in divided doses usually protects the patient, even in cases of maximum stress. • This dose is then tapered to the patient's baseline steroid requirements over a course of time, varying from several days to weeks, dictated by the preoperative steroid dose, the length of preoperative steroid treatment, and the degree of stress induced by the operative procedure and postoperative course. • The dosage equivalents of corticoids are as follows:

Duplicate Systemic Corticosteroids: Equivalent Doses & Relative Potencies

Drug	Equivalent dose (mg)	Relative glucocorticoid potency	Relative mineralocorticoid potency
Short-acting			
Cortisone	25	0.8	0.8
Hydrocortisone	20	1	1
Intermediate-acting			
Prednisone	5	4	0.8
Prednisolone	5	4	0.8
Methylprednisolone	4	5	0.5
Triamcinolone	4	5	0
Long-acting			
Betamethasone	0.6	25	0
Dexamethasone	0.75	25	0

http://www.pharmhs.com/Forms/Formulary%20Preface.doc

ANSWERS:
Question 28: A
Question 29: D

30. A 42-year-old man is found to have an obstructing kidney stone and a 3-cm left adrenal mass found on CT scanning performed when the man presented with a right-sided abdominal pain. Which of the following would be correct management of the adrenal mass?

    A. Laparoscopic resection of the mass

    B. Measurement of serum potassium, 24-hr urine VMA, metanephrine, and catecholamine levels

C. Observation with repeated CT scanning in 6 months

D. Fine-needle aspiration to rule out malignancy

Ref.: 1–3

COMMENTS: Incidental adrenal masses are commonly seen owing to the greater frequency and use of abdominal CT scans. • It is expected that as many as 2% of individuals undergoing abdominal CT scanning will be found to have adrenal masses. • Important aspects about adrenal masses are that (1) benign, clinically inactive adrenocortical adenomas are common autopsy findings; (2) adrenocortical carcinomas are rare, with an annual incidence estimated from 0.06 to 0.17 per 100,000 population; and (3) the adrenal glands are a common site for metastasis. • The differential diagnosis consists of cortical adenoma, adrenocortical carcinoma, pheochromocytoma, ganglioneuroma, cyst, organized hemorrhage or fibrosis, myelolipoma, adenolipoma, or metastasis from a nonadrenal malignancy.

Adrenocortical carcinoma is rare, and size is the most important predictor of malignancy. • In a review of six series, 90% of adrenocortical carcinomas were larger than 6 cm. • Age is also taken into account because the number of adrenal nodules increases in older patients. • Most surgeons advocate surgery for patients with nonfunctioning adrenal masses larger than 6 cm, and some perform adrenalectomy on masses larger than 4 cm. • In younger patients, who have decreased operative risk, adrenalectomy has been recommended for adrenal masses larger than 3 cm.

In asymptomatic patients, one should rule out functional tumors as well as metastatic disease. • Measurement of (1) the serum potassium level should be performed to rule out aldosteronoma; (2) the 24-hr VMA, metanephrine, and catecholamine levels to rule out pheochromocytoma; and (3) the 17-hydroxycorticosteroids and 17-ketosteroids in 24-hr urine levels to rule out Cushing's syndrome.

Tumors that most commonly metastasize to the adrenals are melanoma, hypernephroma, and carcinoma of the lung, breast, and stomach. • Therefore, even patients without a history of malignancy should have, at minimum, laboratory screening studies including stool testing for occult blood, a chest radiograph, and for women a mammogram. • Patients with a history of malignancy should undergo fine-needle aspiration of the adrenal mass. • Any adrenal mass of 3–6 cm with ominous CT characteristics should be resected. • Observation is appropriate for patients 50 years of age and older who have masses between 3 and 6 cm and for all lesions smaller than 3 cm that are not hormonally active. • Such observation consists of serial CT scanning performed at 3-month intervals for the first year and annually thereafter.

ANSWER:
B

31. A 50-year-old woman presents with clinical features of Cushing's syndrome. A CT scan shows a 6-cm right adrenal mass extending into the liver and right kidney. What is the appropriate treatment?

A. Open en bloc surgical resection

B. Laparoscopic surgical resection

C. Radiation therapy and mitotane followed by surgical resection

D. Radiation therapy

E. Transsphenoidal hypophysectomy

Ref.: 1–3

COMMENTS: Adrenocortical carcinoma is a rare but deadly malignancy. • It is more common in women and has a peak incidence in the first and fifth decades of life. • One half are functional tumors producing cortisol, aldosterone, or sex steroids. • Large masses (>6 cm) or those with extra-adrenal invasion are usually malignant. • Most (80%) patients have advanced disease at presentation. • En bloc resection is the only chance for cure and usually is only palliative. • Laparoscopic surgery is contraindicated for malignancies greater than 6 cm, those with accompanying adenopathy, and locally invasive tumors. • Overall, survival is dependent on completeness of resection. • Mitotane is an adrenal cytotoxic agent most commonly used for unresectable and metastatic disease. • It has limited effectiveness. • Radiation therapy has not been effective for adrenocortical carcinoma.

ANSWER:
A

32. Which of the following is the most appropriate approach to resect a 10-cm right adrenal mass that is likely but not confirmed to be benign?

A. Anterior transabdominal

B. Posterior retroperitoneal

C. Laparoscopic transabdominal

D. Laparoscopic retroperitoneal

E. Thoracoabdominal

Ref.: 1–3

COMMENTS: The anterior transabdominal approach allows exploration of the entire peritoneal cavity, including both adrenal glands. • It is indicated for large (>6 cm) adrenocortical cancers and large benign lesions (>10–12 cm). • Very large adrenocortical carcinomas (10–15 cm) may require a thoracoabdominal approach. • The open posterior approach was used in the past for small unilateral tumors but has been replaced by the laparoscopic approach. • The transabdominal laparoscopic approach is the most common approach to small adrenal tumors. • The laparoscopic retroperitoneal approach provides less working space, but it is preferred if the patient has had previous extensive upper abdominal surgery.

ANSWER:
A

33. Which of the following are contraindications to laparoscopic adrenalectomy?

A. Bilateral pheochromocytomas

B. Adrenocortical cancer of 3 cm

C. Adrenocortical cancer with lymphatic spread

D. Previous abdominal surgery

E. A 2-cm, nonfunctioning adrenal incidentaloma

Ref.: 1–3

COMMENTS: Contraindications to laparoscopic adrenalectomy include large (>6 cm) adrenocortical tumors and those invading surrounding lymph nodes or local structures. • A relative contraindication to laparoscopic adrenalectomy is previous surgery in the area of the adrenal gland, specifically, liver resection, splenectomy, or nephrectomy. • Laparoscopy can be used for large incidentalomas requiring surgical intervention, functioning adenomas of less than 10 cm, and bilateral small adenomas.

ANSWER:
C, E

REFERENCES

1. Townsend CM, Beauchamp RD, Evers BM, et al (eds): *Sabiston Textbook of Surgery: The Biological Basis of Modern Surgical Practice*, 17th ed. Saunders, Philadelphia, 2004.

2. Brunicardi FC, Andersen DK, Billiar TR, et al: *Schwartz's Principles of Surgery*, 8th ed. McGraw-Hill, New York, 2004.

3. Greenfield LJ, Mulholland MW, Oldham KT: *Surgery Scientific Principles and Practice*, 3rd ed. Lippincott, Williams & Wilkins, Philadelphia, 2001.

C H A P T E R 31

Esophagus

John D. Christein, M.D., and Keith W. Millikan, M.D.

1. With regard to the vascular supply and innervation of the esophagus, match the following.

   A. Myenteric plexus

   B. Submucosal plexus

   C. Cervical esophagus

   D. Thoracic esophagus

   a. Superior and inferior thyroid arteries

   b. Meissner's plexus

   c. Auerbach's plexus

   d. Aortic branches, intercostals, bronchial, inferior phrenic, and left gastric arteries

   Ref.: 1–3

COMMENTS: The muscular tube of the esophagus consists of two layers. • Between the outer longitudinal and inner circular layers is a rich supply of vessels and lymphatics as well as Auerbach's myenteric neural plexus. • The submucosa of the esophagus is thick and also rich in lymphatics and contains Meissner's neural plexus. • This thick submucosa is the strong layer of the esophagus.

There is a segmental blood supply to the esophagus, and the right and left blood supplies communicate through collateral vessels. • The superior thyroid arteries, off the external carotid artery, and the inferior thyroid artery, off the thyrocervical trunk, both supply the cervical esophagus. • The extensive blood supply to the thoracic esophagus is composed of four to six aortic branches and collateral vessels from the left gastric, inferior phrenic, intercostal, bronchial, and inferior thyroid arteries.

ANSWER:
A-c; B-b; C-a; D-d

2. With regard to the lymphatic drainage of the esophagus, which of the following is/are true?

   A. A lymphatic plexus in the mucosa and submucosa drains the esophagus.

   B. Before draining to adjacent nodes, lymphatic vessels run longitudinally before penetrating the muscularis.

   C. The entire esophagus drains caudad to the perigastric and left gastric artery lymph nodes.

   D. Sites of metastasis from esophageal carcinoma may include internal jugular nodes, pretracheal nodes, subcarinal nodes, perigastric nodes, left gastric artery nodes, and axillary nodes.

   Ref.: 1–3

COMMENTS: The two lymphatic plexuses arise in the mucosa and within the muscularis. • The pattern of spread seen in esophageal carcinoma is due to the unique longitudinal path that the lymphatic vessels take before penetrating the muscularis and draining to their adjacent nodes. • The metastasis of esophageal carcinoma is predictable but can be very diverse. • The upper two thirds of the esophagus drains cranially, whereas the distal one third drains in a caudad direction. • This pattern can give rise to metastatic disease in the gastric, pretracheal, subcarinal, celiac, and internal jugular nodal basins. • There is no direct lymphatic connection to the axillary lymph nodes.

ANSWER:
B

3. With regard to the anatomy of the esophagus, which of the following statements is/are true?

   A. The esophagus is 35 cm long.

   B. The esophagus is divided into four segments.

   C. There are five predictable areas of narrowing: (1) the thyropharyngeus muscle, (2) the thoracic inlet, (3) the left subclavian artery, (4) the left bronchus, and (5) the crossing of the thoracic duct.

   D. The arterial blood is supplied by the splenic, right gastric, pulmonary, and innominate arteries.

   E. The pharyngoesophageal segment of the esophagus consists of three constrictors and the stylopharyngeus muscle.

   Ref.: 1, 2

COMMENTS: See Question 4.

4. With regard to the anatomy of the esophagus, which of the following statements is/are true?

   A. The outer muscular layer of the upper thoracic esophagus lies adjacent to the membranous portion of the trachea.

   B. In patients with cirrhosis with portal hypertension, venous drainage flows through the azygous system.

   C. The cervical and the lowest portion of the thoracic esophagus lie slightly to the left of the midline.

   D. The left and right vagal plexi are intimately attached to the esophagus and emerge as two main anterior and posterior trunks just above the esophageal hiatus.

E. The thoracic duct travels from right to left at the upper third of the esophagus.

Ref.: 1, 2

COMMENTS: Proper surgical management of diseases of the esophagus requires a thorough understanding of esophageal anatomy. • The esophagus is a muscular tube 25 cm long with an inner circular layer and an outer longitudinal layer. • The absence of a serosal covering, which has substantial strength, may contribute to the risk of anastomotic leakage after esophageal resection or repair of transmural esophageal defects. • The esophagus is lined by squamous epithelium except for its distal 2 cm, which is lined by columnar epithelium. • The absence of mucous glands renders it susceptible to peptic acid injury.

For convenience, the esophagus is divided into four segments. • The **pharyngoesophageal** segment is between the laryngopharynx and cervical esophagus and includes the superior, middle, and inferior constrictors and the stylopharyngeus muscle. • The stylopharyngeus muscle is an inferior constrictor and courses obliquely upward. • The cricopharyngeal muscle is believed by some to be part of the inferior constrictor, and its fibers course transversely. • The cricopharyngeal muscle blends intimately with the upper fibers of the cervical esophagus and the lower fibers of the thyroglossus muscle. • Because these fibers have divergent directions, it is believed that a weakness develops, allowing for the development of a Zenker's diverticulum. • The cricopharyngeal muscle serves as the upper sphincter of the esophagus and relaxes when the thyropharyngeus portion of the inferior constrictor contracts to propel a bolus of food.

The **cervical** esophagus is a segment 5–6 cm long. • It begins at the cricopharyngeal muscle and ends at T1.

The **thoracic** esophageal segment begins at T1 and ends at the hiatus.

The **abdominal** esophageal segment varies in length from 1 to 5 cm. • It begins at the hiatus and ends at the cardia.

In its course from the pharynx to the stomach, the esophagus is positioned to the left or the right of the midline at various levels, a condition that influences surgical accessibility. • The cervical esophagus lies behind the trachea and slightly to its left. • The esophagus then deviates to the right in the subcarinal area, gradually returning to the left behind the pericardial sac at the level of the seventh thoracic vertebra. • Since the esophagus lies behind the trachea adjacent to its membranous aspect, it is susceptible to involvement in tracheoesophageal fistulas.

The caliber of the normal esophagus is not uniform. • Rather, it has predictable areas of narrowing at the levels of the cricopharyngeal muscle, the aortic arch, and the diaphragm. • Of these areas, the cricopharyngeal muscle marks the narrowest point of the esophagus.

The **arterial blood supply** of the esophagus is segmental and arises from numerous and abundant terminal sources. • The cervical esophagus receives branches from the superior thyroid and thyrocervical arteries. • The thoracic esophagus is supplied by four to six branches—including the bronchial, inferior phrenic, left gastric, and inferior thyroid arteries—terminating in a fine capillary network before penetrating the musculature, allowing safe, blunt esophagectomy without the need for individual arterial ligation. • The **submucosal venous plexus** of the thoracic esophagus drains into the azygous and hemizygous system, and the venous plexus of the abdominal portion drains into the left gastric vein. • Continuity is established by three submucosal venous plexi.

Lymphatic drainage may extend longitudinally in the wall of the esophagus before continuing on to regional lymph nodes. • This point is important when determining proximal margins at the time of esophagectomy for malignant disease.

The **thoracic duct** courses from right to left behind the upper third of the esophagus and is thus exposed to possible surgical damage.

The **vagus nerves** lie on either side of the esophagus, forming a plexus on its musculature. • Just above the hiatus, they form two major trunks: left anterior and right posterior.

The **esophagogastric junction** is a complex area anatomically and physiologically. • Supportive structures in this area include the diaphragmatic crura and the phrenoesophageal ligament, which is a continuation of the endoabdominal fascia and circumferentially attaches the esophagus to the muscular diaphragm. • The anatomy of the phrenoesophageal membrane is an important factor in the pathophysiology of gastroesophageal (GE) reflux. • It is important to know that it is a continuation of the transversalis fascia of the abdomen.

ANSWERS:
Question 3: B, E
Question 4: A, B, C, D, E.

5. With regard to normal esophageal motility, which of the following statements is/are true?

A. The most common method for measuring pressures employs micropressure transducers.

B. Secondary waves are initiated when the entire bolus of food has not cleared the esophagus.

C. The pressure of the upper esophageal sphincter is higher than that of the lower esophageal sphincter.

D. Normal postdeglutition contraction of both the upper and the lower esophageal sphincters results in pressures greater than the predeglutition resting pressure.

Ref.: 1–3

COMMENTS: Manometric studies have defined normal esophageal motility and characterized anomalies in various pathologic states. • Studies are typically performed with the use of multiple perfused catheter systems and pull-through techniques. • Recently, micropressure transducers have provided an accurate, simple measurement method without using a water-perfused system. • However, since these techniques are expensive and difficult to maintain, they are not used widely. • Two high-pressure zones can be identified within the esophagus: one corresponding to the upper esophageal sphincter (UES) at the level of the cricopharyngeal muscle and another representing the lower esophageal sphincter (LES) near the GE junction. • The UES pressure is greater than the LES pressure.

The normal act of deglutition involves coordination of both voluntary and involuntary movements. • After the act of swallowing, the UES allows a food bolus to enter the esophagus. • A primary peristaltic wave progressively moves the food to the stomach, which is entered after coordinated relaxation of the LES. • After relaxation, a postdeglutition contraction of the sphincters occurs before resumption of a resting pressure. • If the esophagus is not cleared of material by the primary peristaltic wave, secondary peristaltic waves are initiated in the smooth muscle of the lower two thirds of the esophagus. • Tertiary waves are not peristaltic. • Numerous hormonal, neural, pharmacologic, chemical, and mechanical factors can affect esophageal motility, although the mechanisms of control are incompletely defined.

Entry of air into the esophagus with inspiration or swallowing is prevented by the UES, which normally stays closed as a result of tonic contractions of the cricopharyngeal muscle.

ANSWER:
B, C, D

6. With regard to esophageal anatomy and physiology, with of the following is/are true?

   A. The confluence of the cisternae chili forms the thoracic duct.

   B. The thoracic duct travels from left to right in the neck to enter the venous system at the confluence of the right internal jugular and subclavian veins.

   C. Primary peristalsis is progressive and involuntary.

   D. Secondary peristalsis is progressive, involuntary, and triggered by esophageal irritation.

   E. Tertiary contractions are progressive and occur after a voluntary swallow or between swallows.

Ref.: 1–3

COMMENTS: The anatomy and location of the thoracic duct is important because of its proximity to the esophagus. • To the right of the aorta at approximately the twelfth thoracic vertebra, the cisternae chili join to form the thoracic duct. • The duct then travels through the aortic hiatus to the right of the aorta, and, as it courses into the posterior mediastinum, it travels to the left at the level of the fourth thoracic vertebra. • The duct drains into the venous system at the confluence of the left internal jugular and subclavian veins.

    The esophagus functions as a conduit for the passage of food boluses from the oropharynx to the stomach. • Swallowing is accomplished throughout the complex interactions of oral, pharyngeal, and esophageal musculature. • Both primary and secondary peristalsis are progressive in nature. • A voluntary swallow stimulates primary peristalsis, whereas secondary peristalsis occurs in response to irritation or distention of the esophagus. • In a normal physiologic situation, a primary peristaltic wave follows 97% of swallows. • Tertiary contractions are not peristaltic waves. • They are simultaneous contractions that occur in an uncoordinated, nonperistaltic, monophasic manner. • On upper gastrointestinal barium study, tertiary contractions have a "corkscrew" esophagus appearance.

ANSWER:
A, D

7. With regard to the LES which of the following is/are true?

   A. The LES is a distinct band of muscle fibers measuring 3–5 cm in length.

   B. The LES is the only factor important in preventing GE reflux.

   C. Normal resting pressure is 30–40 mmHg.

   D. GE reflux is likely to occur if mean pressures are less than 6 mmHg and the length is less than 2 cm.

Ref.: 1–3

COMMENTS: See Question 8.

8. Of the following, which factors play a role in maintaining the competency of the LES?

   A. Positive intrathoracic pressure

   B. Positive intra-abdominal pressure

   C. Segment of intra-abdominal esophagus

   D. Phrenoesophageal ligament

   E. Length of high-pressure zone greater than 1 cm

   F. Mean pressure greater than 3 mmHg

Ref.: 1–3

COMMENTS: Through the use of manometry, a distal high-pressure zone has been identified that is usually 3–5 cm in length. • The resting pressure of this zone is 10–20 mmHg. • No anatomic band of fibers corresponding to an LES has been identified. • The mechanism of the distal high-pressure zone is complex and multifactorial in preventing GE reflux. • The important factors are a length over 2 cm, a mean pressure greater than 6 mmHg, a segment of intra-abdominal esophagus, and the presence of the phrenoesophageal ligament. • Reflux does occur under normal physiologic conditions, but protective forces of basic saliva and the motility of the esophagus prevent injury.

ANSWERS:
Question 7: D
Question 8: B, C, D

9. For each factor in the left-hand column, select the appropriate effect on the LES pressure from the right-hand column.

   A. Atropine   a. Increased pressure

   B. Coffee   b. Decreased pressure

   C. Metoclopramide   c. No effect

   D. Cigarettes

   E. Gastric acidification

   F. Alcohol

   G. Bacon and eggs

   H. Protein meal

Ref.: 1, 2

COMMENTS: The control of the distal high-pressure zone in the esophagus, which acts as a physiologic sphincter, is complex and is affected primarily by mechanical factors and secondarily by neural, hormonal, and chemical factors. • Therapeutic administration of agents that increase sphincter pressure and avoidance of factors that reduce sphincter pressure are important to the medical management of patients with symptomatic reflux. • Cholinergic agents (e.g., bethanechol), anticholinesterases, and α-adrenergic agents (e.g., metoclopramide) increase sphincter tone, whereas anticholinergic agents (e.g., atropine), α-adrenergic antagonists, and β-adrenergic agonists decrease sphincter pressure. • Nicotine, alcohol, chocolate, and fatty meals have detrimental (pressure weakening) effects on sphincter tone, whereas a high-protein meal increases sphincter tone. • Hormonal influences include the stimulatory effects of gastrin and the inhibitory influences of secretin and cholecystokinin, but it is not clear what effect these hormones have in physiologic doses. • Gastric alkalinization and distention tend to increase LES pressure, whereas gastric acidification decreases sphincter tone.

ANSWER:
A-b; B-b; C-a; D-b; E-b; F-b; G-b; H-a

10. Which of the following are the most important for maintaining competence of the GE junction?

   A. Angle of esophageal entry into the stomach

   B. Orientation of muscle fibers of the LES

C. Small diameter of the esophagus at the hiatus

D. Level of insertion of the phrenoesophageal ligament on the esophagus

E. Intra-abdominal segment of esophagus

Ref.: 1–3, 5

COMMENTS: See Question 11.

11. Which of the following factor(s) play(s) a role in limiting esophageal exposure to acid?

A. Tertiary peristaltic waves

B. Saliva

C. Gastric emptying

D. Gastrin

E. Secretin

Ref.: 1–3, 5

COMMENTS: The anatomic arrangement of the GE junction and the physical means by which competence of the GE junction is maintained to limit esophageal exposure to acid have been studied extensively but are still not completely understood. • In humans, unlike other animals, there is no distinct anatomic muscular sphincter. • Pharmacologic studies in humans, however, have demonstrated variations in background basal tone in response to excitatory and inhibitory neurohumoral exposure, the knowledge of which is being applied clinically to the therapy of reflux. • Among hormones, for example, gastrin, motilin, and bombesin increase the high-pressure zone, whereas secretin, cholecystokinin, glucagon, progesterone, estrogen, and prostaglandins E_1 and E_2 decrease it.

Several anatomic considerations affect the competence of the GE junction, but it is generally agreed that the presence of a segment of esophagus exposed to intra-abdominal pressure is the most important. • The laws of physics pertaining to wall tension and to pressure in hollow tubes of different diameters, as well as many years of clinical experience with various antireflux operations, support this concept. • According to the law of Laplace, the pressure required to distend a pliable tube is inversely proportional to the diameter of the tube. • With a sliding esophageal hiatal hernia, the phrenoesophageal membrane is stretched, thus exerting centrifugal tension on the distal esophagus and increasing its diameter. • Likewise, the rate of reflux varies inversely with the length of the abdominal segment of the esophagus. • In patients with reflux, the attachment of the phrenoesophageal ligament is closer to the stomach, and the intra-abdominal esophagus is shorter. • The critical anatomic factor in maintaining a segment of the esophagus in the intra-abdominal position appears to be insertion of the phrenoesophageal membrane into the esophagus at a point approximately 3–4 cm above the manometrically determined GE junction. • The LES is better named the LES mechanism or distal esophageal high-pressure zone, since no anatomic sphincter exists. • There is no absolute value for the high-pressure zone, but the pressure in it is somewhere between 10 and 20 mmHg. • Patients with no reflux may have low values, and patients with massive reflux may have high values. • This discrepancy results from variations in the aforementioned anatomic characteristics and the evidence that there is an uneven and eccentric pressure around the circumference of the high-pressure zone. • Two other important mechanisms limiting exposure of the distal esophagus to acid are (1) esophageal clearing through primary and secondary peristaltic activity, salivation, and gravity and (2) proper gastric function, such as timely emptying and peptic acid activity. • Patients with symptoms and endoscopic evidence of esophagitis but normal manometric findings and pH should be evaluated for other causes of this condition, such as drug-induced esophagitis, alkaline reflux, and gastric disease.

A N S W E R S :
Question 10: C, D, E
Question 11: A, B, C, D

12. With regard to GE reflux, which of the following statements is/are true?

A. Symptomatic GE reflux does not occur without a hiatal hernia.

B. Reflux occurs less than 7% of the day in all patients, regardless of the presence or absence of hiatal hernia.

C. Most patients with symptomatic GE reflux have hiatal hernia.

D. Patients with columnar epithelium–lined esophagus have reflux 26% of the day.

Ref.: 1–3, 5, 6

COMMENTS: See Question 16.

13. Which of the following tests is the most sensitive for the detection of GE reflux?

A. Barium swallow

B. Manometric testing

C. Acid perfusion (Bernstein) test

D. 24-hr pH monitoring

E. Standard antireflux test (SART)

Ref.: 1–3, 5, 6

COMMENTS: See Question 16.

14. A 50-year-old woman complains of pyrosis, nightly cough, and a sour taste in her mouth. Which of the following are helpful in deciding whether to perform antireflux surgery?

A. Failure of medical therapy to control symptoms

B. Defect of LES

C. Positive Bernstein test results

D. Positive histologic findings

E. Increased esophageal exposure to gastric juice

Ref.: 1–3, 5, 6

COMMENTS: See Question 16.

15. A 45-year-old woman has a history of a previous vagotomy and antrectomy with Billroth II gastroenterostomy for recurrent duodenal peptic ulceration. She now has severe heartburn, nausea, and emesis. Endoscopy reveals severe esophagitis. Which of the following are important before antireflux surgery?

A. Acid perfusion (Bernstein) testing

B. One week of metronidazole (Flagyl) therapy

C. 24-hr pH monitoring.

D. Fiberoptic bile probe

E. Barium swallow

Ref.: 1–3, 5, 6

COMMENTS: See Question 16.

16. The patient described in Question 15 is found to have normal esophageal motility, a normal barium swallow test result, and pH in the basic-to-neutral range as determined by 24-hr monitoring. Which of the following are helpful?

   A. Conversion of a Billroth II anastomosis to a Roux-en-Y anastomosis

   B. Allison procedure

   C. Angelchik prosthesis

   D. Bile-chelating agents

Ref.: 1–3, 5, 6

COMMENTS: Limited acid reflux into the esophagus is a normal physiologic event. • Reflux and its attendant complications are clinically significant when the high-pressure zone at the lower end of the esophagus is of inadequate degree or length. • This condition is not necessarily related to the presence of a sliding hiatal hernia, in which the stomach and transversalis (endoabdominal) fascia protrude through the esophageal hiatus. • Most patients with significant reflux, however, can be demonstrated to have a sliding hernia. • The cause of the reflux is not the hernia per se. • In fact, most patients with sliding hiatal hernias do not have significant or symptomatic reflux.

The overlap between the symptoms of GE reflux and those of other upper abdominal or mediastinal problems necessitates accurate documentation of pathologic reflux before definitive therapy is undertaken. • **Contrast studies** that include the pharynx, esophagus, and stomach can reveal anatomic problems such as diverticula, various types of hiatal hernia, and gastric abnormalities, which help the endoscopist perform safer, more complete endoscopy. • In addition, well-done videofluoroscopic contrast studies detect abnormal peristaltic activity and spontaneous reflux. • Reflux during the Valsalva maneuver can be demonstrated as a matter of course and is not pathologic. • Numerous other tests have been used to identify abnormal reflux. • **Twenty-four hour pH monitoring** is now the gold standard and the most precise measurement of acid reflux. • An electrode probe placed 5 cm above the LES records the frequency and exposure time of pH dips. • To document symptoms and type of activity, the patient keeps a log, and the entries are correlated to the pH recording. • A fiberoptic probe that recognizes bilirubin can measure bile reflux. • It is important to note that both pH and bile probes measure concentration, not the amount of acid or bile present. • Normal acid exposure time in 24 hr is considered to be 4–7%. • Acid exposure time is 12% for mild esophagitis and 26% in those with Barrett's epithelium. • Other tests using the pH probe may be performed in special circumstances.

The SART is a test in which 300 ml of 0.1 *N* hydrochloric acid is instilled in the stomach, and the pH is measured while the patient performs various maneuvers. • The **Bernstein test**, in which 0.1 *N* hydrochloric acid is instilled into the esophagus in an attempt to reproduce symptoms, and acid-clearing tests, which measure the ability of the esophagus to remove instilled acid, are less accurate. • **Endoscopic examination** is useful for assessing anatomic damage produced by reflux, such as esophagitis, ulceration, or stricture, and is critical for ruling out cancer.

Manometric measurements of the esophagus should be performed when a motility disorder is suspected owing to symptoms of dysphagia or reflux. • Manometric testing before antireflux procedures may disclose primary esophageal disease, which could alter plans for the type of procedure employed. • For instance, in a patient with poor peristaltic waves, a partial wrap may be required, whereas a patient with simultaneous contractions or failure of relaxation of the distal esophagus may require a different procedure.

Before embarking on a surgical procedure, the results of endoscopic examination, histologic studies, pH monitoring, and manometric testing are tabulated, and the patient is given a score. • Patients whose test results are negative or equivocal are given scores 0 and 1, respectively. • These patients are not candidates for surgery. • Patients with positive test results but no mucosal damage are given a score of 2. • Patients whose test results are all positive are given a score of 3, and those with severe disease are given a score of 4. • Patients in the latter last three categories are candidates for surgical therapy.

Medical therapy should be attempted for a period of 8–12 weeks in most patients before surgery. • The patient described in Question 15 probably has bile reflux. • Conversion of her Billroth II anastomosis to a Roux-en-Y anastomosis or use of bile-chelating agents is not likely to help. • The Angelchik prosthesis and the Allison procedure are antireflux measures to prevent acid reflux and are not appropriate in this case.

Ref.: 1–5

ANSWERS:
Question 12: B, D
Question 13: D
Question 14: A, B, D, E
Question 15: C, D, E
Question 16: A, D

17. Recognized complications of GE reflux include which of the following?

   A. Ulcer

   B. Aspiration

   C. Columnar epithelium–lined esophagus

   D. Motility disturbance

   E. Zenker's diverticulum

   F. Stricture

   G. Laryngeal inflammation

Ref.: 1–6

COMMENTS: Significant reflux of acid gastric contents into the esophagus can produce mucosal inflammation, ulceration, chronic blood loss, and eventual stricture or shortening from scar contracture. • Pulmonary aspiration of refluxed material can lead to laryngeal edema, bronchospasm, recurrent pneumonia, bronchiectasis, and lung abscess. • The chronic destructive influences of reflux can produce metaplasia of the normal squamous esophageal epithelium, resulting in lining of the esophagus by columnar epithelium, a condition known as Barrett's esophagus. • Abnormal motility disorders, including spasm and disordered peristalsis, can result from chronic reflux or stenosis.

In general, the indications for operative intervention include symptoms or complications intractable to medical management or the desire to escape the need for continual drug treatment. • Medical management consists of mechanical measures—including avoidance of positions or activities that cause reflux, such as total recumbency, by keeping the head of the bed elevated (particularly after meals); weight loss; and avoidance of constricting garments—as well as pharmacologic measures, including simple antacids, alginic acid, H₂-blockers, proton-pump inhibitors (omeprazole), and prokinetic agents (metoclopramide). • Fortunately, medical management is sufficient for most patients with symptomatic GE reflux disease (GERD). • Even the complication of esophageal stenosis can often be effectively treated by esophageal dilatation, but an antireflux procedure should accompany the dilatation to prevent recurrence and irreversible stricture. • Surgery has been demonstrated to be superior to medical management for patients with complications of GERD.

ANSWER:
A, B, C, D, F, G

18. With regard to Barrett's esophagus, which of the following are appropriate?

    A. Histamine antagonist

    B. Proton-pump inhibitor

    C. *Helicobacter pylori* triple therapy

    D. Endoscopic surveillance without biopsy every 12 months

    E. Endoscopic surveillance with biopsy every 2 years

    F. Antireflux procedure

Ref.: 1–3, 7

COMMENTS: Along with stricture and ulcer, Barrett's esophagus is a complication of GE reflux. • Barrett's esophagus occurs when columnar metaplastic epithelium replaces the normal esophageal squamous epithelium. • It is found in 7–10% of patients with long-standing reflux. • Patients with columnar metaplasia have an increased lifetime risk of developing adenocarcinoma of the esophagus.

Barrett's esophagus is thought to be mainly due to refluxed gastric secretions. • However, the metaplasia may be secondary to acid or alkaline reflux. • The complications of Barrett's esophagus include esophageal stenosis, ulceration in the columnar epithelium (Barrett's ulcer), and an increased risk of dysplasia and subsequent development of adenocarcinoma of the esophagus. • This risk may be as high as 40 times the risk in the normal population. • Proton-pump inhibitors are useful in controlling the symptoms of reflux as well as healing esophagitis or esophageal ulcers. • Unfortunately, there is no consensus or absolute documentation of regression of columnar epithelium in the esophagus while on proton-pump inhibitors.

The indications for antireflux operations for Barrett's esophagus not complicated by high-grade dysplasia or malignancy are no different from the indications for any patient with GE reflux. • Operative therapy for reflux is attractive because it not only prevents the reflux of acid and pancreaticobiliary secretions but also provides symptomatic relief. • The literature reports mixed results for operative therapy, but several series show either regression or nonprogression of Barrett's esophagus. • When combined with medical antireflux therapy, the benefit of surgery may be greater.

Recently, ablative procedures, such as thermal or phototherapy, and neodymium:yttrium-aluminum-garnet (Nd:YAG) laser therapy have been used to treat Barrett's esophagus. • To date, there is no good model for this therapy, but it does appear to offer some long-term benefit if surveillance is continued. • Regardless of the treatment offered, patients with Barrett's esophagus and only metaplastic changes should undergo endoscopic surveillance with biopsy at least every 2 years. • If low-grade dysplasia is present, surveillance with biopsy should be as frequent as every 6 months. • If high-grade dysplasia is found, esophagectomy is warranted.

Helicobacter therapy has no role in the treatment of Barrett's esophagus.

ANSWER:
E, F

19. Which of the following principles is/are common to the Belsey, Nissen, Hill, and laparoscopic Nissen antireflux operations?

    A. Effective antireflux procedure

    B. Gastric plication around the distal esophagus

    C. Restoration of normal GE anatomy

    D. Restoration of an intra-abdominal segment of esophagus

    E. Pyloroplasty

Ref.: 1–6

COMMENTS: See Question 21.

20. Match each operative characteristic in the left-hand column with one or more appropriate operations in the right-hand column.

Characteristic	Operation
A. Thoracic approach	a. Belsey
B. Abdominal approach	b. Nissen
C. Median arcuate ligament	c. Hill
D. Prosthetic device	d. Allison
E. Anatomic repair	e. Angelchik
F. Short esophagus	f. Collis gastroplasty
G. Partial wrap	

Ref.: 1–6

COMMENTS: See Question 21.

21. Which is/are true of laparoscopic Nissen fundoplication?

    A. Contraindicated in the presence of short esophagus

    B. Rarely performed

    C. No medical therapy indicated before the procedure

    D. Only history required before the procedure

Ref.: 1–6

COMMENTS: Simple reconstitution of normal GE anatomy, as with the transabdominal **Allison** repair, is not an effective antireflux operation because of the high rate of recurrence of GE reflux. • Several well-conceived, standardized operations have now been devised as effective antireflux procedures. • These operations include the Nissen fundoplication, the Belsey Mark IV operation, and the Hill posterior gastropexy with calibration of the cardia. • Common to all of these procedures are restoration of an intra-abdominal segment of esophagus, a variable degree of gastric plication around the distal esophagus, and reconstitution of the esophageal hiatus. • Certain principles must be adhered to when an antireflux operation is performed. • The procedure should permanently establish an adequate length of esophagus in the abdomen and restore the sphincteric pressure to twice that of the gastric pressure. • The cardia must not be constricted and must be allowed to relax. • In addition, it must not impede the bolus of food from progression when the propulsive force of the esophagus is diminished. • The factors to be considered before a reflux operation are the propulsive force of the esophagus, the presence or absence of concomitant esophageal disorders, the presence of gastric reflux that mimics esophageal reflux symptoms, and the presence of gastroduodenal disorders that may necessitate additional procedures. • The surgical texts referred to in this chapter should be consulted for simple anatomic understanding of the operations.

The **Belsey** operation is difficult to learn. • It is performed only through the chest and involves placement of two layers of plicating sutures between the gastric fundus and the lower esophagus, with subsequent creation of an approximately 280-degree anterior gastric wrap and posterior approximation of the crura.

With the **Nissen** fundoplication, which can be performed via an abdominal or a thoracic approach, a 360-degree circumferential wrap of the gastric fundus around the distal esophagus is created. • Whereas Nissen originally had recommended a 4-cm wrap, the frequent occurrence of the gas bloat syndrome has led surgeons to use a 2-cm "floppy" wrap to achieve better results.

With the **Hill** operation, performed only through the abdomen, posterior approximation of the crura is followed by the anchoring of both the anterior and posterior aspects of the GE junction to the median arcuate ligament adjacent to the aorta, thereby creating a gastric wrap of approximately 180 degrees. • Calibration of the plication by intraoperative manometric measurements is considered critical for success.

All of these operations can effectively prevent GE reflux. • Whether one operation is clearly superior to another is controversial, but most surgeons prefer the Nissen fundoplication for uncomplicated reflux. • When there is insufficient esophageal motility, a partial fundoplication, such as the Belsey Mark IV procedure, may be preferred.

In the presence of a short esophagus, a **Collis** gastroplasty combined with the Belsey Mark IV or Nissen procedure is suggested. • With the Collis gastroplasty, performed through the chest, the esophagus is lengthened by dividing the stomach parallel to the lesser curvature, starting at the angle of His, and then constructing the fundoplication from around the esophagus. • Each procedure has a place in the management of GE reflux, depending on the characteristics of the individual patient, technical considerations, and the surgeon's experience.

The **Angelchik** prosthesis is a horseshoe-shaped Silastic device placed around the distal esophagus, thus keeping this segment in the abdomen. • Its simplicity invites use through the abdominal approach. • Its disadvantages are erosion of the device into the esophagus or stomach and migration. • Its use is not recommended.

Laparoscopic Nissen fundoplication, now performed widely, is a safe and effective procedure that has been tested for several years. • The indications are the same as for the open procedure, but, most important, the presence of a short esophagus must be excluded lest the wrap be placed around the cardia of the stomach, which would lead to complications. • Skilled laparoscopic surgeons have developed techniques for laparoscopic Collis procedures in conjunction with fundoplication, but experience with these operations is relatively limited.

ANSWERS:
Question 19: A, B, D
Question 20: A-a,b,f; B-b,c,d,e; C-c; D-e; E-d; F-f; G-a,c
Question 21: A

22. With regard to paraesophageal hernia, which of the following apply?

A. Type 3 is the most common.

B. The laparoscopic repair should not be done.

C. Excision of the hernia sac is imperative.

D. Antireflux repairs should always accompany the repair.

E. Mesh may reduce recurrence rates in hernias larger than 8 cm.

Ref.: 1–3, 8, 9

COMMENTS: There are two main types of anatomically defined esophageal hiatal hernias: type I (sliding) hernia and type II (paraesophageal) hernia. • Other types of hernia that have anatomic features and complications of both types are described also. • With **type I** (sliding) hiatal hernia (H1), the cardia enters the chest through a widened hiatus and a stretched but intact phrenoesophageal ligament. • Because the phrenoesophageal ligament is intact, abdominal pressure is still applied to the distal esophagus, so that, in most patients, reflux does not develop. • However, most patients with reflux do have a sliding hiatal hernia. • The point of insertion of the phrenoesophageal ligament on the esophagus and lateral tension on the esophagus are factors that may contribute to reflux. • With **type II** (paraesophageal) hiatal hernia (H2), the anatomic problem involves a defect in the phrenoesophageal membrane, with herniation of the stomach into a peritoneum-lined pouch adjacent to the esophagus. • With other hernias, such as **type III** paraesophageal hernia (H3), the esophagogastric junction is in the mediastinum. • With **type IV** paraesophageal hernia (H4), the entire stomach and other viscera are in the mediastinum.

Occult gastrointestinal bleeding from gastritis, ulceration in the herniated portion of the stomach, and gastric volvulus are the most common complications of paraesophageal hernia. • Acute gastric volvulus is a surgical emergency. • It may be manifested by a classic triad of pain, nausea with inability to vomit, and inability to accept passage of a nasogastric tube. • A significant risk of serious complications and a high mortality rate are associated with paraesophageal hernias, even when the patient is asymptomatic. • For this reason, repair is generally indicated when the condition is diagnosed.

The evaluation of a paraesophageal hernia should include a barium esophagram to delineate the anatomy. • Upper endoscopy and biopsy, if indicated, should be done to rule out malignancy. • Manometric testng is usually inconclusive because of the altered anatomy and motility. • Owing to the altered anatomy of the GE junction, reflux is usually present, and therefore pH monitoring does not add to the evaluation.

During operative repair, it is important to reduce the hernia contents, usually stomach, colon, and omentum, although giant hernias may contain other intra-abdominal organs. • After reduction of hernia contents, it is imperative to excise the hernia sac. • The sac excision is done to prevent postoperative fluid collections and/or recurrence. • A cruroplasty is performed as part of the repair. • Others advocate gastropexy and or gastrostomy tube placement to decrease recurrence. • In some series, repair of hernias larger than 8 cm are reinforced with polytetrafluoroethylene (PTFE) mesh, which is added to the cruroplasty to decrease long-term recurrence. • There have been anecdotal reports of mesh erosion, but it has not been reported in more recent, larger series.

The laparoscopic repair is reported to be as durable as traditional open mesh repairs in most large reviews, although it must be understood that a long learning curve is necessary to obtain acceptable results.

Antireflux procedures are variably added to the hernia repair. • Some surgeons advocate the routine addition of an antireflux procedure for several reasons. • First, once a hiatal dissection has been done, several mechanisms to prevent reflux have been altered. • Second, the fundoplication may help to buttress the repair.

ANSWER:
C, E

23. Achalasia can be described by which of the following?

A. It is failure or lack of relaxation of the LES.

B. Dysphagia, regurgitation, and nocturnal asthma are included in the classic triad of symptoms.

C. *Trypanosoma cruzi*, a parasite that causes Chagas' disease, destroys Auerbach's plexus in only the esophagus, resulting in dilation and failure of the LES to relax.

D. Biopsy to rule out carcinoma is not necessary because there is no malignant potential.

E. A barium esophagram may demonstrate a distal "bird's beak" configuration at the GE junction.

F. Manometric evaluation demonstrates failure of LES relaxation, lack of progressive peristaltic waves, and increased resting pressure of the distal high-pressure zone.

Ref.: 1–3

COMMENTS: Achalasia is a motility disorder that affects the entire esophagus. • During the early stages of the disease, the focus is on the failure of relaxation of the LES. • Patients learn what foods to eat in order to minimize their symptoms. • As progression occurs, the esophagus dilates, and foul-smelling, stagnant esophageal contents often regurgitate. • Nocturnal asthma may occur, and pain is a frequent presenting symptom, occurring in up to 90% of patients. • However, the classic triad of presenting symptoms in a patient with achalasia includes dysphagia, regurgitation, and weight loss.

The cause of achalasia is unknown. • An unusual cause is infection by the parasite *T. cruzi,* which occurs primarily in South America. • The histopathologic findings demonstrate destruction of the smooth muscle myenteric Auerbach's plexus. • It is interesting to note that this progressive dilation occurs in other organs, such as the ureters and colon.

The diagnosis of achalasia can be difficult. • In the early stages of the disease, symptoms are vague. • Initially, a barium esophagram shows mild esophageal dilation, which progresses to a redundant, sigmoid-shaped esophagus. • The "bird's beak" is the characteristic taper effect of achalasia seen on the esophagram. • Further confirmation of the diagnosis of achalasia should be done with manometric measurements. • The classic findings include increased pressure in the LES, which fails to relax, and, in late disease, a lack of progressive peristalsis in the proximal esophagus.

After 15–25 years, patients with achalasia have up to a 10% chance of developing carcinoma. • Metaplasia occurs in the setting of prolonged esophageal mucosal irritation. • Screening should occur with upper endoscopy.

A N S W E R :
A, E, F

24. Which of the following is true of the treatment of achalasia?

A. Sublingual nitroglycerin and calcium-channel blockers may improve symptoms.

B. Bougie dilation will not improve symptoms.

C. Pneumatic dilation carries a 10% perforation risk.

D. Esophageal myotomy carries a 1% perforation risk.

E. An esophageal myotomy can only be performed through a laparoscopic or open abdominal approach.

Ref.: 1–3

COMMENTS: Achalasia is a progressive disease for which the treatment is difficult. • The goals of treating achalasia are centered on relieving the functional obstruction at the LES. • In the early stages of achalasia, symptoms may be nonspecific, but benefit can be gained with oral nitroglycerin and calcium-channel blockers.

• As the disease progresses, more invasive procedures may be necessary.

Bougie dilation is successful, but the benefits are short lived. • In patients who undergo pneumatic dilation, 65% have improved symptoms. • During this procedure, a balloon is inflated to approximately 300 torr for 10–15 seconds. • The success of this procedure is counterbalanced by the 4% incidence of esophageal perforation. • The gold-standard treatment of achalasia remains an esophagomyotomy with or without an antireflux procedure. • Of the patients who have received esophagomyotomy, 85% have relief of symptoms, and the risk of perforation is only 1%.

The esophageal myotomy can be performed through a variety of approaches, all of which are similarly efficacious. • The procedure can be performed with a transthoracic approach through the sixth or seventh intercostal space as well as thoracoscopically. • An open abdominal or laparoscopic approach is also possible. • When performing a distal esophagomyotomy for achalasia, it is necessary to divide the thickened LES as well as the esophageal musculature from the inferior pulmonary vein to about 3 cm onto the stomach.

Recently, innovative treatments of achalasia, such as botulism toxin injection, have been advocated, but the long-term results of these methods have not equaled those of esophagomyotomy.

A N S W E R :
A, D

25. A 45-year-old man complains of dysphagia and regurgitation. An esophagram shows a narrow distal esophagus. Manometric studies demonstrate an absence of peristaltic waves and an LES that does not relax with swallowing. Which of the following descriptions apply?

A. Bilateral vagal injury

B. Weight loss

C. Midbrain lesion

D. LES relaxation with deglutition

E. "Bird's beak"

Ref.: 1–3, 5

COMMENTS: See Question 28.

26. Appropriate treatment for the patient described in Question 25 may include which of the following?

A. Botulin neurotoxin

B. Balloon dilatation

C. Cervical esophagomyotomy

D. Distal esophagomyotomy

E. Esophagectomy

Ref.: 1–6

COMMENTS: See Question 28.

27. A 40-year-old woman complains of chest pain and dysphagia. An esophagram is normal. Manometric studies demonstrate simultaneous, moderately high-amplitude contractions with normal relaxation of the LES. Which of the following applies?

A. Nutcracker esophagus

B. Diffuse esophageal spasm

C. "Vigorous" achalasia

D. Scleroderma

E. Coronary angiograph

Ref.: 1–6

COMMENTS: See Question 28.

28. What is the appropriate treatment for the patient described in Question 25 if medical measures fail?

A. Antispasmodics

B. Balloon dilatation

C. Cervical esophagomyotomy

D. Thoracic esophagomyotomy

E. Forceful dilatation

Ref.: 1–6

COMMENTS: Esophageal motility disorders may be primary, or they may be secondary to mechanical obstruction or various neuromuscular disorders. • Ruling out mechanical problems, such as tumor or stricture, and accurate characterization of the type of motility disorder are mandatory before definitive therapy. • Motility disorders often can be differentiated on the basis of the findings of esophagoscopic, esophagographic, and manometric studies and 24-hr pH measurements.

In **achalasia**, the LES fails to relax; the inner circular muscle is greatly hypertrophied, with interstitial fibrosis; and there is absence or degeneration of ganglia in Auerbach's plexus. • Manometrically, there is absence of peristaltic waves late in the disease and simultaneous contractions earlier. • The high-pressure zone demonstrates normal pressure but no relaxation. • The cause of achalasia is not known, but a similar condition is found in Chagas' disease and can be produced experimentally by causing midbrain lesions in cats and vagal nerve dysfunction in dogs. • An esophagram may demonstrate esophageal dilatation and a typical "bird's beak" narrowing of the distal esophagus. • Clinically, patients experience dysphagia, regurgitation, and weight loss. • Although the problem may occur at any age, it is most commonly diagnosed in patients between 30 and 50 years of age and is somewhat more common in men. • Diagnostic tests should exclude cardiac disease, but angiographic study is seldom indicated. • Therapy is focused on destruction of the muscular apparatus of the hypertonic and hypertrophic lower esophageal segment. • This can be effectively accomplished in about 60% of patients by *forceful dilatation* with hydrostatic or pneumatic balloons and in 90% of patients with surgical *myotomy* of the lower thoracic esophagus. • Operative treatment is essentially more effective and carries a lower risk of perforation. • The extent to which the myotomy should be carried down onto the stomach and the need for concomitant performance of an antireflux procedure are controversial features of the surgical management of achalasia, but most surgeons perform complete myotomy with a loose or partial (Dor or Toupet) wrap. • Recently, minimal-access myotomy has been performed through the transabdominal or transthoracic approach with good results. • *Botulin neurotoxin* injected into the LES through flexible endoscopic technique inhibits neural release of acetylcholine and has a favorable effect on patients with achalasia, but effects are usually temporary, and injection may make operative dissection more difficult.

Diffuse esophageal spasm (DES) is manifested with chest pain and dysphagia. • The cause is unclear, although in many patients it is associated with emotional factors and functional gastrointestinal disorders. • Manometric studies demonstrate repetitive simultaneous high-amplitude contractions, although peristalsis

may be observed in the upper, striated portion of the esophagus. • In contrast to achalasia, the LES usually has a normal relaxation response. • Manometric findings may fluctuate, obscuring the diagnosis. • The esophagram frequently is normal, although the classic "corkscrew" esophagus is occasionally demonstrated. • Surgical treatment for diffuse esophageal spasm is less satisfactory than that for achalasia. • For this reason, medical management with antispasmodics, dietary modulation, and psychiatric counseling constitute the initial therapeutic regime. • When surgical therapy is necessary, an extended thoracic esophagomyotomy is indicated.

Nutcracker esophagus is a motor abnormality characterized by chest pain and extremely high-amplitude peristaltic waves up to 400 mmHg. • Twenty-four–hour manometric studies are important for identifying a subgroup of patients with a manometric pattern of DES. • These patients, similar to those with DES and dysphagia, can obtain relief from a long myotomy. • Esophagectomy is occasionally indicated for patients with advanced esophageal dilatation because of motility disorders of any type.

Variants of achalasia and diffuse esophageal spasm may be seen, and precise diagnosis is sometimes difficult. • One example is so-called **vigorous achalasia**, in which the patient may present with symptoms of dysphagia, regurgitation, and chest pain. • Manometric findings are suggestive of diffuse spasm and abnormal relaxation of the LES.

It should be noted that, in any patient with a suspected esophageal motility disorder, organic obstruction and particularly carcinoma must be carefully ruled out.

Scleroderma is a collagen vascular disease resulting in fibrous replacement of the esophageal smooth muscle with secondary lack of peristalsis of the distal esophagus. • There is also a loss of the high-pressure zone, leading to reflux, ulceration, and shortening of the esophagus. • If standard medical therapy fails, an antireflux operation with a partial wrap is performed. • If there is a short esophagus, a Collis gastroplasty with a partial wrap is undertaken.

ANSWERS:
Question 25: A, B, C, E
Question 26: A, B, D
Question 27: B
Question 28: D

29. Which of the following apply to DES?

A. It is associated with retrosternal chest pain

B. It is associated with a sigmoid esophagus.

C. Classic manometric findings include simultaneous, multiphasic, high-amplitude contractions.

D. Psychiatric disorders are common.

E. A long esophageal myomotomy is the gold-standard therapy.

Ref.: 1–3

COMMENTS: The disorder of DES is a hypermotility condition of the esophagus. • The cause and progression of this disease are poorly understood. • Patients most commonly present with dysphagia and retrosternal chest pain similar to that of angina pectoris. • It is interesting to note that, in patients in whom DES has been diagnosed, the most severe episodes tend to coincide with periods of high emotional stress. • Psychiatric disorders are common and are diagnosed in greater than 80% of these patients.

The diagnosis of DES is difficult. • First, cardiac causes of pain must be excluded. • Once this is done, a barium swallow will show the classic "corkscrew" esophagus. • Other diagnostic modalities, including upper endoscopic and manometric studies, are usually performed. • Manometric findings of DES include simultaneous, repetitive, multiphasic, often high-amplitude contractions. • These findings occur spontaneously as well as following normal swallowing.

Once the difficult diagnosis of DES has been confirmed, the treatment should focus on relieving the patient's symptoms. • Any underlying psychiatric disorders should be optimally treated. • First-line medical therapy is similar to that of achalasia and includes oral calcium-channel blockers or antispasmodics. • DES responds variably to the administration of oral nitrates. • Bougie dilations may also relieve symptoms temporarily but seldom offer long-term relief. • The surgical treatment of DES is a long esophageal myotomy, from the GE junction to the aortic arch. • Only about 60% of patients with DES have relief of symptoms after a long esophagomyotomy. • Therefore, this extensive procedure is reserved only for those patients with incapacitating symptoms. • In order to relieve all obstructive symptoms, it is usually necessary to divide all circular muscle fibers of the esophagus and proximal stomach. • However, the addition of an antireflux procedure is controversial.

ANSWER:
A, C, D, E

30. With regard to esophageal diverticula, which of the following is/are true?

    A. There are four types of esophageal diverticula: pharyngoesophageal, parabronchial, epiphrenic, and subdiaphragmatic.

    B. Pulsion diverticula are false diverticula, and traction diverticula are true diverticula.

    C. When treating a pharyngoesophageal diverticulum, surgical options include cervical esophagomyotomy along with resection or pexy of the diverticulum.

    D. Mid-esophageal diverticula are true diverticula, caused by traction as well as pulsion forces.

    E. Epiphrenic diverticula are traction diverticula and are treated with esophagectomy.

    F. A barium esophagram, upper endoscopic studies, and manometric measurements are necessary in order to evaluate a patient with an esophageal diverticulum.

Ref.: 1–3, 10

COMMENTS: A true diverticulum is composed of all layers of the wall of the esophagus. • A false diverticulum is a pouch of mucosa that has protruded through the wall of the esophagus. • Both true and false diverticula can be found in the esophagus. • The pharyngoesophageal and epiphrenic diverticula are pulsion diverticula, classifying them as false diverticula. • The cause of the pulsion diverticula is multifactorial, but the major components are increased intraluminal pressure and incoordination of peristalsis. • The parabronchial diverticulum is a true diverticulum, arises from traction forces on the exterior of the esophagus, and is usually associated with mediastinal pathologic conditions.

Diagnosis of an esophageal diverticulum is first based on history. • Patients complain of dysphagia. • In order to diagnose the cause of a patient's dysphagia, a number of studies must be undertaken. • First, a barium esophagram must be obtained in order to delineate anatomic abnormalities and assess motility. • Upper endoscopic examination is then performed to assess for mucosal disease and exclude malignancy. • To complete the evaluation, a manometric examination is performed to detail a motility disorder.

Pharyngoesophageal (Zenker's) diverticula are the most common esophageal diverticula. • These pulsion, false diverticula arise between the transverse fibers of the cricopharyngeus muscle and the oblique fibers of the thyropharyngeus muscle. • Patients present with dysphagia and halitosis, often complaining of regurgitating pills or undigested food. • The treatment centers on a cervical esophageal myotomy and excision or diverticulopexy to the mastoid bone. • Parabronchial diverticula are true diverticula that arise by traction forces on surrounding pathologic conditions of the mediastinum. • More recently, manometric measurements have demonstrated that a pulsion component, secondary to an underlying motility disorder, is partially responsible for Zenker's diverticula in some of these patients. • Epiphrenic diverticula, like Zenker's diverticula, are pulsion in nature and are false diverticula. • An underlying motility disorder is always present. • If the diverticula are larger than 3 cm or the patient has moderate-to-severe symptoms, surgical excision is recommended. • An esophagomyotomy always accompanies excision, and incompetent LES or hiatal hernias should also be repaired.

ANSWER:
B, C, D, F

31. The causes of oropharyngeal dysphagia include which of the following?

    A. Neuropathy

    B. GE reflux

    C. Esophageal carcinoma

    D. Recurrent laryngeal nerve injury

    E. History of vagotomy

    F. Thyromegaly

    G. Stricture

Ref.: 1–3

COMMENTS: The many disorders of esophageal motility are grouped into general categories based on the anatomic area of the esophagus affected. • Oropharyngeal dysphagia can occur as a result of a functional defect, neoplastic processes, infection, or any anatomic abnormality in the cervical area that may affect the swallowing mechanism.

Neurogenic conditions, usually secondary to an intracranial hemorrhage or cerebral infarction, are treated conservatively with supportive care.

GE reflux can be diagnosed with a pH reflux probe. • Reflux can cause early dysfunction secondary to irritation of the esophagus, resulting in abnormal peristalsis. • A late complication of long-standing GE reflux is a peptic stricture. • In this case, the esophagus is shortened and fibrotic. • Treatment should focus on preventing further reflux with medical therapy with a proton-pump inhibitor. • To aid in swallowing, bougie dilation can act as a first-line therapy, but if it is unsuccessful or recurrence is rapid, more extensive surgical intervention may be necessary.

Carcinoma can cause oropharyngeal dysphagia for a variety of reasons. • Pain is common, and a mass effect or invasion of surrounding structures by a tumor may disrupt the swallowing mechanism.

Recurrent laryngeal nerve injury will prevent abduction of the ipsilateral vocal cord.

A history of a vagotomy associated with a gastric emptying procedure or gastrectomy is not a cause of primary dysphagia. • However, a patient may have reflux secondary to a vagotomy and gastrectomy or emptying procedure, which may interfere with normal peristalsis and swallowing.

The thyroid gland is located anterior to the trachea and inferior to the thyroid cartilage. • Thyromegaly can cause upper aerodigestive tract obstruction secondary to extrinsic compression, resulting in airway obstruction and dysphagia.

ANSWER:
A, B, C, F, G

32. Which of the following are prerequisites for a successful result after cricopharyngeal myotomy?

   A. Adequate function of cranial nerves V, VII, X, XI, and XII and the first, second, and third cervical roots

   B. Occlusion of the nasopharynx by the soft palate

   C. Adequate high-pressure zone

   D. Absence of Zenker's diverticulum

   E. Presence of upper esophageal web

   Ref.: 1–3, 6

COMMENTS: See Question 34.

33. With regard to Zenker's diverticulum, which of the following statements is/are true?

   A. Severity of symptoms is not determined primarily by the size of the diverticulum.

   B. Diagnosis is best established endoscopically.

   C. Cricopharyngeal myotomy alone without diverticulectomy is adequate treatment for small diverticula.

   D. Diverticulopexy is adequate in poor-risk patients with large diverticula.

   E. Endoscopic excision is the preferred method.

   Ref.: 1–3, 6

COMMENTS: See Question 34.

34. Cricopharyngeal myotomy may be an appropriate treatment for which of the following conditions?

   A. Plummer-Vinson syndrome

   B. Incomplete relaxation of the cricopharyngeal muscle

   C. Cerebrovascular accident (CVA) with involvement of nerves V, VII, X, and XI

   D. Decreased compliance of hypopharyngeal muscle

   Ref.: 1–3, 6

COMMENTS: The transfer of food and liquid from the mouth into the upper esophagus is a complicated process and requires proper function of the tongue, pharynx, larynx, epiglottis, and soft palate. • For instance, occlusion of the nasopharynx by the soft palate prevents nasal regurgitation of oral contents. • The upper esophageal sphincter in turn must relax properly to allow food to be transferred into the esophagus. • The function of the cricopharyngeal muscle is believed to prevent air from entering the esophagus during breathing and swallowing.

Symptoms of cervical dysphagia may be manifestations of neurologic, muscular, or mechanical disorders affecting the pharyngoesophageal region. • Proper evaluation of swallowing begins with a thorough neurologic evaluation, and pharyngoesophagographic and cervical manometric studies may be required. • The presence of a Zenker's diverticulum is best established radiographically. • Cranial nerves V, VII, X, XI, and XII and the first, second, and third cervical roots must be intact. • If there is a suspicion of gastrointestinal reflux, 24-hr pH monitoring is required, and, if reflux is found, cricopharyngotomy is not advised. • Endoscopic examination and biopsy may be indicated when mucosal damage is suspected.

Cricopharyngeal myotomy has been used widely with variable success. • Unsuccessful outcomes are often due to inadequate evaluation and improper diagnosis. • A good result can be expected in the surgical therapy of cervical dysphagia when performed for the following conditions: (1) presence of Zenker's diverticulum; (2) incomplete relaxation or discoordinated cricopharyngeal relaxation; (3) poor pharyngeal contraction resulting from a CVA that reduces the ability to transverse the bolus against the cricopharyngeal pressure; and (4) manometrically recorded hypopharyngeal "shoulder pressure" with normal relaxation, resulting from decreased compliance because of restrictive myopathy.

The cause of **Zenker's diverticulum** is not clear. • Manometric findings often are normal but may demonstrate incoordination, failure of relaxation, or restrictive myopathy. • The severity of symptoms is not determined primarily by the size of the diverticulum, except in patients whose diverticulum is completely dependent and obstructs the esophagus. • Cricopharyngeal myotomy alone abolishes symptoms in most patients with Zenker's diverticulum (except in those with a large diverticulum). • Thus, removal of the diverticulum is not necessary in most patients. • If the diverticulum persists, excision is recommended in stable patients. • In poor-risk patients, a diverticulopexy in an upside-down position on the prevertebral fascia can be performed. • Cricopharyngeal myotomy is easily performed, even with the use of local anesthesia.

Cervical dysphagia also occurs in patients with **sideropenic dysphagia** (Plummer-Vinson or Paterson-Kelly syndrome), in which the mechanism is usually an upper esophageal web related to a nutritional deficiency. • The treatment consists of esophageal dilatation and nutritional supplementation.

Esophageal motility problems can occur with **scleroderma** and other collagen vascular diseases, which may present as cervical dysphagia. • The primary disturbance, however, is not specific to the cricopharyngeal region and generally involves motility disturbances of the distal esophagus and incompetence of the GE sphincter.

ANSWERS:
Question 32: B, C
Question 33: A, C, D
Question 34: B, D

35. A 50-year-old healthy conventioneer is brought to the emergency room with retching followed by hematemesis.

   A. Treatment is by balloon tamponade.

   B. Bleeding often stops spontaneously.

   C. It is caused by forceful vomiting.

   D. There is air in the mediastinum.

   E. Diagnosis is made by endoscopic examination.

   Ref.: 1–3

COMMENTS: In 1929, G.K. Mallory and S. Weiss described four cases of gastric bleeding that followed repeated emesis and in which there were linear tears in the esophagogastric mucosa. • The mechanism is similar to that of the Boerhaave syndrome (postemetic esophageal rupture), in which there is associated perforation and vomiting against a closed cardia. • It is diagnosed by endoscopic examination, and the bleeding usually stops spontaneously. • Because the bleeding is arterial, a pressure tamponade does not help and may in fact lead to esophageal disruption. • If bleeding does not stop, gastrotomy and oversewing of the bleeding point is the proper therapy, although various nonsurgical alternatives, such as endoscopic injection of epinephrine and cautery, have been attempted.

ANSWER:
B, C, E

36. A smooth filling defect, 3 cm in its greatest dimension, is found in the middle third of the esophagus. Which of the following statements regarding this lesion is/are correct?

   A. An endoscopic procedure should be performed and a biopsy specimen of the lesion obtained.

   B. It usually presents with hematemesis.

   C. The lesion should be excised by enucleation.

   D. It is composed of spindle cells.

   Ref.: 1–3, 5

COMMENTS: Benign esophageal tumors are far less common than malignant neoplasms. • Often, they are completely asymptomatic, but they may cause dysphagia and pain. • **Leiomyomas** are the most common benign esophageal lesions and are usually found in the lower two thirds of the esophagus, which is composed of smooth muscle. • They are extramucosal lesions that produce a characteristic smooth defect with intact mucosa on radiographic studies. • In contrast to those located in the stomach, they rarely bleed. • Treatment consists of simple enucleation. • Endoscopic examination is indicated, but biopsy should not be performed because the secondary scarring hinders proper enucleation of the leiomyoma.

ANSWER:
C, D

37. With regard to esophageal cancer, which of the following is/are false?

   A. Approximately 1300 patients per year are diagnosed with esophageal cancer in the United States.

   B. African Americans are five times more likely to develop adenocarcinoma than are members of other groups.

   C. The incidence of squamous cell carcinoma is increasing in Western countries.

   D. Twenty-five percent of patients present with lymph node metastasis.

   E. Metaplastic columnar epithelium, when present, warrants esophagectomy.

   Ref.: 1–3, 11, 12

COMMENTS: During 2001, esophageal cancer accounted for 12,500 deaths in the United States. • Traditionally, esophageal cancer has been up to five times more prevalent in African-American men than in Caucasian men. • Worldwide, squamous cell carcinoma is more prevalent than adenocarcinoma.

• Throughout the last two decades, in Westernized countries, the incidence of adenocarcinoma among Caucasian males has been dramatically increasing. • In some series, up to 80% of patients are Caucasian males with adenocarcinoma of the lower third of the esophagus.

The symptoms at presentation in a patient with esophageal cancer are vague. • The majority present with pain and dysphagia in reaction to solids and/or liquids. • Weight loss is common. • On final histologic examination, the majority of patients are at an advanced stage. • In clinical series, up to 60% of patients present with lymph node metastasis. • These patients have a dramatically decreased survival compared to patients without lymph node metastasis. • In a multivariate analysis at Rush University Medical Center in 2001, the presence of lymph node metastasis, intraoperative blood transfusions, and adjuvant therapy were independent predictors of survival.

Columnar metaplasia of the esophageal epithelium is known as Barrett's esophagus. • Barrett's esophagus has malignant potential. • Once it has been diagnosed, patients should undergo biopsies of the involved areas. • If only metaplasia or low-grade dysplasia is present, then surveillance with upper endoscopy and biopsy is continued at 2- to 3-year intervals. • If high-grade dysplasia is found, then esophagectomy is warranted.

ANSWER:
A, B, C, D, E

38. With regard to epidermoid cancer of the esophagus, which of the following statements is/are true?

   A. Incidence is increased among African-American men.

   B. Incidence is increased among American women.

   C. Domestic chickens in Linxian, China, have exhibited the same increased incidence of epidermoid cell cancer as their owners.

   D. Tylosis is associated with a decrease in epidermoid cell cancer.

   E. Incidence is increased as a result of nitrosamine exposure.

   Ref.: 1–3, 5

COMMENTS: See Question 39.

39. Which of the following factors is/are associated with adenocarcinoma of the esophagus?

   A. Achalasia

   B. Barrett's esophagus

   C. Corrosive stricture

   D. Ectopic gastric mucosa

   E. Upper esophageal web

   Ref.: 1–3, 5, 13

COMMENTS: The incidence of **epidermoid cell cancer** of the esophagus varies widely throughout the world and for men varies from 6/100,000 to more than 140/100,000 in some areas of Asia, South Africa, and the former Soviet Union. • In the United States, the highest incidence is among African-American men, at approximately 12/100,000. • In Western countries, a high-risk area is the wine district of southern France (e.g., Bordeaux). • Risk factors have been found to vary from region to region. • In the United States and Western Europe, tobacco use and alcohol use each have been found to be independent risk factors, and together they have a synergistic effect. • In South Africa, tobacco is a more significant risk factor because the tobacco is chewed after it is smoked in pipes. • In Linxian, China, domestic chickens sharing food and water with their owners have a cancer incidence of 175/100,000, whereas among humans the incidence is 142/100,000. • Another risk factor is exposure to nitrosamines, accounting for higher incidence in Kenya and Asia, resulting from pickled vegetables and cured meats. • There is an increased incidence of epidermoid cancer in individuals with achalasia, corrosive esophageal stricture, sideropenic dysphagia, tylosis, or celiac disease. • Most malignant esophageal neoplasms are epidermoid carcinomas.

Adenocarcinoma may occur in the distal esophagus at the columnar-epithelial junction or in other columnar-lined areas of the esophagus, as observed with Barrett's esophagus or ectopic gastric mucosa. • Adenocarcinoma in the distal esophagus may also be seen as an extension of a primary gastric neoplasm. • The incidence of adenocarcinoma of the esophagus and gastric cardia has been increasing from 1976, in contrast to the steady incidence of epidermoid cancer. • The increase among men ranges from 4 to 10% per year, a greater increase than for any other type of cancer. • This phenomenon occurs disproportionately among Caucasian men and, rarely, among women. • Risk factors have not been discovered, and the subject has not been studied well, but Barrett's esophagus is a possible risk factor.

ANSWERS:
Question 38: A, C E
Question 39: B, D

40. Which of the following statements regarding epidermoid esophageal cancer is/are true?

   A. Patients present with dysphagia and weight loss.

   B. Diagnosis is confirmed by a barium esophagogram and endoscopic biopsy.

   C. Lymph nodes are usually not involved.

   D. There is no submucosal spread.

   E. Exploration is the best determinant of resectability.

Ref.: 1–3, 5

COMMENTS: See Question 43.

41. With regard to the use of the colon as an esophageal substitute after complete esophageal resection, which of the following statements is/are true?

   A. Three anastomoses are required.

   B. The colon resists peptic stricture.

   C. The colon is the organ of choice in young patients with benign disease.

   D. It functions best when placed substernally.

   E. The blood supply and venous drainage depend on the marginal vessels.

Ref.: 1–3, 5, 13

COMMENTS: See Question 43.

42. With regard to the use of the stomach as an esophageal substitute after total esophagectomy, which of the following statements is/are true?

   A. The blood supply is derived from the fundal branch of the splenic artery.

   B. It can usually be made to reach the cervical esophagus.

   C. A narrow gastric tube is preferred.

   D. A drainage procedure is always required.

Ref.: 1–3, 5, 13

COMMENTS: See Question 43.

43. Which of the following statements regarding esophagectomy for esophageal cancer is/are true?

   A. It is contraindicated in the presence of liver metastasis.

   B. It is indicated for palliation only if endoscopic intubation is unsuccessful.

   C. It has been observed to have improved results when preceded by chemotherapy and irradiation.

   D. It is potentially curative in about 20% of patients.

Ref.: 1–3, 5

COMMENTS: Esophageal cancer is a disease with a dismal outlook. • The most frequent symptoms of esophageal cancer are dysphagia and weight loss. • Both symptoms occur late, owing to the ability of the esophagus to accommodate. • Any patient with dysphagia should undergo barium esophagography followed by upper endoscopy and biopsy. • It is important to stage these patients because those with distal metastases (e.g., to the lung, liver, or adrenals) are not usually considered candidates for esophagectomy, since their expected survival is less than 12 months. • Local lymphadenopathy does not preclude resection. • Transesophageal ultrasound studies are extremely accurate for detecting depth of invasion and lymphadenopathy, but the computed tomographic (CT) scan is the test most often used. • However, many cancers that are judged unresectable on CT scan are found to be resectable on exploration. • Therefore, exploration is the best method for judging resectability in patients with questionable CT findings. • Bronchoscopic examination is mandatory in upper- and middle-third lesions to rule out tracheobronchial invasion. • The extensive submucosal lymphatic network of the esophagus predisposes patients to early involvement of mediastinal, supraclavicular, and abdominal lymph nodes. • Hematogenous spread to lung and liver also occurs, but less frequently. • Furthermore, these tumors tend to be locally invasive, with involvement of adjacent mediastinal structures, such as the tracheobronchial tree, recurrent laryngeal nerve, aorta, pericardium, and diaphragm. • Submucosal extension proximally is common, which is an important point to remember when proximal surgical margins are obtained. • Although operation for esophageal cancer is most often noncurative, many clinicians consider esophagectomy the best method of providing palliation. • Either pulling up the stomach or using a colon interposition generally accomplishes reconstruction.

There are a number of disadvantages associated with using the colon as an esophageal substitute: (1) the colon has tenuous marginal vessels for blood supply and venous drainage; (2) bacteria are present; (3) three anastomoses are required; and (4) the operation is long. • It is now believed that, for advanced malignant disease, the stomach is the substitute of choice and the colon should be used only when the stomach is not available. • The colon, however, is the preferred substitute when resection is for benign disease of the esophagus (e.g., advanced achalasia and long-standing corrosive or peptic strictures) and for diseases with a favorable outlook (e.g., early cancer, benign tumors, and premalignant conditions). • Many of these conditions are seen among young patients who are healthy and have a long life expectancy. • It is advantageous in these patients to preserve gastric function. • The colon is resistant to peptic stricture, and, when it is anastomosed posteriorly in the stomach and with a partial wrap, reflux is avoided. • The subcutaneous approach has the poorest functional result

The stomach is considered the safest esophageal substitute because only one anastomosis is required. • Its blood supply and drainage are abundant because of the right gastroepiploic vessels, which send anastomotic branches to the lesser curvature through an abundant submucosal network. • The vascular supply and venous drainage of the fundus especially depend on the plexus of the subcardial region. • This information has changed the approach to preparing the fundus for cervical and pharyngeal anastomosis. • It is best to preserve the subcardial plexus in this instance and not try to transect the stomach longitudinally to shape it as a tube (i.e., tubulation), as was formerly done, on the assumption that it would improve vascularity. • The best vascularity is maintained when the whole stomach is used, especially for pharyngogastric anastomosis. • However, partial tubulation of the stomach may be necessary for cervical anastomosis to reduce the bulk of the stomach or to resect the cardia and lesser curvature to ensure margins and nodal removal in malignant disease. • The requirement for an emptying procedure is controversial. • Pyloric obstruction and postoperative gastric dilatation have been reported when an emptying procedure has not been performed. • Pyloroplasty leads to shortening of the gastric tube, and the possibly increased tension of the suture line may increase the risk of anastomotic disruption. • For these reasons, pyloromyotomy may be performed, but conversion to pyloroplasty may be necessary when the duodenal mucosa is perforated. • The trend is toward intraoperative finger dilatation or endoscopic postoperative balloon dilatation when delayed gastric emptying occurs. • The mortality rate after esophagectomy is 2–5%.

Endoscopic intubation of unresectable obstructing esophageal cancers appears to be an attractive technique but has not been uniformly acceptable because of the complications of tube obstruction or dislodgement and because of esophageal perforation. • Placing an esophageal tube, however, may be the preferred method of palliation for the difficult problem of malignant tracheoesophageal fistula. • Use of the stomach or colon for retrosternal bypass of the obstructed esophagus is associated with a high morbidity rate and has not been proved superior to esophagectomy for palliation. • For many patients unsuitable for surgery, irradiation provides palliation, since epidermoid cancer is radiosensitive. • The University of Michigan group used chemotherapy and radiation before blunt esophagectomy with results better than those seen with surgery alone. • D.B. Skinner and associates have demonstrated a similar experience.

ANSWERS:
Question 40: A, B, E
Question 41: A, B, C, D, E
Question 42: B
Question 43: A, C, D

44. Match each surgical approach in the left-hand column with one or more appropriate comments in the right-hand column.

A. Ivor Lewis   a. Two separate incisions

B. Left thoracoabdominal   b. Transect diaphragm

                         c. Inadvertent injury to azygous vein

                         d. Increased incidence of pulmonary complications

                         e. Poor exposure of upper esophagus

                         f. One incision

Ref.: 1–3, 5, 13, 14

COMMENTS: See Question 45.

45. Complications of esophagectomy performed without thoracotomy for esophageal cancer include which of the following?

A. Chylothorax

B. Increased mortality from anastomotic leakage

C. Increased incidence of GE reflux

D. Increased blood loss

E. Pneumothorax

Ref.: 1–3, 5, 15

COMMENTS: Standard approaches to the thoracic esophagus include a left thoracoabdominal incision, a combined abdominal incision and separate right thoracotomy, and, most recently, an esophagectomy without thoracotomy but with the use of abdominal and cervical incisions.

The **abdominal and right thoracic incision**, known as the Ivor Lewis procedure, was described by Ivor Lewis in 1946 in his Hunterian Lecture. • It was intended primarily for middle esophageal lesions. • The advantages of the Ivor Lewis approach are (1) excellent exposure of the entire esophagus, with an improved opportunity to obtain clear margins; (2) ready accessibility to the azygous vein; and (3) the fact that the aortic arch is out of the way and protects the left pleural cavity. • The **left thoracoabdominal approach** gained popularity because it afforded excellent exposure of the distal esophagus, but it provides poor exposure for the upper esophagus. • This approach is associated with high morbidity and mortality as a result of transection of the costal margin and diaphragm, greater risk of injury to the azygous vein during the mobilization (because it is not seen clearly), and poor visualization of the upper esophagus.

The approach more recently popularized involves a **transhiatal blunt** resection of the thoracic esophagus from the abdomen, with subsequent pull-up of the stomach and an esophagogastric anastomosis in the neck. • W. Denk conceived the "blunt," or transhiatal, approach for esophagectomy in 1913 (see Comments, Question 1) and popularized by M.B. Orringer in 1980. • Such an approach violates the dictum of traditional cancer surgery that calls for a **radical en bloc resection** of the affected organ and regional lymph nodes in planes away from the tumor. • Nonetheless, proponents of blunt esophagectomy argue that the avoidance of thoracotomy minimizes morbidity from the operation, leakage from the cervical anastomosis is far less catastrophic than an intrathoracic leakage, postoperative GE reflux is less common than with an intrathoracic anastomosis, the technique has not detrimentally affected survival, and much of the distal esophagectomy is performed under direct vision. • Blunt esophagectomy, however, is not without complications. • Pneumothorax is common, and serious injury to the trachea, recurrent laryngeal nerve, aorta, or thoracic duct can occur. • Randomized prospective clinical trials comparing the blunt technique with standard radical esophagectomy have not been reported.

ANSWERS:
Question 44: A-a; B-b,c,d,e,f
Question 45: A, E

46. A 65-year-old Caucasian male presents with a 60-pack-per-year history of cigarette smoking and GERD. He has dysphagia to solids only and has had a 10-kg weight loss over the past 3 months. Which of the following is/are true?

A. The history is classic for a patient with achalasia.

B. Smoking or alcohol use are major risk factors for esophageal carcinoma.

C. CT is more sensitive than endoscopic ultrasound imaging for staging lymph nodes in the chest.

D. Lymph nodes must be biopsied before enrolling patients in adjuvant chemotherapy trials.

Ref.: 1–3, 11, 15

COMMENTS: The history is classic for a patient with esophageal carcinoma. • Smoking and alcohol use are the major risk factors for esophageal carcinoma. • The patient presents with typical symptoms of dysphagia, pain, and weight loss.

The evaluation of the patient focuses on the symptoms. • If dysphagia is present, the next step is to obtain a barium esophagram. • If a mass lesion is seen, an upper endoscopy with biopsy is imperative. • Once a malignancy is diagnosed, and if a patient is a good surgical candidate, it is typical to begin a metastatic workup.

CT scanning of the chest and abdomen are done in patients with esophageal carcinoma. • A CT scan will help to delineate the tumor itself and to determine the presence of distant pulmonary or hepatic metastasis. • A chest radiograph is routinely done before any major operation.

Endoscopic ultrasound imaging is more sensitive than CT in determining the presence of lymph node metastasis in the chest or celiac axis lymph node basins as well as in establishing the depth of tumor invasion. • Based on this information, a surgeon or medical oncologist may choose to enroll a patient in a trial with neoadjuvant chemoradiation therapy followed by surgery.

ANSWER:
B

47. With regard to the TNM staging of esophageal cancer, which of the following are true?

A. T1 tumors invade the submucosa.

B. T3 tumors invade the longitudinal muscle.

C. T4 tumors invade surrounding structures.

D. N2 lesions involve more than three lymph nodes.

E. M1 disease designates distant metastsis.

Ref.: 1–3

COMMENTS: The most accurate method of staging a patient with esophageal cancer is the Tumor (T), Node (N), and Metastsis (M) classification system. • This system is summarized in the tables.

Stage	Characteristics
Tx	Unable to assess primary tumor
T0	No residual tumor on histopathologic examination
Ti.s.	Carcinoma in situ
T1	Tumor invades submucosa
T2	Tumor invades muscularis
T3	Tumor invades adventia
T4	Tumor invades a surrounding structure
Nx	Unable to assess lymph nodes
N0	No lymph metastasis
N1	Lymph node metastasis
Mx	Unable to assess for metastatic disease
M0	No distant metastasis
M1	Metastatic disease

Stage	Tumor Classification
Stage 0	T0, N0, M0
	Ti.s, N0,M0
Stage I	T1, N0, M0
Stage IIA	T2, N0, M0
	T3, N0, M0
Stage II B	T1, N1, M0
	T2, N1, M0
Stage III	T3, N1, M0
	T4, any N, M0
Stage IV	Any T, any N, M1

ANSWER:
A, C, E

48. Most patients with esophageal cancer present with advanced disease. With regard to the stage of patients with esophageal cancer, which of the following are true?

A. Patients with stage IIB disease have a greater than 50% 5-year survival.

B. Patients with lymph node metastases have a greater than 50% 5-year survival.

C. Patients with tumors invading the muscularis propria have a greater than 50% 5-year survival.

D. After neoadjuvant chemoradiation followed by surgery, up to 25% of patients have T0 disease on final histopathologic examination.

E. Patients with columnar metaplasia are classified as stage 0.

Ref.: 1–3, 11, 17

COMMENTS: Esophageal cancer is diagnosed in about 13,000 patients per year in the United States. • Of these patients, more than 50% present with advanced disease, meaning full-thickness tumor invasion or lymph node metastases. • Due to this stratification of disease, most patients that present for resection have stage IIB or III disease.

Stage 0 patients are usually found through screening endoscopy of patients with Barrett's esophagus. • In this instance, the tumor is in situ or high-grade dysplasia. • No lymph node metastases are present.

Stage I patients represent a group in which the primary tumor has invaded the lamina propria but remains confined to the submucosa. • Lymph node metastases are not present.

Stage IIA is characterized by a primary tumor that has invaded further into the esophageal wall but not into the surrounding structures. • Lymph node metastases are not present.

Stage IIB disease is found when lymph node metastases are diagnosed. • However, the primary tumor has only invaded into the submucosa or muscularis propria of the esophagus. • Patients in this group should not be expected to have a survival of greater than 30% at 5 years.

Stage III is very similar to stage IIB, but, in this case, the primary tumor is found to invade through the esophageal wall into the adventitia and may involve surrounding structures, such as the pericardium, pleura, or aorta.

Stage IV represents the presence of metastatic disease.

Patients with columnar metaplasia alone are not placed into the TNM staging system. • However, this disease is a premalignant condition, and these patients should be screened with upper endoscopy and biopsy every 2 years. • If high-grade dysplasia is found, the patient is classified as T0, and esophagectomy is recommended.

The question of whether a patient should undergo preoperative chemoradiation therapy or surgery alone is still being debated in the literature. • To date, large nonrandomized trials and small randomized trials have been completed comparing patients undergoing neoadjuvant chemoradiation plus surgery to surgery alone for cancer of the esophagus. • In those who complete a neoadjuvant protocol followed by surgery, up to 25% of patients are noted to have a complete histologic response (T0, N0, M0), and these patients have up to a 70% 5-year survival. • More research is needed to select the patients who will benefit from neoadjuvant therapy, although the data are promising. • The table summarizes the 5-year survival rates found by various researchers.

Esophageal Cancer: 5-year Survival Rates

	I	IIA	IIB	III	IV
Skinner et al, 1986	55%	15%	27%	6%	0
Ellis et al, 1993	50.8%	37.5%	16.2%	13.6%	0
Roder et al, 1994	18%	14%	6%	4%	2%
Killinger et al, 1996		50%	38%		10%
Ellis et al, 1997	50.3%	22.5%	22.5%	16.7%	0

ANSWER:
D

49. Regarding patients with advanced esophageal carcinoma, which of the following are options for palliation?

   A. External beam radiation therapy

   B. Esophageal stent

   C. Chemotherapy

   D. Cervical esophagostomy and gastrostomy tube

   E. Neodymium:yttrium-aluminum-garnet (Nd:YAG) laser therapy

   F. Brachytherapy

Ref.: 1–3, 18

COMMENTS: Unfortunately, most carcinomas of the esophagus present at an advanced stage, and palliation may be the only realistic goal for these patients. • More than 70% of esophageal cancer patients present with dysphagia and/or pain. • A variety of treatment modalities to provide palliation for dysphagia have been developed and have evolved in recent years.

External beam radiation therapy alone offers little chance at cure. • However, in high-risk patients with advanced disease, up to 50% can be relieved of dysphagia. • The decision to undergo radiotherapy alone is difficult and is reserved for high-risk patients only. • Benefit can be gained from the addition of chemotherapy, but with this modality the morbidity is significantly increased.

Endoluminal brachytherapy administered with the aid of upper endoscopy is a more recently developed modality in palliating advanced esophageal cancer patients. • The brachytherapy catheters are used to deliver fractionated doses of about 6 Gy over a few weeks. • Up to 30% of patients are dysphagia free at 1 year, but this therapy is time consuming and requires multiple endoscopic evaluations. • Other modalities are less labor intensive and seem to have a better outcome.

Esophageal stent placement is an attractive method for malignant dysphagia palliation. • Rigid plastic or self-expanding metal stents can be placed. • Relief from dysphagia is immediate, and the stent allows for oral nutritional support. • Up to 80% of patients benefit when an esophageal stent is placed. • One disadvantage of esophageal stenting is that an experienced surgeon and/or endoscopist must be available to perform the procedure.

Nd:YAG laser tumor ablation is another method for palliation of malignant dysphagia. • A flexible endoscope is used during the ablation. • Patients benefit from relatively quick relief of symptoms with this method compared to the use of external beam radiation. • However, repeated treatments as frequently as every 2–4 months may be necessary.

ANSWER:
A B, E, F

50. After diagnostic esophagoscopy, a patient complains of odynophagia and chest pain, but results of a water-soluble contrast swallow are negative. Which of the following apply?

   A. Discharge the patient if the electrocardiogram is normal.

   B. Use of barium in the chest is devastating.

   C. Esophageal manometry should be performed immediately.

   D. Repeat the swallow with barium.

Ref.: 1–3, 5

COMMENTS: Chest pain, fever, tachycardia, subcutaneous emphysema, dysphagia, and dyspnea are typical of esophageal perforation. • Perforation may result from iatrogenic operations (e.g., periesophageal endoscopy), external trauma, primary esophageal disease, or postemetic ("spontaneous") esophageal hypertension. • The incidence of mortality from esophageal perforation is clearly related to the time interval between perforation and definitive treatment. • Whenever perforation is suspected, a contrast study should be performed with water-soluble contrast material. • However, if this study does not demonstrate the perforation, it should be repeated with barium. • Although barium is contraindicated in the presence of colonic injuries because of the harmful effects of feces and barium, it does not cause a problem in the chest. • Barium is more accurate than water-soluble contrast media for delineating esophageal leakage. • Contrast studies are important not only for verifying esophageal rupture but also for documenting the level of injury, which has important implications for treatment. • Although endoscopy can be used in cases of suspected esophageal perforation and may enable retrieval of a foreign body, it is usually not required and is associated with the potential hazard of extending the perforation.

ANSWER:
D

51. For each clinical situation described in the left-hand column, choose the most appropriate treatment in the right-hand column.

   A. Septic patient with 48-hr-old perforation of the thoracic esophagus and pneumohydrothorax

   a. Antibiotics, nothing orally, and parenteral nutrition

   B. Stable patient with fever, subcutaneous emphysema, and cervical perforation 2 hr after endoscopy

   b. Emergency esophagectomy

   C. Patient with epidermolysis bullosa, minimal chest pain, and low-grade fever 2 days after endoscopy and an esophagram showing thoracic perforation with limited mediastinal involvement

   c. Pleural drainage, esophageal exclusion, gastrostomy, and cervical esophagostomy

D. Patient with 6-hr-old stab wound, fever of 102°F (38.9°C), left pleural effusion, and thoracic esophageal perforation

d. Primary transthoracic esophageal repair

E. A 65-year-old patient with cancer of the esophagus, chest pain, and pneumohydrothorax 6 hr after endoscopy

e. Transcervical esophageal repair and drainage

f. Emergency esophagectomy

g. Emergency esophagectomy and colon interposition

Ref.: 1–3, 5

COMMENTS: Treatment of esophageal perforation depends on the site and extent of injury, the cause, the presence or absence of underlying esophageal disease, the patient's general status, and the time interval between perforation and diagnosis. • The latter factor is particularly significant.

Cervical perforations usually can be managed with transcervical drainage. • Repair is desirable if technically possible.

Recognized early perforations of the *thoracic* esophagus can be managed successfully by primary esophageal repair, the principles of which include layered closure of the esophagus, buttressing of the repair, and thoracic drainage. The gastric fundus or pleural or pericardial flaps can be useful for buttressing the sutured closure and are important for decreasing postoperative leakage.

Among *septic patients with late perforations*, the mortality rate is high. These patients require aggressive control of the septic focus. • Attempts at primary repair are doomed to failure. Techniques of esophageal exclusion may be useful in this setting. Some surgeons also favor esophagectomy. • In patients with esophageal perforations and underlying esophageal disease, such as obstructing distal lesions, surgical management of the perforation includes definitive treatment of the underlying pathologic process. It may necessitate esophagectomy, for example, in patients with perforation and concomitant esophageal cancer.

There is a subset of patients who may be managed conservatively without operation. • They include stable patients with perforations that are recognized late; patients with epidermolysis bullosa, who often demonstrate asymptomatic limited perforations; patients who are clinically stable and improving; patients in whom perforation is radiographically limited, without pleural extension; and patients with evidence of spontaneous drainage of the periesophageal cavity back into the esophagus.

ANSWER:
A-c; B-e; C-a; D-d; E-b

52. A 4-year-old child is brought to the emergency room 15 minutes after ingesting drain cleaner. The child is hoarse and stridorous. Which of the following apply?

A. Laryngeal ulceration

B. Instillation of vinegar into the stomach

C. Immediate fiberoptic endoscopy

D. Tracheostomy

Ref.: 1–3, 5

COMMENTS: See Question 54.

53. With regard to the role of endoscopy in the acute therapy of a patient who has ingested a corrosive substance, which of the following statements is/are true?

A. It should be performed after 24 hr if the patient is stable.

B. It is contraindicated before esophagography because of the risk of perforation.

C. It is contraindicated if obvious oropharyngeal burns are present.

D. It is used to remove a button-type alkaline battery from the esophagus.

E. The full extent of the injury must be visualized to determine appropriate therapy.

Ref.: 1–3, 5

COMMENTS: See Question 54.

54. Which of the following is/are indications for emergency surgical intervention for corrosive ingestion?

A. Cervical subcutaneous crepitance

B. Presence of alkaline gastric contents

C. Extensive damage to the esophagus and stomach

D. Scattered exudate in the esophagus found on endoscopic examination

Ref.: 1–3, 5

COMMENTS: When caustic alkaline burns of the esophagus are suspected, the ingested agent should promptly be identified and the extent of injury assessed early. • Superficial burns usually heal without complication, whereas deeper injury must be aggressively but judiciously treated to avoid late formation of stricture and yet not cause iatrogenic perforations. • Early endoscopic examination is important for verifying the presence or absence of esophageal injury and for assessing its severity. • It is critical that the endoscope not be advanced any farther than the proximal extent of injury to avoid perforation, and endoscopic examination is contraindicated when perforation is suspected. • The distal extent of injury can be assessed radiographically at a later date when the patient is stable. • Esophagoscopy is contraindicated in patients with evidence of perforation or potential airway obstruction.

Aggressive attempts to neutralize or dilute the corrosive agent are not helpful because the injury is instantaneous, and as little as 1 ml of lye has been known to cause extensive esophageal injury. • Likewise, induced emesis and lavage also are contraindicated because they may aggravate the injury. • Patients who swallow disk-shaped alkaline batteries should have them removed endoscopically if they are lodged in the esophagus.

The child described in Question 52 exhibits laryngeal or epiglottic edema, and preservation of the airway must be the priority of treatment. Endoscopic examination is therefore deferred, and tracheostomy may be required. • When an esophageal burn is confirmed or when the presence or absence of an esophageal injury cannot be verified because of airway considerations, treatment with antibiotics and steroids has been advocated, although there is no statistical evidence that steroids lessen early complications or late stricture formation. • Early esophageal dilatation has been advocated by some clinicians, but this, too, has not been demonstrated to prevent later stricture formation. • Indeed, it may lead to iatrogenic injury. Silastic stents have been beneficial for avoiding strictures when left in for 2–3 weeks. • It may be best to avoid the use of steroids in patients with suspected perforation or acid ingestion. • In such patients, the site of injury is more frequently the stomach than the esophagus, and the addition of steroid therapy may increase the risk of hemorrhage or peptic ulceration.

In most cases, oral intake is allowed after several days, when the edema of the initial injury has subsided and the patient can swallow effectively. • Oral intake, in fact, provides a natural method of esophageal dilatation and may help prevent stricture formation. • Radiographic studies at this time disclose the full extent of the injury. • Swallowing usually is possible for 2–3 weeks, at which time stricturing may begin. • At that time, radiographic studies are repeated to confirm the full anatomy, and dilatation is begun.

The presence or absence of oropharyngeal burns in a patient with suspected corrosive injection is not a reliable indicator of esophageal injury. • In general, acids such as sulfuric acid and nitric acid cause coagulation injuries, whereas alkali substances cause liquefaction injury.

Emergency surgery after ingestion of corrosive substances may necessitate thoracotomy, laparotomy, or both. • Indications for emergency *thoracotomy* are signs and symptoms of mediastinitis or perforation of the esophagus: severe chest pain, tachycardia, cervical subcutaneous crepitance, wide mediastinum, pneumomediastinum, pneumothorax, and pleural effusion. • The only indication for radiopaque contrast studies of the esophagus or stomach at this time is a suspicion of perforation secondary to the burn or to the use of instrumentation. • Indications for *laparotomy* are signs of perforation, free abdominal air, interstitial air in the wall of the stomach, and radiologic confirmation of perforation. • Laparotomy is also indicated if nasogastric intubation was erroneously performed, when advanced injury to the esophagus or stomach is seen on endoscopic examination, or when nasogastric alkali contents from the stomach have been aspirated (once alkali contents have reached the stomach, direct visualization of the stomach is necessary to rule out full-thickness liquification necrosis).

ANSWERS:
Question 52: A, D
Question 53: D
Question 54: A, B, C

55. With regard to the late sequelae of ingestion of corrosive substances, which of the following statements is/are true?

A. Stricture is best treated by botulin neurotoxin injection.

B. Acid ingestion is complicated more commonly by gastric outlet obstruction than by esophageal stricture.

C. Tracheoesophageal fistula is best treated by leaving an excluded segment of esophagus attached.

D. Cancer that develops after corrosive injury carries a better prognosis than does esophageal cancer in general.

Ref.: 1–3, 5

COMMENTS: Late complications of corrosive burns of the esophagus include stricture, GE reflux, malignancy, and, rarely, tracheoesophageal fistula. • Strictures often are multiple and involve the cervical esophagus, the region of the aortic arch, and the cardia. • Spasm of the cricopharyngeal muscle may entrap the corrosive agent in the pharynx, resulting in pharyngeal obstruction and, often, severe laryngeal injury, necessitating permanent tracheostomy. • The standard treatment for stricture is esophageal dilatation, often performed in a retrograde manner through a gastrostomy. • There is limited experience with treatment of localized strictures by direct injection of steroids. • Refractory strictures

may necessitate esophagectomy or a bypass operation. • Direct approach to the repair of tracheoesophageal fistula should be avoided. • It is best to leave a small segment of excluded esophagus attached to the fistula. • For patients in whom severe GE reflux develops as the result of scarring and shortening of the esophagus and hiatal hernia, dilatation of the stricture may necessitate an associated antireflux operation. • Malignant degeneration is a well-recognized complication of corrosive esophageal stricture and should be suspected in any patient with long-standing stricture who exhibits a change in symptoms. • The prognosis of patients with these cancers, however, has been more favorable than that of patients without this predisposing injury or with sporadic epidermoid cancer, and resection may provide cure. • In contradistinction to alkaline ingestion, acid ingestion more commonly produces gastric injury. • This is because the squamous epithelium of the esophagus is somewhat resistant to acid injury and the pylorospasm that accompanies acid ingestion prolongs contact with the stomach.

ANSWER:
B, C, D

REFERENCES

1. Townsend CM, Beauchamp RD, Evers BM, et al (eds): *Sabiston Textbook of Surgery: The Biological Basis of Modern Surgical Practice*, 17th ed. WB Saunders, Philadelphia, 2004.
2. Schwartz SI, Shires GT, Spencer FC: *Principles of Surgery*, 8th ed. McGraw-Hill, New York, 2004.
3. Greenfield LJ, Mulholland MW, Oldham KT: *Surgery: Scientific Principles and Practice*, 3rd ed. Lippincott, Williams & Wilkins, Philadelphia, 2001.
4. Skinner DB: Pathophysiology of gastroesophageal reflux. *Ann Surg* 202:546–556, 1985.
5. Skinner DB, Belsey RHH: *Management of Esophageal Disease*. WB Saunders, Philadelphia, 1988.
6. Stein HJ, DeMeester TR, Hinder RA: Outpatient physiologic testing and surgical management of foregut motility disorders. *Curr Probl Surg* 24:413–555, 1992.
7. Haag S: Regression of Barrett's esophagus: the role of acid suppression, surgery, and ablative methods. *Gastrointest Endosc* 50(2): 229–40, 1999.
8. Bowrey D: Laparoscopic esophageal surgery. *Surg Clin North Am* 80(4):1213–1242, 2000.
9. Frantzides C: A prospective randomized trial of laparoscopic polytetrafluoroethylene (PTFE) patch repair vs. simple cruroplasty for large hiatal hernia. *Arch Surg* 137(6):649–652, 2002.
10. Millikan K, Saclarides T: *Common Surgical Diseases: An Algorithmic Approach to Problem Solving*. Springer-Verlag, New York, 1998.
11. Christein J, Hollinger E, Millikan K: Prognostic factors associated with resectable carcinoma of the esophagus. *Am Surg*: 68(3):258–262, 2002.
12. Katzka DA: Barrett's esophagus: surveillance and treatment. *Gastroenterol Clin North Am* 31(2):481–497, 2002
13. Rüedi TP: State of the Art of Surgery 1991/92 [summaries of the Luncheon Panels held at the 34th World Congress of Surgery of the International Society of Surgery, organized as International Surgical Week in Stockholm, 1991]. Schwabe, Basel, 1992.
14. Weiss GD, Read RC: The Ivor-Lewis procedure. *Surg Rounds* 7:41–48, 1984.
15. Orringer MB: Transhiatal esophagectomy without thoracotomy for carcinoma of the thoracic esophagus. Ann Surg 200:282–288, 1984.
16. Botet JF, Lightdale CJ, Zauber AG, et al: Preoperative staging of esophageal cancer: comparison of endoscopic US and dynamic CT. *Radiology* 181(2):419–425, 1991.
17. Rafaely Y: Multimodal therapy for esophageal cancer. *Surg Clin North Am* 82(4):729–746, 2002.
18. Weigel TL: Endoluminal palliation for dysphagia secondary to esophageal carcinoma. *Surg Clin North Am* 82(4):747–761, 2002.

CHAPTER 32

Stomach and Duodenum

Daniel J. Deziel, M.D.

1. With regard to the blood supply of the stomach, which of the following statements is/are true?

A. The right gastric artery arises from the common hepatic artery and constitutes the major vascular supply to the antrum.

B. The left gastric artery often originates anomalously from the superior mesenteric artery.

C. The gastroepiploic arcade arises from both the gastroduodenal and splenic arteries.

D. Ligation of the splenic artery results in necrosis of the greater curvature of the stomach.

Ref.: 1–3

COMMENTS: The arterial blood supply of the stomach is derived primarily from the celiac trunk, which gives off the hepatic, left gastric, and splenic arteries. • The **left gastric artery** usually arises directly from the celiac trunk and is found at the proximal lesser curvature, where it divides into ascending and descending branches. • An anatomic variation of surgical significance is origination of a left hepatic artery from the left gastric artery. • The **right gastric artery** typically originates from the common hepatic artery distal to the gastroduodenal artery. • This vessel contributes to the pyloroduodenal blood supply and does not generally anastomose widely with the left gastric artery, as is sometimes pictured. • The **right gastroepiploic artery** usually comes from the gastroduodenal artery (occasionally from the superior mesenteric artery), whereas the left gastroepiploic artery arises from the splenic artery. • The extent of connection between the right and left gastroepiploic vessels is variable. • The **vasa brevia**, or **short gastric arteries**, arise from the branches of the splenic or left gastroepiploic artery. • Because of the abundant collateral blood supply present, the stomach is well protected from ischemia and can survive with ligation of all but one of its major vessels. • The splenic artery may also contribute a branch to the posterior fundus, referred to as the **posterior gastric artery**.

ANSWER:
C

2. When the stomach is mobilized for esophageal replacement, the arterial supply is primarily based on which of the following vessels?

A. Left gastric artery

B. Right gastric artery

C. Left gastroepiploic artery

D. Right gastroepiploic artery

E. Superior mesenteric artery

Ref.: 1–3

COMMENTS: The left gastric artery arising from the celiac trunk and the short gastric vessels arising from branches of the splenic artery are routinely divided when the stomach is mobilized for esophageal replacement. • The main blood supply of the gastric interposition is derived from the right gastroepiploic artery. • The gastroduodenal artery, from which the right gastroepiploic vessel originates, must therefore be preserved during dissection. • Under usual circumstances, the right gastric artery and the superior mesenteric artery contribute a less significant proportion of the blood supply to the mobilized stomach.

ANSWER:
D

3. Match each item in the left-hand column with the appropriate vagal innervation-related item in the right-hand column.

A. Right thoracic vagus   a. Anterior abdominal vagus

B. Left thoracic vagus   b. Posterior abdominal vagus

C. Sympathetic innervation   c. Both

D. Hepatic vagal branch   d. Neither

E. Celiac vagal branch

F. Nerve of Latarget

G. "Crow's foot"

H. Criminal nerve of Grassi

Ref.: 1–4

COMMENTS: Parasympathetic innervation of the foregut and midgut is supplied by the vagus nerves (sacral parasympathetic nerves supply the hindgut). • Sympathetic innervation of the stomach travels via the splanchnic nerves (preganglionic) and fibers along branches of the celiac artery (postganglionic). • In the thorax, vagal trunks are right and left of the esophagus. • As the result of embryonic gastric rotation, the vagal trunks assume anterior (left vagus) and posterior (right vagus) positions at the level of the cardia. • The anterior vagus divides into anterior gastric (anterior nerve of

Latarget) and hepatic branches. • A separate pyloric nerve (nerve of McCrea) may arise from the anterior vagus or its hepatic branch. • The posterior vagus divides into posterior gastric (posterior nerve of Latarget) and celiac branches. • The "crow's foot" refers to the distal branches of the gastric vagal divisions in the pyloroantral region where the nerves of Latarget terminate. • The term was first used in reference to the distal branches of the descending left gastric artery. • The vagal branches to the proximal fundus do not originate from a constant level, and, if they are missed, incomplete vagotomy can result. • Indeed, a simple anterior vagus nerve is present in only 60% of patients and a simple posterior one in 40%. • One of those proximal branches, originating from the posterior vagal innervation, is known as the criminal nerve of Grassi. • Selective vagotomy divides the nerves of Latarget below the hepatic and celiac branches. • Highly selective vagotomy divides individual branches of the nerve of Latarget, preserving the "crow's foot."

A N S W E R :
A-b; B-a; C-d; D-a; E-b; F-c; G-c; H-b

4. Match each cell type in the left-hand column with the appropriate secretory product or products in the right-hand column.

A. Parietal cell	a. Intrinsic factor
B. Chief cell	b. Gastrin
C. G cell	c. Pepsinogen
D. Brunner's gland	d. Hydrochloric acid
E. Neck cells	e. Mucus

Ref.: 1–3, 5

COMMENTS: See Question 5.

5. Match the cell types in the left-hand column with their primary anatomic location in the right-hand column.

A. Parietal cell	a. Gastric cardia
B. Chief cell	b. Gastric corpus and fundus
C. G cell	c. Gastric antrum
D. Brunner's gland	d. Duodenum
E. Delta cell	

Ref.: 1–3, 5

COMMENTS: The gastric mucosa consists of surface columnar epithelial cells and glands containing various cell types. • The mucosal cells have various specific secretory functions and anatomic distributions. • These relationships constitute the physiologic foundation on which surgical management of peptic ulcer disease is based. • **Parietal cells** (which produce hydrochloric acid and intrinsic factor) and **chief cells** (which produce pepsinogens) are located predominantly in the fundus and corpus. • The **G cells** of the antrum are the primary source of gastrin. • The duodenum in humans contains 10–20% as much gastrin as does the antrum, and it appears to be physiologically active. • Mucus, for lubrication, is secreted by gastric surface epithelial cells, neck cells of the gastric glands, and **Brunner's glands**. • Brunner's glands are found in the submucosa of the proximal duodenum and are also a source of pepsinogens. • Somatostatin presumably is synthesized and stored by the **delta (antral) cells**. • Other mediators, such as serotonin and prostaglandins, are also produced in the stomach. • Subtotal gastrectomy removes a large portion of the acid-secreting parietal cell mass. • Antrectomy removes the main

source of acid-stimulating gastrin. • The effectiveness of highly selective vagotomy is based on denervation of the parietal cell mass. • After resections of the corpus and fundus, periodic injections of vitamin B_{12} are required to prevent a deficiency caused by lack of intrinsic factor.

A N S W E R S :
Question 4: A-a, d; B-c; C-b; D-c, e; E-e
Question 5: A-b; B-b; C-c, d; D-d; E-c

6. The oxyntic portion of the stomach consists of which anatomic area(s)?

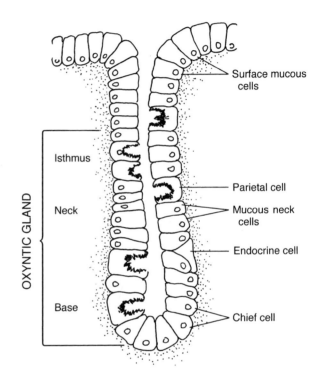

A. Cardia

B. Fundus

C. Corpus

D. Antrum

E. Pylorus

Ref.: 3, 5

COMMENTS: The oxyntic portion of the stomach contains the oxyntic, or parietal, glands, which are the acid-producing glands. • The oxyntic glands, as illustrated, have a characteristic histologic arrangement and contain surface mucous cells and mucous neck cells near the top, scattered parietal cells and enteroendocrine cells, and chief cells at the bottom. • The oxyntic glands occupy the gastric fundus and corpus. • The gastric cardia is the area just distal to the gastroesophageal (GE) junction, and the fundus is above and to the left of the GE junction. • The border between the corpus and more distal antrum is more distinct on histologic than on gross examination. • The pylorus can readily be identified by its thick muscular ring.

A N S W E R :
B, C

7. Which parietal cell receptors stimulate acid secretion?

A. Histamine

B. Gastrin

C. Acetylcholine

D. Prostaglandin E$_2$

E. Somatostatin

Ref.: 1, 3, 5

COMMENTS: See Question 8.

8. The final common pathway of acid secretion by parietal cells involves which one of the following?

A. Adenylate cyclase

B. H$^+$-K$^+$-ATPase

C. Increased intracellular Ca^{2+}

D. Protein kinase

E. Phosphorylase kinase

Ref.: 1, 3, 5

COMMENTS: Understanding the cellular basis for parietal cell acid secretion is important in order to appreciate the pharmacologic control of acid in clinical practice. • The parietal cell has three specific plasma membrane receptors that stimulate acid: histamine, acetylcholine, and gastrin receptors. • These three receptors eventually activate a common proton pump, H$^+$-K$^+$-ATPase, resulting in an exchange of hydrogen ions for potassium. • The mechanisms and second-messenger systems by which this occurs are different for various secretogues. • Histamine activates adenylate cyclase and subsequently a protein kinase that leads to protein phosphorylation and H$^+$-K$^+$-ATPase activation. • Gastrin- and acetylcholine-stimulated secretion depends on specific membrane phospholipases and increases in intracellular calcium levels, with subsequent phosphorylase kinase–induced protein phosphorylation and H$^+$-K$^+$-ATPase activity. • Parietal cells also have somatostatin and prostaglandin receptors that inhibit acid secretion. • Pharmacologic agents act at various sites during this process.

ANSWERS:
Question 7: A, B, C
Question 8: B

9. Gastric acid secretion is stimulated by all but which of the following?

A. Acetylcholine

B. Duodenal gastrin

C. Intraluminal protein

D. Secretin

E. Gastric distention

Ref.: 1–3, 5

COMMENTS: There are cephalic, gastric, and intestinal phases of gastric acid secretion. • As previously mentioned, the parietal cell has receptors for acetylcholine, gastrin, and histamine that stimulate acid secretion. • The **cephalic phase** is primarily mediated by the vagus nerve and by neuropeptides. • Vagal cholinergic stimulation directly releases acid from parietal cells, in addition to releasing gastrin from the antrum. • The **gastric phase** is mediated by gastrin released in response to gastric distention, peptides, and amino acids. • Although the antrum is the predominant source of gastrin, secretion from the duodenal mucosa also occurs, accounting for part of the **intestinal phase** of gastric acid secretion. • An intestinal hormone, entero-oxyntin, has also been implicated as a stimulant of gastric acid secretion during the intestinal phase, but this entity has not been specifically characterized. • Duodenal acidification releases secretin, which blocks gastrin receptors on the parietal cell without affecting histamine or acetylcholine sites. • Antral acidification releases somatostatin, which inhibits acid and gastrin release. • Cholecystokinin and enterogastrones also inhibit acid secretion.

ANSWER:
D

10. Match the intestinal peptide hormone in the left-hand column with its function in the right-hand column.

A. Cholecystokinin	a. Stimulates gastric acid secretion
B. Gastric inhibitory peptide	b. Stimulates intestinal secretion and motility
C. Motilin	c. Inhibits release of gastrin
D. Somatostatin	d. Regulates phase III interdigestive migrating motor complex
E. Bombesin	e. Inhibits gastric acid secretion and potentiates insulin secretion
F. Vasoactive intestinal peptide	f. Stimulates pancreatic exocrine secretion

Ref.: 1–3

COMMENTS: The gastrointestinal (GI) mucosa is rich in endocrine cells that produce single-chain polypeptides to act as hormones and neurotransmitters. • These peptides act in a complex interplay to control GI tract secretion, motility, and absorption and gut growth. • **Cholecystokinin** is produced in the I cells of the duodenum and upper jejunum. • Amino acids and fatty acids in the upper intestine stimulate its release. • The main actions in the GI tract are the stimulation of pancreatic exocrine secretion and gallbladder contraction. • It has two known receptors. • **Gastric inhibitory peptide** (GIP) is found in K cells of the duodenum and jejunum and is released in response to ingested nutrients. • Inhibition of gastric acid secretion and potentiation of glucose-induced insulin release are its two main actions. • Motilin is secreted by M cells in the duodenum, jejunum, and upper ileum. • It regulates the activity front (phase III) of the interdigestive migrating motor complex. • **Somatostatin** is found in greatest concentration in the GI tract in pancreatic islet D cells and in the gastric antrum. • It has a wide range of inhibitory actions on the release of insulin, glucagon, gastrin, secretin, GIP, motilin, neurotensin, and enteroglucagon. • The result of somatostatin release is inhibition of gastric emptying, pancreatic endocrine and exocrine secretion, and gallbladder contraction. • **Bombesin**, or gastric-releasing peptide, is found throughout the enteric and central nervous systems. • It has stimulating effects on intestinal motor activity, pancreatic enzyme secretion, and gastric acid secretion. • **Vasoactive intestinal peptide (VIP)** is mainly a neurotransmitter in the enteric nervous system. • It is a strong stimulus for intestinal secretion and motility.

ANSWER:
A-f; B-e; C-d; D-c; E-a, f; F-b

11. With regard to normal gastric emptying, which of the following statements is/are true?

   A. Emptying of solids is dependent on fundal tone.

   B. The rate of emptying of solids is linear.

   C. Emptying of liquids is dependent on antral propulsion.

   D. The rate of emptying of liquids is exponential.

   E. Patterns of emptying of solids and liquids are similar.

Ref.: 1, 3, 5

COMMENTS: Gastric emptying, regulated by changes in gastric motor activity, is a complicated process influenced by meal composition and by neural and hormonal factors. • Emptying of solids is different from emptying of liquids. • Emptying of solids depends on mechanical action of the pyloroantral region. • Propulsive and retropulsive activity breaks solids into small particles that become mixed with the liquid gastric contents. • The pattern of emptying of solids is linear after an initial lag period. • Gastric emptying of liquids depends primarily on the pressure gradient between the proximal stomach and the pylorus and is largely determined by fundal tone. • The pattern of emptying of liquids is exponential, and the rate is determined by the volume of gastric contents.

ANSWER:
B, D

12. Which of the following clinical conditions is/are associated with rapid gastric emptying?

   A. Hyperglycemia

   B. Hypokalemia

   C. Scleroderma

   D. Gastric resection

   E. Zollinger-Ellison syndrome

Ref.: 1, 3, 5

COMMENTS: Abnormalities in gastric emptying can produce significant and disabling clinical situations. • Most clinically significant problems of gastric motility are related to delayed gastric emptying. • Other than mechanical obstruction, important causes of delayed gastric emptying include drugs (e.g., opiates and anticholinergics), electrolyte imbalances (e.g., hypokalemia and hypocalcemia), metabolic derangements (e.g., myxedema and hyperglycemia), and systemic diseases (e.g., diabetes mellitus and scleroderma). • Disorders of rapid gastric emptying are encountered less frequently and are most commonly a consequence of previous gastric surgery, such as resection. • Other situations associated with rapid gastric emptying include Zollinger-Ellison syndrome, caused by hypergastrinemia and lack of inhibition by duodenal acidification, and conditions producing steatorrhea caused by loss of inhibition of gastric emptying from impaired fat absorption (e.g., from pancreatic insufficiency, short bowel syndrome, or gluten enteropathy). • Duodenal ulcer may be associated with normal or rapid gastric emptying.

ANSWER:
D, E

13. Gastric emptying of solids is best assessed by which one of the following tests?

   A. Saline load test

   B. Serial intubation and aspiration of test meal

   C. Technetium 99m pertechnetate (^{99m}Tc)-labeling radionuclide scintigraphy

   D. Indium 111 (^{111}In)-labeling radionuclide scintigraphy

   E. Barium burger upper GI series

Ref.: 1, 3, 5

COMMENTS: Gastric emptying of solids is most accurately assessed by radionuclide scans after ingestion of ^{99m}Tc-labeled chicken liver or egg white. • The isotope remains bound to the solid phase, and computer quantification of emptying is possible by analysis of appropriately selected windows through use of the geometric mean of the anterior and posterior counts. • The radioisotope ^{111}In remains in the liquid phase of gastric contents and is thus a marker for assessment of liquid emptying. • Traditional radiographic contrast studies provide only a rough qualitative assessment of gastric emptying. • Barium may empty with the liquid phase, and labeling of ingested solids is not an accurate method for determining solid emptying. • The saline load test (whereby 750 ml of saline solution is instilled into the stomach and the residual volume is aspirated 30 minutes later) and other intubation tests involving nonabsorbable markers are inconvenient, less sensitive, and limited to assessment of liquid emptying.

ANSWER:
C

14. With regard to postoperative effects on gastric emptying, which of the following statements is/are true?

   A. Truncal vagotomy delays emptying of liquids.

   B. Truncal vagotomy accelerates emptying of solids.

   C. Parietal cell vagotomy does not affect gastric emptying.

   D. Pyloroplasty accelerates emptying of solids.

   E. Roux-en-Y gastrojejunostomy delays gastric emptying.

Ref.: 1, 3, 5

COMMENTS: Changes in gastric emptying result from operative procedures on the stomach. • These changes occasionally produce clinically significant problems, ranging from delayed emptying to the dumping syndrome. • Resective procedures with Billroth I or Billroth II reconstruction are usually accompanied by more rapid emptying. • Reconstruction by Roux-en-Y gastrojejunostomy can result in impaired emptying of the gastric remnant and the Roux limb of the jejunum, perhaps because of interruption of neural impulses from the duodenal pacemaker. • Vagal denervation of the proximal stomach accelerates emptying of liquids as a result of the loss of receptive relaxation and accommodation. • Parietal cell vagotomy is therefore associated with increased emptying of liquids but normal emptying of solids. • Complete gastric vagotomy, in the form of truncal vagotomy or selective vagotomy, also delays emptying of solids. • The addition of a pyloroplasty initially increases the rate of emptying of solids. • Later, emptying may be delayed or remain rapid. • The pattern of emptying of solids after various types of vagal denervation often normalizes over time.

ANSWER:
D, E

15. Gastric infection with *Helicobacter pylori* has been associated with all but which of the following conditions?

A. Duodenal ulcer

B. Gastric ulcer

C. Chronic gastritis

D. Gastric cancer

E. Eosinophilic gastroenteritis

Ref.: 1, 3

COMMENTS: *H. pylori* (formerly *Campylobacter pylori*) is a gram-negative microaerophilic spiral bacterium that chronically infects the gastroduodenal mucosa in a high percentage of patients with gastroduodenal disorders. • Investigators have demonstrated *H. pylori* infection in most patients with antral gastritis, duodenal ulcer, and gastric ulcer. • Infection may play an etiologic role in these conditions, inasmuch as treatment of *H. pylori* has resulted in healing of gastritis, more rapid healing of duodenal ulcers, and significantly lower recurrence rates for both duodenal and gastric ulcers. • In addition, *H. pylori* has been associated with chronic atrophic gastritis, which in turn is associated with gastric cancer. • *H. pylori* infection may be a cofactor in gastric carcinogenesis. • Colloidal bismuth subcitrate in combination with one or two antibiotics has proved effective in eradicating *H. pylori* infection. • Gastric cancers below the cardia are approximately three times more common in patients with *H. pylori* infection than in noninfected control subjects. • Eosinophilic gastroenteritis is an unusual infiltrative disorder typically affecting the gastric antrum. • Its cause is unknown.

ANSWER:
E

16. Which of the following tests is/are not appropriate for the detection of *H. pylori* in dyspeptic patients?

A. Urea breath test

B. Rapid urease testing (RUT) of a mucosal biopsy specimen

C. Culture and sensitivity testing of a mucosal biopsy specimen

D. Histologic evaluation of a mucosal biopsy specimen

E. Serologic assay for *H. pylori* antibodies

Ref.: 6

COMMENTS: Because of the important role of *H. pylori* in the cause of peptic ulcer disease, it is important to document the presence or absence of the organism in order to optimally treat dyspeptic patients. • Several methods have been developed to detect host colonization with *H. pylori*, but there continues to be debate on the optimal detection strategy. • RUT of mucosal biopsy specimens utilizes a change in pH resulting from the breakdown of urea in culture media caused by a urease enzyme in the bacteria. • It is probably the test of choice because of its accuracy, low cost, simplicity, and rapid availability of results. • Histologic study is the gold standard and should always be performed when endoscopic biopsy specimens are obtained, to confirm RUT results and assess the integrity of the gastric mucosa. • Cultures with sensitivities should also be obtained from the biopsy specimen at the same procedure. • Urea breath tests are reported to be 90–100% sensitive and are indicated when endoscopic examination is not performed. • Serologic tests for the presence of antibodies to the organism have been questioned for all but epidemiologic purposes.

• Polymerase chain reaction methods to detect the organism in biopsy specimens are also available and highly accurate but expensive. • At present, the optimal strategy for detecting *H. pylori* in dyspeptic patients should employ at least two of the above mentioned methods utilizing random biopsy specimens from the antrum and corpus of the stomach.

ANSWER:
E

17. Gastric secretion tests in an unoperated patient demonstrate a basal acid output (BAO) of 2 mmol/hr and a peak acid output (PAO) of 25 mmol/hr. These findings are most consistent with which of the following conditions?

A. Duodenal ulcer

B. Zollinger-Ellison syndrome

C. Normal acid secretion

D. Pernicious anemia

E. Antral G-cell hyperplasia

Ref.: 4

COMMENTS: The normal mean BAO is about 2 mmol/hr (range 0–>5 mmol/hr), and the normal mean PAO is 20–35 mmol/ hr (range <1–60 mmol/hr). • Patients with duodenal ulcer commonly have increased gastric acid output, whereas patients with gastric ulcer typically have outputs in the normal range. • Adults with pernicious anemia are achlorhydric. • Patients with gastric cancer may also be achlorhydric or have subnormal acid outputs. • In contrast, Zollinger-Ellison syndrome and antral G-cell hyperplasia are associated with hypergastrinemia and high gastric acid output. • Gastric secretory studies in gastrinoma patients may demonstrate a BAO of more than 15 mmol/hr and a BAO/maximal acid output ratio that exceeds 60%, although acid secretory studies alone are not reliable for establishing the diagnosis.

ANSWER:
C

18. Elevated serum gastrin levels during fasting are typical in all but which of the following conditions?

A. Pernicious anemia

B. Chronic gastritis

C. Duodenal ulcer

D. Postvagotomy state

E. Gastric outlet obstruction

Ref.: 2, 4

COMMENTS: Hypergastrinemia has a broad differential diagnosis that can be narrowed considerably by consideration of several clinical factors. • Conditions associated with elevated serum gastrin levels *and* increased acid secretion include Zollinger-Ellison syndrome, antral G-cell hyperplasia, retained antrum, renal failure, gastric outlet obstruction, and short bowel syndrome. • In contradistinction, hypergastrinemia is associated with normal or diminished acid production in pernicious anemia, chronic gastritis, gastric cancer, and postvagotomy states and in patients receiving pharmacologic agents for acid suppression. • Serum gastrin levels during fasting are normal in patients with uncomplicated duodenal ulcer but may be excessively elevated postprandially.

• The absolute level of an abnormally elevated serum gastrin level is not necessarily indicative of the cause. • Although marked elevations (>1000 pg/ml) are often associated with Zollinger-Ellison syndrome, the elevations are not always as pronounced and may overlap considerably with those seen in other conditions. • Pernicious anemia can also be associated with high gastrin levels.

ANSWER:
C

19. Match each finding in the left-hand column with the appropriate condition or conditions in the right-hand column.

    A. Serum gastrin level   a. Zollinger-Ellison syndrome
       is elevated.

    B. Gastric acid output   b. Antral G cell hyperplasia
       is elevated.

    C. Secretin stimulation   c. Both
       markedly increases
       gastrin level.

    D. Protein meal markedly   d. Neither
       increases gastrin levels.

    E. Bombesin stimulation
       markedly increases
       gastrin level.

Ref.: 4

COMMENTS: Zollinger-Ellison syndrome, antral G-cell hyperplasia, and retained antrum are conditions causing peptic ulcer that are associated with hypergastrinemia as a cause of elevated gastric acid secretion. • Although these conditions are unusual, they must be differentiated to determine proper therapy. • They can be differentiated on the basis of the serum gastrin response to several provocative tests. • A pronounced increase in serum gastrin level after intravenous infusion of secretin is typical of Zollinger-Ellison syndrome. • Elevations can be seen with other conditions, but they are not as dramatic. • In contradistinction, more marked increases in gastrin levels occur after stimulation by a protein meal in patients with G-cell hyperplasia or retained antrum than in patients with Zollinger-Ellison syndrome. • Bombesin stimulates release of gastrin from the antrum but not from gastrinomas, and bombesin assessments may also aid the differentiation of these entities.

ANSWER:
A-c; B-c; C-a; D-b; E-b

20. With regard to the medical treatment of duodenal ulcer, which of the following statements is/are true?

    A. Antacids alone provide symptomatic relief but have not been demonstrated to promote healing.

    B. Diets have not been demonstrated to promote healing.

    C. Minimal relapse has been observed after an adequate 6-week course of H₂-blockers.

    D. Omeprazole binds to necrotic tissue at the ulcer base to prevent back-diffusion of hydrogen ion.

    E. *H. pylori* infection is usually controlled by antibiotics alone.

Ref.: 1–3

COMMENTS: Much of the traditional medical therapy for duodenal ulcer is unfounded. • Controlled clinical studies have not demonstrated any type of diet or feeding schedule to affect ulcer healing or recurrence, although aspirin, nonsteroidal anti-inflammatory drugs (NSAIDs), and cigarettes should be avoided. • Antacids and H₂-receptor antagonists are equally effective, and both have been demonstrated to promote ulcer healing, in comparison with placebo. • Traditionally, there has been a high rate of relapse after cessation of any medical therapy, and medical treatment has not altered the natural history of the disease. • More recently, however, the combination of antisecretory therapy with antibiotics for eradication of *H. pylori* infection has been shown to reduce dramatically the recurrence of both duodenal and gastric ulcers. • Treatment of *H. pylori* introduces the potential risks of antibiotic side effects and development of resistant organisms. • For these reasons, routine treatment is controversial for first-time ulcer patients, who may respond to antisecretory therapy alone. • However, combination therapy is appropriate when *H. pylori* infection is demonstrated in patients with recurrent peptic ulcer disease.

ANSWER:
B

21. A 45-year-old man requires surgery for intractable duodenal ulcer. Which operation best prevents ulcer recurrence?

    A. Subtotal gastrectomy

    B. Truncal vagotomy and pyloroplasty

    C. Truncal vagotomy and antrectomy

    D. Selective vagotomy

    E. Highly selective (parietal cell) vagotomy

Ref.: 1–4

COMMENTS: See Question 22.

22. Which operation for duodenal ulcer is least likely to produce undesirable postoperative symptoms?

    A. Subtotal gastrectomy

    B. Truncal vagotomy and pyloroplasty

    C. Truncal vagotomy and antrectomy

    D. Selective vagotomy

    E. Highly selective (parietal cell) vagotomy

Ref.: 1–4

COMMENTS: The goal of surgical therapy for duodenal ulcer is to reduce acid in a manner that is safe and has the fewest possible side effects. • Acid can be reduced by eliminating vagal stimulation, removing the antral source of gastrin, and removing the parietal cell mass. • Traditionally, subtotal two-thirds gastrectomy has carried the highest mortality rate. • Truncal vagotomy with antrectomy has the lowest recurrence rate. • Highly selective vagotomy, also known as parietal cell vagotomy or proximal gastric vagotomy, aims to denervate the parietal cell–bearing portion of the stomach but preserve innervation to the pyloroantral region and thus maintain more normal gastric emptying. • This operation carries the lowest mortality rate, the lowest incidence of side effects, but the highest recurrence rate, particularly in patients with prepyloric and pyloric ulcers. • Procedures that involve gastric resection, pyloroplasty, or truncal vagotomy may be complicated by diarrhea, postprandial dumping, or bile reflux. • Selective vagotomy, which preserves the hepatic and celiac vagal branches, has been associated with a lower rate of diarrhea than truncal vagotomy.

A N S W E R S :
Question 21: C
Question 22: E

23. A 75-year-old man on NSAIDs for arthritis presents with an acute abdomen and pneumoperitoneum. His symptoms are 6 hr old, and his vital signs are stable after infusion of 1 L of normal saline solution. What should be the next step in the management of this patient?

    A. Operation

    B. Esophagogastroduodenoscopy

    C. Upper GI contrast study

    D. Antisecretory drugs, antibiotics for gram-negative organisms, and operation if he fails to improve in 6 hr

    E. Antisecretory drugs, antibiotics for *H. pylori*, and operation if he fails to improve in 6 hr

    Ref.: 1–4

COMMENTS: See Question 24.

24. The patient in Question 23 is found to have a perforated duodenal ulcer. Which of the following best describes the required operation?

    A. Suture closure of perforation

    B. Omental patch of perforation

    C. Repair of perforation and highly selective vagotomy

    D. Repair of perforation and truncal vagotomy

    E. Repair of perforation and gastric resection

    Ref.: 1–4

COMMENTS: The preferred treatment for perforated duodenal ulcer is resuscitation and prompt operation. • Nonoperative management is reserved for old contained or fruste–type perforations or for terminally ill patients who otherwise cannot undergo surgery. • The diagnosis is a presumptive one based on clinical grounds and should not be excluded if pneumoperitoneum cannot be demonstrated, since about 20% of patients with perforations do not have this typical radiographic feature. • Operative management requires closure of the perforation, which is generally best accomplished by an omental (Graham) patch. • Following simple repair alone, the traditional natural history has been that about one third of patients have no further ulcer problems, one third have ulcer recurrence amenable to medical management, and one third require a subsequent operation for ulcer disease. • How precisely this concept applies to patients whose ulcer may be due to drugs or *H. pylori* infection is not clear. • It has been suggested that chronicity of symptoms before perforation or operative findings of chronicity increase the advisability of performing a more definitive antiulcer operation at the time a perforation is repaired. • Definitive operations should be performed only on stable patients. • A highly selective vagotomy is an excellent choice. • Truncal vagotomy may be more rapid but has a greater incidence of side effects. • Resective procedures are generally avoided in the setting of perforation owing to higher morbidity. • Following surgery, ulcerogenic drugs should be withheld, and any concomitant *H. pylori* infection should be treated.

A N S W E R S :
Question 23: A
Question 24: B

25. With regard to hemorrhage complicating duodenal ulcer, which of the following statements is/are true?

    A. It is a more common complication of duodenal ulcer than is perforation.

    B. Endoscopic treatment before operation decreases mortality.

    C. Endoscopic treatment decreases the need for operation.

    D. Operative management is indicated only if endoscopic treatment fails.

    E. Operative management should include an acid-reducing procedure.

    Ref.: 1–4

COMMENTS: Hemorrhage is the most common complication of duodenal ulcer. • It usually presents with melena or hematemesis. • There may be massive bleeding from an eroded gastroduodenal artery or one of its tributaries. • Endoscopic examination is critical for diagnosing the site of upper GI hemorrhage. • Endoscopic techniques can be useful for controlling hemorrhage, but whether they decrease mortality rates or the need for subsequent operation has not been universally established. • The most important endoscopic predictor of persistent or recurrent bleeding is active bleeding (arterial spurting) at the time of the endoscopic procedure. • The presence of a "visible vessel" implies a high risk of recurrent bleeding even if the vessel is not bleeding at the time of endoscopy. • When operation is necessary, bleeding is controlled by suture ligation, with attention to proper suture placement for control of the posterior complex of gastroduodenal vessels. • A definitive antiulcer operation should then be performed because of the high risk of recurrent hemorrhage. • Selection of the appropriate definitive procedure is highly dependent on the physiologic status of the patient. • If the patient has been in shock or is otherwise ill, truncal vagotomy and pyloroplasty are advisable. • For fit patients, parietal cell vagotomy or truncal vagotomy and antrectomy are considered.

A N S W E R :
A, E

26. Advanced gastric outlet obstruction is characterized by which of the following metabolic abnormalities?

    A. Hypochloremia and increased urinary chloride levels

    B. Hypokalemia due to urinary potassium loss

    C. Metabolic alkalosis with alkaline urine

    D. Metabolic alkalosis with acid urine

    E. Increased serum ionized calcium levels

    Ref.: 1–3

COMMENTS: The classic metabolic abnormality resulting from gastric outlet obstruction and prolonged vomiting is a hypochloremic, hypokalemic metabolic alkalosis. • Initial loss of hydrochloric acid causes hypochloremia and a mild alkalosis compensated for by renal excretion of bicarbonate. • Therefore, in the early stages the urine is alkaline. • Continued vomiting produces a severe extracellular fluid deficit and sodium deficit from both renal and gastric losses. • The kidneys begin to conserve sodium and, in exchange, excrete hydrogen and potassium cations to accompany bicarbonate. • The kidneys are the predominant site of potassium loss, and the urine is paradoxically acidic. • Urine chloride content is reduced throughout and eventually absent. • Serum ionized calcium levels are decreased because calcium is mildly alkaline and shifts to its nonionized form to reduce alkalosis. • Treatment of this metabolic situation is accomplished primarily by administration of isotonic saline solution, which replenishes the deficits of volume, sodium, and chloride. • Potassium is replaced when renal function has been optimized.

ANSWER:
B, D

27. Concerning the treatment of patients with Zollinger-Ellison syndrome, which of the following statements is/are true?

A. Operative treatment of associated hyperparathyroidism takes precedence over abdominal operation.

B. Pancreatic tumors can be removed by enucleation.

C. Duodenal tumors usually require pancreaticoduodenectomy.

D. Total gastrectomy is indicated if the tumor cannot be localized.

E. Resection of liver metastases is not indicated.

Ref.: 1–4

COMMENTS: The treatment of Zollinger-Ellison syndrome is two-pronged and is aimed at both resecting tumor when possible and protecting the gastric end organ. • Therapy must be individualized. • Patients with known endocrine tumors should undergo careful evaluation for other potential endocrine tumors. • In patients with gastrinoma and hyperparathyroidism, parathyroidectomy should first be performed to eliminate hypercalcemia. • Abdominal operation is not urgent with current antisecretory medications. • Although gastrinomas are often multiple and are usually metastatic, long-term survival is possible. • Aggressive attempts to localize and resect tumors can provide cure in 5–20% of patients and can diminish gastrin secretion in others. • Both pancreatic and duodenal gastrinomas can be resected by enucleation when appropriately located. • Blind pancreatic resections are not generally indicated. • When complete tumor removal is not possible, a gastric operation may be appropriate. • Proximal gastric vagotomy may be useful, but total gastrectomy still provides the best long-term quality of life for some patients. • Lifelong pharmacologic treatment with antisecretory agents may control the ulcer diathesis in some patients, but problems with high doses, compliance, and side effects may occur. • Resection or ablation of metastatic disease, although not curative, can provide important palliation and decrease the need for drug therapy.

ANSWER:
A, B

28. Concerning "stress" bleeding from acute erosive gastritis, which of the following statements is/are true?

A. Polyphylactic treatments with H_2-blockers and with antacids are equally effective.

B. The incidence of such bleeding has been decreasing.

C. The site of hemorrhage is most often in the antrum.

D. There is minimal recurrent bleeding after treatment by oversewing of bleeding sites, vagotomy, and pyloroplasty.

E. Effective surgical treatment necessitates total gastrectomy.

Ref.: 1–3

COMMENTS: Stress bleeding in critically ill patients is best prevented by the use of antacids, with dosage monitored by titration of the gastric pH. • H_2-receptor antagonists alone are not as effective as antacids alone, but use of the two conjointly may decrease the volume of buffer required. • Sucralfate is effective as an acute cytoprotective topical agent, and it works in an acidic environment. • It may decrease oropharyngeal colonization by enteric bacteria and the subsequent rate of pneumonia. • For reasons that are not known, the incidence of major bleeding from acute mucosal erosions has decreased greatly. • However, the lesions should be anticipated in malnourished patients with septic syndrome or septic shock. • Bleeding often begins insidiously, but major bleeding may develop rapidly. • Gastroscopy usually demonstrates acute, superficial lesions that appear first in the proximal stomach (fundus) and then spread distally. • If an operation is indicated for protracted bleeding, gastroscopic findings should dictate the procedure needed. • Total gastrectomy is warranted if the bleeding sites cannot be controlled by means of a lesser operation (vagotomy and pyloroplasty).

ANSWER:
B

29. The pathogenesis of benign type I gastric ulcers is predominantly which one of the following?

A. Hypersecretion of acid as a result of increased parietal cell mass

B. Hypergastrinemia as a result of gastric stasis

C. Antral stasis

D. Defective gastric mucosal barrier

E. Hyperpepsinogenemia

Ref.: 1–3, 5

COMMENTS: Type I gastric ulcers occur along the lesser curvature, typically on the antral side of the junction between the acid-secreting and non–acid-secreting mucosa. • Type II gastric ulcers are those combined with duodenal ulcers. • Type III ulcers are prepyloric. • Type II and III gastric ulcers are similar to duodenal ulcers in terms of acid-secretory behavior and the types of therapy to which they are amenable. • Isolated benign gastric ulcers are thought to result from a defect in the mucosal barrier to hydrogen ion diffusion in the presence of acid. • A variety of factors, such as duodenogastric reflux of bile, mucosa-damaging drugs (e.g., aspirin and NSAIDS), and ethanol, may be involved in the mucosal injury. • The gastric mucous layer primarily acts as a lubricant and is not particularly important in protection from acid. • Dragstedt's theory of antral stasis as the primary cause of gastric ulcer is no longer accepted. • Most patients with gastric ulcer have normal gastric emptying.

ANSWER:
D

30. Match each clinical feature in the left-hand column with the appropriate ulcer type in the right-hand column.

A. Most frequent peptic ulcer   a. Gastric ulcer (type I)

B. More common after 50 years of age   b. Duodenal ulcer

C. Slower healing with medical therapy   c. Both

D. Hemorrhage associated with   d. Neither
   higher mortality rate

E. Malignant transformation
   common

Ref.: 1–4

COMMENTS: In the United States, isolated gastric ulcers are about four times less common than are duodenal ulcers, whereas in Japan gastric ulcers are more common. • Gastric ulcers occur more commonly in older patients, and when they are complicated by bleeding, perforation, or obstruction, the corresponding prognosis is generally worse than it is for patients with duodenal ulcer. • Antisecretory therapy promotes healing of gastric ulcers, but healing is in general slower and therapy is not as effective as for duodenal ulcer. • *H. pylori* infection must be treated. • All gastric ulcers should be examined by biopsy (and repeated biopsy as necessary) to rule out malignancy. • Approximately 5% of benign-appearing gastric ulcers are malignant. • In uncommon cases, cancer develops in the mucosa peripheral to a chronic ulcer.

ANSWER:
A-b; B-a; C-a; D-a; E-d

31. With regard to surgical therapy of gastric ulcer, which of the following statements is/are true?

    A. A type I ulcer at the incisura is effectively treated by distal gastrectomy without vagotomy.

    B. A type I ulcer at the incisura is preferably treated by vagotomy and pyloroplasty.

    C. A type III prepyloric ulcer without obstruction is best treated by parietal cell vagotomy.

    D. Type II (combined duodenal and gastric) ulcers are best treated by subtotal (70–80%) gastrectomy without vagotomy.

    E. A type I ulcer on the lesser curve near the GE junction is best treated by total gastrectomy.

Ref.: 1–4

COMMENTS: Surgical therapy of benign gastric ulcer depends on the type of ulcer and associated acid secretion. • Isolated type I ulcers are usually well treated by antrectomy or hemigastrectomy (including removal of the ulcer) without vagotomy. • Although the addition of vagotomy to distal resection for type I ulcers has not improved outcome, vagotomy is sometimes used because of the possibility of associated duodenal ulcer or when the distinction between a type I ulcer and a type III ulcer is not clear. • Vagotomy with pyloroplasty for type I ulcers has been associated with a higher recurrence rate than has resection and has conferred no advantages. • Limited experience with parietal cell vagotomy for type I ulcers has yielded reasonable clinical results. • Type I ulcers near the GE junction can be treated by modifications of distal gastrectomy that include ulcer excision. • Type II and III ulcers are treated as duodenal ulcers with vagotomy and resection or drainage. • Parietal cell vagotomy is generally not indicated for prepyloric ulcers because of high recurrence rates, although there are data demonstrating that parietal cell vagotomy in combination with a pyloric drainage procedure may be effective therapy in this situation.

ANSWER:
A

32. Malignant gastric ulcers can preoperatively be distinguished from benign gastric ulcers based on which of the following?

    A. Size larger than 2 cm

    B. Location on the greater curvature

    C. Acid secretory studies demonstrating achlorhydria

    D. Multiple biopsies

    E. Failure to heal by 8 weeks

Ref.: 1–3

COMMENTS: Although certain characteristics suggest that an ulcer is malignant (e.g., size, location, and achlorhydria), the only accurate method of distinction is adequate histologic sampling. • Even the visual endoscopic appearance of a malignant lesion can be misinterpreted as that of a benign ulcer. • Multiple (four or more) biopsies at various quadrants increase the accuracy of histologic diagnosis. • Benign gastric ulcers can be slow to heal, especially if they are large, and malignant gastric ulcers also can show partial healing. • Repeated biopsy is advised for ulcers that have not healed after 8–12 weeks of medical therapy.

ANSWER:
D

33. With regard to the epidemiologic characteristics of gastric cancer, which of the following statements is/are true?

    A. The highest incidence is in Japan.

    B. Predominance among males or females varies geographically.

    C. Both incidence and death rates in the United States have decreased.

    D. There is a higher incidence among patients with blood group O.

    E. There is a higher incidence among patients who have undergone gastric resection for duodenal ulcer.

Ref.: 1–4

COMMENTS: The significant geographic variations in the incidence of gastric cancer are likely related to environmental and dietary differences that result in exposure to *N*-nitroso-compounds, polycyclic hydrocarbons, and other potential carcinogens. • The highest incidence is in Japan, where the death rate is about eight times higher than that in the United States. • Gastric cancer occurs more frequently in males in all areas of the world. • Parallel dramatic declines in the incidence and death rates of gastric cancer in the United States have been observed since the early 1940s, although a slight increase may now be occurring, the reasons for which are unknown. • Although most risk factors for gastric cancer are probably exogenous, genetic factors may also be involved, as exemplified by patients with pernicious anemia and by the slightly increased risk among patients with blood group A. • There appears also to be an increased risk 10–15 years after gastric resection for benign disease, perhaps indicating the role of chronic bile reflux.

ANSWER:
A, C, E

34. Which of the following conditions is/are associated with gastric cancer?

 A. Adenomatous gastric polyps

 B. Autoimmune chronic gastritis

 C. Hypersecretory chronic gastritis

 D. Environmental chronic gastritis

 E. Ménétrier's disease

Ref.: 4

COMMENTS: Certain gastric lesions have a significant association with gastric cancer and can be considered precursors to malignancy. • Adenomatous polyps in the stomach have a malignant potential, as do adenomatous polyps of the colon. • Chronic atrophic gastritis, of which several forms are recognized, underlies most gastric cancers. • Epithelial changes of intestinal metaplasia and dysplasia are premalignant. • Autoimmune chronic gastritis (type A gastritis) involves the body and fundus of the stomach. • It is associated with pernicious anemia, parietal cell antibodies, achlorhydria, very high gastrin levels, and a high risk of cancer. • Hypersecretory chronic gastritis (type B gastritis) involves the gastric antrum and is associated with peptic ulcer disease but *not* malignancy. • Environmental chronic gastritis is multifocal, involving the body and antrum, and occurs in geographic areas with a high incidence of gastric cancer. • Ménétrier's disease, one of the hyperplastic gastropathies, characterized by enlarged rugae, is no longer considered premalignant. • Earlier descriptions of cancer in Ménétrier's disease referred to patients with gastric polyposis.

ANSWER:
A, B, D

35. With regard to the prognosis of gastric adenocarcinoma, which of the following statements is/are true?

 A. The polypoid gross type carries a better prognosis than does the diffusely infiltrating type.

 B. The intestinal histologic type carries a better prognosis than does the diffuse type.

 C. The overall 5-year survival rate in the United States is approximately 50% after resection.

 D. Cure rates of 80–90% are obtained for lesions confined to the mucosa.

 E. Length of survival is improved by chemotherapy and radiation therapy after curative resection.

Ref.: 1–4

COMMENTS: Gastric cancers can be classified according to gross and histologic appearances with some correlation between the two. • On gross examination, polypoid, ulcerating, superficial spreading, and diffusely infiltrating (linitis plastica) types are recognized. • The polypoid and superficial spreading types carry a better prognosis, whereas the prognosis of patients with linitis plastica is dismal. • Histologically, Lauren distinguished intestinal and diffuse types. • The intestinal variety, which is decreasing in incidence in the United States, is better differentiated and is associated with longer survival stage for stage than is the diffuse type. • The intestinal pattern predominates in polypoid and superficial spreading tumors. • Resection of stage I tumors, confined to the mucosa, yields excellent survival rates. • However, these lesions

are unusual in the United States in comparison with Japan, where they constitute 20–40% of tumors. • In the United States, the overall 5-year survival rate after treatment is only about 10% because most of the patients have more advanced disease. • Survival rates of 40–50% are found in node-negative patients and even in node-positive patients with intestinal histologic findings. • Adjuvant therapy after potentially curative resection has yielded no clear benefit.

ANSWER:
A, B, D

36. With regard to the surgical treatment of gastric adenocarcinoma, which of the following statements is/are true?

 A. Total gastrectomy for antral lesions results in longer survival than does partial gastrectomy.

 B. Routine splenectomy does not improve survival rates.

 C. Extended lymph node dissection improves survival rates for patients with stage I and II lesions.

 D. Total gastrectomy for palliation is contraindicated.

 E. Linitis plastica should be resected to histologically negative margins.

Ref.: 1–4

COMMENTS: Gastric adenocarcinoma is preferably treated by resection, although resection usually proves to be palliative. • The general strategy for curative resection is to remove as much stomach as necessary to obtain free margins and to perform limited node dissection. • Although data from Japan support the benefit of extended nodal dissections (celiac, mesenteric, hepatic, and paraaortic), studies in the United States have not generally confirmed this benefit. • Furthermore, these extended dissections can be associated with substantial morbidity. • Most resections entail distal subtotal gastrectomy. • Total gastrectomy is appropriate for locally extensive tumors, proximal tumors (to avoid esophageal anastomosis to distal stomach remnant), and even palliation if necessary. • Extending clear margins on a distal tumor by total rather than subtotal gastrectomy is of no benefit. • Resections for linitis plastica are palliative, usually necessitate total gastrectomy, and are carried out to grossly negative margins only. • Splenectomy is performed according to the location of gastric resection, but its routine performance does not improve the survival rate.

ANSWER:
B

37. An upper GI series demonstrates enlarged rugae in the corpus and fundus of the stomach. Which of the following is not included in the differential diagnosis?

 A. Ménétrier's disease

 B. Lymphoma

 C. Pseudolymphoma

 D. Eosinophilic gastroenteritis

 E. Adenocarcinoma

Ref.: 2, 4

COMMENTS: A number of disorders are associated with grossly enlarged gastric folds. • In Ménétrier's disease, mucosal folds of the fundus and corpus may be markedly enlarged as a result of mucous cell hyperplasia. • The condition may be associated with protein-losing enteropathic conditions and typically spares the antrum. • Eosinophilic gastroenteritis, in contrast, is a process characterized by polypoid or diffuse eosinophilic infiltration that occurs in the antrum. • Gastric malignancy, adenocarcinoma, or lymphoma can be manifested by thickened folds. • These radiographic characteristics may also be demonstrated in pseudolymphoma, which represents lymphoid hyperplasia.

ANSWER:
D

38. With regard to primary gastric lymphoma, which of the following statements is/are true?

A. GI bleeding is the most common symptom.

B. Mucosal biopsy can establish the diagnosis in nearly all cases.

C. Primary therapy is surgical resection.

D. Primary therapy is irradiation.

E. The long-term survival rate is equivalent to that for adenocarcinoma.

Ref.: 1–4

COMMENTS: Gastric lymphoma is not common, but the stomach is the most common site of extranodal non-Hodgkin's lymphoma. • Patients usually present with abdominal pain and weight loss. • Endoscopic visualization and biopsy may not establish the diagnosis because the lesion begins as a submucosal process. • Even when ulceration is present, biopsy specimens may yield only nondiagnostic necrotic material. • The primary treatment is surgical resection, for both cure and palliation. • The 5-year survival rate with curative resection is 75%. • Radiation therapy has been used as primary therapy, as an adjunct to resection, and for unresectable tumors. • Although the value of adjuvant radiation has not been fully established, it is often employed, particularly if there is nodal or serosal involvement. • Chemotherapy is also used for patients with unresectable lesions or systemic disease and may be considered for resected tumors with poor prognostic factors, such as nodal disease or transmural involvement.

ANSWER:
C

39. Concerning the Mallory-Weiss syndrome, which of the following statements is/are true?

A. It is a complication of GE reflux.

B. It involves esophageal rupture near the GE junction.

C. Profuse hemorrhage is the most common manifestation.

D. Bleeding can generally be managed medically.

E. Vagotomy is indicated for patients requiring surgical treatment.

Ref.: 1, 2

COMMENTS: Mallory-Weiss syndrome refers to a tear of the mucosa and submucosa near the GE junction that occurs as a result of retching. • The tear is usually on the gastric side and on its lesser curvature. • The bleeding can often be managed medically. • There is profuse hemorrhage in about 10% of cases.

• Should operation be necessary, bleeding can be controlled simply by oversewing the site of the tear. • An acid-reducing operation is not required.

ANSWER:
D

40. With regard to gastric volvulus, which of the following statements is/are true?

A. Symptoms consist of severe nausea with inability to vomit.

B. It is associated with congenital anomalies of gastric fixation.

C. It frequently is relieved simply by passage of a nasogastric tube.

D. It constitutes a surgical emergency.

E. It is associated with an increased incidence of sigmoid volvulus.

Ref.: 2

COMMENTS: Gastric volvulus is a serious complication of paraesophageal hernia. • Two types of gastric volvulus may occur, depending on the axis of rotation. • **Organoaxial volvulus**, the more common type, involves rotation around the axis of a line connecting the cardia and pylorus. • With **mesenterioaxial volvulus**, the axis is approximately at a right angle to the cardiopyloric line. • Combined types have also been described. • Patients generally have severe pain and nausea but are unable to vomit, and a nasogastric tube cannot be passed. • Strangulation can follow. • Hence, gastric volvulus requires prompt reduction.

ANSWER:
A, D

41. Which of the following is the preferred treatment for a symptomatic duodenal diverticulum?

A. Antibiotics for suppression of bacterial overgrowth

B. H$_2$-blockers

C. Surgical excision

D. Gastrojejunostomy

E. Pancreaticoduodenectomy

Ref.: 4

COMMENTS: A duodenal diverticulum is usually an asymptomatic, incidental finding that does not necessitate specific therapy. • In a patient with GI symptoms, other pathologic processes should be carefully sought. • Duodenal diverticula occasionally cause abdominal pain, obstruction, bleeding, bacterial overgrowth, perforation, or pancreaticobiliary problems. • The diverticulum is most commonly located on the medial wall of the second portion of the duodenum near the papilla of Vater. • When treatment is required, surgical excision is recommended. • In general, this can be accomplished after a Kocher maneuver, although transduodenal excision is occasionally necessary. • Care must be taken to identify the bile duct and pancreatic duct.

ANSWER:
C

42. Which of the following conditions is/are associated with an increased risk of duodenal adenocarcinoma?

    A. Heterotopic pancreas

    B. Adenoma of Brunner's glands

    C. Nodular hyperplasia of Brunner's glands

    D. Familial polyposis coli

    E. Gardner's syndrome

Ref.: 4

COMMENTS: A variety of benign and malignant duodenal neoplasms can occur, and surgeons should be familiar with them. • Adenocarcinoma, the most common malignant duodenal neoplasm, has been associated with a number of conditions, including adenomatous polyps, villous adenomas, familial polyposis coli, Gardner's syndrome, and von Recklinghausen's disease. • Heterotopic pancreas is not neoplastic, but it can be manifested as a submucosal duodenal nodule. • Adenomas of Brunner's glands are probably hamartomas. • They are benign but enter into the differential diagnosis of duodenal tumors. • Nodular hyperplasia of Brunner's glands is a diffuse benign process that can be seen in patients on hemodialysis or after renal transplantation.

ANSWER:
D, E

43. An 18-year-old woman presents with abdominal pain and weight loss. Examination reveals a soft, moveable epigastric mass. Endoscopic examination demonstrates a large mass of black hair in the stomach. Which of the following is the most appropriate therapy?

    A. Endoscopic extraction

    B. Oral administration of papain

    C. Psychiatric consultation

    D. Gastrotomy and removal

    E. Gastrojejunostomy

Ref.: 4

COMMENTS: Gastric bezoars caused by ingested hair are termed **trichobezoars**. • They most typically occur in young women. • The hair is not digestible, and endoscopic removal is generally inadequate. • Additional bezoars may be present in the small intestine. • For these reasons, gastrotomy and operative removal are indicated. • **Phytobezoars** are made up of vegetable or fruit fiber. • These are more common in older patients and may occur in association with diabetes, previous gastric surgery, or other causes of delayed gastric emptying. • A unique type of phytobezoar resulting from persimmon fruit (**diopyrobezoar**) may necessitate operation. • Otherwise, most phytobezoars can be treated with liquid diets, enzymatic digestion, and endoscopic manipulation.

ANSWER:
D

44. A spot film from an upper GI study was obtained on a patient who had vague abdominal pain. From the radiographic findings shown in the figure, which of the following is the most likely diagnosis?

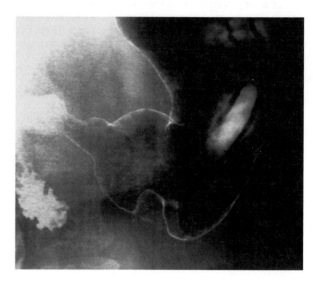

    A. Mucosal polyp

    B. Gastric ulcer

    C. Ectopic pancreas

    D. Adenocarcinoma

Ref.: 4

COMMENTS: Note that there is a mass along the greater curvature portion of the antrum with radiographically smooth mucosa. • The mass makes 90-degree angles with the gastric lumen, which places the mass in the **submucosal** location. • Radiographically, **mucosal** masses produce acute angles with the lumen. • Adjacent masses that push on the stomach to create the image of a mass have angles greater than 180 degrees.

A **mucosal polyp**, either hyperplastic or an adenoma, is unlikely because of the suspected submucosal origin. • Hyperplastic polyps are usually multiple and are found in the fundus and proximal stomach. • Adenomas usually are single, are found in the antrum, and carry the same ominous implications as do adenomas in the colon. • **Leiomyomas** are the most common submucosal masses found in the GI tract, and the radiologic findings shown for the patient described here are compatible with a submucosal mass. • On occasion, if the mass is large, the mucosa ulcerates. • The differential diagnosis between benign leiomyoma and leiomyosarcoma cannot be made on radiographic grounds alone. • Other submucosal masses include neuromas, neurofibromas, hemangiomas, lipomas, and lymphomas. • **Ectopic pancreas** is a rest of pancreatic tissues in an unusual location. • Usually, these rests are found in the gastric antrum or duodenum. • They are submucosal in location, as in this patient. • On occasion, as in this case, there is an aborted pancreatic duct that fills with contrast material (it appears as a white dot in the center of the mass). • The definitive diagnosis is established by excision. • **Gastric carcinoma** destroys the mucosa, which is reflected by an ulceration within the mucosal pattern seen radiographically. • Early gastric cancer may be found as a small lesion that resembles a gastric polyp. • Other appearances of early gastric cancer include a plaque-like area of ulceration that can mimic the appearance of a benign ulcer. • **Lymphoma** is another lesion that can occur submucosally and should be ruled out whenever a submucosal mass is discovered. • Ruling out malignancy in submucosal masses is difficult because endoscopic evaluation with biopsy often reaches only the mucosa. • The endoscopist must therefore be aware of the submucosal nature of the mass. • Repeated biopsies in the same area or surgical excision may be needed to establish the diagnosis.

ANSWER:

C

REFERENCES

1. Townsend CM, Beauchamp RD, Evers BM, et al (eds): *Sabiston Textbook of Surgery: The Biological Basis of Modern Surgical Practice*, 17th ed. Saunders, Philadelphia, 2004.
2. Brunicardi FC, Andersen DK, Billiar TR, et al (eds): *Schwartz's Principles of Surgery*, 8th ed. McGraw-Hill, New York, 2004.
3. Greenfield L, Mullholland MW, Oldham KT, et al (eds): *Greenfield's Surgery: Scientific Principles and Practice*, 3rd ed. Lippincott, Williams & Wilkins, Philadelphia, 2001.
4. Wastell C, Nyhus LM, Donahue PE (eds): *Surgery of the Stomach and Duodenum*, 5th ed. Little, Brown, Boston, 1995.
5. O'Leary JP: *The Physiologic Basis of Surgery*, 2nd ed. Williams & Wilkins, Baltimore, 1996.
6. Burette A: How and when to test for *Helicobacter pylori*. *Acta Gastroenterol Belg* 61:336–343, 1998.

CHAPTER 33

Small Intestine

Marc Brand, M.D.

1. During an operation for presumed appendicitis, the appendix is found to be normal. The terminal ileum, however, is markedly thickened and feels rubbery to firm. Its serosa is erythematous and inflamed, and several loops of apparently normal small intestine are adherent to it. The terminal ileum mesentery is thickened, with fat growing about the bowel circumference. Which of the following is the most likely diagnosis?

A. Crohn's disease of the terminal ileum

B. Perforated Meckel's diverticulum

C. Ulcerative colitis

D. Ileocecal tuberculosis

E. Acute ileitis

Ref.: 1, 2

COMMENTS: Crohn's disease can present acutely, and, when it involves the terminal ileum, it may clinically resemble appendicitis. • Involved segments of bowel may have a characteristic gross appearance. • The mesenteric fat "creeps" over the serosa; the mesentery is thickened, dull, and rubbery; and it may contain lymph nodes as large as 4 cm in diameter. • Not infrequently, partial obstruction of the involved segment can produce dilatation of the proximal bowel. • Enteric fistulas may also be seen to adjacent viscera, such as the bladder, vagina, or bowel.

Acute ileitis may clinically mimic appendicitis and grossly appear as inflammation of the terminal ileum. • The operative findings, however, do not resemble those of advanced Crohn's disease.

Meckel's diverticulitis can clinically mimic appendicitis, but the inflammatory process is located approximately 50 cm proximal to the ileocecal valve, and the bowel wall and mesenteric changes seen with Crohn's disease are not present.

Tuberculosis of the terminal ileum—rare in the United States—can produce scarring and stenosis of the distal ileum and enlargement of the mesenteric lymph nodes. • Demonstration of caseation and acid-fast bacilli on biopsy of a mesenteric lymph node confirms the diagnosis. • There may also be miliary seeding of the peritoneal cavity, seen as tiny disseminated white spots on the serosa and peritoneum.

Ulcerative colitis is confined to the large bowel, and any associated pain can usually be distinguished from that of appendicitis.

A N S W E R :
A

2. During exploratory surgery for presumed appendicitis, the cecum and appendix are found to be normal. The terminal 50 cm of ileum, however, is inflamed, beefy red, and slightly edematous. It is soft, and there is no proximal ileal distention. Which of the following is the most appropriate operative choice?

A. Appendectomy

B. Resection of involved ileum and appendix

C. Placement of irrigation catheters and appendectomy

D. Closure without appendectomy or ileal resection

E. Bypass ileo-ascending colostomy

Ref.: 1, 2

COMMENTS: When **acute regional enteritis** of the terminal ileum is encountered during exploration for presumed appendicitis, the appropriateness of appendectomy is somewhat controversial. • The incidence of enterocutaneous fistula after operation in patients with Crohn's disease is high, but the fistulas usually arise from the diseased ileum, not the appendiceal stump. • In addition, 90% of patients in whom acute regional enteritis is found at operation do not progress to chronic Crohn's disease. • Symptoms resolve without sequelae. • Therefore, if the stump of the appendix is not involved, most surgeons favor performance of an appendectomy. • This step ameliorates the dilemma of the differential diagnosis if right lower abdominal pain develops at a later date. • When acute regional enteritis is encountered, as in this clinical setting (i.e., without evidence of obstruction or fistula formation), the ileum should not be resected.

A N S W E R :
A

3. With regard to Crohn's disease, which of the following statements is/are correct?

A. It is the most common primary disease of the small intestine that requires operation.

B. Black males and males of Mediterranean descent are most commonly affected.

C. The disease involves both the terminal ileum and the right colon in 90% of cases.

D. The disease may involve any portion of the gastrointestinal (GI) tract from the mouth to the anus.

Ref.: 2

COMMENTS: Although uncommon in comparison with other GI diseases, Crohn's disease is the most common primary disease of the small intestine that requires operation. • The incidence is highest in the United States, England, and Scandinavia. • Crohn's disease is three times more common in Jews than in non-Jews, more common in whites than in nonwhites, and slightly more common in males than in females. • It occurs in all age groups but is most frequently diagnosed in young adults. • The distribution of involvement is such that 30% of patients have disease limited to the small intestine and 20% to the colon. • About 50% have both small- and large-intestine involvement. • Diseased segments may be separated by normal bowel (i.e., skip areas). • Isolated involvement of the esophagus, stomach, or duodenum does occur but is rare.

ANSWER:
A, D

---

4. As to the microscopic appearance of Crohn's disease, which of the following statements is/are true?

A. The disease is confined to the mucosa.

B. The disease is confined to the mucosa and submucosa.

C. Granulomas demonstrating caseation without acid-fast bacilli confirm the diagnosis.

D. Submucosal fibrosis occurs secondary to bacterial invasion.

E. Marked lymphangiectasia is a prominent microscopic feature.

Ref.: 1, 2

COMMENTS: Several microscopic features characterize but are nonspecific for Crohn's disease. • These features progress from an early to a late phase of involvement and can be described as a granulomatous fibrotic inflammation progressing through all layers of the bowel wall. • In the **early phase**, edema of the entire bowel wall is seen, accompanied by lymphangiectasia and hyperemia associated with an increased proportion of goblet cells in an otherwise normal mucosa.

In the **intermediate phase**, thickening is caused by fibrosis of the submucosal and subserosal areas of the bowel. • Focal mucosal ulcers become numerous, and, in 60% of patients, sarcoid-like granulomas appear, particularly in the submucosa, subserosa, and regional lymph nodes. • These granulomas contain epithelioid giant cells, do not caseate, and do not contain acid-fast bacilli. • The absence of granulomas does not exclude the diagnosis of Crohn's disease. • Lymphangiectasia remains visible throughout the intermediate and late phases.

In the **late phase**, dense fibrosis exceeds that expected from the simple healing of an inflammatory insult, producing a fixed stenosis and partial obstruction of the lumen. • The mucosa is denuded over wide areas, with occasional islands of intact mucosal cells (pseudopolyps). • Glands deep in the mucosa resemble those of the pyloric region and are termed aberrant pyloric glands or Brunner's gland metaplasia. • The ulcers can be deep, and progression through the bowel wall may occur, sometimes resulting in fistula formation.

ANSWER:
E

---

5. With regard to the cause of Crohn's disease, which of the following statements is/are true?

A. The primary pathologic mechanism is a progressive, obstructive lymphangitis.

B. Crohn's disease is a form of sarcoidosis limited to the GI tract.

C. A mouse-footpad virus has been identified as the etiologic agent.

D. The disease is the result of a local hypersensitivity reaction.

E. The disease is primarily a psychosomatic illness.

F. The cause is unknown.

Ref.: 1, 2

COMMENTS: Despite extensive investigation, the cause of Crohn's disease is unknown. • The possibility of a transmissible agent has emerged as a result of work demonstrating the development of granulomatous lesions in the mouse footpad following injection of intestinal homogenates obtained from patients with Crohn's disease. • These results, however, have been difficult to reproduce, and their precise meaning requires further investigation. • Although the granulomas of sarcoidosis and Crohn's disease are similar, Kveim test results, positive in 80% of patients with active sarcoidosis, are almost always negative in those with Crohn's disease. • It is generally thought that the immunologic alterations and psychosomatic manifestations seen in patients with Crohn's disease reflect responses to the disease rather than indicate its cause.

ANSWER:
F

---

6. Regarding the clinical manifestations of Crohn's disease, which of the following statements is/are true?

A. Most patients present acutely with pain, nausea, and diarrhea.

B. Bloody diarrhea is an infrequent symptom.

C. Bloody diarrhea almost always produces anemia.

D. There is steatorrhea as a result of pancreatic involvement.

E. Fever and signs of systemic toxicity are common.

Ref.: 1, 2

COMMENTS: Only 10% of patients with Crohn's disease present acutely and with symptoms similar to those of appendicitis. • In most instances, the onset is insidious, with intermittent **pain** or discomfort being the most frequent and sometimes the only symptom. • The pain often is precipitated by a dietary indiscretion. • With advanced disease, the pain may become associated with signs and symptoms of partial obstruction. • Constant, localized pain, especially if associated with a palpable mass, suggests the presence of an abscess or bowel fistula.

Diarrhea is the next most frequent symptom, and, unlike the diarrhea of chronic ulcerative colitis, it rarely contains mucus, pus, or blood. • Diarrhea is the result of several factors. • The inflamed segment of small bowel has a decreased capacity to absorb intestinal contents. • In addition, the **obstruction** produced by this involved segment alters the absorptive capacity of the proximal bowel. • **Decreased absorption** of bile salts in the terminal ileum leads to bile salt-induced damage of the absorptive cells of the colonic mucosa, producing a choleretic diarrhea.

One third of patients present with **fever** and one half with **weight loss**, **weakness**, and **easy fatigability**. • Although the diarrhea is usually nonbloody, persistent occult loss of blood frequently produces **anemia**, which may be aggravated by a vitamin B$_{12}$ deficiency. • **Hypoproteinemia** occurs because of increased loss of protein from the inflamed bowel mucosa. • **Vitamin and mineral deficiencies** are the result of decreased ingestion, altered metabolism, and decreased absorption.

ANSWER:
B

7. With regard to the complications of Crohn's disease, which of the following statements is/are true?

   A. When obstruction is present, it usually is partial rather than complete.

   B. Perforation of the bowel wall occurs in 15–20% of patients.

   C. Free perforations into the peritoneal cavity are as common as are confined perforations.

   D. Fistulization rarely occurs in patients who have not had an operation.

   E. Perianal disease rarely occurs in patients with Crohn's disease confined to the small bowel.

   F. Crohn's disease of the small bowel is not associated with an increased risk of malignancy.

Ref.: 1, 2

COMMENTS: Complete obstruction is uncommon in Crohn's disease. • **Partial obstruction** is common, and when it is high grade, an elective operation may be necessary. • **Perforation** occurs in 15–20% of patients, usually resulting in formation of a contained abscess, phlegmon, or an internal **fistula** to the bowel, bladder, or vagina. • Enterocutaneous fistulas rarely occur in patients not previously operated on, but they are common after operation. • **Free perforations** into the peritoneal cavity are rare. • When they do occur, they usually are on the antimesenteric border of the distal ileum, proximal to a stenotic lesion. • Frank hemorrhage is rare, but it can occur if an ulcer erodes into a large blood vessel. • Up to 30% of patients with Crohn's disease of the small bowel develop **perirectal abscesses or fistulas,** usually without evidence of communication with the diseased small bowel.

Patients with Crohn's disease have an increased risk of developing **cancer** in comparison with the general population, but the risk of colon cancer does not approach the level seen in patients with chronic ulcerative colitis. • This difference may be related to the shorter period between diagnosis and colectomy for Crohn's disease compared with ulcerative colitis. • The risk, however, is not considered high enough to warrant prophylactic resection. • Most cases of small-bowel cancer associated with Crohn's disease have occurred in patients with long-standing disease and have appeared in a previously bypassed segment of bowel. • They may also be formed at the site of a small-bowel stricture.

ANSWER:
A, B

8. Regarding the radiographic findings of Crohn's disease of the small intestine, which of the following statements is/are true?

   A. Barium enema with reflux into the terminal ileum is adequate for defining the extent of disease.

   B. The string sign of Kantor is produced by luminal narrowing.

   C. When present, fistulas are almost always seen on small-bowel follow-through studies.

   D. Studies with barium should be avoided because they can convert partial-thickness bowel wall involvement to a full-thickness lesion.

   E. Increased space between bowel loops or deviation of the bowel wall may be due to thickening of the bowel wall and mesentery or to abscess formation.

Ref.: 1, 2

COMMENTS: An upper GI series of x-ray films with small-bowel follow-through studies, as well as a barium enema with reflux into the terminal ileum, should be obtained when evaluating patients suspected of having Crohn's disease. • Barium enema alone is not sufficient for determining the extent of disease. • Luminal narrowing of the terminal ileum as a result of acute edema or chronic fibrosis of the bowel wall produces the string sign of Kantor seen on barium examination. • Thickening of the bowel wall and mesentery increases the space between adjacent loops of bowel and may give the impression of extraluminal abscess formation. • Fistulas may be seen, but they often are obscured by adjacent loops of bowel. • The mucosal pattern may be markedly distorted and skip areas of diseased bowel, and intervening normal bowel segments may also be detected.

ANSWER:
B, E

9. With regard to the medical management of Crohn's disease, which of the following statements is/are true?

   A. Nonabsorbable antibiotics (e.g., sulfasalazine) may alleviate symptoms.

   B. Steroids relieve symptoms and can induce remission but do not alter the natural course of Crohn's disease.

   C. Azathioprine is more effective than a placebo in relieving symptoms or maintaining remission.

   D. 6-Mercaptopurine is more effective than a placebo in decreasing symptoms, healing fistulas, and allowing steroid dosage to be reduced.

   E. Elemental diets and total parenteral nutrition (TPN) do not affect the natural course of Crohn's disease.

   F. Prednisone is most effective for small-bowel involvement, while sulfasalazine is most effective for colonic involvement.

Ref.: 1, 2

COMMENTS: There is no curative therapy for Crohn's disease. • Although certain therapeutic agents can effectively control symptoms, none has been shown to influence the natural course of the disease. • The goal of medical management, therefore, is to control symptoms and to provide nutritional support. • Failure of medical therapy that necessitates operation usually results from progression of the disease at the established site rather than from longitudinal extension along uninvolved bowel. • Most patients with Crohn's disease ultimately require an operation, but, because the rate of recurrence after operation is high, medical management is preferred until a complication makes an operation mandatory. • Occasionally, a patient with an incomplete obstruction or an internal fistula responds to aggressive nonoperative management. • These complications therefore should not be considered absolute indications for operation.

ANSWER:
A, B, C, D, E, F

10. Regarding surgery for Crohn's disease, which of the following statements is/are true?

   A. Operation is curative.

   B. Perirectal disease may respond to resection of diseased small bowel.

   C. The most common indication for operation is obstruction.

   D. The recurrence rate after operation is 15%.

Ref.: 1, 2

COMMENTS: Up to 90% of all patients with Crohn's disease ultimately need an operation. • Because Crohn's disease is panintestinal and typically recurrent, surgery is not curative (all tissue at risk for Crohn's disease cannot be removed). • Therefore, surgery is reserved for treating the complications of Crohn's disease, not to cure the disease. • The most common indications for operation, in decreasing order of frequency, are obstruction, persistent symptomatic abdominal mass, abscess, fistula, perirectal disease that fails to respond to local therapy, and intractability of symptoms despite adequate medical management. • Less common indications are free perforation, hemorrhage, and the blind-loop syndrome. • Whichever operation the surgeon chooses to perform, the foremost goal is preservation of intestinal length whenever possible. • Most surgeons resect only grossly diseased bowel. • Neither the use of frozen-section microscopic examination to assess resection margins nor excision of involved mesenteric lymph nodes has been conclusively shown to improve the long-term course of the disease. • Simple bypass and bypass with exclusion are no longer used routinely. • The bypassed segment often continues to be a source of active disease, and it is prone to the development of bacterial overgrowth, obstruction, perforation, and possibly malignant transformation. • Bypass is reserved for elderly or poor-risk patients, for patients with obstructive gastroduodenal disease (treated with gastrojejunostomy), for patients who have undergone previous extensive small-bowel resection, and for those instances when resection would be too risky because of fixation to adjacent structures. • Multiple fibrotic strictures in a patient who has had previous resections can be treated with strictureplasty in an attempt to conserve bowel length. • Recurrence of symptoms after operation occurs in up to 50% of patients, and the yearly rate for reoperation remains constant at approximately 15%.

A N S W E R :
B, C

11. With regard to tuberculous enteritis, which of the following statements is/are true?

   A. Primary infection usually results from ingestion of nonpasteurized milk contaminated with *Mycobacterium bovis*.

   B. Secondary infection results from the ingestion of bacilli contained in contaminated sputum.

   C. The ileocecal region is the site of involvement in 85% of cases.

   D. Infection may be indistinguishable from Crohn's disease or cancer.

   E. Approximately one half of the patients with colonic or ileocolonic disease may be treated medically without surgery.

Ref.: 3

COMMENTS: Primary enteral tuberculosis is rare in the United States but is still common in underdeveloped countries where ingestion of nonpasteurized milk occurs more commonly. • Usually it causes minimal symptoms, but occasionally it causes stricturing and stenosis in the ileocecal area. • Radiographic findings may be indistinguishable from those of carcinoma of the colon. • Although it may be necessary to resect bowel because of high-grade obstruction, it is not appropriate to do so simply to establish the diagnosis. • This can be accomplished with biopsy alone. • Treatment with isoniazid, para-aminosalicylic acid, and streptomycin usually suffices.

   Ulcerative tuberculosis is a form that develops *secondary* to pulmonary disease and is more common than the primary form of this disease in the United States. • Symptoms are variable, but most often consist of pain and diarrhea. • The diagnosis is made by barium enema examination, and confirmation is obtained by documenting an appropriate response to antitubercular therapy, which may allow healing of the lesion. • Operation may be required for perforation, obstruction, or hemorrhage.

A N S W E R :
A, B, C, D, E

12. Regarding typhoid enteritis, which of the following statements is/are true?

   A. The diagnosis can be made by culturing *Salmonella typhi* from the blood or stool.

   B. Chloramphenicol is the preferred treatment.

   C. Bleeding requiring operative intervention occurs in 10–20% of patients.

   D. Steroids should be used in patients who are toxic and who fail to respond after several days of antibiotic therapy.

Ref.: 2

COMMENTS: Typhoid enteritis, a systemic infection caused by *S. typhi*, is accompanied by fever, headache, cough, maculopapular rash, abdominal pain, and leukopenia. • There are hyperplasia and ulceration of Peyer's patches, mesenteric lymphadenopathy, and splenomegaly. • Chloramphenicol is not the drug of choice because of the emergence of resistant strains of bacteria and the risk of marrow toxicity. • Currently, trimethoprim and sulfamethoxazole are preferred. • Patients who remain toxic after 1 week of therapy often benefit from a short course of prednisone. • Bleeding occurs in 10–20% of patients and is usually treated with transfusion. • Perforation through ulcerated Peyer's patches occurs in 2% of patients and is most often free, solitary, and located in the terminal ileum. • Operative closure and appropriate peritoneal toilet are required. • Occasionally, the perforations are multiple, necessitating intestinal resection with primary anastomosis.

A N S W E R :
A, D

13. With regard to benign tumors of the small intestine, which of the following statements is/are true?

   A. Most are found in the ileum.

   B. Often they produce no symptoms and are difficult to diagnose by either clinical or radiologic examination.

   C. The most common clinical manifestations are bleeding and obstruction.

D. They obstruct the bowel by encroachment on the lumen or by causing intussusception.

Ref.: 1, 2

COMMENTS: The types and relative frequency of benign neoplasms of the small intestine vary among series, but common lesions include leiomyoma, lipoma, adenoma, and hemangioma. • About 15% occur in the duodenum, 25% in the jejunum, and 60% in the ileum, usually the distal third. • These lesions are frequently asymptomatic but may cause vague and nonspecific symptoms. • Bleeding and obstruction are the two most common symptoms. • The bleeding usually is occult and intermittent and may even lead to iron-deficiency anemia. • Leiomyoma and hemangioma are the lesions that most often bleed. • Intussusception in adults usually has an organic cause, with 50% of cases due to benign small-bowel neoplasms. • When small-bowel neoplasms are suspected, barium small-bowel follow-through study is indicated and is usually diagnostic. • Capsule endoscopic evaluation may be diagnostic as well. • When identified, small-bowel tumors should be excised because of the risk of complications, to establish the diagnosis, and to exclude cancer.

ANSWER:
A, B, C, D

14. A 26-year-old man presents to the emergency room with the complaint of recurrent, colicky, midabdominal pain. Physical examination reveals a palpable abdominal mass and several areas of increased pigmentation on his lips, palms, and soles. He states that his father had a colon polyp removed several years ago. Which of the following is the most likely diagnosis?

A. Familial polyposis with malignant degeneration

B. Gardner syndrome with intussusception

C. Peutz-Jeghers (PJS) syndrome with intussusception

D. Symptomatic Crohn's disease

Ref.: 1, 2

COMMENTS: PJS is an autosomal dominant familial disease characterized by intestinal polyposis and mucocutaneous hyperpigmentation. • The polyps are hamartomas that most frequently are located in the jejunum and ileum, but they also can be found in the stomach, duodenum, colon, and rectum. • It is generally believed that their malignant potential is extremely low. • PJS can cause intussusception or hemorrhage. • Up to one third of patients present with abdominal pain and a palpable mass. • An operation is indicated for obstruction or bleeding and should be limited to conservative resection of the involved portion of the bowel rather than attempt to resect all polyps.

ANSWER:
C

15. With regard to malignant small-bowel tumors, which of the following statements is/are true?

A. They account for 2% of all GI malignancies.

B. Carcinoid is the most common malignancy of the small intestine.

C. The 5-year survival rate is highest with adenocarcinoma, followed by lymphoma and leiomyosarcoma.

D. Wide resection with regional lymphadenectomy is the correct operation.

Ref.: 2

COMMENTS: Malignant tumors of the small bowel account for 2% of all GI malignancies. • The most frequent type is adenocarcinoma, followed in decreasing frequency by carcinoid, lymphoma, and sarcoma, principally leiomyosarcoma. • Although adenocarcinoma occurs with equal frequency in the duodenum, jejunum, and ileum, the other types tend to occur most often in the ileum. • Clinical manifestations may include diarrhea, obstruction, or chronic blood loss with anemia. • The preferred therapy is wide resection with regional lymphadenectomy. • For each entity, survival is dependent on a number of factors and is variable, but in general leiomyosarcomas and lymphomas are associated with the highest 5-year survival rates (about 40%) and adenocarcinoma with the lowest (about 20%). • Postoperative chemotherapy and radiation therapy can be useful for treating a patient with lymphoma but are not useful adjuncts for adenocarcinoma or sarcoma. • Histiocytic lymphoma may develop in patients with long-standing celiac sprue and has a worse prognosis than do conventional small-bowel lymphomas. • The Mediterranean-type lymphoma, a variant associated with monoclonal alpha heavy chains and a dense plasma cell tumor infiltration, also carries a bad prognosis.

ANSWER:
A, D

16. Which of the following statements regarding carcinoid tumors is/are true?

A. The cell of origin is the Kupffer cell.

B. The rectum is the most common site of origin.

C. There is a tendency toward multicentricity.

D. Prognosis is related to tumor size, location, and histologic pattern.

Ref.: 1, 2, 4

COMMENTS: The origin of carcinoid tumors is the Kulchitsky cell, which is thought to arise from the neural crest. • Carcinoids can occur anywhere in the GI tract. • The most frequent site is the appendix, followed by the ileum and the rectum. • Extraintestinal sites include the bronchus and ovary. • Small-bowel carcinoid tumors tend to be multiple in 30% of cases, and a second GI tumor of another histologic type can be found in 30%. • The prognosis is a function of the size of the tumor and its site of origin. • Ileal carcinoids tend to metastasize more commonly than do those that originate in the appendix.

Lymph Node Metastasis	Ileum	Appendix
<1 cm	20–30%	0%
1–2 cm	60–80%	0–11%
>2 cm	>80%	30–60%

Recent information suggests that the histologic pattern also may affect prognosis. • Patients with well-differentiated lesions fare better than do those with small-cell, anaplastic lesions.

ANSWER:
C, D

17. With regard to carcinoid tumors and their surgical management, which of the following statements is/are true?

   A. They produce a characteristic luminal deformity seen on barium examination.

   B. They are usually easily palpable on external physical examination of the bowel.

   C. Often their metastases are much larger than the primary tumor.

   D. Resection is not indicated when there is metastatic disease.

   Ref.: 1, 2, 4

COMMENTS: The usual submucosal location of carcinoid tumors often makes them difficult to find on radiographic examination or with cursory palpation during an exploratory laparotomy. • The tumors may incite an intense fibrotic reaction in the surrounding soft tissue and mesentery, which can cause luminal narrowing. • Mesenteric lymph node and liver metastases can be large compared to the primary tumor. • Tumors less than 1 cm in diameter and without demonstrable metastases can be treated by excision or segmental resection. • Those larger than 1 cm or with regional metastases should be excised widely. • This excision should include right hemicolectomy for lesions of the distal ileum and appendix. • For patients with metastases (local or distant) and in whom the carcinoid syndrome is present, debulking can provide significant palliation.

A N S W E R :
C

18. Concerning the clinical manifestations of the carcinoid syndrome, which of the following statements is/are true?

   A. Episodic manifestations include cutaneous flushing, hyperperistalsis, diarrhea, and asthma.

   B. Cardiac manifestations occur early and primarily affect the mitral and aortic valves.

   C. Cutaneous phenomena are the most characteristic and frequently recognized manifestations.

   D. Diarrhea is a significant complaint in fewer than 30% of patients.

   E. Asthmatic attacks occur in most patients.

   Ref.: 1, 2, 4

COMMENTS: Episodic manifestations of the carcinoid syndrome include flushing, diarrhea, and asthma. • The cutaneous manifestations are the most common and consist of episodes of flushing of the face, neck, arms, and upper trunk, occasionally accompanied by vasomotor collapse. • Diarrhea is significant in more than 80% of patients and usually is sudden in onset, watery, and accompanied by cramping pain and borborygmi. • Asthmatic attacks occur in 25% of patients. • Manifestations of long-standing involvement include the development of facial hyperemia with telangiectasias of the cheeks, nose, and forehead; development of the cutaneous lesions of pellagra; and valvular heart disease. • The valves most commonly involved are the tricuspid and pulmonic, although the mitral and aortic valves are sometimes affected. • Peripheral edema is present in about 70% of patients and can occur in the absence of valvular disease.

A N S W E R :
A, C

19. With regard to carcinoid syndrome, which of the following statements is/are true?

   A. Carcinoid tumors, which produce serotonin, consume up to 60% of dietary tryptophan.

   B. The most useful diagnostic test for suspected carcinoid syndrome is the determination of serum serotonin levels.

   C. Patients with normal serotonin levels do not develop carcinoid syndrome.

   D. 5-Hyroxyindoleacetic acid (5-HIAA) is the active form of serotonin.

   Ref.: 1, 2, 4

COMMENTS: Functioning carcinoid tumors divert up to 60% of dietary tryptophan in the production of serotonin, thereby contributing to the development of pellagra and protein deficiency. • Serotonin is metabolized in the liver to 5-HIAA, which is excreted in the urine. • For this reason, the most useful diagnostic test in patients suspected of having a carcinoid tumor is the determination of 5-HIAA in a 24-hr collection of urine. • 5-HIAA is inactive and does not cause the carcinoid syndrome. • The carcinoid syndrome is produced by release of serotonin into the systemic circulation either by liver metastases or by tumors located outside of the portal distribution. • While it is generally believed that patients with carcinoid syndrome have tumors that produce serotonin, the role of serotonin in the mediation of the syndrome is not clear. • Not all patients with elevated production of serotonin have the syndrome. • Some patients with the syndrome have normal levels of 5-HIAA in the urine, and injection of pure serotonin does not create all of the manifestations of the disease. • It is likely that carcinoid tumors have the capacity to produce a number of biologically active peptides, which accounts for the variability of the syndrome and discrepancies between a patient's serotonin levels and the clinical presentation. • Other substances produced by carcinoid tumors include histamine, dopamine, kallikrein, substance P, prostaglandins, and neuropeptide K.

A N S W E R :
A

20. Regarding the treatment of carcinoid syndrome, which of the following statements is/are true?

   A. Exploration is indicated in nearly all patients with malignant carcinoid syndrome.

   B. The antiserotonin agents methysergide, cyproheptadine, and *p*-chlorophenylalanine may be helpful for controlling bowel symptoms.

   C. Phenothiazines and α-adrenergic blockers may ameliorate flushing attacks.

   D. Occasionally, corticosteroid therapy can decrease the symptoms of carcinoid syndrome.

   E. In some patients with carcinoid syndrome and unresectable tumor, a combination of streptozotocin and 5-fluorouracil (5-FU) can provide palliation through their antineoplastic effect.

   Ref.: 2

COMMENTS: As previously stated, exploration may be worthwhile for patients with carcinoid syndrome and noncurable metastasis because debulking may relieve symptoms for prolonged periods. • A number of pharmacologic agents can be used to ameliorate the symptoms. • A combination of streptozotocin and 5-FU alleviates the syndrome in some patients.

ANSWER:
A, B, C, D, E

21. Somatostatin has emerged as a safe and effective agent with a broad range of applications. Which of the following is true for patients with carcinoid tumors?

    A. Somatostatin may be used as a provocative agent before measuring 5-HIAA levels.

    B. Somatostatin receptor scintigraphy is more effective at localizing primary and metastatic carcinoid tumors than is computed tomography (CT) or magnetic resonance imaging (MRI).

    C. Somatostatin is ineffective for management of carcinoid crisis.

    D. Somatostatin therapy improves survival in patients with carcinoid syndrome.

    E. Somatostatin therapy response may be predicted by the results of somatostatin receptor scintigraphy.

Ref.: 1, 4

COMMENTS: Somatostatin was first identified in 1973. • Since then, a great deal of interest has been directed at characterizing and identifying the physiologic effects and the clinical utility of somatostatin and its analogues. • Somatostatin is a 14–amino-acid protein with several analogues of shorter length that maintain clinical effectiveness. • The general effects of somatostatin are those of an *inhibitory* hormone. • Several provocative agents may be used before conducting tests for neuroendocrine tumors, including pentagastrin, secretin, and calcium infusion. • Somatostatin is not effective as a provocative agent.

Somatostatin receptor scintigraphy uses indium-111 and a gamma camera. • This study has several advantages over conventional imaging (CT or MRI). • Its sensitivity is higher (90% versus 70%) for metastatic disease, it is more effective for identifying the primary tumor site, and it visualizes the entire body to detect occult metastases. • Carcinoid tumors visible by somatostatin receptor scintigraphy suggest that these particular tumors have somatostatin receptors and are therefore subject to the inhibitory effects of somatostatin.

Carcinoid crisis is a life-threatening episode that may occur during episodes of flushing, anesthesia, or surgery. • Severe hypotension and bronchospasm may occur during carcinoid crises, and they may be refractory to usual supportive care. • The reported incidence of such crises is variable and is between 2 and 50%. • Somatostatin may be administered preoperatively as a prophylactic agent or during a carcinoid crisis as a therapeutic agent. • It is usually successful in reversing the condition.

Somatostatin has also been found to be highly effective for relieving symptoms of the carcinoid syndrome. • It has even been suggested that chronic octreotide therapy results in longer survival for patients with carcinoid syndrome compared with survival for patients treated with chemotherapy, but this hypothesis remains to be proved by randomized, controlled trials.

ANSWER:
B, E

22. With regard to Meckel's diverticula, which of the following statements is/are true?

    A. They are found in various anatomic forms and clinical presentations in 50% of the population.

    B. They are true diverticula.

    C. Some can be visualized on technetium 99m pertechnetate (^{99m}Tc) scans.

    D. Most complications occur in the elderly.

    E. Diverticulitis is the most common complication.

Ref.: 1, 2

COMMENTS: Meckel's diverticulum is the most frequently encountered diverticulum of the small intestine, occurring in 2–4% of the general population. • It is a true diverticulum, arising from the antimesenteric border of the ileum, 50–75 cm from the ileocecal valve. • Often, there is a persistent band of tissue extending from the tip of the diverticulum to the umbilicus.

The diverticulum may contain ectopic gastric mucosa capable of producing peptic ulceration and bleeding in adjacent ileal mucosa. • This ectopic gastric mucosa can be visualized using ^{99m}Tc scans. • Clinical problems are most often seen in the pediatric population. • The most frequent complications are bleeding, intussusception, and obstruction. • The latter is usually caused by volvulus or kinking around the persistent band. • The least common manifestation is diverticulitis, which presents clinically as lower abdominal pain and usually is diagnosed as appendicitis. • Therapy consists of diverticulectomy for uncomplicated diverticulitis and segmental ileal resection for bleeding or for complicated diverticulitis. • Prophylactic diverticulectomy generally is not performed when a diverticulum is found incidentally unless there is evidence of ectopic gastric mucosa or the neck of the diverticulum is narrow.

ANSWER:
B, C

23. Concerning duodenal, jejunal, and ileal diverticula, which of the following statements is/are true?

    A. Duodenal diverticula are true diverticula.

    B. Duodenal diverticula often are multiple, whereas jejunal diverticula are often solitary.

    C. Asymptomatic duodenal diverticula should be resected to avoid potentially serious complications.

    D. Asymptomatic jejunal diverticula do not require therapy.

Ref.: 2

COMMENTS: Diverticula of the duodenum, jejunum, and ileum are false (pulsion) diverticula containing only mucosa, submucosa, and serosa. • Duodenal diverticula usually are solitary and project medially toward the head of the pancreas. • Although most are asymptomatic, 10% of patients present with nonspecific epigastric symptoms, such as bleeding and perforation. • In instances of perforation, the local site should be drained. • Gastrojejunostomy is the operation most often applicable, although occasionally biliary decompression is necessary. • In instances of bleeding without inflammation, diverticulectomy is indicated, either from a dorsal approach utilizing the Kocher maneuver or via a duodenotomy.

Jejunal and ileal diverticula are often multiple and project from the mesenteric border of the bowel into the leaves of the mesentery. • This type of diverticulum is more common in the jejunum than in the ileum. • The usual treatment for symptomatic diverticula in these areas is segmental resection. • Asymptomatic diverticula of the duodenum, jejunum, or ileum do not require therapy.

ANSWER:
D

24. A 56-year-old woman has a history of pelvic radiation therapy 5 years ago for cervical cancer. Now, 5 days after she underwent a right hemicolectomy for a villous adenoma of the cecum, her surgical wound is red and tender. The surgeon opens her wound, and the initial drainage is obviously purulent. She becomes afebrile. The drainage persists as a continuous brown, liquid discharge. Which of the following is the most likely diagnosis?

   A. Simple wound infection

   B. Clostridial infection

   C. Anastomotic leakage with enterocutaneous fistula

   D. Dehiscence

Ref.: 2

COMMENTS: Most fistulas are iatrogenic and result from anastomotic leakage, inadvertent injury to the bowel during the operation, laceration of the bowel during abdominal closure, or retained foreign bodies. • Fewer than 2% of fistulas are the result of diseased bowel. • When they are, the most common contributing factors are preoperative radiation therapy, intestinal obstruction, and inflammatory bowel disease. • Although small-bowel fistulas occasionally lead to generalized peritonitis, they most commonly produce a walled-off abscess that presents as an infection of the operative incision. • The initial drainage may be purulent, but, if the infection is caused by anastomotic leakage of the small bowel, the drainage becomes enteric within 1–2 days.

ANSWER:
C

25. For the patient described in Question 24, which of the following may be included in appropriate initial management?

   A. Packing of the subcutaneous tissue with wet-to-dry dressings

   B. Packing of the subcutaneous tissue with dry, absorbent dressings

   C. Placing a sump catheter attached to suction

   D. Protecting the skin around the fistula with Stomahesive karaya powder, aluminum paste, or zinc oxide and collecting the draining fluid in an attached plastic bag

   E. Inserting a nasogastric tube and administering appropriate intravenous fluids

Ref.: 2

COMMENTS: The initial management of a small-bowel fistula includes the administration of appropriate intravenous fluids, proximal decompression with nasogastric suction, control and quantification of the fistula output, and protection of the surrounding skin. • Fistulas are classified according to their location and to the volume of their output. • Proximal fistulas tend to have a higher output and lead to more severe electrolyte and fluid imbalances. • Nasogastric suction can be helpful in diminishing the output of proximal intestinal fistulas, but the output of those more distal in the gut may not be influenced by this maneuver. • Sump catheters can provide a means of controlling and quantifying high-output fistulas, especially early in their formation. • Maintaining proper position of the catheter in the wound can be problematic. • Once the fistula tract is established, suction catheters should be promptly replaced with a stoma appliance fixed to the edges of the fistula. • Enteric contents are highly corrosive, and the skin surrounding the fistula opening should be carefully protected. • Gauze dressings are generally ineffective at absorbing all the drainage and protecting the skin. • Therefore, their use is generally avoided. • Most well-established fistulas do not produce sepsis, but in patients with persistent fever, systemic administration of antibiotics and a careful search for an undrained abdominal abscess are indicated.

ANSWER:
C, D, E

26. After the first several days, a diagnostic workup of the patient described in Question 24 should be performed to localize the fistula. Which of the following procedures can be included in the workup?

   A. Upper GI series with small bowel follow-through

   B. Fluoroscopic examination of the colon with contrast material

   C. Instillation of contrast material via a catheter into the fistula

   D. CT scan of the abdomen

Ref.: 2

COMMENTS: Early in the workup of this patient and before the GI tract has been filled with contrast material (from conventional GI radiographs), a CT scan should be performed to look for areas of abscess formation or fluid accumulation. • This may also identify the site of the fistula. • If this does not show the site, a fistulogram is helpful. • If one is concerned about distal obstruction, a small-bowel follow-through may provide information if this issue was not satisfactorily answered by CT or fistulogram. • Fluoroscopic assessment of the colon adds little and is not initially performed.

ANSWER:
A, C, D

27. Diagnostic workup of the woman described in Question 24 reveals that she has a distal ileal fistula that communicates with a small cavity. Which of the following is/are appropriate therapy?

   A. Prompt exploration and interruption of the fistula tract

   B. Prompt exploration and bypass of the fistula

   C. Prompt exploration, with resection of the portion of ileum involved in the fistula and primary reanastomosis

   D. A 4- to 6-week trial of intravenous hyperalimentation

   E. A 4- to 6-week trial of low-residue or elemental enteral alimentation

Ref.: 2

COMMENTS: Knowing the location of the fistula is of important prognostic and therapeutic value. • The overall mortality rate for small-bowel fistulas is 20%, and the rate is higher for jejunal fistulas and lower for those of the ileum. • With proper supportive care, such as intravenous or enteral alimentation, and in the absence of distal obstruction, up to 40% of small-bowel fistulas close spontaneously. • Enteral alimentation has the advantage of avoiding the possible hepatic and septic complications of prolonged TPN. • Even if there is a slight increase in fistula output after the start of enteral nutrition, the fistula still may close. • Fistulas of the proximal jejunum may require transnasal insertion of a long tube through the stomach and duodenum and just beyond the fistula before starting enteral alimentation. • Surgery should be avoided for 4–6 weeks to permit spontaneous closure and to allow local inflammation to subside, thereby facilitating subsequent surgery. • The preferred operation for correcting a persistent fistula is resection of the fistula in continuity with the segment of involved bowel, followed by a primary anastomosis. • Alternative therapies include complete or partial exclusion with primary anastomosis.

ANSWER:
D, E

28. With regard to the blind-loop syndrome, which of the following statements is/are correct?

   A. It manifests as abdominal pain, diarrhea, malabsorption, and vitamin deficiencies.

   B. Bacteria successfully compete for vitamin B_{12}, which may lead to megaloblastic anemia.

   C. Bacterial deconjugation of the bile salts can lead to steatorrhea.

   D. Addition of intrinsic factor in the Schilling test causes urinary vitamin B_{12} excretion to return to normal.

   E. The addition of tetracycline in the Schilling test causes urinary vitamin B_{12} excretion to return to normal.

Ref.: 1, 2

COMMENTS: The blind-loop syndrome is caused by stasis of intestinal contents, with subsequent bacterial overgrowth. • This stasis can be caused by a number of abnormalities, including stricture, stenosis, fistula, diverticula, or the formation of a blind pouch. • The syndrome presents with steatorrhea, diarrhea, anemia, weight loss, abdominal pain, multiple vitamin deficiencies, joint pains, and occasionally neurologic disorders. • The steatorrhea is the result of bile salt deconjugation that takes place in the stagnant fluid in the blind loop of bowel. • Megaloblastic anemia probably is a result of successful competition by the bacteria for vitamin B_{12}. • The Schilling test reveals a type of urinary excretion of vitamin B_{12} similar to that seen with pernicious anemia except that it is corrected, not by addition of intrinsic factor, but by the use of oral tetracycline. • Although the administration of tetracycline and parenteral vitamin B_{12} can correct megaloblastic anemia, only surgical correction of the cause of the bowel stasis is curative.

ANSWER:
A, B, C, E

29. Select the correct statement(s) in regard to the short-bowel syndrome.

   A. Serious nutritional deficits are produced with resection of the entire jejunum.

   B. Abnormal absorption of fat, vitamin B_{12}, electrolytes, and water constitutes the four major nutritional derangements.

   C. Resection of up to 70% of the bowel can be tolerated if the terminal ileum and ileocecal valve are preserved.

   D. Relative gastric hyposecretion, with increased intestinal pH in conjunction with interruption of the enterohepatic bile salt circulation, is the cause of steatorrhea.

Ref.: 2

COMMENTS: The entire jejunum can be resected without adverse nutritional sequelae. • The entire ileum can be resected without harm as long as vitamin B_{12} is replaced postoperatively. • Up to 70% of the small bowel can be safely resected if the terminal ileum and ileocecal valve are left intact. • If they are resected, however, loss of 50–60% of the small bowel can lead to severely compromised nutrition. • The deficiencies created by extensive resection of the small bowel are vitamin B_{12} malabsorption, altered fat absorption, and fluid and electrolyte problems. • Vitamin B_{12} malabsorption leads to vitamin B_{12} deficiency and megaloblastic anemia. • Altered fat absorption produces steatorrhea as a result of several factors. • First, massive small-bowel resection leads to gastric hypersecretion, since decreased bowel pH stimulates the intestine, thereby shortening transit time and interfering with absorption of ingested fat. • Second, interruption of bile salt resorption interferes with micelle formation. • Third, the unabsorbed fats are irritating to the colonic mucosa, thereby increasing the diarrhea and steatorrhea associated with the syndrome. • Fluid and electrolyte problems are a function of the shortened transit time and the diarrhea that results from loss of small-bowel absorptive area.

ANSWER:
B, C

30. With regard to short-bowel syndrome, which of the following statements is/are true?

   A. Initial therapy consists of control of diarrhea, restriction of oral intake, and intravenous administration of nutrients, fluid, and electrolytes.

   B. Diarrhea is best controlled by administration of medium-chain triglycerides.

   C. The administration of oral bile salts is of central importance in controlling steatorrhea.

   D. Vagotomy/pyloroplasty and reversal of a segment of bowel are the two most important operations for early management of short-bowel syndrome.

Ref.: 1, 2

COMMENTS: Treatment of short-bowel syndrome centers on control of diarrhea and parenteral maintenance of nutrition. • With time (2–3 years), the mucosa of as little as 30–45 cm of small bowel may undergo enough hypertrophy to allow withdrawal of intravenous alimentation and the start of carefully modified oral feedings. • Treatment with growth hormone, glutamine, and fiber has had some promising results in terms of gut regeneration. • Diarrhea can be controlled with agents such as Lomotil or codeine, which slow intestinal motility. • Oral calcium carbonate is also useful and acts by neutralizing hydrochloric acid and free fatty acids. • When oral intake is resumed, dietary fat is restricted to 30–50 g daily. • Some patients benefit from the use of medium-chain triglycerides. • Oral bile salts are tolerated and aid in the formation of micelles in some patients, whereas in others they cause increased diarrhea. • Cholestyramine, an agent that sequesters bile acids, is useful in patients who have had less than 100 cm of small bowel resected. • There is no standard approach to the resumption of oral intake, and the treatment must be highly individualized. • Whereas some patients ultimately do well with a modified oral diet, others remain dependent on permanent parenteral nutrition. • There are no operative procedures that reliably correct short-bowel syndrome. • Therefore, operative treatment should be considered only in patients who cannot maintain their body weight within 30% of normal without intravenous supplementation. • Operations that may be useful are reversal of a segment of intestine, creation of a recirculating loop of small bowel, creation of an artificial sphincter, vagotomy and pyloroplasty, correction of bowel obstruction, and placing all bowel in continuity (i.e., reversal of pre-existing stomas). • Vagotomy and pyloroplasty have rarely been performed for short-bowel syndrome since the introduction of H_2 blockers and proton-pump inhibitors. • Allotransplantation of small bowel in humans has been successfully performed but has a high failure rate and remains experimental.

ANSWER:
A

31. The following medications may be used in the medical management of inflammatory bowel diseases. Match each medication in the left-hand column with its possible complication in the right-hand column.

A. Prednisone	a. Neutropenia
B. 5-Acetylsalicylic acid (5-ASA)	b. Peripheral neuropathy
C. Metronidazole	c. Diabetes mellitus
D. Cyclosporine	d. Renal failure
E. 6-Mercaptopurine and azathioprine	e. Watery diarrhea

Ref.: 5

COMMENTS: Systemic corticosteroids are used to manage Crohn's disease and severe ulcerative colitis. • The initial dose of oral prednisone may vary from 40 to 60 mg/day. • Glucose intolerance may complicate steroid therapy, and some patients require insulin therapy while on high doses of prednisone. • The other common side effects are fluid retention, hypertension, mood swings, acne, and, with long-term use, osteoporosis, aseptic necrosis of the hips, and cataracts.
5-ASA products are used to treat Crohn's colitis and ulcerative colitis. • Several oral forms are replacing sulfasalazine to avoid side effects attributed to the sulfa moiety. • One disturbing side effect seen with 5-ASA has been watery diarrhea, which occurs in 15–30% of patients.
Metronidazole is used for Crohn's disease, particularly when perianal disease and fistulas are present. • It has also been used to treat pouchitis after ileoanal anastomosis. • At high doses (>1.5 g/day) metronidazole has been associated with GI upset and peripheral neuropathy. • Use of metronidazole (Flagyl) should be avoided during pregnancy because of its teratogenic effects. • Alcohol should be avoided while using metronidazole, since a disulfiram-like reaction may develop.
Cyclosporine has been used in cases of severe refractory ulcerative colitis and for Crohn's disease. • Renal function deterioration and hypertension can be seen at the recommended doses, which limits its use.

6-Mercaptopurine and azathioprine are immunosuppressive medications whose chief use is to permit a reduction in corticosteroid dose (i.e., steroid-sparing effect). • In particular, 6-mercaptopurine can be used in Crohn's disease patients with fistulas. • The use of these agents to maintain Crohn's remission is controversial. • Neutropenia and bone marrow depression are seen in 2% of patients, and pancreatitis has been described. • Secondary malignancies are rare.

ANSWER:
A-c; B-e; C-b; D-d; E-a

32. Which of the following is/are true regarding the use of corticosteroids in inflammatory bowel disease?

A. Corticosteroids are safe to use in pregnant patients with an acute flare-up of Crohn's disease.

B. Corticosteroids effectively maintain remission of Crohn's colitis and ulcerative colitis.

C. Corticosteroids used in enema (topical) form are not absorbed into the systemic circulation and therefore have no systemic side effects.

D. Every-other-day therapy is effective in these patients.

E. Intravenous corticosteroids and adrenocorticotropic hormone (ACTH) are equally effective in patients with acute severe ulcerative colitis that is refractory to oral treatment.

F. Corticosteroid therapy can be used to control flare-ups, depending on their severity, for 4–8 weeks. The dose is then tapered for another 4–8 weeks, with the goal of discontinuation.

Ref.: 5

COMMENTS: The use of steroids in patients with an acute flare-up of Crohn's colitis or ulcerative colitis during pregnancy has been shown to be not only effective but also safe for the mother and fetus. • The same statements apply to sulfasalazine.
Corticosteroids have never been shown to maintain remission of Crohn's colitis or ulcerative colitis. • Sulfasalazine and the newer 5-ASA products olsalazine and coated 5-ASA are effective in maintaining remission of only ulcerative colitis.
Topical steroids in foam or enema preparations may be absorbed in small amounts (10–20%). • Alternate-day dosing has not been effective in most patients with inflammatory bowel disease.
Intravenous ACTH is preferred to intravenous hydrocortisone by some, but controversy still exists regarding whether ACTH is more effective, even for previously untreated ulcerative colitis. • An ACTH dose of 40–60 units over 8 hr appears to be as effective as 300–400 mg/day of hydrocortisone.
The duration of steroid therapy varies, depending on the severity of the disease, but it should always be tapered on an individual basis, with the goal of discontinuation. • Many patients (10–15%) are kept on a low maintenance dose when complete elimination leads to flare-up. • This situation should not be confused with the incorrect practice of continuing a maintenance dose in patients who have achieved complete remission. • Some consider failure to achieve remission after 2 months of administering more than 15 mg of prednisone an indication for surgery.

ANSWER:
A, E, F

33. In patients with inflammatory bowel disease refractory to medical treatment, nutritional support may influence the course of disease. Which of the following statements is/are true?

A. Bowel rest and parenteral nutrition are primary therapy for Crohn's colitis.

B. Parenteral nutrition helps prevent the need for total colectomy in patients with ulcerative colitis.

C. In patients with Crohn's ileitis, TPN helps maintain lean body mass.

D. In those with Crohn's disease with high-output fistula, TPN promotes fistula closing.

E. Elemental diet is the primary therapy for exacerbation of Crohn's disease.

Ref.: 6

COMMENTS: TPN has no role as primary therapy for ulcerative colitis, but it may help maintain a satisfactory nutritional state during bowel rest. • TPN does not prevent the need for colectomy in refractory cases. • The role of TPN in patients with Crohn's colitis is not well established, but in those with Crohn's colitis and small-bowel involvement, TPN may induce remission and promote fistula closure. • Elemental diets have been shown by some to be effective in inducing remission of active Crohn's disease. • The patient's tolerance may be poor, however, and results are not superior to those obtained with corticosteroids and sulfasalazine. • Peripheral intravenous alimentation rarely provides adequate caloric replacement and may induce venous sclerosis and phlebitis.

ANSWER:
C, D

34. A 30-year-old woman has a bowel obstruction secondary to Crohn's disease. She has had multiple previous small-bowel resections. At laparotomy, multiple strictures throughout the bowel are noted. Which of the following statements is/are true?

A. Strictureplasty should be considered only for cases in which there is an isolated stricture.

B. Strictureplasty is preferred to bowel resection at the initial laparotomy.

C. Anastomotic leak and fistula following strictureplasty have been seen in 50% of cases.

D. Restricture of the strictureplasty site has been seen in fewer than 5% of cases.

E. Because residual disease is left behind, reoperation for Crohn's disease is more likely with strictureplasty than with bowel resection.

Ref.: 7

COMMENTS: Strictureplasty for Crohn's disease was first performed in 1981. • Experience since then has shown it to be a safe alternative to resection in properly selected patients. • Strictureplasty should be considered in any patient who has had extensive previous resections of diseased bowel and in whom further resection might create short-bowel syndrome. • Multiple strictures can be safely treated at a single laparotomy. • The entire small bowel must be inspected to avoid overlooking strictures that are not obvious. • This can be accomplished by passing, via a proximal enterostomy, a long intestinal tube with the balloon inflated to a diameter of 2 cm through the entire length of small bowel. • Ideally, fibrotic rather than acute edematous strictures are treated. • A longitudinal incision is made over the stricture and extended for 2 cm proximally and distally beyond the stricture. • The enterotomy is then closed transversely. • If a stricture is encountered at a patient's first surgery, resection rather than strictureplasty is preferable, since it eliminates diseased bowel and establishes the diagnosis. • Patients treated by strictureplasty have been compared to patients treated by resection. • The need for reoperation at the original site is similar.

Postoperative complications are infrequent. • At the Cleveland Clinic, anastomotic leakage, abscess, or fistula has occurred in 9% of patients treated by strictureplasty. • Restricture of the strictureplasty site occurred in only 2%.

ANSWER:
D

35. With regard to ileostomy physiology, which of the following statements is/are true?

A. Daily output from an established ileostomy is approximately 1500 ml.

B. Ileostomy output can increase by 50% at times of dietary indiscretion.

C. With dehydration, the concentration of the ileostomy sodium output rises.

D. Compared to normal ileal fluid, ileostomy effluent contains a 100-fold increase in the number of aerobes and a 2500-fold increase in the number of coliform bacteria.

Ref.: 7

COMMENTS: The daily output from an established ileostomy is 500–800 ml. • Although there is a great deal of variation in daily output among individuals, the output in a given patient varies only about 20% with changes in diet or with episodes of gastroenteritis. • The usual ileostomy sodium concentration is 115 mEq/L, although the concentration rises and falls with changes in total body sodium. • With dehydration, the sodium concentration falls and the potassium level rises, reflecting the ability of the terminal ileum to conserve sodium in times of salt depletion. • Normally, the sodium/potassium ratio is about 12:1. • The microbiologic flora of ileostomy output is markedly different from that of normal ileal fluid. • The total number of bacteria is 80 times greater, and there are a 100-fold increase in the number of aerobes, a 2500-fold increase in the number of coliform bacteria, and an increase in the number of total anaerobes.

ANSWER:
D

36. Which of the following statements about small-bowel motility is/are true?

A. Oral feeding stimulates production of migrating motor complexes (MMCs).

B. If motility is impaired, absorption of nutrients is similarly affected.

C. The frequency of MMCs returns to normal within 6–24 hr after laparotomy.

D. Vagotomy-induced diarrhea is due to increased secretion secondary to denervation.

E. Segmental bowel resection causes a temporary interruption of the MMCs, but the clinical results are usually insignificant.

***Ref.:* 4**

COMMENTS: MMCs are propagated aboral peristaltic contractions occurring at 90-minute intervals. • Activity fronts of MMCs usually originate high in the stomach, propagate distally, and end in the ileum, usually at the midileal level. • Oral feeding inhibits MMCs, resulting in irregular, nonpropagating contractions throughout most of the small intestine. • This postprandial inhibition may persist for 3–4 hr after a meal and is most pronounced with lipids. • Although this motility pattern is disorganized, there is a distal progression of chyme. • Absorption is not affected by intestinal motility. • Enteral feedings can therefore be safely and efficiently used in postoperative patients in whom motility may be altered.

Both gastric and small-bowel motility can be affected by exogenous conditions. • The small bowel is less sensitive than the stomach to general anesthesia and laparotomy, each of which decreases the frequency of MMCs. • The frequency of MMCs returns to normal within 6–24 hr in the absence of peritonitis or abscess formation. • The tone of the stomach is affected more than that of the small bowel by general anesthesia and laparotomy, at times taking longer than 24 hr to normalize. • This may explain the occurrence of postoperative nausea and emesis. • Vagotomy-induced diarrhea is a result of persistence of the sustained, organized wave of MMCs during the postprandial state.

Segmental small-bowel resection or denervation temporarily reduces the frequency of MMCs, with a resultant temporary impairment of motility. • Resection or denervation does not, however, produce long-term sequelae, provided intestinal length is not sacrificed.

ANSWER:
C, E

37. A 60-year-old alcoholic man presents with a 24-hr history of nausea and vomiting, abdominal pain and distention, and decreased passage of stool and flatus. He had an abdominoperineal resection of the rectum for cancer 18 months ago, with postoperative irradiation and chemotherapy. Examination reveals a distended, diffusely tender, tympanitic abdomen. Which of the following is the least likely diagnosis?

A. Pancreatitis with ileus

B. Adhesive bowel obstruction

C. Bowel obstruction due to extrinsic compression

D. Bowel obstruction due to radiation injury

E. Alcoholic hepatitis with ascites

***Ref.:* 1, 2**

COMMENTS: The classic presentation of bowel obstruction is the triad of nausea and vomiting, crampy abdominal pain, and decreased passage of stool and flatus. • However, nonobstructive conditions may have a similar presentation.

Ileus is temporary paralysis of the bowel due to metabolic or neurofactors. • *Electrolyte disorders* (particularly hypokalemia) may cause paralytic ileus by disrupting the normal electrical activity of intestinal nerves and muscles. • *Neural reflexes* that inhibit intestinal motor activity may be caused by distention of a hollow viscus (ureter), retroperitoneal processes (e.g., hemorrhage, pancreatitis, or spinal fracture), or peritonitis.

Mechanical bowel obstruction may be caused by a process extrinsic to the bowel wall, intrinsic to the bowel wall, or within the lumen of the bowel. • *Extrinsic lesions* cause obstruction by kinking or compression of the lumen of the bowel. • Intra-abdominal adhesions form in up to 90% of patients after abdominal surgery and may also follow intra-abdominal inflammatory conditions (e.g., diverticulitis or abscess). • *Adhesions* may cause a fixed bend in the bowel or a tight band crossing a segment of bowel, or they can act as a focus for the bowel to twist upon itself (volvulus). • Adhesions are the most common cause of small-bowel obstruction in adults. • The other two major categories of extrinsic bowel obstruction are hernias and masses. • *Hernias* may be external (inguinal, femoral, ventral, or perineal) or internal (due to congenital or surgical defects in the mesentery). • Obstructing *masses* may be neoplastic (primary malignancy, carcinomatosis, or desmoid tumor) or inflammatory (phlegmon or abscess). • *Intrinsic lesions* may be congenital (atresia or duplication), anastomotic or inflammatory strictures (Crohn's disease, radiation injury, or recovered ischemic bowel), or neoplastic (adenocarcinoma, melanoma, lymphoma, or sarcoma). • *Intraluminal lesions* may cause bowel obstruction by acting as a lead point for intussusception or by acting as mass-like intraluminal contents (large gallstone, bezoar, inspissated barium, stool, or foreign object).

Although abdominal distention may be due to ascites, its onset is much more gradual than 24 hr, and it is usually painless.

ANSWER:
E

38. Which of the following statements is true regarding the radiographic appearance of small-bowel obstruction?

A. Gas within the small bowel is distinguished from gas within the colon by luminal lines perpendicular to the bowel wall. The small-bowel lines partially cross the lumen, whereas the colonic lines completely cross the lumen.

B. Ileus may be difficult to distinguish from small-bowel obstruction, since both conditions can produce gaseous distention of the bowel with air-fluid levels.

C. The "string-of-pearls" sign refers to a series of radiolucent images in the small bowel representing the gallstones of gallstone ileus.

D. A gasless abdomen seen on plain films rules out a small-bowel obstruction.

E. The distinction between complete and partial small-bowel obstruction may be difficult during the early stages of presentation.

***Ref.:* 1, 2**

COMMENTS: Plain radiographs of the abdomen are useful for evaluating patients with a possible diagnosis of small-bowel obstruction. • Gas-filled loops of small bowel are typically seen in the central portion of the abdomen. • The presence of both dilated (>4 cm) and normal-diameter (<2 cm) small bowel is typical of small-bowel obstruction. • Small-bowel loops are recognized by the valvulae conniventes (plicae circulares), which are visible as lines that completely cross the lumen. • Colonic loops are usually located peripherally and have lines within them that only partially cross the lumen (plicae semilunaris and haustra).

Air-fluid levels are seen with both small-bowel obstruction and ileus. • They are seen only on upright or decubitus views, which allow gravity to be directed perpendicularly to the x-ray beam, with pooling of intestinal fluid in the dependent portion of the bowel.

The "string-of-pearls" sign is a series of small radiolucent circles seen when a small amount of air at the top of an air-fluid level is broken up by several valvulae conniventes in a row.

A gasless abdomen may be seen in the presence of small-bowel obstruction. • It may be the result of decompression of the obstructed proximal bowel by emesis or nasogastric suctioning, or there may be completely fluid-filled bowel with no visible air.

The distinction between partial and complete bowel obstruction is important. • A partial obstruction is present when the patient is able to pass some gas and liquid stool beyond the obstruction. • Radiographically, this condition is recognized by gas seen in decompressed bowel distal to the transition point. • In contrast, complete small-bowel obstruction is manifested as an absence of flatus and stool (obstipation), and no gas is seen distal to the dilated proximal bowel. • Early, complete bowel obstruction may be confused with partial obstruction, since distal gas and stool, present before the obstruction developed, have not yet been evacuated.

ANSWER:
B, E

39. Initial treatment of patients with acute, complete small-bowel obstruction includes which of the following?

   A. Immediate operation is warranted as soon as the diagnosis is made.

   B. Nasogastric decompression for 24 hr allows spontaneous resolution of complete bowel obstruction in most patients.

   C. The presence of fever, tachycardia, localized pain, or leukocytosis suggests strangulation and warrants prompt operation.

   D. All patients with complete small-bowel obstruction require blood and plasma for resuscitation.

   E. If small-bowel resection must be performed, a stoma and mucous fistula are necessary, since anastomosis is unsafe.

Ref.: 1, 2

COMMENTS: Timing an operation for small-bowel obstruction requires significant judgment. • The need for resuscitation must be balanced against the need to prevent gangrene by prompt intervention. • Severe intravascular volume depletion can occur owing to fluid sequestration (as much as 6 L) in the lumen of the bowel and peritoneal cavity. • Sodium, chloride, and potassium depletion frequently accompany bowel obstruction. • Blood loss is unusual unless strangulation is present. • Therefore, before induction of general anesthesia and operation, fluid and electrolyte replacement should be instituted with isotonic saline solution to normalize the heart rate, blood pressure, and urine output. • Potassium repletion should begin once adequate urine output is established. • Operation is delayed until the patient is stabilized and ready for general anesthesia. • Nasogastric decompression is an important component of supportive therapy of small-bowel obstruction. • Nausea and vomiting are controlled by this measure, and the risk of aspiration is reduced. • Swallowed air is evacuated, limiting further intestinal distention.

In cases of adhesive *partial* bowel obstruction without signs of strangulation (i.e., fever, tachycardia, localized abdominal pain, or leukocytosis) a 24- to 48-hr period of bowel rest and nasogastric decompression is warranted. • The likelihood of strangulation is limited. • In most patients, the obstruction resolves spontaneously. • Delay in surgical intervention for *complete* small-bowel obstruction is not recommended (beyond the period of resuscitation), since the possibility of strangulation is much higher than with partial bowel obstruction.

There is no increase in the anastomotic leakage rate of small-bowel anastomoses in urgent versus elective small-bowel resections, provided the bowel used in the anastomosis is healthy.

• Therefore, a proximal stoma and mucous fistula are seldom necessary following small-bowel resection for obstruction.

ANSWER:
C

40. Which of the following statements is/are true regarding PJS?

   A. The cardinal features of PJS are a diffuse intestinal hamartomatous polyposis and mucucutaneous pigmentation.

   B. Patients with PJS do not have an increased risk for cancer.

   C. Diagnosis of PJS requires a family history of intestinal hamartomatous polyposis.

   D. PJS is caused by mutation in the STK-11 gene.

   E. Intraoperative enteroscopy may improve the outcome from surgery.

Ref.: 8, 9

COMMENTS: PJS is an autosomal dominant inherited condition with cardinal manifestations of diffuse intestinal hamartomatous polyposis and melanin deposits, typically on the buccal mucosa, hands, and feet. • The polyps are distributed throughout the digestive system but have a greater preponderance in the small intestine. • Patients with this condition are at increased risk for cancers in multiple locations. • The greatest risk is in the GI tract, but additional risk is present for pancreatic, lung, breast, uterine, ovarian, and testicular tumors. • Although PJS is an inherited condition, the majority of patients do not have a family history of PJS, and this is not necessary for diagnosis of the condition. • PJS has been associated with germ-line mutations in the serine threonine kinase-11 (STK-11) gene on chromosome 19. • Mutations in the STK-11 gene account for 20–60% of PJS cases. • Intraoperative enteroscopy may improve the outcome of surgery. • Additional polyps that were not palpable may be visible, and thus enteroscopic visualization may reduce the frequency with which repeat laparotomy and polypectomy are necessary for small-bowel polyps.

ANSWER:
A, D, E

41. Which of the following statements is/are true regarding the recurrence of Crohn's disease after ileal resection?

   A. The recurrence rates (symptomatic and surgical) are unaffected by the type of anastomosis.

   B. Crohn's disease does not recur after surgery, since surgery is curative.

   C. Ileal Crohn's disease is associated with a higher recurrence rate than are other patterns of Crohn's disease.

   D. Wide margins of resection are necessary to reduce the postoperative recurrence rate.

   E. Smoking cessation is beneficial in reducing postoperative recurrence of Crohn's disease.

Ref.: 10–13

COMMENTS: Crohn's disease is an inflammatory condition of the digestive system that may affect it anywhere from the mouth to the anus. • It is characterized by remissions and exacerbations and recurrence in areas previously unaffected by the condition. • Recurrence after resection of Crohn's disease increases with time from the operation, and it is estimated that one third of patients will require a second surgery within 5 years. • Initial studies have demonstrated decreased recurrence rates with the use of a wide-lumen (75–90 mm) stapled anastomosis compared to a hand-sewn end-to-end anastomosis. • The 5-year symptomatic recurrence rate was reduced from 52 to 32%, and the 5-year surgical recurrence rate was reduced from 20 to 11%.

Several studies have suggested that the distribution of Crohn's disease affects the likelihood of recurrence. • Ileal Crohn's disease is most likely to require reoperation for recurrent Crohn's disease, followed by ileocolic and colonic Crohn's disease. • In a recent study, the median reoperation free period was shortest for ileal disease (37.8 months), followed by ileocolic disease (47.8 months) and colonic disease (54.7 months).

Multiple studies have been conducted to examine the relationship of the margins of resection to postoperative recurrence. • Two prospective studies assessing the length of grossly uninvolved bowel margin and resection fail to demonstrate an advantage of extended resections (2 versus 12 cm, and less than or >5 cm). • Other studies have assessed the relationship of microscopic disease at the margin of resection to postoperative recurrence. • This issue remains controversial, since several studies suggest a benefit from microscopically disease-free margins, while other studies show no difference in recurrence rates.

The relationship between smoking cessation and symptomatic recurrence of Crohn's disease has been evaluated in several retrospective studies. • These studies suggest that smoking cessation may decrease the symptomatic recurrence rate by 50%.

ANSWER:
C, E

42. Which of the following is true regarding capsule endoscopy of the small intestine?

    A. It is a simple, complication-free, outpatient procedure that allows examination of the entire length of small intestine.

    B. Capsule endoscopy is not well tolerated by patients, since the capsule is attached to a thin wire externalized through the nose to power the device and transmit images.

    C. Capsule endoscopy of the small intestine may be completed in 1 day.

    D. The capsule endoscope is reusable.

    E. Endoscopic images are viewed using existing endoscopic imaging systems.

Ref.: 14, 15

COMMENTS: Imaging of the small intestine has been notoriously difficult owing to its length and its location in the mid-portion of the GI tract. • A variety of attempts have been made to improve imaging of the small intestine. • The most recent and technologically advanced technique is capsule endoscopy. • The system consists of a disposable capsule that is swallowed and then passed through the digestive system by peristalsis. • It reaches the colon within 7 hr. • The capsule is self-contained, with a short–focal-length lens, a light-emitting diode, digital imaging technology, and a power source. • The images are transmitted wirelessly to a recorder worn externally on a belt. • The endoscopic images themselves are then viewed at a special work station designed for processing and viewing the images acquired by the capsule and recorder. • The plastic capsule weighs 3.7 g and measures 11 mm in diameter by 26 mm in length. • Due to its small size and weight, as well as its being completely self-contained, the capsule is well tolerated by patients and does not require hospitalization during the conduct of the examination.

• One potential complication is bowel obstruction if the capsule becomes lodged at a narrow point of the GI tract. • The capsule is disposable, and the battery is generally exhausted by the time the capsule leaves the colon.

ANSWER:
A, C

43. Which of the following is/are true regarding small-bowel endoscopy?

    A. Capsule endoscopy has replaced push enteroscopy in the evaluation of the small intestine.

    B. Capsule endoscopy is available only in specialized centers participating in clinical trials.

    C. Intraoperative enteroscopy is a simple, safe technique that eliminates the need for the less sensitive technique of capsule endoscopy.

    D. Push enteroscopy is more sensitive and specific than capsule endoscopy in the area that can be examined by push enteroscopy.

Ref.: 15

COMMENTS: Several techniques have been developed for endoscopic examination of the small intestine. • Techniques currently in use include push enteroscopy, intraoperative enteroscopy, and capsule endoscopy. • **Push enteroscopy** involves the examination of the proximal jejunum by extending the depth of insertion during upper endoscopy with the use of either a colonoscope or an enteroscope. • Push enteroscopy may also be used during colonoscopy after intubation of the ileocecal valve and further retrograde advancement of the colonoscope through the terminal ileum. • The depth of examination is typically 30–50 cm in either direction and does not allow evaluation of the majority of the central portion of the small intestine.

Intraoperative enteroscopy may be performed as described for push enteroscopy, but it is coupled with laparotomy or laparoscopy and surgical assistance in advancing the scope farther into the small intestine to reach greater depths of examination in either direction. • In addition, intraoperative enteroscopy may be performed through an enterotomy in the small intestine, which further enhances the ability to completely examine the length of the small intestine.

Capsule endoscopy involves examination of the full length of the small intestine using a wireless camera contained in a capsule. • However, the endoscopist is not able to control the passage of the capsule and is unable to perform any therapeutic interventions with the capsule.

Push enteroscopy remains a commonly used technique in evaluating the small intestine. • It is more sensitive and specific than capsule endoscopy over the length of intestine that can be examined by push enteroscopy. • It also allows for the performance of biopsies and therapeutic maneuvers. • However, push enteroscopy is not able to examine the full length of the small intestine, as can be done with capsule endoscopy. • Therefore, these two minimally invasive endoscopic examinations of the small intestine are complementary, and neither has made the other obsolete.

Capsule endoscopy is becoming more widely available. • It received the approval of the U.S. Food and Drug Administration in August 2001 and may be used in a clinical setting outside of clinical trials.

Although the entire small intestine may be examined endoscopically by both intraoperative enteroscopy and capsule endoscopy, these two procedures are also complementary.

• Intraoperative enteroscopy requires general anesthesia, a laparotomy or laparoscopy, and complete mobilization of the small intestine from adhesions. • It entails a significantly higher morbidity than does capsule endoscopy. • The findings of capsule endoscopy may provide the indication for intraoperative enteroscopy.

ANSWER:
D

44. Which one of the following conditions is not associated with an increased risk of small-bowel malignancy?

A. Celiac disease

B. Crohn's disease

C. Scleroderma

D. Familial adenomatous polyposis

E. PJS

Ref.: 16

COMMENTS: Cancer in the small intestine is a relatively uncommon occurrence, particularly when one considers that the small bowel contains approximately 90% of the surface of the alimentary tract. • Several conditions are associated with an increased risk of small-bowel cancer. • However, it is difficult to assess the magnitude of the increased risk, since small-bowel cancers are uncommon and the number in any particular series is low.

Celiac disease is a chronic inflammatory condition of the small intestine. • Lymphoma, esophageal carcinoma, and small-bowel adenocarcinoma occur with increased frequency in patients with celiac disease. • The majority of lymphomas occur in the small intestine, and adenocarcinoma is the next most frequent small-bowel cancer in patients with celiac disease.

Crohn's disease is another chronic inflammatory condition affecting the small intestine. • Risk factors associated with Crohn's disease and the development of adenocarcinoma in the small bowel include bypassed (rather than resected) segments of Crohn's disease, chronic fistulas, multiple strictures, long duration disease in a particular segment of bowel, and male gender.

Familial adenomatous polyposis and PJS are both inherited conditions. • There is a strong propensity to develop adenomas in familial adenomatous polyposis and hamartomatous polyps in PJS.

• Both conditions are associated with an increased risk of adenocarcinoma of the small bowel.

ANSWER:
C

REFERENCES

1. Townsend CM, Beauchamp RD, Evers BM, et al (eds): *Sabiston Textbook of Surgery: The Biological Basis of Modern Surgical Practice,* 17th ed. Saunders, Philadelphia, 2004.
2. Brunicardi FC, Andersen DK, Billiar TR, et al (eds): *Schwartz's Principles of Surgery,* 8th ed. McGraw-Hill, New York, 2004.
3. Corman ML: *Colon and Rectal Surgery,* 5th ed. Lippincott, Philadelphia, 2005.
4. Memon MA, Nelson H: Gastrointestinal carcinoid tumors: current management strategies. *Dis Colon Rectum* 40:1101–1118, 1997.
5. Sleisenger MH, Fordtran JS: *Gastrointestinal Disease: Pathophysiology, Diagnosis, Management,* 4th ed. WB Saunders, Philadelphia, 1989.
6. Wilson JD, Braunwald E, Isselbacher KJ, et al: *Harrison's Principles of Internal Medicine,* 12th ed. McGraw-Hill, New York, 1991.
7. Gordon PH, Nivatvongs SH: *Principles and Practice of Surgery for the Colon, Rectum, and Anus.* Quality Medical Publishing, St. Louis, 1999.
8. Scott RJ, Crooks R, Meldrum CJ, et al: Mutation analysis of the STK11/LKB1 gene and clinical characteristics of an Australian series of Peutz-Jeghers syndrome patients. *Clin Genet* 62:282–287, 2002.
9. Edwards DP, Khosraviani K, Stafferton R, et al: Long-term results of polyp clearance by intraoperative enteroscopy in the Peutz-Jeghers syndrome. *Dis Colon Rectum* 46:48–50, 2003.
10. Munoz-Juarez M, Yamamoto T, Wolff BG, et al: Wide-lumen stapled anastomosis vs. conventional end-to-end anastomosis in the treatment of Crohn's disease. *Dis Colon Rectum* 44:20–26, 2001.
11. Borley NR, Mortensen NJ, Chaudry MA, et al: Recurrence after abdominal surgery for Crohn's disease: relationship to disease site and surgical procedure. *Dis Colon Rectum* 45:377–383, 2002.
12. Wolff BG: Resection margins in Crohn's disease. *Br J Surg* 88:771–772, 2001.
13. Rampton DS: Crohn's disease recurrence can be prevented after ileal resection. *Gut* 153–154, 2002.
14. Ginsberg GG, Barkun AN, Bosco JJ, et al: Technology status evaluation report: wireless capsule endoscopy. *Gastrointest Endosc* 56:621–624, 2002.
15. Rossini FP, Pennazio M: Small-bowel endoscopy. *Endoscopy* 34:13–20, 2002.
16. Green PHR, Jabri B: Celiac disease and other precursors to small-bowel malignancy. *Gastroenterol Clin North Am* 31:625–639, 2002.

C H A P T E R 34

Appendix

Heather L. Rossi, M.D., and José M. Velasco, M.D.

1. With regard to the location of the appendix, which of the following is/are true?

   A. The base of the appendix can always be found at the confluence of the cecal taenia.

   B. In the majority of cases, the tip of the appendix is found in the pelvis.

   C. The appendix is often retrocecal and extraperitoneal.

   D. After the fifth gestational month of pregnancy, the appendix is shifted posterior and lateral by the gravid uterus.

   E. The position of the tip of the appendix in appendicitis does not determine the symptoms of the patient.

   Ref.: 1, 2

COMMENTS: The appendix, along with the ileum and ascending colon, is a derivative of the midgut. • Following developmental rotation, the cecum ends fixed in the right lower quadrant and determines the final location of the appendix. • The appendiceal orifice and, therefore, the base of the appendix are always found at the antimesenteric confluence of the cecal teniae. • The anterior one, in particular, may be used as a landmark to find the appendix at operation. • Although the base of the appendix is found in a constant location, the location of the tip varies. • In the majority of patients (65%), the tip of the appendix is found retrocecally and within the peritoneal cavity. • It occurs in the pelvis in approximately 30% of the population and in an extraperitoneal position in approximately 2%. • In pregnancy, the gravid uterus tends to push the appendix superiorly and the tip medially. • The various locations of the tip of the appendix determine the location of physical findings produced by irritation of parietal peritoneum in patients with appendicitis, but any prodromal symptoms remain the same.

ANSWER:
A

2. Which of the following regarding appendiceal innervation is correct?

   A. The innervation of the appendix is from both the autonomic and somatic nervous systems.

   B. In early appendicitis, the autonomic nervous system is responsible for poorly defined periumbilical pain.

   C. The somatic pain fibers are responsible for localization of pain in the periumbilical region.

   D. Both the autonomic and somatic nerve fibers follow midgut embryologic origin.

   E. In cases of ruptured appendicitis, the somatic innervation is disrupted and the patient is often rendered pain free.

   Ref.: 1, 2

COMMENTS: The innervation of the appendix is derived from the autonomic nervous system, which follows midgut embryologic origin. • As with all visceral organs, no somatic pain fibers are found in the appendix. • Early in the course of appendicitis, inflammation leads to poorly localized pain that is referred to the periumbilical region via autonomic innervation. • As appendiceal inflammation worsens, irritation of the parietal peritoneum results in right lower quadrant tenderness via somatic innervation. • There might be a slight decrease in pain with rupture, but a truly pain-free interval is rare.

ANSWER:
B

3. With regard to the function of the appendix, which of the following statements is/are true?

   A. It is a vestigial organ with no known function.

   B. It is a component of the secretory immune system.

   C. Its immunologic function protects against the development of colon cancer.

   D. The infantile appendix is the sole source of maturation for thymus-independent lymphocytes.

   Ref.: 1–4

COMMENTS: Although the appendix is dispensable, it functions as an immunologic organ, being part of the gut-associated lymphoid tissues (GALT) that secrete immunoglobulins. • Lymphoid tissue appears in the appendix during infancy and involutes during adulthood. • A few submucosal lymphoid follicles, present at birth, increase in number to a peak of 200 follicles at age 20. • After age 60, they involute and may totally disappear. • Concurrent with lymphoid atrophy is fibrosis, which obliterates the lumen in many older patients. • Although there has been an increased incidence of colon cancer during the last several decades, there is no evidence that appendectomy predisposes to its development.

It has been postulated that the appendix, the tonsils, and Peyer's patches of the small intestine are sites where the processing of thymus-independent lymphocytes occurs in humans.

ANSWER:
B

4. Which of the following statements regarding the pathogenesis of appendicitis is false?

   A. Luminal obstruction is always the cause of acute appendicitis.

   B. Luminal obstruction leads to increased pressure and distention of the appendix.

   C. Obstruction of venous outflow and then arterial inflow results in gangrene.

   D. Obstruction of the lumen may occur from lymphoid hyperplasia, inspissated stool, or a foreign body.

   E. Viral or bacterial infections can precede an episode of appendicitis.

Ref.: 1, 2

COMMENTS: In most instances of appendicitis, luminal obstruction leads to bacterial overgrowth, active mucus secretion, and increased luminal pressure. • Increased pressures lead to decreased venous return and, later, decreased arterial inflow, which leads to gangrene, bacterial translocation, and perforation. • The midportion of the antimesenteric border of the appendix has the poorest blood supply and most frequently shows evidence of perforation. • The cause of the obstruction is usually lymphoid hyperplasia in younger patients and fecaliths in adults. • Fecaliths are responsible for approximately 30% of cases in adults and have been identified in 90% of patients with gangrenous appendicitis with rupture. • However, luminal obstruction does not occur in all cases, since in some patients the lumen of the appendix is patent on radiologic, gross, and histologic examination. • The pathogenesis in these cases remains unclear. • It is thought that either viral or bacterial infections, such as salmonella, shigella, or infectious mononucleosis, can precede appendicitis, probably secondary to lymphoid hyperplasia in the appendix and subsequent obstruction.

ANSWER:
A

5. With regard to the natural history of acute appendicitis, which of the following statements is/are true?

   A. Rupture occurs most frequently in adolescent girls because of the difficulty in establishing the diagnosis and the consequent delay in operation.

   B. Perforation rates are correlated with the severity of the initial illness.

   C. Acute appendicitis does not resolve spontaneously.

   D. Early antibiotic treatment decreases the incidence of perforation.

   E. None of the above is true.

Ref.: 1, 2

COMMENTS: Although some episodes of acute appendicitis apparently resolve spontaneously and recurrent appendicitis is a recognized entity, the natural history of acute appendicitis is generally one of persistent obstruction leading to gangrene and

perforation. • Perforation occurs more commonly in patients at either end of the age spectrum, but clinical manifestations of the disease are not otherwise correlated with the risk of appendiceal rupture. • Prompt appendectomy therefore is indicated when the diagnosis is made, because it is the only certain way of preventing perforation and its attendant morbidity. • Antibiotics are indicated for prophylaxis of infectious complications. • Nevertheless, antibiotics do not alter the natural history of the disease. • Antibiotics should be directed against aerobic and anaerobic enteric bacteria, since they are most commonly involved in bacterial invasion of the appendix.

ANSWER:
E

6. With regard to the clinical course of appendicitis, which of the following statements is/are true?

   A. The typical history is one of vague abdominal pain, followed by periumbilical pain and, later, right lower quadrant pain.

   B. Nausea and vomiting usually precede the pain.

   C. Gross hematuria and pyuria are quite common.

   D. Most patients present with obstipation.

Ref.: 1, 2

COMMENTS: Classically, abdominal pain, which begins in the periumbilical region and subsequently localizes to the right lower quadrant, is the hallmark of acute appendicitis. • Distention of the appendix stimulates visceral afferent pain fibers, producing vague periumbilical pain of midgut origin. • The inflammatory process eventually involves the serosa and the parietal peritoneum, producing the characteristic shift in pain to the right lower quadrant. • Variations in the location of the appendix account for variations from the classic localization of somatic pain at McBurney's point (e.g., retrocecal appendix may cause flank or back pain). • Atypical abdominal pain occurs in 45% of patients with proved appendicitis and is frequently found in elderly patients and patients receiving steroids or chronic antibiotic therapy. • Anorexia is a fairly constant symptom, and the diagnosis should be questioned if it is not present. • Vomiting occurs in 75% of patients and typically follows the onset of pain. • This sequence has diagnostic significance because, in 95% of patients, anorexia precedes the onset of pain and is followed by vomiting. • Although many patients have vomiting, they have only one or two episodes. • This is in contrast to the profuse and frequent vomiting seen in patients with gastroenteritis. • Variable patterns of bowel function may be seen and are usually not of diagnostic significance. • Indeed, protracted diarrhea accompanied by vomiting is more suggestive of gastroenteritis than of appendicitis.

ANSWER:
A

7. Match each sign in the left-hand column with the appropriate physical finding in the right-hand column.

   A. Dunphy's sign   a. Pain in the right lower quadrant when pressure is applied in the left lower quadrant

   B. Rovsing's sign   b. Pain on extension of the right thigh with the patient lying on the left side

C. Psoas signing

D. Obturator sign

c. Increased pain caused by cough

d. Pain with passive rotation of the flexed right hip

Ref.: 1, 2

COMMENTS: The pain from peritoneal irritation can be worsened with movement (rebound tenderness). • Any movement, including coughing (Dunphy's sign), will exaggerate the pain. • Rovsing's sign is elicited by palpating the left lower quadrant of the abdomen, which causes the pain to be felt in the lower right quadrant, suggesting peritoneal irritation. • The psoas sign is elicited by extension of the right thigh with the patient lying in the left lateral decubitus position. • Pain elicited by the stretched psoas muscle irritating an inflamed overlying appendix suggests appendicitis. • The obturator sign is elicited with passive rotation of the flexed right hip. • If positive, the obturator sign suggests that the inflamed tip is lying in the pelvis.

A N S W E R :
A-c; B-a; C-b; D-d

8. Which of the following imaging studies is/are not a proven useful adjunct in the diagnosis of appendicitis?

A. Abdominal obstructive x-ray series

B. Ultrasound imaging

C. Computed tomographic (CT) scanning

D. Barium enema

E. Positron emission tomographic (PET) scanning

Ref.: 1–5

COMMENTS: The diagnosis of acute appendicitis is usually based on the history and physical findings, particularly when substantiated by leukocytosis. • Abdominal imaging studies are often performed in the evaluation of patients with acute abdominal pain. • They are useful in terms of the differential diagnosis and to demonstrate complications of appendicitis but should not be considered mandatory. • Plain abdominal films may show a fecalith, localized ileus in the right lower quadrant, or loss of the peritoneal fat strip. • The use of graded compression ultrasound imaging has been successfully applied to the diagnosis of appendicitis in equivocal cases of right lower quadrant pain. • The appendix is visualized, and pain is then assessed as gradually increasing pressure is placed on the area of the appendix with the ultrasound probe. • An abnormal appendix is defined as a tubular, immobile, noncompressible image. • On transverse imaging, it is seen as a target with an outer diameter at least 6 mm, a wall thickness at least 2 mm, or hyperechoic submucosa. • Using these criteria, graded compression ultrasound studies have high sensitivity (82%) and specificity (96%), with an overall accuracy of 88%. • False-negative results are frequently associated with nonvisualization of the appendix. • The advantages of this technique include wide accessibility, the ability to identify other pathologic conditions responsible for pain, lack of ionizing radiation (for women of childbearing potential), and limited expense. • Disadvantages include examiner variability and factors related to the patient that limit the study (e.g., obesity, bowel gas, or discomfort). • CT scanning was being used more frequently for patients with an equivocal history, findings on physical examination, and laboratory test results. • Currently, however, CT scanning has become popular among physicians because it has evolved into a quick and accurate examination.

• The correlation between pathologic conditions and CT results remain to be defined. • CT scanning is 90% sensitive, with an approximately 85% positive predictive value in the detection of intra-abdominal inflammation. • Focused 5-mm cuts in the area of the appendix, along with intestinal and/or intravenous contrast, aid in the radiographic diagnosis of appendicitis. • The appendix is considered abnormal when it is thickened by more than 5–7 mm in size or fluid filled. • The wall is circumferentially thickened, and its appearance is referred to as the "target" sign. • Periappendiceal inflammation along with fat stranding, fluid collections, and/or phlegmons are all suggestive of appendicitis. • Barium enemas were primarily used before the advent of ultrasound imaging and CT scanning. • A positive study result may show nonfilling of the appendix. • However, a false-negative result, showing partial filling of the appendix, can occur in about 10% of the cases, with equivocal findings occurring in about 40%. • The barium enema is no longer used routinely in the diagnosis of appendicitis. • There is no defined role for PET scanning in appendicitis.

A N S W E R :
E

9. With regard to acute appendicitis, which of the following statements is/are true?

A. A normal total and differential white blood cell (WBC) count excludes the diagnosis of appendicitis.

B. The presence of white and red blood cells in the urine is not compatible with the diagnosis of appendicitis.

C. The degree of abnormality in the total and differential WBC count is correlated to the degree of appendiceal abnormality.

D. Symptoms of appendicitis and the finding of anemia should raise suspicion of a concomitant cecal neoplasm.

E. All of the above are true.

Ref.: 1, 2

COMMENTS: Moderate leukocytosis, ranging from 10,000 to 18,000/mm³, with a moderate polymorphonuclear predominance, is typical of acute uncomplicated appendicitis. • However, up to one third of patients have a normal WBC count. • The degree of abnormality in the serum WBC count is not correlated with the degree of pathologic findings with uncomplicated appendicitis, although counts higher than 18,000/mm³ are frequently found with a ruptured appendix.

Minimal albuminuria, some WBCs, and even occasional red blood cells can be found in the urine of patients with appendicitis, particularly when the appendix is retrocecal. • Nevertheless, patients with more than 30 red blood cells per field in a specimen of voided urine should be suspected of having urinary tract disease. • The presence of bacteria in the urine does not exclude the diagnosis of appendicitis.

Anemia, particularly in elderly patients, should raise suspicion for a carcinoma of the cecum. • In cases of suspected appendicitis in which the laboratory findings are at variance with the clinical findings, the latter take precedence in terms of diagnostic value.

A N S W E R :
D

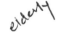

Children

10. With regard to appendicitis in young preschool children, which of the following statements is/are true?

    A. It is more uncommon than in adults because of the relatively larger diameter of the appendiceal lumen.

    B. It is often associated with higher fever and more vomiting than in adults.

    C. There is a high rate of rupture because of commonly delayed diagnosis and more rapid progression of disease.

    D. When rupture occurs, a localized periappendiceal abscess results more often than in adults.

    E. All of the above are true.

Ref.: 1, 2

COMMENTS: Diagnostic accuracy of acute appendicitis in infants and young children is lower than in adults. • First, the patient is unable to give a precise history; second, nonspecific abdominal pain is common in this age group; and third, appendicitis is infrequent in infants (probably because of the larger lumen of the appendix at its base than at the tip before differential growth of the cecum occurs), and therefore it is less often considered a cause of abdominal pain. • Vomiting, fever, and diarrhea are likely early complaints. • On physical examination, abdominal distention is common. • Leukocyte counts are not reliable. • The presence of a fecalith on a plain film of the abdomen in a child with suspicious symptoms should be enough to establish the diagnosis.

    Gangrene and rupture occur more commonly than in adults because of delay in diagnosis, more rapid progression of the disease, and atypical presentation. • The rupture rate varies from 15 to 50%. • In preschool children it is higher, ranging from 50 to 85%.

    Rupture of a gangrenous appendix in children is frequently followed by diffuse peritonitis and multiple intra-abdominal abscesses. • The walling-off process is less efficient than in adults, partly because of the incompletely developed greater omentum. • The mortality rate has traditionally been reported to be as high as 5%. • Recently, low mortality and low morbidity rates have been reported in pediatric centers, perhaps because of the acute awareness of the disease and earlier operation, thorough irrigation of the peritoneal cavity, and the use of antibiotics directed against aerobic and anaerobic organisms.

ANSWER:
B, C

elderly

11. With regard to appendicitis in the elderly, which of the following statements is/are true?

    A. Elderly patients tend to present later in the course of the ailment.

    B. Elderly patients have a lower rate of perforation because of appendiceal atrophy.

    C. Perforation has an associated mortality rate of 50%.

    D. Appendicitis may mimic bowel obstruction.

Ref.: 1, 2

COMMENTS: Acute appendicitis in the elderly may not present with the typical signs and symptoms of appendicitis. • Fever, leukocytosis, and/or right lower quadrant pain may be minimal or absent. • Often, the absence of typical symptoms can lead to a delay in diagnosis, with a 60–90% described rupture rate. • A mortality rate of approximately 15% has been reported for a ruptured appendix in elderly patients. • The atrophic omentum is less capable of walling off a perforated appendix. • Therefore, diffuse peritonitis or a distant intra-abdominal abscess is more common. • Physical examination is characterized by a paucity of findings. • Abdominal distention is prominent, and symptoms and signs mimicking bowel obstruction are not uncommon. • Occasionally, a patient presents with a painless palpable mass in the right lower quadrant due to a black, gangrenous appendix (pseudotumor appendix). • In patients older than 60, the surgeon should always be cognizant that a cancer may be causing a phlegmonous mass that is affecting the cecum. • This situation may necessitate a right hemicolectomy.

ANSWER:
A, D

immune comp

12. With regard to appendicitis in immunocompromised patients, which of the following statements is/are true?

    A. Immunocompromised patients with appendicitis often present with fever, a normal WBC count, and nonspecific abdominal pain.

    B. Typhlitis often mimics acute appendicitis.

    C. CT scanning is particularly useful in immunocompromised patients.

    D. Cytomegalovirus (CMV) infections and Kaposi's sarcoma can occlude the appendiceal orifice and cause acute appendicitis.

    E. None of the above is true.

Ref.: 1, 2

COMMENTS: Appendicitis in immunocompromised patients can be difficult to diagnose. • The patient often has nonspecific findings on abdominal examination, fever, and a normal WBC count. • The differential diagnosis of an immunocompromised patient with abdominal pain includes CMV enteritis, typhlitis, and unusual infections, including those due to mycobacteria, protozoal species, and fungus. • Typhlitis or neutropenic colitis often mimics appendicitis in these patients. • CT scanning can be particularly useful in helping establish the diagnosis. • Acute appendicitis secondary to luminal obstruction in a patient with autoimmune deficiency syndrome (AIDS) may be due to a fecalith, CMV bodies, or Kaposi's sarcoma. • Approximately 30% of acute appendicitis in patients with AIDS is caused by conditions particular to AIDS.

ANSWER:
A, B, C, D

pregnant

13. With regard to appendicitis during pregnancy, which of the following statements is/are true?

    A. Acute appendicitis is the most common cause of an acute abdomen in women after the first trimester of pregnancy.

    B. It may present with right upper quadrant or right flank pain.

    C. It should initially be treated with antibiotics in an attempt to avoid an operation.

    D. It is more common than in nonpregnant women.

    E. A perforated appendix is associated with a fetal mortality rate of 80% and a maternal mortality rate of 10%.

    F. All of the above are true.

Ref.: 1, 2

COMMENTS: Appendicitis is the most common cause of an acute abdomen in pregnant women past the first trimester. • Because during the third trimester the gravid uterus pushes the appendix (and cecum) to a more lateral and cephalad position, the typical location of somatic pain is altered. • Nevertheless, during the first 6 months of pregnancy, symptoms of appendicitis do not differ much from those in nonpregnant patients. • Acute pyelitis and torsion of an ovarian cyst can be difficult to distinguish from appendicitis. • The common occurrence of abdominal pain, nausea, and leukocytosis during the normal course of pregnancy may also make the diagnosis more difficult. • When the diagnosis is strongly suggested, prompt operation is indicated.

The incidence of appendicitis is not increased by pregnancy. • Most cases occur during the second trimester. • Appendicitis during the third trimester is associated with a higher incidence of rupture because of delay in diagnosis. • Furthermore, the omentum cannot wall off the inflamed appendix. • Premature labor occurs in 50% of women who develop appendicitis during the third trimester. • The fetal mortality rate is approximately 2.0–8.5% overall and rises to 35% with rupture. • The prognosis of the fetus is related to the birth weight and the effects of sepsis. • The maternal mortality rate is less than 0.5%.

ANSWER:
A, B

14. With regard to a ruptured appendix, which of the following is/are appropriate management choices?

   A. Drainage and immediate appendectomy for periappendiceal abscess

   B. Drainage and interval appendectomy for periappendiceal abscess if the appendix cannot be removed safely

   C. Antibiotics and nonoperative therapy

   D. Appendectomy, peritoneal lavage, and drainage for diffuse peritonitis

   E. All of the above

Ref.: 1, 2

COMMENTS: A ruptured appendix may result in a localized periappendiceal abscess, diffuse peritonitis, or abscesses at other abdominal sites, notably in the pelvis, in the right subhepatic region, or between loops of bowel. • Unrelenting obstruction of the appendix leads to gangrene and rupture of the organ, which occurs more commonly in pediatric and geriatric patients. • Because the patient is ill, the abdominal pain is more severe and diffuse, and evidence of sepsis is apparent. • Physical signs are more obvious after rupture, depending on the position of the appendix. • With a periappendiceal abscess or phlegmon, a mass is usually felt, and its nature can be further clarified by ultrasound imaging or CT scan examination.

Drainage of the abscess through a transverse or a gridiron incision is indicated. • The appendix should be removed if it is easily identified, particularly in patients younger than 40 years of age. • If it is not removed, about one third have recurrence of appendicitis.

Selected patients presenting with a well-localized abscess identified by ultrasound examination or CT scan may be treated by nonoperative therapy if the symptoms are of several days' duration and subsiding. • Performance of an elective appendectomy within 6–8 weeks is controversial. • The presence of a fecalith or retained barium in the appendix following nonoperative treatment of simple or ruptured acute appendicitis predisposes patients to recurrent attacks within 2–3 years. • If the CT scan is normal after nonoperative treatment, the recurrence rate may be quite low.

• In these cases, colonoscopy is indicated to exclude cecal causes seen on CT scanning, such as polyp or tumor.

A ruptured appendix that is producing a spreading peritonitis warrants prompt surgical exploration. • Drainage of diffuse peritonitis is not warranted and, in truth, is not physically possible. • In most such cases, the subcutaneous tissues and skin should be left open. • Whenever drains are used, they should be exteriorized through counterincisions to minimize wound dehiscence. • Use of antibiotic irrigating solution is not universally accepted. • Nevertheless, antibiotics against aerobic and anaerobic bacteria given preoperatively should be continued after surgery until the patient has no evidence of wound infection or abscess. • Complications occur in as many as 47% of patients, mainly owing to abscess formation and wound infection. • The overall mortality rate for patients with a ruptured appendix is 3%. • In elderly patients, it is about 15%.

ANSWER:
A, B

15. For which of the following patients would nonoperative therapy of appendicitis be appropriate?

   A. A pregnant woman during the third trimester

   B. A 35-year-old patient with subsiding symptoms and a right lower quadrant mass *abscess*

   C. An elderly patient with concomitant cardiac disease

   D. A 20-year-old woman with Crohn's disease

   E. None of the above

Ref.: 1, 2

COMMENTS: When the diagnosis of appendicitis is a strong consideration but not certain, in most instances operation should be undertaken because delay involves the risk of rupture, with its accompanying increased morbidity and mortality. • Operation should not be delayed during pregnancy, because doing so increases the risk to both mother and fetus. • Nor should it be delayed for elderly patients, because they face an increased risk of appendiceal rupture and death.

Although the optimal timing of operation for a ruptured appendix with established periappendiceal abscess has been controversial, most surgeons now favor prompt operation rather than nonoperative treatment and delayed appendectomy. • However, initial nonoperative therapy followed by interval appendectomy in 6–8 weeks may be considered for selected patients whose symptoms are clearly subsiding and in whom a discrete right lower quadrant mass is palpable. • Such expectant treatment consists of intravenous fluids, nasogastric suction, and appropriate antibiotics. • Vital signs, WBC count, and size of the mass are watched closely. • With these measures, most abscesses resolve, but prolonged hospitalization and antibiotic therapy are needed. • Should progression occur, the abscess is drained. • The manifestations of acute regional enteritis often mimic those of appendicitis. • Acute ileitis should be distinguished from Crohn's disease because progression of the former to the latter occurs in only 10% of cases. • If exploration reveals an acutely inflamed ileum and a normal appendix, an appendectomy may be performed, but only if the cecum is normal. • To do otherwise— that is, to perform an appendectomy in the face of cecal inflammation—risks the formation of a fecal fistula.

ANSWER:
B

16. A 20-year-old woman is operated on through a McBurney incision for presumed appendicitis, but the appendix is normal. At this point, which of the following would be appropriate treatment?

    A. Exploration and treatment of any associated pathologic condition, as indicated, without appendectomy

    B. Exploration and, if no pathologic condition is found, closure without appendectomy

    C. Exploration and diverticulectomy if Meckel's diverticulum is present, and it is normal by inspection and palpation

    D. Exploration and ileal resection if the terminal ileum appears acutely inflamed

    E. None of the above

    Ref.: 1, 2

COMMENTS: If appendicitis is not found at the time of operation, a careful exploration for other pathologic conditions must be carried out. • The accuracy of the preoperative diagnosis should be 85%. • In general, appendectomy is performed, except in some cases of Crohn's disease with extensive involvement of the ileum and cecum. • The pelvic organs, gallbladder, colon, and gastroduodenal areas should be inspected to the extent possible. • A laparoscopic approach may allow better evaluation of other areas than can be accomplished through a limited right lower quadrant incision.

Mesenteric lymph nodes are assessed. • If they are enlarged, a biopsy is performed. • The lymph nodes are examined histologically for granulomas (indicating Crohn's disease), and tissue cultures are performed for mycobacteria and *Yersinia*. • Infection with *Yersinia* causes mesenteric adenitis, ileitis, colitis, and acute appendicitis.

The small intestine is inspected in a retrograde manner for evidence of inflammatory bowel disease or an inflamed Meckel's diverticulum. • The incidence of perforation or peritonitis with Meckel's diverticulitis is about 50%. • Resection of Meckel's diverticulum is indicated if diverticulitis is present. • An asymptomatic Meckel's diverticulum found incidentally during a laparotomy in adults should not necessarily be removed. • If acute regional enteritis is discovered, appendectomy alone is indicated, provided the cecum is not involved.

ANSWER:
E

17. A 26-year-old woman presents to the emergency room at the midpoint of her menstrual cycle with right lower quadrant abdominal pain and tenderness, fever to 39°C, mild diarrhea, and two episodes of vomiting. The WBC count is 12,500/mm³. Which of the following is the most likely diagnosis?

    A. Acute appendicitis

    B. Ruptured Graafian follicle

    C. Acute gastroenteritis

    D. Pelvic inflammatory disease

    E. Crohn's disease

    Ref.: 1, 2

COMMENTS: See Question 18.

18. With regard to the patient in Question 17, which of the following is an appropriate course of action?

    A. Laparotomy through a midline incision

    B. Laparoscopy

    C. Appendectomy via McBurney incision

    D. Observation and antibiotics

    E. Ultrasound examination

    Ref.: 1, 2

COMMENTS: Right lower quadrant abdominal pain may be caused by numerous gastrointestinal, genitourinary, and infectious causes, which are best differentiated on the basis of the history, clinical examination, and laboratory findings. • Occasionally, plain abdominal films, radiographic contrast studies of the colon, and ultrasound studies are of use. • To make a correct diagnosis, a laparotomy is sometimes needed. • A false-positive rate of 15% is commonly considered acceptable. • A policy of active surgical intervention on the basis of clinical suspicion reduces both morbidity and mortality associated with appendicitis. • Removal of a normal appendix in appropriate circumstances can never be construed as an unnecessary appendectomy. • Other causes of such symptoms most commonly include acute mesenteric lymphadenitis, acute pelvic inflammatory disease, torsion of an ovarian cyst, ruptured Graafian follicle, acute gastroenteritis, and even no organic pathologic condition.

A negative exploration rate for appendicitis of 32–45% has been reported in women of childbearing age and is compounded by a higher incidence of appendicitis during the latter half of the menstrual cycle than during the first half.

Careful observation is indicated if the pain is atypical, there is no guarding on the right lower quadrant, and fever and leukocytosis are absent.

Salpingitis offers the greatest diagnostic difficulty. • The pain is usually bilateral and low in the abdomen, and pelvic examination may elicit extreme pelvic tenderness (chandelier sign). • Intracellular diplococci may be demonstrable on a smear of purulent vaginal discharge.

Although laparotomy through a midline incision has been advocated in women presenting with equivocal findings, laparoscopy is being used increasingly to ascertain the cause of the process and to perform therapeutic operations. • It allows rapid inspection of the abdominal cavity and assessment of possible intra-abdominal pathologic conditions. • It also directs the surgeon toward the most appropriate incision, if needed. • Many surgeons prefer a McBurney or a transverse (Rockey-Davis) incision in patients with suspected appendicitis. • The transverse approach allows extension of the incision if it becomes necessary to address a pathologic condition in the pelvis and avoidance of a second incision.

ANSWERS:
Question 17: A
Question 18: B, C, E.

19. During evaluation of a male patient with right lower quadrant pain, which of the following should be included in the differential diagnosis?

    A. Acute mesenteric adenitis

    B. Gastroenteritis

    C. Diverticulitis

    D. Epiploic appendagitis

    E. Intussusception

    Ref.: 1, 2

Carcinoid

COMMENTS: The differential diagnosis of appendicitis is basically that of the acute abdomen. • Often, it is impossible to differentiate the entities listed above and other inflammatory processes from acute appendicitis. • An extensive diagnostic workup is usually not warranted. • The surgeon must be prepared to treat other pathologic entities should they be found on exploration for appendicitis.

Acute mesenteric adenitis is most often confused with appendicitis in children. • Often, an upper respiratory tract infection precedes or is present at the onset of a more diffuse abdominal pain. • Tenderness is not localized and may change as the patient assumes various positions. • Generalized lymphadenopathy or relative lymphocytosis, when present, can be of help. • If, after observation, the differentiation is in doubt, an operation is warranted.

Acute **gastroenteritis** is characterized by cramping pain followed by watery stools, nausea, and vomiting. • Laboratory study results are usually normal. • Diagnosis of a specific bacterial infection (e.g., *Salmonella* or typhoid fever) is made by stool culture. • **Diverticulitis** of the cecum or a perforated carcinoma of the cecum may be impossible to distinguish from acute appendicitis. • Both often present as a right lower quadrant mass with evidence of infection and peritonitis. • Frequently, a right hemicolectomy is needed because the diagnosis may be difficult to establish at operation. • Sigmoid diverticulitis may also mimic appendicitis if a mobile, inflamed sigmoid colon is located in the right lower quadrant.

Epiploic appendagitis results from infarction of the appendage due to torsion. • The pain shift is unusual, and the patient does not appear ill. • Tenderness, rebound tenderness, and absence of rigidity over the site are common.

In contrast to the previously mentioned entities, it is important to differentiate **intussusception** from appendicitis. • The patient's age, the type of pain, a palpable mass in the lower quadrant, and the passage of currant-jelly stool may help the diagnosis. • A barium enema offers a diagnostic and therapeutic option for intussusception.

ANSWER:
A, B, C, D, E

Crohn's

20. A patient suspected of having appendicitis underwent exploration. Crohn's disease was found. Which of the following are true?

A. The normal appendix always should be removed.

B. All grossly involved bowel, including the appendix, should be resected.

C. An inflamed appendix, cecum, and terminal ileum should be resected.

D. Perforated bowel and advanced Crohn's disease with obstruction should be resected.

E. All of the above

Ref.: 1, 2

COMMENTS: If a normal appendix is found at the time of laparotomy, other causes should be sought. • If Crohn's disease is encountered and the cecum and base of the appendix are normal, an appendectomy should be performed. • If the base is involved with Crohn's disease and the appendix is normal, appendectomy should not be performed. • If the finding of Crohn's disease is uncomplicated by perforation or obstruction, ileal resection is not indicated. • However, in the case of perforation or Crohn's disease with obstruction, the involved bowel should be resected.

ANSWER:
D

21. With regard to carcinoids of the appendix, which of the following statements is/are true?

A. The ileum is the most common location for gastrointestinal carcinoids.

B. Nearly one third are multiple.

C. Most carcinoid tumors occur at the tip of the appendix.

D. Most appendiceal carcinoids are malignant and produce the carcinoid syndrome.

E. All of the above are true.

Ref.: 1, 2

COMMENTS: The most common locations for gastrointestinal carcinoids are the rectum, ileum, and appendix, in order of increasing frequency. • Appendiceal carcinoids are usually solitary. • About 75% of them occur at the distal tip, and fewer than 10% occur at the base. • They are usually an incidental finding and only rarely cause appendicitis. • Carcinoids of the small bowel are multiple in approximately 30% of the cases. • Carcinoid syndrome occurs most commonly in patients with small-bowel tumors that have metastasized to the liver. • Appendiceal carcinoids less then 1 cm in size are generally considered biologically benign lesions, with approximately 3% found to be metastatic. • If the lesion is found at the tip of the appendix and is smaller than 1 cm, an appendectomy is considered adequate treatment, since these lesions have a higher risk of metastasis. • A right hemicolectomy is indicated if tumor is present at the surgical margins, if there is nodal involvement, and if the lesion is larger than 1 cm.

ANSWER:
C

22. If an incidental appendiceal carcinoid is recognized during simple appendectomy, which of the following statements is/are true?

A. If the tumor is 2 cm in size, the mesoappendiceal lymph nodes are negative, and the resection margins are clear, no further surgical treatment is necessary.

B. Right hemicolectomy is routinely indicated, regardless of nodal status.

C. If mesoappendiceal lymph nodal metastases are present, surgical cure is unlikely and chemotherapy should be initiated.

D. Right hemicolectomy is indicated if tumor is present at the surgical margins or if there is nodal involvement.

E. None of the above is true.

Ref.: 1, 2

COMMENTS: A carcinoid of the appendix is usually found incidentally and is recognized by the presence of a small, firm, circumscribed, yellowish tumor. • The malignant potential is related to the site of origin (foregut, midgut, or hindgut) and the size of the tumor. • Only 3% of appendiceal tumors metastasize, in contrast to 35% of those arising in the ileum. • Tumors less than 1 cm in size rarely metastasize to regional lymph nodes and distant organs, tumors with diameters of 1–2 cm metastasize in 50% of cases, and 80–90% of tumors larger than 2 cm metastasize. • The microscopic growth pattern seems to be correlated with long-term survival as well. • The median survival time for a patient with mixed insular/glandular pattern is 4.4 years, whereas that for a patient with an undifferentiated tumor is 6 months.

• Simple appendectomy and resection of the mesoappendix are considered adequate treatment for carcinoids of the appendix that are small (<1 cm), that do not have regional nodal metastases, and that have been completely resected by appendectomy.

If nodes are involved or the tumor is larger than 2 cm, right hemicolectomy should be performed. • For patients with tumors 1–2 cm in size, the decision to perform a right hemicolectomy must be individualized, since these patients have a substantial risk (50%) of metastasis. • When extensive metastatic disease precludes cure, extensive debulking surgery for palliation is indicated. • Chemotherapy with a combination of 5-fluorouracil and streptozocin has provided some palliation of the carcinoid syndrome in patients with unresectable metastatic disease. • Various antiserotonin agents have also been employed for controlling symptoms in patients with the carcinoid syndrome. • Somatostatin can be used for controlling symptoms and as an antineoplastic agent. • Up to 25% of patients who undergo palliative resections survive 5 years.

ANSWER:
D

23. When a mucocele of the appendix is found at the time of surgery, which of the following is/are appropriate initial therapy?

   A. Incisional biopsy with subsequent appendectomy if malignancy is confirmed by frozen section

   B. Routine right hemicolectomy with lymph node dissection

   C. Needle aspiration of cystic fluid for cytologic examination

   D. Appendectomy

   E. None of the above

Ref.: 1, 2

COMMENTS: Appendectomy is adequate treatment for mucocele, but care must be taken to avoid rupture, since pseudomyxoma peritonei has been reported following rupture and peritoneal dissemination of the appendiceal contents. • Histologically, mucocele can be categorized as a benign type, which is the result of an occlusion of the proximal lumen of the appendix, or a malignant type, which is a variant of a mucous papillary adenocarcinoma. • Treatment of an appendiceal adenocarcinoma is right hemicolectomy.

ANSWER:
D

24. Which of the following statements is/are true regarding laparoscopic versus open appendectomies?

   A. Laparoscopic appendectomy is associated with less postoperative pain, shortened hospital stay, faster recovery, and lower wound infection rates.

   B. Laparoscopic appendectomy is the procedure of choice for appendicitis in most situations.

   C. The operative time for the two procedures is similar.

   D. Conversion from laparoscopic to open appendectomy occurs in approximately 10% of cases.

   E. Laparoscopic appendectomy results in a higher intra-abdominal abscess rate in patients with advanced appendicitis.

Ref..: 1, 2, 6, 7

COMMENTS: Laparoscopic appendectomy has several advantages over the open technique, including shortened hospital stay, faster recovery, and lower wound infection rates. • The wound infection rate for laparoscopic appendectomy is less than one half that for open appendectomy. • The major disadvantages of laparoscopic appendectomy are the longer operative time and the use of disposable instruments, which can increase overall cost. • The rates of conversion are variable but occur approximately 10% of the time. • For patients with advanced appendicitis at presentation, there is a greater tendency for the formation of intra-abdominal abscesses with laparoscopic appendectomy than with the open technique.

ANSWER:
A, D, E

REFERENCES

1. Lally KP, Cox CS, Andrassy RJ: Appendix. In: Townsend CM, Beauchamp RD, Evers BM, et al (eds): *Sabiston Textbook of Surgery: The Biological Basis of Modern Surgical Practice*, 16th ed. Saunders, Philadelphia, 2001.
2. Matthews JB, Hodin RA: Acute abdomen and appendix. In: Greenfield LJ, Mulholland MW, Oldham KT, et al (eds) *Greenfield's Surgery: Scientific Principles and Practice*, 3rd ed. Lippincott, Williams & Wilkins, Philadelphia, 2001.
3. Galindo GM, Fadrique B, Nieto MA, et al: Evaluation of ultrasonagraphy and clinical diagnostic scoring in suspected appendicitis. *Br J Surg* 85:37–40, 1998.
4. Rua PM, Rhea JT, Novelline RA, et al: Effect of computed tomography of the appendix on treatment of patients and use of hospital resources. *N Engl J Med* 338:141–146, 1998.
5. Raptopoulos V, Katsou G, Rosen MP, et al: Acute appendicitis: effect of increased use of CT on selecting patients earlier. *Radiology* 226(2):521–526, 2003.
6. Golub R, Siddiqui F, Pohl D: Laparoscopic versus open appendectomy: a metaanalysis. *J Am Coll Surg* 186:545–553, 1998.
7. Liu SI, Siewert B, Raptopoulos V, et al: Factors associated with conversion to laparotomy in patients undergoing laparoscopic appendectomy. *J Am Coll Surg* 194:298–302, 2002.

CHAPTER 35

Colon and Rectum

Theodore J. Saclarides, M.D.

1. With regard to the anatomy of the colon and rectum, which of the following statements is/are true?

   A. The colon has a complete outer longitudinal and an incomplete inner circular muscle layer.

   B. The haustra are separated by plicae circulares.

   C. The ascending and descending colon are normally fixed to the retroperitoneum.

   D. The anatomic rectum is partially intraperitoneal and partially extraperitoneal.

   Ref.: 1

COMMENTS: A thorough understanding of anatomy is integral to the surgical management of problems of the colon and rectum. • The colon has two muscle layers: an outer longitudinal layer and an inner circular layer. • The **inner** layer completely encircles the colon. • The **outer** layer, unlike in the small intestine, is in the form of three grossly recognizable longitudinal strips, **taeniae coli**, that do not cover the full circumference of the bowel. • At the rectosigmoid junction, the three taeniae coli become broad and fuse together, and the rectum is totally invested with two complete muscle layers.

The **plicae semilunares** are spaced, transverse, crescentic folds that separate the tissue between the taeniae coli, forming haustra. • They produce a characteristic, intermittently bulging pattern that radiologically permits differentiation of the colon from the small intestine, which has circular mucosal folds known as **plicae circulares** or **valvulae conniventes**. • In contrast to the plicae semilunaris, the plicae circulares traverse the full diameter of the small-bowel lumen, facilitating radiographic distinction.

Normally, the ascending and descending portions of the colon are fused to the retroperitoneum, whereas the transverse and sigmoid portions are free. • Developmental anomalies of fixation, as seen with malrotation and in some cases of volvulus, are not uncommon. • Cecal volvulus, for example, could not occur unless incomplete fixation to the retroperitoneum made it possible for a mobile cecum to rotate around a narrow mesenteric pedicle.

Surgeons traditionally have placed the upper border of the rectum at the peritoneal reflection. • An alternative definition is that point where the taeniae have completely merged. • The distal rectum is void of any peritoneal covering, the middle rectum is covered by peritoneum ventrally, and the upper rectum is completely covered by peritoneum, except for a thin strip dorsally where the short mesorectum suspends the rectum to the presacral tissue.

ANSWER:
C, D

2. With regard to the arterial system of the colon and rectum, which of the following statements is/are true?

   A. The ileocolic, right colic, and middle colic arteries originate from the superior mesenteric artery.

   B. The superior and middle rectal arteries originate from the inferior mesenteric artery.   *m iliac*

   C. Approximately 80% of intestinal blood flow circulates to the mucosa and submucosa, and the remaining 20% passes to the muscularis.

   D. The colon and small bowel are equally vulnerable to ischemic injury produced by acute reductions in blood flow.

   E. An increase in the functional motor activity of the colon is accompanied by a corresponding increase in blood flow.

   Ref.: 4, 5

COMMENTS: The total blood flow to the gastrointestinal tract is approximately 25 ml/kg/min, or 20% of the cardiac output. • During a meal, the blood flow to the intestine rises to 50% above normal without a corresponding rise in cardiac output. • Physical exercise, in contrast, doubles cardiac output, with a 20% decrease in superior mesenteric artery flow.

The right and transverse colons are derived from the foregut and receive their blood supply from the superior mesenteric artery via its ileocolic, right colic, and middle colic branches. • The left colon and sigmoid, derived from the hindgut, are supplied by the left colic and sigmoid branches, originating from the inferior mesenteric artery. • In general, there are well-developed collaterals between the mesenteric arteries through a marginal arcade adjacent to the colon. • The rectum, a hindgut structure, is supplied by the superior hemorrhoidal artery, originating from the inferior mesenteric artery, and by the middle and inferior hemorrhoidal arteries, originating from the internal iliac artery or its internal pudendal branch. • The venous and lymphatic drainage systems of the colon and rectum generally parallel the arterial supply, with the exception of the inferior mesenteric vein, which courses directly cephalad to empty into the splenic vein.

Approximately 80% of the blood flow to the colon wall reaches the mucosa and submucosa, and the remaining 20% supplies the muscularis. • Despite the extensive collateral vessels to the colon, it receives only about 50% of the blood flow that the small intestine receives. • The colon therefore is more sensitive to ischemic injury during acute reductions in blood flow.

411

In contrast to other areas of the body, an increase in functional motor activity of the colon does not result in a parallel increase in absolute colonic blood flow.

ANSWER:
A, C

3. Which of the following is/are accepted and effective method(s) of reducing the risk of wound infection in colorectal operations?

   A. Systemic antibiotics alone

   B. Mechanical bowel cleansing alone

   C. Mechanical cleansing plus systemic antibiotics

   D. Mechanical cleansing plus nonabsorbable oral antibiotics

   E. Mechanical cleansing plus nonabsorbable oral antibiotics and systemic antibiotics

Ref.: 1, 2, 6

COMMENTS: The colon contains a higher concentration of bacteria, both aerobic and anaerobic, than any other area of the body, and infectious complications constitute the major morbidity of colorectal operations. • The ability of intestinal antisepsis to lessen these complications has been well established in numerous laboratory and clinical studies, although there are conflicting data as to the best method of providing antisepsis. • Mechanical cleansing of the colon can be achieved by administration of a cathartic in combination with enemas or by peroral lavage with a relatively large volume of solution. • The lavage being used most frequently is a nonabsorbable polyethylene glycol–electrolyte solution administered during the afternoon before surgery. • Metoclopramide, given orally or intramuscularly before the lavage begins, may reduce the relatively commonly associated nausea. • No cathartics are necessary when using a lavage solution. • Such mechanical cleansing clearly is important, but if used alone it does not significantly alter the concentration of bacterial flora, nor does it decrease the incidence of postoperative septic complications. • Wound infections still occur in approximately 50% of cases. • A combination of mechanical preparation with the administration of nonabsorbable oral antibiotics effective against both aerobic and anaerobic colonic flora provides effective protection against infections. • Systemic antibiotics are often combined with lavage and oral antibiotics, but such a combination has not been conclusively demonstrated to confer an advantage over the use of lavage and oral antibiotics alone. • The use of systemic antibiotics in place of oral antibiotics is also an effective method of prophylaxis, and many surgeons have resorted to this regimen in order to avoid the nausea associated with some oral antibiotics. • While reports in the literature disagree as to the best protocol, the standard of care is to mechanically cleanse the colon and provide antibiotics: oral, systemic, or both.

ANSWER:
C, D, E

4. In the United States, what is the most common cause of mechanical obstruction of the colon?

   A. Adhesions

   B. Diverticulitis

   C. Cancer

   D. Volvulus

   E. Inguinal hernia

Ref.: 1, 2

COMMENTS: Whenever a patient presents with signs and symptoms of intestinal obstruction, one first attempts to define the level of obstruction (i.e., small bowel or large bowel). • Colonic obstruction is often suggested by the gas pattern on plain abdominal radiographs and can be confirmed radiographically by a carefully performed enema with a water-soluble contrast medium. • Barium used in this situation has potential hazards. • One concern is causing peritonitis in the presence of a perforating lesion. • Another is inspissation proximal to a partially obstructing cancer or diverticulitis, effectively converting a partial obstruction to a complete one.

In the United States, **colorectal cancer** is by far the leading cause of large-bowel obstruction. • **Diverticulitis** is the next most common cause. • In some parts of the world (e.g., Iran, Iraq, and Pakistan) where there is a high fiber content in the diet, resulting in large volumes of stool and an elongated colon, **volvulus** is the leading cause. • In the United States, sigmoid volvulus is rare and is usually seen in elderly, institutionalized patients. • **Intussusception** is a common cause of colonic obstruction in infants and children but is unusual in adults unless a neoplasm has precipitated an intussusception. • It is highly unusual to have large-bowel obstruction secondary to **adhesions** or **incarceration** within an inguinal hernia, is in contradistinction to an obstruction of the small intestine. • Other causes of large-bowel obstruction include **fecal impaction**, especially in the elderly and infirm, and **benign strictures** secondary to ischemia or inflammatory bowel disease. • A neglected obstruction from any mechanism can be fatal. • Colon obstruction in the presence of a competent ileocecal valve creates a closed-loop phenomenon. • Progressive distention of the colon between the point of obstruction and the ileocecal valve may lead to necrosis and perforation of the gut wall. • Volvulus can behave in the same manner and have the same consequence.

ANSWER:
C

5. Which of the following are the most common causes of massive colonic bleeding?

   A. Cancer

   B. Ulcerative colitis

   C. Diverticulosis

   D. Diverticulitis

   E. Angiodysplasia

Ref.: 2, 7, 8

COMMENTS: Diverticulosis and angiodysplasia are responsible for most cases of massive colonic bleeding, and they occur with equal frequency. • These two entities frequently coexist, and precise identification of the bleeding source may require a combination of endoscopic, radiographic, and histologic methods. • Before the advent of angiography, angiodysplasia was not recognized as a source of colonic hemorrhage. • Its cause is not known but may be related to degenerative changes associated with aging and to intramural muscular hypertrophy that obstructs the submucosal veins, leading to their dilatation and propensity to bleed. • **Diverticulosis** can also cause **massive** bleeding, attributed to ruptured vasa recta at the apex or neck of a diverticulum. • **Diverticulitis** also can cause bleeding as a result of superficial mucosal ulceration, but usually such bleeding is mild. • **Ulcerative colitis** is more likely to cause mild-to-moderate bleeding and frequently is associated with diarrhea and systemic signs of a chronic illness, such as weight loss and failure to thrive. • **Cancer** of the colon usually causes occult rather than massive gastrointestinal bleeding.

ANSWER:
C, E

6. With regard to lower gastrointestinal hemorrhage, match each statement in the left-hand column with the appropriate disease in the right-hand column.

A. At least 50% of cases have bleeding originating in the right colon.	a. Diverticulosis
B. The bleeding is arterial and severe.	b. Angiodysplasia
C. After the first episode, the rate of recurrent bleeding is at least 25%.	c. Both
D. Extravasation of dye during angiography can be seen in most cases.	d. Neither
E. Total colectomy is the procedure of choice.	

Ref.: 3

COMMENTS: Diverticulosis and angiodysplasia account for 90% of cases of **massive lower gastrointestinal bleeding** in patients older than 50 years of age. • Since the advent of angiography for evaluating colonic hemorrhage, angiodysplasia is being recognized as increasingly the most likely cause, although diverticulosis is still known to be responsible for a significant number of cases.

Although 80% of diverticular disease is concentrated in the left and sigmoid colon, 50% of diverticular bleeding originates from the right colon. • Almost all colonic angiodysplasias are located in the cecum and right colon. • The bleeding associated with diverticulosis is secondary to a ruptured vasa recta at the neck or apex of a diverticulum and is arterial and usually severe. • In contrast, bleeding from angiodysplasia is venous and is not as severe. • After the initial episode, diverticular bleeding may recur in 25% of cases, and rebleeding after the second episode occurs in 50%. • The rebleeding rate for angiodysplasia is not known with certainty. • Some sources cite rates as high as 85%, others substantially less.

In most cases of diverticular hemorrhage, angiography reveals the source by demonstrating extravasation of radiopaque contrast material into the intestinal lumen. • In contrast, only 8–10% of bleeding secondary to angiodysplasia exhibits angiographic extravasation. • Other, more common angiographic findings associated with angiodysplasia include a dense, slowly emptying mesenteric vein (92%); a vascular tuft (68%); and an early-filling mesenteric vein (56%).

If preoperative localization studies precisely locate the site of bleeding, a limited resection is preferred. • This preference holds true for bleeding from cecal angiodysplasia, even though asymptomatic sigmoid diverticula are incidentally discovered. • Total colectomy is reserved for cases in which the degree of bleeding warrants surgery but preoperative localizing studies are unsuccessful in pinpointing the site of bleeding.

ANSWER:
A-c; B-a; C-c; D-a; E-d

7. A 68-year-old man is admitted to the hospital having passed three large maroon-colored stools. On arrival at the hospital, he passes more bloody stools as well as clots. He is pale, orthostatic, and tachycardic. Nasogastric aspirates are bilious. After resuscitation is begun, which of the following is the most appropriate initial test?

A. Angiography

B. Nuclear medicine red blood cell scan

C. Rigid proctoscopy

D. Colonoscopy

E. Barium enema

Ref.: 3

COMMENTS: While all of the aforementioned tests may play a role in evaluating a patient with massive loss of blood through the rectum, proctoscopy is the most appropriate initial test. • Proctoscopy may reveal an anorectal source of the bleeding and a diffuse mucosal process, such as ulcerative proctitis.

Proceeding directly to a barium enema examination is ill advised, since the barium obscures details if angiography is subsequently needed. • Furthermore, finding sigmoid diverticula does not prove that they are the source of the bleeding.

Mesenteric angiography is performed if the hemorrhage is brisk and persistent. • A bleeding rate of approximately 1–5 ml/min is necessary to visualize the responsible vessel. • The superior mesenteric artery should be injected first because most bleeding originates in the right colon. • If no abnormalities are found, this step is followed by injecting the inferior mesenteric artery and *finally the celiac axis.* • If a source of the bleeding is found, embolization may be performed using Gelfoam strips or autologous blood clots. • Rebleeding following embolization occurs in approximately 25% of cases. • Embolization may occlude more than the single bleeding vessel and lead to ischemia and even colon infarction, which occurs in approximately 5% of patients. • Therefore, embolization should be reserved for patients who cannot tolerate surgery or vasopressin. • Vasopressin may be selectively infused into the mesenteric vessel. • While it stops the bleeding in many patients, it may also cause cardiac arrhythmias, heart failure, and hypertension. • Cessation of vasopressin may precipitate further bleeding in 30% of patients. • The use of vasopressin gives the physician time to complete resuscitation and to address coexisting medical disorders.

Sulfur colloid nuclear scanning has also been used to assess lower intestinal bleeding. • Unfortunately, the isotope is cleared rapidly by the reticuloendothelial system, and repetitive scanning is not possible. • Alternatively, red blood cells may be tagged with technetium. • This technique detects bleeding at a rate as low as 0.1 ml/min. • Because this isotope is not cleared from the vascular system as rapidly, repeated scanning may be possible over an extended period. • Sensitivity, specificity, and accuracy rates have varied widely among reported series, and the precise role of red blood cell scanning is controversial.

Colonoscopy has emerged as a valuable diagnostic and therapeutic tool for stable patients who are not bleeding briskly. • No bowel cleansing is needed, but the examination must be done by an experienced endoscopist. • Angiodysplastic lesions can be treated successfully by colonoscopic methods.

ANSWER:
C

8. A definitely increased risk of developing colon cancer is associated with which of the following?

A. Diet high in fiber

B. Diet low in animal fat and protein

C. Ulcerative colitis

D. Familial polyposis

E. Previous cholecystectomy

F. Strong family history of colon cancer in several preceding generations

Ref.: 1, 3

COMMENTS: In the United States, colorectal cancer is second only to lung cancer as the leading cause of death from cancer. • Environmental factors, particularly dietary habits, may explain the wide variation in geographic distribution of colon cancer.

Diets low in fiber and high in animal fats and protein are associated with an increased risk of colon cancer. • The mechanisms may include alterations in intestinal transit time and an increase in the formation of carcinogenic compounds as a result of bacterial metabolism of dietary components. • Gallstone disease appears to be more common in areas where colon cancer is prevalent. • Some studies have suggested that cholecystectomy is associated with a higher incidence of subsequent colon cancer, particularly involving the right colon. • A proposed mechanism for this relationship is related to the carcinogenic potential of secondary bile acids, to which the intestinal mucosa is increasingly exposed after cholecystectomy as a result of increased enterohepatic cycling. • Evidence supporting this association is conflicting, however, and any association that may exist is minimal.

Genetic factors play a definite role in carcinogenesis, and mutational abnormalities have been identified in familial polyposis and hereditary nonpolyposis colorectal cancer syndromes (HNPCC). • Almost 100% of patients with familial polyposis develop cancer, usually by age 40, if the colon is left untreated. • In HNPCC, the lifetime risk of developing colorectal cancer approaches 80%. • The aforementioned notwithstanding, familial polyposis, the HNPCC syndrome, and ulcerative colitis account for only a small percentage of the total cases of colorectal cancer.

Risk factors for the development of cancer in patients with ulcerative colitis include disease of long duration (the incidence increases 1–2% per year after 10 years) and total colonic involvement. • An increased risk of cancer has also been seen with Crohn's disease, of both the small and large intestine, particularly in bypassed segments.

A N S W E R :
C, D, F

---

9. With regard to screening and surveillance for colorectal cancer, which of the following is/are true?

    A. Barium enema alone is a cost-effective means of screening asymptomatic patients.

    B. Population-based screening programs using guaiac tests for fecal occult blood have been able to detect a higher than expected number of early, superficial cancers.

    C. The positive predictive value of a positive fecal occult blood test (FOBT) result is approximately 10% for cancer and 30% for adenomas.

    D. When combined with flexible sigmoidoscopy, FOBT reduces mortality from colorectal cancer.

    E. For patients with familial polyposis or hereditary nonpolyposis colorectal cancer, screening is best achieved with FOBT performed alone every 6 months.

Ref.: 6

COMMENTS: Screening asymptomatic, low-risk patients for colorectal cancer must be accomplished with a cost-effective means that encourages patients' compliance. • The test that best accomplishes these goals is annual examination of the stool for occult blood. • This test utilizes the peroxidase-like activity of hemoglobin. • Stools are collected on three separate occasions and smeared on filter paper impregnated with guaiac solution. • Hydrogen peroxide is added, and if hemoglobin is present to catalyze the reaction the colorless guaiac is oxidized to a blue-colored quinone. • Prolonged storage of the test slides may interfere with proper performance of the test. • Normal blood loss in stool is 2 mg of hemoglobin per gram of stool. • FOBT requires a fecal blood loss of 10 mg of hemoglobin per gram of stool to obtain a positive result.

Mass screening programs yield positive results in 1–8% of patients. • The positive predictive value of a positive test result is 10% for cancer and 30% for adenoma. • These programs diagnose a higher percentage of early localized cancers than may be expected otherwise, a fact that lends support to performing FOBT as a matter of routine. • The FOBT is not a perfect test. • For example, small adenomas and cancers not actively bleeding may not yield a positive result. • In fact, in patients with a known cancer, the sensitivity of FOBT is 50–85%. • Furthermore, it is not clear whether the mortality from colorectal cancer is reduced by FOBT alone. • When annual FOBT is combined with periodic flexible sigmoidoscopy, there is evidence to suggest that cancer mortality is reduced. • When used as a screening tool, barium enema is combined with sigmoidoscopy and is performed every 5 years. • Alternatively, colonoscopy may be performed every 10 years.

Current screening practices for asymptomatic patients endorsed by the American Cancer Society consist of the following: annual digital rectal examination with FOBT beginning at age 40 and flexible sigmoidoscopy at age 50. • If the findings are normal, sigmoidoscopy is repeated at 3 to 5 years. • If a polyp is found, the remainder of the colon must be examined with colonoscopy. Alternative screening tests for asymptomatic patients include colonoscopy or the combination of flexible sigmoidoscopy and barium enema.

Screening is not a term that applies to high-risk conditions, such as familial polyposis and HNPCC. • For these conditions, the high likelihood of finding neoplastic lesions, coupled with the increased risk to the patient if the tumors are not found, mandates tests in addition to FOBT. • Beginning at puberty, patients at risk for familial polyposis should be examined at yearly intervals with flexible sigmoidoscopy. • If the disease does not become apparent by age 40, the patient likely does not have it. • Patients at risk for HNPCC should undergo colonoscopy beginning at age 25. • Alternatively, genetic testing can be performed. • If an at-risk individual tests negative, he or she can be spared intense endoscopic surveillance programs and instead undergo screening used for the general population.

A N S W E R :
B, C, D

---

10. Select the most common mode of spread of colon cancer.

    A. Hematogenous

    B. Lymphatic

    C. Direct extension

    D. Implantation

Ref.: 1, 2

COMMENTS: Of the various mechanisms by which colon cancer may spread, the **lymphatic** route to regional mesenteric lymph nodes is the most common. • This fact has surgical importance because it dictates the extent of resection necessary when operating with curative intent. • **Hematogenous** spread from colon cancer is primarily via the portal circulation to the liver. • Cells that escape this effective filter can reach the lung and occasionally the brain.

Rectal cancers can metastasize to the spine via Batson's plexus. • Because the rectum has dual venous drainage—through the portal vein and the inferior hemorrhoidal veins into iliac veins—malignant cells may reach the liver or the lungs. • Distal rectal cancers may spread to the lungs without entering the portal circulation. • **Direct extension** to adjacent structures can occur with or without distant metastases. • With the latter, en bloc resection of portions of these organs may be necessary.

If the colon cancer has broken through the serosal surface, **implantation** on the peritoneal surface, locally or widely, can result, accounting for metastatic deposits in the rectovesical pouch (Blumer's shelf), to the peritoneum under the umbilicus (Sister Joseph's nodule), and to the ovary (Krukenberg's tumor, originally described for metastases from the stomach to the ovary).

ANSWER:
B

11. Which of the following is the most important prognostic determinant of survival after treatment for colorectal cancer?

    A. Lymph node involvement

    B. Transmural extension

    C. Tumor size

    D. Histologic differentiation

    E. DNA content

Ref.: 1–3

COMMENTS: Of the many variables that affect the cure of patients with colon cancer, the status of the **lymph nodes** remains the most important. • Long-term survival for node-positive patients is approximately half that for node-negative patients. • The extent of nodal disease also has an impact on the prognosis. • Patients with four or more positive lymph nodes have a lower 5-year survival rate than do patients with three or fewer positive nodes.

   Transmural extension also has an impact on prognosis, as demonstrated by the decline in 5-year survival rates from Dukes' A to Dukes' B lesions (80% versus 60%, respectively). • The difference, however, is not as pronounced as with the effect of lymph node metastases (35% survival in patients with positive lymph nodes).

   Tumor size in and of itself has no bearing on metastatic potential or prognosis. • The **DNA** content of colorectal tumors has been studied extensively, and aneuploidy seems to correlate well with histologic differentiation, transmural penetration, and the presence of nodal metastases. • DNA content, however, has not been shown conclusively to be an important independent prognostic indicator.

ANSWER:
A

12. Examine the illustration of a colon cancer and select the appropriate stage or stages.

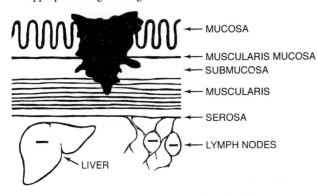

    A. Dukes' A

    B. Astler- Coller A

    C. T2N0M0

    D. T1N0M0

    E. Dukes' B

    F. Astler-Coller B$_2$

    G. Astler-Coller B$_1$

Ref.: 1, 2

COMMENTS: Dukes' classification was the original standardized method of staging colorectal cancer. • In recent years, however, confusion has arisen because of numerous subsequent modifications. • According to the original scheme proposed in 1932 by Cuthbert Dukes, an A lesion was confined to the bowel wall, a B lesion extended through the bowel wall but did not involve lymph nodes, and a C lesion indicated regional node involvement. • It is not uncommon to hear someone refer to a colon cancer with distant metastases as a Dukes D lesion even though that designation was not part of the original classification.

   In 1949, J. W. Kirklin and associates modified Dukes' classification, designating an A lesion as one confined to mucosa and submucosa, a B$_1$ lesion as one extending into but not through the muscularis propria, and a B$_2$ lesion as one extending through the muscularis propria into the pericolonic fat.

   In 1954, V. B. Astler and F. A. Coller modified the Kirklin classification (itself a modification of Dukes' classification) by designating a C$_1$ lesion as one limited to the bowel wall but with positive lymph nodes and a C$_2$ lesion as one invading all layers of the bowel wall with positive lymph nodes.

   In 1978, the staging classification was modified further, with the designation of A for a lesion confined to the mucosa and submucosa, B$_1$ for involvement of the muscularis, B$_2$ for involvement of the serosa, and B$_3$ for involvement of an adjacent organ. • The C lesions are the same with respect to local involvement but with positive lymph nodes. • D lesions are any of the aforementioned but include distant metastases as well.

   The American Joint Committee on Cancer has proposed a TNM classification that also stages a tumor according to the extent of bowel wall involvement and the presence or absence of lymph node involvement (N1 or N0 respectively). • A T1 tumor penetrates only into the submucosa, whereas a T2 tumor demonstrates partial invasion of the muscularis. • Transmural penetration imparts a T3 designation, and a T4 lesion invades adjacent structures. • An N0 lesion has not metastasized to regional nodes, an N1 lesion involves three or fewer positive lymph nodes, and an N2 lesion has metastasized to four or more lymph nodes. • The designations M0 and M1 indicate the absence and presence, respectively, of metastases.

ANSWER:
A, C, G

13. Which of the following is the appropriate operation for a sigmoid cancer that has not metastasized distantly?

    A. Segmental resection of the sigmoid

    B. Resection of sigmoid and distal descending colon, sparing the main left colic artery

    C. Resection of the sigmoid and the descending colon, including the inferior mesenteric artery at its origin

    D. Resection of the entire colon proximal to the lesion with ileorectostomy

    E. Concomitant oophorectomy in women

Ref.: 2, 3

COMMENTS: The respective draining mesenteric lymph nodes and the vascular supply to an area of the colon determine the amount of resection necessary when one is operating with intent to cure. • For a sigmoid cancer without evidence of distal spread, the resection should include, at a minimum, the sigmoid and distal descending colon and the accompanying mesentery to include the sigmoidal and superior hemorrhoidal vessels but sparing the left colic artery. • A more extensive mesenteric resection, with ligation of the inferior mesenteric artery at its origin, is advocated by some, although there is no conclusive evidence that it improves the survival rate. • Resection of the entire intra-abdominal colon can be considered for an obstructing cancer because resection of a dilated stool-laden colon may safely permit an ileorectostomy rather than a colostomy. • Other indications for total colectomy include synchronous cancers in separate segments of the colon or cancer in high-risk (younger) patients who require lifelong surveillance. • Oophorectomy may be considered in postmenopausal women, because approximately 6% of these patients have simultaneous drop metastases to the ovaries. • It has not been established that routine prophylactic oophorectomy improves survival. • Furthermore, only 1.4% of women with colorectal cancer subsequently require an operation for a recurrence in the ovary.

ANSWER:
B

14. Which of the following constitute(s) appropriate operative management of a left colon cancer that is causing a high-grade obstruction?

    A. Resection and primary anastomosis

    B. Resection and intraoperative colonic irrigation followed by primary anastomosis

    C. Initial decompressing colostomy followed by resection within 7–10 days

    D. Primary left colectomy and either a Hartmann procedure or a mucous fistula

    E. Primary subtotal colectomy and ileocolic anastomosis

    Ref.: 1–3

COMMENTS: Cancer is the leading cause of colon obstruction, and left-sided tumors in particular are susceptible to obstruction. • Most **right and transverse colon cancers** presenting with obstruction can be treated safely by primary resection and reanastomosis as a one-stage procedure. • For **left-sided tumors** producing obstruction, the traditional surgical approach has been an initial decompressing transverse colostomy, followed at a second stage by resection within 7–10 days and possibly a third-stage operation for colostomy closure. • Initial treatment by decompressing colostomy only is still appropriate, particularly for poor-risk patients, but resection of the obstructing pathologic entity is more commonly performed today. • A primary colocolostomy remains hazardous in patients with both an unprepared and distended bowel. • Therefore, for many patients with obstructing left-sided tumors, the preferred operation is primary resection accompanied by a Hartmann procedure or creation of a mucous fistula. • The reanastomosis is performed at a second stage. • Some advocate primary subtotal colectomy with an ileocolic anastomosis as a one-stage procedure.

In the absence of peritonitis or perforation, an alternative approach consists of resection followed by intraoperative colonic irrigation and then primary anastomosis. • The irrigation is accomplished with several liters of saline solution administered through a cecostomy or an appendicostomy. • The effluent is discharged through large-caliber tubing inserted into the open end of the left colon. • This operative approach has a clinical leakage rate of 5–7%.

ANSWER:
B, C, D, E

15. In which of the following situations should a combined abdominoperineal resection be performed?

    A. A circumferential villous adenoma beginning at the dentate line and extending proximally 8 cm

    B. A rectal cancer in which a 5-cm distal margin cannot be obtained

    C. A rectal cancer that produces pain and tenesmus

    D. Anastomotic recurrence after low anterior resection of a distal rectal cancer

    E. Palliation of obstructing rectal cancer just above the dentate line with minimal liver metastases

    Ref.: 1, 2

COMMENTS: The Miles abdominoperineal resection is frequently required for cancers of the mid- and distal rectum. • It means, however, a permanent colostomy and the potential morbidity of impotence and bladder dysfunction. • Therefore, it is indicated for malignant rather than benign lesions. • Large and even circumferential rectal adenomas can be removed with a variety of transanal techniques that preserve the sphincter muscle and fecal continence. • Curative resection of cancers in the mid- and even distal rectum can be performed by low anterior resection and colorectostomy or by coloanal anastomosis without the need for permanent colostomy, depending on the exact extent of the lesion, the size of the patient's pelvis, and the skill of the surgeon. • A distal *mural* margin of 2 cm and an adequate mesorectal excision must be obtained. • The end-to-end surgical stapling devices introduced through the rectum have greatly facilitated anastomoses deep in the pelvis. • The traditional attempt to obtain a distal margin of 5 cm may not be necessary, particularly if doing so sacrifices the sphincter. • Resections with distal margins of 2 cm have demonstrated equivalent survival and recurrence rates. • Because stapling devices have increased our capability of performing deep pelvic anastomoses, there is concern that local recurrence rates will be higher as a result of compromising the distal margin. • In fact, distal margins are not compromised, and the ability to obtain an even greater margin is enhanced. • Recurrence rates after stapled and hand-sewn anastomoses are the same.

Abdominoperineal resection is usually performed with curative intent, although it is justified for symptomatic patients with minimal metastatic disease who are expected to survive 6 months or longer. • A cancer that produces pain and tenesmus usually involves the sphincter muscle. • Recurrent cancer following low resection of a distal cancer usually mandates abdominoperineal resection.

ANSWER:
C, D, E

16. With regard to adjuvant chemotherapy, radiation therapy, or both for locally advanced rectal cancer, which of the following statements is/are true?

    A. Postoperative radiation therapy alone decreases local recurrence rates of rectal cancer.

    B. Postoperative radiation therapy alone increases survival rates of patients with rectal cancer.

C. Postoperative combined chemotherapy and radiation therapy yield improved local control and survival rates in comparison with irradiation alone.

D. Side effects of combined postoperative chemotherapy and radiation therapy are few, and 95% of patients are able to complete treatment.

E. Preoperative chemotherapy and radiation down-stage the tumor and improve resectability.

Ref.: 6, 9, 10

COMMENTS: Adjuvant chemotherapy and radiation therapy have been studied in an attempt to determine their impact on survival and recurrence rates for rectal cancer. • The Gastrointestinal Tumor Study Group (GITSG) and the National Surgical Adjuvant Breast and Bowel Protocol R-01 (NSABP) have shown that **postoperative** radiation therapy reduces local recurrence rates, but its impact on survival was not significant. • A randomized Swedish trial showed that a short course of 2550 cGy in five fractions administered **preoperatively** reduced local failure and improved 5-year survival compared with surgery alone. • Another Swedish study compared this preoperative regimen with 6000 cGy in 30 fractions administered postoperatively and showed significantly better locoregional control with the preoperative treatment. • No chemotherapy was administered.

The GITSG and the North Central Cancer Treatment Group (NCCTG) have investigated the **combined** use of 5-fluorouracil and methyl chloroethylcyclohexyl nitrourea (methyl-CCNU) and **postoperative** irradiation for Dukes' B and C cancers of the rectum and found a reduction in the recurrence rates and an improvement in 5-year survival rates. • This combined therapy, however, is accompanied by significant toxicity. • Only approximately 65% of patients are able to complete treatment. • Side effects included diarrhea, leukopenia, and enteritis. • Postoperative regimens now generally omit methyl-CCNU, and tolerance is better.

An encouraging trend in the management of rectal cancer is the use of **preoperative combined** chemotherapy and radiation therapy for T3 tumors or any tumor that has evidence of nodal metastases seen by rectal ultrasonound studies. • This regimen acts to down-stage tumors and improve resectability. • The advocates of this protocol claim that sphincter preservation is likely to be enhanced, but this advantage remains to be seen. • It is of note that up to 30% of patients have a complete response to treatment; that is, no residual tumor is found in the resected specimen. • Preoperative combined therapy is becoming the standard for locally advanced neoplasms.

In summary, (1) **postoperative radiation therapy alone** reduces locoregional recurrence rates but has not shown an effect on survival; (2) **postoperative radiation therapy combined with chemotherapy** reduces recurrence rates, improves survival, and is indicated for Dukes' B and C tumors; (3) **preoperative radiation therapy alone** reduces recurrence rates and may improve survival; and (4) **preoperative radiation therapy combined with chemotherapy** down-stages tumors, improves resectability, and induces a complete response in some patients.

A N S W E R :
A, C, E

17. Hamartomas are found in which of the following situations?

A. Juvenile polyps

B. Peutz-Jeghers syndrome

C. Familial polyposis

D. Gardner's syndrome

E. Chronic ulcerative colitis

Ref.: 1–3

COMMENTS: See Question 18.

18. Match each characteristic in the left-hand column with one or more syndromes in which it appears in the right-hand column.

A. Malignant potential	a. Peutz-Jeghers syndrome
B. Extraintestinal manifestations	b. Familial polyposis
C. Small-bowel polyps	c. Gardner's syndrome
D. Mendelian dominant gene	d. Turcot's syndrome
	e. Cronkhite-Canada syndrome

Ref.: 1, 2, 11, 12

COMMENTS: Hamartomas are lesions in which normal tissue is found in an abnormal structural configuration. • Because the tissue itself is not neoplastic, there is no malignant potential. • **Peutz-Jeghers syndrome** is transmitted as an autosomal dominant trait. • The polyps are hamartomas and are found primarily in the jejunum and ileum, with involvement of the colon and rectum in one third and the stomach in one fourth of the cases. • The polyps may cause obstruction, intussusception, or bleeding. • It is now generally accepted that there is an increased incidence of gastrointestinal cancers associated with Peutz-Jeghers, and polypectomy is advised, particularly if the patient has recurrent colicky pain or anemia. • Colonic lesions are usually treated by polypectomy, and colectomy is generally not needed. • In addition to intestinal polyps, the syndrome is characterized by melanin spots of the oral mucosa, lips, palms of the hands, and soles of the feet. • **Juvenile polyps** are solitary 70% of the time, and in 60% of cases they are located within 10 cm of the anal verge. • Occasionally, a patient is found to have a syndrome of juvenile polyposis characterized by anemia, anergy, hypoproteinemia, and failure to thrive. • Some authors have found a strong association between gastrointestinal malignancy and juvenile polyposis. • In **Cronkhite-Canada syndrome** the polyps, which are hamartomas, are dispersed throughout the gastrointestinal tract. • This entity is characterized by hyperpigmentation of the skin, alopecia, and atrophy of the fingernails and toenails. • **Familial adenomatous polyposis** by itself lacks extraintestinal manifestations. • Turcot's and Gardner's syndromes are types of familial polyposis associated with certain noncolonic manifestations. • **Turcot's syndrome** has the additional characteristic of central nervous system tumors. • Small-bowel polyposis is seen in all of the syndromes listed, with the exception of Turcot's syndrome. • In addition to the polyps, **Gardner's syndrome** is typified by the presence of osteomas, exostoses, and desmoid tumors. • The polypoid lesions observed with chronic ulcerative colitis are inflammatory "pseudopolyps," and the malignant potential of ulcerative colitis is not related to the presence of these lesions.

Of the conditions listed, Cronkhite-Canada syndrome is not inherited and does not have malignant potential. • Familial polyposis, Turcot's syndrome, and Gardner's syndrome may represent different expressions of the same disease. • Patients with familial polyposis, Turcot's syndrome, or Gardner's syndrome must undergo surveillance upper endoscopy at 3- to 5-year intervals. • In the Cleveland Clinic Polyposis Registry, duodenal polyps were found in 33% of patients and gastric polyps in 28%, and,

Handwritten margin notes:

tubular 75% (<1cm: rarely, 1-2cm 10%, >2cm 30%)
villous 10% (40-50%)
tubulovillous 15% (22%)

although most gastric polyps were of the fundic gland type, all duodenal polyps were adenomas. • Following colorectal cancer, the most common cause of death in these patients was cancer of the periampullary region. • An autosomal dominant gene has been proposed for Peutz-Jeghers syndrome, familial polyposis, and Gardner's syndrome, whereas it is believed that Turcot's syndrome is due to an autosomal recessive gene or an autosomal dominant tract with incomplete penetrance.

ANSWERS:

Question 17: A, B

Question 18: A-a,b,c,d; B-a,c,d,e; C-a,b,c,e; D-a,b,c,d

19. With regard to colorectal polyps, which of the following is/are considered precancerous?

    A. Hyperplastic polyp

    B. Tubular adenoma

    C. Tubulovillous adenoma

    D. Villous adenoma

    Ref.: 1, 2

COMMENTS: See Question 21.

20. Match each statement in the left-hand column with the appropriate pathologic entity in the right-hand column.

    A. Most common type of   a. Tubular adenoma
       intestinal polyp

    B. Children and adolescents   b. Hyperplastic polyp

    C. Mitoses at the depths of crypts   c. Both

    D. Mitoses at the surface of crypts   d. Neither

    E. Differentiation into mature
       goblet cells

    Ref.: 1, 2

COMMENTS: See Question 21.

21. Match each statement in the left-hand column with the appropriate response in the right-hand column.

    A. Pedunculated   a. Tubular adenoma

    B. Size usually less than 1 cm   b. Villous adenoma

    C. Rectosigmoid the most   c. Both
       common location

    D. Malignant potential related to size   d. Neither

    E. Malignant potential related
       to location

    Ref.: 1, 2

COMMENTS: Polypoid colorectal lesions can be classified as being neoplastic or nonneoplastic. • The **nonneoplastic polyps** include hyperplastic polyps, pseudopolyps, and hamartomas. • The **neoplastic polyps** include tubular adenomas, tubulovillous adenomas, and villous adenomas. • **Hyperplastic polyps** are the most common type of all polyps. • They result from an imbalance between cell division and cell exfoliation. • They are small, multiple, and sessile, and they occur most frequently in the rectosigmoid. • Although hyperplastic

polyps are nonneoplastic and have no malignant potential, they are nonetheless removed to differentiate them from neoplastic polyps (adenomas), which have varying malignant potential, depending on their size, histologic pattern, and degree of cellular atypia.

The distinction between hyperplastic polyps and adenomatous polyps (tubular, tubulovillous, or villous) is readily made based on the **histologic characteristics** of cellular differentiation and location of cell division. • In normal colonic mucosa and hyperplastic polyps, cell division is limited to the depths of the crypts of Lieberkühn, and differentiation into mature cells occurs as the cells migrate up the crypt to the surface. • In adenomatous polyps, cell division occurs at all levels of the crypt, including the surface, and the differentiation is incomplete.

Neoplastic polyps may be classified by histologic characteristics (tubular versus villous) and morphologic features (sessile versus pedunculated). • **Tubular adenoma** is the most common type of neoplastic polyp, constituting approximately 75% of this group. • Generally, tubular adenomas are asymptomatic, pedunculated, less than 1 cm in size, and (as with all colon polyps) found most commonly in the rectosigmoid region. • The likelihood that a neoplastic polyp contains cancer is directly related to its size and configuration. • Tubular adenomas less than 1 cm in diameter rarely harbor malignancy. • Those of 1–2 cm in diameter are likely to be malignant in 10% of cases, with a 30% malignancy rate for larger lesions. • Sessile adenomas, of all the histologic types, are more likely to harbor an occult cancer than are pedunculated ones. • **Villous adenomas** account for approximately 10% of neoplastic colon polyps. • They generally are sessile, and, compared to tubular adenomas, are larger and more likely to present with symptoms such as rectal bleeding, mucous discharge, or diarrhea. • They also have a significantly higher risk of malignancy. • Overall, approximately 40–50% of villous adenomas contain cancer, and one half of those are invasive.

Approximately 15% of neoplastic colon adenomas exhibit a **mixed histologic pattern**, containing both tubular and villous elements. • They are referred to as tubulovillous adenomas. • The risk of malignancy in tubulovillous adenomas is 22%, greater than that seen with tubular adenomas but less than that reported with villous adenomas. • **Nonneoplastic polyps** also may have a sessile or pedunculated morphology, so this characteristic has limited value in predicting the histologic nature of the polyp. • However, sessile neoplastic polyps are more likely to harbor cancer than are their pedunculated counterparts.

ANSWERS:

Question 19: B, C, D

Question 20: A-b; B-d; C-c; D-a; E-b

Question 21: A-a; B-a; C-c; D-c; E-d

22. A pedunculated 1.5-cm tubular adenoma is removed endoscopically from the sigmoid colon and is found to contain well-differentiated adenocarcinoma extending to, but not beyond, the muscularis mucosa. The margin of resection is free of tumor. Select the best therapeutic option.

    A. Observation and repeat endoscopic examination in 3 months

    B. Endoscopic fulguration of the polypectomy site

    C. Operative colotomy and excision of the polypectomy site

    D. Sigmoid colectomy

    Ref.: 1, 2, 13

COMMENTS: By definition, this lesion is classified as carcinoma in situ and is treated adequately by endoscopic polypectomy. • Since a lymphatic plexus exists just below the muscularis mucosae, lymphatic dissemination is possible only when invasion beyond this structure has occurred. • The muscularis mucosa of the colon wall may extend for a variable distance into the stalk of the polyp and may not even reach the head. • Pedunculated polyps consist of four anatomic levels: level 1 is the head itself, level 2 is the interface between the head and the stalk, level 3 is the stalk, and level 4 is the junction between the stalk and the colonic wall. • Endoscopic polypectomy should be considered adequate treatment of a polyp containing invasive cancer at level 1, 2, or 3 if the carcinoma is well differentiated and does not exhibit invasion of the veins or lymphatics and the resection margins are free of cancer. • For example, endoscopic polypectomy would be sufficient for a tubular adenoma with a well-differentiated cancer extending to level 3 as long as there was no evidence of venous or lymphatic invasion and the margin of resection was free of disease. • A poorly differentiated cancer extending to level 2, however, would require a formal segmental resection. • Similarly, any polyp with cancer extending to level 4 requires segmental resection, regardless of differentiation or vascular invasion.

ANSWER:
A

23. Biopsy of a villous lesion of the rectum beginning 4 cm from the anal verge and extending proximally for 5 cm exhibits cellular atypia. Which of the following steps is the most appropriate for management?

    A. Repeated biopsy

    B. Fulguration

    C. Transanal excision

    D. Abdominoperineal resection

    E. Intracavitary radiotherapy

Ref.: 1, 2

COMMENTS: A villous adenoma of the dimensions given has a 30–50% chance of harboring cancer. • The sigmoidoscopic biopsy represents a limited sample size and is not adequate proof of the lesion's precise histologic characteristics. • In this instance, the finding of atypia suggests a high probability of cancer elsewhere in the adenoma. • Complete full-thickness transanal excision of the lesion should be performed so that, if a carcinoma is present, its depth of penetration can be accurately assessed. • If there is no invasive cancer, the patient is followed by interval endoscopic examinations because the risk of recurrence is approximately 10%, even though the initial lesion was benign. • If invasive cancer is found, the need for further treatment is determined based on the depth of penetration. • A T1 cancer is adequately treated with transanal excision, provided the tumor is well differentiated, it lacks vascular or lymphatic invasion, and the margins of excision are clear. • A T2 cancer should be treated with radical resection. • Alternatively, irradiation with or without chemotherapy may be appropriate, but long-term studies are needed to determine the efficacy of this treatment. • Fulguration of the lesion can be performed in elderly or poor-risk patients in whom precise histologic staging is not essential. • This is not the standard of care for good-risk patients. • If there is a local recurrence after transanal excision, endoscopic fulguration, organ plasma coagulation, or repeat transanal excision may be considered. • Abdominoperineal resection is rarely indicated for benign polyps, since there are so many treatment options that are less radical. • Intracavitary radiotherapy is reserved for superficial malignant lesions and is not the preferred treatment in this case.

ANSWER:
C

24. With regard to ulcerative colitis, which one or more of the following statements is/are true?

    A. In at least half of the cases, the entire colon is involved in a continuous pattern without skip areas.

    B. The characteristic histologic finding of crypt abscesses is the sine qua non of ulcerative colitis and is not seen with other inflammatory conditions of the bowel.

    C. The disease is most commonly a chronic relapsing one, with an acute and fulminant course seen in only 10–15% of patients.

    D. Cancers arising in ulcerative colitis tend to be more evenly distributed throughout the involved colon, are more frequently multicentric, and usually are more aggressive than are similar lesions arising from colons without ulcerative colitis.

Ref.: 1, 2

COMMENTS: Ulcerative colitis is usually limited to the mucosal and submucosal layers of the bowel. • The rectum is almost always involved, with continuous proximal spread to varying lengths of colon. • The entire colon is involved in at least half of the cases. • The characteristic crypt abscesses, containing an infiltration of neutrophils and eosinophils, extend down into the bases of the crypts of Lieberkühn and the lamina propria. • Although crypt abscesses may be seen with other inflammatory conditions of the colon, they are always present with ulcerative colitis and usually in greater numbers. • In contrast to Crohn's disease, in which the supply of goblet cells is preserved, the microscopic appearance of ulcerative colitis characteristically reveals goblet cell depletion. • Ulcerative colitis is most commonly chronic and relapsing in character, although in 10–15% of cases the disease runs an acute and fulminant course.

Cancers arising in colons with past or present ulcerative colitis are usually diagnosed later in their course, because the signs and symptoms may be confused initially with an inflammatory relapse. • For this reason, these cancers are associated with a poorer prognosis. • Studies have shown that, contrary to what has been believed, colitic cancers do not behave more aggressively than do their noncolitic counterparts when similar stages are compared. • Compared to noncolitic cases, cancers arising within a colitic colon are more evenly distributed throughout the colon, have a higher incidence of proximal involvement, and are frequently multiple.

ANSWER:
A, C

25. A 25-year-old woman presents with a history of repeated episodes of bloody diarrhea and general abdominal cramping with lower abdominal pain and weight loss. The presumed diagnosis is ulcerative colitis. Which of the following is/are correct management?

    A. A barium enema radiographic examination is done early to assess the extent and severity of her disease.

    B. Hydrocortisone has been shown to induce remissions, but such steroid-induced remissions are more likely to be followed by a relapse than are spontaneous remissions.

    C. Total parenteral nutrition, if administered early as part of the treatment, may delay or even prevent the need for colectomy.

    D. Maintenance, low-dose steroids are effective in preventing relapses.

E. If medical therapy fails and an abdominal colectomy with ileorectal anastomosis is performed, there is a 15–20% chance that carcinoma will develop in the rectal remnant during the next 30 years.

Ref.: 2

COMMENTS: Endoscopy with biopsy is the most widely used method for diagnosing ulcerative colitis. • **Barium enema** examinations can be performed but should be done with caution and avoided altogether during acute attacks because of the risk of perforation and of precipitating toxic megacolon. • **Prednisone** or **hydrocortisone** is highly effective for treating acute phases of the illness. • However, both drugs have side effects sufficiently adverse that the dose is tapered early when possible. • Administration of low-dose steroids on a maintenance basis has not been shown to prevent relapses. • The risk of relapse is the same whether it follows a steroid-induced remission or a spontaneous remission. • The optimal role of **total parenteral nutrition** for treatment of these patients has not been well defined, but it does not appear to delay the need for surgical intervention. • It should not be used as primary treatment.

Approximately 5–6% of patients with ulcerative colitis develop **cancer**. • Patients with pancolitis or disease of long-standing duration are at highest risk. • When an ileorectal anastomosis is performed, lifetime proctoscopic surveillance for dysplasia or neoplasia is mandatory because the risk of subsequent cancer is approximately 20% after 25 years. • In addition to the cancer risk, proctitis symptomatic enough to require proctectomy is another concern following ileorectostomy for ulcerative colitis. • Approximately 50% of patients undergoing this operation require proctectomy because of cancer, dysplastic changes, or refractory proctitis.

ANSWER:
E

26. Match the clinical comment in the left-hand column with the disease process in the right-hand column.

A. Anal involvement in 50%   a. Crohn's disease

B. Rectal involvement   b. Ulcerative colitis
   frequently seen

C. Small-bowel involvement common c. Both

D. Chronic diarrhea, cramps, and fever d. Neither

E. Curative surgery available

F. Toxic megacolon

Ref.: 2

COMMENTS: In ulcerative colitis, the anus is spared, while in Crohn's disease, **anal** or perianal disease is the first manifestation in 25–30% of cases. • Ultimately, 50–70% of patients with Crohn's colitis develop anal disease. • **Rectal** involvement can be seen with both of these inflammatory diseases of the colon but is more common in ulcerative colitis (95% versus 50%). • The **small bowel** is extensively involved in approximately 50% of patients with Crohn's disease, whereas "backwash ileitis," a nonspecific dilatation of the terminal ileum, occurs in perhaps only 10% of patients with ulcerative colitis and has no prognostic or physiologic implications.

The clinical presentations of these two entities are similar: chronic diarrhea, cramping, abdominal pain, and fever. • Bloody stools, common with ulcerative colitis, are less common with

Crohn's disease. • Total proctocolectomy or colectomy, rectal mucosectomy, and ileal pouch–anal anastomosis eliminate ulcerative colitis, whereas there is no curative operation for Crohn's disease. • Indeed, even after total proctocolectomy for pancolonic involvement with Crohn's disease, its recurrence rate may be as high as 50%. • One third of patients require additional surgery for such recurrence. • A toxic megacolon can be an emergent, life-threatening complication of either ulcerative colitis or Crohn's disease, although it occurs less frequently with the latter.

ANSWER:
A-a; B-c; C-a; D-c; E-b; F-c

27. Match each clinical presentation in the left-hand column with the appropriate clinical condition in the right-hand column.

A. The principal mechanism is   a. Sigmoid volvulus
   twisting of a segment of bowel
   on a narrow mesentery.

B. It is most common in elderly,   b. Cecal volvulus
   debilitated persons with psychiatric
   or neurologic diseases.

C. Nonoperative reduction is   c. Both
   successful in approximately
   70% of patients.

D. It is characterized by abdominal   d. Neither
   distention, pain, and radiographic
   signs of a small-bowel obstruction.

E. Mortality rates are not altered
   whether operating urgently for
   peritonitis or electively after
   successful nonoperative reduction.

Ref.: 1, 2, 11

COMMENTS: The prerequisite for developing a sigmoid or a cecal volvulus is a mobile segment of bowel that can rotate around a mesentery whose points of fixation are in close proximity. • Otherwise, there are surprisingly few similarities between a sigmoid and a cecal volvulus.

Volvulus of the cecum is found most frequently in persons 25–35 years of age, whereas it is unusual for sigmoid volvulus to occur in an active, otherwise healthy individual. • Usually, it is seen in elderly, debilitated persons or in those with psychiatric or neurologic disorders in which immobility, medications that impair bowel motility, and loss of accessory defecatory muscles may lead to constipation and elongation of the colon.

Both types of volvulus typically cause abdominal distention and pain. • With cecal volvulus, there may be radiographic evidence of small-bowel obstruction. • With sigmoid volvulus, the distended twisted loop has a fairly characteristic appearance of a "bent inner tube."

For sigmoid volvulus, endoscopic detorsion and insertion of a rectal tube to evacuate the voluminous fecal contents is the preferred initial therapeutic approach but should be attempted only if the mucosa does not appear gangrenous. • It should not be attempted if the patient has rebound abdominal tenderness or other signs of peritoneal inflammation. • Although nonoperative detorsion is successful approximately 70% of the time, a recurrence rate of 33–60% mandates elective resection of the elongated colon if the patient is believed to be an acceptable operative risk.

Nonoperative colonoscopic reduction of a cecal volvulus is successful in only 25% of cases and should not be attempted in the presence of peritoneal inflammation. • If colonoscopy is unsuccessful or contraindicated (e.g., when there is tenderness), an operation is indicated as soon as the patient can be prepared. • If gangrenous, the cecum must be resected. • In the absence of vascular compromise, a cecopexy with or without cecostomy is sufficient. • The most important determinant of patients' outcome is whether bowel gangrene is present, mortality being highest if surgery is performed for intestinal infarction or perforation. • Mortality is also higher if operating for recurrent volvulus.

ANSWER:
A-c; B-a; C-a; D-b; E-d

---

28. With regard to diverticular fistulas, which of the following statements is/are true?

  A. Colocutaneous fistulas frequently occur spontaneously.

  B. Colovesical fistulas normally present with urinary tract infections that may be accompanied by pneumaturia and fecaluria, and the diagnosis is best confirmed with barium enema.

  C. Coloenteric fistulas may be totally asymptomatic.

  D. Surgical correction should be in staged operations because of the hazards of primary anastomosis in the presence of extensive local prior inflammation.

Ref.: 1, 2

COMMENTS: Fistula formation occurs in 5% of complicated cases of colonic diverticulitis. • Fistulas are usually to adjacent viscera, in the bladder, uterus, vagina, or small bowel. • **Colocutaneous fistulas** rarely form spontaneously. • They are most commonly seen as a postoperative complication, draining through operative incisions or drain tracts. • **Colovesical fistulas** are most commonly the result of diverticular disease, followed in frequency by cancer, Crohn's disease, radiation colitis, and foreign bodies. • Their first symptoms (e.g., fecaluria and pneumaturia) are referable to the urinary tract. • The patient may relate a history of abdominal pain and fever before the development of the fistula. • Although a barium enema may give information regarding the site and extent of involvement of the colon with diverticulosis, the fistula is demonstrated in only half of the cases. • Cystoscopy is more likely to demonstrate the fistula. • Findings may include bullous (edematous) edema of the dome of the bladder. • Computed tomographic (CT) scanning may reveal a constellation of findings including air in the bladder, a thickened loop of bowel lying adherent to the bladder, and enteric contrast in the bladder (before intravenous contrast has been administered). • **Coloenteric fistulas** may cause no symptoms or may present with diarrhea.

  The fistula can be corrected by a one-stage operation in most patients, and thus this procedure is the preferred treatment. • If the bowel preparation is inadequate or if there is extensive local inflammation or abscess formation, staged procedures may be required.

ANSWER:
C

---

29. Match the characteristic features in the left-hand column with the locations of diverticula in the right-hand column.

  A. They are frequently true diverticula   a. Sigmoid
    and therefore are considered congenital
    in origin.

  B. When inflamed, they may be clinically   b. Cecal
    indistinguishable from cancer.

  C. Resection and primary anastomosis   c. Both
    may be hazardous in the presence of
    perforation with frank peritonitis.

  D. Asymptomatic diverticula found   d. Neither
    incidentally on a barium enema should
    be treated operatively because of the
    high incidence of complications.

Ref.: 2

COMMENTS: Sigmoid diverticula lack a muscular component and so are not considered true diverticula. • Right-sided diverticula may occur as part of diffuse colonic diverticulosis and are thus pseudodiverticular and acquired. • Occasionally, isolated, solitary, right-sided diverticula are found and possess all layers of the bowel wall. • They are probably congenital in origin. • Cecal diverticulitis is uncommon, and the correct preoperative diagnosis is rarely made because it is confused with acute appendicitis in 80% of cases and with cancer in approximately 5%. • In rare cases of repeated attacks, the cecal inflammation and subsequent scarring and fibrosis may be indistinguishable from those of cancer. • Similarly, an inflammatory mass of the sigmoid colon may resemble a cancer at laparotomy.

  The surgical options depend on the extent of inflammation. • If inflammation is minimal and limited, segmental resection and anastomosis may be all that is necessary. • If there has been perforation with frank peritonitis, most surgeons hesitate to perform a primary anastomosis and instead resect the involved segment and divert the stool proximally. • For both types of diverticula, surgical therapy is not required if the diverticulum is discovered incidentally and the patient is asymptomatic.

ANSWER:
A-b; B-c; C-c; D-d

---

30. With regard to radiation enterocolitis, which of the following statements is/are true?

  A. Histologically, subintimal foam cells are pathognomonic, and additional changes include a progressive vasculitis of the submucosal arteries.

  B. The rectum is the most common site of injury.

  C. Rectovaginal fistulas secondary to irradiation can be treated only by fecal diversion.

  D. Long segments of strictured small bowel are best treated with resection.

  E. Prior pelvic irradiation predisposes to rectosigmoid cancer.

Ref.: 2

COMMENTS: The incidence of radiation injury to the bowel is dose dependent. • Substantial bowel injury is uncommon at external doses of less than 4000 rad. • In addition to the radiation dose, other factors that may predispose to injury include advanced age, hypertension, arteriosclerosis, diabetes, and adhesions that fix the bowel to a constant location. • After cessation of radiation therapy, the denuded intestinal epithelium regenerates. • The vessels, however, develop a progressive vasculitis, which may lead to thickening of the vessel wall with progressive diminution of the vessel lumen with occlusion or thrombosis (or both).

  The rectum is the most common site of injury because of its proximity to the most frequently targeted organs (i.e., cervix, uterus, and prostate) and its fixed location within the pelvis. • When rectal ulcers occur, they are on the anterior wall about

4–6 cm from the dentate line. • Rectal strictures usually occur at the 8- to 12-cm level.

When faced with a rectovaginal fistula, every attempt should be made to rule out a recurrence of the cancer as the cause of the fistula. • If cancer is present, fecal diversion usually palliates symptoms. • In the absence of recurrent cancer and in selected patients, an attempt can be made to correct the fistula. • Operative correction must interpose nonirradiated tissue between the rectum and the vagina after the fistulous openings have been closed. • When possible, anterior resection or coloanal pull-through, employing nonirradiated intestine for the proximal anastomotic limb, is preferred. • The aforementioned precautions to ensure primary healing notwithstanding, there should be proximal temporary fecal diversion in the form of a colostomy.

Prior pelvic irradiation does predispose to rectosigmoid cancer after a latent period of several years. • For this reason, flexible sigmoidoscopy is advised on a periodic basis.

In summary, when treating radiation enterocolitis, the following principles should be observed: (1) avoid an operation unless no other option exists, (2) resect short segments but bypass long segments of diseased bowel, (3) avoid extensive adhesiolysis, and (4) safeguard an anastomotic leak with a temporary proximal colostomy.

ANSWER:
A, B, E

---

31. With regard to pseudomembranous colitis, which of the following statements is/are true?

   A. Diarrhea that begins 1 week after antibiotics have been discontinued rules out pseudomembranous colitis.

   B. Pseudomembranous colitis does not occur in the absence of antibiotic therapy.

   C. Administration of vancomycin or metronidazole is appropriate treatment.

   D. There is a relapse rate of 50% after treatment.

Ref.: 1, 2

COMMENTS: Pseudomembranous enterocolitis, first described by Theodor Billroth in 1867, has been seen with increased frequency and is associated with the use of many antibiotics. • The disease has not been described with the use of vancomycin or with antimicrobials used to treat mycobacteria, fungi, or parasites. • There is evidence that antibiotics change the intracolonic flora, allowing overgrowth of *Clostridium difficile*, which then produces enterocolitis. • There is also evidence, however, that pseudomembranous colitis is infectious and is spread by patient-to-patient or staff-to-patient contact.

Pseudomembranous colitis should be suspected in any patient who develops diarrhea during or up to 3 weeks after the cessation of antibiotic therapy. • The diagnosis is established endoscopically by visualizing the characteristic raised mucosal plaques or by a cytotoxic assay for *C. difficile* exotoxin, which usually has a positive result in cases of pseudomembranous colitis.

Therapy should begin with prompt cessation of the offending antibiotic. • Vancomycin (500 mg 4 times a day for 10 days) or metronidazole (500 mg 4 times a day for 10 days) has been used to treat this condition successfully. • However, the relapse rate is 20% for vancomycin and 23% for metronidazole. • Surgery is rarely necessary, except in cases of toxic colitis or perforation.

ANSWER:
C

---

32. With regard to carcinoid tumors of the colon and rectum, which of the following statements is/are true?

   A. They occur with equal frequency at these two sites.

   B. The incidence of invasive malignancy and metastases correlates with carcinoid size.

   C. They frequently cause the carcinoid syndrome.

   D. Superficial, small rectal lesions should be excised transanally.

   E. Invasive rectal lesions larger than 2 cm are best treated by abdominoperineal resection.

Ref.: 6

COMMENTS: Carcinoid (neuroendocrine) tumors of the colon and rectum represent a wide and diverse group of neoplasms that range from completely benign lesions to poorly differentiated cancers with an extremely dismal prognosis. • These lesions share the capability of storing large amounts of an amine precursor (5-hydroxytryptophan), and, through the amine precursor uptake and decarboxylation (APUD) system, these lesions produce several biologically active amines. • The gastrointestinal tract is the most common site for carcinoid formation. • In decreasing order of frequency, the most common locations are the appendix, ileum, rectum, stomach, and colon. • Colon carcinoids account for only 2.5% of all gastrointestinal carcinoids, while rectal carcinoids account for 12–15%. • The incidence of invasive malignancy and metastases to regional lymph nodes correlates well with the size of the carcinoid for both colonic and rectal lesions. • For example, when rectal carcinoids are larger than 2 cm, only 5–10% are benign, whereas a lesion less than 2 cm is malignant only approximately 5% of the time.

Because rectal carcinoids less than 2 cm rarely demonstrate invasion of the muscularis or lymph node metastases, they may be excised transanally. • Lesions larger than 2 cm and located in the rectum are best treated by abdominoperineal resection or low anterior resection, if possible. • If malignant, colon carcinoids should be treated by a formal segmental resection with the accompanying lymph node-bearing tissue. • Up to two thirds of patients with carcinoids of the colon have either local spread or systemic metastases at the time of diagnosis. • If there is disseminated disease, resection of the primary lesion is still recommended to alleviate symptoms and avoid the potential for bleeding and obstruction. • Carcinoids of the colon and rectum infrequently produce the carcinoid syndrome unless systemic metastases have occurred.

ANSWER:
B, D, E

---

33. With regard to amebiasis, which of the following statements is/are true?

   A. Approximately 10% of the people in the United States are asymptomatic carriers.

   B. *Entamoeba histolytica* antibodies are detectable in the serum of more than 90% of those with active amebiasis.

   C. Acute amebic dysentery closely resembles fulminant ulcerative colitis and should be treated aggressively with steroids.

   D. Amebic abscess of the spleen is the most common complication of amebic colitis.

   E. Colon perforation with peritonitis occurs in approximately half of the patients with an acute presentation.

Ref.: 1, 2

COMMENTS: Amebic colitis is caused by the protozoan *E. histolytica*, which infests primarily the colon and rectum and, secondarily, other organs, such as the liver. • It has been estimated that 10% of the American population are asymptomatic carriers. • Transmission of the disease is through food or water contaminated with feces containing *Entamoeba* cysts. • The disease can assume an acute and a chronic form.

Acute amebic dysentery is seen with contamination of the water supply and has a presentation similar to that of acute ulcerative colitis (i.e., fever, cramps, and bloody diarrhea). • The distinction between these two entities is important. • Steroids are given routinely on a short-term basis to treat ulcerative colitis but are contraindicated in the therapy of amebic dysentery. • The desired effect of steroids—muting of the inflammatory response—would mask the clinicopathologic progression of amebic colitis. • In a typical case, proctosigmoidoscopy should reveal extensive ulceration of the intestinal epithelium, and warm saline preparation of the stool usually demonstrates numerous trophozoites containing ingested erythrocytes. • The diagnosis is strengthened by a serologic test for *E. histolytica* antibodies, which has a positive result in 90% of patients with active amebiasis. • Treatment is with metronidazole 750 mg 3 times a day for 10 days.

Perforation of the colon during the acute form of the disease is rare. • Amebic abscess of the liver is the most common complication of amebic colitis, which may in turn rupture into the pleura, pericardium, or peritoneum.

Chronic amebic dysentery is more common than the acute form and is characterized by three to four foul-smelling bowel movements per day, along with abdominal cramping and fever. • The diagnosis of chronic amebic dysentery is more difficult to establish because cysts or trophozoites are not always demonstrable in stool preparations and findings on sigmoidoscopy are normal in up to 30% of such individuals. • *E. histolytica* antibodies, however, should be detectable. • The treatment is diiodohydroxyquin 650 mg 3 times a day for 20 days and metronidazole or diloxamide furoate 500 mg 3 times a day for 10 days.

ANSWER:
A, B

34. Match each disease in the left-hand column with the appropriate drug or drugs that may be used for their treatment in the right-hand column.

A. Actinomycosis	a. Hydrocortisone
B. Lymphogranuloma venereum	b. Metronidazole
C. Tuberculous enteritis	c. Penicillin
D. Yersinia infection	d. Tetracycline
	e. Streptomycin

Ref.: 1–3

COMMENTS: Actinomycosis is a suppurative, granulomatous disease caused by *Actinomyces israelii*, an anaerobic, gram-positive bacterium that produces chronic inflammatory induration and sinus formation. • Although the causative organism is part of the normal oral flora, infections may occur in the cervicofacial area, thorax, or abdomen. • The cecal region is the most frequent site of abdominal infection, producing a pericecal mass, abscesses, and sinus. • Rectal strictures have been reported as well. • Treatment consists of surgical drainage and penicillin or tetracycline.

Lymphogranuloma venereum is a sexually transmissible disease due to *Chlamydia trachomatis*. • It is seen most frequently in the homosexual population, in which it starts as proctitis and produces tenesmus, discharge, and bleeding. • Perianal and rectovaginal fistulas may develop, as may rectal strictures. • The diagnosis is made by the Frei intracutaneous test when the test is available. • Otherwise, the diagnosis may be confirmed by a complement fixation test. • Tetracycline is curative, and steroids have been recommended.

Tuberculous enteritis is seen most commonly in the ileocecal region and occasionally leads to stenosis of the distal ileum, cecum, and ascending colon, producing endoscopic and radiographic features that may be indistinguishable from those of Crohn's disease. • Surgery is reserved for patients with obstruction. • Triple-drug therapy of isoniazid, paraaminosalicylic acid, and streptomycin usually heals the intestinal lesions.

Yersinia infections are caused by a gram-negative rod that is transmitted through food contaminated by feces or urine. • It produces a clinical picture frequently indistinguishable from that of acute appendicitis. • *Yersinia* may also cause acute gastroenteritis, which affects primarily the ileocecal region. • *Yersinia* responds to treatment with tetracycline, streptomycin, ampicillin, or kanamycin.

ANSWER:
A-c,d; B-a,d; C-e; D-d,e

35. With regard to ischemic colitis, which of the following statements is/are true?

A. The most common symptoms are lower abdominal pain and bright-red rectal bleeding.

B. Occlusion of the major mesenteric vessels is responsible for producing the ischemia in most cases.

C. The splenic flexure and descending colon are the most vulnerable areas, although any segment of colon may be involved.

D. Nonoperative management is not justified because, in a significant percentage of such cases, perforation and peritonitis eventually develop.

Ref.: 1–3, 11

COMMENTS: Ischemic colitis should be considered in the differential diagnosis of any elderly patient who presents with left lower quadrant pain. • It can also be found in individuals of any age in association with periarteritis nodosa, systemic lupus erythematosus, rheumatoid arthritis, polycythemia vera, and scleroderma.

Ischemic colitis may present as three distinct clinical syndromes depending on (1) the extent and duration of vascular occlusion, (2) the adequacy of collateral circulation, and (3) the extent of septic complications. • Mild or transient ischemia is compensated for by collateral blood flow. • There may be a partial, reversible mucosal slough that heals in 2–3 days. • Transmural ischemia may predispose to a stricture if healing takes place without perforation. • If these ischemic changes progress to full-thickness gangrene, perforation and peritonitis will ensue.

Ischemic colitis appears to be a disease of the small arterioles. • Occlusion of the major mesenteric vessels does not adequately explain the cause of this disease. • For example, patients with frank ischemic colitis may have angiographic evidence of patent major arteries. • Moreover, ligation of these vessels (e.g., when ligating the inferior mesenteric artery during aortic aneurysmectomy) may not cause ischemic colitis. • Although this disease can occur in any segment of the large bowel, it is seen most commonly in the splenic flexure or distal sigmoid colon, a plausible explanation being the suboptimal blood flow in areas positioned between two vascular systems ("watershed areas"), which rely on an intact but meandering artery for their blood supply. • **Sudeck's point** is the area between the blood supply from the last sigmoid artery and the superior rectal artery. • The clinical significance of Sudek's point is questionable because of retrograde flow from the middle and inferior rectal arteries. • **Griffith's point** is the vulnerable area at the splenic flexure that is positioned between areas perfused by the left branch of the middle colic artery and the ascending branch of the left colic artery.

The diagnosis is made by endoscopic examination, which reveals cyanotic, edematous mucosa that may be covered by exudative membranes, or by barium enema, which may show the typical "thumbprinting" of the bowel wall. • If gangrenous colitis is suspected on the basis of ominous physical findings, these studies are contraindicated and prompt laparotomy is mandatory.

Transient ischemic colitis usually responds to nonoperative management. • Ischemic strictures may be electively resected with primary anastomosis after the initial ischemic episode has subsided. • If surgery is needed for peritonitis and gangrenous colitis, resection with end colostomy is the preferred operation.

ANSWER:
A, C

36. With regard to the operation that includes proctocolectomy, formation of an ileal reservoir, and ileoanal anastomosis, which of the following statements is/are true?

　　A. It is indicated for either ulcerative colitis or Crohn's disease, provided the rectum is minimally involved.

　　B. Bladder and sexual function are preserved postoperatively.

　　C. The need for a permanent ileostomy is avoided.

　　D. Construction of an ileal pouch proximal to the anastomosis increases intestinal storage capacity and decreases stool frequency.

Ref.: 1, 2

COMMENTS: Patients who require total proctocolectomy and permanent ileostomy for ulcerative colitis may be eligible for a sphincter-preserving procedure. • Proctocolectomy, ileal reservoir, and ileoanal anastomosis offer advantages over proctocolectomy and permanent ileostomy because, not only is the diseased mucosa eliminated, but so is the need for a permanent abdominal stoma. • The operative technique was described by Mark Ravich and David Sabiston in 1947 and has undergone certain modifications, most notably, construction of an ileal pouch proximal to the ileoanal anastomosis. • The pouch may be S-shaped or J-shaped, increasing intestinal storage capacity and decreasing stool frequency. • A temporary diverting ileostomy is usually required for 2–3 months while the pouch heals. • The procedure is currently recommended for selected patients with ulcerative colitis and those with familial polyposis. • It is not indicated for Crohn's disease because of the risk of recurrence within the pouch, which may lead to complex fistulas and septic complications. • Although advanced age is not an absolute contraindication, elderly patients with multiple comorbid conditions may be better served with a permanent ileostomy. • Similarly, patients with preexisting fecal incontinence from anorectal surgery or obstetric injuries should probably avoid an ileoanal anastomosis. • For appropriately selected patients, functional results are good, with preservation of the parasympathetic innervation to the bladder and genitalia. • Fecal sensation and continence are retained in most of these patients.

ANSWER:
B, C, D

37. With regard to megacolon, which of the following statements is/are true?

　　A. The common feature of congenital megacolon (Hirschsprung's disease) and acquired megacolon is chronic partial distal obstruction.

　　B. Hirschsprung's disease is due to the congenital absence of ganglion cells in the myenteric plexus.

　　C. There is a transition zone from the dilated nondiseased colon to normal-caliber aganglionic bowel.

　　D. Acquired megacolon may be seen in patients whose colon is infested with *Trypanosoma cruzi* and in patients with neurologic disorders, such as paraplegia and poliomyelitis.

　　E. The surgical importance of megacolon is in its formation of chronic bowel dilatation, elongation, and a propensity to volvulus formation.

Ref.: 1, 2

COMMENTS: Megacolon may be congenital or acquired. • Both forms are characterized by dilatation, elongation, and hypertrophy of the colon proximal to a segment of nonperistaltic collapsed bowel, causing obstruction. • Both have an increased risk of volvulus.

Hirschsprung's disease is caused by the congenital absence of ganglion cells in the myenteric plexus of the bowel, resulting in loss of peristaltic activity in that segment of intestine. • The rectosigmoid region is most frequently involved, with variable extension of the disease proximally. • There is a transition zone from the normal bowel, which is dilated, to the abnormal bowel, which is aganglionic, aperistaltic, and of normal or decreased caliber. • Although primarily a disease of infants and children, occasionally Hirschsprung's disease does not manifest until later in life if an ultra-short segment of distal rectum is involved. • In these cases, patients relate a history of constipation dating back to infancy. • The diagnosis is apparent during the first 24 hr of life if the infant fails to pass meconium. • A rectal biopsy is diagnostic. • In adolescents and young adults, Hirschsprung's disease can be diagnosed using anal manometric measurements. • If the disease is present, the normal relaxation of the internal sphincter, which is the expected response to rectal distention, is lost. • The treatment of Hirschsprung's disease is primarily surgical, utilizing a coloanal anastomosis.

Acquired megacolon may be seen in protozoal colon infections with *T. cruzi*, which is endemic in South and Central America. • *T. cruzi* causes widespread destruction of the intramural nervous system. • Acquired megacolon is seen also in patients with colonic dilatation as a result of chronic constipation due to the loss of voluntary defecatory muscles (e.g., in paraplegia), extreme inactivity (e.g., in poliomyelitis), or voluntary inhibition of defecation (e.g., in psychotic disorders). • Resection of the excessive redundant colon is occasionally justified in the latter group of patients.

ANSWER:
A, B, C, D, E

38. With regard to the polyposis coli syndromes, which of the following statements is/are true?

　　A. Screening family members at risk should begin at puberty and consists of an annual complete colonoscopy.

　　B. Death from colon cancer that develops in these patients occurs at a significantly earlier age than in nonpolyposis patients with colon cancer.

　　C. The risk of the development of colon cancer is approximately 100%.

D. Abdominal colectomy and ileoproctostomy eliminate the risk of carcinoma.

E. Periampullary tumors are an important cause of death.

Ref.: 1, 2, 11, 12

COMMENTS: Most reports of polyposis syndromes reflect experience in American and European populations, but these diseases have been identified in Africans and Asians as well. • There probably is no race or geographic area that is exempt. • The polyposis syndromes occur in approximately 1 of every 12,000 births. • Thus, 300 new patients are diagnosed each year in the United States. • The disease is transmitted as an autosomal dominant trait, and therefore approximately 50% of the offspring of an afflicted individual have the disease. • About 30–40% of patients do not have a family history of polyposis, and these cases represent spontaneous mutations at the polyposis locus.

The polyps are not present at birth but first appear usually at puberty and gradually increase in number so that by age 21 the colon and rectum are carpeted by thousands of polyps. • If the polyps are left untreated, the risk of developing cancer of the colon is approximately 100%, with death from colon cancer occurring at an average age of 41.5 years.

Subtotal colectomy with ileoproctostomy has been advocated by some authors. • If this procedure is performed, close surveillance of the rectal remnant is mandatory and is accomplished with proctoscopy performed at 6-month intervals. • The incidence of rectal cancer after ileorectostomy varies widely among reported series, with one study reporting an incidence as high as 59% at 23 years. • Other reports estimate the risk to be 5–15% and the chance of dying from rectal cancer extremely low. • In fact, patients are less likely to die of rectal cancer than from periampullary tumors or desmoids. • Nevertheless, the importance of surveillance proctoscopy cannot be overemphasized. • Extensive carpeting of the rectum with polyps should dissuade one from recommending ileorectostomy.

Mucosal proctectomy with ileoanal anastomosis removes all neoplastic mucosa while avoiding the need for permanent ileostomy.

Screening asymptomatic family members at risk should begin at puberty. • Because colon polyps rarely if ever develop in the absence of rectal polyps, sigmoidoscopy is adequate for screening. • If polyps are found, a biopsy is recommended to verify the presence of adenomatous tissue. • Upper endoscopic examination should be done at the time of diagnosis to document the involvement of the stomach and duodenum. • Alternatively, a family may choose genetic screening for members at risk. • If genetic testing is negative, that individual may avoid annual flexible sigmoidoscopy.

ANSWER:
B, C, E

39. With regard to colonic fluid and electrolyte absorption, which of the following statements is/are correct?

A. The colon protects against hyponatremia by actively absorbing sodium against both concentration and electrical gradients.

B. Under normal conditions, absorption of sodium and water in the right colon is the same as in the rectum.

C. Chloride and bicarbonate ions participate in an exchange mechanism, and chloride is actively absorbed from the colonic lumen.

D. The colon is not involved in urea metabolism.

E. The maximal absorptive capacity of the colon is 5–6 L/day.

Ref.: 14

COMMENTS: In healthy subjects, the colon normally absorbs 1–2 L of water and up to 200 mEq of sodium and chloride per day. • This absorptive capacity can increase up to 5–6 L/day, thereby protecting the person against severe diarrhea. • Lack of a colon may lead to enteric losses of sodium and chloride.

Absorption of sodium is an active process and continues even when luminal concentrations are as low as 15–25 mM. • Sodium absorption also takes place against a potential (electrical) gradient of 35–50 mV (mucosa negative). • Colonic absorption varies regionally. • The cecum and right colon absorb sodium and water the most rapidly, while the rectum is impermeable to sodium and water.

Chloride ions are actively absorbed at the expense of bicarbonate, which is secreted in exchange. • Absence of luminal chloride inhibits bicarbonate secretion. • When the sigmoid colon is used as a urinary conduit, urinary chloride is actively absorbed. • As a consequence, bicarbonate is secreted, leading to the common and predictable complication of chronic acidosis. • The ileal mucosa, in contrast, absorbs chloride less avidly, making it more suitable as a urinary conduit.

The daily urea production exceeds urinary excretion by 25%. • The excess is metabolized by the colon. • Through the mesenteric vessels, circulating urea reaches the mucosa, where bacterial ureases convert urea to ammonia, which is then reabsorbed.

ANSWER:
A, C, E

40. Match each physician in the left-hand column with the contribution to the management of colorectal cancer in the right-hand column.

A. John B. Murphy   a. Posterior approach to the rectum with division of the sphincter muscle

B. Nicholas Senn   b. Instrumental in the suturing of anastomoses with a continuous inverting suture

C. Arthur Dean Bevan c. Internal stent for constructing intestinal anastomoses

D. Claude E. Dixon   d. Low anterior resection

E. W. Ernest Miles   e. Abdominoperineal resection

Ref.: 3

COMMENTS: Before the advances in critical care and blood bank technology, the most frequently performed operations for rectal cancer were through transperineal or transsacral approaches. • **Paul Kraske** (1851–1930) removed the coccyx and a portion of the sacrum (while preserving the sphincter) before resecting accessible rectal cancers. • If intestinal continuity could not be restored, a sacral anus was created. • Extension of the paracoccygeal incision down to and through the sphincter was first advocated by **Arthur Dean Bevan** (1861–1943). • Bevan, who was a graduate of Rush Medical College in 1883 and subsequently appointed Chairman of Surgery at the same institution in 1909, used this approach "for small carcinomas of the rectum without any radical involvement." Because proximal lymphatic spread was not addressed by this method, **W. Ernest Miles** (1869–1947) concluded that the approaches used by Kraske and Bevan were inadequate operations for rectal cancer. • Miles contended that all areas of potential lymphatic spread must be removed along with the anus, rectum, and a portion of the sigmoid. • The abdominoperineal resection was reported by Miles in 1908. • His operation lasted approximately 30 minutes. • An alternative approach to the Miles operation is low anterior resection and primary anastomosis for properly selected patients. • Fear of anastomotic leak and sepsis prompted **John B. Murphy** (1857–1916), a professor of surgery at Rush Medical College, to create in 1892 his "button," which by acting as an internal stent helped to coapt ends of intestinal tissue without the need for suturing. • Primary anastomosis of the intestine was perfected by several surgical researchers, including William Halsted, A. Lembert, and Nicholas Senn. • **Nicholas Senn** (1844–1908) was one of the first surgeons in the Western hemisphere to appreciate the importance of the animal laboratory for refining surgical technique. • Senn, a professor of surgical pathology at Rush Medical College, worked with F. Gregory Connell in perfecting the continuous inverting suture for intestinal anastomoses. • **Claude E. Dixon** (1893– 1968), head of the Section of General Surgery at The Mayo Graduate School from 1928 to 1957, was one of the first advocates of low anterior resection and primary anastomosis without colostomy.

ANSWER:
A-c; B-b; C-a; D-d; E-e

41. Colonoscopy is indicated for which of the following applications?

   A. Determining the extent of ulcerative colitis in a patient admitted to the hospital for an acute exacerbation

   B. Screening family members at risk for familial adenomatous polyposis

   C. Evaluation of an equivocal finding on barium enema

   D. If an adenomatous polyp is found in the upper rectum on screening sigmoidoscopy

   E. Evaluating gastrointestinal symptoms such as bleeding or pain when radiographic studies fail to reveal the cause

Ref.: 3

COMMENTS: Colonoscopy is contraindicated in cases of acute peritoneal inflammation, such as acute diverticulitis, peritonitis, or perforation. • Also, colonoscopy should not be performed during acute presentations of inflammatory bowel disease because of the potential for colonic perforation. • Colonoscopy is also contraindicated in patients immediately after an acute myocardial infarction (because of the possibly adverse sequelae associated with a vasovagal reflex), in patients with marked splenomegaly (traction on the splenic flexure may precipitate splenic bleeding), and during pregnancy (if fluoroscopy is to be used).

Because colonic polyps in patients with familial polyposis rarely develop in the absence of rectal polyps, screening family members at risk for polyposis is best accomplished with proctosigmoidoscopy.

Colonoscopy may confirm or refute suspected or equivocal radiographic findings during a barium enema examination. • If the barium enema fails to reveal the cause of a patient's anemia, pain, or bleeding, colonoscopy is indicated.

If an adenomatous polyp or cancer is discovered during screening sigmoidoscopy, colonoscopy is indicated to exclude the possibility of primary synchronous polyps (30%) or cancers (4–8%).

Colonoscopy is indicated for sigmoid volvulus and pseudoobstruction of the colon, provided there are no signs of peritoneal inflammation. • Decompression of the distended colon can be achieved successfully with minimal patient preparation.

ANSWER:
C, D, E

42. For medical management of toxic megacolon, which of the following is/are true?

   A. Nasoenteric decompression should be employed early.

   B. Endoscopy is necessary for the correct diagnosis.

   C. The patient should be rolled into a prone position on a flattened bed several times daily.

   D. Intravenous steroids have no role in this condition.

Ref.: 11, 15

COMMENTS: Toxic megacolon is seen in patients with ulcerative colitis (1–13%) and less frequently in Crohn's colitis. • Rapid fluid resuscitation and blood product transfusion are essential. • A nasogastric tube should be inserted to help minimize the accumulation of swallowed air in the colon. • Air usually gathers in the transverse colon, and such accumulation is promoted in patients lying supine. • Therefore, it is suggested to have patients roll into the prone position for 10–15 minutes every 2 hr. • Whether this promotes resolution of the problem is debatable.

There is little need to confirm the diagnosis with endoscopy. • In fact, intubation of the colon above the peritoneal reflection may cause perforation. • In patients with a fulminant presentation and no previous history of inflammatory bowel disease, a proctoscope, if inserted, should be advanced carefully to 10–15 cm and with little insufflation. • It helps confirm suspected inflammatory bowel disease and rules out anorectal causes of blood per rectum, such as hemorrhoids. • The diagnosis of toxic megacolon is based on clinical findings of fever, tachycardia, and abdominal bloating, combined with radiographs of the abdomen showing colonic distention. • Response to medical management is assessed with serial abdominal radiographs. • Prompt administration of steroids is an important factor when inducing a response. • Broad-spectrum antibiotics are also used. • Even if medical therapy is successful, most patients do not have a satisfactory long-term outcome, and ongoing symptoms and even recurrent toxic colitis continue to be concerns.

Worsening colonic distention, fever, and leukocytosis are indications for surgery. • In these instances, the operative choice is abdominal colectomy without proctectomy. • This procedure allows sphincter-preserving surgery to take place once health has been restored.

ANSWER:
A, C

43. Match each colitic process in the left-hand column with the appropriate statement in the right-hand column.

   A. Backwash ileitis   a. Responds to short-chain fatty acid instillation

   B. Diversion colitis   b. Metronidazole used to treat this condition

   C. Microscopic (lymphocytic) colitis   c. Seen in some cases of ulcerative colitis

   D. Acute ileitis   d. Good response to sulfasalazine

   E. Pseudomembranous colitis   e. *Yersinia* infection

Ref.: 15

COMMENTS: Backwash ileitis consists of nonspecific inflammation and dilatation of the ileum in patients with ulcerative colitis involving the entire colon. • There is no thickening or narrowing, as seen in Crohn's disease. • Its presence does not imply a pre-Crohn's disease condition, nor does it imply a poor outcome following the ileal pouch–anal anastomosis procedure.

Diversion colitis is found in segments of defunctionalized bowel. • The instillation of short-chain fatty acids ameliorates the condition, supporting the concept that these substances (being primary nutrients for the colonic mucosal cells) are deficient in this condition, leading to chronic inflammation. • Preliminary trials concerning idiopathic ulcerative proctocolitis have shown a response to short-chain fatty acid enemas. • Following reversal of the fecal diversion, the endoscopic findings of diversion colitis usually resolve.

Microscopic colitis (also known as **lymphocytic colitis**) is characterized by a history of watery diarrhea and microscopic inflammation of colonic mucosa. • The colitis often responds favorably to sulfasalazine. • **Collagenous colitis** (which exhibits a collagenous band under the surface epithelium of the colon on microscopic examination) may be a variant of this condition because patients present with similar symptoms and respond to sulfasalazine. • Spontaneous remission of these two conditions is common. • Most of these patients have been incorrectly labeled for years as having irritable bowel syndrome. • Colonoscopy with biopsy may yield the correct diagnosis.

Acute inflammatory ileitis presents with right lower quadrant pain and is commonly confused with appendicitis or Crohn's disease. • Acute ileitis, often due to *Yersinia enterocolitica* infection, is capable of producing self-limited, acute ileitis and colitis, sometimes with a granulomatous reaction.

Antibiotic-induced colitis (also known as **pseudomembranous colitis**) presents with watery diarrhea, which is rarely bloody and is due to *C. difficile* proliferation. • The diagnosis is best made by detecting the *C. difficile* toxin in the stool. • Either oral vancomycin or metronidazole is used to treat this condition. • The latter is less expensive and is therefore used more often.

ANSWER:
A-c; B-a; C-d; D-e; E-b

44. Colonoscopy is strongly indicated in which of the following groups of patients?

   A. In patients with Crohn's colitis to monitor the efficacy of treatment

   B. In patients with an 8- to 10-year history of ulcerative colitis

   C. In patients with recurrent anal fistula and fissures

   D. In patients with suspected colovaginal or colovesical fistulas

   E. Patients with colorectal cancer in first-degree relative(s)

Ref.: 11, 15

COMMENTS: Endoscopy is not indicated simply for the purpose of monitoring the response of Crohn's disease to medical therapy. • It can be performed on a clinical basis alone.

Patients with a history of ulcerative colitis for more than 8–10 years are at higher risk of having adenocarcinoma of the colon and should undergo surveillance colonoscopy with multiple-site biopsies for the determination of dysplasia. • This procedure should be done even if the disease is in remission. • Thereafter, if results are negative, surveillance should probably be done at least annually. • Patients with pancolitis appear to be at higher risk for cancer than do patients with limited left-sided disease, but the latter group should also undergo surveillance. • In patients with Crohn's disease, there is no guideline for cancer surveillance.

Patients with recurrent or multiple anal fistulas and fissures should undergo colonoscopy to exclude Crohn's disease. • If the ileum is not intubated, a small-bowel radiograph should be obtained.

The presence of a colovaginal or colovesicle fistula is difficult to demonstrate endoscopically or radiographically. • With either fistula, the colon must be assessed, and, even if a fistula is not demonstrated, indirect evidence with regard to its cause can be obtained. • For example, diverticular disease, cancer, or inflammatory bowel disease can be responsible for fistula formation and should be seen. • A barium enema is probably preferable to colonoscopy for workup of a colovesicle or colovaginal fistula because of its lower risk and cost and the enhanced total image of the colon and its flexures. • Also, a fistula is more likely visualized with a contrast enema than with endoscopy.

At-risk patients in families with HNPCC must undergo colonoscopy beginning at age 25. • First-degree relatives of patients with sporadic colorectal cancer have a two- to threefold increased risk of developing cancer, especially if the family member was younger than age 55 at the time of cancer diagnosis. • The age at which to begin screening first-degree relatives with colonoscopy is controversial, but it has been suggested that screening begin at an age 10 years younger than the age of the relative when cancer was diagnosed.

ANSWER:
B, C, E

45. Match each type of radiation therapy used for treatment of rectal cancer in the left-hand column with the appropriate feature or features in the right-hand column.

   A. Preoperative   a. Minimizes or avoids radiation damage to the small intestine

   B. Intraoperative   b. Capable of improving local control by treating tumor cell spillage during surgery

   C. Postoperative   c. When combined with chemotherapy, has demonstrated benefit in local control and survival

      d. Capable of down-staging the tumor

Ref.: 6

COMMENTS: All of the forms of radiation therapy listed are capable of improving local control and lowering recurrence rates by treating potential tumor cell spillage. • **Preoperative radiation** lowers recurrence rates, and there is evidence to suggest that it improves survival. • Resectability rates may be improved and tumors may be down-staged by ablating metastatic lymph nodes. • When preoperative radiation is combined with chemotherapy, complete response rates of 20–30% have been noted for cancers in the distal rectum. • Because the rectum fills the pelvis, the small bowel can be potentially spared, owing to its mobility and lack of fixation within the pelvis. • The radiation dose has varied widely in reported series. • The dose most frequently used is 40–45 Gy over 4–6 weeks, with a 6-week hiatus before surgery.

Intraoperative irradiation is used to treat tumors or tumor beds where gross residual or microscopic disease remains. • This technique allows some radiosensitive structures, such as the small bowel, to be shielded from the radiation beam, thereby minimizing damage to normal tissue. • A single dose of 10–20 Gy is given, and patients are also usually treated with postoperative external-beam radiation therapy as well. • Results have not shown an improvement in survival, and a significant portion of patients develop ureteral obstruction and sacral neuritis.

Postoperative irradiation is considered for rectal tumors at high risk for local recurrence, such as those demonstrating transmural penetration or lymph node metastases. • When combined with chemotherapy, improved local control and survival have been noted. • The main advantage of administering radiation postoperatively is that the exact stage of the cancer is known. • Patients with early lesions or those whose tumor has spread beyond the confines of the pelvis are spared treatment. • The current trend, however, is to administer radiation and chemotherapy preoperatively. • A randomized controlled trial comparing similar radiation doses for high-risk tumors only has not been done.

A N S W E R :
A-a,b,c,d; B-a,b; C-b,c

46. Pouchitis can frequently complicate the ileal pouch–anal anastomosis procedure. With regard to this condition, which of the following is/are true?

    A. It occurs with equal frequency in patients with familial polyposis and ulcerative colitis.

    B. It is found more frequently in patients with capacious S-shaped pouches than in those with J-shaped pouches.

    C. Most patients can be treated successfully with oral metronidazole.

    D. The responsible pathogen is usually *Bacteroides*.

    E. Recurrent persistent pouchitis invariably necessitates pouch excision.

Ref.: 6

COMMENTS: Pouchitis is a nonspecific inflammation of the ileal reservoir following the ileal pouch–anal anastomosis procedure. • It occurs in up to 50% of patients. • The cause is not precisely known, but pouchitis is seen more frequently in patients with ulcerative colitis than in those with familial polyposis. • Pouchitis is not related to pouch design, stasis within the pouch, or a specific aerobic or anaerobic bacterial pathogen. • Pouchitis is manifested clinically by increased stool output and frequency, malaise, cramps, and arthralgias. • Most cases respond to oral metronidazole, and hospitalization or pouch excision is rarely required.

A N S W E R :
C

47. Match each type of rectal cancer in the left-hand column with one or more appropriate operations in the right-hand column.

    A. Fixed, circumferential adenocarcinoma just above the dentate line

    a. Abdominoperineal resection

    B. Ulcerating adenocarcinoma whose lower edge is 7 cm from the dentate line, with infiltration and expansion of the second hypoechoic layer seen on ultrasound imaging

    b. Low anterior resection with descending colorectostomy

    C. A 2-cm, mobile adenocarcinoma arising in a villous adenoma 3 cm from the dentate line, with an intact second hyperechoic band seen on ultrasound imaging

    c. Low anterior resection with coloanal anastomosis

    D. Circumferential adenocarcinoma 12 cm from the anal verge

    d. Local excision

    E. A 3.5-cm carcinoid at 4 cm from the dentate line

Ref.: 6

COMMENTS: The most important determinant of which operation to perform for a rectal cancer is the location of the lesion within the rectum. • Tumors located 0–5 cm from the anal verge, especially those that involve the sphincter muscle and are producing pain, are best treated by abdominoperineal resection. • Approximately 10–15% of tumors within this region, however, can be considered for local excision if they satisfy strict selection criteria. • They should be no larger than 3–4 cm, exhibit minimal penetration of the rectal wall as seen on rectal ultrasound imaging, lack lymphovascular invasion, and be well differentiated. • Occasionally, a coloanal anastomosis can be performed in thin patients, especially if there has been a significant reduction in the size of the tumor from preoperative radiation and chemotherapy.

Lesions in the upper rectum (10–15 cm) are amenable to anterior resection with restoration of intestinal continuity by descending colorectostomy.

Lesions located in the midrectum (5–10 cm) are treated by a variety of operations, depending on the skill of the surgeon and the patient's body habitus. • Most cancers in this region can be treated by low anterior resection with colorectostomy (which has been facilitated by use of surgical staplers) or coloanal anastomosis. • In the latter case, a proximal temporary colostomy is constructed to divert stool away from the anastomosis. • Impaired fecal continence has been noted in 10–35% of patients after coloanal anastomosis. • However, construction of a colonic J-pouch or performing a coloplasty may avoid frequent stools and incontinence. • The decision with regard to the appropriateness of sphincter preservation must be individualized, and safety is a primary concern. • If the patient is obese or the pelvis is narrow and a satisfactory anastomosis cannot be done, abdominoperineal resection or low anterior resection with coloanal anastomosis is an option for midrectal cancers. • Also, if the patient preoperatively has sphincter impairment due to age or previous surgery, a low anastomosis should be avoided.

For low rectal carcinoids larger than 2 cm, transabdominal surgery with lymphadenectomy should be performed. • An abdominoperineal resection would likely be indicated for the patient described in E, but low anterior resection with coloanal anastomosis could be considered as well.

A N S W E R :
A-a; B-b,c; C-d; D-b; E-a,c

48. Regarding HNPCC (Lynch's syndrome), which of the following is/are true?

    A. It is inherited as an autosomal dominant trait.

    B. Most cancers are in the right colon.

    C. There is a greater likelihood of multiple, synchronous lesions.

    D. Most patients are under 50 years of age.

    E. Up to 40% of patients develop metachronous colorectal cancers within 10 years.

    F. There is a high frequency of endometrial, ovarian, breast, and gastric cancers.

Ref.: 6, 16

COMMENTS: HNPCC syndrome occurs in two varieties: (1) site-specific colorectal cancer (**Lynch's syndrome I**) and (2) colorectal cancer associated with other forms of cancer (e.g., endometrial, ovarian, breast, and gastric; **Lynch's syndrome II**). • Accounting for approximately 5–6% of all colorectal cancers, HNPCC is due to mutations in mismatch repair genes that normally repair errors in DNA replication. • It is inherited as an autosomal dominant trait and may affect multiple generations in succession. • Afflicted individuals show a predominance of right-sided cancers (72.3%), are likely to have multiple carcinomas (18.1%), are usually young (mean age 44.6 years), and often develop metachronous colorectal cancers (40% risk over 10 years). • It is interesting to note that these individuals may have an improved survival compared to those with sporadic cancers.

Family members at risk should undergo biannual colonoscopy beginning at age 25. • Women should have an annual pelvic examination with endometrial biopsy every 3 years. • Mammograms should be obtained earlier than usually advised. • Alternatively, a family may choose to undergo genetic screening to identify members who have inherited the mutation.

If a new cancer is found in an HNPCC family, consideration should be given to subtotal colectomy because of the risk of metachronous tumors. • If a woman has completed childbearing, one may also consider hysterectomy and bilateral salpingo-oophorectomy.

A N S W E R :
A, B, C, D, E, F

49. Match the gene in the left-hand column with the applicable statement in the right-hand column.

A. Adenoma polyposis coli (APC)
B. *p53*
C. *hMSH2*
D. *DCC*
E. *K-ras*

a. Tumor-suppressor gene located on chromosome 17
b. Late-occurring alteration resulting in loss of cell-to-cell contact, thereby enhancing metastases
c. Located on chromosome 5
d. Most common mutation found in HNPCC
e. Oncogene that, when mutated, codes for a protein that cannot regulate cell growth and differentiation

Ref.: 16

COMMENTS: The **adenoma polyposis coli (APC)** gene is located on chromosome 5, is large (consisting of approximately 15 exons), and encodes for a cytoplasmic protein of 2843 amino acids. • APC mutations occur in both sporadic colorectal cancers and familial polyposis, are frequent, are comparable in incidence between adenomas and carcinomas, and occur early in the development of cancer. • The protein product of the APC gene is normally involved in maintaining cellular adhesions and suppressing neoplastic growth, but the mutant protein may not be capable of serving this function. • The APC gene thereby acts as a tumor-suppressor gene. • Approximately 35% of sporadic cancers and up to 75% of polyposis cancers have APC mutations that can occur at variable points within the gene. • This may explain the various phenotypes associated with the polyposis syndromes.

The **p53 gene** is a tumor-suppressor gene located on chromosome 17. • Mutations of this gene are the most common genetic abnormality found in various human cancers. • The gene encodes for a nuclear phosphoprotein that regulates transcription and negatively influences cellular proliferation by binding at specific DNA sites. • For example, cells damaged by ultraviolet light or radiation are kept from replicating by the wild-type (natural) P53 protein. • Mutant P53 binds to wild-type P53, preventing specific binding to DNA, thereby permitting tumor growth.

Mismatch repair genes correct errors of DNA replication. • Alterations in these genes have been implicated in the pathogenesis of hereditary nonpolyposis colorectal cancer. • The identified genetic sequences are (1) *hMSH2* on chromosome 2 (mutation of this gene may account for up to 40% of the genetic alterations seen in HNPCC families); (2) *hMLH1* on chromosome 3, which may act as a tumor-suppressor gene; (3) *hPMS1* on chromosome 2; and (4) *hPMS2* on chromosome 7. • Mutations of the latter two genes account for only 10% of the mutations seen in HNPCC families. • Germ-line mutations of *hMSH2* and *hMLH1* genes by themselves are not enough to produce the HNPCC phenotype. • A somatic mutation of the remaining wild-type allele is also necessary.

The **DCC gene** is located on chromosome 18 and encodes for a protein involved in cell-to-cell contact. • Deletions of this gene have been found in 73% of colorectal cancers but only 11% of adenomas, suggesting that gene loss occurred late during tumorigenesis. • Cancers with a loss of the DCC gene are more likely to present as advanced disease (compared to tumors maintaining this gene), and patients' survival is consequently compromised.

The **K-ras gene**, an oncogene found on chromosome 12, encodes for a plasma membrane–based protein involved in transduction of growth and differentiation signals. • Approximately 50% of colorectal cancers have *ras* mutations. • Large adenomas and adenomas with small areas of invasive cancer have nearly the same incidence of *ras* mutations, suggesting that genetic alterations in the *ras* gene occurs early (but not as early as APC mutations) during tumorigenesis. • It has yet to be proved if *ras* mutations have any prognostic significance.

A N S W E R :
A-c; B-a; C-d; D-b; E-e

50. Which of the following are accepted applications of endorectal ultrasound imaging?

A. Assessing sphincter integrity in patients complaining of fecal incontinence

B. Determining whether a rectal cancer is suitable for local excision

C. Ruling out recurrent cancer

D. Evaluating anal fistulas

Ref.: 17

COMMENTS: Endorectal ultrasound imaging has had significant impact on the diagnosis and management of a variety of anorectal diseases. • The initial use of ultrasound instrumentation was for staging **rectal cancers**. • The depth of penetration and presence of abnormal lymph nodes was used to determine the stage of the cancer and its suitability for transanal, local excision. • Generally, tumors that demonstrate deep penetration of the rectal wall have an increased likelihood of lymph node metastases and are not suitable candidates for transanal excision because of the unacceptably high recurrence rates associated with local excision of these advanced neoplasms. • Recently, the use of ultrasound imaging for staging rectal cancers has been expanded to determine whether a lesion is advanced enough to warrant preoperative radiation therapy and chemotherapy. • Ultrasound imaging can be used to assess the rectal wall and the extraluminal tissue for any sign of recurrent cancer following surgery. • In this respect, it has distinct advantages over other imaging modalities, such as CT scanning, in that the probe is placed in direct contact with the area of maximal interest, namely, the operative site. • Resolution capabilities are much better with ultrasound imaging than with CT scanning.

Regarding **benign diseases** of the anus and rectum, the endorectal ultrasound device can also be used to image the sphincter mechanism in patients complaining of fecal incontinence. • In fact, before any patient is given a diagnosis of idiopathic or neurogenic incontinence, an ultrasound scan must be done to inspect the integrity of the sphincter. • Although most anorectal abscesses and fistulas can be managed without elaborate imaging studies, ultrasound imaging has proved useful for determining the extent laterally and in a cephalad direction of abscess collections. • Furthermore, the tract of the fistula in relationship to the sphincter muscle can be assessed using ultrasound imaging, whereby the internal opening can be identified as a hypoechoic disruption of the internal sphincter muscle. • In some instances, hydrogen peroxide has been injected into the fistula tract during ultrasound scanning to further delineate the fistula tract.

ANSWER:
A, B, C, D

51. Which of the following is/are true regarding anorectal ultrasound imaging?

A. Sedation is required.

B. The bowel must be prepared as if for colonoscopy or colectomy.

C. Scanning is best performed with a 3.0-MHz crystal.

D. Imaging of lesions more than 10 cm from the anus is not possible.

E. Image-guided needle biopsy of extraluminal nodules is safe.

Ref.: 17

COMMENTS: Anorectal ultrasound imaging is generally performed as an office procedure without the need for sedation or a formal bowel preparation. • Frequently, a single enema is given 1–2 hr before the examination to remove any stool from the rectal vault. • Because minimal penetration of the rectal wall and perirectal tissues is required, a high-frequency ultrasound crystal is used (i.e., 7 or 10 MHz). • High resolution of the superficial structures is thus obtained. • With lower frequencies, there would be better penetration of the deeper structures, but the information obtained from assessing the deep structures of the pelvic cavity has little bearing on the clinical management of anorectal diseases. • It is possible to image lesions in the mid and upper rectum, but, to be certain that the ultrasound probe is in contact with neoplasms at this level, it is necessary to insert the probe under direct vision through a commercially available 2-cm wide proctoscope. • The proctoscope is advanced under direct vision to the desired level, and, once the lesion is identified, the ultrasound probe is inserted through the shaft of the proctoscope directly to the area of interest. • Image-guided needle biopsy of extraluminal nodules is a safe

procedure and can be performed with the ultrasound probe used by the urologist for imaging the prostate. • Suspicious perirectal nodules can be biopsied in this fashion, although one must be careful with the interpretation of these biopsy data. • If adipose tissue or skeletal muscle is obtained, one cannot assume that the nodule in question does not contain cancer. • Only if the nodule contains benign lymphoid tissue can it be assumed that the nodule in question is truly free of cancer.

ANSWER:
E

REFERENCES

1. Townsend CM, Beauchamp RD, Evers BM, et al (eds): *Sabiston Textbook of Surgery: The Biological Basis of Modern Surgical Practice*, 17th ed. Saunders, Philadelphia, 2004.
2. Brunicardi FC, Andersen DK, Billiar TR, et al (eds): *Schwartz's Principles of Surgery*, 8th ed. McGraw-Hill, New York, 2004.
3. Corman ML: *Colon and Rectal Surgery*, 5th ed. JB Lippincott, Philadelphia, 2005.
4. Kaleya RN, Boley SJ: Colonic ischemia. *Perspect Colon Rectal Surg* 3(1):62–81, 1990.
5. Taylor I: Intestinal blood flow. *Perspect Colon Rectal Surg* 1(2):49–57, 1988.
6. Gordon PM, Nivatvongs S: *Principles and Practice of Surgery for the Colon, Rectum and Anus*, 2nd ed. Quality Medical Publishing, St. Louis, 1999.
7. Boley SJ, Brandt LJ, Frank MS: Severe lower intestinal bleeding: diagnosis and treatment. *Clin Gastroenterol* 10:65–91, 1981.
8. Browder W, Cerise EJ, Litwin MS: Impact of emergency angiography in massive lower gastrointestinal bleeding. *Ann Surg* 204:530–536, 1986.
9. Diaz-Canton EA, Pazdur R: Adjuvant therapy for colorectal cancer. *Surg Clin North Am* 77:211–228, 1997.
10. Fleshman JW, Myerson RJ: Adjuvant radiation therapy for adenocarcinoma of the rectum. *Surg Clin North Am* 77:15–26.
11. Mazier WP, Levien DH, Luchtefeld MA, et al: *Surgery of the Colon, Rectum and Anus*. Saunders, Philadelphia, 1995.
12. Fazio VW (ed): *Current Therapy in Colon and Rectal Surgery*. BC Decker, St. Louis, 1990.
13. Gordon MS, Cohen AM: Management of invasive carcinoma in pedunculated colorectal polyps. *Oncology* 3:99–105, 1989.
14. Pemberton JH, Phillips SF: Colonic absorption. *Perspect Colon Rectal Surg* 1(1):89–103, 1988.
15. Sleisenger MH, Fordtran JS: *Gastrointestinal Disease: Pathophysiology, Diagnosis and Management*, 4th ed. Saunders, Philadelphia, 1989.
16. Howe JR, Guillem JG: The genetics of colorectal cancer. *Surg Clin North Am* 77:175–196, 1997.
17. Staren ED: *Ultrasound for the Surgeon*. Lippincott-Raven, Philadelphia, 1997.

CHAPTER 36

Anus and Perianal Disease

Theodore J. Saclarides, M.D.

1. Match each of the following anatomic structures or landmarks with its proper location in the coronal view of the anorectal area (only one side shown).

A. Levator ani

B. Valve of Houston

C. Superficial external sphincter

D. Ischiorectal fossa

E. Deep external sphincter and puborectalis

F. Internal hemorrhoidal plexus

G. Internal sphincter

H. Columns of Morgagni

I. External hemorrhoidal plexus

J. Dentate line

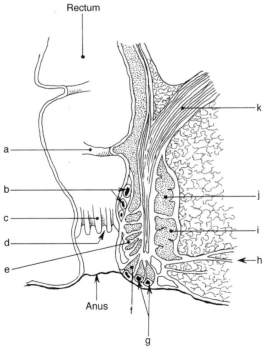

Ref.: 1, 2

COMMENTS: See Questions 2 and 3.

2. With regard to the anal sphincteric mechanism, which of the following statements is/are true?

A. The longitudinal muscle of the rectal wall eventually forms the internal anal sphincter.

B. The internal sphincter is made up of smooth muscle and surrounds the distal two thirds of the anal canal.

C. The external sphincter is made up of striated muscle and is voluntary.

D. The puborectalis is a part of the levator ani muscle.

E. The anorectal ring is composed entirely of the palpable deep portion of external sphincter.

Ref.: 1, 2

COMMENTS: The teniae of the colon fuse at the upper border of the rectum to completely invest the rectum with longitudinal muscle in addition to an inner circular muscle layer. • In the anal canal, the longitudinal muscle forms the **conjoined longitudinal muscle**, which descends in the plane between the internal and external sphincter. • The circular muscle of the rectum thickens to form the involuntary **internal sphincter**, which is smooth muscle and surrounds the distal two thirds of the anal canal. • The lowest edge of the internal sphincter is 1.0–1.5 cm below the dentate line and just above the lowest portion of the external sphincter. • The **external sphincter** is formed of three parts—subcutaneous, superficial, and deep—which are striated muscles and under voluntary control. • Clinically, these components of the external sphincter are not distinguishable as separate layers. • The **puborectalis muscle** is fused with the deep portion of the external sphincter and is not part of the levator muscle. • The puborectalis originates from the posterior surface of the symphysis pubis and runs in a posterior direction to form a U-shaped loop around the rectum. • Contraction of the puborectalis muscle pulls the rectum forward, thereby establishing a resting anorectal angle of 90–110 degrees. • Unhindered defecation requires relaxation of the puborectalis. • Inappropriate contraction during straining renders the anorectal angle more acute, thereby impairing defecation. • The puborectalis muscle and the deep portion of the external sphincter, along with the upper portion of the internal sphincter, form the palpable anorectal ring.

See Question 3.

3. With regard to the anatomy of the anal canal, which of the following statements is/are true?

A. The dentate line lies above the columns of Morgagni.

B. Anal gland ducts open into the anal crypts.

C. Anal glands are frequently found in the ischiorectal space.

D. The columns of Morgagni overlie the internal hemorrhoidal plexus.

E. The epithelium above the dentate line is innervated by the autonomic nervous system.

Ref.: 1, 2

COMMENTS: The dentate line is at the level of the anal crypts. • Above it are vertical mucosal folds, the columns of Morgagni, which overlie the internal hemorrhoidal plexus. • The anal mucosa proximal to the dentate line is supplied by the autonomic nervous system and is insensitive to most painful stimuli. • The anoderm distal to this is supplied by somatic nerves and is sensitive to painful stimuli. • Anal glands, 6–10 in number, usually lie in the intersphincteric space or the internal sphincter, and their ducts open into the anal crypts.

ANSWERS:
Question 1: A-k; B-a; C-f; D-h; E-j; F-b; G-e; H-c; I-g; J-d
Question 2: B, C
Question 3: B, D, E

4. With regard to perirectal spaces, which of the following statements is/are true?

A. The supralevator space is situated above the levator muscle and is connected with the contralateral side anteriorly.

B. The retrorectal space lies between the rectum and the sacrum above the rectosacral fascia.

C. The deep postanal space lies between the levator ani and the superficial external sphincter posteriorly.

D. The perianal space and the superficial postanal space lie deep to the superficial anal sphincter.

E. The intersphincteric space lies within the conjoined longitudinal muscle.

Ref.: 2

COMMENTS: The **supralevator space** is located above the levator ani on both sides and communicates with the contralateral side posteriorly. • This space is bounded superiorly by the peritoneum, laterally by the pelvic wall, medially by the rectum, and inferiorly by the levator ani. • Infection in this space can arise from a pelvic source (e.g., diverticulitis or pelvic inflammatory disease) or as an upward extension from an anorectal source. • The **retrorectal space** lies above the rectosacral fascia between the upper two thirds of the rectum and sacrum. • The fascia runs downward and forward from the sacrum to the anorectal junction. • The retrorectal space contains loose connective tissue and is a site for the formation of tumors arising from embryologic remnants (i.e., dermoids, teratomas, and chordomas). • The retrorectal space is bounded anteriorly by the rectum, posteriorly by the presacral fascia, laterally by the pelvic side wall, superiorly by the peritoneal reflection, and inferiorly by the rectosacral fascia, below which is the supralevator space. • The **ischiorectal space** lies below the levator muscle, above the transverse septum of the ischiorectal fossa, and between the external sphincter and lateral pelvic wall. • This space communicates posteriorly through the **deep postanal space,** which lies between the levator ani and the superficial external sphincter. • The lower border of the deep postanal space is the anococcygeal ligament, which originates from the superficial portion of the external sphincter in the posterior midline. • This communication allows a deep postanal space abscess to extend to both ischiorectal spaces (horseshoe abscess). • The **perianal space** (the most common

space involved in abscesses) lies superficial to the superficial external anal sphincter. • The **intersphincteric space** lies within the conjoined longitudinal muscle, where the anal glands also are located. • The perianal, ischiorectal, and supralevator spaces may each connect posteriorly with their counterparts on the contralateral side, forming a horseshoe connection in any of these spaces.

ANSWER:
B, C, E

5. With regard to hemorrhoids, which of the following statements is/are true?

A. Internal hemorrhoids are vascular cushions above the dentate line and are covered by anoderm.

B. Prolapsing hemorrhoids are external hemorrhoids covered by anoderm.

C. Bleeding internal hemorrhoids are best managed by surgical excision.

D. Thrombosed hemorrhoids are best treated by hemorrhoidectomy, with the patient under general anesthesia.

E. Recurrence is uncommon after surgical hemorrhoidectomy.

Ref.: 1, 2

COMMENTS: **Internal** hemorrhoids are exaggerated submucosal vascular cushions normally located above the dentate line and are therefore covered by the transitional mucosa of the anal canal and not by anoderm. • **External** hemorrhoids are the dilated veins of the inferior hemorrhoidal plexus located below the dentate line and are covered by anoderm. • **Prolapsing** hemorrhoids are internal hemorrhoids that prolapse beyond the dentate line. • **Bleeding** is the main manifestation of smaller internal hemorrhoids and is managed initially by rubber banding, infrared coagulation, or injection sclerotherapy. • Surgery is reserved for internal hemorrhoids that do not respond to these conservative measures. • Surgery is the best initial therapy for prolapsing internal hemorrhoids that require manual reduction or for those that are incarcerated. • **Thrombosed** hemorrhoids are best treated by incising the overlying anoderm with evacuation of the thrombus. • **Recurrence** should be rare after surgical hemorrhoidectomy. • When it occurs, it is usually related to inadequate removal of the rectal mucosa and hemorrhoidal tissue.

ANSWER:
E

6. With regard to anal fissure, which of the following statements is/are true?

A. It is located above the dentate line.

B. It is located at the posterior midline in more than 90% of patients.

C. The operation of choice for a midline fissure is excision of the fissure and posterior internal sphincterotomy.

D. Lateral partial subcutaneous sphincterotomy is the operation of choice for nonmidline fissures.

E. Treatment should consist of fissurectomy and lateral partial subcutaneous external sphincterotomy.

Ref.: 1, 2

COMMENTS: Anal fissure, a tear of the skin-lined part of the anal canal, is located at or below the dentate line. • Gentle spreading of the buttocks is frequently all that is needed to reveal the fissure.

• About 90% of fissures (acute or chronic) are located at the posterior midline, an area where the anoderm is least supported by the sphincter. • Fissures located laterally should arouse suspicion of Crohn's disease, ulcerative colitis, syphilis, tuberculosis, leukemia, or other causes, and therapy is directed toward the underlying disease. • The initial treatment of a midline fissure is conservative, involving lubricants and bulk laxatives. • Operative treatment is a lateral subcutaneous partial internal sphincterotomy to relax the internal sphincter, with the sphincterotomy carried up to the dentate line. • A major cause of nonhealing is inadequate sphincterotomy. • Posterior fissurectomy and sphincterotomy can lead to a keyhole defect and constant soiling. • It can be avoided by performing the sphincterotomy in the lateral location.

A N S W E R :
B

7. With regard to perirectal suppuration, which of the following statements is/are true?

A. The pathophysiology of perirectal abscess is related to infection of the perianal skin.

B. A horseshoe abscess begins as a posterior midline infection of the anal canal.

C. An intersphincteric abscess causes pain deep in the rectum without external manifestations.

D. Most perianal abscesses can be drained with the use of local anesthesia and without immediate concern for subsequent formation of fistula in ano.

E. Ischiorectal abscesses should be drained with the patient under general anesthesia, and the fistula must be identified and treated.

Ref.: 1, 2

COMMENTS: A **perirectal abscess** starts in the anal glands lying in the intersphincteric space. • **Horseshoe abscesses** include bilateral ischiorectal, supralevator, or perianal abscesses that communicate. • Horseshoe abscesses usually start from infection of the posterior midline and glands. • A horseshoe ischiorectal abscess starts in the deep postanal space and extends in a U-shaped manner into each ischiorectal space. • The patient is treated in the operating room under regional or general anesthesia and by incising the skin from the external sphincter to the coccyx. • This step exposes the superficial external sphincter, which is split longitudinally but not transected. • The incision provides access to the deep postanal space. • A probe is inserted into the posterior midline crypt and then into the deep postanal space. • A rubber seton is placed in this space and wrapped around the internal sphincter and superficial external sphincter. • Small counterincisions are made laterally along the extensions of the abscess. • Sequential tightening of the seton should result in minimal, if any, sphincter impairment. • An **intersphincteric abscess** usually presents with pain and bulging inside the rectum but with no external swelling. • Treatment consists of transanally laying open the internal sphincter, beginning at the lower edge of the abscess and extending cephalad to the top of the abscess cavity. • Most **perianal abscesses** can be drained with the use of local anesthesia, but if the patient has a high fever or significant leukocytosis or is immunocompromised, treatment in the operating room under general anesthesia is preferable. • Identification of a fistula may be deferred until there are clinical signs that a fistula is present, namely, nonhealing of an abscess wound or recurrence of the abscess at the same location.

A N S W E R :
B, C, D

8. With regard to the management of patients with fistula in ano, which of the following statements is/are true?

A. All internal openings of fistulas are located posteriorly, according to Goodsall's rule.

B. The most common type of fistula is intersphincteric.

C. Excision of the entire fistulous tract is necessary for cure.

D. High fistulas can be managed by means of a seton suture.

E. A horseshoe fistula can be treated by opening of the deep postanal space, placement of a seton, and curetting (but not laying open) the lateral extensions.

Ref.: 1, 2

COMMENTS: Anal fistulas are classified as intersphincteric (most common), transsphincteric, suprasphincteric, and extrasphincteric. • **Goodsall's rule** states that, if the external opening is anterior to an imaginary line drawn between the ischial tuberosities, the fistula usually runs directly into the anal canal, and, if the external opening is posterior, the tract curves to the posterior midline. • Anal fistulotomy and establishment of adequate drainage constitute sufficient therapy. • Excision of the tract is unnecessary and prolongs healing. • High transsphincteric fistulas can be managed by means of a seton suture. • Alternatives include the use of fibrin glue or a rectal advancement flap to close the internal opening. • With the latter, the internal opening is excised, and a flap consisting of mucosa, submucosa, and circular muscle is raised, advanced, and sutured. • A horseshoe fistula, which starts with infection at the posterior midline anal glands, is best treated by opening the deep postanal space and identifying and curetting the lateral extensions. • Laying open the fistula extensions could be done but would result in large, gaping wounds that may require a long time to heal. • The external opening in the posterior midline can be managed by placement of a seton drain.

A N S W E R :
B, D, E

9. Anal incontinence associated with rectal prolapse is caused primarily by which one of the following?

A. Levator diastasis

B. Loss of the rectal angle

C. Stretching of the anal sphincter

D. Stretching of the pudendal nerve

E. Loose endopelvic fascia

Ref.: 1, 2

COMMENTS: Anal and urinary incontinence in advanced cases of prolapse is due to entrapment and stretching of the pudendal nerve, resulting in neuromuscular dysfunction. • It is important, therefore, to repair rectal prolapse before incontinence develops. • Chronic stretching of the sphincter by the prolapse itself may lead to sphincter impairment as well. • Repair of the prolapse improves continence in approximately 50% of patients. • The other defects listed are associated with the prolapse but are not the cause of incontinence. • Their correction therefore does not cure the problem of incontinence.

A N S W E R :
C, D

10. Match each of the anal conditions in the left-hand column with the most appropriate initial therapy in the right-hand column.

A. Bowen's disease   a. Local excision

B. Paget's disease   b. Local excision and postoperative radiotherapy

C. Basal cell carcinoma   c. Abdominoperineal resection

                            d. External beam radiotherapy

                            e. Chemotherapy and radiotherapy

Ref.: 1, 2

COMMENTS: **Bowen's disease** is an intraepidermal squamous cell carcinoma. • It rarely metastasizes but can be locally recurrent. • Local excision with clear margins is adequate. • **Paget's disease** of the perianal skin is a malignant neoplasm of the intraepidermal portion of the apocrine glands. • It usually appears as an eczematoid perianal lesion in women and is intensely pruritic. • Paget cells stain with periodic acid–Schiff stain, which differentiates them from bowenoid cells. • Invasion occurs late, and metastases are rare. • Wide local excision with adequate margins is the procedure of choice. • Both Bowen's and Paget's diseases have been associated with other cutaneous or visceral malignancies, but this association is controversial. • **Basal cell carcinoma** is usually noninvasive and nonmetastasizing. • Local excision with adequate margins virtually ensures a cure.

A N S W E R :
A-a; B-a; C-a

11. In comparison with squamous cell cancers of the anal margin, which of the following statements is/are generally true of squamous cell cancers of the anal canal?

A. They are more common in women.

B. They are more often associated with benign anal conditions.

C. They are more advanced when diagnosed.

D. They are more frequently associated with basaloid histology.

E. They are associated with a better prognosis.

Ref.: 1, 2

COMMENTS: The **anal canal** is generally considered to be the region from above the dentate line to the top of the anorectal ring. • The **anal margin** is distal to the dentate line. • Squamous cell cancers of the anal canal are more common in women. • Because they are often mistaken for benign anal disorders, they are usually advanced at the time of diagnosis and therefore have a worse prognosis. • Basaloid and cloacogenic carcinomas are a histologic variant of squamous cell cancer of the anal canal. • Conversely, perianal (anal margin) squamous cell carcinoma is four times more common in men and is usually slow growing and late to metastasize. • Basaloid features are uncommon. • Wide local excision with a 2-cm margin may be adequate therapy for superficial squamous cell cancers of the anal margin, whereas squamous cell cancers of the anal canal generally necessitate multimodality therapy, involving irradiation and chemotherapy.

A N S W E R :
A, C, D

12. There is general agreement that survival after treatment for squamous cancer of the anus is related to which of the following?

A. Tumor size

B. Depth of invasion

C. Basaloid versus squamous histologic features

D. Lymph node involvement

Ref.: 1, 2

COMMENTS: The poor prognosis of squamous cell carcinoma of the anal canal is related to delay in diagnosis. • Poor prognostic factors include large tumor size, deeply invasive lesions, and lymph node metastases. • In basaloid cancers, there is good correlation between histologic differentiation and the 5-year survival rate (90% for well-differentiated, 50% for moderately differentiated, and 0% for anaplastic lesions). • The presence of basaloid histologic features versus squamous histologic features alone has not been conclusively shown to affect prognosis.

A N S W E R :
A, B, D

13. With regard to the management of inguinal lymph nodes in patients with squamous cell cancer of the anus, which of the following statements is/are true?

A. Prophylactic groin dissection is indicated when abdominoperineal resection is performed.

B. Groin dissection for synchronously and that for metachronously appearing nodes yield equivalent survival rates.

C. Metachronously appearing metastatic lymph nodes should be treated with radiation therapy, since groin dissection in this setting improves salvage only minimally.

D. Combined irradiation and chemotherapy may be applied to clinically normal inguinal lymph nodes with benefit.

Ref.: 2, 3

COMMENTS: Prophylactic inguinal lymph node dissection in every case yields positive nodes in only 10–30%. • Therefore, the morbidity of this operation does not justify its performance on a routine basis. • Synchronous inguinal lymph node metastasis is an ominous sign. • In contrast, metachronous nodal disease carries a better prognosis (up to 75% of patients survive 5 years). • Synchronous metastatic inguinal nodes are treated with radiation and chemotherapy simultaneously with treatment of the primary tumor. • Metachronous-appearing metastatic nodes are treated with groin dissection, since, in most instances, the groins have already been radiated. • When a combination of chemotherapy and irradiation is used as the initial treatment for the anal disease, prophylactic irradiation of clinically negative inguinal nodes reduces the incidence of lymph node involvement to less than 5% from a rate of 15–25% without such treatment.

A N S W E R :
D

14. Which of the following may be appropriate initial therapy for a 3-cm cancer of the anal canal with invasion of the internal sphincter and no inguinal adenopathy?

A. Local excision

B. Abdominoperineal resection

C. Combined external beam alone

D. Combined chemotherapy and radiotherapy

Ref.: 1, 2, 10

COMMENTS: The optimal management of a small (<5 cm) squamous cell cancer of the anal canal without palpable groin lymph nodes is usually multimodal, involving radiation therapy and chemotherapy. • The effect of chemotherapy is believed to be radiopotentiating. • External radiation therapy alone can be used for small lesions, and doses up to 60–65 Gy have been used. • The addition of chemotherapy lowers the dose of radiation necessary to control the tumor. • In Norman Nigros' original protocol, a dose of 30 Gy was used. • Most centers use a dose of 45–50 Gy. • The cure rate without abdominoperineal resection approaches 80–85%. • Local excision of anal neoplasms is reserved for anal margin cancers that do not approach the dentate line or involve the sphincter. • Similarly, local excision of anal canal cancers is indicated only for well-differentiated lesions that have not invaded the sphincter. • Abdominoperineal resection is reserved for patients who have persistent cancer after chemoradiation or in whom the lesions recur.

ANSWER:
C, D

15. With regard to the results of initial combined radiation therapy with 5-fluorouracil (5-FU) and mitomycin C for squamous cell cancer of the anus, which of the following statements is/are true?

A. Complete regression of gross tumor has been observed in most patients.

B. Patients may be followed without abdominoperineal resection if posttreatment biopsies reveal no tumor.

C. Anal sphincter function may be preserved in at least one half of patients.

D. Randomized prospective trials demonstrate improved survival compared with abdominoperineal resection alone.

Ref.: 1, 2

COMMENTS: A combination of radiation therapy and chemotherapy with 5-FU and mitomycin C results in regression of gross tumor in all cases and microscopic disappearance of tumor cells in more than 80% of patients. • It is estimated that the anal sphincter can be saved in 85% of patients. • Abdominoperineal resection, therefore, is reserved for patients with gross or microscopic persistent tumor or for those with treatment failure, recurrent disease, or anal complications of treatment. • Based on the excellent results of multimodal therapy, randomization with abdominoperineal resection alone is not justified.

ANSWER:
A, B, C

16. With regard to anal infection with condyloma acuminatum, which of the following statements is/are true?

A. The causative agent appears to be human papillomavirus.

B. Podophyllin, administered in a 25% solution, causes resolution of warts in 80% of patients, and recurrence rates are less than 10%.

C. Immunotherapy with autologous condyloma is used as initial treatment for small condyloma.

D. Carcinoma frequently develops in untreated condyloma.

Ref.: 3

COMMENTS: Anal infection with papillomavirus is responsible for condyloma acuminatum, which appears as a group of cauliflower-like masses on the perianal skin and anal canal. • The disease is transmitted by close contact and is seen in both heterosexuals and homosexuals. • It is especially prevalent in anal-receptive homosexual men, and in this population it is seen more often than genital warts. • Another high-risk condition is immunosuppression after organ transplantation. • Podophyllin, a cytotoxic agent available in 10 and 25% solutions, must be applied by a physician. • Results have been disappointing. • Clearance of the warts has been noted in 22–77% of patients, with recurrence rates as high as 65%. • Podophyllin may cause skin burns and cannot be used within the anal canal. • Multiple treatments may be necessary. • Failure to treat intraanal lesions may cause higher recurrence rates.

Autologous vaccine prepared from the condyloma is injected weekly for 6 weeks. • No adverse reactions have been seen, and resolution of the lesions has been noted in up to 95% of cases. • At present, such therapy is considered for extensive, persistent, or recurrent cases of condyloma. • Although malignant transformation can occur, few cases have been reported to date.

ANSWER:
A

17. With regard to anal and perianal Crohn's disease, which of the following statements is/are true?

A. It is the first sign of the disease in 50% of patients.

B. Anal involvement is more common in patients with small-bowel rather than colonic disease.

C. Multiple fistulas are the most common anal manifestation.

D. One third of low fistulas may demonstrate spontaneous healing.

E. Healing after fistulectomy is correlated with the absence of rectal disease and Crohn's activity elsewhere in the gastrointestinal tract.

Ref.: 3

COMMENTS: Anal or perianal disease is the first sign of Crohn's disease in approximately 10% of patients. • Ultimately, up to 30% of Crohn's disease patients manifest anal disease. • The anus is more likely to be involved with distal gastrointestinal involvement. • Approximately 50% of patients with Crohn's colitis have anal involvement, compared to 25% of patients with Crohn's disease of the small intestine.

The most common anal manifestation is edematous, thickened skin tags 1–2 cm in size. • They can cause pain and difficulty in achieving satisfactory local hygiene. • Fistula in ano is the second most common anal manifestation. • Most fistulas are low and simple. • Approximately one third demonstrate spontaneous healing. • If a fistula is symptomatic and persistent, fistulotomy can be performed, but healing may not occur. • Preoperatively, every attempt should be made to control proximal disease within the gastrointestinal tract. • Failure to do so results in a higher incidence of nonhealing perineal involvement. • The absence of rectal disease is well correlated with successful healing after fistulotomy. • Surgery for perianal Crohn's disease should be directed at relieving symptoms and should include such measures as draining of abscesses, gentle dilatation of strictures, and promoting drainage of fistula tracts with curettage or placement of noncutting seton sutures.

ANSWER:
D, E

18. With regard to rectovaginal fistulas, which of the following is/are true?

    A. Repaired obstetric tears of the rectum and vagina dehisce in 10% of cases, and 30–60% of fistulas due to obstetric trauma heal spontaneously.

    B. Low rectovaginal fistulas may be treated with fistulectomy.

    C. High rectovaginal fistulas are best treated through a transabdominal approach.

    D. Rectovaginal fistulas associated with Crohn's disease usually necessitate proctectomy.

    E. Radiation-induced fistulas generally necessitate a colostomy.

Ref.: 3

COMMENTS: Rectovaginal fistulas are classified according to location and cause, which influence the type of corrective surgery required. • *High* fistulas require an abdominal approach, whereas *low* or *mid*-fistulas can be repaired through a transvaginal, transperineal, or transrectal approach. • The causes of these fistulas include obstetric injuries, irradiation for pelvic cancers, recurrent cancer, inflammatory bowel disease, violent trauma, or infection (e.g., tuberculosis or lymphogranuloma venereum).

Episiotomy with a third- or fourth-degree rectal tear occurs in about 5% of deliveries. • Approximately 10% of the repairs disrupt, leading to impaired fecal control and, potentially, a rectovaginal fistula. • Approximately 30–60% of fistulas heal spontaneously. • Therefore, if the patient's symptoms are not disabling, a 3- to 6-month wait is recommended. • This waiting period also allows tissue inflammation and edema to subside before any surgical intervention. • Repair of a fistula secondary to an obstetric injury can be accomplished with a local procedure that usually involves excision of the fistula tract with a layered closure. • A diverting colostomy is not required unless multiple previous surgical attempts have failed. • An *anovaginal* fistula may be treated with fistulotomy, but rectovaginal fistulas, even distal ones, should not be treated by this method. • Partial or total incontinence may result if the fistula tract is divided.

High rectovaginal fistulas are best treated through a transabdominal approach so that coexisting pathologic conditions, such as diverticulitis, cancer, or inflammatory bowel disease, can be addressed. • If local tissues are normal, the rectovaginal septum is mobilized, the fistula is divided, the rectum and vagina are closed separately, and normal tissue, such as omentum, is interposed. • If tissue is not normal as a result of inflammation or irradiation, bowel resection is usually necessary.

Fistulas secondary to *Crohn's disease* do not necessitate a proctectomy if symptoms are minimal, the rectum is relatively healthy, and continence is normal. • In such cases, an advancement flap can result in healing. • Refractory rectal Crohn's disease (especially the structuring form) or incontinence usually necessitates proctectomy. • Radiation-induced fistulas usually necessitate a colostomy as sole therapy in a poor-risk patient, in a patient with recurrent cancer, or to divert stool from an anastomosis after resection of diseased bowel.

ANSWER:
A, C, E

19. For patients with rectal cancer, radiation therapy is recommended in which of the following settings?

    A. Preoperatively in patients whose primary tumors have extended transmurally and become fixed to adjacent structures

    B. Postoperatively with chemotherapy for patients with T3–4 cancers and lymph node metastases

    C. Postoperatively after low anterior resection for T2N0 adenocarcinoma of the rectum with negative margins

    D. All of the above

    E. None of the above

Ref.: 4, 5, 6, 7, 8

COMMENTS: Preoperative radiation therapy may down-stage and shrink a tumor and is invaluable in rendering a fixed tumor resectable. • Pretreatment staging by endorectal ultrasound imaging will identify T3 or T4 cancers or those with suspiciously enlarged lymph nodes. • These lesions should be treated before surgery with radiation and chemotherapy. • Studies from Sweden and published meta-analyses have shown lower recurrence rates and down-staging of cancers. • The response rate is variable, and complete response rates of approximately 20–25% have been reported. • In addition, preoperative radiation with chemotherapy may increase sphincter preservation. • A dose of 45–50 Gy is delivered to the pelvis. • The reported local failure rate is low, ranging from 1–17%, and sphincter function is good to excellent in most patients. • Since at least 80–90% of patients with stage I rectal carcinoma survive 5 years with surgery alone, neoadjuvant treatment is not recommended. • Postoperative chemotherapy and radiation became the standard of care in 1991 for patients with either transmural disease or lymph node metastases, but the trend now is to administer such treatment before surgery. • If therapy was not given before surgery, it is indicated for the conditions described above. • Improved survival and lower recurrence rates were noted in the North Central Cancer Treatment Group and the Gastrointestinal Tumor Study Group.

ANSWER:
A, B

20. The theoretic advantages of preoperative radiation therapy of rectal cancers include which of the following?

    A. Radiation treatment to the tumor bed, the regional lymphatics, or both may be initiated without delay.

    B. Tumor cells are more sensitive to the effects of radiation administered preoperatively than to those of radiation administered postoperatively.

    C. It results in improved wound healing over that seen with postoperative irradiation.

    D. It results in improved ease of tumor resectability.

Ref.: 9

COMMENTS: The rationale for preoperative radiation therapy includes elimination of microscopic disease beyond the margins of surgical resection and improving the ease of tumor resectability. • Another advantage is the elimination of viable cells that could exfoliate at the time of surgery. • Moreover, treatment may begin immediately without delay for postoperative recovery, during which time remaining tumor cells may be multiplying. • Tumor cells are likely more sensitive to the effects of neoadjuvant therapy, presumably because they are better vascularized and oxygenated than in the postoperative setting. • A potential disadvantage is that surgical staging information is not available before initiation of treatment, but this issue may be less significant with accurate ultrasound imaging. • Some studies have demonstrated an increased incidence of wound healing complications with preoperative irradiation. • However, with proper technique and doses of 45–50 Gy, the effect should be minimal.

ANSWER:
A, B, D

21. The theoretic advantages of postoperative radiation therapy include which of the following?

  A. Higher doses of radiation are given postoperatively than those given preoperatively.

  B. Gastrointestinal function, the number of daily bowel movements, and continence are better.

  C. The altered vascularity of the postoperative tumor bed leads to greater radiosensitivity of any remaining cancer cells.

  D. The stage of disease is precisely known, and one can avoid treating patients with stage I or IV disease.

Ref.: 9

COMMENTS: Postoperative irradiation is used to eliminate any residual locoregional disease. • Patients with stage I disease and those with distant metastases discovered at the time of surgery can be spared treatment. • Radiation doses are similar in the United States whether radiation is given before or after surgery. • However, the altered vascularity of the surgical bed may render tumor cells more hypoxic and, as a result, more resistant to radiation. • Bowel function is generally better after preoperative radiation, since the radiated tissue is largely removed and the anastomosis and proximal bowel are not exposed.

ANSWER:
D

22. Regarding the medical treatment of anal fissures, which of the following is/are true?

  A. Glyceryl trinitrate (GTN) ointment relaxes the internal sphincter by acting as a nitric oxide donor.

  B. GTN heals fissures in approximately 65% of patients at doses of 2% applied four times a day.

  C. The main side effect of GTN is orthostatic hypotension.

  D. Topical calcium-channel blockers reduce resting anal pressure and heal fissures.

  E. Botulinum toxin is an accepted form of therapy and should be injected directly into the internal sphincter.

Ref.: 10

COMMENTS: Internal sphincterotomy for anal fissures, while highly effective, may cause problems with fecal soilage or control of flatus. • As a result, nonoperative forms of treatment have been pursued as initial management. • GTN acts as a nitric oxide donor, which induces relaxation of the internal sphincter. • It is applied topically to the anoderm at doses of 0.2% two to three times a day. • Its main side effect is headache. • Topical calcium-channel blockers, such as nifedipine or diltiazem, are capable of causing significant reductions in anal canal resting pressures and are capable of healing fissures in up to 90% of patients. • Botulinum toxin (Botox) is a powerful inhibitor of neuromuscular transmission. • When injected directly into the internal anal sphincter on either side of the fissure, healing has been noted, although success rates are variable.

ANSWER:
A, D, E

23. Regarding the use of infliximab (Remicade) for Crohn's disease, which of the following is/are true?

  A. It is a monoclonal antibody to tumor necrosis factor-α (TNF-α), which has been implicated in the pathogenesis of Crohn's disease.

  B. Approximately 90% of patients will achieve complete remission of disease.

  C. Adverse side effects include serum sickness, sepsis, autoimmune phenomena, and opportunistic infections.

  D. Endoscopic appearance of the bowel is not correlated with response to infliximab.

  E. Before beginning therapy, it is advised that patients be skin-tested for tuberculosis and have a chest x-ray.

Ref.: 10

COMMENTS: TNF-α has been implicated in the pathogenesis of Crohn's disease. • An antibody to TNF-α, infliximab has been studied extensively and has shown great promise in active disease. • Overall, approximately two thirds of patients respond, and one third enter remission. • The majority of patients maintain their response for several weeks. • Infliximab is better suited to fistulizing Crohn's disease (30–60%, including rectovaginal fistulas, heal) than for stricturing Crohn's disease, where symptoms can actually worsen. • Infliximab can cause all of the side effects mentioned and activate tuberculosis. • Consequently, it is advised that patients be skin-tested and have a chest x-ray before beginning treatment.

ANSWER:
A, C, E

REFERENCES

1. Brunicardi FC, Andersen DK, Billiar TR, et al (eds): *Schwartz's Principles of Surgery*, 8th ed. McGraw-Hill, New York, 2004.
2. Townsend CM, Beauchamp RD, Evers BM, et al (eds): *Sabiston Textbook of Surgery: The Biological Basis of Modern Surgical Practice*, 17th ed. Saunders, Philadelphia, 2004.
3. Gordon PH, Nivatvongs S: *Principles and Practice of Surgery for the Colon, Rectum and Anus*. Quality Medical Publishing, St. Louis, 1999.
4. Minsky BD: Preoperative radiation therapy followed by low anterior resection with coloanal anastomosis. *Semin Radiat Oncol* 8:30–35, 1998.
5. Martensen JA, Gunderson LL: Colon and rectum. In: Perez CA, Brady LW (eds) *Principles and Practice of Radiation Oncology*, 3rd ed. Lippincott-Raven, Philadelphia, 1998.
6. Gastrointestinal Tumor Study Group: Prolongation of the disease-free interval in surgically treated rectal carcinoma. *N Engl J Med* 312:1465–1472, 1985.
7. Krook JE, Moertel CG, Gunderson LL, et al: Effective surgical adjuvant therapy for high-risk rectal carcinoma. *N Engl J Med* 324:709–715, 1991.
8. NIH Consensus Conference: Adjuvant therapy for patients with colon and rectal cancer. *JAMA* 264:1444–1450, 1990.
9. Perez CA, Brady LW, Roti Roti JL: Overview. In: Perez CA, Brady LW (eds) *Principles and Practice of Radiation Oncology*, 3rd ed. Lippincott-Raven, Philadelphia, 1998.
10. Corman ML: *Colon and Rectal Surgery*. Lippincott, Philadelphia, 2005.

CHAPTER 37

Liver

Jonathan Myers, M.D.

1. Which of the following statements about the anatomy of the liver is/are true?

   A. The right lobe extends to the umbilical fissure and falciform ligament.

   B. The left lobe extends to the right of the falciform ligament.

   C. The quadrate lobe is a portion of the medial segment of the left lobe.

   D. The left lobe contains the anterior and lateral segment.

   Ref.: 1–3

COMMENTS: See Question 2.

2. The lateral segment of the left lobe of the liver in the American system consists of which anatomic segment(s) in the French system?

   A. Segments II and III

   B. Segment IV

   C. Segments V and VI

   D. Segments V and VIII

   E. Segments VI and VII

   Ref.: 1–3

COMMENTS: The surgical anatomy of the liver is based on the distribution of the hepatic veins and portal structures and has been modified several times. • It is divided into right and left lobes by a vertically angled plane that extends from the gallbladder to the left of the inferior vena cava. • This plane, called the portal fissure, or Cantlie's line, contains the middle hepatic vein. • In the American system, the liver is further broken down into four segments. • In the French system, developed by C. Couinaud, it is further broken down into eight segments. • According to the American system, the right lobe of the liver consists of a posterior and anterior segment. • The left lobe consists of a medial segment (quadrate lobe) and a lateral segment divided by the falciform ligament (continuous with the umbilical fissure). • The caudate lobe can be considered anatomically independent from the right and left lobes because it receives portal and arterial blood supply from both sides and has venous drainage directly into the inferior vena cava.

   According to the French system, the liver is divided into four sectors by the planes (scissurae) of the right, middle, and left hepatic veins and is further divided into segments by the branching of the portal structures. • The caudate lobe is called segment I. • The lateral sector of the left lobe consists of a superior segment (II) and an inferior segment (III). • The medial sector of the left lobe is segment IV. • The left hepatic vein divides segments II and III from segment IV. • The right lobe consists of anteromedial and posterolateral sectors divided by a vertical plane containing the right hepatic vein. • The anteromedial sector is made up of segment V (inferior) and segment VIII (superior), and the posterolateral sector is made up of segment VI (inferior) and segment VII (superior).

ANSWERS:
Question 1: B, C
Question 2: A.

3. Which of the following statements is/are true about the hepatic arterial supply?

   A. Aberrant hepatic arterial anatomy is present in almost half of all patients.

   B. The cystic artery usually is a branch off the proper hepatic artery.

   C. A "replaced" right hepatic artery arises from the superior mesenteric artery.

   D. The hepatic artery provides 75% of blood flow to the liver.

   Ref.: 1–3

COMMENTS: The hepatic arterial supply normally is derived from the celiac axis by way of the common hepatic artery, which becomes the proper hepatic artery after giving off the gastroduodenal branch and subsequently bifurcates into right and left hepatic branches. • The cystic artery generally is a branch of the right hepatic artery. • There is, however, significant variability in hepatic arterial anatomy in up to 50% of patients. • In approximately 15% of individuals, the right hepatic artery arises from the superior mesenteric artery (replaced right hepatic artery) and is found in the right posterior border of the hepatoduodenal ligament. • In roughly 10% of individuals, the left hepatic artery originates from the left gastric artery and is located in the gastrohepatic ligament. • These commonly encountered variants can have important surgical implications during upper abdominal operations. • The arterial blood supply accounts for only 25% of hepatic blood flow, with the remainder supplied by the portal vein.

ANSWER:
A, C

4. Which of the following statement(s) about the anatomy of the hepatic veins is/are true?

A. The left hepatic vein drains the entire left lobe.

B. Veins from the caudate lobe enter the inferior vena cava directly.

C. The middle hepatic vein usually drains into the right hepatic vein.

D. There are no valves in the hepatic venous system.

Ref.: 1–3

COMMENTS: The hepatic veins begin in the liver lobules as the central veins and coalesce to form the right, left, and middle hepatic veins, which drain into the inferior vena cava and are of considerable surgical importance because they define the three vertical scissura of the liver. • The **right vein**, which is generally the largest, drains most of the right lobe. • The **left vein** drains the lateral segment of the left lobe and a portion of the medial segment as well. • The **middle vein** drains the inferoanterior portion of the right lobe and the inferomedial segment of the left lobe. • This vein joins the left hepatic vein in 80% of individuals and enters the inferior vena cava directly in the remainder. • There are also smaller veins, particularly those draining the caudate lobe posteriorly, which enter directly into the inferior vena cava. • There are no valves in the human hepatic venous system.

ANSWER:
B, D

5. Which of the following statements is/are true about the anatomy of the portal vein?

A. It is formed by the junction of the inferior mesenteric vein and splenic vein.

B. It is the most posterior structure in the hepatoduodenal ligament.

C. It contains the valves of Mirizzi.

D. The right portal vein typically branches sooner than does the left portal vein.

Ref.: 1–3

COMMENTS: The portal vein is usually formed dorsal to the neck of the pancreas by the junction of the superior mesenteric vein and splenic veins. • It ascends dorsal to the common bile duct and hepatic artery in the hepatoduodenal ligament. • These three structures make up the portal triad. • There are no valves in the portal venous system. • (Pablo Mirizzi described valves in the common hepatic duct that do not exist.) • The portal vein bifurcates just outside the liver. • The right portal vein has anterior and posterior branches that typically come off only a short distance from the bifurcation and then quickly dive into the liver parenchyma. • The left portal vein has a longer transverse portion (pars transversus) and then angulates anteriorly in the umbilical fissure (pars umbilicus), where it gives off medial branches to segment IV and lateral branches to segments II and III.

ANSWER:
B, D

6. Which of the following hepatic resection(s) involve(s) dissection in the plane of the falciform ligament or umbilical fissure?

A. Right lobectomy

B. Right trisegmentectomy

C. Left lobectomy

D. Left lateral segmentectomy

E. None of the above

Ref.: 1–3

COMMENTS: Hepatic resections can be broken down into (1) anatomic resections, (2) nonanatomic resections (wedge resections), and (3) enucleation procedures. • Anatomic resections are based on either the American or French segmental system. • Right lobectomy includes segments V, VI, VII, and VIII. • Right trisegmentectomy also includes segment IV. • Left lobectomy includes segments II, III, and IV. • Left lateral segmentectomy includes only segments II and III. • The umbilical fissure is the segmental plane between the medial and lateral segments of the left lobe of the liver. • A portion of the left branch of the portal vein, known as the pars umbilicus, runs in the inferior portion of the umbilical fissure. • Dissection is therefore never carried out directly in the segmental fissure. • During left lateral segmentectomy, the plane of the parenchymal dissection is to the left of the fissure, whereas with right trisegmentectomy, the parenchyma is divided to the right of the fissure. • Both right and left lobectomies involve dissection well to the right of this plane.

ANSWER:
E

7. Which of the following characteristics is/are typically seen on ultrasound imaging of the hepatic portal vein branches?

A. Hyperechoic vessel walls

B. Hepatofugal blood flow

C. Diastolic reversal of blood flow

D. Location between hepatic segments

Ref.: 4

COMMENTS: The portal veins and hepatic veins can be readily differentiated from each other based on their distinctive sonographic features. • The portal vein and its branches have prominent hyperechoic-appearing walls. • This appearance has been attributed to the accompanying intrahepatic branches of the hepatic artery and bile duct, which generally are not individually seen by external ultrasound imaging. • In contrast, the hepatic veins appear to be essentially "wall-less." • They are anechoic or hypoechoic tubular structures that are vertically oriented and increase in caliber as they course toward the inferior vena cava. • The portal veins are more transversely oriented and of larger caliber centrally. • The portal vein branches are located within the anatomic liver segments, and the hepatic veins are found between the segments. • Doppler ultrasound study permits characterization of flow patterns in the hepatic vessels. • Under normal circumstances, portal vein flow is toward the liver (hepatopedal). • Flow in the portal vein is usually of fairly low velocity, with minor undulations and continued forward flow during diastole. • Flow in the hepatic veins is hepatofugal and varies according to the cardiorespiratory cycle.

ANSWER:
A

8. Ultrasound imaging demonstrates a hyperechoic liver with a geographic hypoechoic area adjacent to the gallbladder. What does this picture likely represent?

 A. Duplication of the gallbladder

 B. Reverberation artifact

 C. Focal fatty sparing

 D. Hepatic abscess

 E. Bowel gas

Ref.: 4

COMMENTS: Fatty infiltration of the liver is a common finding that produces a hyperechoic parenchymal pattern on ultrasound scans. • It is not unusual to have focal areas of fatty sparing within an otherwise steatotic liver. • These areas typically appear as zonal hypoechoic regions and are usually found adjacent to the gallbladder or anterior to the porta hepatis. • Duplication of the gallbladder is a rare occurrence. • Reverberation artifacts are echoes within cystic structures. • The sonographic appearance of hepatic abscesses is variable, depending on the cause and duration. • Pyogenic abscesses are usually complex, with cystic characteristics and internal echoes due to debris or septations. • Bowel gas is highly reflective and impedes ultrasound imaging.

ANSWER:
C

9. The hepatocytes most susceptible to hypoxic injury are located in which of the following areas?

 A. Acinar zone I

 B. Acinar zone II

 C. Acinar zone III

 D. Central lobular region

Ref.: 1, 3

COMMENTS: The functional histologic unit of the liver is the acinus. • At the center of the acinus is a portal triad, which consists of a terminal branch of the portal vein (portal venule) along with an hepatic arteriole and bile ductule. • Blood from the terminal portal venule goes into hepatic sinusoids, around which the hepatocytes are located. • Eventually, the blood returns to the central vein leading to the terminal hepatic venules at the periphery of the acinar unit. • The central vein is at the center of the histologic hepatic lobule. • Each hepatic lobule is thus surrounded by several peripheral acini. • The hepatocytes of the acinus are divided into three zones, with zone I being closest to the afferent portal venule and zone III being nearest the efferent central vein and hepatic venule. • Zone II is between these two points. • Within the acinus, there is a gradient of solute concentration and oxygen tension that is greatest near the portal venules at the center of the acinus. • The hepatocytes in zone I are therefore exposed to more oxygen and are less subject to hypoxia than are the hepatocytes near the periphery of the acinus (zone III). • This explains the histologic pattern of centrilobular necrosis that occurs following ischemia.

ANSWER:
C, D

10. Alkaline phosphatase is primarily located in which portion of the hepatocyte plasma membrane?

 A. Sinusoidal membrane

 B. Basolateral membrane

 C. Canalicular membrane

 D. None of the above

Ref.: 1, 3

COMMENTS: The plasma membrane of the hepatocyte has different regions, or domains, with ultrastructures designed for various functions. • The sinusoidal membrane is the domain that borders the perisinusoidal space of Disse. • It is covered with microvilli that project into the perisinusoidal space. • These microvilli increase the absorptive area in contact with sinusoidal blood, allowing proteins, solutes, and other substances to be transported across this border of the hepatocyte. • The flat basolateral membrane connects the adjacent hepatocytes and is important for attachment and cellular interactions. • The canalicular membrane is a specialized section of the hepatocyte membrane that is involved in bile formation and in the transport of various substances into bile. • The canalicular regions are separated from the pericellular space by tight junctions. • The canalicular membrane contains enzymes such as alkaline phosphatase and 5°-nucleotidase. • Thus, high levels of alkaline phosphatase are noted with extrahepatic bile duct obstruction.

ANSWER:
C

11. During fasting, the liver provides energy substrates by all but which of the following mechanisms?

 A. Glycogenolysis

 B. Glycolysis

 C. Gluconeogenesis from alanine

 D. Gluconeogenesis from lactate

 E. Formation of ketone bodies from fatty acids

Ref.: 1, 3, **5**

COMMENTS: The liver plays a pivotal role in energy metabolism. • In the fed state, glucose is converted to glycogen for storage. • The liver itself obtains its energy primarily from ketoacids rather than glucose, although it can use glycolysis during periods of glucose excess (fed state). • During fasting, the liver provides glucose by breakdown of the stored glycogen (glycogenolysis). • Glucose is a critical energy source for red blood cells, the central nervous system, and the kidney. • Because glycogen stores are depleted after about 48 hr, the liver generates glucose from other sources. • Alanine, other amino acids, lactate, and glycerol can serve as carbon sources for gluconeogenesis. • Lipolysis occurs during prolonged fasting, and the fatty acids released from adipose stores are oxidized in the hepatocytes to form ketone bodies. • Ketone bodies are an important alternative fuel source for brain and muscle.

ANSWER:
B

12. The reticuloendothelial function of the liver is primarily dependent on which of the following cells?

A. Hepatocytes

B. Kupffer cells

C. Histiocytes

D. Ito cells

Ref.: 1, 3, 5

COMMENTS: The reticuloendothelial system (RES) functions to clear the circulation of particulate matter and microbes. • The RES consists of fixed phagocytic cells, located primarily in the liver, spleen, and lung. • Kupffer cells are responsible for the reticuloendothelial function of the liver. • Located along the lining of the hepatic sinusoids (along with the sinusoidal endothelial cells), they are uniquely positioned to phagocytize and process gut antigens from the splanchnic and systemic circulation. • Kupffer cells have an important role in the production and control of various cytokines and inflammatory regulators. • Histiocytes are macrophages in connective tissue. • Ito cells are perisinusoidal cells involved in collagen and vitamin A metabolism.

ANSWER:
B

13. Which of the following proteins is/are not primarily synthesized in the liver?

A. Albumin

B. Fibrinogen

C. von Willebrand factor

D. Transferrin

E. Factor VII

Ref.: 1, 3, 5

COMMENTS: The liver is the primary or sole source of numerous plasma proteins, including albumin, α-globulins and an array of other transport proteins, such as transferrin, hepatoglobulin, ferritin, and ceruloplasmin. • Eleven proteins involved in hemostasis are synthesized in the liver, including fibrinogen (factor I); the vitamin K–dependent factors (II, VII, IX, and X); and all of the procoagulation factors except for von Willebrand factor, which is synthesized by vascular endothelial cells. • Because factor VII has the shortest half-life, of 5–7 hr, measurements of factor VII levels are useful for determining liver failure.

ANSWER:
C

14. The cytochrome P-450 system transforms compounds by which of the following mechanisms?

A. Oxidation

B. Hydrolysis

C. Conjugation

D. Reduction

Ref.: 1, 3, 5

COMMENTS: The liver is responsible for biotransformation of many endogenous and exogenous substances. • For the most part, this process detoxifies potentially injurious substances and facilitates their elimination. • In some instances, however, hepatic biotransformation produces more toxic metabolites. • There are two general mechanisms by which the liver accomplishes biotransformation. • The cytochrome P-450 enzyme system catalyzes phase I reactions, which are primarily oxidation, reduction, and hydrolysis. • The second mechanism involves an array of enzymes that conjugate substances with other endogenous molecules. • These reactions are referred to as phase II reactions, and their purpose is to convert hydrophobic compounds to hydrophilic ones that are water soluble and can thus be eliminated in bile or urine. • The liver is also the principal site of conversion of ammonia to urea via the urea cycle, which is a separate process.

ANSWER:
A, B, D

15. The liver is integral to which of the following steps in vitamin D metabolism?

A. Intestinal absorption

B. 1-Hydroxylation

C. 25-Hydroxylation

D. All of the above

Ref.: 1, 3

COMMENTS: The absorption, metabolism, and storage of vitamins is dependent on hepatic events. • Intestinal absorption of the fat-soluble vitamins—A, D, E, and K—requires bile salts synthesized in the liver. • Vitamin D undergoes 25-hydroxylation in the liver and subsequent 1-hydroxylation in the kidney to arrive at the metabolically active form. • The liver is an important storage site for fat-soluble vitamins and is the only site of storage of vitamin A. • Excessive vitamin A is hepatotoxic. • The liver also produces a number of transport proteins required for vitamin metabolism.

ANSWER:
A, C

16. During typical obstructive jaundice, marked elevations might be expected in which of the following?

A. Alkaline phosphatase

B. Alanine aminotransferase (ALT)

C. γ-Glutamyltransferase (GGT)

D. Transferrin

E. Leucine aminopeptidase

Ref.: 1

COMMENTS: AST (serum glutamic oxaloacetic transaminase, or SGOT), ALT (serum glutamate pyruvate transaminase, or SGPT), and lactate dehydrogenase (LDH) are indicators of the integrity of the cell membrane, and elevated levels reflect hepatocyte injury with leakage. • Levels of these enzymes usually are only mildly or moderately elevated in pure obstructive jaundice. • Other enzymes, including alkaline phosphatase, 5′-nucleotidase, leucine aminopeptidase, and GGT, reflect the excretory capacity of the liver. • Levels of these enzymes are typically elevated in the presence of extrahepatic bile duct obstruction or intrahepatic cholestasis. • Elevations are also seen in hepatic parenchymal disease or liver tumors. • Transferrin and albumin levels decrease with liver disease, since they reflect changes in liver function and nutritional status.

ANSWER:
A, C, E

17. Which of the following statements is/are true regarding the management of patients undergoing major hepatic resection?

    A. Removal of more than 80% of the liver is not compatible with life.

    B. Postoperative hyperglycemia resulting from intraoperative release of glycogen stores is a common finding.

    C. Postoperative coagulopathy reflects vitamin K deficiency and is best treated by parenteral vitamin K.

    D. Transient postoperative elevations of serum ammonia levels are expected and are treated by lactulose and administration of branched-chain amino acids.

    E. Intra-abdominal abscess formation and sepsis are common complications of major liver resection.

    Ref.: 1–3

COMMENTS: Operations that involve removal of one or more anatomic segments of the liver are considered major resections. • The operative mortality rate for elective major hepatic resection is now 1% or less, reflecting refinements in surgical technique and advances in preoperative preparation and postoperative support. • Preoperative preparation involves correction of reversible defects, such as anemia, malnutrition, and vitamin K deficiency, as well as adequate fluid resuscitation. • Unfortunately, there is no single test of liver function that accurately predicts the adequacy of the remaining liver. • Removal of up to 80% of the liver is compatible with life. • Postoperative metabolic complications include liver and renal failure, hypoglycemia (treated by infusion of 10% dextrose), hypoproteinemia (treated with exogenous albumin), and coagulopathy (treated by administration of fresh whole blood or platelets and fresh-frozen plasma). • Patients with preexisting liver disease, suggested by increased bilirubin levels and depressed synthetic parameters, are at greater risk for liver failure after major resection. • Transient elevations of alkaline phosphatase, bilirubin, or transaminase levels are not uncommon, but, even with extensive hepatic resection, blood ammonia levels usually remain normal. • Complications such as abscess formation and sepsis are the most frequent problems after major resection and occur in 20–30% of cases.

ANSWER:
A, E

18. Which of the following techniques is/are appropriate to limit blood loss during major hepatic resection?

    A. Portal triad clamping

    B. Normothermic total hepatic vascular isolation

    C. Total hepatic vascular isolation with venovenous bypass

    D. Low central venous pressure anesthesia

    Ref.: 6

COMMENTS: Hemorrhage is one of the major hazards during liver resection. • Troublesome bleeding is most likely to occur during division of the hepatic parenchyma, and life-threatening hemorrhage is most commonly from the hepatic veins and their branches. • A variety of intraoperative techniques have been employed in efforts to avoid this problem. • A disadvantage of any vascular occlusion, however, is the potential for ischemic injury to the liver, particularly in patients with underlying hepatocellular disease. • Occlusion of the portal triad (Pringle maneuver) can be useful for limiting bleeding from the hepatic artery and portal vein branches. • It has generally been suggested that periods of occlusion not exceed 20 minutes and perhaps should be shorter. • Total hepatic vascular isolation requires occlusion of the inferior vena cava above and below the liver in addition to the Pringle maneuver. • Such management can be complex and is not well tolerated by some patients. • Venovenous bypass, which has commonly been used during hepatic transplantation, has also been applied to major hepatic resections at some centers. • Attempts to protect the liver during vascular occlusion using local hepatic hypothermia or systemic steroids have not been uniformly practiced or successful. • Low central venous pressure anesthesia minimizes hepatic venous bleeding by fluid restriction, head-down positioning, and the vasodilatory effects of standard anesthetics. • This technique has been successful in nearly 500 patients at Memorial Sloan-Kettering Cancer Center in New York. • Low central venous pressure anesthesia during major hepatic resection has obviated the need for perioperative blood transfusion in two thirds of patients and has a reported mortality rate of 4% and only a 3% rate of clinically important postoperative increases in serum creatinine levels.

ANSWER:
A, B, C, D

19. Resection of hepatic metastases has most clearly benefited patients with which of the following cancers?

    A. Colon

    B. Breast

    C. Stomach

    D. Pancreas

    E. Lung

    Ref.: 1 3

COMMENTS: Resection of hepatic metastases from colorectal cancer provides a clear survival advantage compared to any other treatment and should be performed whenever possible. • The 5-year survival rate is approximately 25% and is as high as 40% in favorable subgroups. • Resection of metastatic neuroendocrine tumors (e.g., carcinoid, insulinoma, and gastrinoma) can be valuable for controlling symptoms of excessive endocrine secretion. • Experience with hepatic resection for metastases from other portal sites (e.g., stomach, pancreas, and biliary) or nonportal sites (e.g., lung, breast, melanoma, gynecologic, head and neck, and renal) has been more limited, and results have not generally been as encouraging. • Occasionally, a patient with a noncolorectal primary malignancy is cured when he or she undergoes resection of the isolated hepatic metastasis. • However, the natural history of noncolorectal primary malignancies is such that patients rarely develop metastases isolated to the liver. • Hepatic resection for direct, contiguous growth of the primary tumor (e.g., stomach and biliary) into the liver sometimes produces long-term survivors.

ANSWER:
A

20. A 50-year-old woman is found to have a 4-cm hepatic cyst with no internal echoes on ultrasound imaging. Which of the following would be the most appropriate management?

    A. Observation if the cyst is asymptomatic

    B. Tamoxifen to prevent enlargement

    C. Resection because of the risk of hemorrhage

    D. Percutaneous aspiration for cytologic study

    Ref.: 1, 3, 5

COMMENTS: Simple, nonparasitic hepatic cysts are presumed to be congenital. • They may be single or multiple, are more common in women, and are usually asymptomatic. • The absence of internal echoes is diagnostic of a simple rather than a complex cyst, a cystic neoplasm, or a solid lesion. • No further intervention is indicated for asymptomatic liver cysts when the diagnosis is secure, which can be ascertained by ultrasound imaging, computed tomographic (CT) scanning, or magnetic resonance imaging (MRI). • Complications such as hemorrhage or infection are rare, and these lesions are not premalignant. • Exogenous hormones are not recognized to be harmful, nor is antihormonal therapy indicated. • Occasionally, large cysts are symptomatic, primarily due to local pressure, which may cause biliary obstruction. • Treatment of symptomatic cysts is by operative resection or unroofing. • This may be performed using an open or a laparoscopic technique. • Percutaneous drainage or injection of alcohol or other sclerosing agents does not suffice and is not recommended. • If the cyst is found to communicate with the bile ducts, either excision or Roux-en-Y cystojejunostomy may be performed.

ANSWER:
A

21. Polycystic liver disease in adults is associated with which of the following?

    A. Polycystic kidney disease

    B. Intracranial aneurysms

    C. Hepatic fibrosis and portal hypertension

    D. Increased risk of malignancy

    Ref.: 1, 3, 5

COMMENTS: Adult polycystic disease is an autosomal dominant disorder. • About half of patients with liver cysts also have cystic involvement of the kidneys or rarely other organs, such as the pancreas, spleen, or adrenal glands. • Intracranial arterial aneurysms occur in up to 30% of patients. • The number of cysts varies, and most are asymptomatic, requiring no treatment. • Complications of the liver cysts are infrequent and include rupture, hemorrhage, and infection. • When the cysts are symptomatic, pain is the predominant problem. • Operations to unroof or excise superficial cysts and fenestrate deeper cysts may provide the best symptomatic relief, although the benefit may be temporary. • These procedures can be accomplished laparoscopically. • Cyst aspiration or sclerosis is ineffective because of recurrence. • Infantile polycystic kidney disease often results in death from renal failure, and congenital hepatic fibrosis may be present. • Hepatic fibrosis also occurs in association with multiple dilatations of the intrahepatic biliary tree (Caroli's disease). • Polycystic liver disease is not a premalignant condition, but Caroli's disease is associated with malignancy.

ANSWER:
A, B

22. Select the type of hepatic abscess in the right-hand column that is best described by each statement on the left.

    A. Patients have fever, chills, abdominal pain, and weight loss.

    B. Diagnosis requires serologic testing for confirmation.

    C. Transmission may be hematologic or via the biliary tree.

    D. Primary treatment is pharmacologic.

    E. Preferred treatment is drainage and antibiotics.

    a. Amebic liver abscess

    b. Pyogenic liver abscess

    c. Both

    d. Neither

    Ref.: 1–3

COMMENTS: The clinical signs and symptoms of pyogenic (bacterial) and amebic liver abscesses may be similar, consisting predominantly of fever and pain, but it is important to differentiate between the two for therapeutic purposes. • *Escherichia coli* or other gram-negative bacteria are the organisms most commonly isolated from pyogenic abscesses. • *Streptococcus* spp. and anaerobes such as *Bacteroides* are also common. • Today, the most frequent source of pyogenic abscess is contiguous infection in the biliary tract, such as with cholangitis. • Other sources include infectious foci within the portal venous drainage system, direct extension from perihepatic sites, and hematogenous spread. • The right lobe is most commonly involved, which has been attributed to a streaming effect on the portal vein. • Approximately 20% of pyogenic abscesses are cryptogenic. • Diagnosis is based on the clinical presentation and hepatic imaging and may be confirmed by fine-needle aspiration. • Treatment of pyogenic abscess requires eradication of both the abscess and the source. • Treatment of the abscess usually requires drainage by operative or percutaneous approaches. • Antibiotic therapy alone may suffice for treatment of multiple small abscesses.

Amebic abscesses are caused by the protozoan *Entamoeba histolytica*, which is spread by the fecal-oral route. • Diagnosis requires hepatic imaging (usually ultrasound imaging or CT scanning) and serologic testing for the presence of *E. histolytica* antibodies. • The organisms reach the liver from the intestine via the portal vein and produce a liquefaction necrosis responsible for the classic "anchovy paste" appearance. • Protozoa are not usually isolated from the abscess, since they are located in the peripheral rim of tissue. • Hepatic amebiasis is treated primarily by the administration of amebicidal drugs, with metronidazole as the drug of choice. • Percutaneous aspiration may be indicated if the patient does not respond to medical management, and percutaneous or operative drainage is indicated in the presence of secondary bacterial infection, which occurs in about 10% of amebic abscesses.

ANSWER:
A-c; B-a; C-b; D-a; E-b

23. What is the preferred treatment for a patient with a 5-cm, calcified cystic lesion containing daughter cysts in the right lobe of the liver?

    A. Pericystectomy

    B. Percutaneous catheter drainage

    C. Transperitoneal surgical drainage

D. Metronidazole

E. Liver resection

Ref.: 1–3

COMMENTS: The helminth *Echinococcus granulosus* is responsible for most hydatid disease of the liver. • It is usually a unilocular process involving the right lobe, although it may present as multiple cysts. • Complications include intrabiliary, intraperitoneal, or intrapleural rupture; secondary infection; anaphylaxis; and mass replacement of the liver. • These lesions often have a calcified wall and can be diagnosed serologically by indirect hemagglutination tests, complement fixation tests, serum immunoelectrophoresis, and, formerly, by the Casoni skin test. • CT scanning and ultrasound imaging may demonstrate characteristic daughter cysts or hydatid sand within the cyst.

Treatment is primarily surgical. • Percutaneous aspiration or drainage is contraindicated because of the risk of intraperitoneal dissemination. • The principles of surgical therapy are to avoid spillage and to remove the entire germinal layer. • The cyst consists of an inner germinal layer (endocyst) and an outer fibrous membrane layer (pericyst). • Resection is usually accomplished by pericystectomy. • Anatomic hepatic resection is not generally required but may be utilized. • Surgery in addition to preoperative and postoperative benzimidazole has been shown to be very effective. • Metronidazole is used for the treatment of amebic liver abscesses. • Because 20% of echinococcal cysts have biliary communication, assessment by preoperative endoscopic retrograde cholangiopancreatography or intraoperative cholangiography is important in any patient with jaundice, cholangitis, elevated liver enzyme levels, or bile noted during resection. • Scolicidal agents should be used with caution because of the risk of sclerosing the bile ducts in the event that the agent finds its way into the ductal system.

ANSWER:
A, E

24. Match the characteristics in the left-hand column with the correct hepatic neoplasms in the right-hand column.

A. Clearly associated with oral contraceptive use	a. Hepatic adenoma (HA)
B. High risk of hemorrhage	b. Focal nodular hyperplasia (FNH)
C. Malignant potential	c. Both
D. Pathology displays a central stellate scar	d. Neither
E. Contains Kupffer cells	

Ref.: 1–3, 5

COMMENTS: HA and FNH are benign neoplasms with important differentiating clinical and histologic features and therapeutic implications. • Both occur most commonly in women of childbearing age. • HA is associated with use of oral contraceptives and anabolic steroids and is also seen in certain glycogen storage diseases. • The relationship of FNH to steroid use is questionable and not completely settled. • HA is usually symptomatic (80% of cases) and is associated with rupture and bleeding in a substantial proportion of patients. • Malignant transformation of HA is recognized. • The risk of malignancy in FNH is unlikely but uncertain. • Histologically, HA consists of hepatocytes without bile ducts or

Kupffer cells. • FNH contains Kupffer cells along with a central stellate scar surrounded by fibrous tissue. • Scanning for Kupffer cell activity with technetium 99m (^{99m}Tc)-labeled sulfur colloid is thus useful in differentiating the lesions.

ANSWER:
A-a; B-a; C-a; D-b; E-b

25. A 25-year-old woman on oral contraceptives develops right upper quadrant abdominal pain. A CT scan demonstrates a hypodense, 6-cm mass in the right lobe of the liver. A ^{99m}Tc scan reveals a defect in the area of the mass. Angiographic study reveals a hypervascular tumor with a peripheral blood supply. Which of the following is the appropriate management?

A. Discontinuation of oral contraceptives and observation with serial CT scans

B. Percutaneous needle biopsy

C. Hepatic resection

D. Arterial embolization

E. Radiation therapy

Ref.: 1–3, 5

COMMENTS: The imaging characteristics described are typical of HA. • Because HA does not contain Kupffer cells, it does not take up radioisotope. • This point may be useful for differentiating HA from FNH but not necessarily from other mass lesions of the liver. • Percutaneous biopsy of suspected HA is not advisable because of the risk of hemorrhage. • HAs associated with oral contraceptives tend to be larger and have a higher risk of bleeding. • Regression does not reliably occur with cessation of oral contraceptives. • However, for lesions smaller than 4 cm, a trial of cessation of contraceptives or steroids with observation may be attempted. • Resection is indicated for most suspected HAs, particularly for symptomatic lesions, for patients not on oral contraceptives, and if the diagnosis is uncertain. • Embolization may be useful for treating hemorrhage in a patient whose HA is inoperable. • Irradiation has no role in the management of HA.

ANSWER:
C

26. An asymptomatic 45-year-old woman is found to have a 7-cm liver mass. A CT scan demonstrates an initial hypodense lesion with peripheral-to-central enhancement by contrast material. MRI shows a dense T2-weighted phase. Which of the following is the appropriate management?

A. Arteriography

B. Observation

C. Percutaneous needle biopsy

D. Resection

E. Radiation therapy

Ref.: 1–3, 5

COMMENTS: Hemangiomas are the most common benign liver tumor, occurring in 7% of the population. • They are characterized by collections of dilated blood vessels that can be diagnosed by their appearance on noninvasive imaging studies. • Contrast CT scanning reveals a typical pattern of enhancement. • A dense T2-weighted image on MRI is a sensitive (although not specific) finding. • Radiolabeled red blood cell scans can also diagnose hemangiomas. • Angiography would also be diagnostic but is not necessary. • These lesions are usually asymptomatic and simply can be observed. • They do not have a high risk of spontaneous rupture. • Percutaneous biopsy is contraindicated because of the risk of bleeding. • Resection by enucleation is appropriate for symptomatic lesions, for enlarging lesions, or if the diagnosis is uncertain. • There is no established role for such treatments as arterial ligation, embolization, or irradiation.

ANSWER:
B

27. Hepatocellular carcinoma is epidemiologically associated with which of the following?

   A. Hepatitis A infection

   B. Hepatitis B infection

   C. Hepatitis C infection

   D. Cavernous hemangioma

   E. Alcoholic cirrhosis

Ref.: 1, 3

COMMENTS: Primary hepatocellular cancer, although less common in North America, is the most common malignant neoplasm worldwide. • Endemic areas include sub-Saharan Africa, Southeast Asia, and Japan. • The primary risk factors are chronic liver disease with cirrhosis (from essentially any cause), chronic infection with hepatitis B or C virus, and various hepatotoxins. • Hepatocellular carcinoma can develop in patients with liver disease related to alcohol abuse, hemochromatosis, α-1-antitrypsin deficiency, hepatic adenomas, and other conditions. • Exogenous risk factors include dietary aflatoxins (found in grain, dairy products, and peanuts), oral contraceptives, anabolic steroids, vinyl chloride, and certain pesticides. • Hepatitis A virus or cavernous hemangiomas are not associated with hepatocellular cancer.

ANSWER:
B, C, E

28. Marked elevations of α-fetoprotein (AFP) levels (>400 ng/ml) may be found with which of the following?

   A. Normal 6-week-old infant

   B. Hepatocellular carcinoma

   C. Colon cancer

   D. Acute viral hepatitis

   E. Teratocarcinoma

Ref.: 1, 3

COMMENTS: AFP is an oncofetoprotein that is useful diagnostically in regard to hepatocellular carcinoma. • It is abundant during fetal development but decreases rapidly after birth. • Approximately 75% of patients with hepatocellular cancer and cirrhosis have levels above 400 ng/ml, whereas AFP levels are elevated in only about one third of patients with hepatocellular cancer and a noncirrhotic liver. • Other conditions that may be associated with pronounced elevations of serum AFP levels include teratocarcinomas, yolk sac tumors, and occasionally metastatic pancreatic or gastric carcinoma. • Milder elevations may be found in patients with chronic liver disease, acute viral hepatitis, and metastatic cancer. • Interval measurements of AFP (every 3 months) in combination with ultrasound imaging have been effective in screening high-risk patients for the development of hepatocellular cancer.

ANSWER:
B, E

29. Which of the following best approximates the 5-year survival rate after complete resection of a hepatocellular cancer?

   A. 5%

   B. 30%

   C. 50%

   D. 75%

Ref.: 1, 3

COMMENTS: Resection is the only potentially curative treatment for hepatocellular cancer. • Unfortunately, most lesions are not resectable because of tumor spread or underlying cirrhosis. • Prognostic factors that influence long-term survival following resection include tumor size, tumor multiplicity, encapsulation, completeness of resection, portal or hepatic vein invasion, and histologic differentiation. • The 5-year survival rate after resection ranges from 26.4 to 58.8%. • Higher survival rates are dependent on surgical margins of more than 1 cm. • Liver transplantation for hepatocellular cancer in cirrhotic patients who cannot undergo partial hepatic resection has also been utilized. • Tumor recurrence most frequently is in the liver following either resection or transplantation.

ANSWER:
B

30. Match the clinical characteristics in the left-hand column with the appropriate type of hepatocellular tumor in the right-hand column.

   A. AFP level usually elevated   a. Standard hepatocellular cancer

   B. Female predilection   b. Fibrolamellar cancer

   C. Associated with hepatitis A   c. Both

   D. Associated with cirrhosis   d. Neither

Ref.: 1, 3

COMMENTS: The fibrolamellar variant of hepatocellular cancer is relatively uncommon but has clinical and pathologic features that distinguish it from standard hepatocellular cancer. • Histologically, it consists of sheets of well-differentiated hepatocytes separated by fibrous tissue. • It tends to be well localized and occurs in younger patients, often less than 35 years old. • Standard hepatocellular cancers have a distinct male predominance, but fibrolamellar tumors are as common or perhaps even more common in females. • Unlike typical hepatocellular cancer, the fibrolamellar variant is not commonly associated with hepatitis B infection, cirrhosis, or elevated AFP levels (all <10%). • These tumors are more often resectable, and the prognosis following resection is considerably better. • Neither tumor is associated with hepatitis A.

ANSWER:
A-a; B-b; C-d; D-a

31. Which of the following statements is/are true regarding intra-hepatic cholangiocarcinoma?

A. Survival following resection is generally lower than for distal bile duct cancer.

B. Resection is contraindicated unless histologically negative margins can be obtained.

C. Best survival is obtained with liver transplantation.

D. Adjuvant chemotherapy improves survival following resection.

Ref.: 1, 7

COMMENTS: Cholangiocarcinoma arises from the bile duct epithelium and can occur anywhere along the biliary tract. • It comprises 5–20% of primary liver carcinoma. • Tumors arising from the extrahepatic bile ducts differ from those located intrahepatically in terms of their presentation, therapy, and prognosis. • Tumors of the extrahepatic bile ducts typically present with biliary obstruction. • Intrahepatic tumors present as a liver mass with absent or vague symptoms, such as pain, weight loss, nausea, and anorexia. • The treatment of choice is surgical excision, which is associated with a 15–20% 5-year survival rate. • The prognosis is best for tumors of the distal bile ducts that can be resected by pancreaticoduodenectomy. • Tumors involving the bifurcation of the bile duct (Klatskin's tumor) are less often resectable. • Tumor size and the presence of satellite nodules are correlated with outcome. • Histologically negative margins are always desirable, but prolonged survival can be attained even with microscopically involved margins. • If the tumor cannot be resected, improved survival has been noted with bypass or stenting procedures. • The results of liver transplantation for cholangiocarcinoma have been associated with frequent recurrence and have not generally been encouraging. • Adjuvant chemotherapy has not typically been useful for bile duct cancer.

A N S W E R :
A

32. In which of the following situations would resection of an isolated hepatic segment for malignancy be contraindicated?

A. Primary hepatocellular cancer

B. Malignant tumor in a noncirrhotic liver

C. Malignant tumor in a patient with extrahepatic metastases

D. Metastatic colorectal cancer

Ref.: 8

COMMENTS: The surgical anatomy of the liver, based on the branching of the portal structures, permits anatomic resections of single or multiple hepatic segments. • These resections allow conservation of hepatic parenchyma and may be appropriate for patients with cirrhosis, those undergoing multiple or bilobar resections, or those undergoing repeat liver resection. • The segmental vascular pedicle is isolated and divided before parenchymal division. • In appropriate patients, the rate of margin positivity does not exceed that of nonanatomic wedge resections and may be lower. • Disease recurrence is usually elsewhere in the liver and not at the resection margin. • It must be emphasized that safe performance of these resections requires an experienced hepatic surgeon who is thoroughly familiar with hepatic anatomy and dissection techniques. • Metastatic extrahepatic disease is a general contraindication to any type of hepatic resection.

A N S W E R :
C

33. Which of the following is/are contraindications for resection of colorectal hepatic metastases?

A. Synchronous metastases

B. Bilobar metastases

C. Advanced cirrhosis

D. Extrahepatic metastases

E. Size greater than 5 cm

Ref.: 1, 3

COMMENTS: See Question 34.

34. Prognosis following resection of colorectal hepatic metastases is influenced by which of the following?

A. Portal metastatic spread versus systemic metastatic spread

B. Resection margin greater than 1 cm

C. Adjuvant hepatic arterial chemotherapy

D. Primary tumor biologic features

E. Adjuvant radiation therapy

Ref.: 1, 3, 9

COMMENTS: Resection is currently the preferred treatment for liver metastases from colorectal cancer, provided the patient has adequate liver reserve and does not have extrahepatic metastases, total hepatic involvement, advanced cirrhosis, or vena cava or portal vein invasion. • The goal is to resect all hepatic disease. • Survival is adversely affected by margins that are positive for cancer or are less than 1 cm. • As long as the resection margin is adequate, the specific type of liver resection (anatomic versus "wedge") does not influence survival. • Synchronous lesions discovered at the initial operation for colorectal cancer may be removed at the original operation if the length of original procedure, general condition of the patient, extent of hepatic resection, and experience of the surgeon allow for this. • Otherwise, resection can be performed at a later date.

Many parameters have been evaluated for their prognostic importance following resection of colorectal metastases. • Although long-term survival is not as good for patients with four or more tumors or lesions greater than 5 cm, resection, when possible, still provides some longevity. • Factors that have not consistently been found to influence survival include synchronous versus metachronous lesions (although some reports state that patients with metachronous lesions fare better than those with synchronous lesions), tumor distribution (unilobar versus bilobar), and stage of the primary tumor (although patients with positive mesenteric nodes are more likely to develop extrahepatic metastases). • Better prognosis is associated with tumors that are well differentiated or divide more slowly and with portal metastatic spread versus systemic spread. • Most patients undergoing hepatic resection for colorectal metastases eventually have a recurrence at some site.

Hepatic arterial infusion of chemotherapeutic agents has a higher response rate than does systemic administration, although adjuvant chemotherapy has not prolonged survival following hepatic resection in randomized studies. • Irradiation is not useful for hepatic metastases. • The role of ablative therapy such as cryosurgery or hyperthermia (radiofrequency or laser) for hepatic metastases is under evaluation. • These approaches appear useful for patients who cannot undergo resection, but they cannot yet be considered appropriate alternative treatment for otherwise resectable tumors.

ANSWERS:
Question 33: C, D
Question 34: A, B, D

35. Which of the following is the most accurate method for identifying hepatic metastases?

 A. Transabdominal ultrasound imaging

 B. CT scanning

 C. Laparoscopy

 D. Intraoperative palpation

 E. Intraoperative ultrasound imaging

Ref.: 4

COMMENTS: Transabdominal ultrasound imaging is as accurate as CT scanning for detecting liver tumors that are 2 cm in size or larger. • For somewhat smaller lesions, CT scanning is more accurate, although it can miss the smallest lesions (<1 cm). • Laparoscopy is useful for identifying small metastases on the liver or peritoneal surfaces that escape discovery by noninvasive preoperative imaging modalities. • Laparoscopy has been incorporated in the staging workup of a variety of intra-abdominal malignancies, including those of the liver. • However, one of its limitations is its ability to assess the interior structure of solid organs. • It is now well recognized that intraoperative ultrasound imaging is the most accurate method for detecting and assessing hepatic tumors. • Not only does intraoperative ultrasound imaging discover more lesions than any other modality (including palpation), but it also clearly demonstrates the anatomic relationship of tumors to important vascular structures, which is a critical determinant of resectability and the extent of resection necessary. • Intraoperative ultrasound imaging can be performed with handheld or laparoscopic transducers. • Experience with intraoperative ultrasound imaging for liver tumors has shown that the sonographic findings affect the surgical management of one third to one half of patients. • Intraoperative ultrasound imaging has become an indispensable component of hepatic surgery.

ANSWER:
E

36. Which of the following should be used for initial treatment of a patient in hepatic coma?

 A. Reduction of dietary protein to 50 g/day or less

 B. Control of active bleeding

 C. Lactulose

 D. Systemic antibiotics

 E. Nutritional supplementation with branched-chain amino acids

Ref.: 1–3

COMMENTS: The treatment of hepatic encephalopathy and coma is aimed at limiting the nitrogen that the liver must metabolize by eliminating nitrogenous materials from the gastrointestinal tract and by inhibiting their absorption. • At the same time, precipitating causes are sought and treated. • Nutritional support is important and can be initiated with standard amino acids and restriction of dietary protein. • Cessation of any gastrointestinal bleeding from varices is an important step in reducing the conversion of intraluminal blood into ammonia. • Lactulose acts as a cathartic and also inhibits absorption of ammonia by acidifying the colon. • Nonabsorbable antibiotics, such as neomycin and kanamycin, reduce the colonic flora and the production of ammonia. • Systemic antibiotics may be useful for treating specific infections that precipitate encephalopathy but are not indicated empirically. • Because the colon is the major site of ammonia absorption, colonic resection or exclusion has been suggested to improve encephalopathy but is not a widely employed therapeutic measure. • Although alterations in the balance of aromatic amino acids and branched-chain amino acids have been demonstrated in patients with hepatic disease and encephalopathy, there is no evidence that administration of branched-chain amino acids significantly alleviates encephalopathy.

ANSWER:
A, B, C

37. The initial management of ascites associated with cirrhosis should include which of the following?

 A. Therapeutic large-volume paracentesis

 B. Sodium restriction

 C. Diuretic administration

 D. Fluid restriction

 E. Diagnostic paracentesis

Ref.: 10

COMMENTS: Ascites is the most common major complication of hepatic cirrhosis. • It is associated with a 2-year survival rate of 50%, and its onset in a cirrhotic patient should prompt an evaluation for liver transplantation. • The treatment of ascites depends on its cause, and therefore diagnostic paracentesis is required after a history and physical examination. • Abdominal ultrasound imaging can confirm the presence of ascites if it is not certain by examination. • The serum-ascites albumin gradient is useful diagnostically. • A high gradient (1.1 g/dl) indicates portal hypertension and suggests that the patient will be responsive to medical management consisting of sodium restriction (2000 mg/day) and oral diuretics. • Usually, both spironolactone and furosemide are administered to produce fluid loss and natriuresis. • Spironolactone alone may cause hyperkalemia, and furosemide alone is less effective. • Fluid restriction is not necessary unless the patient has pronounced hyponatremia (<120 mmol/L). • Medical therapy controls ascites in about 90% of patients. • When the ascites is refractory, serial therapeutic paracenteses (with or without administration of albumin or other plasma volume expanders) is indicated. • Liver transplantation is the ultimate treatment. • A peritoneovenous shunt is an option for patients with refractory ascites who are not transplantation candidates or who cannot undergo repeated paracenteses. • These shunts are fraught with potential complications, however, and do not prolong survival compared to medical management. • Transjugular intrahepatic portosystemic shunts or operative side-to-side type portosystemic shunts may control ascites in selected patients.

ANSWER:
B, C, E

38. Which of the following is/are relative contraindication(s) to peritoneovenous shunting for intractable ascites?

A. History of variceal bleeding

B. Oliguria

C. Bacterial peritonitis

D. Uncorrectable coagulopathy

E. Malignant intra-abdominal disease

Ref.: 1, 3

COMMENTS: Patients with significant ascites due to cirrhosis or malignancy who do not respond to medical management may be candidates for peritoneovenous shunting. • The shunts decrease ascites and increase cardiac output and renal blood flow. • Some degree of coagulopathy, usually transient, occurs in nearly all patients with cirrhotic ascites. • Uncorrectable coagulopathy is considered a contraindication to shunting. • Patients with portal hypertension and previous variceal bleeding may rebleed following shunting because of the increase in circulating blood volume. • Other contraindications to shunting in patients with cirrhotic ascites include bacterial peritonitis, liver failure, and cardiac failure. • Patients undergoing peritoneovenous shunts for malignancy have a higher incidence of shunt occlusion. • Relative contraindications include the presence of bloody ascitic fluid or fluid with high protein content.

ANSWER:
A, C, D

39. Which of the following statements is/are true regarding spontaneous bacterial peritonitis (SBP)?

A. Diagnosis can be made clinically without paracentesis.

B. Infection is most commonly polymicrobial.

C. Antibiotic therapy is reserved for patients with positive findings on ascitic fluid culture.

D. Gram-negative enteric bacteria are often present.

Ref.: 3, 10

COMMENTS: SBP is a potentially lethal complication of ascites that affects about 10% of patients with cirrhotic ascites. • Fever and abdominal pain are common manifestations, but the presentation may be subtle. • Diagnosis requires paracentesis with demonstration of an elevated ascitic fluid polymorphonuclear neutrophil (PMN) count (>250 cells/mm³) or, eventually, positive findings on culture. • Antibiotic therapy should be instituted promptly based on an elevated ascitic fluid PMN count or on symptoms even if the PMN count is lower. • Infection is usually from one organism, most commonly *Escherichia coli*, *Klebsiella*, and pneumococci. • A third-generation cephalosporin is typically the preferred antibiotic. • Differentiation from secondary bacterial peritonitis due to a surgical condition is critical. • Patients with SBP typically respond to appropriate antibiotics within 48 hr, and ascitic PMN counts decrease. • Failure to improve; the presence of polymicrobial infection; or ascitic fluid with a total protein level greater than 1 g/dl, an LDH level greater than serum level, or a glucose level less than 50 mg/dl suggests secondary peritonitis. • Risk factors for SBP include previous SBP, variceal hemorrhage, and low-protein ascites (<1.0 g/dl). • Short or long-term prophylactic antibiotics may be appropriate for high-risk patients.

ANSWER:
D

40. With regard to hernias in patients with ascites, which of the following statements is/are true?

A. Increased abdominal pressure is one cause of umbilical hernias in patients with ascites.

B. The umbilical hernia recurrence rates for patients with and without ascites are the same.

C. Patients with asymptomatic groin hernias should be treated expectantly.

D. Preoperative paracentesis is a helpful strategy for electively repairing these hernias.

Ref.: 11

COMMENTS: Umbilical, and less frequently inguinal, hernias occur in approximately 20% of patients with ascites. • They occur because of increased intra-abdominal pressure, muscle wasting, fascial thinning, and nutritional deficits. • The recurrence rate following repair of umbilical hernias in patients with ascites may be as high as 73%. • Because of the high complication rate following hernia repair, it should not be entertained for the asymptomatic hernia. • Preoperative optimization with paracentesis helps to decrease intra-abdominal pressure. • Ascites leak following a surgical procedure should be treated aggressively, and early wound exploration and repair of fascial dehiscence is necessary. • Diuretic therapy alone is ineffective in this situation.

ANSWER:
A, C, D

41. With regard to the liver injury scale of the American Association for the Surgery of Trauma (AAST), which of the following statements is/are true?

A. A grade I liver hematoma is subcapsular, nonexpanding, and smaller than 10 cm.

B. A grade II liver laceration is greater than 5 cm in parenchymal depth.

C. A parenchymal injury involving 50% of an hepatic lobe is classified as a grade IV liver laceration.

D. Hepatic avulsion is classified as a grade VI liver injury.

Ref.: 12

COMMENTS: The Organ Injury Scaling Committee of the AAST created the hepatic injury classification system in 1989 and updated it in 1994. • This classification standarized the description of hepatic injuries. • The liver injury scale is as follows:

Grade	Injury Description
I hematoma	Subcapsular, nonexpanding, <10 cm
I laceration	Capsular tear, nonbleeding, <1 cm parenchymal depth
II hematoma	Subcapsular, nonexpanding, 10–50% surface area; intraparenchymal, nonexpanding, <10 cm
II laceration	Capsular tear, active bleeding; 1–3 cm parenchymal depth, <10 cm in length
III hematoma	Subcapsular, >50% surface area or expanding; ruptured subcapsular hematoma with active bleeding; intraparenchymal hematoma >10 cm or expanding
III laceration	>3 cm parenchymal depth
IV hematoma	Ruptured intraparenchymal hematoma with active bleeding
IV laceration	Parenchymal disruption involving 25–75% of hepatic lobe or 1–3 Couinaud's segments within a single lobe
V laceration	Parenchymal disruption involving >75% of hepatic lobe or >3 Couinaud's segments within a single lobe
V vascular	Juxtahepatic venous injuries (retrohepatic, vena cava, central major hepatic veins)
VI vascular	Hepatic avulsion

ANSWER:
A, C, D

42. Patients with which of the following blunt hepatic injuries are candidates for nonoperative management?

    A. A grade IV liver laceration in a hemodynamically stable patient

    B. A grade II liver laceration in a patient requiring the transfusion of 8 units of packed red blood cells in 24 hr

    C. A grade I liver hematoma in a patient with peritonitis

    D. A grade III liver laceration based on CT scanning in a hemodynamically stable patient with a Glasgow Coma Scale classification of 8

Ref.: 12

COMMENTS: Criteria for nonoperative management of adult blunt hepatic injuries are (1) absence of peritoneal signs, (2) precise CT delineation and grading of the injury, (3) no associated intra-abdominal or retroperitoneal injuries on CT scan that require operative intervention, and (4) avoidance of excessive liver injury–related blood transfusion. • Patients who are not neurologically intact are candidates for nonoperative management of their liver injury if they meet these criteria. • The initial belief that nonoperative management should be reserved for patients with grade I–III hepatic injuries has generally been replaced with data showing that the hemodynamic status of the patient is the most important indicator of the need for operative intervention. • The success of nonoperative management has been reported at 96%. • The most common complications of this type of treatment are hemorrhage (3.3%), biloma (3.0%), and abscess (0.7%). • The use of angiography has also been utilized in patients who are hemodynamically stable, with CT scan findings of a "blush" or "pooling of contrast material" indicating ongoing arterial bleeding. • Regardless of the extent of injury, patients should be adequately prepared for operative intervention with frequent monitoring of vital signs, physical examination, and hemoglobin and hematocrit measurements during the observation period. • Follow-up CT scan in stable patients has not been shown to affect outcome.

ANSWER:
A, D

43. Important steps in dealing with the operative management of complex hepatic injuries include which of the following?

    A. Use of the Pringle maneuver

    B. Bimanual compression

    C. Avoidance of débridement of hemostatic nonviable liver parenchyma

    D. Open drainage of grade III–V injuries

    E. Placement of an omental pedicle into the wound

Ref.: 12

COMMENTS: Operative management of complex hepatic injuries should be addressed with a sequential algorithmic approach. • In unstable patients with hemoperitoneum found to have liver injuries on exploration, bimanual compression with resuscitation followed by portal triad occlusion (Pringle maneuver) are appropriate initial steps. • If the bleeding can be controlled, finger fracture to the site of injury with repair or ligation of injured structures is then performed. • This is followed by débridement of nonviable parenchyma and placement of an omental pack and closed suction drains in patients with grade III–V injuries.

• The use of open drains has been associated with a higher incidence of postoperative abscess formation. • In a patient who continues to bleed after compression and portal triad occlusion, the wound should be packed. • If the bleeding is controlled, the packing can be left in place and the abdomen temporarily closed to take the patient for rewarming and resuscitation to correct any coagulopathy. • The patient is then re-explored in 18–36 hr, and the packs are removed. • If bleeding continues despite packing, retrohepatic IVC or hepatic venous injury should be considered, and vascular isolation with intracaval shunt may be necessary.

Hepatic resection is associated with a high mortality rate and is used more frequently abroad than in the United States. • It may be considered when (1) there is total destruction of normal hepatic parenchyma, (2) the extent of injury precludes perihepatic packing, (3) a clean resection line lessens the likelihood of postoperative bleeding, necrosis, or abscess formation, (4) the injury has virtually performed the resection, or (5) it is the sole method of controlling hemorrhage. • Mesh hepatorrhaphy has also been used with limited success. • Wrapping the liver with mesh in a similar fashion as that used for splenic injuries serves to control bleeding through a tamponading effect. • However, data ares still lacking concerning the appropriate population of patients for this method.

ANSWER:
A, B, E

44. Other modalities used in the treatment of unresectable liver lesions include which of the following?

    A. Percutaneous ethanol injection

    B. Radiofrequency ablation (RFA)

    C. Cryoablation

    D. Orthotopic liver transplantation

    E. Transarterial chemoembolization

Ref.: 1, 13

COMMENTS: While resection is the preferred treatment for liver lesions, if the disease cannot be safely resected with adequate remaining healthy liver parenchyma or if a patient cannot tolerate a major resection, there are several other modalities available. • Data are inconclusive as to the effectiveness of these modalities, but survival may be increased with their use. • Percutaneous ethanol or acetic acid injection has been used in Asia on hepatocellular carcinoma in cirrhotics. • It appears to be effective on small lesions, but recurrence is a problem. • RFA and cryoablation are ablative techniques that utilize intraoperative ultrasound guidance and work by local tumor necrosis through the use of heating and freezing probes, respectively. • Orthotopic liver transplantation has been used in patients with cirrhosis and hepatocellular carcinoma. • Transarterial chemoembolization is a technique in which a chemotherapeutic agent (frequently doxorubicin, cisplatin, or mitomycin) is suspended in ethiodized oil and iodine ethyl ester and then injected through a catheter in the hepatic artery toward the tumor.

ANSWER:
A, B, C, D, E

45. Indications for using RFA of liver tumors include which of the following?

    A. Unresectable lesions in close proximity to major vascular structures

    B. Multiple lesions

    C. Very large lesions

D. In conjunction with liver resection

E. Patients with hepatocellular carcinoma or metastatic colon cancer

Ref.: 13, 14

COMMENTS: RFA is a technique in which a needle electrode is inserted into a malignant liver tumor. • A radiofrequency generator is connected to the electrode, which produces localized tumor destruction with coagulative necrosis as the temperature of the tissue exceeds 50°C. • The introduction of the electrode can be performed through a laparotomy incision, laparoscopically, or even percutaneously, with the use of ultrasound guidance. • This method has been utilized for patients with hepatocellular carcinoma as well as those with metastatic colon and rectal cancer. • Some institutions combine the treatment with resection when multiple lesions are involved and resection alone would not leave enough viable hepatic parenchyma for survival. • RFA works well when lesions are close to major vascular structures. • The maximum-sized lesion that can be ablated by RFA is unclear because multiple applications can be utilized, but it does appear to be more effective on smaller lesions (<5–6 cm).

ANSWER:
A, B, D, E

46. Eight weeks after open-heart surgery with transfusions, a 56-year-old man notes dark urine, fatigue, and anorexia. An examination discloses only mild, tender hepatomegaly. Laboratory investigations reveal a bilirubin level of 2 mg/dl; an SGOT level of 540 IU/L; an SGPT level of 620 IU/L; an alkaline phosphatase level of 1120 IU/ L; and negative assay results for hepatitis B surface antigen (HBsAg), hepatitis B core antibody (anti-HBc), immunoglobulin M anti-hepatitis A virus antibody (IgM anti-HAV), and anti-hepatitis C virus antibody (anti-HCV). Which of the following is the most likely explanation for the patient's clinical condition?

A. Acute viral hepatitis A

B. Acute viral hepatitis B

C. Acute viral hepatitis C

D. Acute viral hepatitis D

E. Acute viral hepatitis E

Ref.: 1, 3

COMMENTS: Posttransfusion non-A, non-B hepatitis is mostly the result of hepatitis C infection. • The incubation period is usually 5–10 weeks, and the mean peak aminotransferase levels are 500–1000 IU/L. • Anti-HCV antibody is commonly not detectable until 18 weeks after illness onset. • Approximately 70% of patients with acute hepatitis C progress to chronic hepatitis and potentially cirrhosis. • The negative serologic study results exclude acute infection with hepatitis A and B. • Hepatitis D (delta) virus (HDV) is capable of infecting only patients who also have HBsAg, because HDV is an incomplete RNA virus. • Hepatitis E (epidemic) virus is rare, except in association with water-borne epidemics in India, the Middle East, and South America.

ANSWER:
C

47. Which of the following clinical conditions is indicated by the presence of serum antibodies against hepatitis B surface antigen (anti-HBs) and hepatitis B core antigen (anti-HBc) in the absence of HBsAg?

A. Active, acute infection with the hepatitis B virus

B. Normal response to vaccination with the hepatitis B vaccine

C. Chronic active hepatitis due to the hepatitis B virus

D. Recovery with subsequent immunity following acute hepatitis B

E. Asymptomatic chronic carrier of the hepatitis B virus

Ref.: 1, 3

COMMENTS: The pattern of negative HBsAg, positive anti-HBs, and positive anti-HBc assays is seen during the recovery phase following acute hepatitis B and clearance of HBsAg from the liver. • This antibody pattern may persist for years and is not associated with liver disease or infectivity. • Vaccination with the hepatitis B vaccine (genetically manufactured HBsAg particles *without* HBcAg or HBV DNA) is associated with the development of anti-HBs antibody alone. • Active, ongoing infection with the hepatitis B virus, whether acute hepatitis, chronic active hepatitis, or asymptomatic chronic carrier state, is manifested by the presence of HBsAg and anti-HBc in the serum.

ANSWER:
D

REFERENCES

1. Townsend CM, Beauchamp RD, Evers BM, et al (eds): *Sabiston Textbook of Surgery: The Biological Basis of Modern Surgical Practice,* 16th ed. Saunders, Philadelphia, 2001.
2. Schwartz SI, Shires GT, Spencer FC: *Principles of Surgery,* 7th ed. McGraw-Hill, New York, 1999.
3. Greenfield LJ, Mulholland M, Oldham T, et al: *Surgery: Scientific Principles and Practice,* 3rd ed. Lippincott, Williams & Wilkins, Philadelphia, 2001.
4. Deziel DJ: Hepatobiliary ultrasound. *Probl Gen Surg* 14:13–24, 1997.
5. O'Leary JP: *The Physiologic Basis of Surgery,* 3rd ed. Lippincott, Williams & Wilkins, Philadelphia, 2002.
6. Melendez JA, Arslan V, Fischer ME, et al: Perioperative outcomes of major hepatic resections under low central venous pressure anesthesia: blood loss, blood transfusion and the risk of postoperative renal dysfunction. *J Am Coll Surg* 187:620–625, 1998.
7. Roayaie S, Guarrera JV, Ye MQ, et al: Aggressive surgical treatment of intrahepatic cholangiocarcinoma: predictors or outcome. *J Am Coll Surg* 187:365–372, 1998.
8. Billingsley KG, Jarnagin WR, Fong Y, et al: Segment-oriented hepatic resection in the management of malignant neoplasms of the liver. *J Am Coll Surg* 187:471–481, 1998.
9. Lorenz M, Muller HH, Schramm H, et al: Randomized trial of surgery versus surgery followed by adjuvant hepatic arterial infusion with 5-fluorouracil and folinic acid for liver metastases of colorectal cancer. *Ann Surg* 228:756–762, 1998.
10. Runyon BA: Management of adult patients with ascites caused by cirrhosis. *Hepatology* 27:264–272, 1998.
11. Rosemurgy AS, Statman RC, Murphy CG, et al: Postoperative ascitic leaks: the ongoing challenge [see Comments]. *Surgery* 111:623–625, 1992.
12. Mattox KL, Feliciano DV, Moore EE: *Trauma,* 4th ed. McGraw-Hill, New York, 2000.
13. Curley SA, Izzo F, Ellis LM, et al: Radiofrequency ablation of hepatocellular cancer in 110 patients with cirrhosis. *Ann Surg* 232:381–391, 2000.
14. Wong SL, Edwards NJ, Chao C, et al: Radiofrequency ablation for unresectable hepatic metastases. *Am J Surg* 182:552–557, 2001.

C H A P T E R **38**

Portal Venous System

Daniel J. Deziel, M.D.

1. With regard to portal venous anatomy, which of the following is true?

   A. The main portal vein is formed by the junction of the splenic vein and inferior mesenteric vein.

   B. The portal vein is the most anterior structure in the hepatoduodenal ligament.

   C. The extrahepatic portal vein contains valves.

   D. The intrahepatic branches are intrasegmental.

   Ref.: 1, 2

COMMENTS: The portal vein is formed by the junction of the splenic vein and superior mesenteric vein behind the neck of the pancreas. • It is valveless. • In the hepatoduodenal ligament, the portal vein is posterior to the bile duct and hepatic artery. • The portal vein enters the liver at the porta hepatis and divides into the main right and left portal veins. • The right portal vein divides into anterior and posterior branches and subsequently branches to each liver segment on the right. • The left portal vein has an initial transverse or horizontal portion and then turns anteriorly to form the ascending (umbilical) portion. • Branches to each liver segment on the left come off the left portal vein. • The portal vein branches are primarily intrasegmental, while the hepatic vein branches are intersegmental. • One exception is the ascending portion of the left portal vein, which is located between the medial and lateral segments of the left lobe. • Variations or anomalies in the anatomy of the main portal vein are relatively uncommon. • Occasionally, the right portal vein is absent, so that the bifurcation of the main portal vein is essentially a trifurcation. • There are some variations in the number and arrangement of the intrahepatic segmental branches.

ANSWER:
D

2. Which of the following is the most common cause of portal hypertension?

   A. Increased portal venous blood flow

   B. Post-sinusoidal obstruction

   C. Sinusoidal obstruction

   D. Extrahepatic obstruction

   Ref.: 1

COMMENTS: Portal hypertension can result from either increased resistance to portal venous flow or from increased flow alone. • By far the most common cause is increased resistance to flow due to obstruction. • The site of obstruction may be prehepatic, intrahepatic, or posthepatic. • Furthermore, hepatic obstruction may be characterized as presinusoidal, sinusoidal, or postsinusoidal, depending on the particular condition. • Often, more than one hepatic level is involved. • Portal hypertension due to increased flow alone is rare but can occur in conditions such as massive splenomegaly or splanchnic arterial venous fistula.

ANSWER:
C

3. In which of the following disorders does the pathophysiology of portal hypertension involve presinusoidal obstruction?

   A. Budd-Chiari syndrome

   B. Alcoholic cirrhosis

   C. Posthepatitic cirrhosis

   D. Schistosomiasis

   Ref.: 1, 2

COMMENTS: It is useful to consider the level of obstruction leading to portal hypertension, since patients with presinusoidal obstruction may have normal liver function, whereas patients with sinusoidal or postsinusoidal obstruction usually have hepatocellular damage. • Schistosomiasis is an important worldwide cause of portal hypertension and is associated with presinusoidal fibrosis of terminal portal vein branches. • Technically, prehepatic obstruction, as in portal vein thrombosis, may also be considered presinusoidal. • Hepatic cirrhosis is associated with sinusoidal and postsinusoidal obstruction. • The level of obstruction is primarily posthepatic in Budd-Chiari syndrome (hepatic vein obstruction) and also in constrictive pericarditis or right heart failure.

ANSWER:
D

4. A patient with hepatic cirrhosis has a portal systemic pressure gradient of 8 mmHg (portal pressure minus free hepatic venous pressure). This indicates which one of the following?

   A. The patient does not have portal hypertension.

   B. The site of obstruction is presinusoidal.

C. Variceal hemorrhage is unlikely.

D. Variceal hemorrhage is inevitable.

Ref.: 1, 2

COMMENTS: Normal portal venous pressure is about 5–8 mmHg. • Portal pressure can be measured indirectly by hepatic venous wedge pressure. • In cases of presinusoidal obstruction, however, the wedge pressure will be normal. • The clinical consequences of elevated portal pressure are often due to increased flow through the many portosystemic collateral pathways that develop. • The most prominent clinical manifestation is bleeding from esophagogastric varices. • It has been estimated that two thirds of patients with portal hypertension will develop varices and that one third to one half of those will bleed. • A number of factors have been identified as risk factors for variceal hemorrhage, although none alone is a reliable independent predictor. • However, variceal bleeding does not typically occur when the pressure gradient is less than 12 mmHg.

ANSWER:
C

5. The risk of bleeding from esophageal varices is related to all but which of the following?

A. Absolute portal pressure

B. Size and structure of the varix

C. Presence of a red spot

D. Child's classification

Ref.: 1–3

COMMENTS: Esophageal varices are thought to bleed by rupture rather than by erosion. • Although varices are rarely found if the portal pressure gradient is less than 12 mmHg, not all patients with higher gradients develop varices, and there is a poor correlation of the actual portal pressure and the risk of bleeding. • Variceal pressure, size, wall tension (LaPlace's Law), and wall thickness are all factors. • Endoscopic features of varices, such as size, structure, coloration, and markings, are also correlated to the risk of rupture. • Patients with poor liver function, as reflected by Child's classification, are more likely to have a first bleed.

ANSWER:
A

6. The Child-Pugh classification of hepatic dysfunction includes all but which of the following?

A. Serum bilirubin level

B. Serum aspartate aminotransferase (AST) level

C. Prothrombin time

D. Serum albumin level

E. Assessment of ascites

Ref.: 1, 2, 4

COMMENTS: Hepatic functional reserve can be clinically estimated based on Child's classification, which incorporates a combination of five clinical and biochemical parameters. • The Child-Pugh modification includes the parameters of serum bilirubin level, serum albumin level, prothrombin time, ascites, and the presence of a neurologic disorder (encephalopathy). • The Child-Turcotte modification has the same parameters except that it includes assessment of nutritional status rather than prothrombin time. • The Child's classification system categorizes patients into A, B, or C status, although there is frequent overlap. • The operative mortality rate associated with portosystemic shunt procedures (and other major operations) and long-term prognosis are correlated with the Child's status. • For example, the respective operative mortality rates for Child's A, B, and C patients are 0–5%, 10–15% and 25–50%.

ANSWER:
B

7. A 51-year-old man presents to the emergency room with hematemesis and a systolic blood pressure of 80. After initial fluid resuscitation, his blood pressure is 120/80, and his pulse rate is 100. His file contains the radiograph shown. What is the next step in the management of this patient?

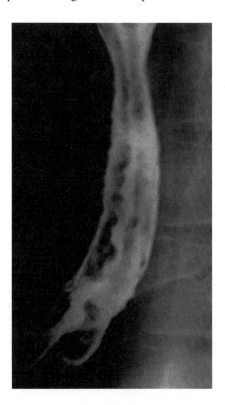

A. Flexible upper endoscopic examination

B. Administration of vasopressin

C. Administration of a proton-pump inhibitor

D. Placement of a Sengstaken-Blakemore tube

Ref.: 1, 2

COMMENTS: The principles of managing acute gastrointestinal (GI) hemorrhage are resuscitation, diagnosis, and control. • Volume is restored by infusion of isotonic crystalloid solutions, blood is typed and crossmatched, and the patient's volume status is monitored with vital signs, placement of a Foley catheter for urinary output, and central venous pressure measurements as necessary. • When the patient has been stabilized, endoscopy is performed to identify the source of bleeding. • The x-ray picture here shows esophageal varices. • Although variceal hemorrhage is certainly a likely diagnosis in the patient described, it is also possible that his bleeding is from another source that would require different therapy.

ANSWER:
A

---

8. Esophagogastroduodenoscopy in the patient described in Question 7 shows large esophageal varices with overlying clot. What is the next step in the management of this patient?

   A. Administration of vasopressin or octreotide

   B. Balloon tamponade

   C. Endoscopic sclerotherapy or variceal ligation

   D. Transjuglar intrahepatic portosystemic shunt (TIPS)

   E. Emergency portocaval shunt

Ref.: 1, 2, 5

COMMENTS: Variceal hemorrhage is the most lethal complication of portal hypertension. • The mortality rate for each bleeding episode is 25–40% and even higher for patients with hepatic decompensation. • The initial priority is to control the bleeding. • Once this is achieved, the ultimate treatment will depend on multiple factors, including the cause of portal hypertension, functional hepatic reserve, site of hemorrhage, and specific venous anatomy. • Variceal hemorrhage can be diagnosed endoscopically if active bleeding or other stigmata of recent hemorrhage are seen. • Endoscopic management by injection of sclerosing agents or band ligation can control acute bleeding in 80–90% of patients. • This method of local control is considered first-line therapy and, with proper personnel, can be performed at the time of the initial diagnostic endoscopy if bleeding esophageal varices are diagnosed. • However, it should be noted that endoscopic methods are not usually effective for bleeding gastric varices. • Pharmocologic agents that reduce splanchnic blood flow can also control acute variceal hemorrhage alone (50–70%) and are a useful adjunct to endoscopic therapy. • Vasopressin is given as an intravenous bolus of 20 units over 20 minutes, followed by a continuous infusion at 0.2–0.4 units/min. • Octreotide, an analogue of somatostatin, is given as a 50-g IV bolus, followed by continuous infusion 25–50 g/hr. • Octreotide appears to have fewer side effects than does vasopressin. • Balloon tamponade is effective for controlling acute bleeding, but there is a high rate of recurrent bleeding, and it has been associated with serious complications, including esophageal rupture, aspiration, and asphyxiation. • It is no longer a first-line treatment, but it is an important temporizing measure if other therapies fail or cannot be performed. • Emergency TIPS can control acute hemorrhage in 90% of patients but is reserved for those in whom less invasive measures have failed, particularly for those with hepatic decompensation who may be candidates for liver transplantation or for whom an emergency shunt operation entails prohibitive risk. • Emergency operations for acute variceal bleeding are also best limited to patients in whom other therapies have failed or cannot be applied. • The mortality rate for emergency shunt procedures is high, especially for decompensated patients.

ANSWER:
C

---

9. Both vasopressin and octreotide cause which of the following?

   A. Variceal vasoconstriction

   B. Splanchnic vasoconstriction

   C. Systemic vasoconstriction

   D. Dilutional hyponatremia

Ref.: 1, 2

COMMENTS: Pharmacotherapy with vasopressin or octreotide is effective in variceal bleeding because splanchnic arteriolar vasoconstriction reduces portal venous blood flow. • Neither agent directly affects the bleeding varices, which do not have smooth muscle. • Vasopressin also causes systemic vasoconstriction but can therefore also cause hypertension, diminished cardiac output, and coronary vasoconstriction. • These effects can be ameliorated to some extent by the simultaneous infusion of nitroglycerin. • Other potential side effects of vasopressin include cramping abdominal pain and diarrhea, peripheral extremity ischemia, and dilutional hyponatremia (antidiuretic effect).

ANSWER:
B

---

10. A patient develops recurrent upper GI bleeding after chronic sclerotherapy for esophageal varices. Endoscopic examination demonstrates that the mucosa of the gastric fundus and body is granular, with multiple red spots. What is the likely diagnosis?

   A. Enterochromaffin-like hyperplasia

   B. Hypertrophic gastritis

   C. Portal hypertensive gastropathy (PHG)

   D. Gastric varices

   E. Splenic vein thrombosis

Ref.: 1, 6

COMMENTS: PHG is a condition other than varices that can cause bleeding in patients with portal hypertension. • PHG and varices often occur together, and PHG may be more common following variceal sclerotherapy. • Unlike esophageal varices, bleeding from PHG is not usually successfully treated by endoscopic methods. • Initial control may involve pharmacotherapy or an emergent TIPS or surgical shunt procedure if medical management fails.

ANSWER:
C

---

11. Which of the following treatments most effectively prevents recurrent variceal hemorrhage?

   A. Endoscopic sclerotherapy

   B. Endoscopic variceal ligation

   C. Propranolol

   D. TIPS

   E. Surgical portal systemic shunt

Ref.: 1, 3, 7, 8

COMMENTS: The majority of patients with variceal hemorrhage will rebleed (60–75%), and the mortality rate associated with each episode remains high. • Long-term management of patients who have bled from varices is directed at preventing rebleeding while maintaining hepatic function. • Unfortunately, surgical portal systemic shunts, which are the most effective method of preventing bleeding, may do so at the expense of hepatic function. • Long-term treatment with the β-adrenergic blocker propranolol (possibly in combination with nitrites) may decrease rebleeding, but the reduction of portal pressure does not seem to correspond to a reduction in pulse rate, as monitored clinically, and rebleeding rates remain high. • Chronic endoscopic sclerotherapy is currently the most common treatment, but rebleeding occurs in one third to one half of patients. • Endoscopic variceal ligation may be more effective than sclerotherapy and has fewer complications. • TIPS, although effective in the initial control of bleeding, has a high incidence of late failure due to stenosis or thrombosis. • At this time, it is best suited to short-term decompression for patients who will undergo liver transplantation or for those whose survival is limited by advanced hepatic dysfunction. • Evolving technical improvements in TIPS materials may be expected to improve patency rates.

ANSWER:
E

12. Which of the following is appropriate for prevention of variceal hemorrhage in a patient with varices that have never bled?

    A. Propranolol

    B. Endoscopic sclerosis

    C. TIPS

    D. Surgical selective shunt

    E. None of the above

Ref.: 1, 3, 9

COMMENTS: Prophylactic therapy for patients with varices is best predicated on the ability to identify patients at greater risk for bleeding (since a substantial proportion of patients with varices will not bleed) and on the availability of therapy that is safe, effective, and minimally invasive. • Of the currently available therapies—pharmacologic, endoscopic and shunting—only treatment with β-adrenergic blockade may be appropriate. • Most studies have shown some decrease in the incidence of bleeding with prophylactic propranolol. • Endoscopic sclerotherapy as prophylaxis has not yielded consistent benefit and may be detrimental to some patients. • Early trials evaluating surgical therapy in the form of portacaval shunts as prophylaxis showed a decreased risk of bleeding in operated patients but an increased risk of hepatic failure and encephalopathy and decreased survival. • Clearly, invasive and potentially morbid therapies are not indicated for bleeding prophylaxis in patients with varices who, although at risk, may never bleed.

ANSWER:
A

13. Which of the following statements is true regarding TIPS?

    A. Procedure mortality prohibits routine use.

    B. It physiologically functions as a selective shunt.

    C. Rates of variceal rebleeding are lower than with endoscopic sclerotherapy.

    D. It is contraindicated in patients with significant ascites.

Ref.: 1, 5

COMMENTS: TIPS is a vital and evolving technology in the modern management of patients with portal hypertension. • Its efficacy has been established for control of acute variceal hemorrhage, for prevention of recurrent hemorrhage in refractory patients, and for the management of intractable ascites or pleural effusions. • The procedure involves transjugular catheterization of the right (usually) hepatic vein, needle puncture of the portal vein, and placement of a sheath, followed by dilatation of the tract and stent placement. • Specific procedure-related mortality is about 2% and procedure-related morbidity 10–15%. • Contraindications include heart failure, pulmonary hypertension, severe liver failure, encephalopathy, and sometimes mechanical obstacles, such as liver masses or portal vein thrombosis. • Controlled trials have demonstrated lower rebleeding rates with TIPS than with endoscopic sclerotherapy. • However, stenosis rates remain substantial, and stenosis leads to rebleeding. • Since TIPS functions as a nonselective shunt, encephalopathy occurs in 25–50% of patients. • Developments in shunt design and construction will likely improve future patency rates. • In some centers, TIPS have all but replaced surgical portal systemic shunts for patients with portal hypertension who require shunts.

ANSWER:
C

14. Which of the following is considered a selective portal systemic shunt?

    A. End-to-side portacaval

    B. Side-to-side portacaval

    C. Distal splenorenal

    D. Central splenorenal

    E. TIPS

Ref.: 1

COMMENTS: Physiologically, portal systemic shunts can be classified as nonselective (total) shunts, which deprive the liver of blood flow, or as selective shunts, which aim to maintain portal perfusion of the liver. • The end-to-side portacaval shunt (Eck fistula) completely diverts portal flow away from the liver. • However, even side-to-side type shunts that maintain continuity between the portal vein and the liver produce a total physiologic shunt because the portal vein acts as an outflow tract from the high-pressure system and flow is diverted away from the liver. • Some of the side-to-side or lateral shunts that behave nonselectively are the side-to-side portacaval, mesocaval, mesorenal, and central splenorenal. • These shunts can be constructed by direct venovenous anastomosis or with the use of interposition grafts. • TIPS also function as nonselective shunts. • Selective shunts aim to decompress the gastroesophageal region while preserving portal flow to the liver. • Examples are the distal splenorenal (Warren shunt) and the left gastric (coronary) caval shunt (Inokuchi). • Function as a selective shunt depends on adequate division of collateral vessels when the shunt is constructed. • Even then, however, additional collaterals may develop over time, thus decreasing hepatic flow and limiting the selectivity of the shunt. • The degree to which this occurs appears to depend on both the underlying cause of portal hypertension and the extent of interruption of collateral vessels at the time of operation.

ANSWER:
C

---

15. Which of the following statements is true regarding small-diameter (8–10 mm) portacaval interposition shunts?

    A. They are intended to function as nonselective shunts.

    B. They are intended to only partially reduce portal venous pressure.

    C. Survival is superior to that associated with larger-diameter shunts.

    D. The incidence of thrombosis is similar to that associated with TIPS.

    Ref.: 1, 2, 10

COMMENTS: The goal of smaller-diameter interposition portacaval shunts is to partially reduce portal pressure by decompressing varices while maintaining hepatic perfusion. • Thus, these shunts are designed to function as partial shunts that are physiologically similar to selective shunts rather than as nonselective shunts, like their larger-diameter counterparts. • Division of collateral vessels is also performed. • Studies to date have suggested a lower failure rate than with TIPS. • Compared to larger-diameter shunts, the incidence of encephalothopy has been lower, and survival is similar. • Whether these shunts evolve toward a nonselective hemodynamic pattern over time remains to be seen.

ANSWER:
B

---

16. In patients with alcoholic cirrhosis, the advantages of a distal splenorenal shunt compared to a standard portacaval shunt include which of the following?

    A. Technically easier to perform

    B. Improved survival

    C. Better prevention of variceal hemorrhage

    D. Reduced risk of encephalopathy

    E. Better control of ascites

    Ref.: 1, 2

COMMENTS: A number of controlled trials have compared the selective distal splenorenal shunt to the nonselective portacaval shunt in patients with alcoholic cirrhosis. • Efficacy in controlling variceal hemorrhage and long-term survival are equivalent. • Half of the trials found a lower rate of encephalopathy in selectively shunted patients, and half found no difference in postoperative encephalopathy. • The distal splenorenal shunt is a more technically demanding operation. • When an emergency operation is necessary (which is relatively uncommon today), a portacaval shunt is therefore preferred. • A distal splenorenal shunt should be avoided in patients with intractable ascites because it can make it worse. • Results of selective splenorenal shunts in patients with nonalcoholic cirrhosis or portal hypertension secondary to portal vein thrombosis may differ from those in patients with alcoholic cirrhosis. • Data on the former is more limited, but some experience

has suggested less risk of encephalopathy and better overall survival.

ANSWER:
D

---

17. Which of the following is an appropriate initial treatment for hepatic ascites?

    A. Water restriction and diuretics

    B. Sodium restriction and diuretics

    C. Large-volume paracentesis

    D. Antibiotics and paracentesis

    Ref.: 1, 2, 5

COMMENTS: In portal hypertension, fluid transudation from both the liver and the intestines leads to the accumulation of ascites. • This is a sign of advanced disease, since the average survival of patients is only 2 years once ascites develops. • The intravascular fluid deficit that develops leads to secondary hyperaldosteronism. • Initial medical management consists of restriction of sodium and the use of spironolactone, an aldosterone antagonist that acts on the distal tubule. • Many patients will benefit from the addition of a thiazide or a loop diuretic (furosemide) that acts on the proximal nephron and is natriuretic. • Initial medical management will suffice for the vast majority of patients. • For those with persisting problems, large-volume paracentesis can be useful. • Antibiotics are not indicated for the initial treatment of ascites but are used when spontaneous bacterial peritonitis occurs as a complication.

ANSWER:
B

---

18. A Child's C cirrhotic patient has intractable ascites and esophageal varices that have not bled. Which of the following is the best treatment?

    A. Peritoneovenous shunt

    B. TIPS

    C. Side-to-side portacaval shunt

    D. End-to-side portacaval shunt

    Ref.: 1, 2

COMMENTS: Medically intractable ascites occurs in patients with end-stage liver disease. • The definitive treatment in this situation is liver transplantation. • As a prelude, TIPS is probably the preferred option today. • It is quite effective in controlling ascites, although it has an important associated rate of encephalopathy. • In the past, peritoneovenous shunts were used, but the results were often less than satisfactory. • Peritoneovenous shunts do not prolong survival compared to medical management and can lead to problems with shunt malfunction, bacterial peritonitis, coagulopathy, variceal hemorrhage, and heart failure. • Any shunt procedure for ascites requires a nonselective, side-to-side arrangement (end-to-side portacaval or distal splenorenal shunts are therefore contraindicated). • Surgical shunts are not indicated for treatment of ascites alone in a patient who has not had bleeding varices.

ANSWER:
B

19. Which of the following veins is not divided during a distal splenorenal shunt?

A. Left adrenal vein

B. Inferior mesenteric vein

C. Superior mesenteric vein

D. Coronary vein

E. Pancreatic branches of splenic vein

Ref.: 1, 2

COMMENTS: The selective distal splenorenal shunt is performed by end-to-side anastomosis of the distal end of the divided splenic vein to the left renal vein, thereby decompressing gastroesophageal collaterals through the short gastric vessels. • The left adrenal vein and inferior mesenteric vein are ligated during dissection of the renal vein and splenic vein, respectively. • Vessels are divided to separate the gastrosplenic portion of the splanchnic circulation from the superior mesenteric portion. • For this reason, the left gastric vein (coronary vein) and right gastroepiploic vein are divided. • In addition, it has been recognized that pancreatic branches of the splenic vein should be divided to prevent the late development of peripancreatic collaterals, which would divert hepatic portal blood flow and negate the selectivity of the shunt.

ANSWER:
C

20. Which of the following technical situations would be least likely to interfere with construction of a portacaval shunt?

A. Portal vein thrombosis

B. Large caudate lobe of liver

C. Previous splenectomy

D. Previous operations for biliary stricture

Ref.: 1, 2

COMMENTS: Selection of the appropriate type of shunting operation for a particular patient must consider the cause of the portal hypertension, the clinical manifestations, the status of the liver and the technical demands of each operation. • Portacaval shunts can be difficult or not possible when there are extensive adhesions from previous right upper quadrant operations. • The presence of a large caudate lobe may prevent direct approximation of the portal vein and inferior vena cava. • This can sometimes be circumvented by placing an interposition graph. • Previous splenectomy has no bearing on technical construction of a portacaval shunt but would preclude performance of a selective distal splenorenal shunt.

ANSWER:
C

21. A 45-year-old man with chronic pancreatitis presents with hematemesis. Endoscopic examination demonstrates gastric varices with clot and no other abnormality. Which of the following is the most appropriate treatment?

A. Splenectomy

B. Pancreatic resection

C. TIPS

D. Portacaval shunt

E. Distal splenorenal shunt

Ref.: 1

COMMENTS: Left-sided or sinistral portal hypertension is caused by splenic vein thrombosis, which, in turn, is most commonly associated with pancreatitis or pancreatic tumors. • This can lead to gastric varices without an esophageal component. • Portal venous pressure is not elevated. • Splenectomy should solve the problem.

ANSWER:
A

22. A 28-year-old woman with portal venous thrombosis has rebled from esophageal varices after repeated endoscopic attempts at management. Angiography demonstrates thrombosis of the portal, splenic, and superior mesenteric veins. Which of the following interventions would be least appropriate?

A. Esophageal transection and reanastamosis alone

B. Esophageal resection and intestinal interposition

C. Esophageal transection, extensive esophagogastric devascularization, and splenectomy

D. Splenectomy alone

Ref.: 1, 2, 11, 12

COMMENTS: Numerous nonshunt operations have been devised and performed for esophagogastric varices. • The goal of these procedures is to interrupt communication between the high-pressure splanchnic circulation and the varices and/or to ablate the varices. • Worldwide, these operations have been applied to different types of patients with varying results. • They were more commonly considered before the availability of endoscopic treatments for patients with poor hepatic reserve because of the risk of hepatic failure and encephalopathy if a shunt was performed. • Currently, in the United States, nonshunt operations may be useful for patients with failed endoscopic management and lack of suitable vessels for shunting when the patients are not imminent candidates for liver transplantation. • Esophageal or gastric transection and reanastomosis with stapling devices may be the simplest approach but has a high rebleeding rate. • The results of the more extensive Sugiura procedure (esophageal transection, extensive devascularization of the distal esophagus and proximal stomach, and splenectomy) have not been consistent and seem to be dependent on the population of patients undergoing the procedure. • Esophageal resection with jejunal or colonic interposition can be effective but also has not been widely practiced. • Splenectomy alone will not decompress esophageal varices.

ANSWER:
D

23. With regard to portal hypertension in children, which of the following is true?

A. Congenital hepatic fibrosis is the most common cause.

B. Variceal bleeding is the most common cause of massive hematemesis in children.

C. Acute variceal hemorrhage usually requires operation.

D. Portosystemic shunts are contraindicated because of the long-term risk of encephalopathy.

Ref.: 2, 13

COMMENTS: Unlike portal hypertension in adults, portal hypertension in children is most commonly caused by extrahepatic portal venous thrombosis. • Other causes include liver disease due to hepatitis, metabolic defects, and congenital hepatic fibrosis. • Although bleeding from esophageal varices accounts for less than 15% of upper GI bleeding in adults, it is the most common cause of massive upper GI hemorrhage in children. • Serial endoscopic management has become the mainstay of treatment. • Liver transplantation is indicated for progressive liver disease or for correction of the underlying inherited defect. • Shunt procedures may be indicated when endoscopic management fails or when compliance and follow-up are an issue. • The results of surgical shunts are excellent in children without underlying liver disease. • The technical details of shunt construction depend on vein size and anatomy, and numerous options are available.

ANSWER:
B

---

24. In Budd-Chiari syndrome, portal hypertension results from which of the following?

A. Massive splenomegaly

B. Cavernous hemangioma of the liver

C. Hepatic vein obstruction

D. Arterial venous fistula

Ref.: 2, 5

COMMENTS: Budd-Chiari syndrome is an unusual and challenging condition resulting from obstruction of hepatic venous outflow from the liver. • Clinically, this causes hepatomegaly, pain, and ascites. • Patients may present with a chronic indolent course, end-stage liver disease, or acute fulminant hepatic failure. • Hepatic outflow obstruction may be due to many causes but most commonly involves thrombosis due to hematologic or coagulation disorders. • It can occur in women during the postpartum period or who are on oral contraceptives. • Other causes include mechanical obstruction by tumor or membranous webs in the inferior vena cava and veno-occlusive disease of the terminal hepatic venules.

ANSWER:
C

---

25. Which of the following information is not necessary in determining therapy for Budd-Chiari syndrome?

A. Albumin content of ascitic fluid

B. Protein C levels

C. Findings on liver biopsy

D. Results of an inferior venacavagram

E. Wedged hepatic venous pressure

Ref.: 2, 5

COMMENTS: Treatment of Budd-Chiari syndrome depends on the underlying cause, the status of the liver, and the anatomy and hemodynamics of the portal system and inferior vena cava. • Patients with advanced liver disease or acute fulminant hepatic failure are candidates for liver transplantation. • Histologic findings on liver biopsy are crucial. • TIPS may be a temporizing measure for these patients. • For patients in whom liver function is preserved, treatment is a nonselective, lateral-type shunt. • A mesocaval interposition graft is preferred by some experts because the caudate lobe (which drains into the inferior vena cava independently of the other hepatic veins) is typically hypertrophied and would interfere with a portacaval shunt. • Also, a mesocaval shunt may be less problematic later if the patient eventually needs a liver transplant. • Patients with Budd-Chiari syndrome can have inferior vena cava obstruction at suprahepatic or intrahepatic levels. • If caval pressure is as high as portal pressure, a standard portal systemic shunt alone would be inadequate. • Assessment of the anatomy of the inferior vena cava and hepatic veins and pressure measurements are critical to determining this. • Albumin content of ascitic fluid tends to be high in Budd-Chiari syndrome compared to normal cirrhotic ascites. • While this is of diagnostic interest, it does not affect treatment.

ANSWER:
A

---

26. Initial management of a patient with hepatic encephalopathy should include which one of the following?

A. Protein restriction to 25 g/d

B. Administration of lactulose

C. Administration of neomycin

D. Infusion of branched-chain amino acids

Ref.: 1, 5, 14

COMMENTS: The first step in the management of hepatic encephalopathy is to identify and treat any of the common precipitating factors: GI bleeding, infection, hypokalemia, dehydration, sedatives, or other medications. • Lactulose, a nonabsorbable disaccharide, is given to acidify the colonic environment, thus decreasing absorption of ammonia and inhibiting growth of the bacteria that produce ammonia. • Lactulose is also an osmotic cathartic that helps eliminate toxic substances. • The recommended protein intake for patients with liver disease is 1–1.5 g/kg/day. • If response to lactulose is not satisfactory, temporary mild protein restriction (minimum 40 g/day) may be useful, but more severe restriction is not consistent with positive nitrogen balance and may be detrimental. • Neomycin is active against intestinal bacteria that produce urease. • Because it can cause nephrotoxicity and ototoxicity, it has been recommended that it be added only if lactulose and protein restriction are not sufficient. • Neomycin is not indicated on a chronic basis. • Oral or infused branched-chain amino acids may be useful in refractory patients, but efficacy has not been conclusively established. • Many other treatment modalities have been investigated but are not first-line therapies, including administration of a nonurease-producing bacteria, treatment for *Helicobacter pylori* infection, sodium benzoate, and benzodiazepine-receptor antagonists. • Patients with postshunt encephalopathy (surgical or TIPS) may occasionally require occlusion of the shunt or of major collateral vessels.

ANSWER:
B

27. All but which of the following may be appropriate in the management of portal venous injury?

A. Direct venorrhaphy

B. Portal vein ligation

C. End-to-end anastamosis

D. Grafted interposition

E. Portal vein ligation with portal systemic shunt

Ref.: 1

COMMENTS: Portal vein injuries generally result from penetrating trauma and is associated with a high fatality rate. • The preferred method of management is some form of repair, by lateral venorrhaphy, when possible, or by reanastomosis or graft interposition. • If repair is not possible, the portal vein may be ligated. • Portal systemic shunting is not advocated. • It is more dangerous than ligation alone and entails a risk of hepatic encephalopathy.

ANSWER:
E

REFERENCES

1. Townsend CM Jr., Beauchamp RD, Evers BM, et al (eds): *Sabiston Textbook of Surgery: The Biological Basis of Modern Surgical Practice,* 16th ed. Saunders, Philadelphia, 2001.
2. Greenfield LJ, Mulholland M, Oldham T, et al (eds): *Surgery: Scientific Principles and Practice,* 2nd ed. Lippincott-Raven, Philadelphia, 1996.
3. D'Amico G, Pagliaro L, Bosch J: The treatment of portal hypertension: a meta-analytic review. *Hepatology* 22:332–354, 1995.
4. Pugh RN, Murray-Lyon IM, Dawson JL, et al: Transection of the esophagus for bleeding esophageal varices. *Br J Surg* 60:646–649, 1973.
5. Cameron JL (ed): *Current Surgical Therapy,* 7th ed. CV Mosby, St. Louis, 2001.
6. D'Amico G, Montalbano L, Traina M, et al: Natural history of congestive gastropathy in cirrhosis. *Gastroenterology* 99:1558–1564, 1990.
7. Laine L, Cook D: Endoscopic ligation compared with sclerotherapy for treatment of esophageal variceal bleeding: a meta-analysis. *Ann Intern Med* 123:280, 1995.
8. Rikkers LF: The changing spectrum of treatment for variceal bleeding. *Ann Surg* 228:536–546, 1998.
9. Grace ND: Prevention of initial variceal hemorrhage [Review]. *Gastroenterol Clin North Am* 21:149, 1992.
10. Sarfeh IJ, Rypins EB: Partial versus total portacaval shunt in alcoholic cirrhosis: results of a prospective randomized clinical trial. *Ann Surg* 219:353–361, 1994.
11. Dagenais M, Langer B, Taylor BR, et al: Experience with radical esophagogastric devascularization procedures (surgical) for variceal bleeding outside Japan [Review]. *World J Surg* 18:222–228, 1994.
12. Sugiura M, Futagawa S: Esophageal transection with paraesophagogastric devascularization in the treatment of esophageal varices. *World J Surg* 8:673–679, 1984.
13. Hassall E: Nonsurgical treatments for portal hypertension in children [Review]. *Gastrointest Endosc Clin North Am* 4:223–258, 1994.
14. Riordan SM, Williams R: Treatment of hepatic encephalopathy: a review article. *N Engl J Med* 337:473–479, 1997.

C H A P T E R 39

Biliary System

Daniel J. Deziel, M.D.

1. During palpation of the hepatoduodenal ligament, a pulsation is felt behind and slightly to the right of the common bile duct. Which of the following does this pulsation most likely represent?

A. Normal common hepatic artery

B. Normal right hepatic artery

C. Replaced right hepatic artery

D. Gastroduodenal artery

Ref.: 1, 2

COMMENTS: The most common variation in hepatic arterial anatomy is the origination of the right hepatic artery from the superior mesenteric artery. • This is a replaced hepatic artery and not simply an accessory vessel that can be sacrificed with impunity. • When an operation is performed in the right upper abdomen, the pulsations encountered in the porta hepatis and gastrohepatic ligaments should be assessed. • If the hepatic artery is absent or small, the surgeon must be alert to the possibility of a replaced hepatic vessel. • When the right hepatic artery originates from the superior mesenteric artery, it courses posterior to the head of the pancreas and the portal vein and is usually identified posterolateral to the common bile duct. • Only rarely does a replaced right hepatic artery course through the pancreas. • A replaced left hepatic artery originates from the left gastric artery and is located in the gastrohepatic ligament, where it is frequently encountered during operations on the stomach and gastroesophageal junction.

A N S W E R :
C

2. With regard to the blood supply to the common hepatic and common bile ducts, which of the following statements is/are true?

A. Blood supply to the supraduodenal bile duct has a primarily longitudinal pattern.

B. Blood supply to the bifurcation of the common hepatic duct is the least constant, which explains the high frequency of hilar strictures.

C. Blood supply to the common bile duct is derived primarily from the common hepatic artery.

D. The segmental end-artery arrangement of the blood supply contributes to the occurrence of bile duct stricture.

Ref.: 1–3

COMMENTS: Ischemia is an important contributing factor to the development of postoperative bile duct stricture. • The blood supply to the area of the bile duct bifurcation and the distal retropancreatic duct is primarily lateral in arrangement, whereas the blood supply to the supraduodenal portion of the bile duct has a primarily axial or longitudinal pattern. • The so-called 3 and 9 o'clock arteries and other small vessels arise from the right hepatic artery and the retroduodenal artery, which is a branch of the gastroduodenal artery, and form the skeleton of a pericholedochal plexus of vessels. • An additional source of blood supply to the common bile duct can be the retroportal artery. • This vessel arises from the celiac axis or the superior mesenteric artery and generally joins the retroduodenal artery; but in approximately one third of individuals it ascends the back of the common bile duct to the right hepatic artery. • The portion of the bile duct supplied by the longitudinal vessels receives most of its arterial blood supply from below, rendering the proximal portion of the duct subject to ischemia after injury or transection.

A N S W E R :
A

3. Match the numbered layers (1–3) of the gallbladder wall with the following.

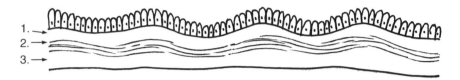

1. →
2. →
3. →

A. Lamina propria

B. Smooth muscle

C. Muscularis mucosa

D. Submucosa

E. Subserosa

Ref.: 1

COMMENTS: The histologic structure of the gallbladder consists of five layers: (1) epithelium, (2) lamina propria, (3) smooth muscle, (4) subserosal connective tissue, and (5) serosa. • Unlike the bowel, there is no submucosa or muscularis mucosa. • The epithelium is composed of columnar cells. • The lamina propria has nerves, vessels, lymphocytes, and supportive connective tissue. • The smooth muscle is thin, loosely arranged, and not well defined.

ANSWER:

1-A; 2-B; 3-E

4. Which of the following statements best describes the anatomy of the bile duct shown in this cholangiogram?

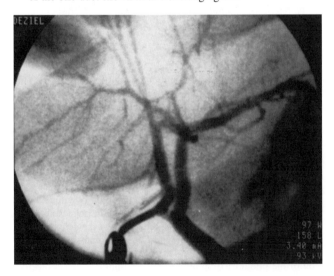

A. Normal "textbook" pattern

B. Accessory right hepatic duct

C. Separately inserting right sectoral duct

D. "Crossover" right hepatic duct

Ref.: 2–4

COMMENTS: Variations in the anatomy of the extrahepatic bile ducts occur commonly. • The surgeon must be cognizant of these variations and learn to recognize and identify them in order to prevent inadvertent injury of the bile ducts during cholecystectomy. • Approximately two thirds of individuals have the "textbook" anatomy, with the anterior (segments V and VIII) and posterior (segments VI and VII) sectoral ducts from the right joining to form a main right hepatic duct, which then joins the main left hepatic duct to form the common hepatic duct. • In 15–25% of individuals, the anterior or posterior duct from the right inserts separately into the common hepatic duct. • When the posterior duct inserts separately, it is usually at a greater distance caudally from the junction of the left duct and the other right duct than when the anterior duct inserts separately. • This duct is therefore at risk of injury during cholecystectomy if the anatomy is not recognized.

One of the most common variations in cystic duct anatomy is direct insertion into one of these separately inserting right hepatic ducts, as the pictured cholangiogram demonstrates. • The terms *crossover duct* and *accessory duct* are misnomers for this arrangement. • True accessory ducts are rare and occur when there is embryologic duplication of the bud that forms the bile ducts and liver. • True accessory ducts may enter the gallbladder or the bile ducts but are small and can be ligated. • Use of the term *aberrant ducts* should be discouraged, since these are common normal anatomic variations.

ANSWER:

C

5. Identify the structures labeled in this *longitudinal* laparoscopic ultrasound scan of the hepatoduodenal ligament.

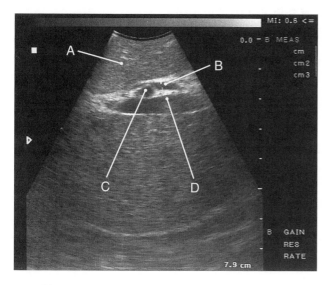

a. Liver

b. Portal vein

c. Right hepatic artery

d. Common bile duct

Ref.: 5

COMMENTS: See Question 6.

6. Identify the structures labeled in this *transverse* laparoscopic ultrasound scan of the hepatoduodenal ligament.

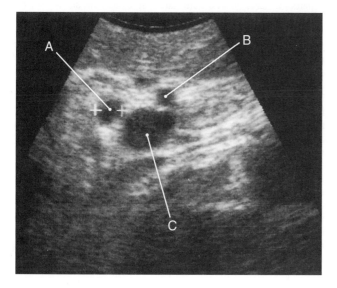

a. Common bile duct

b. Portal vein

c. Right hepatic artery

d. Common hepatic artery

Ref.: 5, 6

COMMENTS: A general principle of ultrasonography is that any structure visualized in one plane should also be examined in a second plane at a 90-degree angle to the first view to ascertain where and what the structure is. • Intraoperative ultrasound imaging, whether laparoscopic or open, is an accurate method of assessing the bile duct for stones during cholecystectomy. • The longitudinal and transverse scans of the hepatoduodenal ligament in Questions 5 and 6 depict typical anatomy. • In the longitudinal plane, the common bile duct appears as a hypoechoic, tubular structure parallel and anterior to the portal vein. • The normal upper-limit diameter of the duct at this location is 6 mm by ultrasound imaging criteria. • In other words, a nondilated duct should not exceed one half the diameter of the neighboring portal vein. • The right hepatic artery most commonly crosses behind the bile duct and is viewed in cross section on the longitudinal scan. • In the transverse plane, the structures of the hepatoduodenal ligament have a "Mickey Mouse" configuration. • The cross sections of the bile duct and common hepatic artery appear as smaller hypoechoic circles anterior to the larger portal vein.

ANSWERS:
Question 5: A-a; B-d; C-c; D-b
Question 6: A-a; B-d; C-b

7. With regard to the composition of hepatic bile, which of the following statements is/are true?

A. It contains 90% water.

B. The concentration of bicarbonate is lower than in plasma.

C. The primary organic solute is conjugated bilirubin.

D. The osmolarity of hepatic bile is similar to that of plasma.

Ref.: 2, 3, 7

COMMENTS: Hepatic bile is composed of 90% water and 10% electrolytes and organic solutes. • The inorganic electrolyte composition is similar to that of plasma, although the concentration of sodium, potassium, calcium, and bicarbonate is somewhat higher and that of chloride somewhat lower. • The osmolarity of hepatic bile is approximately 300 mOsm, which is also similar to that of plasma. • Bile acids make up approximately two thirds of the organic solute composition. • The remainder is approximately 20% phospholipid, 4–5% cholesterol, 4–5% proteins, and less than 1% bilirubin, which is predominantly in conjugated form. • Other organic solutes, including drugs, hormones, and dyes, may be present as well.

ANSWER:
A, D

8. For which of the following functions is bile essential?

A. Triglyceride absorption

B. Vitamin D absorption

C. Bilirubin excretion

D. Cholesterol excretion

E. Lipase transport

Ref.: 3

COMMENTS: Bile has a number of critical functions related to the digestion and absorption of fats and the elimination of various endogenous and exogenous substances. • Bile interacts with pancreatic lipase and colipase in the intraluminal hydrolysis of dietary triglycerides. • It subsequently solubilizes the monoglycerides and fatty acids produced by triglyceride metabolism by forming mixed micelles. • The micelles facilitate mucosal uptake of triglycerides by permitting transport across the water barrier adjacent to the enterocyte membrane. • Although bile therefore plays an important role in triglyceride absorption, a substantial amount of triglycerides can be absorbed, even in the absence of bile, because of the long length of the intestine. • The same is not true for fat-soluble vitamins A, D, E, and K, which are minimally water soluble and are not absorbed in any substantial amount in the absence of micelles. • Patients with long-standing cholestasis generally require supplementation of these fat-soluble vitamins to prevent the clinical effects of deficiency. • Bile is the sole pathway for elimination of bilirubin and cholesterol from the body. • Bilirubin is secreted into hepatic bile by an active transport mechanism following hepatic uptake and conjugation. • Cholesterol is eliminated both by synthesis of bile acids from cholesterol and by solubilization of cholesterol in bile during secretion.

ANSWER:
B, C, D

9. What change(s) in bile flow would be expected in a patient with an external biliary fistula?

   A. Increased total canalicular flow

   B. Decreased bile acid–dependent canalicular flow

   C. Increased bile acid–dependent canalicular flow

   D. Decreased bile acid–independent canalicular flow

   E. Increased bile acid–independent canalicular flow

Ref.: 2, 3

COMMENTS: Approximately 600 ml of hepatic bile is produced daily. • Seventy-five percent of hepatic bile is formed by bile canaliculi, and the remainder is secreted by the ducts. • **Canalicular** bile can be divided into approximately equal bile acid–dependent and bile acid–independent fractions. • The **bile acid–dependent** fraction results from active secretion of bile acids by the hepatocyte. • This secretion depends on intestinal absorption and enterohepatic circulation of bile acids. • Patients with external bile losses therefore have reduced bile acid–dependent canalicular flow and therefore reduced total canalicular flow. • The **bile acid–independent** portion of canalicular flow is the result of secretion of inorganic electrolytes. • **Ductular secretion** modifies canalicular bile flow by adding fluid and inorganic electrolytes.

ANSWER:
B

10. Which of the following is/are primary bile acids in humans?

   A. Cholic acid

   B. Deoxycholic acid

   C. Chenodeoxycholic acid

   D. Lithocholic acid

   E. Ursodeoxycholic acid

Ref.: 1–3, 8

COMMENTS: The primary bile acids cholic acid and chenodeoxycholic acid are synthesized from cholesterol in the liver. • The secondary bile acids deoxycholic acid and lithocholic acid

are formed in the intestine as the result of bacterial enzyme activity. • 7-Ketolithocholic acid is also a secondary bile acid. • It is converted to the tertiary bile acid ursodeoxycholic acid in the liver.

ANSWER:
A, C

11. Match each metabolic step of enterohepatic bile acid circulation in the left-hand column with the appropriate anatomic site or sites in the right-hand column.

   A. Bile acid conjugation with glycine or taurine
   B. Bile acid deconjugation
   C. Conversion of primary bile acids to secondary bile acids
   D. Active intestinal transport of bile acid
   E. Passive intestinal resorption of bile acids

   a. Liver
   b. Bile ducts
   c. Gallbladder
   d. Small intestine
   e. Colon

Ref.: 1, 3–5

COMMENTS: See Question 12.

12. With regard to enterohepatic circulation of bile acids, which of the following is/are true?

   A. Bile secreted by the liver contains both primary and secondary bile acids.

   B. Ninety-five percent of bile acids are reabsorbed in the intestine.

   C. Interruption of enterohepatic circulation increases hepatocyte secretion of bile acids.

   D. Bile acid deficiency results in vitamin C malabsorption.

Ref.: 1–3, 8

COMMENTS: Enterohepatic cycling of bile acids begins at the hepatocyte level. • Bile acids are conjugated in the liver with glycine or taurine, secreted into the biliary system, concentrated and stored in the gallbladder, and then delivered to the duodenum after gallbladder contraction. • Most bile acids are efficiently resorbed in the intestine. • The site and mechanism of intestine absorption differs according to the form of the bile acid and its corresponding lipid solubility. • Conjugated bile acids are predominantly ionized in the intestinal pH range and are relatively lipid insoluble. • Conjugated forms are therefore absorbed by an active transport mechanism in the terminal ileum. • This mechanism accounts for approximately 70–80% of the enterohepatic circulation. • Bacterial deconjugation of bile acids occurs in the colon and small intestine, as does conversion of primary bile acids to secondary forms. • Deconjugation raises the pKa of bile acids and enables resorption by passive nonionic diffusion, which occurs predominantly in the colon but to some extent in the small intestine as well. • Both primary and secondary bile acids are resorbed and taken back to the liver. • Unconjugated forms are then reconjugated and resecreted. • Hepatic bile therefore contains both primary and secondary bile acids, with the primary bile acids normally constituting 60–90% of the total bile pool. • Hepatic synthesis of new bile acids approximates fecal losses of 300–600 mg/day.

The bile acid pool cycles four to eight times per day, and hepatic secretion is dependent on enteral return. • Disruption of this cycle therefore diminishes bile acid secretion. • Clinical conditions that may be associated with bile acid malabsorption include ileal disease or resection, small-bowel dysmotility or obstruction, and blind-loop syndrome. • Clinical consequences of this disordered physiology may include fat malabsorption, deficiencies of fat-soluble vitamins (A, D, E, and K), choleretic diarrhea caused by impaired colonic water absorption by bile acids, and gallstones.

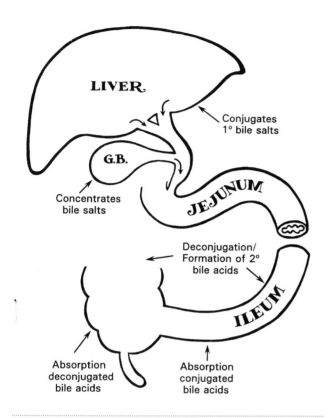

ANSWERS:
Question 11: A-a; B-d,e; C-d,e; D-d; E-d,e
Question 12: A, B

13. Normal functions of the gallbladder epithelium include all but which of the following?

 A. Absorption of water

 B. Absorption of sodium and chloride

 C. Absorption of conjugated bile acids

 D. Secretion of hydrogen iron

 E. Secretion of glycoproteins

Ref.: 1, 8

COMMENTS: The primary functions of the gallbladder are to concentrate and store bile between feedings. • The gallbladder epithelium absorbs solutes and water across concentration gradients by both active and passive mechanisms. • The main concentrating force is active absorption of sodium (coupled to chloride transport), which leads to passive absorption of water. • Abnormalities in gallbladder absorption are part of the pathophysiologic process of gallstone formation. • Absorption of organic solutes is normally minimal and depends on their lipid solubility. • Unconjugated bile acids are more lipid soluble than are their conjugated forms. • Absorption of unconjugated bile acids that form in the presence of bacteria or inflammation damages the mucosa, thereby promoting absorption of other solutes and destabilizing cholesterol in solution. • The gallbladder epithelium is also secretory. • Secretion of hydrogen ion lowers the pH of gallbladder bile in relationship

to hepatic bile. • Mucin glycoproteins secreted by the mucosa may have both a protective function and a critical role as a nucleating factor during gallstone formation.

ANSWER:
C

14. Which of the following usually produces gallbladder contraction?

 A. Cholinergic stimulation

 B. Adrenergic stimulation

 C. Cholecystokinin (CCK)

 D. Vasoactive intestinal peptide (VIP)

 E. Somatostatin

Ref.: 1

COMMENTS: Gallbladder function is subject to many neurohormonal influences. • Historically, parasympathetic vagal nerves have been considered responsible for gallbladder contraction, and stimulation of sympathetic nerves from the celiac ganglion has been thought to cause gallbladder relaxation. • Regulation of gallbladder function is actually a much more complex process that involves the interaction of various neural, hormonal, and peptidergic stimuli on various receptors located on the gallbladder muscle, blood vessels, and nerves. • Cholinergic stimuli (including vagal) and CCK cause contraction. • CCK receptors can be found on both gallbladder smooth muscle cells and intrinsic cholinergic nerves. • Adrenergic stimulation (sympathetic) usually causes relaxation, but selective stimulation of certain adrenergic receptors can cause contraction. • VIP and somatostatin inhibit gallbladder contraction, which can account for clinical biliary manifestations in patients with tumors that secrete those substances or in patients being administered somatostatin agonists. • Many other peptides, hormones, and neurotransmitters may also affect gallbladder function, although their clinical significance is unknown.

ANSWER:
A, C

15. Gallbladder emptying is influenced by all but which of the following?

 A. Sphincter of Oddi resistance

 B. Common bile duct peristalsis

 C. Postprandial CCK

 D. Fasting motilin

Ref.: 1, 8

COMMENTS: Bile flow in the biliary tract varies according to the *fasting* or *fed* state of the individual. • CCK, which is released by the duodenum in response to ingestion of food substances, is the most important postprandial stimulant of gallbladder contraction and relaxation of the sphincter of Oddi, permitting bile delivery to the intestine. • Normal contraction of the gallbladder in response to meals results in approximately 80% emptying in 2 hr. • The common bile duct is for the most part a passive conduit in humans and is not thought to play an active role in biliary motility. • Filling of the gallbladder after it has emptied depends on neural and hormonal factors that relax the gallbladder and increase resistance of the sphincter of Oddi. • During the interdigestive period, the gallbladder gradually fills, but this filling is interrupted by cyclic periods of emptying, during which time approximately one third of the gallbladder volume is dispensed. • This cyclic pattern during fasting is correlated to the interdigestive myoelectric migratory complex of the intestine and seems to be related to increased levels of plasma motilin. • Motilin is a 21–amino-acid peptide, and plasma motilin levels vary cyclically during the fasting period.

ANSWER:
B

16. Which of the following levels of enzyme activity is most likely to be present in a nonobese individual with cholesterol gallstones?

A. Increased 3-hydroxy-3-methylglutaryl coenzyme A (HMG-CoA) reductase activity

B. Decreased HMG-CoA reductase activity

C. Increased 7α-hydroxylase activity

D. Decreased 7α-hydroxylase activity

Ref.: 3

COMMENTS: Cholesterol solubility in bile depends on the concentration of cholesterol relative to bile acids and phospholipids. • Whereas an increase in hepatocyte cholesterol synthesis and secretion has been implicated in obese patients with gallstones, a relative deficiency of bile acid secretion is thought to be responsible for gallstone formation in many nonobese patients. • HMG-CoA reductase catalyzes the conversion of HMG-CoA to mevalonate and is the early rate-limiting enzyme in cholesterol synthesis. • The primary bile acids are formed from cholesterol, and the rate-limiting enzyme in this process is 7α-hydroxylase. • Relative imbalances in the activities of these enzymes therefore affect cholesterol solubility in bile.

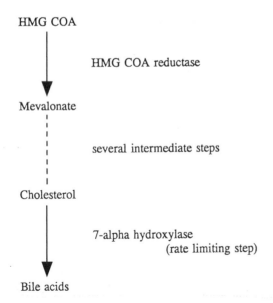

ANSWER:
D

17. Which of the following is/are decreased following cholecystectomy?

A. Size of the bile acid pool

B. Rate of enterohepatic recycling

C. Rate of bile acid secretion

D. Cholesterol solubility in bile

Ref.: 2

COMMENTS: The total size of the bile acid pool is diminished by cholecystectomy as a result of loss of the gallbladder reservoir. • However, cholecystectomy produces a more continuous flow of bile into the intestine, which increases the frequency of enterohepatic cycling and stimulates bile acid secretion. • For these reasons, even though the size of the bile acid pool is diminished, cholecystectomy improves cholesterol solubility in bile. • The solubility of cholesterol in bile depends on the relative molar concentration of cholesterol in relation to the concentrations of bile acids and the phospholipid lecithin. • This relationship, described by W. Admirand and D.M. Small in 1969, is graphically depicted by this familiar diagram.

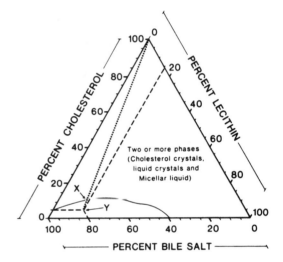

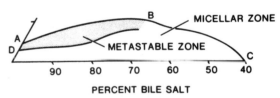

The three biliary lipids plotted as mole percentages on triangular coordinates. On the upper diagram, point Y represents a bile with 15% phospholipid (lecithin), 80% bile salt, and 5% cholesterol that is within the micellar zone. The dotted line connecting Y to the apex of the triangle intersects at point X, the line of maximum solubility of cholesterol, as defined by Admirand and Small. To calculate the saturation index of the bile represented by Y, the actual mole percent cholesterol (5) is divided by the mole percent cholesterol at point X (9), to give a value of 0.56. The expanded lower diagram shows a line DBC that indicates the true equilibrium solubility line of bile. Bile with a lipid composition represented by a point between ABC and DBC lies within a metastable zone where cholesterol may require nucleating factors to precipitate from solution. It is usual to calculate the saturation index using the line DBC and not ABC. (From Way LW, Pellegrini CA: *Surgery of the Gallbladder and Bile Ducts.* Saunders, Philadelphia, 1987.)

ANSWER:
A

18. Which of the following is the primary form in which cholesterol is transported in bile?

A. Dissolved as free cholesterol

B. Dissolved as conjugated cholesterol

C. Attached to a protein carrier

D. Solubilized in mixed micelles

E. Solubilized in phospholipid vesicles

Ref.: 1, 8

COMMENTS: Cholesterol is insoluble in water, and bile is a solution composed of 90% water. • The solubility of cholesterol in bile depends on the presence of bile acids and the phospholipid lecithin. • These molecules aggregate into physicochemical structures that shelter cholesterol within a nonpolar, hydrophobic center and thus permit dissolution. • For many years, the mixed micelle was recognized as the structure principally responsible for cholesterol solubility. • Subsequently, it has been found that most cholesterol is usually solubilized in larger bilayered lipid structures known as vesicles. • The balance between micelles and vesicles is a dynamic process. • Recognition of these vesicles is particularly important because crystallization of cholesterol to form stones is thought to occur from this phase.

ANSWER:
E

19. Which of the following is/are not part of the process of cholesterol gallstone formation?

A. Cholesterol supersaturation of bile

B. Bilirubin deconjugation

C. Crystal nucleation

D. Glyocalyx production

E. Stone growth

Ref.: 1, 2, 7, 8

COMMENTS: Cholesterol gallstone formation is a complex physicochemical process. • The requisite steps in the genesis of cholesterol stones can be conceptually simplified as cholesterol saturation, nucleation, and stone growth. • The cholesterol content of bile must exceed the capacity for bile to solubilize cholesterol in vesicles and micelles. • Cholesterol supersaturation alone, however, is not sufficient to cause stones, since this process can occur in normal individuals. • Nucleation must also take place; that is, cholesterol monohydrate crystals must form and aggregate. • Finally, the crystals must enlarge by fusion or continued solid deposition to produce a stone large enough to be clinically relevant. • Bacterial infection is thought to be an important pathogenetic factor in the development of some pigment stones but not generally in cholesterol stones. • Bacterial infection is associated with deconjugation of bilirubin and subsequent formation of insoluble calcium bilirubinate complexes. • Bacterial infection can also result in the production of glycocalyx, an adhesive glycoprotein that may play a role in pigment stone formation.

ANSWER:
B, D

20. Nucleation during cholesterol gallstone formation appears to involve all but which of the following?

A. Mixed micelles

B. Biliary vesicles

C. Biliary calcium

D. Gallbladder stasis

E. Mucus secretion

Ref.: 1, 8

COMMENTS: Nucleation, the formation and aggregation of solid cholesterol monohydrate crystals, is a critical step in gallstone formation. • Although the process is not entirely understood, it has been determined that there are important factors that promote nucleation and some antinucleating factors that may protect against stone formation. • Mucin glycoproteins secreted by the gallbladder epithelium are thought to be key nucleating factors. • Increased mucus secretion occurs whenever there is stasis, which precedes the development of crystals. • Prostaglandins stimulate mucus production in animal models, and prostaglandin inhibitors can prevent stones. • Nucleation appears to be associated with the vesicular fraction of bile rather than with the mixed micelles. • Biliary calcium also plays a role in the formation of both cholesterol and pigment stones. • Calcium levels in gallbladder bile are increased during cholesterol stone formation. • Calcium affects the absorptive function of the gallbladder epithelium and may also promote nucleation from vesicles. • An understanding that the events of vesicle fusion, nucleation, and stone growth occur *in* the gallbladder is a basic foundation for cholecystectomy as definitive treatment for cholesterol gallstone disease.

ANSWER:
A

21. Which of the following is/are associated with an increased incidence of cholesterol gallstone formation?

A. Obesity

B. Rapid weight loss

C. Total parenteral nutrition

D. Exogenous estrogen

E. Ileal resection

Ref.: 1, 2

COMMENTS: Changes in bile composition that either increase the relative concentration of cholesterol or decrease the relative concentration of bile acids favor cholesterol gallstone formation. • Situations that lead to increased hepatocyte cholesterol secretion include obesity, rapid weight loss, diets high in calories and polyunsaturated fats, and estrogen therapy. • Drugs that inhibit HMG-CoA reductase are used to treat hypercholesterolemia and may prevent gallstone formation. • Theoretically, a relative decrease in the size of the bile acid pool would predispose a person to cholesterol gallstone formation in situations in which there were excessive bile acid losses (e.g., ileal disease or resection) or decreased bile acid synthesis (e.g., decreased 7α-hydroxylase activity). • Stones associated with ileal disease or resection are of the pigment type, however. • Total parenteral nutrition is also associated with pigment gallstones in a high proportion of patients, depending on the duration of therapy.

ANSWER:
A, B, D

22. Which of the following is the main chemical component of pigment gallstones?

   A. Cholesterol

   B. Calcium bilirubinate

   C. Calcium carbonate

   D. Calcium phosphate

   E. Calcium oxalate

Ref.: 2, 8

COMMENTS: Pigment gallstones are composed primarily of calcium precipitated with bilirubin, carbonate, phosphate, or palmitate anions. • Two relatively distinct types of pigment gallstones are recognized: black-pigment gallstones and brown-pigment gallstones. • There are differences between black- and brown-pigment gallstones in terms of gross appearance, chemical composition, pathogenesis, and clinical implications. • **Black-pigment gallstones** are small and spiculated. • They contain calcium bilirubinate primarily in polymerized form, as well as calcium carbonate or phosphate. • **Brown-pigment gallstones** are soft and yellow-brown, are also composed primarily of calcium bilirubinate, but contain more calcium palmitate (fatty acid derived from lecithin) and cholesterol than do black stones. • The oxalate salts of calcium play no role in gallstone disease.

ANSWER:
B

23. Match each item in the left-hand column with the appropriate item in the right-hand column.

   A. Associated with cirrhosis   a. Black-pigment gallstones
   B. Most commonly associated   b. Brown-pigment gallstones
      with bile infection
   C. Found more often in the   c. Both
      common bile duct than the
      gallbladder
   D. Surgical treatment requires   d. Neither
      drainage procedure

Ref.: 1, 2, 8

COMMENTS: There are some important clinical differences between patients with black-pigment gallstones and those with brown-pigment gallstones. • It is postulated that these stones form by different pathogenic mechanisms. • Stasis and infection are critical factors in the formation of **brown-pigment gallstones.** • Bile culture results are positive in most patients with brown-pigment gallstones, and scanning electron microscopy demonstrates bacterial colonies or casts within the stones. • Brown-pigment gallstones are found more frequently in the common bile duct than in the gallbladder. • They occur in older patients with stasis and in post-cholecystectomy patients.

   Black-pigment gallstones are thought to have a metabolic cause. • They typically occur in patients with cirrhosis or hemolysis. • The precise role of stasis and infection in black stone formation remains unclear. • Approximately 20% of patients with black-pigment gallstones have positive bile culture results, and some investigators have demonstrated bacteria in black stones. • A subset of patients with gallstones has combined features of both black- and brown-pigment gallstones. • The important therapeutic implication in differentiating black- from brown-pigment gallstones is that patients with brown-pigment gallstones may require a definitive biliary drainage procedure to prevent recurrence, whereas patients with black-pigment gallstones may not.

ANSWER:
A-a; B-b; C-b; D-b

24. Which of the following sonographic findings are necessary to diagnose gallstones?

   A. Hyperechoic intraluminal structure

   B. Movement of structure

   C. Posterior shadowing

   D. Posterior acoustic enhancement

Ref.: 5

COMMENTS: External ultrasound imaging has a sensitivity of about 95% for the diagnosis of gallstones. • The three sonographic criteria for gallstones are (1) the presence of a hyperechoic intraluminal focus, (2) shadowing posterior to that focus, and (3) movement of the focus with positional changes of the patient. • Problems in interpretation arise when all of these criteria are not fulfilled. • For example, small stones may not shadow well, and impacted stones do not move. • Ultrasound imaging may also fail to diagnose stones if the gallbladder cannot be visualized well because it is contracted or close to excessive bowel gas. • For an optimal elective ultrasound scan, the gallbladder should be examined after the patient has fasted for about 6 hr. • Posterior acoustic enhancement is a sonographic feature of hypodense structures such as cysts. • The signals behind the structure are "whiter" because the sound wave energy is less attenuated as it passes through. • The gallbladder itself is a cystic structure and demonstrates this phenomenon, whereas gallstones do the opposite.

ANSWER:
A, B, C

25. Ultrasound imaging reveals gallstones in an asymptomatic 50-year-old woman. Which of the following is the recommended treatment?

   A. Observation

   B. Laparoscopic cholecystectomy

   C. Open cholecystectomy

   D. Ursodeoxycholic acid (UDCA)

   E. Extracorporeal shock wave lithotripsy (ESWL)

Ref.: 1, 2, 7, 8

COMMENTS: The appropriate management of asymptomatic cholelithiasis is sometimes controversial. • First, the physician must determine whether the patient is in fact asymptomatic, because gastrointestinal complaints other than pain may be attributable to biliary tract disease. • It was formerly thought that most patients with silent gallstones would eventually develop symptoms and that the risk of subsequent complications was high. • Subsequent studies suggest that symptoms develop in about 1–2% of patients each year and that serious complications are relatively infrequent. • The morbidity, mortality, and cost of intervention in these patients may exceed that of expectant therapy. • The availability of laparoscopic cholecystectomy has not yet changed the basic indications for surgery, although it likely has altered the symptomatic threshold for surgical referral. • Nonoperative pharmacologic dissolution and ESWL are neither definitive nor cost-effective.

Currently, therefore, the incidental finding of asymptomatic cholelithiasis is not an indication for therapy in most situations. • Circumstances that may be exceptions and that merit consideration on an individual basis include (1) a transplant patient with anticipated immunosuppression because of the risk of sepsis; (2) anticipated long-term parenteral nutrition, because of associated stasis and sludge formation; (3) anticipated pregnancy, because of the possibility of becoming symptomatic as gallbladder emptying is impaired and because of the potential risk imposed on both mother and fetus if complicated cholelithiasis occurs; (4) concurrent abdominal operation for an unrelated problem, because of the relative ease and safety of incidental cholecystectomy in most situations and in consideration of the potential for postoperative cholecystitis otherwise; and (5) coincident with antiobesity surgery, because of the high incidence of gallstones associated with obesity and during rapid weight loss. • In patients requiring massive intestinal resection, concomitant cholecystectomy has been recommended even when the gallbladder is normal because disease will likely develop during parenteral nutrition.

ANSWER:
A

26. For which of the following conditions is early elective cholecystectomy for symptomatic gallstones indicated?

A. Elderly status

B. Diabetes mellitus

C. Child's C cirrhosis

D. Total parenteral nutrition (TPN)-induced gallstones

E. None of the above

Ref.: 1

COMMENTS: Patients with certain medical conditions are often considered to be at higher risk for morbidity and mortality from gallstone disease. • Elderly patients more frequently develop complications of cholelithiasis, such as sepsis, perforation, and choledocholithiasis. • They also have a higher mortality rate during emergent operations. • Elective cholecystectomy can usually be performed safely in the elderly and is recommended for symptomatic patients. • Although the supportive evidence has not always been conclusive, diabetic patients may also be at increased risk, particularly if emergency intervention is required, and therefore should be considered for early elective cholecystectomy. • A high proportion of patients on long-term TPN develop gallstones, and reports suggest that complications, emergency operations, and mortality are more frequent in this population as well. • Early cholecystectomy is therefore indicated. • Patients with hepatic cirrhosis, however, have high morbidity and mortality rates related to cholecystectomy. • This is particularly true for patients with more advanced hepatocellular dysfunction and portal hypertension. • Cholecystectomy should be approached with great caution under these circumstances and is usually reserved for patients with complications of cholelithiasis or for patients with substantial symptoms and less advanced hepatic disease.

ANSWER:
A, B, D

27. A patient with episodic abdominal pain has a CCK-stimulated HIDA scan that demonstrates 25% gallbladder emptying. Ultrasound imaging of the gallbladder is normal. What is true regarding cholecystectomy in this situation?

A. Not indicated, since persistent or recurrent symptoms are likely

B. Indicated only if duodenal drainage yields cholesterol crystals or bilirubinate granules

C. Can alleviate symptoms in most patients if pain is episodic and in the right upper quadrant

D. Improves symptoms in most patients, regardless of pain location or characteristics

Ref.: 1, 9

COMMENTS: Surgeons are often confronted with the challenge of evaluating patients for abdominal pain that may or may not be of biliary origin. • If the symptoms are typical of biliary "colic" and ultrasound imaging demonstrates gallstones, the situation is straightforward. • However, when the symptoms are less typical (even the presence of gallstones) or when ultrasound imaging does not identify any abnormality, further evaluation is necessary to determine whether cholecystectomy is warranted. • Other diagnoses must be excluded, and additional investigations may be appropriate, depending on the specific circumstances (e.g., esophagogastroduodenoscopy, computed tomographic [CT] scanning, endoscopic retrograde cholangiopancreatography, gastrointestinal contrast studies, and colonoscopy).

CCK-stimulated cholescintigraphy can be useful for identifying patients who may have symptoms due to motility disorders of the gallbladder. • However, the test does not always reliably predict the long-term outcome of cholecystectomy. • If the symptoms are more typical of biliary origin and findings on CCK scintigraphy are abnormal (<30% ejection), data suggest that most patients (>70%) can benefit from cholecystectomy. • Pathologic abnormalities of the gallbladder are found in a reasonable number of these patients. • If the symptoms are less typical, the results of cholecystectomy cannot be expected to be as favorable, even though emptying is abnormal. • Additional specific tests for the gallbladder, such as repeated ultrasonography, duodenal drainage with CCK cholecystography, or even oral cholecystocystography are sometimes useful for evaluating these patients.

ANSWER:
C

28. Laparoscopic cholecystectomy is most strongly contraindicated in which of the following situations?

A. Pregnancy

B. Prior upper abdominal surgery

C. Known common bile duct stones

D. Chronic obstructive pulmonary disease

E. Gallbladder cancer

Ref.: 1, 10, 11

COMMENTS: When laparoscopic cholecystectomy was first introduced worldwide during the late 1980s, there were a number of circumstances in which it was more or less strongly contraindicated. • Today, most contraindications are relative, and in fact the laparoscopic approach is preferred when possible in certain situations that were initially considered contraindications (e.g., acute cholecystitis, choledocholithiasis, and obesity). • Basically, the surgeon must be adequately trained and the patient reasonably fit for an operation and give informed consent that includes the possibility of laparotomy. • Although usually performed under general anesthesia, the operation has even been accomplished with thoracic epidural anesthesia. • It must be recognized that there are patients for whom the potential physiologic consequences of a CO_2 pneumoperitoneum are more important, but the presence of underlying disease itself does not prohibit a laparoscopic approach. • In fact, laparoscopic cholecystectomy may be more beneficial to the postoperative course of a compromised patient. • Pregnancy is not a contraindication with appropriate precautions, although the physiologic effects on the fetus are not completely known. • Perhaps the strongest contraindication currently is for patients with suspected or known gallbladder cancer, because of the risk of dissemination.

ANSWER:
E

---

29. Most major bile duct injuries during laparoscopic cholecystectomy occur in patients under which one of the following circumstances?

    A. Acute cholecystitis

    B. Gallstone pancreatitis

    C. Choledocholithiasis

    D. Elective cholecystectomy

    E. Conversion of a laparoscopic procedure to an open procedure

    Ref.: 12, 13

COMMENTS: There are several risk factors for bile duct injury during laparoscopic cholecystectomy. • Pathologic risk factors include severe acute or chronic inflammation. • Several studies have found a statistical correlation between the rate of duct injury and the presence of acute cholecystitis. • Bleeding has long been implicated as a factor predisposing to duct injury during open or laparoscopic cholecystectomy. • Injuries are sometimes attributed to the "anomalous" anatomy of the bile ducts. • More often than not, however, such "anomalies" are simply common anatomic variations that the surgeon must recognize in order to prevent injury (see Question 4). • The surgeon's experience, or the "learning curve," is clearly a risk factor, since higher rates of duct injury have been well documented among less experienced surgeons. • It is interesting to note that there is no convincing evidence that duct injury is more frequent during cases involving laparoscopic management of common bile duct stones, possibly because these procedures are performed by more experienced surgeons. • Unfortunately, most major bile duct injuries during laparoscopic cholecystectomy have occurred in elective and otherwise uncomplicated cases. • Despite the presence or absence of risk factors, the primary problem resulting in duct injury is misidentification of the anatomy. • The most frequent mechanism of injury is when a major bile duct is mistaken for the cystic duct and is clipped and cut. • This pitfall is best avoided by correct operative strategy (i.e., appropriate retraction and adequate dissection) and by the surgeon's alertness to the visual misperceptions that can occur during laparoscopic cholecystectomy.

ANSWER:
D

---

30. The surgeon encounters difficulty during an elective laparoscopic cholecystectomy in a healthy 25-year-old woman and opens the patient. The 4-mm common hepatic duct has been transected 1 cm below the bifurcation. What is the appropriate therapy?

    A. Perform duct-to-duct anastomosis over a T-tube.

    B. Perform duct-to-duct anastomosis without a stent.

    C. Perform Roux-en-Y hepaticojejunostomy.

    D. Perform hepaticoduodenostomy.

    E. Place drains and transfer patient to a referral center.

    Ref.: 12, 13

COMMENTS: When a transection or resection injury of the extrahepatic biliary tree is discovered at the time of cholecystectomy, the surgeon must make some careful decisions. • Repair at the time would be preferable, provided a successful repair could be ensured. • Unfortunately, the body of evidence indicates that most primary repairs by the initial operating surgeon have failed, necessitating repeat operations and other interventions. • The first repair of a major duct injury has the best chance for long-term success. • Therefore, unless the surgeon is experienced with anastomosis of nondilated ducts, most would advise that it is in the patient's best interest that a definitive repair not be attempted. • Rather, drains should be placed and transfer arranged to an appropriate hepatobiliary surgeon. • If repair at the time is appropriate, the standard reconstruction for this type of injury is a Roux-en-Y hepaticojejunostomy. • Duct-to-duct repairs virtually always fail in this situation. • Hepaticoduodenostomy is not recommended for an injury at this level.

ANSWER:
C or E

---

31. How would the bile duct injury described above in Question 30 be classified?

    A. Bismuth type 1

    B. Bismuth type 2

    C. Bismuth type 3

    D. Bismuth type 4

    E. Bismuth type 5

    Ref.: 3

COMMENTS: The Bismuth level classification of bile duct injuries and strictures essentially relates the site of injury to the bifurcation of the main right and left hepatic ducts. • Higher injuries are more difficult. • They require a greater degree of technical skill and expertise to reconstruct, and reconstructions have a lower long-term success rate. • Many of the injuries resulting from laparoscopic cholecystectomy have been higher than those seen with open cholecystectomy. • Also many injuries, initially lower, end up being higher when repaired because of the need to débride unhealthy ductal tissue consequent to ischemia or inflammation and infection caused by bile leakage. • With a type 1 injury, 2 cm or more of the common hepatic duct is preserved below the bifurcation. • With a type 2 injury, less than 2 cm remains. • A type 3 injury involves the hilum, with preserved continuity between the right and left sides. • A type 4 injury involves destruction of the hepatic confluence, with separation of the right and left hepatic ducts. • A type 5 injury involves a separate inserting sectoral duct with or without injury of the common duct.

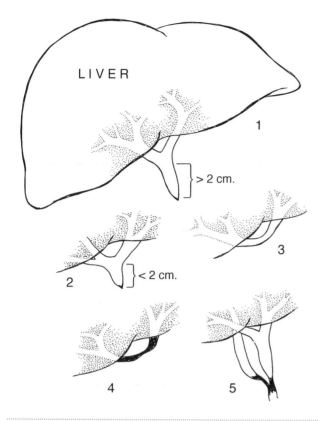

LIVER

1

> 2 cm.

2

< 2 cm.

3

4

5

ANSWER:
B

32. On the second postoperative day after elective laparoscopic cholecystectomy, a 40-year-old woman complains of nausea and abdominal pain. Examination shows a fever of 100°F (37.8°C), a pulse of 100, mild abdominal distention, and moderate right upper quadrant tenderness. What should be done next?

A. Ultrasound imaging of the abdomen

B. CT scan

C. HIDA scan

D. Endoscopic retrograde cholangiopancreatography (ERCP)

E. Percutaneous transhepatic cholangiography (PTC)

Ref.: 13, 14

COMMENTS: Serious delays in the postoperative diagnosis of bile duct injuries can compound a patient's problems. • A patient should be investigated promptly when the clinical course suggests anything other than the anticipated straightforward recovery that most patients experience. • The primary concern is development of a bile leak, which occurs in 1–2% of patients. • Other problems, such as retained bile duct stones or intestinal injury, can occur as well, although they are less frequent.

The various imaging studies can provide complementary information. • A HIDA scan shows an ongoing bile leak and is often the most reasonable initial investigation after the patient is examined. • Ultrasound imaging or CT scanning can demonstrate fluid collections or intrahepatic bile duct dilatation. • If a fluid collection is seen, percutaneous aspiration can determine whether the fluid is bile. • If a bile leak is confirmed, cholangiography is necessary to establish the site of leakage and to help determine further therapy. • Endoscopic cholangiography is generally the first

choice and may be all that is necessary for bile leaks that originate from lateral injuries, the cystic duct stump, or the gallbladder fossa. • Percutaneous transhepatic cholangiography is necessary for complete anatomic definition in patients with transection or resection injuries or injuries to sectoral hepatic ducts that may not be in continuity with the rest of the extrahepatic bile ducts.

ANSWER:
A, C

33. A stable patient has this endoscopic cholangiogram following laparoscopic cholecystectomy two days previously. What should be done next?

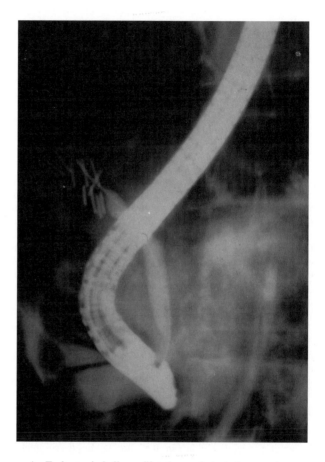

A. Endoscopic balloon dilatation and stent placement

B. Percutaneous transhepatic cholangiography

C. Urgent reoperation for bile drainage

D. Urgent reoperation for bile duct reconstruction

Ref.: 12, 13

COMMENTS: The endoscopic cholangiogram demonstrates complete occlusion of the supraduodenal common bile duct without extravasation of dye. • A classic mechanism of major bile duct injury during laparoscopic cholecystectomy involves clipping the distal common bile duct and resecting a portion of the extrahepatic ductal system. • The proximal level of injury is variable but typically high. • Patients present with bile leak or obstruction, depending on the status of the proximal ducts. • The first priority when managing these injuries is to control sepsis and ensure adequate drainage of any bile leak. • Generally, this can be accomplished by nonoperative percutaneous or endoscopic methods. • Urgent reoperation for bile drainage is not typically necessary. • Complete cholangiographic definition of the injury is essential before definitive repair. • For resection or transection injuries, as depicted here, PTC is required to assess the status of the proximal ducts. • Endoscopic cholangiography alone may be adequate for lateral injuries when the continuity of the ducts is preserved. • Occasionally, a "fistulagram" done through a percutaneous drainage catheter may visualize the proximal ducts. • After complete cholangiography, long-term success is best achieved by an elective, expert reconstruction.

ANSWER:
B

34. Which of the following is/are true regarding the role of intraoperative cholangiography (IOC) in bile duct injury during laparoscopic cholecystectomy?

    A. IOC prevents duct injury.

    B. IOC increases the rate of duct injury.

    C. IOC can limit the severity of injury.

    D. IOC increases the diagnosis of injury.

Ref.: 15

COMMENTS: As long as there are imaging studies to assess the bile ducts intraoperatively, the debate between proponents of routine versus selective use of such studies will continue. • Proponents of IOC argue that its routine or liberal use can be advantageous in terms of bile duct injury, but there is no convincing evidence that IOC actually lowers the rate of duct injury. • Cholangiograms can be incomplete or misinterpreted, or injuries can occur after an IOC has been done. • However, properly performed IOC does not lead to duct injuries. • There is a compelling argument that IOC may limit the severity of duct injury, for example, when IOC allows a surgeon to recognize that the cholangiogram catheter has been placed in the common duct and not the cystic duct before transection of the common duct. • Some evidence suggests that the number of high ductal injuries and anastomotic repairs required to remedy duct injuries has been lower when IOC was performed. • The use of IOC clearly appears to increase the rate of intraoperative recognition of injury. • About 70–90% of injuries have been identified intraoperatively when IOC has been performed, compared to only 15–25% when IOC has not been done. • Failure to interpret the IOC correctly can account for missed injuries. • The two primary reasons for misinterpreting an IOC are failure to completely visualize the proximal ducts (including both right anterior and posterior ducts) and extravasation of dye of uncertain origin.

ANSWER:
C, D

35. Which of the following is/are not considered primary events in the pathophysiology of acute calculous cholecystitis?

    A. Increased biliary lysolecithin

    B. Gallbladder ischemia

    C. Bacterial infection

    D. Cystic duct obstruction

Ref.: 1, 7, 8

COMMENTS: Acute cholecystitis is thought to be initiated by gallbladder obstruction and activation of various inflammatory mediators, which leads to mucosal damage, gallbladder distention,

and eventual ischemia. • Bacteria can be identified in the bile of about 50% (30–70%) of patients with acute cholecystitis, but bacterial infection is a secondary phenomenon. • The primary pathophysiology depends on biochemical events. • Some of the mediators that may be involved in the inflammatory process of acute cholecystitis are bile acids, lithogenic bile, pancreatic juice, prostaglandins, phospholipids, and lysolecithin. • Lysolecithin is formed from lecithin by the enzyme phospholipase, and levels are elevated in acute cholecystitis. • The role of prostaglandins as mediators in this process has also received considerable attention.

ANSWER:
B, C

36. Which of the following is most accurate in the diagnosis of acute cholecystitis?

    A. Plain abdominal radiograph

    B. Ultrasound imaging

    C. Oral cholecystography

    D. Technetium 99m pertechnetate (^{99m}Tc) iminodiacetic acid scan

Ref.: 1, 2, 7

COMMENTS: Radionuclide scanning with ^{99m}Tc iminodiacetic acid agents normally allows visualization of the liver, gallbladder, and extrahepatic biliary tree. • In the presence of acute cholecystitis, the gallbladder cannot be seen because of cystic duct obstruction. • This finding is present in approximately 98% of patients with acute cholecystitis. • Cholescintigraphy is not necessary in most patients with acute cholecystitis, since the diagnosis is founded on clinical examination and demonstration of gallstones by ultrasound imaging. • However, it can be quite useful in less typical situations and to exclude acute cholecystitis (by normal gallbladder uptake) in patients with other diagnoses. • Ultrasound imaging of acute cholecystitis may demonstrate gallstones, pericholecystic fluid, thickening of the gallbladder, intramural edema, or a positive sonographic Murphy's sign, but the morphologic findings are not specific. • Although oral cholecystography fails to allow visualization of the gallbladder in acute cholecystitis, this technique is not as diagnostically reliable as a radioisotope study because of the high frequency of gallbladders that cannot be visualized as a result of impaired dye absorption, hepatic uptake, or the presence of chronic cholecystitis. • Plain abdominal radiographs reveal up to 15% of gallstones and demonstrate emphysematous cholecystitis but otherwise play no specific role in the diagnosis of acute cholecystitis.

ANSWER:
D

37. A ^{99m}Tc iminodiacetic acid scan in a fasting patient demonstrates the following: normal liver activity, no gallbladder visualization at 60 minutes, intestinal activity present at 60 minutes, and gallbladder visualization at 120 minutes. These findings are most consistent with which of the following situations?

    A. Normal study results

    B. Acute calculous cholecystitis

    C. Acute acalculous cholecystitis

    D. Chronic cholecystitis

    E. Partial bile duct obstruction

Ref.: 1, 2

COMMENTS: Since the mid-1970s, technetium-labeled derivatives of iminodiacetic acid (i.e., HIDA, PIPIDA, and DISIDA) have been important in the evaluation of biliary tract disease. • After intravenous injection, these radioisotopes are taken up by the liver and excreted into the biliary tract. • Characteristics of a normal study include visualization of the gallbladder within 60 minutes in fasting patients and the appearance of radioisotope in the duodenum by about the same time. • In nonfasting patients, gallbladder visualization may be delayed. • The hepatic phase of the study may demonstrate mass lesions or diminished uptake when there is hepatic dysfunction. • Such results are similar to those of a liver scan. • With both calculous and acalculous acute cholecystitis, the gallbladder is not visualized owing to cystic duct obstruction. • No visualization or delayed visualization is common with chronic cholecystitis. • The distinction between acute and chronic cholecystitis therefore depends on the clinical presentation, not simply abnormal scan results. • Bile duct obstruction may cause delayed or absent clearance of isotope from the liver or delayed hepatic uptake. • Radioisotope scans can be useful in the clinical assessment of disorders other than cholecystitis, including biliary motility, biliary enteric anastomosis, bile fistulas or leaks, and enterogastric reflux.

ANSWER:
D

38. What is the preferred treatment for acute calculous cholecystitis?

    A. Early laparoscopic cholecystectomy

    B. Delayed laparoscopic cholecystectomy

    C. Early open cholecystectomy

    D. Delayed open cholecystectomy

Ref.: 1, 2, 7

COMMENTS: The former debate over early versus late cholecystectomy for acute cholecystitis has for the most part been put to rest. • Prospective studies have demonstrated that early cholecystectomy is not associated with higher morbidity or mortality, and delayed treatment requires longer hospitalization, is more expensive, and risks recurrent biliary problems before definitive therapy. • Most patients are effectively treated by stabilization, administration of antibiotics, and prompt operation. • From a technical standpoint, cholecystectomy is often easier during the first day or two of the patient's illness, when the inflammation tends to be more edematous than necrotic and hyperemic, as it becomes when the process progresses. • Laparoscopic cholecystectomy is the preferred treatment in most circumstances, although conversion to an open procedure is required more often (20–30%) than when the procedure is performed electively for nonacute symptoms (5%).

ANSWER:
A

39. With regard to acalculous cholecystitis, which of the following statements is/are true?

    A. It most commonly affects elderly patients in an outpatient setting.

    B. The primary pathophysiologic feature involves gallbladder stasis.

    C. HIDA scan results are usually normal.

    D. Ultrasound imaging of the gallbladder is usually normal.

    E. Treatment requires cholecystectomy.

Ref.: 1, 2, 7

COMMENTS: Approximately 5–10% of acute cholecystitis cases occur in patients without gallstones. • The primary predisposing factor is gallbladder stasis, with subsequent distention and ischemia. • Acalculous cholecystitis typically develops in hospitalized patients, often after trauma, unrelated surgery, or other critical illnesses. • Factors present in these patients that may contribute to biliary stasis include hypovolemia, intestinal ileus, absence of oral nutrition, multiple blood transfusions, narcotic use, and positive-pressure ventilation. • Because of the clinical situation in which acute acalculous cholecystitis occurs, the diagnosis may not be readily apparent. • The patient may present with fever or unexplained sepsis, and abdominal signs may not be initially appreciated. • Imaging study results are generally abnormal. • As a result of stasis and functional obstruction of the cystic duct, HIDA scanning fails to allow visualization of the gallbladder, and ultrasonography may demonstrate sludge, gallbladder wall thickening, or pericholecystic fluid. • None of these findings is specific for the presence of acute acalculous cholecystitis, however, and the diagnosis must rely on clinical suspicion.

Standard surgical treatment consists of cholecystectomy (or cholecystostomy for patients who are too infirm to withstand general anesthesia). • Percutaneous cholecystostomy can be a valuable technique for establishing gallbladder decompression in these critically ill patients. • Later cholecystectomy may not be required if stones are not present and if subsequent cholangiography demonstrates a patent cystic duct. • Cholecystectomy is the only effective treatment if the gallbladder is necrotic or gangrenous.

ANSWER:
B

40. The pertinent area of a plain x-ray film of the abdomen obtained on a 78-year-old diabetic man with severe right upper quadrant pain is shown. Which of the following is the appropriate next step?

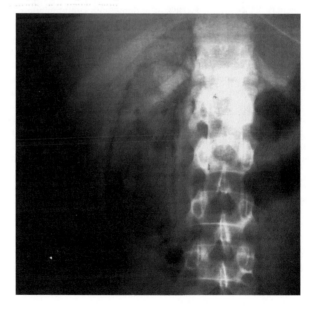

    A. Ultrasound imaging of the gallbladder

    B. CT scanning

    C. HIDA scanning

    D. Cholecystectomy

    E. ERCP

Ref.: 1, 2, 7

COMMENTS: Emphysematous cholecystitis occurs most typically in elderly diabetic men. • Curvilinear lucencies in the right upper quadrant have the configuration of the gallbladder, are in the location of the gallbladder, and are diagnostic for gas in the gallbladder wall. • In their totality, they are pathognomonic of emphysematous cholecystitis. • Gas may also be seen in the gallbladder lumen. • This condition is associated with a high incidence of gallbladder necrosis, perforation, and sepsis. • Unnecessary diagnostic examinations would only delay prompt surgical therapy and possibly affect the outcome adversely. • Urgent operation is needed. • An ultrasound study of an emphysematous gallbladder would show highly reflective shadows as a result of the gas. • Differentiation from bowel gas may be difficult, although usually the diagnosis is evident. • About one third of patients do not have stones. • A CT scan would show the abnormal gas in the gallbladder wall, lumen, or both. • HIDA scans would fail to allow visualization of the gallbladder. • ERCP is unnecessary.

ANSWER:
D

41. With regard to choledocholithiasis, which of the following statements is/are true?

    A. Common duct stones are present in one third of patients undergoing cholecystectomy.

    B. The incidence of common duct stones is highest in elderly patients.

    C. Most common duct stones are composed of calcium bilirubinate.

    D. Common duct stones are found more frequently when cholecystectomy is performed for chronic cholecystitis than for acute cholecystitis.

Ref.: 1, 2, 7

COMMENTS: About 8–18% of patients with symptomatic gallstones have choledocholithiasis, which has a spectrum of clinical presentations. • Approximately 6% of patients undergoing cholecystectomy have common bile duct stones that were completely unsuspected. • Proper recognition of common duct stones is important because of the associated risk of biliary tract obstruction and cholangitis. • The incidence of choledocholithiasis increases with each decade over age 60. • Most common duct calculi originate in the gallbladder and are therefore of the cholesterol variety. • Friable "earthy" stones (brown-pigment gallstones) contain calcium complexed with bilirubinate and other anions and arise de novo in the common duct in association with biliary stasis and infection. • Choledocholithiasis occurs as often with acute cholecystitis as with chronic cholecystitis. • Therefore, appropriate evaluation of the patient for potential choledocholithiasis is mandatory.

ANSWER:
B

42. Which of the following is the best indication for preoperative ERCP in a patient with gallstones?

    A. Obstructive jaundice

    B. Gallstone pancreatitis

    C. History of jaundice

    D. Elevated alkaline phosphatase to twice normal

    E. A 10-mm common bile duct seen on ultrasonography

Ref.: 16

COMMENTS: The rationale for preoperative ERCP is to identify and remove common bile duct stones so that patients may subsequently undergo laparoscopic cholecystectomy and, it is hoped, avoid the need for an open operation or for operative treatment of the common bile duct. • However, since endoscopic evaluation of the bile duct entails its own risks, it should be selected for patients at the highest risk for choledocholithiasis. • Unfortunately, there are no absolute predictors of common bile duct stones. • The yield of ERCP in identifying common bile duct stones is highest in patients presenting with obstructive jaundice or clinical cholangitis or when a duct stone is actually seen on the ultrasound scan. • In all other circumstances, most patients have negative endoscopic cholangiograms, and the examination was not necessary for most of these patients. • As the number of parameters suggestive of common bile duct stones increases, however, so does the likelihood of finding stones. • There is no substitute for good clinical judgment in the utilization of preoperative ERCP. • It is an unquestionably valuable tool for diagnosing and removing common bile duct stones, but its *overuse* is dangerous and must be discouraged.

ANSWER:
A

43. An intraoperative cholangiogram obtained during laparoscopic cholecystectomy shows several 2- to 3-mm filling defects in the distal common duct. What should be done next?

    A. Perform a complete laparoscopic cholecystectomy and perform ERCP postoperatively.

    B. Open the patient and perform common bile duct exploration.

    C. Administer glucagon and flush the common bile duct.

    D. Laparoscopically dilate the cystic duct and perform transcystic choledochoscopy.

    E. Perform laparoscopic choledochotomy.

Ref.: 17

COMMENTS: Choledocholithiasis discovered intraoperatively can often be managed laparoscopically, depending on a number of considerations, such as the size, number, and location of the stones and the size and anatomy of the bile ducts. • When approaching common bile stones laparoscopically, one should start with simple techniques and progress to more complex maneuvers as necessary. • Small stones can often be cleared by flushing the common duct through a transcystic catheter after glucagon has been given to relax the choledochoduodenal sphincter. • Other transcystic manipulations can be used if the cystic duct is dilated or dilatable (with hydrostatic balloons) and provided there is a relatively direct course between the cystic duct and the common bile duct. • These techniques include retrieval with balloon catheters or stone baskets under fluoroscopic or choledochoscopic visualization. • Experienced laparoscopic surgeons can perform choledochotomy when the common bile duct is sufficiently large and when simpler efforts have failed. • In general, the surgeon should not leave common duct stones untreated but may elect to terminate the procedure when (1) the stones are very small or questionable, (2) the common bile duct is narrow, (3) laparoscopic clearance is not feasible, and (4) the morbidity of an open common bile duct exploration is judged to be too high for a particular patient. • Intraoperative endoscopic retrieval of common bile duct stones has been successful but may be logistically impractical. • Relying on postoperative endoscopy for intentionally neglected stones carries the risk that endoscopic removal may fail. • A traditional open common bile duct exploration is a safe, reliable fallback for most patients when laparoscopic methods are unsuccessful and the duct is not too small.

ANSWER:
C

---

44. In general, which of the following is the best treatment for a patient with choledocholithiasis 3 years after cholecystectomy?

A. Transhepatic infusion of mono-octanoin

B. Percutaneous transhepatic stone extraction

C. Endoscopic sphincterotomy and stone extraction

D. Common bile duct exploration and T-tube placement

E. Common bile duct exploration and choledochoduodenostomy

Ref.: 1, 2, 7

COMMENTS: Most common bile duct stones found in patients after cholecystectomy can be successfully treated by nonoperative methods. • Stone extraction through a T tube or endoscopically after endoscopic sphincterotomy if the patient does not have a T tube in place results in successful duct clearance with a low complication rate in more than 90% of patients. • By definition, bile duct stones occurring more than 2 years after cholecystectomy are considered primary common duct stones. • These are pigment gallstones related to biliary stasis and infection rather than the typical cholesterol stones found in the gallbladder. • In addition to stone removal, some type of ductal drainage procedure therefore also is indicated in most of these patients to prevent stone recurrence.

When performed by experienced clinicians, endoscopic sphincterotomy is successful in more than 90% of patients and, when combined with endoscopic extraction with the use of balloon catheters or baskets, results in stone clearance in 85–90% of patients. • Contact dissolution of duct stones with mono-octanoin is successful in certain patients with retained cholesterol stones, but this medium-chain diglyceride is not an effective solvent for pigment stones. • Duct stones have been successfully removed via the percutaneous transhepatic route when endoscopic approaches are unsuccessful. • Neither transhepatic instillation of contact solvents nor transhepatic extraction alone provides long-term biliary drainage, however.

A number of situations may make endoscopic clearance of bile duct stones difficult or unsuccessful, including large impacted stones, the presence of a distal bile duct stricture, previous gastrectomy with gastroenterostomy or Roux-en-Y anastomosis, complications of endoscopic sphincterotomy before stone extraction, or the presence of a duodenal diverticulum. • If access to the bile duct can be achieved endoscopically, adjuvant modalities, such as intracorporeal fragmentation techniques (i.e., mechanical, electrohydraulic, or laser lithotripsy) or extracorporeal shock wave lithotripsy, may allow successful removal of even difficult stones. • Reoperation on the biliary tract for clearance of duct stones is reserved for physiologically fit patients in whom other extraction techniques are unsuccessful.

ANSWER:
C

---

45. Which of the following is the most appropriate initial test for the evaluation of obstructive jaundice?

A. HIDA scanning

B. Ultrasound imaging

C. CT scanning

D. PTC

E. ERCP

Ref.: 1, 2, 7

COMMENTS: All of the abovementioned imaging modalities may be useful for evaluating a patient with obstructive jaundice. • Overall, ultrasound imaging is the most cost-effective initial examination. • It permits identification or visualization of ductal dilatation, suggests the level of obstruction, and provides information about the liver, the pancreas, and the presence or absence of calculous disease. • **CT or magnetic resonance imaging (MRI)** may best delineate the anatomy of mass lesions in the hepatobiliary pancreatic region and assist in the preoperative assessment of resectability. • Magnetic resonance cholangiography can provide precise delineation of the ductal anatomy and is increasingly important in the evaluation of malignant disease. • **PTC** can demonstrate the **proximal** extent of obstruction and is useful for assessing the suitability of the proximal hepatic ducts for anastomosis. • **ERCP** is particularly useful in cases of **distal** biliary tract obstruction and allows evaluation of the ampullary region. • Both PTC and ERCP allow cytologic or histologic sampling, and both can be used to place catheters to decompress the obstructed biliary tract. • Although ^{99m}Tc-iminodiacetic acid scans can demonstrate ductal obstruction, they do not provide sufficient anatomic definition to determine cause or assist in making therapeutic decisions.

ANSWER:
B

---

46. Two weeks following hepaticojejunostomy for treatment of a benign bile duct stricture, a patient has a serum bilirubin level of 6 mg/dl. The patient was jaundiced for 4 weeks before the operation and had a preoperative serum bilirubin level of 12 mg/dl. Which of the following is the most likely explanation for this current serum bilirubin level?

A. Anastomotic stricture

B. Persistent δ-bilirubinemia

C. Postoperative hepatitis

D. Normal expected decline after relief of any obstructive jaundice

Ref.: 3, 7

COMMENTS: After relief of biliary obstruction, there is a prompt increase in bile flow, and normal bile acid secretion resumes within several days. • Serum bilirubin levels decline approximately 50% by 36–48 hr after surgery and 8% per day thereafter. • This rate varies, depending on the duration of jaundice. • δ-Bilirubin is a form of bilirubin that is covalently bonded to albumin and is measured as a part of the direct bilirubin fraction. • As such, it is not filtered by the kidney and has the same serum half-life as albumin, approximately 18 days, which accounts for the slow decline in serum bilirubin levels observed in patients following relief of long-standing jaundice. • Whereas 90% of patients who had jaundice for 1 week or less have a normal serum bilirubin level 3–4 weeks postoperatively, only one third of patients who had jaundice for 4 weeks or longer obtain normal levels by the same time. • Anastomotic stenosis does not usually present early during the postoperative period. • Postoperative hepatocellular dysfunction as a result of hepatitis or other causes can occur early in the postoperative period, but it is a less likely cause of hyperbilirubinemia in a patient whose serum bilirubin levels are gradually declining and who would be anticipated to have persistent δ-bilirubinemia.

ANSWER:
B

47. Which of the following is the most likely explanation for a serum bilirubin level of 40 mg/dl in a patient with obstructive jaundice?

    A. The patient has complete biliary obstruction.

    B. The duration of obstruction has exceeded 2 weeks.

    C. The patient has associated renal dysfunction.

    D. The patient has malignant biliary obstruction.

Ref.: 3

COMMENTS: In the presence of complete biliary obstruction, serum bilirubin levels generally plateau at 25–30 mg/dl. • At this point, the daily bilirubin load equals that excreted by the kidneys. • Situations in which even higher bilirubin levels can be found include renal insufficiency, hemolysis, hepatocellular disease, and, rarely, a bile duct–hepatic vein fistula. • Hyperbilirubinemia tends to be more pronounced in patients with obstruction caused by malignant disease than with obstruction resulting from benign causes. • However, malignant obstruction in the absence of the previously enumerated factors does not produce this degree of hyperbilirubinemia.

ANSWER:
C

48. The pathophysiology of acute renal failure in a patient with biliary obstruction is related to which of the following conditions?

    A. Systemic hypotension

    B. Hyperbilirubinemia

    C. Endotoxemia

    D. Bile acidemia

Ref.: 3

COMMENTS: Acute renal failure is a common and commonly fatal complication of biliary sepsis. • A number of factors contribute to the development of this complication. • Renal hypoperfusion occurs as a result of bacteremia, systemic hypotension, and hypovolemia. • Circulating bacterial endotoxins also are nephrotoxic. • Patients with biliary obstruction are at higher risk for renal failure than are patients with sepsis from other causes. • Evidence suggests that circulating bile acids themselves may induce tubular damage and exacerbate the effects of renal ischemia. • Therapy for patients with biliary sepsis must focus on adequate fluid and vasopressor support, antibiotic coverage, and biliary decompression to prevent renal failure. • Additional treatment, such as the administration of bile acids to minimize gut absorption of bacterial endotoxins, has also been used. • Little evidence exists to indicate that renal damage is caused by bilirubin, even though it may predispose the tubular cells to ischemia.

ANSWER:
A, C, D

49. Which of the following conditions is usually associated with the highest incidence of positive bile culture results?

    A. Acute cholecystitis

    B. Chronic cholecystitis

    C. Choledocholithiasis

    D. Postoperative bile duct stricture

    E. Bile duct malignancy

Ref.: 2, 3

COMMENTS: The recognition of clinical situations in which bacteria are likely to be present in bile is important because the presence of bacteria in the bile is correlated with the risk of postoperative infectious complications. • Prophylactic antibiotics have decreased infectious morbidity in patients older than 50 years of age and in those with jaundice, acute cholecystitis, or choledocholithiasis and cholangitis. • Bile cultures are positive in approximately 5–40% of patients with chronic cholecystitis, 30–70% of patients with acute cholecystitis, 60–80% of patients with choledocholithiasis, and nearly all patients with bile duct stricture. • Bacterial infection of bile occurs in 25–50% of patients with malignant obstruction. • Bile culture results are expected to be positive in any patient with an indwelling biliary tube.

ANSWER:
D

50. Which of the following organisms is/are most commonly isolated from bile?

    A. *Escherichia coli*

    B. *Clostridium* spp.

    C. *Bacteroides fragilis*

    D. *Pseudomonas* spp.

    E. *Enterococcus* spp.

Ref.: 2, 3, 7, 8

COMMENTS: All of the abovementioned organisms are found in the biliary tract, but gram-negative aerobic organisms, particularly *E. coli* and *Klebsiella*, are found most frequently. • Other gram-negative aerobic bacteria that can be cultured are *Proteus*, *Pseudomonas*, and *Enterobacter* spp. Gram-positive organisms, especially *Enterococcus* spp. and *Streptococcus faecalis*, are also frequently observed. • Anaerobes are now recognized in 25–30% of cases, most commonly *B. fragilis*, followed by *Clostridium* spp. • Polymicrobial infection occurs in approximately 60% of cases. • Effective prophylactic or therapeutic antibiotic therapy must be effective against the anticipated organisms. • Serious biliary sepsis is usually treated with broad-spectrum or combination antibiotics that are effective against gram-negative organisms, anaerobes, and enterococci.

ANSWER:
A

51. Which of the following is the most common mechanism leading to bacterial infection in the bile?

    A. Ascending infection from the duodenum

    B. Hematogenous portal venous spread

    C. Hematogenous arterial spread

    D. Lymphatic spread

Ref.: 2, 3

COMMENTS: Bile is usually sterile. • There are various routes by which bacteria can reach the biliary tract, and, although not proved, dissemination from the portal venous system via the liver is currently favored as the most common mechanism. • Ascending infection from the duodenum does not occur to a significant extent. • Also, evidence suggests that the direction of lymphatic flow is from the liver downward, rather than in the reverse direction. • Hematogenous dissemination via hepatic arterial flow is a mechanism of hepatic abscess formation and may lead to bactibilia but is thought to be less common than portal venous spread.

ANSWER:
B

52. Which of the following conditions is sufficient to cause cholangitis with bacteremia?

    A. Bacteria in bile

    B. Partial bile duct obstruction

    C. Complete bile duct obstruction

    D. None of the above

Ref.: 2, 7, 8

COMMENTS: The pathophysiology of cholangitis requires both bacterial infection of bile and bile duct obstruction with elevated intraductal pressure. • Neither the presence of bacteria in bile nor biliary obstruction alone is sufficient to produce bacteremia. • When bacteria are present in the bile and common duct pressures exceed 20 cmH$_2$O, cholangiovenous and cholangiolymphatic reflux occur, resulting in systemic bacteremia. • Partial or complete bile duct obstruction may produce cholangitis if bacteria are present. • In fact, cholangitis occurs more commonly with partial obstruction because it is more frequently associated with stone disease, whereas complete obstruction is more often found with malignancy. • Calculous disease is the most common cause of cholangitis, which is understandable because it is associated with both bile duct obstruction and bacterial infection.

ANSWER:
D

53. If an antibiotic is effective against the bacteria present in the bile, which of the following is the most important consideration for effective therapy of biliary tract infection?

    A. Serum concentration of the antibiotic

    B. Bile concentration of the antibiotic in an unobstructed biliary tract

    C. Bile concentration of the antibiotic in an obstructed biliary tract

    D. Potential renal toxicity of the antibiotic

Ref.: 2, 3

COMMENTS: The most important pharmacologic considerations pertaining to selection of antimicrobial agents for the treatment of biliary sepsis are the antibacterial activity spectrum of the agent and the achievement of adequate serum levels of the drug. • Therapy cannot be adequate if the agents selected are not effective against the anticipated organisms (i.e., gram-negative Enterobacteriaceae, enterococci, and anaerobes) or if dosing does not produce sufficient serum levels. • The significance of biliary levels of antibiotics is often discussed, but they are of little clinical importance. • High bile levels of an antibiotic are meaningless if the agent is not effective against the bacteria present. • Moreover, agents that achieve high concentrations in the normal biliary tract may not reach such levels in the presence of biliary obstruction. • The aminoglycoside gentamicin, for example, has traditionally been an effective agent against the gram-negative organisms that cause biliary sepsis, but it is not concentrated in the bile. • The potential nephrotoxicity of an antibiotic is an important consideration, because the risk of renal compromise already exists in a patient with sepsis and biliary obstruction. • This has encouraged the use of nonaminoglycoside drugs for gram-negative coverage, but this consideration is not as important as the activity spectrum and adequate serum levels of the drugs.

ANSWER:
A

54. Which of the following is/are necessary in the initial treatment of a patient with acute cholangitis?

    A. Intravenous antibiotics

    B. Percutaneous transhepatic drainage

    C. Endoscopic sphincterotomy and drainage

    D. T-tube decompression of the common bile duct

    E. Choledochoduodenostomy

Ref.: 2, 7, 8

COMMENTS: Charcot's triad, which consists of fever, jaundice, and upper abdominal pain, is the clinical hallmark of acute cholangitis. • When accompanied by shock and changes in mental status, it is referred to as Reynold's pentad. • Cholangitis varies widely in severity, and treatment must be individualized according to the patient's condition. • Initial therapy consists of fluid resuscitation and antibiotics that are effective against gram-negative organisms, enterococci, and anaerobes. • Approximately 5–10% of patients present with severe toxic cholangitis and the manifestations of Reynold's pentad. • Patients who fail to improve or who deteriorate despite antibiotic and fluid support require urgent biliary decompression. • This generally can be accomplished nonoperatively by percutaneous transhepatic or endoscopic approaches, depending on the suspected location of the obstruction based on ultrasonographic findings and on the availability of local expertise in these procedures. • The ability to decompress the biliary tract nonoperatively in these cases has been advantageous because it not only allows stabilization of a high percentage of patients but also permits diagnostic cholangiography to be performed when the patient has stabilized. • When initial operative decompression of the biliary tract was the only approach for these critically ill patients, the mortality rate was high, and there was a frequent need for subsequent reoperation on the biliary tract because of the inability to identify or deal with the underlying pathologic condition at the time of the initial operation. • If effective nonoperative drainage of the biliary tract is not possible, surgery should not be delayed in these critically ill patients. • T-tube decompression of the common bile duct is performed. • Choledochoduodenostomy is not performed in critically ill patients but can be considered if the common bile duct is dilated to 15 mm or more, the patient is physiologically stable, and other conditions permit a safe anastomosis. • The current mortality rate of acute cholangitis is approximately 5%. • Poor prognostic factors include renal failure, liver abscess, cirrhosis, and proximal malignant obstruction.

ANSWER:
A

55. A 30-year-old woman is found at the time of cholecystectomy to have hydrops of the gallbladder and a firm, yellow nodule in the cystic duct. Which of the following is the most likely diagnosis?

　A. Cholesterolosis

　B. Carcinoid tumor

　C. Adenocarcinoma

　D. Granular cell myoblastoma

　E. Sarcoidosis

Ref.: 2

COMMENTS: Benign tumors of the gallbladder include papillary adenomas, nonpapillary adenomas, and a host of relatively uncommon neoplasms derived from various connective tissues. • These lesions are usually incidental findings in patients who are undergoing cholecystectomy. • Granular cell myoblastomas are neuroectodermally derived benign tumors that can occur at many sites. • In the biliary tract, they occasionally occur in the gallbladder, in the common duct, or as obstruction of the gallbladder, with symptoms indistinguishable from those of cholelithiasis. • No treatment beyond cholecystectomy is required. • Cholesterolosis is a condition in which deposits of cholesterol are found in macrophages known as foamy histiocytes in the lamina propria of the gallbladder wall. • This condition is often referred to as "strawberry gallbladder" because of the gross appearance of speckled, yellow cholesterol deposits on the background of an erythematous mucosa. • Cholesterolosis is often generalized, although a localized collection may form a "cholesterol polyp." Carcinoid tumors may occur in the gallbladder, but they are rare and usually incidental findings and are not associated with the carcinoid syndrome. • Adenocarcinoma of the gallbladder usually occurs in elderly individuals and does not appear on gross examination as a yellow nodule. • Sarcoidosis is a systemic disorder that may produce granulomatous inflammation of the liver but is not associated with a specific biliary tract lesion.

ANSWER:
D

56. Ultrasound studies of the gallbladder demonstrate a single 5 mm-hyperechoic focus along the gallbladder wall that does not move or shadow and that has a "comet tail" echo pattern behind it. What is the most likely diagnosis?

　A. Adenomatous polyp

　B. Cholesterol polyp

　C. Gallstone

　D. Adenomyomatosis

　E. Fibroxanthogranulomatous inflammation

Ref.: 5

COMMENTS: The term *hyperplastic cholecystosis* describes a group of benign proliferative conditions of the gallbladder, including cholesterolosis and adenomyomatosis, or adenomatous hyperplasia. • These conditions can be symptomatic and are often diagnosed based on their sonographic features. • **Cholesterolosis** consists of deposits of cholesterol in foamy histiocytes in the gallbladder wall. • A localized collection of such cholesterol-laden cells covered by a normal layer of epithelium and connected to the mucosa by a small pedicle is known as a cholesterol polyp. • Ultrasound imaging shows hyperechoic foci with a "comet tail" artifact. • Unlike gallstones, the foci do not move or produce acoustic shadowing. • **Adenomatous hyperplasia** is a proliferative lesion characterized by increased thickness of the mucosa and muscle, with mucosal diverticula known as Rokitansky-Aschoff sinuses. • Segmental, diffuse, and localized forms of adenomyomatous hyperplasia have been described. • Of these, a localized form involving the fundus of the gallbladder is most frequently encountered. • Ultrasound imaging demonstrates a mass lesion or "pseudotumor." **Adenomatous polyps** are true neoplasms derived from the glandular epithelium of the gallbladder. • **Fibroxanthogranulomatous inflammation** is a condition in which foamy histiocytes are found in conjunction with inflammatory cells and a fibroblastic vascular reaction, often with mucosal ulceration.

ANSWER:
B

57. With regard to adenomyomatosis, which of the following statements is/are true?

　A. It can be a premalignant lesion.

　B. It results from chronic inflammation.

　C. It may cause right upper quadrant pain in the absence of gallstones.

　D. It is rarely associated with cholelithiasis and cholecystitis.

Ref.: 1, 2

COMMENTS: Adenomyomatosis is a hyperplastic abnormality of the gallbladder that is not related to inflammation or neoplasia. • Approximately one half or more of patients with adenomyomatosis also have cholelithiasis and cholecystitis, but the relationship is not causal. • Adenomyomatosis is not a premalignant lesion. • The hyperplastic conditions of adenomyomatosis and cholesterolosis may be associated with functional abnormalities of the gallbladder, as evidenced by motility disturbances or hyperconcentration during oral cholecystography. • These abnormalities may be the cause of biliary tract symptoms in patients with hyperplastic cholecystoses in the absence of cholelithiasis. • Cholecystectomy can relieve symptoms in these patients.

ANSWER:
C

58. Of the fistulas in the left-hand column, select the most common type of biliary enteric fistula, and match it with its most common cause in the right-hand column.

　A. Cholecystocolic　　　　a. Cholelithiasis
　B. Cholecystoduodenal　　b. Malignancy
　C. Cholecystoduodenocolic　c. Peptic ulcer
　D. Choledochoduodenal　　d. Congenital
　E. Choledochogastric　　　e. Traumatic

Ref.: 2, 3, 7

COMMENTS: Almost all internal biliary fistulas are acquired communications between the extrahepatic biliary tree and the intestinal tract. • In rare instances, acquired or congenital bronchobiliary or acquired pleurobiliary fistulas occur. • Biliary enteric fistulas most commonly involve the gallbladder and the duodenum (70-80% of cases) and are the result of chronic inflammation caused by gallstone disease. • The second most common fistula occurs between the gallbladder and colon; infrequently, the stomach or multiple sites (cholecystoduodenocolic) are involved. • Occasionally, the biliary site of the fistula is the common bile duct. • Choledochoduodenal fistulas are most frequently caused by penetrating peptic ulcers, but they might occur in patients with choledocholithiasis and prior cholecystectomy. • Other, less common causes of biliary enteric fistulas are malignancy and penetrating trauma.

ANSWER:
B-a

59. With regard to the management of a patient with gallstone ileus, which of the following statements is/are true?

   A. Initial tube decompression and nonoperative management allow spontaneous stone passage in one third of patients.

   B. Operative treatment attempts to displace the stone into the colon without enterotomy.

   C. Operative treatment is by enterotomy proximal to the site of obstruction.

   D. Cholecystectomy and fistula repair at the time of stone removal are contraindicated.

   E. Standard treatment is initial laparotomy for stone removal and mandatory reoperation for cholecystectomy when the patient is stable.

Ref.: 2, 3, 7

COMMENTS: Gallstone ileus is mechanical obstruction of the gastrointestinal tract caused by a gallstone that has entered the intestine via an acquired biliary enteric fistula. • Although gallstone ileus accounts for only 1–3% of all small-bowel obstructions, it is associated with a higher mortality rate than other nonmalignant causes of bowel obstruction because it tends to occur in the elderly population, and typical cases are characterized by diagnostic delay due to waxing and waning of symptoms ("tumbling obstruction"). • Pathopneumonic radiologic features include a gas pattern of small-bowel obstruction with pneumobilia and an opaque stone outside the expected location of the gallbladder. • Not all of these radiologic features are usually present, however. • The most common site of obstruction is in the terminal ileum. • Infrequently, sigmoid obstruction occurs in an area narrowed by intrinsic colonic disease.

   Initial therapy is appropriate resuscitation followed by surgery. • Spontaneous passage is a rare phenomenon, and nonoperative management is associated with a prohibitive mortality rate. • Stone removal is best accomplished by an enterotomy placed proximal to the site of obstruction. • Care must be taken to search for additional intestinal stones, which are present in 10% of patients. • Attempts to extraluminally crush the stone or to milk it distally are contraindicated because they may cause bowel injury. • In rare instances, small-bowel resection is necessary if there is ischemic compromise or bleeding at the site of impaction.

   The main controversy regarding surgical treatment of gallstone ileus is whether a definitive biliary tract operation with cholecystectomy, fistula repair, and possible common duct exploration should be performed at the time of stone removal. • This decision must be based on sound surgical judgment, considering the underlying physiologic status of the patient and the anatomic status of the right upper quadrant. • Up to one third of patients who do not undergo definitive biliary surgery experience recurrent biliary symptoms, including cholecystitis, cholangitis, and recurrent gallstone ileus. • Furthermore, the rate of spontaneous fistula closure is open to question. • For these reasons, a definitive one-stage procedure should be considered in physiologically fit patients if the right upper quadrant dissection does not prove unduly hazardous from a technical standpoint, particularly if residual

stones can be demonstrated in the right upper quadrant. • In properly selected patients, a definitive one-stage procedure is not associated with higher operative morbidity or mortality rates. • However, because most of these patients are elderly and have a high incidence of comorbid disease, surgical therapy has been limited to stone removal in most instances. • Interval cholecystectomy should be considered for patients with postoperative biliary symptoms and for those with residual right upper quadrant stones, provided they are physiologically fit. • In reality, because of the compromised underlying status of many of these patients, interval elective procedures are not commonly performed.

ANSWER:
C

60. Which of the following is the preferred management of a type I choledochal cyst?

   A. Cyst excision

   B. Cyst duodenostomy

   C. Cyst jejunostomy

   D. External drainage

   E. Endoscopic sphincterotomy

Ref.: 2, 7

COMMENTS: Cystic disease of the biliary tract may involve the intrahepatic ducts, extrahepatic ducts, or both. • The most common form of involvement is a cystic dilatation of the extrahepatic bile duct (type I). • Combined intrahepatic and extrahepatic cysts (type IV) are next in frequency of occurrence. • A diverticulum of the common bile duct (type II), a "choledochocele" extending from the distal duct into the duodenum (type III), and cystic disease confined to the intrahepatic ducts (type V) are less common. • Bile duct cysts may be associated with jaundice, abdominal pain, and cholangitis in both adult and pediatric patients. • Furthermore, their association with biliary tract malignancy and with anomalous relationships between the pancreatic duct and bile duct are well recognized. • For these reasons, complete cyst excision with Roux-en-Y hepaticojejunostomy is the preferred treatment. • Internal drainage procedures are followed by a high rate of recurrent jaundice, cholangitis, and stricture. • In some instances, because of the intrahepatic or retroduodenal extent of disease or because of technical considerations, complete excision may not be feasible, and the surgeon may have to settle for partial excision. • Endoscopic treatment by sphincterotomy or resection is occasionally appropriate for the rarely occurring choledochocele.

ANSWER:
A

61. With regard to balloon dilatation of biliary strictures, which of the following statements is/are true?

   A. Dilatation can be performed by the transhepatic or endoscopic route.

   B. Repeat dilatations are not often required.

   C. Bleeding and sepsis are the most frequent complications.

   D. Better success is obtained with primary duct strictures than with anastomotic strictures.

   E. The long-term success rate is better than that with surgical repair.

Ref.: 1, 2

COMMENTS: Nonoperative dilatation of biliary strictures via endoscopic or percutaneous transhepatic access is an alternative to surgery that may be appropriate for some patients. • Repeat dilatations are often required, but overall success rates of 70–80% at 2–3 years of follow-up have been reported. • Success has generally been somewhat higher for patients with primary ductal strictures than for those with strictures of biliary enteric anastomoses. • Bleeding and sepsis have been the most frequent complications and can be life threatening. • Data on long-term results are limited. • Comparison between balloon dilatation and surgery has demonstrated better long-term results (approximate mean follow-up at 5 years) with surgery, with no difference in overall morbidity, hospitalization, or cost between the two therapies. • It cannot be ensured that treatment groups are comparable, however. • Nonoperative dilatation of biliary strictures may be appropriate as initial treatment for a strictured biliary anastomosis or for patients in whom surgical repair is deemed excessively difficult or dangerous. • The decisions about how a biliary stricture is initially treated and when nonoperative maneuvers are abandoned in favor of surgery should be made in consultation with a skilled endoscopist, an interventional radiologist, and an experienced hepatobiliary surgeon.

ANSWER:
A, C, D

62. A 40-year-old man presents with fluctuating jaundice, pruritus, and fatigue. Liver enzyme levels demonstrate cholestasis. Ultrasound imaging does not show gallstones or bile duct dilatation. What diagnostic test should be performed next?

    A. Measurement of serum antimitochondrial antibodies

    B. CT scanning

    C. HIDA scanning

    D. ERCP

    E. Liver biopsy

    Ref.: 1–3, 7

COMMENTS: The presentation described is fairly typical of sclerosing cholangitis, which also can be discovered in asymptomatic patients based on their cholestatic liver enzyme levels. • Sclerosing cholangitis is a disease of undetermined cause characterized by inflammatory fibrosis and stenosis of the bile ducts. • The process can be considered primary when no specific etiologic factor is identified or secondary when associated with specific causes, such as bile duct stones, operative trauma, hepatic arterial infusion of chemotherapeutic agents, or intraductal instillation of various irritants for the treatment of echinococcal disease. • Primary sclerosing cholangitis may be an isolated finding or may occur in conjunction with a variety of other disease processes, most commonly ulcerative colitis and pancreatitis. • Although the cause of primary sclerosing cholangitis is unknown, most attention has focused on an autoimmune or infectious cause. • Evidence of an autoimmune cause is largely inferential and is based on the association of sclerosing cholangitis with a variety of autoimmune diseases. • Abnormal immunologic parameters can be found in the serum of some patients with sclerosing cholangitis, but there are no specific serologic markers for the disease. • Antimitochondrial antibodies are generally associated with primary biliary cirrhosis. • The diagnosis is usually made following ERCP showing multiple strictures and dilatations, giving a "beaded" appearance to the ducts. • Typically, sclerosing cholangitis is a diffuse process affecting both the intrahepatic and extrahepatic bile ducts. • In some cases, more limited involvement of the distal bile duct, the intrahepatic ducts, or the area of the bifurcation can be seen. • Liver biopsy

may show fibroobliterative cholangitis or cirrhosis as the disease progresses.

ANSWER:
D

63. Definitive treatment for a patient with sclerosing cholangitis and biliary cirrhosis involves which of the following?

    A. Ursodeoxycholic acid

    B. Corticosteroids

    C. Endoscopic balloon dilatation and stenting

    D. Extrahepatic bile duct resection and transhepatic stenting

    E. Hepatic transplantation

    Ref.: 1–3, 7

COMMENTS: Once sclerosing cholangitis has progressed to cirrhosis, the only definitive treatment is hepatic transplantation. • The results of transplantation are generally similar to those obtained when it is performed for other indications. • Before the development of cirrhosis, a number of medical and surgical therapies have been tried. • Pharmacologic approaches have included the use of immunosuppressants, bile acid binding, and antifibrotic and antimicrobial drugs. • Unfortunately, there is little evidence that any medical therapy has been effective in slowing progression. • Some hopeful results have been reported with ursodeoxycholic acid, which may improve liver enzyme test results and liver histologic study results. • Dominant strictures can be treated operatively or by nonoperative dilatation via endoscopic or percutaneous transhepatic approaches. • The long-term efficacy of nonoperative approaches has often been limited, however. • Selected patients with predominantly extrahepatic or bifurcation strictures have been successfully treated with bile duct resection followed by Roux-en-Y reconstruction and long-term anastomotic stenting.

ANSWER:
E

64. Adenocarcinoma of the gallbladder extending into the subserosa is discovered incidentally following cholecystectomy. Recommended treatment includes which of the following?

    A. Nothing further at this time

    B. External beam irradiation

    C. Irradiation and chemotherapy

    D. Reoperation for liver resection and lymphadenectomy

    E. Reoperation for performance of pancreaticoduodenectomy

    Ref.: 18, 19

COMMENTS: When gallbladder cancer is discovered postoperatively during pathologic examination of the specimen, the depth of tumor invasion is an important determinant of further therapy. • (The layers of the gallbladder wall are described in Question 1.) Tumors limited to the mucosa (pT1a) or muscular layer (pT1b) are usually cured by cholecystectomy alone. • (It should be noted, however, that recurrence and death have occasionally been reported following cholecystectomy alone for pT1b lesions. • Therefore, further treatment could be considered in this situation, depending on the individual circumstances.) Patients with tumors extending into the subserosal connective tissue layer (pT2) are those most likely to benefit from resection of the adjacent liver segments (IV and V) and hepatoduodenal lymphadenectomy. • A substantial proportion of patients with pT2 lesions can be found to have lymph nodes positive for cancer or residual disease. • Reoperation may increase the 5-year survival rate to 70–90%, compared to 40% for cholecystectomy alone. • More extensive invasion through the serosa (pT3) or more than 2 cm into the liver (pT4), with or without adjacent organ invasion, may be recognized by the surgeon at the time of cholecystectomy, but this is not always the case. • Cholecystectomy is inadequate for cure of these lesions. • Radical resection of these cancers may certainly benefit some patients, but the morbidity and mortality may be high, and conclusive evidence of benefit to many patients is lacking. • Other pathologic findings in the gallbladder specimen that favor reoperation are a cancer-positive cystic duct margin (in which case bile duct resection must be considered) or a cancer-positive cystic duct lymph node. • Irradiation and chemotherapy have generally been ineffective for treatment of gallbladder cancer.

ANSWER:
D

65. Ultrasound imaging demonstrates a 15-mm polypoid lesion in the gallbladder of an asymptomatic 60-year-old patient. Which of the following best describes the recommended treatment?

   A. Observation with repeat ultrasound studies in 6 months

   B. Cholecystectomy

   C. Cholecystectomy if the patient is female

   D. Cholecystectomy only if symptoms develop

   E. Cholecystectomy only if the patient also has gallstones

Ref.: 20, 21

COMMENTS: Polypoid lesions of the gallbladder may be benign, premalignant, or malignant. • Inflammatory polyps and cholesterol polyps are benign, nonneoplastic lesions. • Benign adenomas are neoplasms that have a malignant potential similar to that of adenomas arising in other areas of the gastrointestinal tract. • Polypoid lesions are typically diagnosed by ultrasound imaging and occasionally by other imaging modalities, such as CT scanning. • The indications for cholecystectomy for treatment of a polypoid lesion are (1) symptoms and (2) possible malignancy.

The risk of malignancy is related to the size of the lesion and is higher for lesions that are 10 mm or larger and quite substantial for lesions of 15 mm. • Therefore, cholecystectomy is performed if the patient has biliary tract symptoms—regardless of polyp size or the presence or absence of gallstones—or if the lesion is larger than 10 mm. • Polypoid lesions in patients 60 years of age or older are also more frequently malignant. • The use of laparoscopic cholecystectomy for polypoid lesions is controversial. • Proponents hold that the laparoscopic approach is appropriate, since most polyps are benign and even limited cancers may be cured by cholecystectomy alone. • However, gallbladder leakage is common during laparoscopic cholecystectomy, and consequent dissemination of otherwise "curable" early cancers has been reported. • The long-term results of radical resection following laparoscopic cholecystectomy for gallbladder cancers are unknown. • Until more information becomes available, it is generally advised that open cholecystectomy be performed for patients considered at risk for gallbladder cancer.

ANSWER:
B

66. Which of the following is/are contraindications for resection of the bile duct cancer?

   A. Tumor location in distal common bile duct

   B. Tumor location at bifurcation of bile duct

   C. Peritoneal metastases

   D. Invasion of right portal vein and right hepatic artery

   E. None of the above

Ref.: 1, 3

COMMENTS: Cancers of the extrahepatic bile ducts usually carry a poor prognosis because these tumors are often beyond the confines of surgical resection at the time of diagnosis. • Substantial palliation often can be achieved by therapy directed at the relief of biliary obstruction. • Prognosis is related to tumor location, resectability, and histologic pattern. • Proximal lesions at or near the hepatic bifurcation are most common but also are least often resectable and therefore have a less favorable prognosis. • In some centers, aggressive resection of proximal lesions, usually including hepatic resection, has produced improved survival with morbidity not exceeding that of nonoperative treatment. • Hilar cancers are considered unresectable if there is metastatic disease, bilateral vascular involvement, or bilateral extension of the tumor to second-order biliary radicles. • Hepatic transplantation for otherwise unresectable tumors has had poor results. • Distal lesions resectable by pancreaticoduodenectomy have the best prognosis, with a 5-year survival rate of approximately 30%. • Palliative decompression can be achieved by surgical anastomosis, surgical intubation, or endoscopic or percutaneous catheter placement. • The most appropriate method of palliative decompression for a particular patient depends on the tumor location and extent, the patient's underlying condition, the expertise of the surgeon, and the anticipated complications of each technique. • Nonoperative decompression is preferred for patients who are demonstrated to have metastasis or otherwise unresectable disease before operation.

ANSWER:
C

67. How is a contusion of the gallbladder from blunt abdominal trauma best managed?

   A. Drain placement

   B. Cholecystostomy tube

   C. Suture imbrication of the contusion

   D. Cholecystectomy

Ref.: 7

COMMENTS: The gallbladder may be injured as a result of blunt or penetrating trauma. • Penetrating injury is the most common. • Most injuries of the gallbladder and extrahepatic biliary tree are associated with involvement of other organs, such as the liver, small bowel, and colon. • Blunt injuries, including contusion, avulsion, and rupture, are treated by cholecystectomy. • Penetrating injuries occasionally cause isolated injury to the gallbladder. • The treatment in such instances usually is cholecystectomy, although cholecystostomy or simple closure and drainage are conceivable. • In general, the prognosis following a nonoperative injury of the biliary tract is related to the significance of the associated injuries.

ANSWER:
D

REFERENCES

1. Mullholland MW, Lillemoe KD, Doherty GM, et al (eds): *Greenfield's Surgery: Scientific Principles and Practice*, 4th ed. Lippincott, Williams & Wilkins, Philadelphia, 2006.
2. Townsend CM, Beauchamp RD, Evers BM, et al (eds): *Sabiston Textbook of Surgery: The Biological Basis of Modern Surgical Practice*, 17th ed. Saunders, Philadelphia, 2004.
3. Blumgart LH: *Surgery of the Liver and Biliary Tract*, 2nd ed. Churchill-Livingstone, Edinburgh, 1994.
4. Yoshida J, Chijiwa K, Yamaguchi K, et al: Practical classification of the branching types of the biliary tree: an analysis of 1,094 consecutive direct choler programs. *J Am Coll Surg* 182:37–40, 1996.
5. Deziel DJ: Hepatobiliary ultrasound. *Probl Gen Surg* 14:13–24, 1997.
6. Staren ED, Arregui ME: *Ultrasound for the Surgeon*. Lippincott-Raven, Philadelphia, 1997.
7. Brunicardi FC, Andersen DK, Billiar TR, et al (eds): *Schwartz's Principles of Surgery*, 8th ed. McGraw-Hill, New York, 2004.
8. O'Leary JP: *The Physiologic Basis of Surgery*, 2nd ed. Williams & Wilkins, Baltimore, 1996.
9. Canfield AJ, Hetz SP, Schriver JP, et al: Biliary dyskinesia: a study of more than 200 patients and review of the literature. *J Gastrointest Surg* 2:443–448, 1998.
10. Fong Y, Brennan MF, Turnbulla A, et al: Gallbladder cancer discovered during laparoscopic surgery. *Arch Surg* 128:1050–1054, 1993.
11. Shirai Y, Ohtani T, Hatakeyama K: Is laparoscopic cholecystectomy indicated for early gallbladder cancer? *Surgery* 122:120–121, 1997.
12. Stewart L, Way LW: Bile duct injuries during laparoscopic cholecystectomy: factors that influence the results of treatment. *Arch Surg* 130:1123–1129, 1995.
13. Lillemoe KD, Martin SA, Cameron JL, et al: Major bile duct injuries during laparoscopic cholecystectomy. *Ann Surg* 225:459–471, 1997.
14. Deziel DJ: Complications of cholecystectomy. *Surg Clin North Am* 74:809–823, 1994.
15. Woods MS, Traverso LW, Kozarek RA, et al: Biliary tract complications of laparoscopic cholecystectomy are detected more frequently with routine intraoperative cholangiography. *Surg Endosc* 9:1076–1080, 1995.
16. Barkun AN, Barkun JS, Fried GM, et al: Useful predictors of bile duct stones in patients undergoing laparoscopic cholecystectomy. *Ann Surg* 220:32–39, 1994.
17. Petelin J: Laparoscopic approach to common duct pathology. *Am J Surg* 165:487–491, 1993.
18. Shirai Y, Yoshida K, Tsukada K, et al: Inapparent carcinoma of the gallbladder: an appraisal of a radical second operation after simple cholecystectomy. *Ann Surg* 215:326–331, 1992.
19. Bartlett DL, Fong Y, Fortner JG, et al: Long-term results after resection for gallbladder cancer: implications for staging and management. *Ann Surg* 224:639–646, 1996.
20. Kubota K, Bandai Y, Noie T, et al: How should polypoid lesions of the gallbladder be treated in the era of laparoscopic cholecystectomy? *Surgery* 117:481–487, 1995.
21. Shirai Y, Ohtani T, Hatakeyama K: Is laparoscopic cholecystectomy recommended for large polypoid lesions of the gallbladder [letter]? *Surg Laparosc Endosc* 7:435, 1997.

C H A P T E R 40

Pancreas

Daniel J. Deziel, M.D.

1. With regard to the vascular relationships of the pancreas, which of the following statements is/are true?

   A. The portal vein is formed by the confluence of the splenic vein and the inferior mesenteric vein behind the pancreatic neck.

   B. The portal vein generally has no anterior tributaries behind the neck of the pancreas.

   C. The arterial supply of the pancreatic head is derived primarily from the splenic artery.

   D. The inferior pancreaticoduodenal artery is the first branch of the superior mesenteric artery.

   E. Anomalous hepatic and middle colic arteries may be intimately associated with the pancreatic head.

   Ref.: 1–3, 5

COMMENTS: The relationship of the pancreas to neighboring organs and to critical vascular structures is of great surgical significance. • The arterial supply to the head of the gland is derived from both the gastroduodenal and superior mesenteric arteries via anterior and posterior pancreaticoduodenal arcades. • For the most part, the head of the pancreas and the duodenum have a shared blood supply, so they generally must be resected together. • However, techniques for "duodenal-sparing" resection of the pancreatic head or "pancreatic-sparing" duodenectomy are appropriate in select circumstances.
    The body and tail of the gland receive their blood supply mainly from multiple branches of the splenic artery, which also connect with superior mesenteric sources. • Variations in major arteries—such as the origin of the right hepatic artery from the superior mesenteric artery and the origin of the middle colic artery from the superior mesenteric artery or dorsal pancreatic artery—place these vessels in close proximity to the head and neck of the pancreas, where they are subject to injury during pancreatectomy. • The junction of the splenic vein and superior mesenteric vein to form the portal vein lies behind the neck of the pancreas. • Usually these vessels do not have large anterior tributaries in this area, but appropriate caution must nonetheless be exercised when developing this plane during pancreatic operations.

ANSWER:
B, D, E

2. Which of the following statements regarding heterotopic pancreas is/are true?

   A. It can be histologically distinguished from normally located pancreatic tissue based on the absence of islet cells.

   B. Most patients with heterotopic pancreas have no related symptoms.

   C. Heterotopic pancreas is associated with an increased risk of pancreatic cancer.

   D. Resection of heterotopic pancreas is appropriate when it is discovered coincidentally at operation.

   Ref.: 1, 2, 5

COMMENTS: Heterotopic pancreas is pancreatic tissue located at sites other than the normal location of the gland. • Ectopic pancreatic tissue has been described at many anatomic locations but typically is found in the stomach, the duodenum, or a Meckel's diverticulum. • Theories of origin include metaplasia (the favored theory) and transplantation. • Histologic findings range from those of a rudimentary structure to a fully formed gland. • Most heterotopic rests contain ducts, and both endocrine and exocrine elements may be present. • This entity is not uncommon, being described in 1–2% of autopsies. • It is usually asymptomatic. • When symptoms occur, they are related to the location of the ectopic site and include obstruction (due to intussusception), ulceration, and bleeding. • Although malignancy has been reported, there is no evidence that heterotopic pancreatic tissue is predisposed to cancer. • The typical gross appearance is a submucosal nodule, often with a central umbilication. • Resection is indicated for symptomatic lesions and is appropriate diagnostically for incidental lesions discovered during operations for other reasons.

ANSWER:
B, D

3. The embryologic ventral pancreas forms which area(s) of the fully developed gland?

   A. Superior head

   B. Neck

   C. Uncinate process

   D. Body

   E. Tail

   Ref.: 1–3

COMMENTS: The pancreas is formed from two outpouchings of the primitive gut. • The dorsal pancreas originates from the duodenum, and the ventral pancreas begins as a bud from the hepatic diverticulum, which itself is an outpouching of the duodenum. • Other outgrowths from the hepatic diverticulum mature into the liver, gallbladder, and bile ducts. • During normal fetal development, the ventral pancreas rotates along with the primitive gut and fuses with the dorsal component. • The ventral pancreas constitutes the uncinate process and the inferior portion of the head of the gland in the fully developed state, and the dorsal pancreas forms the remainder of the gland. • Abnormalities in this developmental process result in recognized congenital anomalies that can be clinically important. • An understanding of this embryologic development is also important to recognizing the relationship of the pancreas to adjacent vascular structures during pancreatic operations.

ANSWER:
C

4. Which of the following correctly describe(s) the anatomic location of the uncinate process of the pancreas?

   A. Ventral to portal vein

   B. Ventral to aorta

   C. Ventral to left renal vein

   D. Dorsal to superior mesenteric artery

   E. Caudal to third portion of duodenum

Ref.: 1–5

COMMENTS: The pancreas can be divided into various parts: head, uncinate, neck, body, and tail. • The uncinate process is the portion of the gland that extends to the left behind the portal vein and superior mesenteric artery and in front of the aorta and inferior vena cava. • The uncinate process is located below and ventral to the left renal vein and above the distal duodenum. • Understanding the extent and location of the uncinate is important during resection of the head of the pancreas. • The blood supply of the uncinate is from numerous short branches of the superior mesenteric artery and portal vein. • Bleeding from these branches must be carefully controlled during resection.

ANSWER:
B, C, D

5. What is the recommended treatment for an adult with duodenal obstruction caused by annular pancreas?

   A. Endoscopic division of associated duodenal web

   B. Gastrojejunostomy

   C. Duodenojejunostomy

   D. Surgical division of annular tissue

   E. Pancreaticoduodenectomy

Ref.: 1, 2, 5

COMMENTS: Annular pancreas is a congenital anomaly involving a band of pancreatic tissue encircling the second portion of the duodenum. • The annular tissue appears to originate from the embryologic ventral pancreas. • Causal theories include abnormal fixation of the ventral pancreatic primordium (extramural type) or development of heterotopic pancreatic tissue in the duodenum (intramural type). • Approximately one half of these cases are diagnosed in infants and the remainder in adults, with a peak during the fourth decade of life. Most patients are asymptomatic. • Clinical presentations are obstruction in infants and children and obstruction, ulceration, or pancreatitis in adults. • Associated anomalies include duodenal stenosis or atresia and Down's syndrome. • Treatment of symptomatic patients is surgical bypass by duodenoduodenostomy or duodenojejunostomy. • Gastrojejunostomy can also alleviate obstruction but risks marginal ulceration. • Resection or division of the annular band is not advised, since it risks pancreatic fistula and may fail to relieve the obstruction.

ANSWER:
C

6. Which of the following developmental anomalies best characterizes pancreas divisum?

   A. Aplasia of the dorsal pancreatic anlage

   B. Aplasia of the ventral pancreatic anlage

   C. Incomplete rotation of the ventral pancreatic anlage

   D. Failed fusion of the ventral and dorsal pancreatic parenchyma

   E. Failed fusion of the ventral and dorsal pancreatic ducts

Ref.: 1, 2, 4

COMMENTS: See Question 7.

7. The diagnosis of pancreas divisum can be made by which one or more of the following?

   A. Ultrasound imaging

   B. Computed tomographic (CT) scanning

   C. Pancreatic scintigraphy

   D. Endoscopic retrograde cholangiopancreatography (ERCP)

   E. Glucose tolerance testing

Ref.: 2

COMMENTS: *Pancreas divisum* currently refers to congenital variations of the pancreatic ducts that result from failed or incomplete fusion of the embryologic ventral and dorsal ductal systems. • (Historically, the term may also refer to the rare failure of parenchymal fusion.) There may be complete separation of the ducts, an absent or minimal ventral duct, or only a few meager connections between the systems. • As a consequence, most of the pancreatic duct drainage is through the dorsal duct joining the duodenum at the minor papilla. • Any existing ventral ducts (Wirsung) drain only the uncinate process and the caudal head of the gland, rather than draining the bulk of the gland at the major papilla, as when normally developed. • Some variation of pancreas divisum is present in about 10% of the population. • In some individuals, it is clinically significant if the relatively stenotic minor papilla imposes an obstruction to ductal flow. • This can potentially result in recurrent abdominal pain, acute pancreatitis, or even chronic pancreatitis. • The diagnosis of pancreas divisum requires ERCP to visualize the ductal anatomy.

ANSWERS:
Question 6: E
Question 7: D

8. Which of the following may be appropriate treatment(s) for a patient with pancreas divisum, chronic abdominal pain,

a dilated dorsal pancreatic duct, and an enlarged, calcified pancreatic head?

A. Endoscopic dorsal sphincterotomy

B. Endoscopic dorsal duct stenting

C. Operative dorsal sphincterotomy

D. Longitudinal pancreaticojejunostomy

E. Pancreaticoduodenectomy

Ref.: 1, 2

COMMENTS: The true relationship between the anatomic diagnosis of pancreas divisum and any clinical symptoms is difficult to determine. • Symptomatic patients with pancreas divisum require thorough evaluation of the nature of their symptoms and for any other causes of abdominal pain or pancreatitis. • When it is reasonable to suspect that a stenotic lesser papilla is the cause of recurrent abdominal pain or recurrent acute pancreatitis, therapeutic considerations include endoscopic sphincterotomy or stenting (or both) or operative sphincterotomy and sphincteroplasty. • The long-term results of endoscopic treatment have not always been encouraging, and operative sphincterotomy is considered the definitive intervention when sphincter ablation is appropriate. • Occasionally, there are patients (as described in this question) with established findings of chronic pancreatitis and pancreas divisum. • Sphincter operations are not indicated in this setting. • Rather, surgical treatment, when indicated, must be directed at pancreatic decompression or resection, both of which may be appropriate for the patient described.

ANSWER:
D, E

9. Which of the following is/are more characteristic of pancreatic centroacinar cells than acinar cells?

A. Carbonic anhydrase

B. Zymogen granules

C. Golgi apparatus

D. Rough endoplasmic reticulum

E. Contractile proteins

Ref.: 2, 4

COMMENTS: The twofold function of the exocrine pancreas—to secrete bicarbonate-rich fluid and to synthesize digestive enzymes—is accomplished by two cell types. • The **acinar cells**, which elaborate and secrete digestive enzymes, are designed for protein synthesis. • They contain abundant rough endoplasmic reticulum, Golgi apparatus, and secretory zymogen granules. • Contractile proteins also are abundant near the apical membrane of the cell and facilitate exocytosis of the enzyme bundles into the ductal lumen. • The **centroacinar cells** are part of the ductal system. • They secrete bicarbonate and therefore contain carbonic anhydrase, which dissociates carbonic acid into bicarbonate and hydrogen ion:

$$H_2O + CO_2 \rightarrow H^+ + HCO_3^-.$$

Some ductal cells also contain synthetic and secretory organelles for production of mucoproteins.

ANSWER:
A

10. Which of the following is/are true regarding regulation of pancreatic fluid and electrolyte secretion?

A. Secretin is the primary stimulant.

B. Cholecystokinin (CCK) is the primary stimulant.

C. Bicarbonate concentration increases with the secretory rate.

D. Bicarbonate concentration decreases with the secretory rate.

E. Sodium and potassium concentrations are relatively constant.

Ref.: 1, 3, 4

COMMENTS: The centroacinar cells secrete a bicarbonate-rich solution by an active transport mechanism, primarily in response to secretin. • CCK is the primary stimulant of enzyme secretion from the acinar cells. • The bicarbonate and chloride contents of pancreatic juice are reciprocally related. • As ductal flow rates increase, bicarbonate concentration increases, and chloride concentration decreases. • This is the result of two processes: (1) changes in passive exchange of intraductal bicarbonate for intracellular chloride and (2) changes in the relative contribution of acinar cell secretion. • Acinar cells secrete fluid high in chloride in addition to digestive enzymes. • In contradistinction to anion concentrations, the concentrations of sodium and potassium in pancreatic duct secretion remain relatively constant, despite the flow rate, and are similar to the concentrations in plasma.

ANSWER:
A, C, E

11. Which of the following normally activates pancreatic trypsinogen?

A. Pancreatic amylase

B. pH greater than 7.0

C. Lysosomal hydrolase

D. Duodenal enterokinase

E. Pancreatic enterokinase

Ref.: 1, 3–5

COMMENTS: The pancreatic acinar cells secrete digestive enzymes for fats, carbohydrates, and proteins. • With the exception of amylase, these enzymes are secreted in inactive forms to protect the pancreas from autodigestion. • Activation of the proenzyme trypsinogen to trypsin is the primary event that leads to activation of the other various proteases and phospholipases. • It occurs in the duodenum via the action of enterokinase. • Trypsinogen activation can also occur in acidic environments (pH<7.0). • With acute pancreatitis, intraglandular activation can occur when the inactive enzymes are exposed to lysosomal hydrolases.

ANSWER:
D

12. Match the islet cell type in the left-hand column with the peptide hormone produced in the right-hand column.

A. A cell   a. Pancreatic polypeptide

B. B cell   b. Glucagon

C. D cell   c. Insulin

D. F cell   d. Somatostatin

Ref.: 1, 3–5

COMMENTS: See Question 13.

13. Match the pancreatic peptide in the left-hand column with the physiologic effect(s) in the right-hand column. Each answer may be used more than once or not at all.

A. Insulin	a. Stimulates lipolysis
B. Glucagon	b. Inhibits lipolysis
C. Somatostatin	c. Inhibits pancreatic exocrine secretion
D. Pancreatic polypeptide	d. Marker for pancreatic endocrine tumors

Ref.: 1, 3–5

COMMENTS: The endocrine pancreas is composed of various cells located in the islets of Langerhans, approximately 1 million of which are interspersed with the acinar and ductal elements throughout the gland. • The hormonal peptides produced by the islets effect a wide range of metabolic and physiologic actions. • The primary function of the endocrine pancreas is to regulate glucose homeostasis. • The B cells, which are the most numerous, produce insulin. • Insulin promotes glucose transport, stimulates protein synthesis, and inhibits glycogenolysis and lipolysis. • The A cells secrete glucagon, which counterbalances insulin by stimulating hepatic glycogenolysis, gluconeogenesis, ketogenesis, and lipolysis. • Glucagon also inhibits intestinal motility and gastric acid and pancreatic exocrine secretion. • Somatostatin, produced by the D cells, has a broad range of inhibitory effects on the gastrointestinal tract, including inhibition of secretion of other pancreatic peptides; inhibition of gastric, biliary, intestinal, and pancreatic exocrine secretions; and inhibition of gastrointestinal motility. • The F, or PP, cells are the source of pancreatic polypeptide. • Pancreatic polypeptide inhibits pancreatic exocrine secretion and biliary motility, and it may play a role in glucose homeostasis, although its physiologic function has not been fully elucidated. • Clinically, deficiency of pancreatic polypeptide has been linked to diabetes following resection of the pancreatic head or chronic pancreatitis. • Pancreatic polypeptide has been used as a marker for pancreatic endocrine tumors. • Since postprandial secretion of pancreatic polypeptide is dependent on vagal innervation, it has been used to assess completeness of vagotomy.

ANSWERS:
Question 12: A-b; B-c; C-d; D-a
Question 13: A-b; B-a,c; C-c; D-c,d

14. Which is the principal cell type located at the center of the islets of Langerhans?

A. A cell

B. B cell

C. D cell

D. F cell

E. Varies according to the location of the islet in the pancreas

Ref.: 1, 3

COMMENTS: Each islet of Langerhans is composed of an average of 3000 cells, with the major types as listed above and discussed in the preceding Comments. • The B cells are located at the core and make up about 70% of the islet. • The other cell types are located at the periphery of the islet. • This cellular anatomy has potential functional implications that are as yet not well understood. • The distribution of cell types within the islet varies in various areas of the gland. Islets in the uncinate process derived from the embryologic ventral

pancreas contain F cells but few A cells. • Islets in the body and tail of the gland have abundant A cells but no F cells.

ANSWER:
B

15. Which of the following statements is/are true regarding the microvasculature of the pancreas?

A. The islet cells receive a greater proportion of pancreatic blood flow than exocrine elements.

B. CCK and secretin regulate secretion by altering blood flow.

C. Fragile anastomotic networks predispose the gland to ischemia.

D. Arterioles supply both the islets and the acinar tissue.

E. Blood draining from islets perfuses acinar tissues.

Ref.: 2–4

COMMENTS: The microcirculation of the pancreas is complex and has important correlations with the endocrine and exocrine functions of the gland. • The rich anastomotic supply from various sources makes pancreatic ischemic unusual. • The islets receive a disproportionately large amount of total pancreatic blood flow (10–25%) relative to their mass (1–2%). • Both the islets and the exocrine tissue have arteriolar blood supply. • The acinar tissue is also perfused by blood that drains from the islets, a mechanism referred to as the islet-acinar or insuloacinar portal system. • This system is the structural basis for endocrine regulation of exocrine function. • Insulin receptors are present on acinar cells, and the density of receptors is higher on acini located near the islets. • Since the islets themselves often have a central-to-peripheral pattern of perfusion, insulin from the centrally located B cells can influence the other peripheral islet cell types. • Also, some islets are apparently perfused in a peripheral-to-central pattern. CCK and secretin have relatively little effect on blood flow and so exert their stimulatory effects independently. • Pancreatic blood flow is maintained relatively constant, despite changes in arterial pressure.

ANSWER:
A, D, E

16. Which of the following events occur in the acinar cell with acute pancreatitis?

A. Accelerated extrusion of zymogen granules

B. Impaired extrusion of zymogen granules

C. Fusion of lysosomes and zymogen granules

D. Fusion of mitochondria and zymogen granules

E. Impaired protein synthesis

Ref.: 2–4

COMMENTS: The pathogenesis of pancreatitis involves intrapancreatic activation of digestive enzymes that normally are secreted in inactive form. • It results in "autodigestion" of the gland. • Although the mechanisms by which the various causes of clinical pancreatitis leading to this state are incompletely understood, experimental observations have identified certain derangements in acinar cell biology that may be the underlying common pathway to pancreatic injury. • The primary defects involve blocked extrusion of zymogen granules containing inactive digestive enzymes and alterations in intracellular transport that result in fusion of zymogen granules with lysosomes to form large cytoplasmic vacuoles. • This sequence results in colocalization of digestive enzymes and lysosomal hydrolases. • Lysosomal enzymes, such as cathepsin B, activate trypsinogen and initiate a cascade of intracellular digestive enzyme activation. • Amino acid uptake and protein synthesis are not impaired during this process. • These cellular events have been observed in experimental models of acute pancreatitis. • The extent to which they reflect the cellular change that occurs in human acute pancreatitis is not known.

ANSWER:
B, C

---

18. The mechanism of alcohol-induced acute pancreatitis is thought to involve which of the following?

    A. Pancreatic ductal obstruction

    B. Pancreatic exocrine hypersecretion

    C. Hypertriglyceridemia

    D. Acetaldehyde toxicity

    E. Impaired trypsin inhibition

Ref.: 1, 3

COMMENTS: Ethanol is the prevalent etiologic factor in acute pancreatitis. • The mechanisms by which alcohol-induced pancreatic injury occurs are not precisely known, but there are several plausible theories. • Ethanol causes pancreatic ductal hypertension by increasing ampullary resistance and by intraductal deposition of stone proteins. • Concomitantly, ethanol stimulates gastric acid secretion and increases pancreatic exocrine secretion via secretin release. • The combination of ductal obstruction with stimulated secretion may result in enzyme extravasation. • Acetaldehyde, the metabolic product of ethanol, injures acinar cells by increasing membrane permeability and disrupting the microtubule structure. • Elevated levels of serum triglycerides induced by alcohol are a source of cytotoxic free fatty acids. • Alcohol also impairs normal trypsin inhibition and reduces pancreatic blood flow. • All of these effects may contribute to intraglandular enzyme activation and the development of acute alcoholic pancreatitis.

ANSWER:
A, B, C, D, E

---

18. Hyperamylasemia is diagnostic of acute pancreatitis when associated with which of the following laboratory findings?

    A. Hyperlipasemia

    B. Increased urinary amylase levels

    C. Amylase/creatinine clearance ratio greater than 5%

    D. Hypocalcemia

    E. None of the above

Ref.: 1–3, 5

COMMENTS: The diagnosis of acute pancreatitis is based on the clinical presentation, supported by biochemical findings and morphologic abnormalities on imaging studies such as CT scans. • No biochemical feature is pathognomonic for acute pancreatitis. • Hyperamylasemia, hyperlipasemia, and elevations in urinary amylase levels and in the amylase/creatinine clearance ratio are typical of acute pancreatitis but are not specific or sensitive, and

they can occur with other abdominal and extra-abdominal disorders. • Hypocalcemia may occur as a consequence of pancreatitis, but it also is nonspecific. • There is no absolute level of serum amylase or lipase that is diagnostic of acute pancreatitis. • Marked elevations are more indicative of pancreatitis but are not themselves diagnostic. • Both amylase and lipase levels may be elevated in a number of conditions that can be confused with acute pancreatitis, such as acute cholecystitis, perforated peptic ulcer, and intestinal infarction. • Moreover, severe pancreatitis can occur without substantial elevations in these serum enzymes.

ANSWER:
E

---

19. A patient with abdominal pain is found to have a serum amylase level of 1200 IU/L, a normal urinary amylase level, and an amylase/creatinine clearance ratio (ACCR) of less than 2%. Based on these findings, the likely diagnosis is which of the following conditions?

    A. Acute pancreatitis

    B. Chronic pancreatitis

    C. Renal failure

    D. Choledocholithiasis without pancreatitis

    E. Macroamylasemia

Ref.: 2

COMMENTS: Elevations in serum and urinary amylase levels and in the ACCR, as determined by the following equation, are typical of acute pancreatitis.

$$ACCR = U_{amy}/S_{amy} \times S_{cr}/U_{cr} \times 100$$

where U = urine; S = serum; amy = amylase; and cr = creatinine. • Elevation of the ACCR above the normal 2–5% range is not specific for pancreatitis, but a normal ratio in the presence of hyperamylasemia suggests that the hyperamylasemia results from something other than pancreatitis. • Serum and urinary amylase levels and the ACCR may be normal in the presence of chronic pancreatitis or elevated during an acute exacerbation. • Renal disease may be associated with low urinary amylase levels and an elevated ACCR. • Common duct stones may produce hyperamylasemia without true pancreatitis. • The urinary amylase level is elevated, although the ACCR may be normal. • With macroamylasemia, amylase forms complexes with serum proteins too large for glomerular filtration. • The serum amylase level is therefore elevated, but urinary amylase levels and the ACCR are low. • The diagnosis can be confirmed by electrophoresis. • Abdominal pain has been reported in more than one half of patients with macroamylasemia, although the biochemical abnormality probably is not etiologically related to the pain. • Hyperamylasemia predominantly caused by salivary amylase also may be associated with a low urinary amylase level and ACCR because the salivary isoenzyme is cleared more slowly by the kidneys than the pancreatic isoenzyme.

ANSWER:
E

---

20. Which of the following conditions are unfavorable prognostic criteria for acute alcoholic pancreatitis?

    A. White blood cell (WBC) count higher than 16,000/ml

B. Serum calcium level of less than 8 mg/dl during the initial 48 hr

C. Serum amylase level on admission more than 1200 IU/L

D. Serum lipase level more than three times normal

E. Serum blood urea nitrogen (BUN) level elevated over 2 mg/dl during the initial 48 hr

Ref.: 1, 2, 3

COMMENTS: Several prognostic systems have been devised to gauge the severity of acute pancreatitis. • These systems involve multiple clinical, biochemical, and sometimes radiologic criteria. • The most widely used system in the United States, developed by Ranson, was based on retrospective analysis and subsequent prospective verification. • Ranson's criteria include 11 parameters determined at the time of admission or during the subsequent 48 hr. • Patients with three or more criteria have more severe disease and are at increased risk of septic complications and death. • The criteria reflect the patient's underlying status, the severity of the retroperitoneal inflammatory process, and the effects on renal and respiratory function. • Ranson's criteria originally were developed for alcoholic pancreatitis and have been modified somewhat for gallstone pancreatitis. • For example, a rise in serum BUN level of more than 2 mg/dl is one of the 10 criteria for gallstone pancreatitis, but the rise must be more than 5 mg/dl to meet the criteria for alcoholic pancreatitis (a subtle point). • Other physiologic scoring systems, such as the APACHE II, may also be useful prognostically although they are not designed specifically for assessment of acute pancreatitis.

ANSWER:
A, B

21. Routine initial treatment of a patient with alcoholic pancreatitis and five Ranson's criteria should include which of the following measures?

A. Gastric decompression

B. Intravenous antibiotics

C. Peritoneal lavage

D. Octreotide

E. Laparotomy

Ref.: 1, 2

COMMENTS: The diagnosis of acute pancreatitis initially is a presumptive one. • Patients presenting with acute abdominal symptoms require careful clinical, biochemical, and radiologic evaluation to exclude other intra-abdominal problems, such as bowel obstruction, perforated viscus, mesenteric ischemia, cholecystitis, and others. • Immediate laparotomy may be indicated. • In a patient with acute pancreatitis, the initial treatment is nonoperative and focuses on fluid resuscitation; maintenance of ventilation, oxygenation, and renal perfusion; and prevention of complications.

Gastric decompression is indicated because of associated paralytic ileus and delayed gastric emptying. • Although decompression may theoretically decrease pancreatic stimulation, controlled studies have not shown that decompression alters the course of alcoholic pancreatitis.

Controlled studies also have failed to demonstrate the benefit of routine use of antibiotics in the prevention of infectious complications, but these trials included patients with mild pancreatitis. • Patients with more severe pancreatitis, based on established indexes (more than three of Ranson's signs), are at greater risk for

pancreatic infection, and experienced pancreatic surgeons generally advocate antibiotics for these patients. • A randomized study of intravenous imipenem has shown that it decreased pancreatic sepsis in treated patients. • Selective decontamination of the gut has also been reported to decrease mortality in patients with severe pancreatitis. • Antibiotics are commonly used for patients with biliary pancreatitis.

Various inhibitors of pancreatic enzymes and secretion have been tried without benefit. • Octreotide, a long-acting analogue of somatostatin, has received attention in clinical trials but has not been proved beneficial and could potentially be detrimental by decreasing pancreatic blood flow.

Peritoneal lavage can decrease the early mortality of severe pancreatitis in patients who do not respond to standard supportive measures. • A small study suggested that longer periods of lavage (up to 2 weeks) may decrease septic complications and overall mortality.

Planned early operative intervention to accomplish pancreatic resection in patients with acute pancreatitis has a higher mortality than does nonoperative therapy. • Operation is therefore delayed unless prompted by complications such as infection or hemorrhage.

ANSWER:
A, B

22. What is the leading cause of death from acute pancreatitis?

A. Hemorrhage

B. Pseudocyst rupture

C. Secondary pancreatic infection

D. Biliary sepsis

E. Renal failure

Ref.: 6

COMMENTS: Formerly, death from acute pancreatitis often occurred early in the course of the disease owing to the acute effects of hypovolemia and inadequate resuscitation. • In the current era, about 80% of deaths are attributed to secondary pancreatic infection, which develops in about 10% of patients with acute pancreatitis. • Fatal pancreatic sepsis typically progresses to multisystem organ failure, and deaths occur later in the course of the disease. • To have an impact on this disease, therapeutic efforts have therefore focused on the prevention and early diagnosis of pancreatic infection and on more effective methods of surgical therapy.

ANSWER:
C

23. Which of the following complications of acute pancreatitis is associated with the highest mortality rate?

A. Peripancreatic abscess

B. Infected pancreatic pseudocyst

C. Infected pancreatic necrosis

D. Sterile pancreatic necrosis

Ref.: 2, 6

COMMENTS: Retroperitoneal infection is a serious, often fatal complication of acute pancreatitis. • Early literature pertaining to the local infectious sequelae of pancreatitis may be confusing because of the nonselective use of the term *pancreatic abscess* to describe infectious complications, which vary in severity. • *Pancreatic abscess* best describes a localized collection of drainable pus in or around the pancreas. • Pancreatic abscess and infected pseudocyst can be treated effectively by external drainage, and anticipated mortality for each is about 5%. • Pancreatic necrosis is a manifestation of severe pancreatitis. • When accompanied by infection, it has been associated with a mortality rate that may exceed 40%, which is higher than the mortality rate for noninfected necrosis. • Infected pancreatic necrosis is treated by operative débridement and open or closed retroperitoneal drainage. • Patients with sterile necrosis may require operative intervention as well but are generally treated nonoperatively with intensive support as long as their condition permits.

ANSWER:
C

24. An alcoholic patient has acute pancreatitis with five of Ranson's criteria. He gradually improves over a 14-day hospitalization but then develops a pulse of 120 bpm, a temperature of 39°C, and abdominal distention. A CT scan is obtained, and the results are shown below. The next most appropriate therapy is which of the following measures?

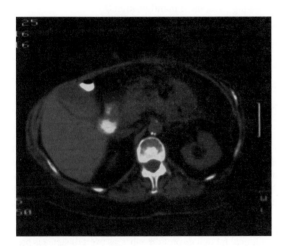

A. Antibiotics

B. Percutaneous catheter drainage

C. Peritoneal lavage

D. Laparoscopy

E. Operative drainage

Ref.: 2, 6

COMMENTS: Pancreatic infection complicating acute pancreatitis should be suspected based on the clinical course of any patient who fails to improve following supportive medical therapy or improves but then demonstrates deterioration. • Pancreatic infection occasionally occurs early during the chronologic course of the disease, but typically it presents later, as in the patient described. CT scanning is the best method for imaging the pancreas. • It should be used serially in patients with severe pancreatitis. • Results of CT of this patient demonstrate air in the pancreas, which is characteristic of pancreatic infection. • The technique of dynamic pancreatography can identify ischemic areas of pancreas and is useful for evaluating patients who may have pancreatic necrosis. • Dynamic pancreatography is performed by serially imaging the pancreas after bolus injection of an intravenous contrast medium. • Percutaneous needle

aspiration of fluid collections or necrotic areas found on CT imaging can be performed to identify the presence of infection and guide therapeutic decisions about the need for drainage. • When pancreatic infection is present, operative drainage and débridement are indicated. • Percutaneous catheter drainage does not permit adequate egress of necrotic tissue. • Interest has focused on the selection of closed or open methods of operative drainage and on whether nonoperative or operative therapy is best for patients with noninfected pancreatic necrosis.

ANSWER:
E

25. Most patients with acute gallstone pancreatitis are best treated by which of the following measures?

A. Urgent (within 24 hr) cholecystectomy and common bile duct exploration

B. Urgent ERCP and subsequent laparoscopic cholecystectomy

C. Initial supportive therapy with cholecystectomy during the same admission

D. Initial supportive therapy with cholecystectomy within 6–8 weeks

E. Initial supportive therapy with cholecystectomy only if symptoms recur

Ref.: 1, 2

COMMENTS: Gallstone pancreatitis is related to passage of stones through the ampulla of Vater. • Patients with smaller gallstones have an increased risk of developing this manifestation. • Cholecystectomy is indicated because gallstone pancreatitis is a recurrent problem for 30–50% of patients if surgery is not performed. • The traditional controversy has been in regard to the timing of operation. • Proponents of immediate intervention have found a higher incidence of choledocholithiasis but have not demonstrated that this approach is safer than delayed operation or that it is necessary for most patients. • Most surgeons advise initial nonoperative therapy until the patient's signs and symptoms subside (most do within 2–3 days) and then elective cholecystectomy with cholangiography and common duct exploration, as necessary, during the same hospitalization. • Laparoscopic cholecystectomy is a safe, effective treatment. • Operative evaluation of the common bile duct with intraoperative cholangiography, laparoscopic ultrasonography, or both should be undertaken.

The role of urgent ERCP and endoscopic sphincterotomy for management of biliary pancreatitis has been controversial. • It should be remembered that most (97%) patients with gallstone pancreatitis have only mild pancreatitis that improves rapidly. • ERCP finds common duct stones in only a small percentage of patients and is *not* indicated routinely. Some randomized trials comparing urgent ERCP and sphincterotomy to traditional treatment have suggested benefit for patients with severe pancreatitis, but this has not been consistently observed. • ERCP can understandably be useful with patients with pancreatitis and concomitant and persisting biliary obstruction or with patients deemed unfit for surgery. • For the small proportion of patients with severe biliary pancreatitis, early cholecystectomy should be avoided. Treatment in this group is directed at resolution of the pancreatitis and its complications. • When pancreatitis has subsided, delayed cholecystectomy is indicated.

ANSWER:
C

26. Which of the following forms of nutritional support should be avoided in a patient with acute alcoholic pancreatitis?

    A. Enteral fat

    B. Parenteral hypertonic dextrose

    C. Parenteral fatty acids

    D. Parenteral amino acids

    E. Parenteral combination of amino acids, glucose, and fat

    Ref.: 2, 7

COMMENTS: Nutritional support is an important component of the successful management of patients with moderate or severe pancreatitis. • The mortality rate is lowered for patients achieving a positive nitrogen balance. • Effects of specific nutrients and administration routes have been studied. • Feeding fat into the stomach and duodenum stimulates pancreatic exocrine secretion and should be avoided. • Jejunal feeding of nutrients does not produce the same degree of stimulation. • Parenteral administration of fats, glucose, and amino acids alone or in combination does not stimulate the exocrine pancreas. • Total parenteral nutrition with intravenous lipid infusions has not been associated with a detrimental outcome and has been critical for reversing nutritional defects and preventing essential fatty acid deficiency. • For patients with acute pancreatitis due to hyperlipidemia, however, there is scarce information about the effect of intravenous lipid administration.

A N S W E R :
A

27. In North America, chronic pancreatitis is most commonly related to chronic alcohol ingestion. Which of the following is the second most common consideration?

    A. Gallstones

    B. Drugs

    C. Infections

    D. Malnutrition

    E. Idiopathic cases

    Ref.: 3

COMMENTS: In the Western world, alcohol use accounts for about 75% of cases of chronic pancreatitis. • Approximately 20% of cases are considered idiopathic. • In parts of Africa and Asia, protein malnutrition is an important etiologic factor. • Other, less common causes of chronic pancreatitis include pancreatic duct obstruction (due to stenosis or pancreas divisum), hyperparathyroidism, trauma, cystic fibrosis, and hereditary causes. • Unlike acute pancreatitis, calculous biliary disease is not a typical cause of chronic pancreatitis. • Certain infections (particularly viral) and drugs are among the many factors that can produce acute, rather than chronic, pancreatitis.

A N S W E R :
E

28. With regard to the histologic characteristics of chronic pancreatitis, all but which of the following are observed?

    A. Increased interstitial connective tissue

    B. Loss of acinar cells

    C. Loss of islet cells

    D. Decrease in nerve tissue

    E. Damaged perineurium

    Ref.: 2

COMMENTS: Chronic pancreatitis is characterized on histologic examination by loss of exocrine acinar cells and a marked increase in interstitial fibrous connective tissue. • The islets of Langerhans are preserved and constitute a relatively greater proportion of pancreatic tissue. • Hyperplasia of islet cells also is seen. • The size and number of nerves are increased, but the protective perineural sheath is damaged, and nerves are found in proximity to inflammatory foci. • There appear to be selective increases in certain peptidergic nerves. • These histologic observations may be related to the cause of pain in chronic pancreatitis.

A N S W E R :
C, D

29. Pain is the predominant clinical manifestation of chronic alcoholic pancreatitis. Most patients also have which of the following associated manifestations?

    A. Clinical diabetes mellitus

    B. Hypoglycemia

    C. Steatorrhea

    D. Subclinical fat malabsorption

    E. Hepatic cirrhosis

    Ref.: 1, 3, 5

COMMENTS: Recurrent or persistent abdominal pain is the predominant symptom of chronic pancreatitis. • Patients usually have variable degrees of nausea, anorexia, and weight loss. • Mechanisms that may contribute to pain include ductal obstruction, parenchymal hypertension, acute inflammation, and perineural inflammation. • About two thirds of patients have abnormal glucose tolerance tests and subclinical fat malabsorption, whereas overt diabetes is present in perhaps 30–50% and frank steatorrhea in only 10–15%. • Endocrine and exocrine insufficiency progresses during the course of the disease. • Diabetes mellitus may be related to impaired insulin release because the islet cells themselves are relatively preserved. • Despite the common etiologic factor of ethanol, most patients with chronic pancreatitis do not have hepatic cirrhosis.

A N S W E R :
D

30. Appropriate management of frank steatorrhea may include all except which of the following choices?

    A. Fat restriction to 75 g/day

    B. Nonencapsulated pancreatic enzymes

    C. Encapsulated pancreatic enzymes

    D. Nonencapsulated pancreatic enzymes and an H₂ blocker

    E. Encapsulated pancreatic enzymes and an H₂ blocker

    Ref.: 2, 3

COMMENTS: Gross steatorrhea and diarrhea occur when pancreatic exocrine function is reduced to about 10% of normal.

• Therapy involves limitation of fat intake and administration of adequate amounts of exogenous pancreatic enzyme preparations to provide at least 10% of normal lipolytic activity in the duodenum at the time the food substrate is present. • Various commercial formulations of pancreatic enzymes are available. • Nonencapsulated forms may improve the malabsorption but can be ineffective due to inactivation in the stomach when the pH falls below 4. • The addition of H_2 blockers may then be useful. • Enteric-coated preparations release their enzymes at a pH above 5. • Therefore, they are useful for patients whose gastric pH remains low to ensure that the enzyme is not released until it reaches the duodenum. • Use of encapsulated forms with H_2 blockers is counterproductive because the enzyme is released in the stomach and is then inactivated if pH falls. • In addition, enteric-coated preparations are microspheres of varying size, and the larger ones do not empty into the duodenum until after the food substrate does.

ANSWER:
E

31. A 58-year-old woman with jaundice underwent ERCP (results shown below) as part of her diagnostic workup. On the basis of this radiograph, what diagnosis is considered the most likely?

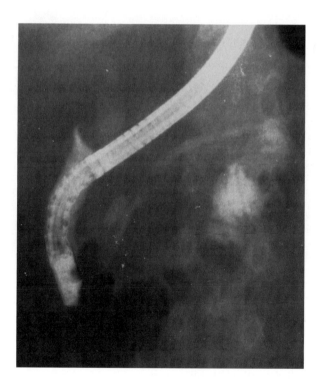

   A. Chronic pancreatitis

   B. Pancreatic neoplasm

   C. Cholangiocarcinoma

   D. Pancreas divisum

Ref.: 1, 5

COMMENTS: This ERCP study shows the classic "double duct sign": dilatation of the biliary system above an area of abrupt narrowing and abrupt termination of the main pancreatic duct. • These findings place the primary abnormality in the geographic location of the pancreatic head, and it is not uncommon for a **pancreatic neoplasm** to involve both ducts. • **Chronic pancreatitis** may cause biliary obstruction, but the obstruction in the biliary systems is usually more distal. • Likewise, no coexistent changes, such as irregular beading of the pancreatic duct, are present in this patient to suggest that there has been chronic pancreatitis. • **Cholangiocarcinoma** may be responsible for the stenosis in the biliary system, but cholangiocarcinomas rarely become large enough to involve the pancreatic duct. • With **pancreas divisum**, injection of the major papilla opacifies only a short, tapering ventral duct draining the caudal portion of the pancreatic head and uncinate process. • Injection of the minor papilla demonstrates the dorsal duct draining the major portion of the gland.

ANSWER:
B

32. A 45-year-old nondiabetic patient with chronic alcoholic pancreatitis and intractable abdominal pain has a 10-mm pancreatic duct. Which of the following choices constitute(s) the best treatment?

   A. Sphincteroplasty

   B. Lateral pancreaticojejunostomy

   C. Caudal (tail) pancreatectomy

   D. Total pancreatectomy

   E. Continued nonoperative therapy

Ref.: 1, 2, 8

COMMENTS: Pain is the primary indication for surgery in patients with chronic pancreatitis. • Selecting the best operation for a particular patient must include consideration of the anatomy of the gland, preexisting endocrine or exocrine dysfunction, compliance and the rehabilitative capacity of the patient, postoperative endocrine or exocrine deficiency, and the likelihood of postoperative pain relief. • Patients with a dilated duct (>6 mm) are treated by ductal drainage, with lateral pancreaticojejunostomy being the best choice of these procedures. • It is important to achieve adequate decompression of the pancreatic head and uncinate process during drainage procedures. • Sphincteroplasty does not have a role in the management of patients with established chronic pancreatitis.

Patients with small duct disease are treated by resection if surgery is necessary. • Resection of the pancreatic head in properly selected patients generally has yielded better long-term results for pain relief than tail resection. • The head of the pancreas is often enlarged and bulky in chronic pancreatitis and has been considered to be the "pacemaker" of the disease. • A number of operative techniques are available for pancreatic head resection. • Total or near-total 95% resections have higher long-term morbidity and mortality rates related to postoperative endocrine insufficiency. • Autotransplantation is investigational for chronic pancreatitis. • Although endocrine and exocrine function tends to deteriorate with time in chronic pancreatitis, some evidence suggests that pancreaticojejunostomy halts or delays this decline better than nonoperative therapy.

ANSWER:
B

33. Biochemical characteristics of pancreatic ascites include which of the following laboratory values?

   A. Fluid amylase level higher than serum amylase level

B. Fluid amylase level lower than serum amylase level

C. Fluid protein level higher than 3 g/dl

D. Fluid protein level lower than 3 g/dl

Ref.: 1, 5

COMMENTS: Pancreatic ascites can be differentiated from ascites of other causes by the characteristic high amylase and protein content of the peritoneal fluid. • Pancreatic ascites and pleural effusion are the results of a disruption in the pancreatic duct, usually consequent to pancreatitis. • The ascites may resolve with conservative management consisting of paracentesis (thoracentesis), total parenteral nutrition, and administration of a somatostatin analogue to inhibit pancreatic exocrine secretion. • Otherwise, an operation is required for internal drainage of the pancreatic duct fistula or pseudocyst.

ANSWER:
A, C

34. CT scan demonstrates a 5-cm peripancreatic fluid collection in a patient 3 weeks after an episode of acute pancreatitis. The patient is eating and does not have clinical signs of infection. What is the recommended treatment?

A. Expectant management without intervention

B. Nothing by mouth and total parenteral nutrition

C. Percutaneous catheter drainage of fluid collection

D. Operation for external drainage of fluid collection

E. Operation within 3 weeks for internal drainage of fluid collection

Ref.: 1, 2, 9

COMMENTS: Peripancreatic fluid collections can be found in about 20% of patients with acute pancreatitis. • Many of them resolve spontaneously and should not be mistaken for pancreatic pseudocysts. • If the patient is stable, can eat, and does not have clinical evidence of infection or other complications, expectant management is indicated. • The fluid collection can be followed with ultrasonography or CT scans in 1–3 months. • If the patient has persistent pain and is unable to eat, parenteral nutrition may be instituted for several weeks to allow resolution or maturation of the collection into a pseudocyst. • If the patient has a symptomatic or complicated fluid collection that requires early intervention, some method of external drainage must be used. • If the fluid is thin, percutaneous catheter drainage may suffice. • Operative drainage is preferred if there is substantial necrotic debris, as there often is, or if there is concern about infection.

ANSWER:
A

35. Which of the following is the most important determinant of the need for drainage of a pancreatic pseudocyst?

A. Pseudocyst symptoms

B. Pseudocyst size

C. Pseudocyst duration

D. Associated chronic pancreatitis

Ref.: 1, 2, 9

COMMENTS: Historically, pancreatic pseudocysts larger than 5 to 6 cm in size and present for longer than 6 weeks were thought to have a low rate of spontaneous resolution and a high rate of complications. • They were therefore treated by operative drainage. • Current understanding of the natural history of pseudocysts is that the rate of spontaneous resolution is higher and the rate of complications lower than previously thought. • Pseudocyst size and duration are therefore no longer absolute criteria for intervention. • Rather, pseudocyst-related symptoms are the primary indication for treatment. • Large pseudocysts are more likely to be symptomatic and less likely to resolve spontaneously than are small pseudocysts. • Also, pseudocysts in patients with chronic pancreatitis are unlikely to resolve but may not require intervention if they are stable, asymptomatic, and uncomplicated.

ANSWER:
A

36. A patient with chronic pancreatitis is unable to eat because of persistent postprandial pain. The CT scan is shown. What is the recommended treatment?

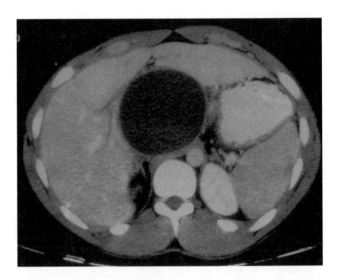

A. Nothing by mouth and total parenteral nutrition for 4–6 weeks

B. Percutaneous catheter drainage

C. Endoscopic drainage

D. Operative internal drainage

E. Operative external drainage

Ref.: 1, 2, 9

COMMENTS: Pseudocysts that develop in patients with chronic pancreatitis can be considered mature when they are discovered unless there also has been a recent episode of acute pancreatitis. • The indications for treatment of a pancreatic pseudocyst are (1) persistent symptoms (pain, inability to eat, or biliary or gastrointestinal obstruction); (2) enlargement; or (3) onset of a pseudocyst-related complication (infection, hemorrhage, or rupture). • Operative internal pseudocyst drainage into the stomach, jejunum, or duodenum is generally the preferred treatment, depending on the location of the pseudocyst. • With patients with chronic pancreatitis, it is critical also to evaluate the pancreatic duct to determine whether a concomitant duct drainage procedure is necessary. • Cyst gastrostomy can be accomplished laparoscopically in some situations. • Pseudocysts in the tail of the gland are sometimes best treated with distal pancreatectomy. • Percutaneous or endoscopic drainage of established pseudocysts is still much debated. • These techniques can successfully treat pseudocysts in some circumstances but have definite limitations and potential complications. • Selection of the most appropriate approach depends on numerous considerations.

ANSWER:
D

37. Which of the following risk factors is most strongly associated with ductal adenocarcinoma of the pancreas?

   A. Chronic pancreatitis

   B. Diabetes mellitus

   C. Cigarette smoking

   D. Coffee consumption

   E. Alcohol consumption

Ref.: 1–3

COMMENTS: Epidemiologic studies have identified numerous demographic, medical, environmental, and dietary factors that have some relationship to pancreatic cancer. • The most firmly established risk factor is cigarette smoking. • Experimentally, nitrosamines have been found to be carcinogenic. • Also, carcinogens in cigarettes have been related to K-*ras* oncogene mutations, which are frequent in pancreatic cancer. • Alcohol has not been demonstrated conclusively to be a risk factor independent of cigarettes. • The previously reported association of pancreatic cancer with coffee consumption is questionable. • Diets high in fats and meat may be associated with pancreatic cancer, whereas diets high in fruits and vegetables may be protective. • Certain occupational and industrial exposures have an increased risk. • There may be some association with diabetes mellitus and certain forms of chronic pancreatitis, but the relationship is not considered causal. • Previous gastrectomy has been associated with an increased risk, whereas tonsillectomy may be protective.

ANSWER:
C

38. A jaundiced, otherwise healthy patient has a 3-cm mass in the head of the pancreas on CT scan. No other disease is apparent. Which of the following is the most appropriate next step?

   A. Endoscopic placement of a biliary stent

   B. Operative exploration for resection

   C. Percutaneous fine-needle aspiration

   D. Angiography

   E. Endoscopic ultrasound imaging

Ref.: 1, 2, 5

COMMENTS: When the clinical situation suggests a resectable pancreatic neoplasm in a good-risk patient with biliary obstruction, operation for potential resection is generally indicated without additional tests. • Routine preoperative biliary decompression is not advantageous in this setting and may increase the morbidity associated with resection. • Endoscopic biliary decompression is invaluable, of course, for palliation of obstruction in patients deemed inoperable or if operation must be delayed for treatment of a serious concomitant medical problem. • Percutaneous pancreatic biopsy is unnecessary for patients who are to be explored and should be discouraged. • Although percutaneous fine-needle aspiration is usually safe, it occasionally causes complications that could prohibit curative resection. • Angiography was formerly popular for preoperative staging of pancreatic cancer, but its accuracy for determining resectability has limitations, and it generally adds little to good quality contrast-enhanced CT scans. • Endoscopic ultrasound imaging has emerged as an adjunct to CT for assessing vascular invasion and can be useful for identifying small tumors that are inapparent on CT. • Some surgeons would perform laparoscopy before laparotomy on the patient described to identify small liver or peritoneal metastases (which would eliminate the need for resection). • Laparoscopic ultrasound imaging has also become a useful tool for improving the accuracy of laparoscopic staging. • If it is determined that the patient is best served by operative palliation because the tumor is found to be unresectable, laparoscopy is unnecessary, although skilled laparoscopic surgeons can perform cholecystojejunostomy and gastrojejunostomy without laparotomy.

ANSWER:
B

39. In which one or more of the following situations is resection of a pancreatic tumor contraindicated?

   A. Patient age greater than 70 years

   B. Tumor located in body of pancreas

   C. Inability to verify malignancy histologically before resection

   D. Tumor invading portal vein

   E. Presence of small peritoneal metastases

Ref.: 1–3, 5

COMMENTS: Resection of a pancreatic malignancy offers the only chance for cure. • Most commonly, resection of ductal carcinomas involves pancreaticoduodenectomy, since most potentially resectable tumors are located in the head or uncinate process of the gland. • Tumors originating in the body or tail of the pancreas are often not diagnosed until they are beyond the confines of surgical resection. • However, location alone does not contraindicate resection because, stage for stage, tumors in the body have the same survival as tumors in the head. • Resection is indicated for physiologically fit patients (age alone is not a contraindication) who do not have metastases beyond the field of resection. • Histologic or cytologic confirmation of malignancy can often be obtained intraoperatively but is not necessary before resection if the clinical circumstances suggest cancer and the surgeon is appropriately experienced. • Tumors with local vascular invasion are often considered unresectable, but en bloc resection with reconstruction of involved vessels is appropriate for some patients if a tumor-free resection can be accomplished. • Positive lymph nodes outside the resection site, peritoneal metastases, and liver metastases contraindicate resection for adenocarcinoma of the exocrine pancreas. However, tumor "debulking" and resection of liver metastases can be beneficial for patients with functioning tumors of the endocrine pancreas.

ANSWER:
E

40. Which of the following operations would not be appropriate for a 3-cm adenocarcinoma in the head of the pancreas?

A. Pancreaticoduodenectomy (Whipple) with hemigastrectomy

B. Pancreaticoduodenectomy (Whipple) with preservation of stomach and pylorus

C. Duodenum-sparing pancreaticoduodenectomy

D. Total pancreaticoduodenectomy

Ref.: 1–3, 5

COMMENTS: A standard Whipple-type resection with gastrectomy or a pyloric and gastric-preserving resection is indicated for a resectable cancer in the head of the pancreas. • Each of these operations yields a long-term survival rate of approximately 15–20%. • There is a higher incidence of initial delayed gastric emptying with pyloric-preserving operations. • However, long-term studies demonstrate normal emptying and good nutritional outcomes. • Likewise, the postprandial gastrin and acid responses are normal despite the loss of duodenal inhibitory factors, and marginal ulcer has not been a prohibitive problem. • Additional advantages of the pyloric-preserving technique are shorter operative time and lower operative blood loss. • Of course, preservation of the stomach and most proximal duodenum is not appropriate for patients with tumors in close proximity if the margins would be compromised. • Duodenum-sparing resection of the pancreatic head has been used in some centers for patients with chronic pancreatitis and has been reported to better maintain enteropancreatic hormonal relationships and glucose homeostasis. • This operation is not indicated for cancer.

Total pancreaticoduodenectomy is not advocated for pancreatic cancers that can be resected otherwise. • It has been used based on the grounds that it produces better clearance of lymph nodes and possible multicentric disease and avoids a pancreatic anastomosis. • However, long-term survival is not improved, and total pancreatectomy is associated with a higher rate of both early and late complications. • Extended pancreaticoduodenectomy involves removal of more retroperitoneal soft tissue and regional lymph nodes. • Some centers have favored this procedure, but improved survival has not yet been conclusively demonstrated, and operative complications may be higher.

ANSWER:
C, D

41. At laparotomy, a jaundiced patient is found to have an unresectable pancreatic cancer obstructing the bile duct. Which of the following statements regarding biliary decompression is/are correct?

A. Preferred management is to close the patient and place an endoscopic stent postoperatively.

B. Cholecystectomy and T-tube placement is preferred management.

C. Choledochoduodenostomy is contraindicated.

D. Cholecystojejunostomy should not be performed if the patient has cholelithiasis.

E. Roux-en-Y choledochojejunostomy is not appropriate because of limited life expectancy.

Ref.: 1–3, 5

COMMENTS: Most patients with pancreatic cancer do not have resectable disease. • Palliative treatment is directed to relieve obstruction of the bile duct and duodenum and to alleviate pain. • For lesions demonstrated to be unresectable before laparotomy,

nonoperative relief of biliary obstruction can be achieved by the endoscopic (preferred) or transhepatic route. • Surgical bypass with some form of biliary enteric anastomosis generally provides more durable relief with less need for further intervention. • It is preferred for patients when unresectability is determined at the time of laparotomy. Cholecystojejunostomy, choledo(hepatico)jejunostomy, and choledochoduodenostomy are each appropriate for management of distal bile duct obstruction. • If there is extensive disease at the porta hepatis, the left hepatic duct is sometimes useful for anastomosis. Otherwise, transhepatic U tubes can be placed, or nonoperative decompression can be attempted. T tubes are inadequate when the obstruction is proximal.

Choledochojejunostomy usually provides the most durable relief, although it is somewhat more involved technically. • A Roux-en-Y configuration is preferred by many surgeons, although a simple loop (with or without distal enteroenterostomy) also suffices. • **Cholecystojejunostomy** is relatively simple but should be avoided if the gallbladder is diseased or when cystic duct patency cannot be demonstrated or may be jeopardized by tumor proximity. • It is sometimes taught that **choledochoduodenostomy** should be avoided with malignant obstruction because of possible tumor growth and eventual reobstruction. • In reality, choledochoduodenostomy can be an effective solution provided the common bile duct is sufficiently dilated and the duodenum is pliable.

ANSWER:
D

42. When should gastrojejunostomy be performed at the time of biliary bypass in a patient with unresectable pancreatic cancer?

A. Always

B. Never

C. Only if symptomatic duodenal obstruction is present at the time of operation

D. Selectively based on tumor extent and anticipated life expectancy

Ref.: 1–3, 5

COMMENTS: In addition to biliary obstruction, pancreatic cancers can obstruct the duodenum. • Traditionally, many surgeons have favored routine "double bypass" for operated patients because the rate of duodenal obstruction that develops later in patients treated by biliary bypass alone has been cited to be 5–30%. • However, most patients do not develop duodenal obstruction, and gastrojejunostomy is sometimes associated with serious problems, such as bleeding or delayed gastric emptying. • The selective approach therefore seems appropriate. • Certainly, patients with obstructive symptoms or impending obstruction due to tumor location should undergo gastrojejunostomy. • Gastrojejunostomy is probably also advisable for patients with an anticipated longer survival, such as those whose lesions are not resected because of local tumor invasion rather than because of hepatic or peritoneal metastases.

ANSWER:
D

43. A 45-year-old woman who is not an alcoholic presents with a septated 10-cm cystic mass in the head of the pancreas. Which of the following statements constitute appropriate advice?

A. The lesion is benign and requires no intervention.

B. The lesion is malignant and likely incurable.

C. Pancreaticoduodenectomy is indicated.

D. Percutaneous needle biopsy is indicated.

E. Drainage by Roux-en-Y cyst jejunostomy is indicated.

Ref.: 1–3, 5

COMMENTS: Cystadenoma and cystadenocarcinoma are cystic neoplasms of the pancreas that most commonly present as mass lesions in middle-aged women. • Serous and mucinous types are recognized, and the risk of malignancy is significant in the mucinous variety. • Cystadenoma is more common than its malignant counterpart, but malignant transformation may occur. • Without resection, exclusion of malignancy can be difficult. • Internal drainage of cystic neoplasms is not appropriate therapy. • Complete excision should be carried out whenever possible. • Five-year survival after resection of cystadenocarcinoma is approximately 50%. • Occasionally, islet cell tumors, ductal adenocarcinomas, or other unusual tumors (e.g., papillary and cystic pancreatic neoplasms) present with cystic components.

ANSWER:
C

44. Whipple's triad includes which of the following characteristics?

A. Fasting hypoglycemia (<50 mg/dl)

B. Symptoms of hypoglycemia

C. Jaundice

D. Hyperamylasemia

E. Symptoms of hypoglycemia relieved by glucose administration

Ref.: 1, 3, 5

COMMENTS: See Question 45.

45. Which of the following is/are true regarding the diagnosis of insulinoma?

A. Whipple's triad is pathognomonic.

B. The serum insulin/glucose ratio exceeds 0.3.

C. An oral glucose tolerance test permits differentiation from reactive hypoglycemia.

D. The tolbutamide test is useful for excluding factitious hyperinsulinemia.

E. A CT scan is the most accurate preoperative method for tumor localization.

Ref.: 1, 3, 5

COMMENTS: Whipple's triad clinically establishes hypoglycemia, the differential diagnosis of which requires further evaluation. • The biochemical diagnosis of insulinoma is based on the findings of fasting hypoglycemia (<50 mg/dl) and hyperinsulinemia (>20 μU/ml), yielding an insulin/glucose ratio higher than 0.3. • The use of tolbutamide or leucine as a provocative test to release insulin may be dangerous and is not required. • C peptide is cleaved from insulin before its release, and determination of C-peptide levels may be useful for excluding factitious hyperinsulinemia. • Serial blood sampling results following oral glucose administration and subsequent fasting demonstrate persistent hypoglycemia and hyperinsulinemia in the case of organic hyperinsulinism. • With reactive hypoglycemia, insulin levels initially rise and glucose levels fall, but the levels become normal after several hours. • Most insulinomas are small. • Arteriography or selective venous sampling may provide useful preoperative localization. • Endoscopic and intraoperative ultrasonography also can aid identification.

ANSWERS:
Question 44: A, B, E
Question 45: B, C

46. Which of the following statements is/are true regarding the treatment of insulinoma?

A. Diazoxide, which inhibits insulin release, is the preferred initial method of management.

B. Simple enucleation is acceptable for localized pancreatic lesions.

C. Because most lesions are multiple or diffuse, total or near-total pancreatectomy is usually necessary.

D. Because most lesions are malignant, adjuvant streptozocin is usually indicated.

E. Parathyroid adenoma should be excluded or treated before pancreatic resection.

Ref.: 1, 3, 5

COMMENTS: Insulinomas are usually single and benign and are rarely ectopic. • Localization of an insulinoma can be difficult, and preoperative imaging along with thorough mobilization and exploration of the pancreas are mandatory. Intraoperative ultrasonography is indispensable. • For localized lesions, simple enucleation is the preferred treatment, but the integrity of the pancreatic duct must be ascertained. • If the lesion cannot be identified and the biochemical basis of the diagnosis is firm, blind distal pancreatic resection with careful histologic examination of the specimen may be necessary. • Intraoperative monitoring of serum glucose levels also has been used. • Diazoxide inhibits insulin release from β cells and is occasionally used for preoperative control or for patients with recurrent postoperative hypoglycemia. • For patients with metastatic malignant insulinoma, tumor debulking may be beneficial, as is the use of streptozocin and 5-fluorouracil. • Gastrinoma, not insulinoma, is the most common pancreatic adenoma associated with multiple endocrine adenomatosis type I syndrome. • Parathyroid disease should be excluded or treated before surgical intervention for gastrinoma.

ANSWER:
B

47. Match each item in the left-hand column with the appropriate response in the right-hand column to compare the characteristics of Zollinger-Ellison syndrome with those of Verner-Morrison syndrome.

A. Diarrhea   a. Zollinger-Ellison syndrome

B. Decreased gastric acid   b. Verner-Morrison syndrome
   secretion

C. Increased gastric acid   c. Both
   secretion

D. Hypercalcemia   d. Neither

E. Malignancy

Ref.: 1, 3, 5

COMMENTS: Both of these syndromes are produced by islet cell tumors, which in the case of Zollinger-Ellison syndrome secrete gastrin and in the case of Verner-Morrison syndrome secrete vasoactive intestinal peptide. • Zollinger-Ellison syndrome is associated with a marked increase in gastric acid secretion and with diarrhea. • Hypercalcemia may occur because of associated parathyroid abnormalities. • The Verner-Morrison syndrome is characterized by watery diarrhea, hypokalemia, and achlorhydria. • Hypercalcemia may occur, but the parathyroids are usually normal. Both syndromes are frequently associated with malignant tumors.

ANSWER:
A-c; B-b; C-a; D-c; E-c

48. Which of the following is/are characteristic of the clinical syndrome associated with glucagon-producing islet cell tumors?

 A. Skin rash

 B. Diabetes

 C. Seizures

 D. Hypoglycemia

 E. Anemia

Ref.: 1, 3, 5

COMMENTS: Patients with glucagon-secreting tumors present with diabetes, anemia, weight loss, venous thrombosis, glossitis, and a characteristic cutaneous lesion known as "necrolytic migratory erythema." • The lesion is rare and often metastatic at the time of diagnosis. • Treatment is directed at achieving as complete a resection as possible. • Postoperatively, chemotherapy with dacarbazine or streptozocin may be useful for residual or recurrent disease.

ANSWER:
A, B, E

49. Which of the following statements is/are true about pancreatic trauma?

 A. It most often occurs secondary to blunt abdominal injury.

 B. It is the most common cause of pancreatic pseudocyst.

 C. Hyperamylasemia is pathognomonic.

 D. Negative peritoneal tap effectively excludes a diagnosis of significant pancreatic injury.

 E. Exclusion requires exploration of all central retroperitoneal hematomas.

Ref.: 1, 3, 5

COMMENTS: Most pancreatic injuries are the result of penetrating trauma, although the gland is vulnerable to blunt trauma because of its fixed position anteriorly over the vertebral column. • The presence of significant pancreatic injury following blunt trauma is not always immediately apparent. • Hyperamylasemia in the serum or peritoneal fluid suggests the diagnosis, but a negative peritoneal tap result does not exclude significant retroperitoneal injury. • Retroperitoneal hematomas in the upper abdomen should be explored to exclude pancreatic ductal injury. • Pancreatitis is the most common cause of pseudocyst, although about 25% occur as a result of trauma.

ANSWER:
E

50. During surgical exploration for blunt abdominal injury, a patient is found to have complete transection of the pancreatic neck. There is no associated injury. Appropriate treatment includes which of the following?

 A. Drainage alone

 B. Distal pancreatectomy and oversewing of the proximal duct

 C. Roux-en-Y pancreaticojejunostomy to the distal pancreas and oversewing of the proximal duct

 D. Roux-en-Y pancreaticojejunostomy of both proximal and distal segments

 E. Pancreaticoduodenectomy with Roux-en-Y pancreaticojejunostomy to the distal duct

Ref.: 1, 3, 5

COMMENTS: Pancreatic contusions or lacerations without ductal disruption are managed by drainage alone. • The pancreatic neck is a frequent site of pancreatic injury when it occurs with blunt trauma. • Distal pancreatectomy with identification and closure of the proximal duct and drainage is safe, and resections involving up to 80% of an otherwise normal gland can be accomplished without subsequent endocrine insufficiency. • Roux-en-Y pancreaticojejunostomy may be desirable in theory to preserve pancreatic tissue but is not advisable for the management of acute injuries because of the risk of a pancreatic anastomosis and the need to open the gut. • Pancreaticoduodenectomy is indicated only for patients with severe combined duodenal, pancreatic, and bile duct injuries.

ANSWER:
B

REFERENCES

1. Townsend CM, Beauchamp RD, Evers BM, et al (eds): *Sabiston Textbook of Surgery: The Biological Basis of Modern Surgical Practice,* 17th ed. Saunders, Philadelphia, 2004.
2. Howard J, Idezuki Y, Ihse I, et al: *Surgical Diseases of the Pancreas,* 3rd ed. Williams & Wilkins, Baltimore, 1998.
3. Mullholland MW, Lillemoe KD, Doherty GM, et al (eds): *Greenfield's Surgery: Scientific Principles and Practice,* 4th ed. Lippincott, Williams & Wilkins, Philadelphia, 2006.
4. O'Leary JP: *The Physiologic Basis of Surgery,* 2nd ed. Williams & Wilkins, Baltimore, 1996.
5. Brunicardi FC, Andersen DK, Billiar TR, et al (eds): *Schwartz's Principles of Surgery,* 8th ed. McGraw-Hill, New York, 2004.
6. Sarr MG: Acute necrotizing pancreatitis. *Probl Gen Surg* 13(4), 1996.
7. Pisters PWT, Ranson JHC: Nutritional support for acute pancreatitis. *Surg Gynecol Obstet* 175:275, 1992.
8. Prinz, RA, Deziel DJ: Chronic pancreatitis. *Probl Gen Surg* 15(1), 1998.
9. Deziel DJ, Prinz RA: Drainage of pancreatic pseudocysts: indications and long-term results. *Dig Surg* 13:101–108, 1996.

CHAPTER **41**

Spleen

José M. Velasco, M.D., and Edie Chan, M.D.

1. Regarding the surgical anatomy of the spleen, which of the following statements is/are true?

   A. The average weight of the spleen in the adult is 150 g.

   B. The splenic suspensory ligaments usually are relatively avascular, except for the gastrosplenic ligament.

   C. The first major branches of the splenic artery are the short gastric vessels.

   D. Accessory spleens are most commonly located in the greater omentum.

   E. The spleen must be triple in size before it becomes palpable.

Ref.: 1–4

COMMENTS: Embryologically, the spleen arises from mesenchymal differentiation in the dorsal mesogastrium next to the anlagen of the left gonad during the fifth week of gestation. • The remnants of the embryologic ventral mesogastrium constitute the gastrohepatic ligament and the falciform ligament. • The spleen is the second-largest organ in the reticuloendothelial system. • In adults, the spleen weighs 75–300 g and resides in the posterior aspect of the left upper quadrant adjacent to the diaphragm, colon, stomach, and left kidney. • Several ligaments, including the gastrosplenic, gastrocolic, splenorenal, splenoomental, and phrenosplenic ligaments, suspend the spleen. • The suspensory ligaments are usually avascular except for the gastrosplenic ligament, which contains the short gastric vessels. • In certain disease states, such as portal hypertension or myeloproliferative disorders, the ligaments become vascularized and can be a significant source of operative hemorrhage. • The splenic pedicle enters the hilum of the spleen and contains artery, vein, lymphatics, and often the tail of the pancreas. • The splenic artery (a direct branch off the celiac) furnishes the arterial supply, along with the short gastric arteries, which originate off the gastroepiploic, and occasionally the splenic, artery. • The artery divides into three to five segmental branches that enter along the trabeculae of the spleen, thus forming the anatomic basis for partial splenectomy. • The first major branch of the splenic artery is the superior polar artery, not the short gastric vessels. • Accessory spleens occur in 15–35% of individuals (the percentage is higher in the presence of hematologic disease). • The most common location is in the splenic hilum, followed by, in decreasing frequency, the gastrosplenic, splenocolic, gastrocolic, and splenorenal ligaments; the greater omentum; and the mesentery. • Uncommonly, accessory spleens may be found in the pelvis along the left ureter or adjacent to the left gonad.

ANSWER:
A, B

2. Regarding the anatomy of the spleen, which of the following statement is/are true?

   A. The splenic blood supply is of a segmental end-artery type.

   B. Because of intervening splenic cords, splenic pulp pressure is not a true reflection of the portal venous pressure.

   C. The splenic microcirculation is predominantly a closed system with direct arteriovenous channels.

   D. Cellular elements of the blood pass directly from red pulp cords to sinuses.

   E. The splenic capsule contains smooth muscle, which facilitates mobilization of blood cells.

Ref.: 1–4

COMMENTS: The splenic blood supply arises from the major splenic artery and the short gastric vessels. • The anatomy of the spleen is segmental. • An artery and a vein that enter the splenic trabeculae supply each segment. • The parenchyma between the trabeculae contains a small area of periarterial white pulp, a marginal zone, and a larger red pulp that makes up 75% of the parenchyma. • The capsule does not contain smooth muscle, in contrast to the anatomy in other mammals. • The trabecular arteries give off central arteries, which are surrounded by a lymphatic sheath containing T lymphocytes and follicles with B cells. • During antigen stimulation, the lymphatic sheath expands. • The red pulp contains cords (cords of Billroth) with intervening sinuses. • These cords are made of fibroblasts and macrophages. • The sinuses are filled with erythrocytes. • The blood flow to the spleen is approximately 5% of the cardiac output. • The arterial blood flow within the spleen follows two paths: the fast flow and the slow flow, or open circulation. • Nearly 90% of the flow enters the open system through the red pulp, where filtration occurs.

ANSWER:
A, D

3. Normal splenic function in humans includes all but which of the following?

A. A reservoir for platelets

B. A site of hematopoiesis throughout life

C. Removal of abnormal intracellular erythrocyte particles and senescent erythrocytes

D. Site for antibody production in the germinal follicles

E. Production of tuftsin and opsonins

Ref.: 1–4

COMMENTS: The spleen has a number of important functions, particularly its immunologic and phagocytic activities. • In humans, the spleen is a reservoir for circulating platelets but not an important reservoir for red blood cells (RBCs), lymphocytes, and reticulocytes, except in some disease states. • In the presence of splenomegaly, as occurs with portal hypertension, RBC pooling, with increased destruction, occurs. • In general, erythrocytes survive 120 days, 2 days of which are spent passing through the spleen. • In the fetus, the spleen is one of the primary sites of hematopoiesis. • This function is minimized after birth but can become significant again in the presence of certain pathologic conditions, such as myeloid metaplasia. • Because of the microvascular anatomy of the spleen, it is an effective filter for old or damaged blood elements and for bacteria and particulate antigens. • In concert with its filtering ability, the spleen has an important role in the phagocytosis of these elements. • The splenic reticuloendothelial tissue located in the splenic cords provides this phagocytic function. • Cell morphologic features, surface characteristics, and splenic pulp pressure affect the filtering and phagocytic functions of the spleen.

Pitting is the process by which the spleen removes abnormal intracellular particles, such as Howell-Jolly bodies (nuclear remnants), Heinz bodies (denatured hemoglobin), and Pappenheimer bodies (iron granules) from RBCs with deformable membranes. • **Culling** is the removal of RBCs with abnormal, less deformable membranes. • Immunologically, the spleen produces **opsonins**, including **tuftsin** (a peptide that stimulates phagocytosis of leukocytes) and **properdin** (involved in the alternative pathway of complement). • The spleen also produces antibodies (particularly immunoglobulin M [IgM]). • The spleen also has a role in recycling iron released from destroyed RBCs.

ANSWER:
B

4. Which of the following hematologic or immunologic changes is/are anticipated following splenectomy?

A. Howell-Jolly bodies in blood suggest the presence of accessory spleen or splenosis.

B. Asplenic patients maintain normal complement activation via the alternative pathway.

C. Levels of properdin and tuftsin fall after splenectomy.

D. The spleen can only remove cells coated with immunoglobulin A (IgA).

E. Asplenic patients have a normal response to reimmunization.

Ref.: 1, 2, 4

COMMENTS: The spleen may serve as storage for platelets. • It is estimated that 30% of all platelets reside in the spleen.

• Based on the filtering, phagocytic, and immunologic functions of the spleen, a number of changes can be expected related to loss of these functions following splenectomy. • Hematologically, circulating RBCs with abnormal forms (target cells) and abnormal cytoplasmic inclusions (e.g., Howell-Jolly bodies) are seen. • However, RBC survival may improve dramatically in hereditary spherocytosis and warm-antibody acquired hemolytic anemia, whereas RBC volume and survival generally remain unchanged. • In addition to increases in the number of circulating white blood cells (WBCs) and platelets, sometimes the RBC volume increases because more reticulocytes are permitted to remain in the circulation. • Immunologically, decreases in serum IgM, tuftsin, opsonin, and properdin are seen. • Bacterial clearance and antibody response to intravenous antigens are impaired, and T-cell function also may be altered.

The most important function of the spleen is its mechanical filtration. • The spleen can clear unopsonized bacteria and microorganisms for which the body has no antibodies. • It can also clear organisms contained within erythrocytes, such as malaria and *Bartonella*. • Asplenic patients have a normal immunologic response to reimmunization but have a decreased response to a new antigen after splenectomy. • Patients require significantly higher levels of antibodies to clear organisms, especially the encapsulated bacteria.

Accessory spleens (mesenchymal splenic remnants that did not fuse) are found in 15–30% of people. • **Splenosis** may result from autotransplantation of splenic fragments from a traumatized spleen. • Even though both are capable of performing some reticuloendothelial function, it should be noted that accessory spleens and splenic remnants or transplants do not necessarily perform all or even part of the functions of the whole spleen. • Evidence suggests that 30–50% of normal splenic volume is required for full function, including protection from postsplenectomy sepsis. • Absence of Howell-Jolly bodies after splenectomy suggests the presence of an accessory spleen.

Properdin and tuftsin are important opsonins manufactured in the spleen. • *Properdin* helps initiate the alternative pathway of complement activation, which helps destroy bacteria, particularly encapsulated organisms. • *Tuftsin* enhances the phagocytic activity of granulocytes. • The spleen is the major site of cleavage of tuftsin from the heavy chain of immunoglobulin G (IgG). • The spleen removes cells coated with IgG. • Therefore, autoimmune diseases, such as autoimmune hemolytic anemia, immune thrombocytic purpura, and probably Felty syndrome, lead to cell destruction in the spleen. • Besides being the site of clearance of antibody-coated bacteria, the spleen is the initial site of IgM synthesis in response to bacteria.

ANSWER:
C, E

5. Which of the following congenital hemolytic anemias is/are caused primarily by RBC membrane defects?

A. Thalassemia

B. Sickle cell anemia

C. Hereditary spherocytosis

D. Hereditary elliptocytosis

E. Hereditary pyropoikilocytosis

Ref.: 1–4

COMMENTS: **Thalassemia** and **sickle cell anemia** are hereditary disorders of hemoglobin synthesis. • **Hereditary spherocytosis, elliptocytosis,** and **pyropoikilocytosis** are abnormalities of

RBC membrane synthesis. • **Hereditary spherocytosis** is primarily an autosomal dominant inherited disorder, although 20–25% of cases appear spontaneously. • The membrane defect results from a deficiency in *spectrin* and *ankyrin* (elements of the RBC membrane skeleton). • The severity of its presentation is variable and is characterized by anemia, jaundice, cholelithiasis (in up to 55% of patients), and moderate splenomegaly. • Diagnosis is made by the presence of spherocytes in the peripheral blood, reticulocytosis, increased osmotic fragility, and a negative Coombs' test result.

Splenectomy is indicated in all patients and usually should be deferred until age 4. • For younger patients, partial splenectomy is beneficial. • Preoperative ultrasound imaging should be done to detect gallstones. • Cholecystectomy, combined with splenectomy, should be performed in patients with gallstones. • **Elliptical RBCs characterize hereditary elliptocytosis.** • The predominant abnormality changes spectrin, which exists as a dimer instead of a tetramer. • A deficiency of protein 4.1 has been identified in these patients as well. • It usually produces a mild anemia, with most patients being asymptomatic. • Clinical and laboratory findings in symptomatic patients are similar to those in patients with hereditary spherocytosis except that the RBCs are elliptical in appearance. • Results of splenectomy in symptomatic patients are uniformly good. • Cholecystectomy should be performed in patients with gallstones.

Hereditary pyropoikilocytosis is rare. • It is associated with severe alterations of RBC morphology. • It occurs primarily in African-Americans. • The RBCs are severely deformed, and nearly all RBCs are affected. • As with hereditary spherocytosis and elliptocytosis, jaundice is frequently present. • Splenectomy reduces hemolysis.

ANSWER:
C, D, E

6. For which of the following congenital hemolytic anemias is splenectomy primarily indicated?

   A. Thalassemia

   B. Hereditary spherocytosis

   C. Pyruvate kinase deficiency

   D. Glucose-6-phosphate dehydrogenase deficiency (G6PD)

   E. Sickle cell anemia

Ref.: 1–4

COMMENTS: Splenectomy is the sole effective therapy for **hereditary spherocytosis**, which is the most common congenital anemia for which splenectomy is indicated. • Cholelithiasis (pigment stones) is seen in up to 55% of patients and should be sought by ultrasound imaging before splenectomy. • If cholelithiasis is identified, concomitant cholecystectomy is appropriate. • Splenectomy can generally be delayed until the fourth year of life, at which time the risk of postsplenectomy sepsis is decreased. • Splenectomy can also be an effective therapy for **hereditary elliptocytosis**. • Patients can become symptomatic when ovalocytes constitute 50–90% of the RBC population. • In such cases, splenectomy is indicated. • The **thalassemia** patient has defective hemoglobin synthesis with intracellular precipitates that lead to increased RBC destruction. • The patient presents with anemia, splenic infarctions, intercurrent infection, leg ulcers, and gallstones. • Splenectomy may be beneficial in decreasing the rate of hemolysis and consequent transfusion requirements and may be indicated in some cases of splenic infarction with pain and infection. • Deficiencies in RBC enzymes, such as **pyruvate kinase** and **G6PD,** result in hemolysis because the RBCs are unable to utilize glucose. • Because the spleen is not always the primary site of hemolysis, the benefit from splenectomy is not predictable and so usually is not required. • In severe cases of pyruvate kinase deficiency, splenectomy may be worthwhile, but it is not beneficial in G6PD deficiency. • Splenectomy usually is not necessary for **sickle cell anemia** because of the splenic infarction and "autosplenectomy" that eventually occurs in many of these patients. • Occasionally, however, patients with sickle cell diseases other than sickle cell anemia (e.g., sickle thalassemia or sickle cell disease) may develop chronic hypersplenism. • In such cases, if increased RBC sequestration can be demonstrated, splenectomy may be helpful.

ANSWER:
B

7. Regarding thalassemia and sickle cell disease, which of the following statements is/are true?

   A. Thalassemia is transmitted as an autosomal recessive trait.

   B. Thalassemia major is characterized by an increase in hemoglobin A and F levels.

   C. Heterozygous α-thalassemia is associated with more severe and debilitating symptoms than is heterozygous β-thalassemia.

   D. Splenectomy usually is indicated for adult patients with sickle cell disease.

   E. Patients with sickle cell disease have an increased risk of infectious complications due to autosplenectomy from splenic infarction.

Ref.: 1–4

COMMENTS: Gene pairs are responsible for synthesis of alpha, beta, gamma, and delta chains of the hemoglobin molecule. • Reduction in the production of one of these chains leads to an imbalance in these units, with resultant unstable hemoglobin molecules. • Reduction in the beta chain of β-thalassemia is the most common form in North America.

Thalassemia major is a homozygous expression of this genetic defect and is transmitted as an autosomal dominant trait. • It becomes apparent during the first year of life and is characterized by pallor, retarded body growth, and enlargement of the head. • The characteristic features of this disease are persistence of hemoglobin F (fetal hemoglobin) and decreased hemoglobin A. • The primary treatment for thalassemia major is blood transfusion and iron chelation therapy. • Splenectomy occasionally lessens the hemolytic process, hence decreasing the number of required annual transfusions. • In some patients, splenomegaly or symptomatic repeated splenic infarction constitutes an indication for splenectomy. • Most patients with thalassemia major die by the second decade of life from hemosiderosis (iron excess), in contradistinction to patients with **thalassemia minor** (heterozygous thalassemia), who generally are able to lead normal lives and accommodate to a slightly reduced level of hemoglobin. • **α-Thalassemia** may present in a homozygous or a heterozygous form. • Homozygous α-thalassemia is not compatible with life, although symptoms of heterozygous α- and β-thalassemia are minor and similar.

In **sickle cell disease**, normal hemoglobin A is replaced by abnormal sickle hemoglobin (hemoglobin S). • Under conditions of reduced oxygen tension, hemoglobin S undergoes crystallization, producing sickling of RBCs, which leads to increased blood viscosity and microvascular stasis. • Repeated episodes of splenic infarction may lead eventually to autosplenectomy, with subsequent symptoms of hyposplenism, including increased risk of infectious complications. • In patients with sickle cell anemia (homozygous state for hemoglobin S), an acute crisis of splenic sequestration may lead to massive enlargement of the spleen. • In these cases, an urgent splenectomy is indicated.

ANSWER:
E

8. Regarding idiopathic thrombocytopenic purpura (ITP), which of the following statements is/are true?

   A. Acute ITP predominantly affects adult males.

   B. The diagnosis of ITP requires a platelet count below 50,000/mm³.

   C. Detection of IgG antiglobulin on the platelet surface verifies the diagnosis of ITP.

   D. Anemia secondary to hypersplenism is frequently found in ITP patients.

   E. Splenic IgG production is increased in patients with ITP.

Ref.: 1, 2, 4

COMMENTS: ITP is characterized by cutaneous and mucosal bleeding, a platelet count below 100,000/mm³, normal bone marrow, and the absence of other causes of thrombocytopenia, such as a lymphoproliferative disorder, connective tissue disorder, or exposure to drugs or bacteria. • In patients with human immunodeficiency virus (HIV), a disease virtually identical to ITP has been noted. • Acute ITP affects children, usually under the age of 8, after a viral illness. • The disease is usually self limited, and spontaneous remission occurs in about 80% of the cases. • Emergency splenectomy is required in the case of intracranial bleeding. • Chronic ITP is more common in women between the ages of 20 and 40. • Only 2% of patients with ITP will have a palpable spleen. • Leukopenia and anemia are rarely associated with ITP, and if present, they are due to hypersplenism in the presence of splenomegaly.

For the diagnosis of ITP to be considered, the platelet count must be below 100,000 mm³, but bleeding generally does not occur unless the count is below 50,000/mm³. • The pathophysiologic mechanism of ITP is the development of an IgG antibody directed against the platelet fibrinogen receptor. • The spleen may be the site of initial antibody production, it is the site of continued antibody genesis, and it is the primary site of platelet destruction. • Overall production of IgG from the spleens of ITP patients is increased. • After splenectomy, the amount of IgG produced in the spleen is decreased. • The macrophages, located in the cords of Billroth, have receptors for the fibrinogen (Fc) portion of IgG and will bind and phagocytose the coated platelets. • IgG and the newest drug, Rho(d) immunoglobulin, saturate the macrophage Fc receptors, hence decreasing macrophage phagocytosis.

ANSWER:
C, E

9. Match the clinical situations listed in the left-hand column with the most appropriate management listed in the right-hand column.

   A. A 5-year-old boy with ITP and acute intracranial bleeding
   B. An 8-year-old boy with ITP following recent infection with varicella virus
   C. A 30-year-old woman with HIV and a platelet count of 20,000/mm³ following high-dose steroids and γ-globulin

   a. Bed rest, high-dose steroids, and possibly immunoglobulin
   b. Elective splenectomy
   c. Observation
   d. Emergency splenectomy

   D. A 30-year-old woman with ITP and a platelet count of 100,000/mm³ following high-dose steroids
   E. A 30-year-old woman who is 5 months pregnant with ITP, a platelet count of 25,000/mm³ following steroid and immunoglobulin therapy, and vaginal bleeding

Ref.: 1–4

COMMENTS: The treatment of ITP is dictated by the severity of the disease process. • Intracranial hemorrhage is an absolute indication for emergency splenectomy. • The initial goal in the treatment of ITP patients is to induce remission and to achieve platelet counts greater than 100,000/mm³ by using high-dose corticosteroids. • This management initially is effective in approximately 75% of patients within 24 hr, but complete remission is maintained in only 15–25% of them. • If platelet counts remain low, intravenous IgG is indicated, even though it usually does not induce complete remission. • IgG also is helpful in the management of patients with acute bleeding, in preoperative patients with platelet counts less than 20,000/mm³, and in pregnant patients before delivery. • The mechanism of action of IgG is saturation of the Fc receptors of the splenic macrophages. • The newest drug, Rho(d) immunoglobulin, specifically targets the Fc receptors. • Plasmapheresis and chemotherapy have also been tried in the past, mainly for patients whose disease failed to respond to splenectomy. • Indications for splenectomy include refractory thrombocytopenia despite medical treatment, patients requiring toxic doses of steroids, or recurrence of thrombocytopenia after tapering of steroids.

Special consideration should be given to children with ITP. • It is usually a self-limiting disease that resolves in 6–12 months. • Treatment consists of bed rest, steroids, and intravenous gamma globulin. • Splenectomy is indicated in children who do not experience a spontaneous remission after 1 year.

Ten percent of patients with HIV develop an ITP-like syndrome, with platelet counts less than 100,000/mm³. • Treatment is similar to that for ITP and consists of a course of high-dose steroids. • Splenectomy is indicated in those patients who have persistent thrombocytopenia during steroid dose tapering. • Women with ITP who are in the second trimester of pregnancy are considered for a splenectomy if they have persistent platelet counts less than 10,000/mm³ after medical management or have bleeding with platelet counts less than 30,000/mm³.

ANSWER:
A-d; B-a; C-b; D-c; E-b

10. Regarding the management of patients with ITP, which of the following statements is/are true?

    A. Splenectomy is indicated for patients who fail to improve with initial steroid therapy.

    B. Splenectomy is more often necessary for children with ITP than for adults.

    C. Splenectomy is not indicated in the absence of splenomegaly.

    D. Preoperative platelet transfusions are recommended for patients with platelet counts under 50,000/mm³.

    E. The sole reason for splenectomy for ITP is to remove the source of platelet phagocytization.

Ref.: 1–4

COMMENTS: ITP is an autoimmune disease. • As such, the initial treatment is with steroids. • Splenectomy is recommended for patients who do not respond, for those whose required dose for response is excessive even for a few months, or for those requiring chronic steroid therapy (1 year or longer). • Only 25% of adults respond to medical management, and up to 88% have relief after splenectomy. • The response is better in patients who are younger, with a shorter disease course, and possibly a response to steroid treatment. • Nuclear medicine studies based on indium-labeled platelets are useful in predicting which patients will benefit from splenectomy. • A 96% complete remission has been observed in those cases where the tagged platelets tracked to the spleen, whereas the success rate has been only 8% in those patients where the tagged platelets tracked predominantly to the liver. • Spontaneous remission occurs in most children (80%), and few need splenectomy unless intracranial bleeding occurs.

The diagnosis of ITP is one of exclusion, which requires careful search for possible precipitating factors, such as drugs. • The diagnosis also requires a normal to hypercellular megakaryocyte count in the bone marrow. • Splenomegaly is rare in ITP, its presence suggesting another source for thrombocytopenia, such as hemolytic disease.

Generally, platelet transfusions are not required, despite low platelet counts, unless they are needed to control bleeding. • Platelets should be withheld intraoperatively until just after the spleen is removed. • If given before that time, they simply are consumed and confer minimal benefit. • Immunoglobulin may increase the efficacy of transfused platelets and is frequently used to prepare patients for operations. • Splenectomy is useful not only for removing the organ responsible for phagocytizing platelets but also for decreasing the immunologic response causing ITP in the first place, as evidenced by the lower IgG levels (especially antiplatelet antibody levels) seen following splenectomy.

ANSWER:
A

11. The primary pathophysiologic mechanism of thrombotic thrombocytopenic purpura (TTP) involves which of the following characteristics?

    A. Circulating antiplatelet antibodies

    B. Venous thrombosis

    C. Arteriolar and capillary occlusion

    D. Intravascular activation of the coagulation cascade

    E. Autoimmune response to endothelial cell antigen

Ref.: 1–4

COMMENTS: TTP is characterized by occlusion of arterioles and capillaries by hyaline deposits composed of aggregated platelets and fibrin. • Presumably, this occurs on an immunologic basis. • The classic clinical features include the pentad of fever, purpura, anemia, neurologic manifestations, and renal dysfunction. • Unchecked, the disease runs a fulminant course resulting in death, most commonly secondary to intracerebral hemorrhage or renal failure. • Current primary therapy for TTP involves high-volume plasmapheresis, fresh-frozen plasma replacement, and often high-dose corticosteroids. • Approximately 50% of the patients survive. • Splenectomy no longer is an initial treatment modality, but for patients who fail to respond to plasmapheresis, it can be salvage therapy in combination with steroids, and aspirin and dextran as antiplatelet agents. • The majority of long-term survivors with TTP have undergone splenectomy. • The mechanism

by which the spleen participates in the pathogenesis of TTP is not precisely known.

ANSWER:
C, E

12. Regarding hypersplenism, which of the following statements is/are true?

    A. Hypersplenism results from multiple splenic implants, generally seen after traumatic rupture of the spleen.

    B. The thrombocytopenia resulting from secondary hypersplenism caused by hepatic disease generally requires splenectomy.

    C. Primary hypersplenism rarely responds to steroids, and splenectomy is curative.

    D. Gaucher's disease and Felty's syndrome may cause primary hypersplenism.

    E. Hypersplenism in patients with Gaucher's disease mandates splenectomy.

Ref.: 1–5

COMMENTS: Hypersplenism is a syndrome characterized by any combination of neutropenia, anemia, and thrombocytopenia caused by splenic cellular sequestration. • It is associated with bone marrow hyperplasia and splenomegaly. • The diagnosis of **primary hypersplenism** is one of exclusion and is confirmed by a clinical response to splenectomy. • Corticosteroids rarely affect the course of this disease. • **Secondary hypersplenism** most often is the result of hepatic disease or extrahepatic portal vein obstruction, leading to anemia, leukopenia, or thrombocytopenia, singly or in any combination. • In this circumstance, no correlation exists between the degree of cellular depression and symptoms. • Splenectomy usually is not necessary in those patients with liver disease, especially in light of their frequent lack of symptoms (e.g., petechiae). • **Gaucher's disease** (a familial disorder characterized by disordered lipid metabolism leading to splenomegaly) and **Felty's syndrome** (splenomegaly, hepatomegaly, and adenopathy associated with rheumatoid arthritis) are examples of diseases causing secondary hypersplenism. • Secondary hypersplenism also can be caused by splenic hypertrophy from an immune response and RBC destruction, venous congestion, myeloproliferation, infiltration, and neoplastic proliferation within the spleen. • Gaucher's disease is characterized by a defect in the acid β-glucosidase. • The most common symptoms are related to hypersplenism and massive splenomegaly. • Enzyme replacement therapy with a recombinant β-glucosidase has replaced total or partial splenectomy as the treatment of choice for these patients. • **Splenosis** is the term used to refer to the condition of multiple splenic implants, generally following traumatic injury to the spleen. • It does not lead to hypersplenism.

ANSWER:
C

13. Match the anatomic involvement with Hodgkin's disease in the left-hand column with the appropriate clinical stage of the disease in the right-hand column.

A. Right axillary lymph nodes	a. Stage I
B. Epigastric lymph nodes; liver	b. Stage II
C. Left cervical lymph nodes and right mediastinal lymph nodes	c. Stage III
D. Left cervical lymph nodes, epigastric lymph nodes, and spleen	d. Stage IV

E. Left cervical lymph nodes and left
   axillary lymph nodes with an adjacent
   extranodal focus

e. Stage IIE

Ref.: 1–4

COMMENTS: See Question 14.

14. Regarding staging laparotomy of patients with Hodgkin's
    disease, which of the following statements is/are false?

    A. Lymphangiography, computed tomographic (CT) scanning,
       and positron emission tomographic (PET) scanning have
       eliminated the need for a staging laparotomy in most patients.

    B. The operative technique of a staging laparotomy is different
       for women than it is for men.

    C. Partial splenectomy is adequate for staging and has helped
       lower the incidence of postsplenectomy sepsis.

    D. Laparotomy for purposes of splenectomy is indicated,
       because it enhances the quality and duration of response to
       chemotherapy.

    F. Staging laparotomy results in a change in the stage of
       Hodgkin's disease in 30–40% of cases.

Ref.: 1–4

COMMENTS: The treatment and prognosis of Hodgkin's disease
is related to the histologic type and clinical stage at the time of
presentation. • Hodgkin's disease is commonly staged as follows
(Ann Arbor classification): stage I, one area or two contiguous areas
of lymph node involvement on the same side of the diaphragm;
stage II, two noncontiguous areas on the same side of the
diaphragm; stage III, involvement on each side of the diaphragm
(for purposes of this classification the spleen is considered a lymph
node); and stage IV, involvement of liver, bone marrow, lung, or
any other non–lymph-node tissue, exclusive of the spleen. • The
superscript E signifies extranodal involvement adjacent to involved
lymph nodes. • In addition, patients are subcategorized as asymptomatic (A) or having constitutional symptoms such as night
sweats, fever (>38°C), or 10% weight loss within 6 months (B).

Accurate staging is critical if one is to avoid the consequences
of over- or undertreatment. • Historically, pathologic staging was
accomplished by performing staging laparotomy. • In most
reported clinical series, the preoperative stage of the disease changes
in 30–40% of patients following laparotomy. • Slightly more
cases are up-staged (and need more aggressive therapy) than are
down-staged. • It should be stated that, in few of these reports,
all patients were studied by CT scanning. • In women of childbearing age wishing to remain fertile, oophoropexy (repositioning
the ovaries to the midline) should be performed to move them away
from the radiation field in the event irradiation of the iliac lymph
nodes becomes necessary. • Advances in imaging techniques,
such as helical CT scanning, lymphangiography, and PET scanning, have improved nonoperative staging. • Staging laparotomy
and splenectomy may still be appropriate for selected patients with
an early stage of disease (IA and IIA), who typically receive radiation therapy. • Even in this subset of patients, the trend is not to
perform a laparotomy because of the increasing use of combination
chemotherapy in all cases. • Furthermore, the ultimate outcome
is the same whether these patients undergo staging laparotomy
or are initially treated with radiation therapy, even if a relapse
occurs. • Patients who undergo splenectomy are at high risk
for overwhelming postsplenectomy sepsis (OPSI), and they may
even have a tenfold increased risk for the development of acute

nonlymphocytic leukemia. • Partial splenectomy is not sufficiently accurate for staging to justify its use.

A N S W E R S :
Question 13: A-a; B-d; C-b; D-c; E-e
Question 14: C, D

15. Which one or more of the following statements concerning
    splenectomy for hematologic diseases is/are false?

    A. Indicated to relieve symptoms of splenomegaly

    B. Indicated to relieve pancytopenia

    C. Treatment of choice for hairy-cell leukemia

    D. Indicated during the blast phase of chronic myelogenous
       leukemia (CML)

    E. Highly successful in the treatment of hypersplenism in
       patients with chronic lymphocytic leukemia (CLL)

Ref.: 1–4

COMMENTS: Splenectomy can play a role in the management
of hematologic malignancies. • It can be performed to stage
Hodgkin's disease, to relieve symptoms from splenomegaly, and to
correct pancytopenia from secondary hypersplenism. • In general,
it is recommended for patients who have failed medical therapy
and who have anemia requiring frequent transfusions or who have
thrombocytopenia with bleeding. • Finally, splenectomy is highly
successful in relieving compressive symptoms due to massive
splenomegaly.

Hairy-cell leukemia, so named because of the characteristic
cellular appearance under a light microscope, was thought best
treated initially by splenectomy, with good expectation for long-
term survival and good initial resolution of symptoms and blood
counts in 80–90% of patients. • However, most patients experienced a recurrence in the first year. • Therefore, splenectomy was
supplanted by α_2-interferon therapy, which induced a stable remission in some patients. • Recently, the purine analogues pentostatin
(2-doxycoformycin) and 2-chlorodoxyadenosine have been able to
induce complete remission in close to 80% of patients. • Conversely,
a-interferon therapy achieved complete remission in only 11% of
treated patients. • Currently, splenectomy is best reserved for those
who fail to improve after such medical management. • Splenectomy
is primarily palliative for the remainder of the disorders that follow.

CLL, characterized by abnormal lymphocytes, lymphadenopathy, splenomegaly, and lymphocytosis, often follows an indolent
course. • Splenectomy is performed primarily for the hematologic
consequences of hypersplenism or for palliation in symptomatic
splenomegaly. • It is a highly successful treatment, resulting in
close to 100% resolution of anemia and 85% resolution of thrombocytopenia. • Patients who are younger and have larger spleens
tend to have a better outcome with a splenectomy, even resulting in
improved survival.

This is also true for **non-Hodgkin's lymphoma**. • Because
most patients with non-Hodgkin's lymphoma have disseminated
disease at the time of diagnosis, splenectomy is performed much
less often as a staging procedure and more often for palliation.
• Less than 1% of patients present with splenomegaly without
peripheral lymphadenopathy. • Splenectomy may be indicated in
the diagnosis and staging of patients who present with isolated
splenic disease. • Survival has been noticed to be significantly
improved when a splenectomy is performed in these patients.

CML, with its high leukocyte counts and the characteristic
Philadelphia chromosome, may require splenectomy to alleviate
thrombocytopenia, anemia, or pain from splenomegaly. • Death
often occurs from myeloblastic crisis. • Splenectomy is palliative

and does not delay blastic transformation, does not improve survival after blastic transformation, and does not generally prolong survival. • However, splenectomy can resolve symptoms of splenomegaly and hypersplenism in one third of patients during the blast or acute phase of this disease with a low mortality. • Selected patients in the later stages of CML with extensive transfusion needs or symptomatic splenomegaly benefit from splenectomy. • The course of **myeloid metaplasia** is likewise not altered by splenectomy, although significant palliation may be obtained.

ANSWER:
C

16. Partial, rather than total, splenectomy may be the operation of choice for all but which of the following conditions?

   A. Felty's syndrome

   B. Gaucher's disease

   C. Thalassemia major

   D. Splenic hemangioma

   E. Hereditary spherocytosis in a 3-year-old child

Ref.: 1–5

COMMENTS: Gaucher's disease is an inherited metabolic disorder in which deficiency of acid β-glucosidase activity results in the accumulation of glycosyl ceramide in reticuloendothelial cells of the liver, bone, and spleen. • Traditionally, splenectomy had been the therapy for patients with this condition, who develop hypersplenism or mechanical symptoms due to splenomegaly. • More recent experience has shown that partial splenectomy can be beneficial for these patients. • Also, because accelerated bone disease and an increased risk of malignancy have been observed in patients with Gaucher's disease following total splenectomy, it has been suggested that partial splenectomy may be the procedure of choice. • However, most patients with Gaucher's disease are treated with recombinant β-glucosidase.
   Felty's syndrome describes the clinical association of rheumatoid arthritis, splenomegaly, and neutropenia. • Patients are plagued by recurrent infections. • Because neutropenia is secondary to both antibody and splenic destruction, a good and lasting response to total splenectomy can occur. • Granulomatous involvement of the spleen by sarcoidosis can produce anemia and thrombocytopenia and occasionally require total splenectomy.
   Splenic hemangiomas constitute the most important benign neoplasm of the spleen. • For the most part, they are asymptomatic and require no therapy. • If the hemangioma is large, it may be associated with thrombocytopenia and pancytopenia or even rupture. • In such instances, a total or a partial splenectomy is appropriate. • Because of OPSI, a splenectomy should be delayed until the age of 4 in patients suffering from hereditary spherocytosis. • The recent trend is to perform partial splenectomy in children younger than 4 years of age for hematologic diseases such as thalassemia major.

ANSWER:
A

17. Regarding the role of splenectomy in the treatment of acquired immune hemolytic anemias, which of the following statements is/are true?

   A. Splenectomy is indicated only after failure of steroid therapy.

   B. Splenectomy may be indicated for warm-antibody–type acquired immune hemolytic anemia.

   C. Splenectomy may be indicated for cold-antibody–type acquired immune hemolytic anemia.

   D. Splenectomy is contraindicated for acquired immune hemolytic anemias.

   E. Postoperative thromboembolic complications are more common when splenectomy is performed for acquired immune hemolytic anemias.

Ref.: 1–4

COMMENTS: Splenectomy may be beneficial for certain acquired immune hemolytic anemias, just as it is beneficial for certain congenital anemic disorders. • The acquired immune hemolytic anemias can be divided into cold- and warm-antibody types. • In the **warm-antibody type**, IgG antibody binds to cell membranes, and the RBCs are subsequently removed by the spleen. • There is no complement fixation or direct hemolysis. • Corticosteroids constitute the first line of therapy, but 30–40% of patients do not respond, or they sustain relapse. • Approximately 80% respond to splenectomy. • Splenectomy is not indicated for treatment of the **cold-antibody–type** immune hemolytic anemias. • These anemias are mediated by IgM antibody and complement fixation to direct intravascular cell lysis. • Postoperative morbidity following splenectomy for acquired hemolytic anemia is no higher than that with other hematologic disorders. • An increase in thromboembolic complications has been observed, however, following splenectomy for myeloproliferative disorders.

ANSWER:
A, B

18. Which of the following patients is least likely to develop OPSI?

   A. A 3-year-old child with hereditary spherocytosis

   B. An 11-year-old boy with hereditary spherocytosis

   C. A 3-year-old child with a grade V injury

   D. A 40-year-old man with a grade V injury

   E. A 20-year-old man with stage IIA Hodgkin's disease

Ref.: 1–4, 7

COMMENTS: OPSI is an uncommon but well-recognized potential complication of splenectomy. • The risk of postsplenectomy sepsis depends on the age of the patient and the indication for splenectomy. • It occurs in 0.3% of adults and 0.6% of children and is more common when splenectomy is performed for hematologic disease. • Postsplenectomy sepsis is uncommon in adults undergoing splenectomy for trauma. • The mortality rate associated with postsplenectomy sepsis exceeds 50% in children and approximates 30% in adults. • Most episodes occur within the first 2 years after splenectomy, although they can occur later. • In one recent series, most infection cases occurred more than 2 years after splenectomy, and 42% of them occurred 5 years later. • The typical onset of this clinical syndrome is often insidious, marked by nonspecific symptoms of malaise, headache, nausea, and confusion. • It can progress rapidly to shock and death within 48–72 hr. • The most common organisms are encapsulated bacteria, such as *Streptococcus pneumoniae* (50% of cases), *Haemophilus influenzae, Neisseria meningitidis, Escherichia coli, b-hemolytic streptococci,* and *Pseudomonas.*

ANSWER:
D

19. Appropriate steps to prevent OPSI include which of the following measures?

A. Administration of polyvalent vaccines before splenectomy in childhood

B. Avoidance of splenectomy in children under 4 years of age

C. Routine prophylactic antibiotics after splenectomy

D. Splenic preservation by splenorrhaphy

E. Autotransplantation of splenic fragments when splenectomy is necessary

Ref.: 1–4

COMMENTS: Preventive measures against OPSI include the use of pneumococcal vaccine or polyvalent vaccines, in the case of children. • Vaccines should be given 2 weeks before splenectomy if possible. • *Haemophilus* flu vaccine is now given to *all* children as part of routine immunization. • *Meningococcus* vaccine is not routinely given unless the patient is immunosuppressed. • Prophylactic antibiotics are recommended for children under age 5 years (but compliance is often inadequate). • Prophylactic antibiotics also should be considered for immunosuppressed patients. • The administration of antibiotic prophylaxis in other individuals has not been shown to decrease the risk of postsplenectomy sepsis. • Because the risk of this syndrome is greatest in children, elective splenectomy should be postponed if possible until the child is 4–10 years old. • Concerted attempts at splenic preservation by nonoperative therapy or splenorrhaphy for young children with splenic injury also are appropriate. • Perhaps one of the most important methods for preventing OPSI is to evaluate patients having splenectomy and have them seek prompt medical consultation with the first signs of illness.

Although our understanding of the precise requirements for relatively normal splenic function is incomplete, experimental findings permit certain observations. • Evidence suggests that, with partial splenectomy, at least one third of functioning splenic tissue is necessary for immunologic protection. • Blood flow is also critical, in that immunologic protection is lost following splenic artery ligation. • Finally, it should be kept in mind that, although it is laudable to attempt splenic preservation to avoid OPSI, this syndrome is uncommon. • Excessive concern with preservation should not compromise the welfare of the trauma patient during the operation.

Autotransplantation of splenic fragments has been investigated as an attempt to preserve critical splenic function. • Following autotransplantation, immunologic function in the form of increased IgM and serum complement levels can be demonstrated, as has resumption of filtering function, evidenced by the disappearance of target cells and Howell-Jolly bodies. • These functions are apparently subnormal, however, and do not provide protection against postsplenectomy sepsis.

ANSWER:
A, B, D

20. In regard to splenic cysts, which of the following is/are true?

A. Primary true cysts account for 45% of nonparasitic cysts.

B. Most true cysts smaller than 8 cm are asymptomatic.

C. Splenectomy must be done for symptomatic cysts or cysts larger than 8 cm.

D. Parasitic (echinococcal) cysts are best treated by injection of 3% sodium chloride solution, followed by cyst marsupialization.

E. Splenic pseudocysts smaller than 4 cm warrant observation.

Ref.: 1, 4

COMMENTS: Splenic cysts are classified as true cysts, which may be parasitic or nonparasitic, and pseudocysts. • Primary true cysts account for 10% of all nonparasitic cysts of the spleen. • Most nonparasitic cysts are pseudocysts secondary to trauma. • True cysts are lined by a squamous epithelium, which often stain positive for CA 19-9 and CEA. • Patients with true cysts may have elevated serum levels of these markers. • Most true cysts are asymptomatic, particularly if smaller than 8 cm in size. • Operative intervention is indicated for cysts that are symptomatic or large. • Usually, either partial splenectomy, cyst wall resection, or partial excision of the capsule can be performed successfully. • Most true cysts are parasitic, due to *Echinococcus* spp. • They should be treated by splenectomy after sterilization with 3% NaCl solution, alcohol, or 0.5% silver nitrate solution. • Traumatic pseudocysts account for up to 80% of all nonparasitic cysts. • CT scanning can demonstrate calcifications in up to 50% of the cases. • Most small (<4 cm) asymptomatic pseudocysts can be safely observed, since they may undergo spontaneous resolution. • Symptomatic pseudocysts can be treated by image-guided percutaneous drainage, partial splenectomy, or splenectomy if necessary.

ANSWER:
B, E

21. All but which of the following statements regarding splenic abscesses are true?

A. Metastatic hematogenous spread is the most common route.

B. Most splenic abscesses are solitary and unilocular.

C. The most common organisms cultured are enteric organisms.

D. Complications of splenic abscesses include rupture into the abdominal cavity or rupture into an intra-abdominal organ, resulting in a fistula.

E. Broad-spectrum antibiotics are the mainstay of treatment, with an initial success rate of 85–90%.

Ref.: 1, 2, 4

COMMENTS: Splenic abscesses are relatively rare. • They usually present with fever, vague abdominal pain, and bacteremia. • They are more common in males and immunocompromised patients. • They are generally classified according to the likely pathogenesis. • The most common cause is usually hematogenous spread from infective endocarditis, intravenous drug abuse, or intra-abdominal infections. • Other causes are trauma; secondary infection from splenic infarction, as seen in sickle cell disease; contiguous spread from adjacent organs; or infection in immunocompromised patients. • Most splenic abscesses are solitary and unilocular. • They can be detected by both ultrasound imaging and CT scan, but CT scanning is significantly more sensitive. • The most common organisms cultured are enteric organisms, which account for two thirds of the cases. • Complications are rare but include splenic rupture into the abdominal cavity or rupture into a contiguous organ resulting in a fistula.

Treatment depends on whether the abscess is unilocular or multilocular. • Image-guided percutaneous drainage with concomitant antibiotic use can be attempted for patients with unilocular abscesses, with about a 75% success rate. • However, if there is no clinical improvement postdrainage, the patient should undergo a splenectomy. • Most multilocular abscesses will require a splenectomy along with antibiotic use. • The mortality rate for splenic abscess ranges from 90% for multilocular abscesses in immunocompromised patients to 20% in previously healthy patients with unilocular abscesses.

A N S W E R :
E

---

22. During the performance of a left hemicolectomy, an actively bleeding 2-cm laceration at the inferior pole of the spleen is identified. Appropriate initial management includes which of the following measures?

    A. Splenorrhaphy with topical hemostatic agents, suture repair, or both

    B. Partial splenectomy

    C. Splenectomy

    D. Drainage of the left upper quadrant

    E. Argon beam coagulator and fibrin glue application

Ref.: 1, 2, 4

COMMENTS: Iatrogenic splenic injuries incurred during the course of unrelated abdominal operations are particularly amenable to splenorrhaphy rather than splenectomy because of the generally limited nature of such injuries. • An additional concern has been the increased risk of postoperative complications and even long-term septic sequelae reported in patients undergoing incidental splenectomy. • Simple techniques, such as compression, cautery, and the use of topical hemostatic agents, alone or in combination with simple suture repair are adequate for more than 90% of mild or moderate splenic injuries, including most iatrogenic injuries. • Partial splenectomy is reserved for a small percentage of patients in whom a substantial segment of spleen can be salvaged in an otherwise extensively injured organ. • Most iatrogenic injuries, because of their limited nature, should not require splenectomy. • However, if the surgeon is not able to control the bleeding, splenectomy may be necessary. • Complications related to splenorrhaphy following splenic injury are uncommon. • The overall rate of rebleeding following splenorrhaphy for any reason is less than 2%. • Drainage of the left upper quadrant generally is not necessary. • Argon beam coagulation and fibrin glue application constitute helpful adjuncts to control bleeding from the injured spleen.

A N S W E R :
A

---

23. Match the grade of splenic injury in the left-hand column with the degree of laceration or extent of hematoma in the right-hand column.

    A. II   a. Laceration involving a trabecular vessel
    B. V   b. Subcapsular hematoma less than 10% of surface
    C. III   c. Hilar vessel involvement
    D. IV   d. Hilar vessel disruption
    E. I   e. 5-cm subcapsular hematoma

Ref.: 6

COMMENTS: The grading system for splenic injuries depends on the degree of splenic laceration and the magnitude of the subcapsular hematoma if present. • The American Association for the Surgery of Trauma has summarized the classification as shown in the table.

AAST Organ Injury Scale for Spleen

Grade	Hematoma	Laceration
I	Subcapsular, nonexpanding, <10% surface area	Capsular tear, nonbleeding, <1 cm parenchymal depth
II	Subcapsular, nonexpanding, 10%–50% surface area; intraparenchymal, nonexpanding, <5 cm in diameter	Capsular tear, active bleeding, 1–3 cm parenchymal depth, not involving a trabecular vessel
III	Subcapsular, >50% surface area or expanding; ruptured subcapsular hematoma with bleeding; intraparenchymal, >5 cm or expanding	>3 cm parenchymal depth or active involving trabecular vessels
IV	Ruptured intraparenchymal hematoma with active bleeding	Laceration involving segmental or hilar vessels producing major devascularization (>25% of spleen)
V	Completely shattered spleen	Hilar vascular injury that devascularizes spleen

A N S W E R :
A-e; B-d; C-a; D-c; E-b

---

24. Regarding the ruptured spleen, which of the following statements is/are true?

    A. The spleen is the organ most commonly injured during blunt abdominal trauma.

    B. The spleen is the organ most commonly injured during penetrating abdominal trauma.

    C. Spontaneous rupture is most commonly associated with hematologic, rather than infectious, disease.

    D. Nonoperative management of splenic injury has increased the frequency of delayed splenic rupture.

    E. A splenic "vascular blush" on CT scanning predicts increased failure rate of nonoperative management.

Ref.: 1, 2, 4

COMMENTS: The spleen is the most frequently injured organ during blunt trauma to the abdomen or lower thorax. • In up to 70% of cases, there is associated injury to other organ systems, including, in decreasing order of frequency, the ribs, kidney, spinal cord, and liver. • Penetrating trauma, however, results in small-bowel and liver injuries far more commonly than splenic injuries. • **Spontaneous splenic rupture** is most often caused by complications of malaria and infectious mononucleosis, but it also can occur with sarcoidosis, leukemia, hemolytic anemia, and polycythemia vera. • General signs of splenic rupture include pain at the left shoulder as a result of diaphragmatic irritation (Kehr's sign) and a mass or fixed dullness in the left upper quadrant (Ballance's sign). • Kehr's sign is elicited by manual compression of the left upper quadrant after placing the patient in the Trendelenburg position for several minutes. • The occurrence of Kehr's sign is inconsistent, seen in 15–70% of patients. • Ballance's sign is rare. • In patients with a ruptured spleen, the hematocrit is usually 10–30% below normal, and there is mild leukocytosis. • Diagnostic peritoneal lavage, ultrasound imaging, and CT scanning are accurate tools. • Of these, CT scanning is probably the most accurate. • However, ultrasound imaging, using the FAST (focused assessment with sonography in trauma) technique, has rapidly become the screening test of choice for these patients. • Furthermore, ultrasound imaging is extremely useful in the follow-up of splenic injury when nonoperative management is chosen.

"Delayed" rupture of the spleen was thought to occur in 10–15% of cases of blunt splenic trauma. • The length of the delay, as originally described by Jean Baudet in 1907 (*period de latence*) was less than 2 weeks in 75% of these cases. • Delayed rupture usually represents rupture of false aneurysms, which can be identified by the presence of a "vascular blush" on CT scan examination. • In fact, the presence of such a sign has been associated with two thirds of failures in patients that are managed nonoperatively. • Patients whose spleens contain vascular blushes representing false aneurysms should undergo selective angiography and subsequent embolization. • Approximately 30–50% of vascularized splenic tissue is necessary for normal splenic functions. • This fact is pertinent when trying to salvage inadequate fragments of a traumatized spleen. • In such instances, total splenectomy is more expeditious and safer.

ANSWER:
A, E

25. Which of the following patients is a candidate for nonoperative treatment of splenic injury?

    A. A patient with a grade III splenic injury, a pulse of 80 beats/min, and a blood pressure of 110/70

    B. A patient with a grade III splenic injury with a drop in hematocrit from 45 to 30

    C. A patient with a grade III splenic injury with a pooling of contrast seen on CT scanning

    D. A patient with a grade V splenic injury and left upper quadrant pain

    E. A patient with coronary artery disease and grade III injury

Ref.: 1, 2, 4, 7

COMMENTS: In the last 20 years, there has been a resurgence of interest in splenic preservation, especially in the trauma literature. • Currently, 70–90% of children with splenic injuries are successfully managed nonoperatively, and 40–50% of adult patients also are eligible for nonoperative treatment in trauma centers. • This difference between children and adults is probably due to the different mechanisms of injury and the severity of injury in adult patients. • Peritonitis-associated injuries requiring an operation, severity of injury, hemodynamic instability, and ongoing blood loss are the primary factors considered in the management of these patients. • Furthermore, old age generally has been considered a contraindication to nonoperative management. • Most patients with isolated grade I–III splenic injuries can be observed safely. • Patients with grade IV–V splenic injuries may be managed nonoperatively, provided they are admitted to a large-volume trauma center. • The frequency and need for follow-up imaging studies is controversial. • It is felt that sequential CT scanning may be essential in identifying splenic false aneurysms, since up to 74% of these aneurysms are seen only in studies performed after the initial 24 hr. • The main benefit of a spleen-preserving procedure is reducing the risk of OPSI, which carries mortality rates of greater than 50%. • Criteria for splenic preservation include hemodynamic stability, CT scan documentation of grade of injury, absence of pooling contrast seen on CT scanning, absence of other intra-abdominal injury necessitating operative intervention, and a transfusion requirement of less the 2 units of blood.

ANSWER:
A

26. Which of the following statements regarding laparoscopic splenectomy is false?

    A. Laparoscopic splenectomy can be completed successfully approximately 90% of the time in carefully selected patients.

    B. Postoperative recovery appears to be decreased with laparoscopic splenectomy.

    C. Conversion to open surgery is usually secondary to bleeding, lack of surgical experience, extensive adhesions, or significant splenomegaly.

    D. Laparoscopic splenectomy for ITP parallels the hematologic response and long-term cure rates achieved with open splenectomy.

    E. Laparoscopic splenectomy results in a higher incidence of splenosis.

Ref.: 1, 2, 4

COMMENTS: Laparoscopic splenectomy was first described in 1992 and has been evaluated extensively in comparison to the open technique. • Most retrospective studies have shown that the average operative time is slightly longer than with the open splenectomy, but postoperative recovery and mean duration of hospitalization is significantly shorter. • Conversion to open splenectomy is usually secondary to bleeding, but lack of surgical experience, extensive adhesions, obesity, and splenomegaly also contribute. • Open splenectomy can be performed in 100% of patients with a hospital mortality rate of less than 1%. • In comparison, laparoscopic splenectomy can be performed 90% of the time with a comparable mortality rate.

    The most important aspect of laparoscopic splenectomy that needs to be considered is the long-term cure rate of hematologic disease. • This has yet to be established in long-term follow-up, since the technique is still relatively new. • However, short-term follow-up in most studies has shown success rates of 76–100%. • The most significant cause of failure is attributed to accessory spleens. • The incidence of accessory spleens in the literature is approximately 15%. • The failure is likely secondary to the fact that accessory spleens are more easily felt than seen, and they can be easily mistaken for lymph nodes. • The use of sturdy retrieval bags permits morcellation of the spleen and its safe procurement.

ANSWER:
D

REFERENCES

1. Townsend CM, Beauchamp RD, Evers BM, et al (eds): *Sabiston Textbook of Surgery: The Biological Basis of Modern Surgical Practice,* 16th ed. Saunders, Philadelphia, 2001.
2. Cameron JL: *Current Surgical Therapy,* 7th ed. CV Mosby, St. Louis, 2001.
3. Schwartz SI, Shires GT, Spencer FC, et al (eds): *Schwartz's Principles of Surgery,* 7th ed. McGraw-Hill, New York, 1999.
4. Greenfield LJ, Mulholland MW, Oldham KT, et al (eds): *Greenfield's Surgery: Scientific Principles and Practice,* 3rd ed. Lippincott, Williams & Wilkins, Philadelphia, 2001.
5. Fleshner PR, Aufses AM Jr, Grabowski GA, et al: A 27-year experience with splenectomy for Gaucher's disease. *Am J Surg* 161:69–75, 1991.
6. American Association for Surgery of Trauma (AAST): Organ Injury Scales for Liver, Biliary Tract, Diaphragm, and Spleen: Trauma and thermal injury. In: *ACS Surgery: Principles and Practice.* www.acssurgery.com.
7. Cullingford GL, Watkins DM, Watts ADS, et al: Severe late postsplenectomy infection. *Br J Surg* 78:716–721, 1991.

CHAPTER 42

Hernia, Abdominal Wall, and Retroperitoneum

Keith W. Millikan, M.D.

1. Components of Hesselbach's triangle include which of the following anatomic landmarks?

A. Pectineal ligament

B. Medial border of the rectus sheath

C. Cooper's ligament

D. Inguinal ligament

E. Inferior epigastric vessels

Ref.: 1–3

COMMENTS: The inferior epigastric vessels serve as the supero-lateral border of Hesselbach's triangle. • The medial border of the triangle is formed by the rectus sheath, and the inguinal ligament serves as its inferior border. • Hernias occurring within Hesselbach's triangle are considered direct hernias, whereas hernias occurring lateral to the triangle are indirect hernias. • The original description of Hesselbach's triangle defined the inferior border as Cooper's ligament or the pectoral ligament. • The borders were subsequently modified, substituting the inguinal ligament for Copper's ligament or the pectoral ligament to allow an easier identification of the area by surgeons who use the traditional anterior approach for herniorrhaphy.

ANSWER:
B, D, E

2. Which of the following statements is/are true regarding the iliopubic tract?

A. Extends from the anterosuperior iliac spine to the pubis

B. Is a condensation of transversalis fascia

C. Is of anatomic interest but has little clinical significance

D. Is synonymous with the shelving portion of Poupart's ligament

E. Many branches of the lumbar plexus run inferior to the iliopubic tract

Ref.: 1–3

COMMENTS: The transversalis fascia is the portion of the endo-abdominal fascia that underlies the transversus abdominis muscle.

• It has several thickenings, the most important of which is the iliopubic tract, arising from the iliopectineal arch, inserting on the anterosuperior iliac spine, and extending over the femoral vessels to the pubis. • Proper utilization of the transversalis fascia during repair of an inguinal hernia is important to the success of operations not utilizing prosthetic materials. • The iliopubic tract has particular significance because of its importance as a landmark to the laparoscopic surgeons. • Many of the branches of the lumbar plexus run inferior to the tract, and damage to these nerves may be the result of aggressive dissection or the placement of tacks or staples to affix a prosthesis below this structure.

ANSWER:
A, B, E

3. Which of the following statements is/are true regarding the incidence of abdominal wall hernias?

A. Two thirds of all inguinal hernias are classified as indirect.

B. Femoral hernias are more common in females than in males.

C. Direct hernias are common in females.

D. Hernias generally occur with equal frequency in males and females.

E. Premature babies have a 10% incidence of having inguinal hernia.

Ref.: 1–3

COMMENTS: Approximately three fourths of all abdominal wall hernias occur in the inguinal region, and roughly two thirds of them are indirect inguinal hernias. • The incidence of inguinal hernias in premature babies is approximately 10%. • In general, hernias are considered to be at least five times more common in males than in females. • The most common hernia in each gender is the indirect variety. • It has been estimated that 25% of males and 2% of females develop inguinal hernias during their lifetime. • Hernias therefore constitute a significant economic problem in terms of loss of time from work.

ANSWER:
A, B, E

4. According to the Nyhus classification of groin hernias, which of the following statements are true?

   A. A type II indirect hernia has a dilated internal ring and extends into the scrotum.

   B. A type IIIa hernia is a classically described direct hernia.

   C. A femoral hernia is classified as type IIIc.

   D. Type IV hernias are recurrent hernias.

   E. Type V hernias are spigelian hernias.

Ref.: 2

COMMENTS: Groin hernias may be primary or recurrent. • Hernias are classified as inguinal and femoral, the inguinal hernias being further subdivided into direct and indirect hernias. • Lloyd Nyhus further subdivided groin hernias according to their characteristics. • Type I hernias are indirect hernias with a normal-size internal ring, occurring typically in infants, children, and small adults. • Type II hernias are indirect hernias with a dilated internal ring and an intact posterior wall and do not extend into the scrotum. • Type III hernias are posterior wall defects. • Type IIIA are direct hernias regardless of size. • Type IIIB are indirect hernias with a dilated internal ring encroaching on Hesselbach's triangle (massive scrotal, sliding, or pantaloon type). • Type IIIc are femoral hernias. • Type IV are recurrent hernias of direct, indirect, femoral, or a combined type. • There are no type V hernias according to the Nyhus classification.

ANSWER:
B, C, D

5. Which of the following statements is/are true regarding direct inguinal hernias?

   A. The most likely cause is destruction of connective tissue resulting from physical stress.

   B. Direct hernias should be repaired promptly because of the risk of incarceration.

   C. A direct hernia may be a sliding hernia involving a portion of the bladder wall.

   D. A direct hernia may pass through the external inguinal ring.

   E. Colon carcinoma is a known cause of direct inguinal hernias.

Ref.: 1–3

COMMENTS: Destruction of connective tissue resulting from the physical stress of intra-abdominal pressure, smoking, aging, connective tissue disease, and systemic illnesses reduces the strength of the transverse aponeurosis and fascia. • Direct inguinal hernias, therefore, are acquired from the "wear and tear" of daily life, including straining to urinate or defecate, chronic coughing, and heavy lifting. • Because generally there is a diffuse weakness in the area of Hesselbach's triangle without a narrow-neck sac, the risk of incarceration is low. • Rarely, incarceration results when the direct hernia passes through the external ring posterior to the cord structures. • The involvement of the urinary bladder as a sliding component on the medial wall of a direct hernia sac usually does not cause a problem because the sac can be simply reduced unopened. • The notion that carcinoma of the colon is a cause of inguinal hernia is incorrect.

ANSWER:
A, C, D

6. A sliding inguinal hernia on the left side is likely to involve which of the following?

   A. Jejunum composing the posterior wall of the sac

   B. Ovary and fallopian tube in a female infant

   C. Omentum

   D. Sigmoid colon composing the posterior wall of the sac

   E. Cecum composing the anteromedial wall of the sac

Ref.: 1–3

COMMENTS: A sliding hernia is one in which the visceral peritoneum of an organ makes up part of the wall of the hernia sac. • If the hernia is indirect, it most commonly involves the cecum on the right or the sigmoid colon on the left. • In females, especially infants and children, portions of the female genital tract often are involved. • Recognition of the presence of a sliding hernia and the position of the visceral component is important to avoid injury of the involved organs during repair.

ANSWER:
B, D

7. Which of the following statements is/are true regarding femoral hernias?

   A. Femoral hernias can be approached through an infrainguinal dissection.

   B. Femoral hernias are more common in females than in males.

   C. Femoral hernias are more common than inguinal hernias in females.

   D. Prosthetic material should always be used for large femoral hernias.

   E. All of the above

Ref.: 1–3, 4

COMMENTS: Although femoral hernias are found more often in females than in males, inguinal hernias are still more common than femoral hernias. • Femoral hernias with small orifices in women are repaired from below the inguinal ligament with a few sutures or plugged with a cone of polypropylene mesh because they are rarely associated with hernias above the inguinal ligament. • Large femoral hernias can be repaired by the McVay Cooper's ligament repair or even better by a preperitoneal permanent prosthesis placed either laparoscopically or by an open preperitoneal approach.

ANSWER:
A, B

8. Correct statements regarding the management of an incarcerated groin hernia include which of the following?

   A. Immediate or urgent surgical repair is always required for incarcerated groin hernias.

   B. Evaluation of the hernia sac contents is a required step in the repair of an incarcerated hernia.

   C. Contents within an incarcerated hernia can be omentum, intestine, or an ovary.

D. A hydrocele may mimic an incarcerated hernia.

E. All of the above

Ref.: 1–3

COMMENTS: Incarceration and subsequent strangulation of small bowel are serious complications of groin hernias. • If the patient has an incarcerated inguinal hernia and strangulation is not suspected, an attempt at reduction by using sedation, Trendelenburg positioning, and gentle sustained pressure over the groin mass is appropriate. • If there is any indication of strangulation, reduction should not be attempted preoperatively. • Rather, the sac should first be opened before reduction to inspect the viability of the contents. • Delayed repair following successful reduction may permit resolution of edema. • A hydrocele can mimic an incarcerated hernia. • One can get above a hydrocele with examining fingers. • Also, a hydrocele will transilluminate clearly, but a hernia will not. • The contents of an incarcerated inguinal hernia may be omentum, intestine, or an ovary.

ANSWER:
B, C, D

9. Which of the following statements about management of inguinal hernias in infants and children is/are true?

A. Repair should be delayed until a child reaches school age, since most inguinal hernia defects spontaneously close.

B. Repair usually requires a Bassini procedure.

C. The distal sac should be removed to prevent formation of a secondary hydrocele.

D. Contralateral inguinal exploration is indicated routinely because of the high risk of bilaterality.

E. Intubation of the clinically apparent hernia sac with a laparoscope is one method of examining the contralateral side.

Ref.: 1–3

COMMENTS: Inguinal hernias in infants and children are nearly always indirect, resulting from failure of obliteration of the processus vaginalis. • Effective treatment requires only high ligation and transection of the sac with or without excision of the distal component. • Repair need not be delayed unless the infant has associated medical problems. • In fact, bowel obstruction and gonadal or intestinal infarction as a result of strangulation are most likely to occur during the first 6 months of life. • Therefore, repair should be performed soon after the diagnosis is made. • Exploration of the opposite side in children who present with a unilateral inguinal hernia is controversial. • The incidence of a contralateral hernia following unilateral inguinal herniorrhaphy in children has been reported to be 10–30%. • Contralateral exploration should be performed routinely in the subset of patients most likely to have a clinically occult hernia: patients less than 2 years old, girls less than 3 years old (higher bilateral rate), patients with ventriculoperitoneal shunts, and patients less than 2 years old with a left-sided hernia. • This last recommendation is based on the fact that most (60%) pediatric hernias are right sided. • Intubation of the clinically apparent hernia sac with a laparoscope is one method of examining the contralateral side.

ANSWER:
E

10. Which of the following statements is/are true regarding the preperitoneal or posterior approach for the repair of groin hernias?

A. It may be appropriate for repair of both direct and indirect hernias.

B. It may be appropriate for repair of femoral hernias.

C. It is performed through the same skin incision as for the anterior approach.

D. The preperitoneal approach is not indicated for bilateral or recurrent hernias.

E. Laparoscopic hernioplasty is an extension of the preperitoneal approach.

Ref.: 1–3

COMMENTS: The preperitoneal approach, utilizing a transverse skin incision three finger breadths above the pubic tubercle, has been especially successful in the repair of femoral hernias. • Both direct and indirect inguinal hernias also can be approached in this manner, although many surgeons have reported higher recurrence rates for direct hernias when using this approach. • A Cooper's ligament repair is carried out in the same way as for an anterior approach. • The ligament is approximated to the transversus abdominis aponeurosis medially with a transition suture between the transversus aponeurosis, the iliopubic tract, and Cooper's ligament, with completion laterally by approximation of the iliopubic tract and transversus aponeurosis. • This approach as originally described has not achieved widespread use. • Modifications of the preperitoneal approach utilizing prosthetic material have become more popular, particularly for repair of bilateral and recurrent hernias. • General or regional anesthesia is necessary. • Postoperative paralytic ileus is not infrequent. • Laparoscopic hernioplasty is an extension of the preperitoneal concept. • In most of the laparoscopic repairs, the prosthesis is placed in the preperitoneal space.

ANSWER:
A, B, E

11. Which of the following statements is/are true regarding the mesh-plug hernioplasty?

A. It can be performed under local anesthesia with intravenous sedation.

B. It is associated with a 1% or lower recurrence rate.

C. It may be appropriate for indirect, direct, femoral, and recurrent hernias.

D. A 10- to 14-day recovery is necessary before patients can assume normal daily activities.

E. Manual labor is restricted for 1 month postoperatively.

Ref.: 4, 5

COMMENTS: In the 1990s, I. M. Rutkow and A. W. Robbins introduced the mesh-plug hernioplasty. • In over 3000 reported hernioplasties, a 1% overall recurrence rate has been documented for all varieties of inguinal hernias. • Although Rutkow and Robbins perform the mesh-plug hernioplasty under epidural anesthesia, subsequent reports have described the procedure being performed under local anesthesia with intravenous sedation. • In over 1000 mesh-plug hernioplasties reported by K. W. Millikan and coworkers, a 0.1% recurrence rate was documented, with 96% of patients returning to normal activities within 3 days. • In this series, all manual laborers returned to work without restrictions on postoperative day 14. • During the last decade, the mesh-plug hernioplasty has become the most popular prosthetic hernia repair in the United States.

ANSWER:
A, B, C

12. Which of the following statements concerning the Lichtenstein repair is/are true.

    A. It is performed in an outpatient setting under local anesthesia.

    B. Polytetrafluoroethylene is the most common prosthetic material used for repair.

    C. The medial edge of the mesh is sutured to transversalis fascia, while the lateral edge is sutured to the inguinal ligament.

    D. To reduce recurrence rates, the most cephalad tails of the mesh should extend 2–4 cm beyond the internal ring.

    E. To reduce recurrence rates, the most caudal aspect of the mesh should extend at least 2 cm over the pubic tubercle.

Ref.: 1–3, 6

COMMENTS: As commonly performed, the open herniorrhaphy technique is the tension-free repair popularized by Irving L. Lichtenstein and colleagues. • The Lichtenstein repair is routinely performed in an outpatient setting with local anesthesia. • A polypropylene mesh is sutured medially to the conjoined tendon, with the internal oblique overlapped by approximately 2 cm. • The latter edge of the mesh is sutured to the inguinal ligament. • To reduce recurrence rates, Parvis Amid has described overlapping the mesh at least 2 cm over the pubic tubercle and 2–4 cm lateral to the internal ring. • Lichtenstein encouraged patients to rapidly resume activities. • The Lichtenstein repair was one of the first prosthetic repairs to achieve approximately an overall 1% or lower recurrence rate in the United States.

ANSWER:
A, D, E

13. Which of the following is/are true with regard to the McVay Cooper's ligament repair?

    A. It is appropriate for indirect and direct hernias but not for femoral hernias.

    B. Exposure of Cooper's ligament and the medial border of the femoral sheath is accomplished by excision of the medial portion of the iliopubic tract.

    C. Relaxing incisions are mandatory.

    D. The conjoined tendon is sutured to the Cooper's ligament from the pubic tubercle laterally to the femoral canal.

    E. Using a transition stitch, the surgeon sutures the conjoined tendon to the inguinal ligament lateral to the femoral canal.

Ref.: 1–3

COMMENTS: The Cooper's ligament hernioplasty repairs the three most vulnerable areas for herniation in the myopectineal orifice—the deep ring, Hesselbach's triangle, and the femoral canal—and is therefore indicated for the three common types of hernias of the groin. • In the McVay repair, the conjoined tendon is sutured to Cooper's ligament laterally. • Exposure of Cooper's ligament is

accomplished by excision of the medial portion of the iliopubic tract. • Relaxing incisions are mandatory because there is otherwise too much tension on the suture line. • A transition stitch is necessary to suture the conjoined tendon to the inguinal ligament beyond the femoral canal. • The internal inguinal ring is recreated with adequate laxity to allow the passage of the tip of a Kelly clamp adjacent to the cord structures.

ANSWER:
B, C, D, E

14. Which of the following hernias is most likely to recur after primary repair?

    A. Epigastric hernia

    B. Spigelian hernia

    C. Indirect hernia

    D. Femoral hernia

    E. Incisional hernia

Ref.: 1–3

COMMENTS: Primary repair of incisional hernias can be associated with a 30–50% or higher recurrence rate, depending on the size of the hernia. • Except for small incisional hernias, prosthetic mesh is necessary to reduce recurrence rates to 10% or possibly less. • Patients with incisional hernias usually have predisposing factors, such as obesity, chronic debilitating illness, diabetes, advanced age, and smoking. • The predisposing factors also play a role in the failure of primary repair. • The recurrence rates after the other listed hernia repairs should all be 5% or less.

ANSWER:
E

15. Which of the following developments has led to a decrease in recurrence rates after groin hernia repair?

    A. Modifications of the Bassini repair

    B. Routine use of prosthetic materials

    C. Widespread acceptance of the "tension-free" concept

    D. Use of preperitoneal space for hernia repair

    E. Use of laparoscopy in hernia repair

Ref.: 1–3

COMMENTS: Recurrence rates for groin hernias vary from less than 1% to 30%. • True recurrence rates are difficult to establish because of inadequate patient follow-up. • The Bassini repair and its modifications (Shouldice and McVay) all create tension at the suture line and have been found to have recurrence rates between 10 and 30% when performed outside specialized centers. • Several developments in the latter half of the twentieth century significantly influenced the currently accepted level of recurrence rate of less than 5%. • The routine use of prosthetic materials to perform a tension-free hernia repair became accepted by surgeons after being popularized by Lichtenstein in the 1980s. • Others, such as Rutkow, Robbins, R. D. Kugel, A. Gilbert, G. Wantz, R.E. Stoppa, and Nyhus, have used multiple prosthetic materials and approaches to continue to reduce the recurrence rate to below 1%. • The most popular prosthetic materials are polypropylene, Mersilene, and polytetrafluoroethylene. • The use of the preperitoneal space also helped lower recurrence rates by allowing for larger pieces of prosthetic material to be used and incorporating intra-abdominal pressure to aid in keeping the mesh in place. • Laparoscopy has not helped lower recurrence rates, but it has given the surgeon another option for accessing the preperitoneal space.

ANSWER:
B, C, D

16. Which of the following is/are true regarding laparoscopic hernia repair?

    A. Local anesthesia with sedation is the most common form of anesthesia used.

    B. It is a cost-effective approach.

    C. Transabdominal preperitoneal or total extraperitoneal approaches are commonly used.

    D. Fixation devices for the mesh should not be placed below the iliopubic tract.

    E. It is best suited for recurrent and bilateral hernias.

    Ref.: 1–3, 7

COMMENTS: Laparoscopic techniques for repair of inguinal hernias were introduced in the 1990s and have gained mild-to-moderate acceptance, with less than 10% of all inguinal hernia repairs being performed by these approaches. • The repairs are usually performed under general anesthesia and have been reported to cost twice as much as those performed with an open approach under local anesthesia. • Although there is controversy regarding its use for unilateral, newly diagnosed hernias, it seems ideally suited for recurrent and bilateral hernias, where the disability and technical difficulty associated with open (conventional) repairs cannot be overlooked. • Laparoscopy can be performed totally extraperitoneally by dissecting within the preperitoneal space or transabdominally. • In either case, a preperitoneal repair is performed. • Mesh fixation devices placed below the iliopubic tract risk injury to the genitofemoral nerve and the lateral femoral cutaneous nerve. • Fixation device placement is also avoided below the internal inguinal ring in an area known as the "triangle of doom." • This triangle is bordered laterally by the spermatic vessels and medially by the vas deferens. • Located within this triangle are the external iliac artery and vein and the femoral nerve.

ANSWER:
C, D, E

17. Which of the following is/are true statements regarding umbilical hernias?

    A. They are the embryonic equivalent of a small omphalocele.

    B. Repair in infants is usually deferred until approximately 4 years of age.

    C. Repair in adults is usually indicated.

    D. The "vest-over-pants" type of repair is stronger than simple approximation of fascial margins.

    E. They are most common in Caucasian infants.

    Ref.: 1–3

COMMENTS: Umbilical hernias are the result of a patent umbilical ring, whereas an omphalocele is the result of failure of abdominal wall closure in the midline during early intrauterine life. • Umbilical hernias are said to be present in 40–90% of African-American infants. • Incarceration is rare in infants. • Unless the defect is large, most surgeons defer repair until the child is approximately 4 years of age, because spontaneous closure does occur. • In adults, however, repair should be carried out promptly because of the risk of incarceration. • There is no convincing evidence that a "vest-over-pants" type of repair is structurally superior to simple approximation of fascial margins. • Repair in adults may require use of a prosthetic material, such as polypropylene, if the fascial defect is large or if there is tension.

ANSWER:
B, C

18. Which of the following hernias represent an incarceration of a limited portion of small bowel?

    A. Spigelian hernia

    B. Grynfeltt's hernia

    C. Petit's hernia

    D. Richter's hernia

    E. Littre's hernia

    Ref.: 1–3

COMMENTS: Spigelian, Grynfeltt's, and Petit's hernias are abdominal or lumbar hernias in unusual anatomic locations. • A spigelian hernia occurs at the lateral border of the rectus at the linea semicircularis. • A Petit's hernia occurs at the inferior lumbar triangle bordered by the latissimus dorsi, external oblique, and iliac crest. • A Grynfeltt's hernia occurs at the superior lumbar triangle where the internal oblique inserts on the twelfth rib. • Richter's and Littre's hernias represent incarceration of a limited portion of small bowel. • Littre's hernia has an incarcerated Meckel's diverticulum or the appendix as its contents. • A Richter's hernia has noncircumferential incarceration of small bowel, usually only the antimesenteric portion. • It is important to recognize Richter's and Littre's hernias because vascular compromise may occur without evidence of intestinal obstruction.

ANSWER:
D, E

19. Which of the following statements are true with regard to the Kugel mesh repair for inguinal hernias?

    A. A less than 1% recurrence rate has been documented.

    B. The mesh is placed in the preperitoneal space.

    C. The mesh is sutured to the conjoined tendon and the inguinal ligament.

    D. The repair can be performed on all varieties of inguinal hernias.

    E. The procedure is performed utilizing general anesthesia.

    Ref.: 8

COMMENTS: The minimally invasive Kugel mesh hernia repair is a preperitoneal hernia repair. • The procedure is usually performed under local or epidural anesthesia through an oblique skin incision approximately 2–3 cm above the internal ring. • A pocket is developed in the preperitoneal space, and an oval mesh with a semirigid ring is placed covering the femoral, direct, and indirect defects of all varieties of inguinal hernias. • The mesh is usually not sutured in place. • Occasionally, a suture may be placed in

Cooper's ligament for large direct hernias. • In a series of 808 repairs, Kugel reported a 0.62% recurrence rate over a 54-month period.

ANSWER:
A, B, D

20. Which of the following items represents the optimal convalescent period required before returning to manual labor after inguinal mesh herniorrhaphy?

   A. 6–8 weeks

   B. 4–5 weeks

   C. 2–3 weeks

   D. 1 week

   E. Less than 1 week

Ref.: 1–3, 4

COMMENTS: Traditionally, patients who engage in strenuous activities have been allowed periods of 6–8 weeks to recuperate after traditional open herniorrhaphy. • Studies have shown that collagen maturation and tensile strength in a hernia wound require months to reach maximal states. • Tension-free repair utilizing prosthetic materials has allowed patients to return to normal activities sooner. • These repairs, including mesh-plug, Kugel, and laparoscopic procedures, have allowed patients to perform any activity they choose as soon as they feel comfortable, which is usually within 2–3 weeks. • In a study of mesh-plug repairs, 465 manual laborers returned to work without restriction on postoperative day 14.

ANSWER:
C

21. The cause of neuropathic postherniorrhaphy inguinodynia includes which of the following?

   A. Formation of scar tissue

   B. Transection of the ilioinguinal, iliohypogastric, or the genitofemoral nerves

   C. Suture entrapment of nerves

   D. Staple entrapment of nerves

   E. Periosteal reaction

Ref.: 9

COMMENTS: Postherniorrhaphy inguinodynia may result from such nonneuropathic causes as periosteal reaction (due to suture or staple into pubic tubercle), scar tissue formation, and mechanical pressure from rolled-up or wadded mesh and folded prosthetic material. • Neuropathic pain can be caused by compression of the nerve by perineural fibrosis, suture material, staples, or prosthetic material or by actual nerve injury caused by partial or complete transection of nerves due to accidental cutting of the nerves, excessive traction of the nerves, or injury from electrocautery.

ANSWER:
B, C, D

22. Which of the following statements are true with regard to incisional ventral hernia?

   A. Primary repairs are associated with a 30–50% recurrence rate.

   B. The incidence of incisional hernia is between 2 and 11% after laparotomy.

   C. Prosthetic mesh repairs have reduced the recurrence rate to 10% or less.

   D. All types of mesh can be placed safely in the intra-abdominal cavity.

   E. Comorbidities, such as diabetes, hypertension, and obesity, are uncommon in patients with incisional hernias.

Ref.: 10

COMMENTS: In the United States each year, approximately 2 million laparotomies are performed, resulting in a reported incisional ventral hernia rate of between 2 and 11%. • The population of patients in which wound dehiscence occurs tends to be obese, with comorbidities of smoking history, hypertension, and diabetes. • Primary incisional ventral hernia repairs have been associated with recurrence rates up to 50%. • Prosthetic mesh repairs have lowered recurrence rates to less than 10%. • Recently, it has been found that a bilayer prosthesis composed of both polypropylene and polytetrafluoroethylene can be safely placed in the abdominal cavity without the occurrence of bowel obstruction or entereocutaneous fistulas. • The intra-abdominal placement of mesh allows for the greatest underlay of the fascial defect, enabling the greatest amount of tissue ingrowth to occur. • When polypropylene alone is placed in the intra-abdominal cavity, bowel obstruction, entereocutaneous fistula, and difficult reentrance to the abdomen occur with an unacceptable frequency.

ANSWER:
A, B, C

23. Which of the following statements is/are true regarding hematomas of the rectus sheath?

   A. They usually result from rupture of the epigastric vessels.

   B. The only recognized etiologic factor is trauma.

   C. They are characterized by a palpable mass that is not influenced by tensing of the rectus abdominis muscle (Fothergill's sign).

   D. Their treatment is usually operative drainage.

   E. They occur mainly in males.

Ref.: 1–3

COMMENTS: Although rectus sheath hematomas most commonly follow trauma, they also can follow minor straining or result from certain infectious diseases (e.g., typhoid fever), collagen vascular diseases, blood dyscrasias, coagulopathies, and anticoagulation therapy. • They usually are the result of rupture of the epigastric artery or vein, rather than a tear of the rectus muscle. • In addition to Fothergill's sign, a bluish discoloration of the skin is also diagnostic, but it may take a few days to develop. • Sonographic studies can be helpful for establishing the diagnosis. • Treatment usually is nonoperative. • Operation may be indicated in cases of an expanding hematoma or if the diagnosis is in doubt, in which case evacuation without entering the peritoneal cavity and closure without drains are standard.

ANSWER:
A, C

24. Which of the following statements is/are true regarding desmoid tumors?

  A. They occur more commonly in women.

  B. They are benign fibrous growths often found within or deep to the lower anterior abdominal musculature.

  C. Because of their benign nature, they are unlikely to recur following excision.

  D. If they are located within the abdominal wall, the proper treatment is enucleation.

  E. They are found in conjunction with juvenile polyposis.

Ref.: 1–3

COMMENTS: Desmoid tumors fall in the middle of a spectrum of fibromatoses ranging from benign fibroma to aggressive fibrosarcoma. • Although considered benign, they have the malignant property of local invasiveness, and, when excised incompletely, they have a propensity to recur. • They usually present as a painless mass within or deep to the anterior abdominal wall musculature. • They occur most frequently in women of childbearing age and are also seen in patients with Gardner's syndrome. • In these cases, the desmoids are located within the small-bowel mesentery and may cause obstructive symptoms and potentially death. • Although local irradiation may have a role in the therapy of some abdominal wall desmoid tumors, the appropriate treatment is wide resection to include the contiguously invaded structures. • Nonsteroidal anti-inflammatory drugs and antiestrogens have achieved tumor regression. • Indomethacin combined with ascorbic acid has also caused regression. • The mesenteric desmoids found with Gardner's syndrome are capable of acting in a highly aggressive fashion. • Because of their propensity to grow rapidly following surgery, resection is not advised. • Instead, these desmoids are treated with Clinoril, tamoxifen, or both. • In refractory or extremely aggressive cases, cytotoxic chemotherapy may be indicated.

ANSWER:
A, B

25. Which of the following statements characterizes retroperitoneal fibrosis?

  A. Reactions to methysergide, ergotamine, hydralazine, methyldopa and β-adrenergic-blocking agents have been implicated.

  B. Two thirds of the cases are idiopathic.

  C. It is two to three times more common in women.

  D. Symptoms generally are related to partial inferior vena caval obstruction.

  E. The most definitive noninvasive diagnostic test is intravenous pyelography (IVP).

Ref.: 1–3

COMMENTS: Retroperitoneal fibrosis is one of a constellation of processes of "systemic idiopathic fibrosis" that can involve the mediastinum, the thyroid gland (Riedel's struma), or the biliary tract (sclerosing cholangitis). • Hypersensitivity to methysergide is one of the few etiologic factors. • Ergotamine, hydralazine, methyldopa, and β-adrenergic-blocking agents have also been implicated. • Two thirds of the cases are idiopathic. • Its incidence is two to three times higher in men than in women. • Although the

inferior vena cava may be compressed by the fibrotic stage of the process, symptoms are usually related to genitourinary tract involvement (specifically, entrapment of the ureters) and lymphatic obstruction. • The characteristic findings of hydronephrosis and medial deviation of the ureters on IVP are highly diagnostic of this entity. • The disease is usually bilateral and symmetrical. • High-grade ureteral obstruction accompanied by infection may require urgent nephrostomy. • Otherwise, mild disease is treated with cessation of potentially responsible medications and institution of corticosteriod therapy. • Surgery is indicated when renal function is compromised. • Options include freeing the encased ureters and wrapping them with omentum or renal autotransplantation.

ANSWER:
A, B, E

26. Which of the following statements is/are true regarding mesenteric lymphadenitis?

  A. It is frequently preceded by a sore throat or upper respiratory tract infection.

  B. It occurs more commonly in children than in adults.

  C. It is easily distinguishable clinically from appendicitis.

  D. Culture specimens taken at the time of operation usually show the presence of coliform bacteria.

  E. The disease process tends to be self-limiting and it rarely recurs.

Ref.: 1–3

COMMENTS: A disease primarily of children and adolescents, mesenteric lymphadenitis is characterized by vague and at times migratory abdominal pain. • It is commonly preceded by a recent sore throat or upper respiratory tract infection. • Frequently, it is difficult to distinguish from appendicitis. • The inability to localize the site of maximal tenderness precisely and the change in that site often are helpful signs. • The small amount of free peritoneal fluid found in these patients is usually sterile. • The disease process is self-limiting, although approximately one fourth of patients have additional episodes during their childhood years.

ANSWER:
A, B

27. Tumors of the mesentery are characterized by which of the following statements?

  A. Two thirds of mesenteric tumors are found in the small-bowel mesentery.

  B. Primary and metastatic tumors of the mesentery occur with approximately equal frequency.

  C. Of the primary mesenteric tumors, most are cystic.

  D. Of the solid primary tumors of the mesentery, most are malignant.

  E. Malignant mesenteric tumors tend to occur near the root of the mesentery, whereas benign tumors are more often peripheral in location.

Ref.: 1–3

COMMENTS: Primary mesenteric tumors are rare and are more often cystic than solid, frequently representing developmental defects of embryonic rests. • Most tumors within the mesentery represent metastases to the mesenteric lymph nodes. • Two thirds of the primary mesenteric tumors are located in the small-bowel mesentery, most commonly in the ileum. • Among the solid primary tumors, most are benign and frequently occur in the periphery of the mesentery. • Malignant mesenteric tumors (most often liposarcoma and leiomyosarcoma) are usually found near the root of the mesentery, which significantly increases both the hazards of resection and the likelihood of subsequent recurrence.

ANSWER:
A, C, E

---

28. Regarding retroperitoneal tumors in general, which of the following statements is/are true?

A. They are tumors of young adulthood.

B. Malignant tumors predominate, the most common of which is liposarcoma.

C. Patients' complaints usually are vague, but on clinical examination, a palpable mass almost always is present.

D. Ultrasound imaging or computed tomographic (CT) scanning provides valuable information.

E. These tumors are locally aggressive but rarely metastasize.

Ref.: 1–3

COMMENTS: Considering all histologic types of retroperitoneal tumor, it tends to be a disease of the fifth and sixth decades, although 15% of these lesions are found in children. • Malignant tumors predominate over benign ones, the most common being lymphoma, followed by liposarcomas, fibrosarcoma, and then the other sarcomas. • These tumors are locally aggressive but rarely metastasize. • The clinical history usually is one of vague back or abdominal pain. • Because the tumor is palpable only when it reaches significant size, surgeons rely heavily on imaging techniques. • Thus, CT scanning and ultrasound imaging have been valuable for delineating the extent of the tumor and its relationship to contiguous structures.

ANSWER:
D, E

---

29. Which of the following statements accurately characterize retroperitoneal sarcomas?

A. The operative approach to them is best achieved through a flank incision.

B. The tumors have a well-defined capsule and can easily be shelled out of the tumor bed with excellent results.

C. They respond to chemotherapy and radiation as the primary treatment.

D. Local recurrence rates range from 60–80%.

E. The 5-year disease-free survival rate is about 10%.

Ref.: 1–3

COMMENTS: Retroperitoneal sarcomas can grow to a large size and typically invade contiguous structures. • A midline incision affords the greatest exposure and is the approach of choice. • These tumors have limited response to chemotherapy and radiation, and therefore surgical excision is the treatment of choice. • The tumors are surrounded by a pseudocapsule and, although the tumors can be shelled out along this capsular plane, in such instances there

is virtually always residual tumor. • Avoiding this situation requires wide excision, frequently en bloc excision with the attached organs (e.g., kidney, bowel, or abdominal wall). • Because of the frequent proximity of these tumors to nonresectable structures, complete excision is possible in only about 25% of patients. • For the same reasons, local recurrence rates may be as high as 50%. • The recurrence rate and their potential for distant metastasis, result in 5-year disease-free survival as low as 10%.

ANSWER:
E

---

30. Tumors of the omentum are characteristic by which of the following statements?

A. Some omental cysts are true cysts.

B. Omental cysts are usually symptomatic.

C. The most common solid omental tumor is liposarcoma.

D. Primary solid tumors of the omentum are fairly common and most often malignant.

E. Omentectomy for metastatic carcinoma has a role in the management of certain tumors.

Ref.: 1–3

COMMENTS: Omental cysts may be "true cysts" (presumably caused by congenital lymphatic obstruction) or neoplastic dermoid cysts, or they may be pseudocysts resulting usually from fat necrosis, trauma, or a foreign-body reaction. • Unless they undergo torsion, most are asymptomatic. • The rest produce vague, nondescript symptoms. • Most solid omental tumors represent metastatic carcinoma, and, in the case of ovarian carcinoma, omentectomy can contribute to improved disease control, despite the presence of metastases elsewhere. • Primary solid omental tumors are rare, and only one third are malignant. • Ultrasound imaging can be valuable for bolstering a clinical diagnosis and determining the cystic or solid nature of a tumor. • At present, percutaneous needle or catheter drainage of presumed omental cysts is too hazardous.

ANSWER:
A, E

---

31. Regarding the physiologic characteristics of the peritoneal membrane, which of the following is/are true?

A. Air that enters the peritoneal cavity during laparotomy is present in diminishing amounts for 10–14 days.

B. Intraperitoneal blood is generally not absorbed, and the few red blood cells that are absorbed are nonviable.

C. Intraperitoneal hypertonic fluids can cause a large shift of fluid from the intravascular space (300–500 ml/hr), causing hypotension and possible shock.

D. The following substances can be removed by peritoneal dialysis: ammonia, calcium, iron, lead, and lithium.

E. The following substances are not removed by peritoneal dialysis: opiates, digitalis, diazepam, antidepressants, and hallucinogens.

Ref.: 1–3

COMMENTS: After an initial equilibration phase, isotonic saline solution is absorbed at a rate of 30–35 ml/hr. • The presence of a hypertonic solution, however, causes movement of fluid from the intravascular space into the peritoneal cavity. • Such movement is driven by the osmolar gradient. • Flow rates up to 300–500 ml/hr have been described and can cause hypotension and shock. • Approximately 70% of intraperitoneal blood is absorbed, albeit at a slower rate than for saline solution, and occurs primarily through fenestrated lymphatic channels on the undersurface of the diaphragm. • Absorbed red blood cells have a normal survival time in the circulation. • Leaving blood in the peritoneal cavity is not advised, since it may potentiate infection. • Air and gases are also similarly absorbed. • Air that enters the peritoneal cavity during laparotomy is present in diminishing amounts for 4–5 days. • Peritoneal dialysis is capable of removing a variety of medications and elements, including those listed. • However, it is not capable of eliminating some medications that carry potential morbidity from overdose.

ANSWER:
C, D, E

32. With regard to tuberculous peritonitis, which of the following statements is/are true?

   A. The mortality rate is greater than 5%.

   B. The majority of patients have radiographic evidence of pulmonary tuberculosis.

   C. Diagnosis is made by the tuberculin skin test.

   D. Fever, ascites, abdominal pain, and weakness are common clinical manifestations.

   E. The tubercle bacillus can gain entry to the peritoneal cavity by transmural migration through diseased bowel, from tuberculous salpingitis, or from the bloodstream.

Ref.: 1–3

COMMENTS: Tuberculous peritonitis has decreased in frequency, and at present the mortality rate is less than 5%. • The tubercle bacillus presumably gains entry to the peritoneal cavity by one of three mechanisms: transmurally from diseased bowel, from tuberculous salpingitis, or from the bloodstream. • The majority of patients do not have radiographic evidence of pulmonary or gastrointestinal tuberculosis. • Common clinical manifestations of the disease include fever, ascites, abdominal pain, and weakness. • Diagnosis may be made most reliably by open or closed peritoneal biopsy and culture. • Treatment is generally nonoperative and includes appropriate antituberculous therapy.

ANSWER:
D, E

33. Which of the following statements is/are true with regard to mesenteric cysts?

   A. They are due to congenital vascular anomalies that gradually enlarge.

   B. They present as asymptomatic abdominal masses.

   C. They display a characteristic medial mobility on examination.

   D. They are treated most approximately by percutaneous radiologically guided needle aspiration.

   E. At laparotomy, they are commonly confused with duplication cysts of the intestine.

Ref.: 1–3

COMMENTS: Mesenteric cysts are most often due to congenital lymphatic spaces that gradually enlarge as they fill with lymph. • Mesenteric cysts usually present as abdominal masses accompanied by pain, nausea, and vomiting. • They may display a characteristic lateral mobility. • They are treated most appropriately by surgical excision. • At operation they may be confused with duplication cysts of the intestine.

ANSWER:
E

REFERENCES

1. Townsend CM, Beachamp RD, Evers BM, et al (eds): *Sabiston Textbook of Surgery: The Biological Basis of Modern Surgical Practice,* 16th ed. Saunders, Philadelphia, 2001.
2. Greenfield L, Mulholland MW, Oldham KT, et al (eds): *Surgery: Scientific Principles and Practice,* 3rd ed. Lippincott, Williams & Wilkins, Philadelphia, 2001.
3. Schwartz SI, Shires GT, Spencer FC (eds): *Principles of Surgery,* 7th ed. McGraw-Hill, New York, 1999.
4. Robbins AW, Rutkow IM: Mesh plug repair and groin hernia surgery. *Surg Clin North Am* 78:1007–1028, 1998.
5. Millikan KW, Cummings B, Doolas A: The Millikan modified mesh-plug hernioplasty. *Arch Surg* 138:525–530, 2003.
6. Amid PK: How to avoid recurrence in Lichtenstein tension-free hernioplasty. *Am J Surg* 184:259–260 2002.
7. Millikan KW, Deziel DJ: The management of hernia: considerations in cost effectiveness. *Surg Clin North Am* 76:105–116, 1996.
8. Kugel RD: Minimally invasive nonlaparoscopic preperitoneal and sutureless inguinal herniorrhaphy. *Am J Surg* 178:298–302, 1999.
9. Amid PK: Surgical treatment for postherniorrhaphy neuropathic inguinodynial triple neurectomy with proximal end implantation. *Comtemp Surg* 59(6):276–280, 2003.
10. Millikan KW, Baptista M, Amin B, et al: Intraperitoneal underlay ventral hernia repair utilizing bilayer expanded polytetrafluoroethylene and polypropylene mesh. *Am Surg* 69(4):287–292, 2003.

C H A P T E R   **43**

Pediatric Surgery

Mark R. Edwards, M.D., and Daniel J. Deziel, M.D.

1. Daily fluid requirements vary by age and weight. Which of the following statements are true?

A. Premature infants weighing less than 2 kg may require up to 150 ml/kg/day.

B. Neonates and infants of 3–10 kg require 200 ml/kg/day.

C. Infants and children of 10–20 kg require 1000 ml/day + 30 ml/kg/day for every kilogram over 10.

D. Children over 20 kg require 1500 ml/day + 20 ml/kg/day for every kilogram over 20.

Ref.: 1–3

COMMENTS: Premature infants require up to 150 ml/kg/day because of their inability to achieve conservation of heat and high insensible losses through immature skin. • Newborn term infants during the first 24 hr of life require 80–90 ml/kg/day due to hypervolemia from transfusion of fluid via placenta at birth. • Diuresis occurs during the first week of life. • Neonates less than 30 days of age require 110 ml/kg/day. • Individuals from more than 30 days of age to adulthood require 100 ml/kg/day for the first 10 kg, plus 50 ml/kg/day for 10–20 kg, plus 20 ml/kg/day for every kilogram over 20.

ANSWER:
A, D

2. Which fluid regimen listed below is the most appropriate a 6-kg infant?

A. Lactated Ringer's solution at 15 ml/hr

B. Dextrose 5% in water (D_5W) + 0.5% normal saline solution + potassium chloride (KCl) 20 mEq/L at 15 ml/hr

C. D_5W + 0.25% normal saline solution + KCl 20 mEq/L at 25 ml/hr

D. D_5W + 0.5% normal saline solution + KCl 15 mEq/L at 25 ml/hr

E. D_5W + 0.25% normal saline solution + KCl 15 mEq/L at 50 ml/hr

Ref.: 1–3

COMMENTS: Understanding maintenance fluid and electrolyte requirements is critical for management of infant surgical patients.

• Free-water maintenance requirements include replacement of insensible losses from the skin and lungs and the free water necessary to clear metabolic solutes in the urine. • It does not include treatment for preexisting deficits or ongoing fluid losses. • Numerous formulas are applicable to the calculation of maintenance requirements. • The most widely used formula is based on weight, although the one based on body surface is equally accurate. • The 24-hr requirement is approximately 100 ml/kg for infants up to 10 kg, plus an additional 50 ml/kg for those 10–20 kg, plus an additional 20 ml/kg in those over 20 kg. • Estimations based on body surface area give equivalent results. • Daily electrolyte requirements include sodium (Na) 2–5 mEq/kg and potassium (K) 2–3 mEq/kg. • For term infants during the first week of life, the maintenance needs are less, ranging from 50 to 90 ml/kg/day. • Dextrose is administered to provide a glucose substrate. • Complete caloric support without enteral supplement requires parenteral nutrition solutions.

ANSWER:
C

3. A 5-week-old boy has a 5-day history of vomiting and a resultant weight loss of 0.4 kg (from 4.0 kg to 3.6 kg). Examination finds his anterior fontanelle flattened and his mucous membranes dry. Laboratory data are as follows (mEq/L): Na 132, K 3.2, Cl 91, and CO_2 28. His capillary pH is 7.48. Which of the following statements about this infant is/are false?

A. It is crucial to determine whether the emesis is bilious.

B. Palpation of the abdomen may reveal the diagnosis.

C. Ultrasound imaging of the abdomen may confirm the diagnosis.

D. The diagnosis is intussusception.

E. The condition should be corrected promptly by operation.

Ref.: 1–3

COMMENTS: Age at the time of symptom manifestation is important in the pediatric population. • Duodenal atresia, for example, is manifested only in newborns. • Pyloric stenosis typically produces symptoms in infants between 3 and 12 weeks of age. • Intussusception, in contrast, most commonly occurs in children between 3 and 18 months of age. • The symptoms of pyloric stenosis usually start with nonbilious vomiting, which progressively becomes projectile in nature. • Dehydration and electrolyte imbalance are usually a function of the length of time the baby has been symptomatic. • If the condition is diagnosed early, fluid and electrolyte levels are mostly normal. • If it is diagnosed late, infants are more likely to present with a hypochloremic, hypokalemic alkalosis and more severe dehydration. • Physical examination can reveal an olive-sized mass in the upper abdomen to the right of the midline that is pathognomonic. • Sometimes gastric waves are seen through the abdominal wall. • If the pyloric mass cannot be palpated by an experienced examiner, ultrasound imaging, an upper gastrointestinal series with contrast, or both may be undertaken to confirm the diagnosis. • Preoperative preparation to correct fluid and electrolyte imbalances is important. • When, but not before, correction is achieved, surgery can be performed. • The Ramstedt pyloromyotomy is the preferred treatment. • Laparoscopic pyloromyotomy is an *alternative* approach.

ANSWER:
D, E

4. For the infant in Question 3, the laboratory data reflect which of the following?

   A. Normal acid-base balance

   B. Metabolic alkalosis

   C. Respiratory alkalosis

   D. Combined metabolic and respiratory alkalosis

   E. Compensated metabolic alkalosis

Ref.: 1, 3

COMMENTS: Gastric outlet obstruction with sufficient loss of gastric contents produces a hypochloremic, hypokalemic metabolic alkalosis. • The ability to compensate by hypoventilation is limited. • In fact, infants and children who are crying are hyperventilating and have additional respiratory alkalosis.

ANSWER:
B

5. Which of the following solutions is/are appropriate for initial intravenous therapy of the infant described in Question 3?

   A. Lactated Ringer's solution at 25 ml/hr

   B. D_5W + 0.5% normal saline solution + KCl 20 mEq/L at 15 ml/hr

   C. D_5W + 0.25% normal saline solution + KCl 30 mEq/L at 30 ml/hr

   D. D_5W + 0.5% normal saline solution + KCl 30 mEq/L at 25 ml/hr

   E. D_5W + 0.1% normal hydrochloride (HCl) at 30 ml/hr

Ref.: 1–3

COMMENTS: Appropriate fluid therapy in this situation requires maintenance in addition to replacement for estimated deficit and for ongoing losses. • Estimated initial volume replacement for the first 24 hr includes maintenance of 100 ml/kg = 360 ml/24 hrs and replacement of approximately half of the estimated deficit. • Weight loss is 40 g, or 10%, and one half of this deficit would be 200 ml/24 hr. • The initial rate of fluid replacement is only an estimate, however, and should be adjusted to maintain urine output of 1–2 ml/kg/hr. • An initial bolus of normal saline solution 20 ml/kg may be appropriate for severely dehydrated patients.

• As far as electrolytes are concerned, sodium, potassium, and chloride must be supplied for both maintenance and replacement of gastric losses. • They can be supplied by a solution of 5% dextrose with 0.5% normal saline solution and KCl (approximately 30 mEq/L). • Ongoing assessment of serum electrolytes should be performed and electrolyte replacement adjusted as necessary. • The operation should proceed only after appropriate fluid and electrolyte correction.

ANSWER:
D

6. Match the appropriate kilocalories and protein requirements in the left-hand column to age in the right-hand column.

Kilocalories (kcal/kg)/Protein (g/kg)	Age (years)
A. 30–60/1.5	a. 0–1
B. 60–75/2	b. 1–7
C. 90–120/2.5–3.5	c. 7–12
D. 75–90/2–2.5	d. 12–18

Ref.: 1–3

COMMENTS: Infants require an average of 110 kg/day, and if stressed they may require protein up to 2.5–3.5 g/kg/day. • Appropriate weight gain for a neonate is 1% body weight per day. • As children age, their caloric needs decrease, as do their protein needs. By the time they reach adolescence, they require approximately 50% of their neonatal needs.

ANSWER:
A-d; B-c; C-a; D-b

7. All but which of the following concerning pediatric trauma are true?

   A. Trauma is the leading cause of death for children between 1 and 15 years of age.

   B. Intraosseous access is an acceptable means for delivering intravenous fluids or blood in a child less than 6 years of age.

   C. If evidence of hypovolemic shock persists after two boluses of crystalloid fluid, a blood transfusion is warranted.

   D. Indications for operative intervention include computed tomographic (CT) documentation of injury to the spleen or liver.

Ref.: 1, 2

COMMENTS: For children between the ages of 1 and 15 years, trauma is the leading cause of death. • Motor vehicle accidents, falls, bicycle accidents, and child abuse are the most common causes of traumatic deaths. • The priorities of resuscitation are airway, breathing, and circulation. • Fluid resuscitation is given as 20-ml/kg boluses. • If intravenous access cannot be obtained, a specially designed needle can be used to deliver fluids through an intraosseous route. • Under sterile conditions, the needle is placed 1 to 2 cm below the tibial tuberosity through the anteromedial surface of the tibia. • If hypovolemic shock is refractory to two crystalloid boluses, then a blood transfusion should be initiated. • CT scanning is commonly used to evaluate pediatric trauma patients. • While injuries to the liver and spleen are common, the need for operative intervention is not. • In these circumstances, indications for laparotomy include persistent hemodynamic instability, the need for blood transfusion in a volume greater than half of the child's calculated blood volume within the first 24 hr, or extravascular blush seen on CT scanning.

ANSWER:
D

---

8. A 6-month-old infant requires blood transfusion after injury. Which of the following regimens is the most appropriate initial replacement?

A. 10–20 ml/kg packed red blood cells (PRBCs)

B. 30–40 ml/kg PRBCs

C. 10–20 ml/kg PRBCs + 10–20 ml/kg platelets

D. 10–20 ml/kg PRBCs + 20 ml/kg fresh frozen plasma

Ref.: 1, 2

COMMENTS: Blood volume for infants is usually estimated at 80 ml/kg of body weight. • When blood transfusions are required, PRBCs are typically utilized, and the initial replacement is based on 10–20 ml/kg. • While replacement of coagulation products is not necessary with an initial transfusion, coagulation deficits develop rapidly in infants who require more blood replacement. • Plasma and platelets can be given in the volumes stated in the answers.

ANSWER:
A

---

9. During a history and physical examination in the emergency room, a 2-month-old boy is found to have an acute, nonreducible mass in the right groin. Which of the following are possible diagnoses?

A. Incarcerated inguinal hernia

B. Testicular torsion

C. Acute hydrocele

D. Inguinal lymphadenopathy

E. Testicular teratoma

Ref.: 1–3

COMMENTS: When an infant presents with an acute inguinoscrotal mass, it should be diagnosed as soon as possible. • An incarcerated inguinal hernia in an infant can usually be reduced if the infant is placed in a warm, calm environment and adequately sedated. • After successful reduction, the child is admitted to the hospital, and herniorrhaphy is performed within 24–48 hr. • If the hernia cannot be reduced, an emergency operation is indicated. • Incarceration of an inguinal hernia risks not only intestinal ischemia but testicular ischemia and subsequent atrophy as well. • In girls, the hernia sac may contain the ovary and tube, but ovarian ischemia is not common unless there is associated torsion.

Testicular torsion usually manifests suddenly as a mass in the scrotal area with swelling and edema of that side of the scrotum. • The testis on that side rides high and is extremely tender. • The differential diagnosis usually is epididymitis or torsion of the appendix testis. • A nuclear scan can be helpful, but if there is any doubt, immediate surgical exploration via scrotal raphe is indicated. • If testicular torsion is found, orchidopexy should be performed (for both the affected testis and the contralateral testis).

If differentiation between nonreducible indirect inguinal hernia and acute hydrocele is unclear, prompt surgical exploration and repair should be performed. • Not infrequently, acute inguinal lymphadenopathy manifests as a nonreducible inguinal mass and may be difficult to differentiate from an incarcerated indirect inguinal hernia. • Of all the conditions listed, only testicular teratoma does not have an acute onset.

ANSWER:
A, B, C, D

---

10. Which of the following is the indicated treatment for a noncommunicating hydrocele in a 2-month-old infant?

A. Observation

B. Aspiration

C. Hydrocelectomy through a groin incision

D. Hydrocelectomy through a scrotal incision

Ref.: 1–3

COMMENTS: Most noncommunicating hydroceles in young children are asymptomatic and will resolve as the fluid is absorbed. • If the hydrocele persists past 12 months of age, there is likely a peritoneal communication, and operation for hydrocelectomy and ligation of the processus vaginalis is indicated. • In children, these operations are performed through the groin. • Aspiration of the hydrocele is not recommended. • If it is a noncommunicating hydrocele, it will resolve, and thus aspiration is unnecessary. • If it is a communicating hydrocele, the fluid will reaccummulate, and operation will eventually be necessary.

ANSWER:
A

---

11. Appropriate management of an inguinal hernia in a healthy infant may include all but which of the following?

A. Observation until 12 months of age

B. Routine contralateral groin exploration

C. Laparoscopic evaluation of the contralateral groin

D. High ligation of the hernia sac without repair of the inguinal floor

Ref.: 1–3

COMMENTS: Repair of inguinal hernias in infants is recommended at the time of diagnosis because the patent processus vaginalis does not close after birth and there is a significant risk of incarceration. • Exceptions include the case of a premature or ill infant for whom repair is deferred until the infant's other difficulties have stabilized. • High ligation and excision of the hernia sac is adequate treatment, and routine repair of the inguinal floor is unnecessary. • In patients with a large internal ring, it is advisable to place sutures to narrow it somewhat. • The distal part of the hernia sac should be widely opened to prevent postoperative hydrocele. • Operative management of a clinically normal contralateral groin has long been controversial. • Routine contralateral exploration was once more common, but the trend has evolved to a more selective approach. • Laparoscopic examination of the contralateral groin using an angled scope inserted through the hernia sac can identify a patent processus vaginalis in approximately one half of patients. • Not all patients with a patent processus vaginalis will progress to a clinically significant hernia, but certainly patients without a patent processus vaginalis do not require contralateral exploration.

ANSWER:
A

12. Which of the following statements is/are false with regard to sacrococcygeal teratomas?

    A. Approximately 90% are benign at birth.

    B. They have great potential to become malignant.

    C. α-Fetoprotein is a good tumor marker.

    D. Affected children require close follow-up observation for years.

    E. The coccyx is not actually connected with the tumor.

Ref.: 1, 3

COMMENTS: Sacrococcygeal teratoma is a lesion encountered most often during the first year of life, and it predominates among females (80–85%). • In 90% of cases, there is an exophytic component that makes the diagnosis obvious at birth. • The other 10% grow within the pelvis or abdominal cavity, making the diagnosis more difficult unless it is suspected. • The behavior of such tumors is unique among childhood neoplasms. • When identified and operated on before infants are 2 months of age, 90% of these tumors qualify as benign teratomas. • If they are removed after infants are 2 months of age, the pathologic diagnosis in 90% of cases is a malignant teratoma. • Because of the attachment of the tumor to the coccyx, coccygectomy should always be part of the surgical technique for removal of the tumor. • Malignant lesions do not respond well to radiotherapy or chemotherapy. • α-Fetoprotein is the marker used to make the diagnosis in utero as well as during the follow-up period after operation. • Because of late recurrence, affected infants should be observed closely throughout their entire childhood.

ANSWER:
E

13. At the time of operation, a mass is found in the mesentery of the ileum adjacent to the bowel wall. Which of the following may represent the diagnosis?

    A. Intestinal duplication

    B. Meckel's diverticulum

    C. Mesenteric cyst

    D. Segmental malrotation

Ref.: 2, 3

COMMENTS: Intestinal duplications are a misnomer. • Most such masses are enteric cysts and occur most commonly within the abdomen. • They are manifested as cystic or tubular masses next to the bowel wall between the mesenteric leaves and contain elements of intestinal wall. • Mesenteric cysts are also located within the mesentery, but they do not contain any muscular wall. • Meckel's diverticulum is a type of omphalomesenteric duct remnant and, although found in the terminal ileum, is located on the antimesenteric side of the bowel.

ANSWER:
A, C

14. Which of the following is the most common malignancy found in childhood?

    A. Lymphoma

    B. Leukemia

    C. Wilms' tumor

    D. Neuroblastoma

    E. Rhabdomyosarcoma

Ref.: 1–3

COMMENTS: Malignancy is second only to trauma as the leading cause of death during childhood. • In infants, malignant disease is the third most frequent cause of death after prematurity and congenital anomalies. • Approximately 40% of childhood malignancies are leukemias. • The most common solid tumor in children under 2 years of age is neuroblastoma. • In children older than 2 years, it is Wilms' tumor.

ANSWER:
B

15. All but which of the following statements concerning biliary atresia are true?

    A. Those diagnosed with biliary atresia generally survive 5 years without treatment.

    B. Histologic characteristics of biliary atresia are distinct from those of neonatal hepatitis.

    C. In the most common variant of biliary atresia, there is fibrosis in both the proximal and distal bile ducts.

    D. The prognosis is much worse if the diagnosis and subsequent surgical correction are delayed past 90 days of life.

    E. Key elements of the diagnostic workup of biliary atresia include ultrasound imaging of the liver and gallbladder and percutaneous liver biopsy.

    F. Approximately 30% of infants who undergo the Kasai hepatoportoenterostomy before 60 days of life will not need a liver transplant.

Ref.: 1, 2

COMMENTS: Biliary atresia is typified by progressive, irreversible fibrosis of the extrahepatic and intrahepatic bile ducts. • There is no proven medical therapy. • If surgical correction is not performed, the obliterative process proceeds, and the infant develops biliary cirrhosis and portal hypertension, followed by death by 2 years of age. • Severe cholestasis, bile duct proliferation, and inflammatory cell infiltration are pathologic findings seen in biliary atresia. • These findings are distinct from the hepatocellular necrosis seen in neonatal hepatitis. • Varying forms of biliary atresia exist, with fibrosis of the proximal and distal ducts being the most common, followed by fibrosis of the proximal ducts with distal patency and proximal patency with distal fibrosis, respectively. • Early recognition and management of an infant with an abnormal direct hyperbilirubinemia are extremely important for this disease, since surgical correction performed after 90 days has been correlated to worse outcomes than surgery undertaken before 60 days of life. • The workup of suspected biliary atresia should include ultrasound imaging of the liver and gallbladder. • In biliary atresia, the extrahepatic bile ducts cannot be pinpointed with ultrasound imaging, and the gallbladder is diminutive or absent. • Ultrasound imaging should be followed by percutaneous liver biopsy to help confirm the diagnosis. • The Kasai procedure involves resection of the extrahepatic bile ducts and gallbladder with Roux-en-Y hepaticojejunostomy. • If performed before 60 days of life, 30% of infants will have a long-term successful outcome. • Those with bridging fibrosis and older children generally require liver transplantation.

ANSWER:
A

16. With regard to hepatoportoenterostomy (Kasai procedure) for treatment of biliary atresia, which of the following statements is/are true?

  A. Hepatoportoenterostomy is most successfully performed after patients are 3 months of age, when the bile ducts are larger.

  B. When successful, hepatoportoenterostomy is rarely complicated by cholangitis.

  C. Hepatoportoenterostomy is not indicated as the initial surgical procedure if hepatic transplantation is available.

  D. Hepatic cirrhosis and portal hypertension remain problems despite successful hepatoportoenterostomy.

Ref.: 1–3

COMMENTS: Biliary atresia occurs as part of a spectrum of anomalies known as infantile obstructive cholangiopathy. • Although the cause of these anomalies is unknown, it has been related to in utero viral infection. • A hepatic HIDA scan and ultrasound imaging of the bile ducts are the mainstays among imaging tests to support the diagnosis. • Variable patterns of ductal involvement may occur, although the extrahepatic bile ducts are commonly obliterated and replaced by fibrous cords. • Both the intrahepatic and extrahepatic biliary tree may be involved, although in only 10% of patients is the disorder solely extrahepatic. • The goals of treatment are to provide biliary drainage and prevent late complications of biliary cirrhosis with secondary hepatic failure. • Hepatoportoenterostomy is most successful in establishing bile drainage when performed during the patient's first 2 months of life. • The success rate falls dramatically after 3 months of age. • Cholangitis, biliary cirrhosis, hepatic failure, and portal hypertension remain as late problems, despite the fact that bile drainage is achieved. • Hepatic transplantation has been successful in the treatment of this problem but has not replaced an attempt at biliary enteric anastomosis as the initial procedure. • An unsuccessful hepatoportoenterostomy does not preclude later hepatic transplantation. • Attempts to minimize later cholangitic complications include prompt use of antibiotics coupled with steroids during the initial phase of recovery to minimize inflammation and infection.

ANSWER:
D

17. Which of the following statements is/are false concerning the diagnosis of imperforate anus?

  A. This anomaly is defined as high or low, according to the relationship between the rectum and the anal sphincter complex.

  B. High anomalies are associated with a perineal fistula.

  C. Most affected female infants require an initial colostomy.

  D. Imperforate anus may be associated with esophageal atresia and tracheoesophageal fistula.

  E. Pull-through techniques are successful in preserving continence in low lesions.

Ref.: 1–3

COMMENTS: Imperforate anus is a type of anorectal agenesis in which the anus is absent and the rectum ends at varying levels in relationship to the puborectalis muscle. • The blind rectum may end in a fistula, which, with **high lesions**, usually opens into the prostatic urethra in males and the vagina in females. • **Low lesions** are manifested by a perineal fistula, which often is seen in the median scrotal raphe of males and the posterior vaginal fourchette of females. • The level of the anomaly is the critical determinant of the type of correction required.

High lesions are initially treated by colostomy, followed by a definitive reconstructive procedure aimed at bringing the rectum through the anal sphincter complex to achieve continence. • Low lesions, which are suspected in the presence of a perineal fistula, can be corrected by a simple perineal approach. • Most cases of imperforate anus in females are of the low variety. • The posterior sagittal anoplasty (described by Penã) achieves continence in those with low lesions and in 65–75% of those with high lesions. • Imperforate anus may be part of the VATER syndrome (vertebral anomalies, imperforate anus, tracheoesophageal fistula, esophageal atresia, and radial and renal anomalies). • These conditions, as well as associated genitourinary and occasional cardiac anomalies, must be evaluated before reparative surgery is undertaken.

ANSWER:
B

18. Which of the following always requires surgical correction during infancy?

  A. Imperforate anus

  B. Hypoplastic left colon

  C. Meconium plug syndrome

  D. Hirschsprung's disease

  E. Meconium ileus

Ref.: 1–3

COMMENTS: Choices A–E present as distal bowel obstruction. • Large-bowel obstruction cannot be differentiated from small bowel obstruction in infants based on plain radiographs because of the lack of haustral markings. • Hirschsprung's disease is caused by congenital absence of colonic ganglion cells and should be suspected whenever an infant fails to pass meconium within the first 24 hr of life. • The rectum and rectosigmoid areas are the regions most commonly affected, although longer segments may be involved. • In rare cases, total colonic aganglionosis may be present. • All types require surgical correction. • Hypoplastic left colon syndrome is often seen in infants of diabetic mothers. • Infants with meconium plug syndrome may have clinical and radiographic characteristics similar to those of Hirschsprung's disease. • Both of these conditions usually can be treated with hypertonic water-soluble radiographic contrast enemas. • The diagnosis of cystic fibrosis must be considered in patients with meconium ileus and an associated microcolon (unused colon). • In 80–90% of cases, a Gastrograffin enema relieves the obstruction without need for operation. • Anorectal anomalies rarely present with neonatal intestinal obstruction because 80% present with a fistula to the genitourinary tract. • All require surgical intervention.

ANSWER:
A, D

19. Which of the following statements is/are true concerning Hirschsprung's disease?

   A. It is more common in males.

   B. It may be complicated by enterocolitis.

   C. Barium enema study results may be normal.

   D. It is best diagnosed by rectal biopsy.

   E. The initial treatment may involve colostomy.

Ref.: 2, 3

COMMENTS: The primary clinical manifestation of Hirschsprung's disease is that of intestinal obstruction with failure to pass meconium in newborn male infants or chronic constipation in older infants and children. • Infants with Hirschsprung's disease are prone to develop enterocolitis, which, although not pseudomembranous, still carries a high mortality rate if not recognized and treated promptly. • In newborns, in whom dilatation of the bowel proximal to the aganglionic segment may not yet have developed, a barium enema study result may be normal. • Anal manometric measurements demonstrate a characteristic failure of sphincter relaxation in a response to rectal distention. • This finding, however, is not diagnostic. • A definitive diagnosis is based on the rectal biopsy, which demonstrates an absence of ganglion cells in the Aurbach's and Meisner's plexi, hypertrophied nerve endings, and an abundance of acetylcholinesterase as determined by histochemical techniques. • Infants with Hirschsprung's disease may be treated with single stage pull-through if the infant was full term with no enterocolitis is present. • All others are treated with colostomy at the level of ganglionosis, followed by pull-through 3–6 months later. • Anastomosis of normally innervated colon to the anus is the basis of all three pull-through procedures (Swanson, Duhamel, and Soave).

ANSWER:
A, B, C, D, E

20. A previously well 3-week-old infant exhibits the sudden onset of bilious vomiting. Which of the following is the most likely diagnosis?

   A. Pyloric stenosis

   B. Tracheoesophageal fistula, H type

   C. Hirschsprung's disease

   D. Duodenal atresia

   E. Malrotation of midgut

Ref.: 1–3

COMMENTS: See Question 21.

21. For the scenario described in Question 20, which test listed below would initially be the most appropriate?

   A. Abdominal radiograph

   B. CT scan

   C. Upper gastrointestinal contrast study

   D. Barium enema study

   E. Esophageal pH studies

Ref.: 1–3

COMMENTS: In any infant with the sudden onset of bilious vomiting, malrotation of the midgut with volvulus should be assumed to be the cause until proven otherwise. • In 50% of children with malrotation and volvulus, the presentation is during the first few weeks of life. • Immediate treatment is mandatory if the risk of complete necrosis of the midgut is to be lessened. • Pyloric stenosis is seldom present with bilious vomiting. • Infants with tracheoesophageal fistula, H type, also seldom vomit. • The main symptoms usually are difficulty feeding and recurrent pneumonia. • The main symptom of Hirschsprung's disease is constipation, but the disease may progress to bowel obstruction with bilious emesis. • Duodenal atresia may mimic malrotation in the first 24–48 hr of life, but at 3 weeks of age duodenal atresia should have been already diagnosed and treated. • There is a strong association between duodenal atresia and malrotation of the midgut. • If immediately available, an upper gastrointestinal series may be done, since malrotation is suggested by a cutoff at the duodenum or absence of the ligament in Treitz in the left upper quadrant. • A barium enema can be misleading in the presence of malrotation because the cecum may look normally placed. • As soon as a diagnosis is made, the infant should be taken immediately to surgery to undergo resuscitation and operation simultaneously. • If studies cannot be done immediately, an operation is justified on clinical suspicion alone, inasmuch as delay only increases the chances of intestinal necrosis.

ANSWERS:
Question 20: E
Question 21: C

22. In addition to detorsion, which of the following procedures should be included for the operative treatment of midgut volvulus with viable bowel?

   A. Cecopexy in the right lower quadrant

   B. Appendectomy

   C. Repositioning the small bowel in the right side of the abdomen

   D. Repositioning the colon in the left side of the abdomen

Ref.: 1–3

COMMENTS: The operative management of malrotation involves counterclockwise reduction of a midgut volvulus when present. • Nonviable bowel is resected. • If viability is in question or the presence of necrosis not certain, the bowel may be returned to the abdomen in the hope that some or all of it will survive and bowel length may be preserved. • In this case, a second-look laparotomy should be performed 24 hr later to reassess and treat the intestine appropriately. • Peritoneal bands (Ladd's bands) between the cecum and the abdominal wall are divided, and the duodenum is mobilized so that the small bowel can be positioned in the right side of the abdomen and the colon in the left side of the abdomen. • Appendectomy is routinely performed. • Intraluminal duodenal obstruction can occur with malrotation as a result of an associated web or stenosis. • Ability to pass a nasogastric tube into the proximal duodenum and, after injection of saline solution through the tube, rapid filling of the jejunum usually rule out an intrinsic duodenal obstruction.

ANSWER:
B, C, D

23. Match each clinical characteristic in the left-hand column with the appropriate diagnosis or diagnoses in the right-hand column.

A. Anterior mediastinal mass   a. Esophageal duplication

B. Respiratory distress   b. Bronchogenic cyst

C. Middle mediastinal mass   c. Mediastinal teratoma

D. Benign   d. Thoracic neuroblastoma

E. Posterior mediastinal mass

Ref.: 1–3

COMMENTS: Respiratory distress and dysphagia are symptoms common to all mediastinal masses regardless of location. • Masses in the anterior mediastinum are much more frequently teratomas than thymic tumors. • They are or may become malignant and should always be resected. • The younger the child at the time of resection of teratomas, the better the prognosis. • Esophageal duplication and bronchogenic cysts are of a benign nature but are removed for obstructive symptoms and the risk for malignant degeneration. • In newborns, both entities can be responsible for airway obstruction, usually resulting from a mass. • Bronchogenic cysts may arise within the wall of the bronchus and produce life-threatening respiratory distress without producing an obvious mass. • Neuroblastomas, like teratomas, are or may become malignant. • Masses arising from the posterior mediastinum are almost exclusively neuroblastomas or ganglioneuromas.

ANSWER:
A-c; B-a, b, c, d; C-b, c; D-a, b; E-d

24. Advising parents of an infant with a unilateral undescended testicle, which of the following statements would apply?

A. The problem should be corrected promptly.

B. Descent may occur spontaneously, but if this has not happened by age 2 years, descent should be performed surgically.

C. Orchiopexy should be performed to prevent malignancy.

D. Orchiopexy may prevent infertility.

Ref.: 1–3

COMMENTS: An undescended testicle must first be differentiated from a retractile testicle, which on careful examination can be brought into the scrotum and does not require surgical treatment. • In instances of bilateral undescended testicles, serum gonadotropin determinations and chromosomal studies may be helpful for establishing the presence of testicular tissue. • In many infants with undescended testicles, descent occurs spontaneously during the first year or so of life. • If it does not, an orchiopexy should be performed by the time the child is 2 years old. • There is evidence that, in patients with undescended testicles after the age of 2 years, spermatogenesis is impaired. • Orchiopexy before this time may lessen the chance of infertility, although among patients with bilateral cryptorchidism in particular the incidence of infertility continues to be high. • Cryptorchidism is associated with an increased risk of testicular cancer (predominantly seminoma). • Orchiopexy, however, does not diminish this risk, and affected patients require periodic examination throughout their adolescent years. • Approximately 10% of testicular tumors arise in undescended testicles. • The chance that an undescended testicle will undergo malignant transformation is approximately 1 in 4000. • Additional reasons to perform orchiopexy include psychological considerations, an increased incidence of testicular torsion, and the possibility of testicular trauma when the testicle is at the level of the pubic tubercle.

ANSWER:
B, D

25. If, during a scheduled orchiopexy in a 2-year-old child, the undescended testicle cannot be brought down into the scrotum, which of the following procedures would be the most appropriate treatment?

A. Orchiectomy

B. Attachment to the pubic tubercle and reoperation in 1 year

C. Division of the spermatic artery and vein to provide additional length

D. Termination of the procedure and treatment with chorionic gonadotropin

Ref.: 1–3

COMMENTS: In most cases of cryptorchidism, particularly if the testicle is palpable, the testicle can be brought down into the scrotum without difficulty. • The approach is through a herniorrhaphy incision. • The cord is carefully dissected, and an associated hernia sac, which is usually present, is dissected free and ligated at the internal ring. • The testicle is secured in a subcutaneous pouch in the scrotum after passage through the dartos fascia. • For the occasionally encountered instance in which the testicle is in a higher retroperitoneal position and adequate length cannot be obtained for scrotal positioning, various approaches have been used, including staged orchiopexy with reoperation in 6 months and division of the spermatic vessels, preserving the testicular blood supply along the vas deferens. • In postpubertal teenagers with this condition, orchiectomy is the appropriate treatment. • Human chorionic gonadotropin has been used as a nonoperative method of producing testicular descent. • It is more successful in patients with bilateral undescended testicles than in those with unilateral undescended testicles, but the success rate is nevertheless modest.

ANSWER:
B, C

26. The most common cause of duodenal obstruction at birth is which of the following?

A. Duodenal atresia

B. Choledochal cyst

C. Malrotation

D. Annular pancreas

Ref.: 1–3

COMMENTS: Vomiting within the first 24 hr of life in the absence of abdominal distention suggests high obstruction in the neonate. • Among the various causes of duodenal obstruction beyond neonatal age, malrotation is the most common and potentially the most serious. • The duodenal obstruction generally is caused by extrinsic compression by the peritoneal bands that extend from the abdominal wall to the anomalously located cecum in the right upper quadrant. • The catastrophic complication of malrotation is midgut volvulus and intestinal infarction, which occur because of torsion about the narrow mesenteric pedicle by which the midgut is suspended. • Choledochal cyst and annular pancreas may cause duodenal obstruction but are rare.

ANSWER:
A

27. Regarding jejunoileal atresia, which of the following statements is/are false?

    A. The cause is failure of embryologic recanalization of the gut, and therefore the atresias usually are multiple.

    B. Passage of meconium does not exclude the diagnosis.

    C. Associated anomalies are more common with jejunoileal atresia than with duodenal atresia.

    D. Disparity in lumen size is common but is rarely a technical problem.

Ref.: 1–3

COMMENTS: Intestinal atresia is thought to result from an in utero vascular accident. • In approximately 10% of patients, the atresias are multiple. • A variety of forms may be seen, ranging from a simple web or stenosis to complete separation of bowel ends with varying degrees of mesenteric defect. • With the most severe type, most of the small-bowel mesentery is absent, and the remaining distal small bowel is supplied by the ileocolic artery. • Intestinal atresia is usually manifested by bilious vomiting and abdominal distention. • The passage of meconium does not exclude the diagnosis. • There may be a considerable disparity in size between the proximal bowel and the distal bowel. • This has led to the development of a number of operative techniques for achieving a functional anastomosis. • Associated anomalies are not seen as commonly as they are with duodenal atresia, which, in as many as one third of cases, is associated with trisomy 21 (Down's syndrome).

ANSWER:
A, C

28. Excessive drooling and mild respiratory distress are seen 8 hr after birth. An abdominal radiograph shows complete lack of air in the gastrointestinal tract. What is the most likely diagnosis?

    A. Hirschsprung's disease

    B. Tracheoesophageal fistula, H type

    C. Pyloric atresia

    D. Choanal atresia (bilateral)

    E. Esophageal atresia without tracheoesophageal fistula

    F. Esophageal atresia with distal tracheoesophageal fistula

Ref.: 1–3

COMMENTS: See Question 29.

29. What is the most common type of esophageal atresia and tracheoesophageal fistula?

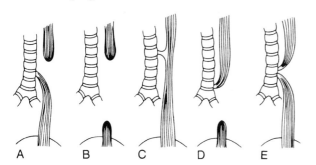

A   B   C   D   E

Ref.: 1–3

COMMENTS: It is necessary to remember that at birth neonates have a completely gasless gastrointestinal tract. • Soon after birth, they start swallowing air, and within 6–12 hr, this air reaches the colon. • A tracheoesophageal fistula does not prevent swallowed or inspired air from reaching the stomach and small bowel. • About 85–90% of patients with esophageal atresia and tracheoesophageal fistula have a blind proximal pouch with a distal tracheoesophageal fistula. • Esophageal atresia without an associated fistula is the second most common form. • Esophageal atresia is suggested when an infant has excess saliva or spits up during attempted feedings. • In the presence of esophageal atresia, a fistula is manifested as air in the gastrointestinal tract, respiratory symptoms with feedings, or both. • When an orogastric tube is passed in an infant with esophageal atresia, a chest radiograph shows the tube coiled in the blind pouch. • Contrast studies and bronchoscopy may be useful in selected cases to confirm the diagnosis and demonstrate the location of a tracheoesophageal fistula. • Recognition of the anatomy of the anomaly is important for establishing appropriate initial treatment and definitive repair. • Hirschsprung's disease is characterized by congenital lack of ganglion cells in the wall of the bowel, most commonly in the distal colon. • Thus, air should be present in the stomach and small bowel. • Pyloric atresia, a rare congenital anomaly, prevents air from going to the duodenum and small bowel, but radiographic studies show extreme distention of the stomach, with air-fluid levels. • Neonates, being obligatory nasal breathers, have major respiratory problems when born with bilateral choanal atresia but do not have difficulty swallowing air.

ANSWERS:
Question 28: E
Question 29: A

30. A 3000-g infant with esophageal atresia and distal tracheoesophageal fistula is born. If the infant does not exhibit respiratory distress and an associated anomaly is not present, which of the following is the preferred treatment?

    A. Gastrostomy, cervical esophagostomy, and delayed repair

    B. Gastrostomy, sump tube drainage of proximal pouch, and delayed repair

    C. Fistula ligation and delayed esophageal repair

    D. Division of the fistula with primary esophageal anastomosis

    E. Primary repair with colon interposition

Ref.: 1–3

COMMENTS: The timing of surgical intervention for esophageal atresia and tracheoesophageal fistula is influenced by the maturity of the infant and the presence or absence of associated cardiorespiratory problems or other congenital anomalies. • Mortality from primary repair is directly related to the risk group to which the infant belongs. • Otherwise healthy infants weighing more than 2500 g are treated by primary repair with fistula division, closure of its tracheal end, and end-to-side anastomosis of the esophageal segments. • Infants who are not well enough for primary repair are treated by gastrostomy and drainage of the blind proximal pouch. • Repair is accomplished after complicating cardiorespiratory problems have been corrected. • The presence of the tracheoesophageal fistula can cause problems with dissipation of ventilatory pressure into the stomach or can allow aspiration of gastric contents into the lung.

ANSWER:
D

31. Repair of esophageal atresia and tracheoesophageal fistula can be complicated with which of the following problems?

A. Esophageal stricture

B. Anastomotic leakage

C. Gastroesophageal reflux

D. Recurrent fistula

E. Empyema

Ref.: 1–3

COMMENTS: Gastroesophageal reflux is a common complication after operation for esophageal atresia and tracheoesophageal fistula in infants and frequently requires later fundoplication. • The cause of reflux may be related to underlying esophageal dysmotility and to dysfunction of the lower esophageal sphincter, which often is displaced cephalad after repair. • Stricture or anastomotic leakage and subsequent recurrent fistula can also occur but are less common. • The morbidity of potential anastomotic leakage can be minimized by use of an extrapleural approach. • If leakage does occur, it usually remains extrapleural.

A N S W E R :
A, B, C, D, E

32. All but which of the following statements concerning necrotizing enterocolitis (NEC) are true?

A. The initial insult in NEC is to intestinal mucosa.

B. The terminal ileum is the most frequently involved site.

C. Operative intervention is indicated in most cases of NEC.

D. Disease progression can occur even after surgical therapy.

Ref.: 1, 2

COMMENTS: NEC is a disease that affects the intestinal tract of the neonate. • Clinical and experimental data have shown that the cause of NEC is multifactorial, since it has developed in the presence of a wide variety of clinical conditions ranging from perinatal stress to maternal cocaine use. • The initial injury in NEC is observed in the intestinal mucosa. • The spectrum of severity ranges from isolated mucosal injury to transmural bowel necrosis. • While the terminal ileum and right colon are the most commonly affected sites, the disease can be segmental or affect the entire gastrointestinal tract. • The overwhelming majority of infants with NEC (90%) can be treated medically with nasogastric decompression, bowel rest, and broad-spectrum antibiotics. • Attention to intravenous fluid management and parenteral nutrition is particularly important in these infants. • Operative intervention, such as a bowel resection with proximal enterostomy, is indicated to treat severe complications of NEC, which include intestinal necrosis, perforation, or stricture. • Operative intervention, however, does not prevent the progression of the disease, which can continue after resection and may require additional surgical therapy.

A N S W E R :
C

33. A premature infant with a history of neonatal respiratory distress requiring ventilatory support is being fed oral formula. Abdominal distention develops, and blood-streaked stool is passed. Appropriate management includes which of the following?

A. Anoscopy for probable neonatal fissure

B. Barium enema to rule out intussusception

C. Restriction of oral intake to clear fluids to prevent mucosal injury

D. Antibiotics only if specific pathogens are cultured from the stool

E. Cessation of all oral feedings, institution of nasogastric drainage, intravenous antibiotics, total parenteral nutrition, and serial abdominal examinations and radiographic studies

Ref.: 1–3

COMMENTS: See Question 34.

34. Which of the following are indications for operation in an infant with NEC?

A. Pneumatosis intestinalis

B. Portal venous gas

C. Pneumoperitoneum

D. Erythema and edema of the abdominal wall

E. Progressive acidosis and thrombocytopenia

F. Abdominal mass with fixed bowel loops

Ref.: 1–3

COMMENTS: The diagnosis of NEC should be considered whenever a premature infant exhibits the findings listed above, and it is the most likely diagnosis in this infant. • NEC is a disease of premature infants and infants subjected to neonatal stress. • The pathophysiologic processes involve mucosal ischemia, bowel necrosis, perforation, peritonitis, and sepsis. • NEC nearly always occurs in affected infants after the start of oral feedings. • Clinical manifestations initially are intolerance of formula, abdominal distention, blood-streaked stools with progression to frank peritonitis, and signs of systemic sepsis, including acidosis, disseminated intravascular coagulation, and thrombocytopenia. • Initial treatment is directed at the prevention of both further mucosal injury and septic complications. • The initial therapy for NEC is medical. • Oral feedings are stopped, tube decompression is instituted, broad-spectrum antibiotics are administered, and fluid and electrolyte support is provided. • Close monitoring is mandatory, involving not only physical examination but also serial radiographs every 6–8 hr and serial biochemical assessment to detect signs of deterioration. • Pneumatosis intestinalis is a characteristic radiographic finding in NEC, caused by invasion of the bowel wall by gas-forming organisms. • Similarly, portal venous gas indicates the presence of gas-forming organisms that have been transported in the portal circulation. • Neither of these radiographic findings alone, however, is an absolute indication for operation.

Indications for surgical intervention are signs of perforation, peritonitis, and progressive clinical deterioration despite nonoperative therapeutic measures. • These signs include pneumoperitoneum; an abdominal mass with fixed bowel loops, which may be suggestive of abscess; tenderness; erythema and edema of the abdominal wall; and progressive acidosis or thrombocytopenia. • When operation is performed, necrotic bowel is resected, abscesses are drained, and the ends of the retained bowel are brought out as enterostomies. • Persistent acidosis and decreased platelet counts are signs of a poor outcome. • The mortality rate associated with NEC ranges from 30 to 60%, according to various reports.

A N S W E R S :
Question 33: E
Question 34: C, D, E, F

35. All but which of the following statements concerning extracorporeal life support (ECLS) are true?

   A. Meconium aspiration syndrome is the most common indication for ECLS in neonates.

   B. Both the alveolar-arterial oxygen gradient and the oxygen index are useful indicators for predicting survival without ECLS.

   C. Exclusion criteria for ECLS include prematurity (<24 weeks gestation), cyanotic congenital heart disease, severe coagulopathy, and significant intracranial hemorrhage.

   D. For venoarterial bypass, the right internal jugular vein and right common carotid artery are most commonly cannulated.

   E. Venovenous bypass provides both respiratory and cardiac support.

Ref.: 1, 2

COMMENTS: ECLS began in the 1970s and has evolved into the standard of care for neonatal respiratory failure that is refractory to conventional management. • It is a type of heart-lung bypass that can be utilized as short-term supportive care for life-threatening respiratory and cardiac failure. • Meconium aspiration syndrome is the most common indication for the use of ECLS. • Other indications include persistent pulmonary hypertension, respiratory distress syndrome, congenital diaphragmatic hernia, and sepsis. • Generally, an infant must have 80% predicted mortality with continued maximal conventional management to justify its use. • Two formulas have proven useful to predict mortality in these situations. • The alveolar-arterial oxygen gradient ($AaDO_2$) is calculated as (atmospheric pressure $- 47$) $- (Pao_2 + Paco_2)$. • An $AaDO_2$ greater than 620 for 12 hr or an $AaDO_2$ greater than 620 for 6 hr that is associated with extensive barotraumas and severe hypotension requiring the use of inotropes is considered acceptable criteria for ECLS. • Oxygen index (OI) is calculated as (fraction of inspired oxygen) $\times$ (mean airway pressure $\times$ 100) $+ PaO_2$. • For an OI greater than 40, one can assume a mortality of 80%. • Exclusion criteria include gestational age less than 24 weeks, severe coagulopathy or hemorrhage, sonographic evidence of greater than grade I intraventricular hemorrhage, and more than 10–14 days of high-pressure ventilatory support. • Venoarterial bypass provides respiratory and cardiac support. • The vessels cannulated typically are the right internal jugular and the common carotid. • Venovenous bypass provides only respiratory support.

ANSWER:
E

36. During treatment of an infant with congenital diaphragmatic hernia, which of the following may be required?

   A. Tube thoracostomy

   B. Extracorporeal membrane oxygenation (ECMO)

   C. Nitric oxide

   D. High-frequency oscillatory ventilation (HFOV)

   E. Immediate operation

   F. Repair via abdominal approach

   G. Patches of synthetic material for repair

Ref.: 1–3

COMMENTS: The primary physiologic disturbance in infants with respiratory distress caused by congenital posterolateral diaphragmatic hernia is related to pulmonary hypoplasia and the high resistance that develops in the pulmonary vasculature because of constriction of pulmonary arterioles. • The initial resuscitation must be rapid to avoid stress such as hypoxia, metabolic acidosis, and hypothermia, which increase pulmonary vasoconstriction. • High resistance in the pulmonary circulation produces right-to-left shunting via the patent ductus arteriosus, further compromising the infant's cardiopulmonary status. • Initial treatment involves endotracheal intubation in infants experiencing respiratory distress, placement of an orogastric tube with suction, and maintenance of adequate vascular volume. • Ventilated infants are prone to developing pneumothorax, and tube thoracostomy may be required. • Inhaled nitric oxide is a pulmonary vascular dilator and the primary treatment, along with HFOV when required to provide gentle ventilation while recruiting alveoli. • The use of ECMO has salvaged infants who have remained critically ill despite conventional ventilator support. • Definitive surgical repair is usually carried out via an abdominal approach. • Synthetic material such as Gore-Tex may be used to repair the deficit if insufficient diaphragm muscle is present. • The possibility of mortality depends on the severity of lung hypoplasia and persistent pulmonary hypertension. • Resuscitation and stabilization of pulmonary status are attempted before surgical repair.

ANSWER:
A, B, C, D, F, G

37. Which one or more of the following characteristically causes respiratory distress at birth?

   A. Diaphragmatic hernia

   B. Pulmonary sequestration

   C. Tracheoesophageal fistula

   D. Congenital lobar emphysema

Ref.: 1–3

COMMENTS: Persistence of the pleuroperitoneal canal of Bochdalek produces the common congenital diaphragmatic hernia. • Displacement of the abdominal contents into the chest results in pulmonary hypoplasia and high-resistance pulmonary arterioles. • Infants often present with low Apgar scores and respiratory distress at birth. • Some of these infants initially remain stable and then deteriorate. • Other causes of immediate respiratory distress after delivery include pneumothorax, airway obstruction, and aspiration. • With congenital lobar emphysema, immediate respiratory distress may occur, but progressive respiratory distress more commonly develops as a result of overexpression of the affected lobe. • Patients with tracheoesophageal fistula may have difficulty handling salivary secretions because of esophageal atresia, and respiratory symptoms commonly develop with attempted feeding. • The usual complication of pulmonary sequestration is infection.

ANSWER:
A, C, D

38. With regard to defects of the abdominal wall, which statement is correct?

   A. With gastroschisis, the herniated bowel contents are covered with a membrane.

   B. Both omphalocele and gastroschisis are frequently associated with other malformations.

C. Chromosomal abnormalities are often present with omphalocele.

D. The initial treatment of omphalocele is always surgical closure of the fascial defect.

Ref.: 1, 2

COMMENTS: Both omphalocele and gastroschisis are neonatal abdominal wall defects. • With an omphalocele, the abdominal wall contents protrude directly through the umbilicus and are usually covered by a membrane composed of peritoneum and amnion. • In contrast, the herniated abdominal contents in gastroschisis are present to the right of the umbilical ring and are never covered with a membrane. • With gastroschisis, the umbilical cord is intact. • Approximately 50% of infants born with an omphalocele have another malformation, and 30% have chromosomal abnormalities as well. • Anomalies associated with gastroschisis are rare, with the major exception being intestinal atresia. • The initial management of an omphalocele consists of nasogastric decompression, intravenous fluids, and broad-spectrum antibiotics. • The sac should be covered with a sterile dressing, and the infant should be transferred to a pediatric surgery facility. • The abdominal contents are covered by a membrane so that repair may be delayed to allow complete evaluation and resuscitation of the infant.

A N S W E R :
C

39. Match each clinical characteristic in the left-hand column with the appropriate abdominal wall defect or defects in the right-hand column.

A. Associated anomalies	a. Omphalocele
B. May close spontaneously	b. Gastroschisis
C. Requires operation in the newborn	c. Umbilical hernia
D. Associated heat and fluid losses	d. None of the above
E. Closure may require prosthetic material	
F. Midline lesion	
G. Lateral to umbilical cord	
H. Absence of sac	

Ref.: 1–3

COMMENTS: Despite the similarities among these lesions, there are also major differences. • Omphalocele results from failure of embryonic development of a portion of the anterior abdominal wall. • It manifests as a truly midline sac-covered defect and frequently is associated with other anomalies. • The umbilical cord always forms part of the omphalocele sac. • An omphalocele always is covered by a sac devoid of skin and may be ruptured at birth. • If the omphalocele is large, it is not unusual for a major portion of the liver to protrude into the sac, although this is unusual with gastroschisis. • If the omphalocele is small, primary closure usually is possible. • If it is large, a silo of Dacron sheet coated with Silastic (Silon) or Gore-Tex sheet is fashioned around the sac. • At subsequent sessions, the silo is progressively made smaller until the contents are reduced. • In contrast, gastroschisis is thought to occur as the result of an umbilical vein vascular accident and is manifested by eviscerated bowel through a defect without a sac. • It usually appears on the right side of a normal cord. • The exposure of the extraperitoneal viscera to amniotic fluid and

subsequently to the postnatal environment results in a burn-type physiologic manifestation, with significant fluid and heat losses that must be compensated for during resuscitation of the infant. • Gastroschisis can be repaired in one stage, but if this is not possible, a Silastic or Gore-Tex silo similar to that for an omphalocele can be used. • Umbilical hernias result from failure of closure of the linea alba at the umbilical ring and may close spontaneously. • If spontaneous closure has not occurred, herniorrhaphy is performed usually when patients are older than 3 years.

A N S W E R :
A-a; B-c; C-a, b; D-a, b; E-a, b; F-a, c; G-b; H-b

40. A 6-month-old infant has a history of acute onset of crampy abdominal pain and leg withdrawal of 12 hr duration. Rectal examination shows guaiac-positive stool. Which of the following is the most likely diagnosis?

A. Bleeding Meckel's diverticulum

B. Acute appendicitis

C. Kidney stone

D. Infected urachal cyst

E. Intussusception

Ref.: 2, 3

COMMENTS: See Question 42.

41. Which of the following statements is/are true regarding the operative management of intussusception?

A. Resection should be performed without an attempt at intra-operative reduction if reduction by barium enema has been unsuccessful.

B. Primary ileocolic anastomosis may be performed if bowel resection is necessary.

C. After successful reduction by barium enema, delayed operation should be performed because of the risk of recurrence.

D. After successful reduction by barium enema in a child over 3 years of age, exploration is indicated to rule out associated pathologic processes.

Ref.: 2, 3

COMMENTS: See Question 43.

42. Contraindications to attempted barium enema reduction of an intussusception in a child include which of the following?

A. Pneumoperitoneum

B. Peritonitis

C. "Currant jelly" stool

D. Recurrence after precious hydrostatic reduction

E. Patient's age over 5 years

Ref.: 1–3

COMMENTS: Ileocolic intussusception should be strongly suspected in a child between the ages of 3 and 18 months with the symptoms described in Question 41. • Barium enema should be performed promptly for diagnosis and for reduction of the intussusception by hydrostatic pressure. • It is successful in approximately 80% of children, usually being the only therapy that is needed. • An attempt at hydrostatic reduction is contraindicated in the presence of perforation or peritonitis. • In such cases, prompt operation is required. • When nonviable bowel is encountered at the time of exploration, resection is carried out without an attempt at reduction. • Otherwise, reduction by gentle digital pressure pushing the intussusceptum proximally is attempted. • Resection is performed if the intussusception is not reducible by this means. • Primary anastomosis can generally be performed. • In cases of successful manual reduction at operation, an appendectomy is usually performed. • Contrast studies usually are sufficient to rule out significant associated pathologic processes that would require operation in older children. • The passage of the characteristic "currant jelly" stool seen may occur as the result of mucosal venous congestion and does not necessarily indicate necrosis. • Thus, it does not contraindicate an attempt at nonoperative reduction. • Recurrence (in 5% of patients after hydrostatic or open reduction) is no longer considered an absolute indication for surgery, and a second and third attempt should be successful. • Age alone does not mandate operation, although a leading point such as a polyp, Meckel's diverticulum, or tumor (lymphoma) is more likely to be found in older children and is more likely to necessitate an operation. • Acute appendicitis and nephrolithiasis can occur in this age group but are extremely rare. • Infected urachal cyst is also infrequent, and symptoms are mainly related to sepsis. • Bleeding Meckel's diverticulum usually is painless, and frank blood is seen in the stools.

ANSWERS:
Question 40: E
Question 41: B
Question 42: A, B

---

43. Cystic hygromas are most commonly complicated by which of the following?

A. Infection

B. Hemorrhage

C. Respiratory distress

D. Malignancy

Ref.: 1–3

COMMENTS: Cystic hygroma is a congenital lymphangiomatous malformation commonly occurring in the posterior region of the neck or the axilla, groin, or mediastinum. • These lesions can reach large size, and all of the complications listed above have been described except malignant degeneration. • Infection, however, is the most common complication.

ANSWER:
A

---

44. Progressive abdominal distention and bilious vomiting develop in a newborn. Radiographic studies reveal distended bowel loops of varying size with air-fluid levels and a "soap suds" appearance in the right lower quadrant. Which of the following procedures should be performed next?

A. Laparotomy

B. Sweat chloride test

C. Gastrograffin lower gastrointestinal radiographic studies

D. Gastrograffin upper intestinal radiographic studies

E. Paracentesis

Ref.: 1–3

COMMENTS: The postnatal development of signs of intestinal obstruction with classic radiographic findings described above suggests a diagnosis of meconium ileus. • Nearly all affected infants have cystic fibrosis with a deficiency of pancreatic enzymes, which produces a thick meconium plug that causes obstruction in the distal ileum. • With uncomplicated meconium ileus, as described in this clinical presentation, administration of a Gastrograffin enema may be both diagnostic and therapeutic. • The detergent and hyperosmolar effects of the contrast material may relieve the obstruction. • Operation is indicated if the obstruction does not respond to the Gastrograffin enema or if complications such as peritonitis or perforation are present. • In such instances, the usual operative treatment entails resection of impaired bowel and creation of an external vent to allow postoperative irrigation with *N*-acetylcysteine. • Later, gastrointestinal continuity is reestablished. • A sweat chloride test should be performed in all of these infants. • Paracentesis or lavage may be helpful for diagnosing perforated NEC, a condition mandating prompt operation.

ANSWER:
C

---

45. The "double-bubble" sign seen in some neonates undergoing abdominal radiographic study is indicative of which of the following conditions?

A. Duodenal atresia

B. Normal newborn right after delivery

C. Malrotation of the midgut

D. Annular pancreas

E. Meconium ileus

Ref.: 1–3

COMMENTS: The double-bubble sign has always been thought to be pathognomonic of duodenal atresia, but other entities are manifested by a similar picture, and it is difficult to differentiate among them. • Infants are born with a gasless abdomen. • After taking the first few breaths, they start swallowing air. • This column of air usually takes 6–12 hr to reach the distal colon. • Therefore, an abdominal film taken a few minutes after delivery might show a double bubble and yet be normal. • Annular pancreas and duodenal atresia are clinically similar entities, and, although they both necessitate surgical repair, they are not operative emergencies. • In contrast, and most important, a double bubble on a radiograph may be indicative of malrotation of the midgut with volvulus, in which case an operation is mandatory as soon as the diagnosis is made. • Any delay increases the chance of vascular obstruction and necrosis of the entire small bowel. • Radiographic assessment of high obstruction in neonates can be performed with simple injection of air into the stomach. • Contrast dyes are usually not necessary. • Meconium ileus is a distal small-bowel obstruction in neonates with cystic fibrosis. • The radiographic findings are multiple, variably sized loops of small bowel ("soapsuds" appearance) in the right lower quadrant.

ANSWER:
A, B, C, D

46. The treatment of choice for duodenal atresia is which of the following?

    A. Duodenojejunostomy

    B. Gastrojejunostomy

    C. Roux-en-Y enterostomy

    D. Duodenostomy with delay repair

    E. Duodenoduodenostomy

Ref.: 1–3

COMMENTS: Once diagnosis is made, surgery can be deferred until all other pertinent systems can be studied and other anomalies excluded. • Duodenoduodenostomy is the preferred operation because it provides physiologic continuity to the gastrointestinal tract. • A windsock diaphragm and intraluminal or partial webs should be sought, otherwise, the obstruction may persist. • It is mandatory to identify the common bile duct and the ampulla of Vater to obviate any damage to these structures. • Postoperatively, the infant is kept on gastric suction until peristalsis resumes, after which oral feedings can be started. • Excellent results (in 95% of patients) can be expected from this operation.

ANSWER:
E

47. Match each characteristic in the left-hand column with the appropriate pediatric hepatic tumor or tumors in the right-hand column.

    A. More common   a. Hepatoblastoma

    B. Better prognosis   b. Hepatocarcinoma

    C. Bimodal age distribution

    D. Primary treatment surgical

Ref.: 1–3

COMMENTS: Hepatoblastoma and hepatocarcinoma are the two most common types of hepatic malignancy in pediatric age groups. • Hepatoblastoma is found most frequently in children under 3 years of age. • Hepatocarcinoma occurs in young infants and during late childhood to early adolescence. • Hepatoblastoma is the more common of the two lesions and has the more favorable prognosis (overall 5-year survival rate of 30–50%), whereas the rate of survival with hepatocarcinoma is approximately 15%. • α-Fetoprotein is a useful biochemical marker for hepatic malignancies. • Therapy of these tumors involves a multimodality approach, although surgical resection offers the best chance of cure.

ANSWER:
A-a; B-a; C-b; D-a, b

48. Which of the following tests is the most reliable for establishing the diagnosis of gastroesophageal reflux in pediatric patients?

    A. Esophagram

    B. Upper gastrointestinal contrast study

    C. Nuclear scanning after ingestion of radioactive milk

    D. Esophagoscopy with biopsy

    E. Monitoring the pH of the esophagus for 12–24 hr

Ref.: 1–3

COMMENTS: All of the studies listed above are used for diagnosis of gastroesophageal reflux, but the test of choice is 12- to 24-hr pH monitoring of the esophagus.

ANSWER:
E

49. Match each characteristic in the left-hand column with the appropriate pediatric solid tumor or tumors in the right-hand column.

    A. More common during first   a. Wilms' tumor
        2 years of life

    B. Usually manifests as an   b. Neuroblastoma
        asymptomatic mass

    C. Calyceal distortion on an
        intravenous pyelogram (IVP)

    D. Elevated vanillylmandelic
        acid (VMA) level

    E. Primary treatment surgical

    F. Overall 5-year survival rate >75%

Ref.: 1–3

COMMENTS: Neuroblastoma and nephroblastoma (Wilms' tumor) are common solid malignancies in children. • Neuroblastoma is the second most common solid tumor after brain tumors. • The clinical presentation is often similar for abdominal involvement, the most common site for both. • The diseases are manifested as an asymptomatic mass in children during the first years of life. • Wilms' tumor, which is an embryonal tumor arising from the kidney, typically produces distortion of the renal collecting system, as seen on IVP. • The lungs are the most common site of metastatic disease. • Neuroblastoma arises from cells of neural crest origin, typically occurring in the adrenal or posterior mediastinum. • IVP differentiates adrenal neuroblastoma from Wilms' tumor by demonstrating renal displacement but not calyceal distortion. • Neuroblastoma may extend through the intervertebral foramen, and, because of this feature, magnetic resonance imaging of the spine should be performed on all these patients. • Because of continued catecholamine turnover, VMA levels are elevated in most patients with neuroblastoma and have been a useful biochemical marker. • Horner's syndrome is a common finding in children with cervical neuroblastoma, attributed to the origin of this tumor at the site of the stellate ganglia. • Neuroblastoma most commonly metastasizes to the liver and bone. • The primary treatment of both of these lesions is complete surgical excision, which is more often possible with Wilms' tumor. • Both chemotherapy and radiotherapy are used but have been more useful for enhancing the survival of patients with Wilms' tumor than those with neuroblastoma. • The overall cure rate for Wilms' tumor is approximately 80%, compared with 30% for neuroblastoma. • Younger children with neuroblastoma have a better prognosis, and infants under 1 year of age may attain a survival rate of 80%.

ANSWER:
A-b; B-a, b; C-a; D-b; E-a, b; F-a

50. Which of the following statements concerning branchial cleft sinuses is/are true?

    A. A branchial cleft sinus is a small painless opening in the anterior border of the sternocleidomastoid muscle and may be associated with a cyst or infection.

B. The first branchial cleft sinus routinely drains into the internal auditory canal and is associated with chronic otitis media.

C. Second branchial cleft sinuses, when complete, track through the carotid bifurcation and into the tonsillar fossa.

D. Differential diagnosis includes cystic hygroma, dermoid, lipoma, neurofibroma, and lymphadenitis.

Ref.: 1–3

COMMENTS: The first branchial cleft sinus ends in the external auditory canal if complete. • When it is infected, it is associated with a draining sinus located anterior to the ear. • During excision, risk includes injury to the facial nerve.

ANSWER:
A, C, D

REFERENCES

1. Townsend CM, Beauchamp RD, Evers BM, et al (eds): *Sabiston Textbook of Surgery: The Biological Basis of Modern Surgical Practice*, 17th ed. Saunders, Philadelphia, 2004.
2. Brunicardi FC, Andersen DK, Billiar TR, et al (eds): *Schwartz's Principles of Surgery,* 8th ed. McGraw-Hill, New York, 2004.
3. Rowe MI, O'Neill IA, Grosfied IL, et al (eds): *Essentials of Pediatric Surgery*. CV Mosby, St. Louis, 1995.

CHAPTER 44

Vascular

A. Vascular Surgery Principles

Christopher Bulger, M.D., Alain Domkam, M.D., and Walter J. McCarthy, M.D.

1. Which of the following is/are not independent risk factors for the development of coronary and peripheral atherosclerosis?

   A. Cigarette smoking

   B. Hypercholesterolemia

   C. Diabetes mellitus

   D. Hypertension

   E. Hypercoagulable conditions

Ref.: 1, 4, 5

COMMENTS: Hypercoagulable conditions are associated with increased risk of thrombosis, but they have not been associated as an independent risk factor for atherosclerosis. • Smoking is a risk factor owing to the release of oxidative free radicals, which damage the vascular endothelium. • Hypercholesterolemia with total serum levels greater than 200 mg/dl and elevated low-density lipoprotein (LDL) fractions are also associated with increased risk. • Diabetes mellitus and hypertension are independent risk factors in proportion to their severity.

ANSWER:
E

2. Which of the following statements regarding claudication is/are true?

   A. The term *claudication* originated from the Latin root word meaning "to limp."

   B. Without intervention, the risk of limb loss approaches 50% at 5 years.

   C. It can be alleviated significantly with cilostazol.

   D. It can be managed successfully without arteriography, balloon angioplasty, or operation in most cases.

   E. The optimal treatment is cessation of smoking and exercise consisting of 1 hr of walking per day.

Ref.: 1–5

COMMENTS: Claudication is derived from the Latin verb meaning "to limp." The risk of limb loss for all claudicant patients is 5%

over 5 years. • The risk of limb loss drops substantially, from 12% to 2%, if a patient successfully stops smoking. • Claudication usually can be treated safely with medication. • Several medications, including pentoxifylline and cilostazol, have been shown to improve walking distance. • "Stop smoking and keep walking" are five words that sum up the treatment strategy for most patients. • A regular, organized walking program generally doubles walking distance.

ANSWER:
A, C, D, E

3. Which of the following describe(s) chronic leg ulcers?

   A. The cause of ulcers often can be determined by their location on the leg.

   B. Venous ulcers are seldom located on the foot.

   C. Arterial ulcers are seldom located on the leg.

   D. Leg ulcers affect diabetic patients less often than other patient groups.

Ref.: 1–3

COMMENTS: Chronic venous insufficiency causes characteristic skin changes, including hyperpigmentation, thickened skin, and ulceration in the gaiter region, named for an item of clothing that covers the leg from the ankle to the knee. • **Venous** ulcers usually occur at the medial malleoli but seldom extend below the ankles. • **Arterial** ulcers form at the distal aspect of the region that has compromised arterial circulation. • They usually result in ulcers of the toes or foot, but islands of ischemia can occur more proximally on the leg, especially the anterior leg. • Diabetic patients can form **neurotrophic** ulcers. • The neuropathy that afflicts patients with long-standing diabetes causes wasting of the muscles of the foot and collapse of the standard architecture of the foot, causing pressure points between the toes and at the metatarsal heads. • Strict avoidance of weight-bearing is essential in order for these pressure ulcers to heal when the arterial circulation is adequate. • If the arterial circulation is compromised, these patients usually need arterial leg bypass operations, rather than balloon angioplasty, to heal these ulcers.

ANSWER:
A, B

4. Which of the following is/are characteristic of ischemic extremity rest pain?

A. Initially occurs mostly at night

B. Can be relieved by placing the involved extremity in the dependent position

C. Is usually located at the toes

D. Can be relieved by intravenous heparin

E. Can be relieved with cilostazol (Pletal)

F. Is characterized as nocturnal calf cramping

Ref.: 1, 2, 4, 5

COMMENTS: Extremity angina occurs most commonly at night because, when patients with severe lower-extremity arterial insufficiency lie supine, they lose the added benefit of gravity for perfusing the lower extremity. • Patients with nocturnal ischemic rest pain quickly discover that walking, standing, or sleeping in a chair relieves this pain, which is centered over the metatarsal heads, not the toes. • Pain in the toes suggests gout or an infection. • Intravenous heparin causes vasodilation by promoting the release of nitric oxide, thereby improving extremity arterial circulation. • Intravenous heparin can relieve rest pain until the arterial circulation can be improved with a bypass operation. • Cilostazol improves claudication-impaired distance walking but has not been shown to be effective for treating ischemic rest pain. • Nocturnal calf cramping afflicts one in five adults and is not indicative of extremity ischemia.

ANSWER:
A, B, D

5. Which of the following characteristics of leg swelling due to venous insufficiency or lymphedema is/are true?

A. Edema forms when the hydrostatic pressure in the interstitium is lower than that in the lymphatic or venule.

B. Venous insufficiency causes pigmentation and hypertrophic changes in the skin over the ankle, causes late lymphedema, and is nonpitting with fibrosis.

C. Lymphedema can be diagnosed by ultrasound imaging.

D. Operative intervention can treat venous insufficiency but is not commonly used for lymphedema.

Ref.: 1, 4, 5

COMMENTS: Edema formation is governed by the balance between hydrostatic and oncotic pressure in the interstitium versus the lymphatics and venules. • Hyperpigmentation and cicatrix formation in the gaiter region (legs from ankle to knees) is pathognomonic of venous insufficiency and is caused by the breakdown of extravascular red blood cells and subcutaneous scar tissue (liposclerosis). • With severe cases of untreated chronic venous insufficiency, such scar tissue formation can cause local destruction of leg lymphatics and secondary formation of lymphedema. • Any severe hypoproteinemia can cause lymphedema. • Lymphedema may present early as a pitting form, but after subsequent protein deposition in the extremity and damage to the lymphatics, the adipose tissue fibroses and the skin thickens. • Venous insufficiency can be recognized clinically by filling of varices but also on color Doppler imaging. • Due to the size of the lymphatics, they are not visible on ultrasound imaging, and only nonspecific subcutaneous edema may be visible. • Operations for lymphedema are generally not performed. • Operations for venous insufficiency include perforator vein ligation, varicose vein ligation and stripping, and deep vein valve transplantation.

ANSWER:
A, B, D

6. A patient with severe peripheral vascular disease underwent aortobiliac bypass grafting 9 months ago and now presents with hematochezia and a syncopal episode. Along with the administration of intravenous antibiotics, appropriate treatment or diagnostic modalities include which of the following?

A. Upper endoscopy (EGD) and computed tomographic (CT) scanning

B. Angiography and tagged red blood cell scanning

C. Bilateral axillofemoral bypass and delayed removal of the graft

D. Removal of the graft and unilateral axillofemoral and femorofemoral bypass

E. Colonoscopy

Ref.: 1, 5

COMMENTS: The general approach to the treatment of aortoenteric fistulas and infections involves prompt diagnosis, antibiotics, removal of the entire prosthesis, and reestablishment of vascular continuity through noncontaminated fields. • Magnetic resonance imaging (MRI) has the highest sensitivity for graft infections but is ill suited to unstable patients, while CT scans are fast and abnormal 91% of the time in patients with aorto-enteric fistula (AEF). • Abnormal CT findings include perigraft fluid, gas, and tissue inflammation. • They actually demonstrate AEF in only 33% of cases. • While arteriography may help in planning the site of distal anastomosis, it rarely demonstrates the fistula and can take considerably longer. • Colonic ischemia is more common in the immediate postoperative period.

In hemodynamically unstable patients, EGD of the third and fourth portion of the duodenum should be performed first, with aggressive resuscitation and rapid transfer to the operating room. • Extraanatomic routes of axillofemoral or femorofemoral grafts permit revascularization through a clean field distal to the original site. • In situations requiring revascularization through a contaminated area, autologous tissue using superficial femoral vein can be used. • Bilateral axillofemoral grafts should be used as a secondary option because of the diminished outflow compared to unilateral axillofemoral and femorofemoral grafts. • Delayed excision of the graft is recommended only in patients who are hemodynamically stable and do not demonstrate a false aneurysm at the site of the fistula.

ANSWER:
A, D

7. Fasciotomy should be performed in patients with which of the following signs or symptoms?

A. Tense fullness of the compartment in an otherwise asymptomatic patient

B. Extremity ischemia for greater than 6 hr

C. Postoperative revascularization patients with progressively worsening neurologic signs

D. Combined traumatic crush injuries of the popliteal artery and vein

E. Compartmental pressure higher than 35 mmHg and unreliable findings on physical examination

F. None of the above

Ref.: 1, 4, 5

COMMENTS: Compartmental syndromes occur whenever tissue pressure within a confined anatomic space becomes sufficiently elevated to impair venous return. • It can be due to bleeding within a compartment or to reperfusion edema. • There is no absolute pressure above which the syndrome invariably occurs, but nutrient blood flow in the muscle ceases between 30 and 40 mmHg. • In addition, a difference between the diastolic blood pressure and intercompartmental pressure greater than 30 mmHg is indicative of impaired blood flow. • At minimum, such elevated pressures mandate close follow-up neurovascular examinations in reliable patients. • Successful treatment is based on early, accurate diagnosis. • Prolonged ischemia is associated with compartment syndrome due to the reperfusion injury and release of free radicals. • Diminished or absent pulses is a late finding, after which irreversible neurologic damage may have occurred. • All the aforementioned symptoms and signs are important, and compartmental syndromes are best diagnosed by a high index of suspicion. • A tense compartment alone in the absence of elevated pressures or physical findings is not an absolute indication for fasciotomy.

A N S W E R :
B, C, D, E

8. In a low-resistance arterial vascular system, at which percent diameter reduction does a stenosis become flow limiting?

A. 10%

B. 20%

C. 40%

D. 50%

E. 80%

Ref.: 2, 6

COMMENTS: In low-resistance arterial systems, such as the internal carotid artery, total blood flow across a stenosis does not decrease until the diameter is reduced by approximately 50%. • This corresponds to a 75% reduction in cross-sectional area. • Total blood flow is maintained by increasing the velocity. • Shear stress (drag) and viscosity limit further increases in velocity once the diameter reduction exceeds 50%. • This hemodynamic fact is the reason for not repairing short stenoses of less than 50%, since total blood flow is not altered. • A longer stenosis increases the shear stress and causes a lesser degree of stenosis over a long length to be flow limiting.

A N S W E R :
D

9. Which of the following characterize duplex ultrasound imaging?

A. It is a combination of Doppler and B-mode ultrasound imaging.

B. Lower frequencies (e.g., 3 MHz) are better suited for deep abdominal imaging, and higher frequencies (e.g., 7 MHz) are better for more superficial structures, such as in-situ vein grafts.

C. High-frequency ultrasound waves have higher energy than do low-frequency ultrasound waves.

D. Diagnosis of deep venous thrombosis (DVT) is made by absence of color flow imaging alone.

E. Calcification within a diseased artery usually is severe enough to prevent an adequate vascular ultrasound examination.

Ref.: 2, 3, 6

COMMENTS: Duplex ultrasound imaging consists of the B-mode image (picture) and Doppler shift, which measures the velocity of the flowing blood. • High-frequency transducers (7–10 MHz) are used for superficial structures, with applications such as saphenous vein mapping and in-situ vein bypasses or pedal bypasses. • These higher-frequency transducers have greater resolution but lower energy and cannot penetrate deeper tissues, as can lower-frequency, higher-energy transducers (3 or 5 MHz). • Since venous flow velocity is slower than arterial flow, artifacts can be more easily introduced by transducer movement when performing a venous examination, especially to rule out a DVT. • For these reasons, a more accurate venous examination to look for a DVT is one without color that demonstrates a dilated uncompressible vein. • The black-and-white image allows better assessment of vein compressibility and is not confused by an artifact introduced by transducer movement. • Absence of flow in that segment of vein with augmentation and lack of respiratory variation confirm the diagnosis. • Arterial wall calcium occasionally interferes with vascular ultrasound scans by blocking ultrasound wave transmission, but it is unusual that one cannot perform an adequate vascular examination of the carotid or other structure because of severe calcification.

A N S W E R :
A, B

10. The advantages of lower-extremity arterial Doppler examinations performed with waveform analysis compared to the ankle-brachial index (ABI) alone include which of the following?

A. Calcification of the artery by diseases such as diabetes mellitus and chronic renal failure make the arterial wall incompressible, causing the ABI to be artificially elevated and unreliable.

B. Inflow disease can be recognized by the delay in the upstroke of the waveform.

C. The loss of reversal of flow when the arterial waveform transforms from triphasic to biphasic is observed with exercise or with moderate atherosclerosis.

D. The ABI can be used to diagnose an arteriovenous fistula.

E. The ABI can be used to diagnose a DVT.

Ref.: 2, 3, 6

COMMENTS: The ABI is a measurement for quantifying extremity ischemia, based on the assumption that the flow in the limb is proportional to the blood pressure in the limb. • The ABI is obtained with a blood pressure cuff and a hand-held Doppler instrument. • The cuff is applied at the point at which the pressure measurement is desired. • The Doppler device is placed over any vessel distal to the cuff, but routinely it is the radial artery in the upper extremity or the posterior tibial or dorsal pedal artery in the lower extremity. • The cuff is inflated to a pressure greater than the systolic pressure. • The pressure at which the arterial Doppler signal returns as the cuff is deflated is the pressure used to calculate the ABI. • Diabetes and renal failure cause calcification of the axial extremity arteries, which makes the arteries noncompressible. • The ABI is artificially elevated with these conditions.

When the ABI is unreliable (ABI > 1.2), one must depend on the Doppler waveform to assess the degree of extremity ischemia. • Waveforms become monophasic in diseased arteries regardless of whether the vessels are compressible. • The degree of arterial inflow disease (above the inguinal ligament) can be assessed by examining the femoral artery waveform. • An arterial upstroke prolonged to more than 180 ms is consistent with significant iliac disease. • Digital artery pressures are useful for quantifying ischemia in patients with diabetes and renal failure, since these vessels are usually compressible even under such conditions. • Toe pressures of less than 30 mmHg are consistent with severe ischemia in nondiabetic patients, and those less than 50 mmHg are consistent with severe ischemia in diabetic patients.

Reversal of blood flow direction is caused by vascular resistance. • Exercise causes vasodilation in the muscular beds and decreases resistance, resulting in the loss of flow. • The first change one observes in waveform morphology due to mild atherosclerotic disease is the loss of flow reversal when the waveform goes from triphasic to biphasic. • Duplex imaging is required to diagnose arteriovenous fistulas and DVTs. • The ABI alone is inadequate for diagnosing these conditions.

A N S W E R :
A, B, C

11. When performing duplex ultrasound imaging of the carotid arteries, what factors help distinguish the external carotid artery from the internal carotid artery?

   A. The internal carotid artery has continuous forward flow, and the external carotid artery has reversal of flow during diastole.

   B. The external carotid artery is larger.

   C. The internal carotid artery is generally seen first.

   D. The superior thyroid artery is the first branch of the internal carotid artery and aids in identifying the internal carotid artery.

Ref.: 2, 3

COMMENTS: The external carotid artery is usually found anteromedially on the duplex examination, whereas the internal carotid artery is usually found posterolaterally. • The external carotid artery is usually the first artery seen. • It has triphasic flow, not continuous flow, as is found in the internal carotid artery. • The first branch of the external carotid artery is the superior thyroid artery. • The internal carotid artery has monophasic continuous flow because it feeds the brain, a low-resistance system. • The external carotid artery has triphasic flow with flow reversal because it feeds the face and its musculature, all high-resistance systems. • Both arteries are approximately the same size in their proximal aspects. • The internal carotid artery has no branches in the neck, in contrast to the external carotid artery.

A N S W E R :
A

12. Which of the following statements regarding percutaneous transluminal balloon angioplasty (PTA) for the treatment of occlusive atherosclerotic arterial blockages or stenoses is/are true?

   A. The rates of intimal hyperplasia following PTA in a small artery (<5 mm) exceed those observed following operative repair of arteries of a similar size.

   B. The short- and long-term results of balloon angioplasty for lesions longer than 10 cm are better than those for operative intervention.

   C. Balloon angioplasty has demonstrated excellent results for stenotic lesions of the common iliac artery, but the results are not as good for occlusive lesions of the external iliac artery.

   D. Complications of PTA include dissection, thrombosis, and atheroembolization.

Ref.: 2, 3, 6

COMMENTS: PTA is performed via the percutaneous intravascular passage of balloon-tipped catheters. • During balloon dilation, the atherosclerotic intima is ruptured and compressed, allowing the media to become overstretched. • PTA works best for short stenoses or occlusions in large arteries, such as may be found in the common iliac artery. • The success rates for PTA of the common iliac artery are 80% at 1 year. • The results of PTA of the external iliac artery fall off to approximately 55% at 2 years.

Myointimal hyperplasia affects all blood vessels that have undergone intervention, but this process exerts its greatest influence on small arteries, with diameters less than 5 mm. • Stents have been introduced to combat this problem, but they have not eliminated this complication of PTA. • Myointimal hyperplasia can lead to failure rates of up to 40% at 6 months for small arteries that have undergone PTA, with the outcome being recurrent stenosis or thrombosis. • PTA of long superficial femoral artery lesions has a success rate of only 22% at 1 year, whereas femoropopliteal bypass has a patency rate of 90% at 1 year. • PTA of the renal artery works well for fibromuscular dysplasia but not as effectively for atherosclerotic lesions. • The patency rate following PTA of the renal artery is only 60% at 2 years. • Atheroembolization, dissection, and thrombosis can complicate any attempted percutaneous intervention and can lead to limb loss.

A N S W E R :
A, C, D

13. What is the most common cause of a congenital hypercoagulable disorder?

   A. Protein S deficiency

   B. Protein C deficiency

   C. Antithrombin III deficiency

   D. Activated protein C resistance (APC-R; factor V Leiden mutation)

   E. Homocysteinemia

Ref.: 2, 3, 6

COMMENTS: Hemostasis is a finely tuned balance between coagulation and fibrinolysis. • The existence of a congenital defect in the procoagulant or anticoagulant proteins can shift this balance and cause increased bleeding or increased thrombotic tendencies, respectively. • Hypercoagulable states are the most common cause of early bypass graft failure in young adults who require vascular interventions for limb salvage. • More than 50% of patients under the age of 50 who require a lower-extremity bypass and experience early graft thrombosis have a hypercoagulable state.

Protein C, protein S, and antithrombin III deficiencies have been known to exist for years, but until recently a specific inherited hypercoagulable state could not be identified in as many as 80% of patients.

It is now known that **APC-R** is the most common inherited hypercoagulable state, existing in more than 50% of patients with inherited thrombosis tendencies. • The cause of APC-R is an amino acid substitution in factor V of glutamine for arginine 506. • Patients with activated protein C resistance have a poor anticoagulant response to activated protein C, a vitamin K–dependent anticoagulant protein. • When protein C is activated, it normally degrades activated clotting factors Va and VIIa. • The altered factor V, or Leiden mutation (named for the Dutch city where it was first found), is resistant to the degrading action of APC. • The altered, activated factor V retains its procoagulant activity, and the hemostatic balance is shifted toward thrombosis.

Antithrombin III is the major plasma inhibitor of thrombin. • Heparin performs its anticoagulant function by forming a trivalent molecule of heparin–antithrombin III–thrombin to inactivate thrombin. • This deficiency is rare, with an incidence of only 1:5000. • Thrombotic events are usually triggered by trauma, operation, or pregnancy.

Proteins C and S are both vitamin K–dependent *anticoagulant* proteins synthesized by the liver. • The incidence of congenital protein C deficiency is 1:200. • Protein C and S deficiencies are found in 20% of patients under the age of 50 with arterial thrombosis, but the combined incidence is much less than the incidence of APC-R.

The treatment for antithrombin III, protein C, and protein S deficiency is lifelong warfarin anticoagulation. • Heparin must be given before initiating warfarin anticoagulation in these patients to protect against warfarin-induced skin necrosis. • *All* patients with thrombosis who are to receive warfarin therapy should receive heparin during the first 3–4 days of warfarin therapy because the half-life of the anticoagulation protein C is much less, since it is degraded much faster than the procoagulant vitamin K–dependent factors II, IX, and X.

Mild homocysteinemia exists in 5–7% of the population. • Elevated levels of homocysteine occur because of a defect in the pathway that metabolizes methionine. • The treatment for homocysteinemia is the B vitamin folate 1–5 mg/day.

ANSWER:
D

14. What is the most common cause of an acquired hypercoagulable state?

A. Smoking

B. Heparin-induced thrombocytopenia (HIT)

C. Antiphospholipid antibody (e.g., lupus anticoagulant)

D. Warfarin

E. Oral contraceptives

Ref.: 2, 3, 6

COMMENTS: Smoking is the most common cause of acquired hypercoagulability. • Smoking is the most important factor that determines the short- and long-term results of any vascular intervention. • The mechanisms of action of smoking are multiple and include both vasoconstriction and a measurable elevation of plasma fibrinogen levels, which itself is a risk factor for thrombosis.

The next most common cause of acquired hypercoagulability is **HIT**. • This condition affects 2–3% of all patients who receive heparin. • Antibodies form to heparin because it is obtained from bovine or porcine sources. • The clinical manifestations are a falling platelet count, increasing resistance to anticoagulation with heparin, and new paradoxical thrombotic events while receiving heparin treatment. • Although low–molecular-weight heparin is responsible for a lower incidence of HIT than is standard heparin, 25% of patients with HIT who receive low–molecular-weight heparin manifest the heparin allergy. • The treatment for HIT is cessation of all heparin. • Warfarin-induced skin necrosis is unusual as long as heparin is given for the first 3 days that warfarin is given.

The antiphospholipid syndrome (APS) is common, affecting 1–5% of the population. • Specific types are lupus anticoagulant and anticardiolipin antibodies. • Since the incidence of APS increases with age, 50% of patients over the age of 80 have APS. • This syndrome is recognized by prolongation of the baseline partial thromboplastin time (PTT). • Brain thromboplastin is the reagent used for triggering the intrinsic clotting system when the PTT is measured. • Patients with APS have serum antibodies that consume this reagent, resulting in a prolonged PTT. • This is an unforgiving hypercoagulable state with an incidence of thrombotic complications approaching 50%.

Warfarin and **oral contraceptives** are less common causes of hypercoagulability.

ANSWER:
A

15. A 70-year-old male who had undergone endovascular abdominal aneurysm repair 1 year ago collapses and complains of back and abdominal pain. His blood pressure is 90/40. The patient denies a history of peptic ulcer or alcohol abuse. What is the most likely diagnostic?

A. Aortoenteric fistula

B. Bleeding duodenal ulcer

C. Ruptured abdominal aortic aneurysm (AAA)

D. Pancreatitis

E. Diverticulitis

Ref.: 7

COMMENTS: The diagnostic of ruptured AAA must be considered in a patient with abdominal pain, back pain, and hypotension. • After endovascular repair, up to 50% of patients develop an endoleak (persistent flow within an aneurysm sac despite an excluded aneurysm). • Type 1 endoleak occurs when a persistent channel of blood flow develops owing to inadequate or ineffective seal at the graft ends. • Type 2 endoleak occurs when there is persistent collateral blood flow into the aneurysm sac flowing retrograde from patent lumbar arteries, or the inferior mesenteric artery. • Type 3 is a graft a defect endoleak, such as when the sections pull apart. • Type 4 is a graft-fabric porosity endoleak. • Only about 1% of patients with stent graft repair of AAAs have a late rupture.

ANSWER:
C

16. Which of the following is the most common symptom of thoracic outlet syndrome (TOS)?

A. Arm pain with exercise

B. Pain or paresthesia in the ulnar nerve distribution

C. Pain or paresthesia in the median nerve distribution

D. Hyperhydrosis

E. Arm discoloration and swelling with exercise

Ref.: 7

COMMENTS: TOS represents a spectrum of disorders caused by mechanical compression of neurovascular structures as they traverse the costoclavicular space. • Pain is the most common presenting symptom of neurogenic TOS, involving the neck, shoulder, and hand, in descending order of frequency. • Paresthesia (numbness and tingling) are a common symptom and typically involve the fingers, hand, or forearm, usually in an ulnar distribution. • Symptoms are initially intermittent, but they progress to continuous patterns and are commonly aggravated by arm elevation. • Symptoms of arm ischemia with TOS are uncommon, since arterial compromise occurs in only 1–3% of cases. • Symptoms of venous insufficiency are likewise uncommon, as is the so-called effort thrombosis of the subclavian vein (Paget–Von Schrotter syndrome).

ANSWER:
B

17. Which of the following statements concerning fibromuscular dysplasia of the carotid arteries is/are true?

A. The incidence in males and females is approximately equal.

B. Atherosclerosis is common when fibromuscular dysplasia is present.

C. Patient should undergo operative dilatation before transient ischemic attacks (TIAs) or stroke occurs.

D. The process can also occur in the subclavian, internal iliac, and mesenteric vessels.

E. Approximately 25% of patients have associated intracranial aneurysms.

Ref.: 7

COMMENTS: Fibromuscular dysplasia occurs predominantly in females and can also involve the renal, external iliac carotid, and vertebral arteries. • The subclavian and mesenteric vessels are not involved. • Symptomatic patients may undergo graded intraluminal dilatation through arteriotomy in the common carotid artery. • Asymptomatic patients may be followed.

Approximately 13–35% of patients have atherosclerosis of the carotid bifurcation. • The incidence of intracranial aneurysm is 23%.

ANSWER:
E

REFERENCES

1. Townsend CM Jr, Beauchamp RD, Evers BM, et al (eds): *Sabiston Textbook of Surgery: The Biological Basis of Modern Surgical Practice,* 17th ed. WB Saunders, Philadelphia, 2004.
2. Moore WS: *Vascular Surgery,* 5th ed. WB Saunders, Philadelphia, 1998.
3. Yao STJ, Pearce WH: *Practical Vascular Surgery.* Appleton & Lange, Stamford, CT, 1999.
4. Brunicardi FC, Andersen DK, Billiar TR, et al (eds): *Schwartz's Principles of Surgery,* 8th ed. McGraw-Hill, New York, 2004.
5. Ernst CB, Stanley JC: *Current Therapy in Vascular Surgery,* 4th ed. CV Mosby, St. Louis, 2001.
6. Porter JM, Taylor LM Jr: *Basic Data Underlying Clinical Decision Making in Vascular Surgery.* Quality Medical Publishing, St. Louis, 1994.
7. Rutherford R: *Vascular Surgery,* 6th ed. Elsevier-Saunders, Philadelphia, 2005.

B. Cerebrovascular Disease

Christopher Bulger, M.D., and Walter J. McCarthy, M.D.

1. The most common cause of cerebral ischemia involves which one of the following?

   A. Extracranial arterial stenosis

   B. Intracranial arterial thrombosis

   C. Arterioarterial embolization (atheroembolization)

   D. Cardioarterial embolization

   Ref.: 1, 2

COMMENTS: Atherosclerosis is the most common cause of ischemic stroke. • Arterioarterial embolization of plaque fragments from degenerative plaques or platelet fibrin aggregates from a thrombogenic plaque surface are believed to be responsible for the neurologic injury. • A small proportion of ischemic strokes may be caused by processes other than atherosclerosis, such as emboli from cardiac sources, fibromuscular hyperplasia, occlusive arteritis of the aortic arch vessels (Takayasu's disease), dissecting thoracic aortic aneurysms, and trauma.

ANSWER:
C

2. What percentage of patients with cerebral ischemia have a surgically accessible lesion?

   A. 95%

   B. 75%

   C. 50%

   D. 25%

   E. 5%

   Ref.: 2

COMMENTS: Of the patients with cerebrovascular ischemia who are studied by four-vessel angiography (common carotid and vertebral arteries), 75% are found to have significant extracranial disease that is surgically accessible. • In the carotid vessels, lesions characteristically involve the carotid bifurcation and the proximal 1–2 cm of the internal carotid artery. • In patients with vertebral basilar insufficiency, plaques or stenotic lesions characteristically occur near the origin of the vertebral arteries from the subclavian vessels. • Because stroke is the third leading cause of death in the United States and because the responsible lesions are often surgically accessible, endarterectomy benefits a significant proportion of patients with symptoms of cerebral ischemia.

ANSWER:
B

3. In which patients is carotid endarterectomy indicated?

   A. Acute stroke, 70% carotid stenosis, rapid recovery, and negative head CT scan

   B. Forty-five percent carotid stenosis with continued or worsening TIAs while the patient was treated with aspirin and Plavix

   C. Transient neurologic deficit (<24 hr) and 70% stenosis

   D. Completed stroke and totally occluded internal carotid artery

   E. Eighty-five percent stenosis, completed stroke, mild deficit, and ulcerated carotid plaque

   Ref.: 1–3

COMMENTS: Among patients with symptoms of cerebrovascular ischemia and greater than 50% stenosis, those with TIAs are optimal candidates for carotid endarterectomy because their risk of subsequent stroke is decreased significantly by operative intervention. • Endarterectomy may also benefit patients with a completed stroke if the neurologic deficit is not severe and there is no evidence of a stroke on CT scan. • A large stroke evident on CT scan means that the patient should wait 6 weeks for endarterectomy. • Endarterectomy of the internal carotid artery has no benefit for a patient who has had a completed stroke with total occlusion of the artery. • The role of carotid endarterectomy in an acute or evolving stroke is controversial. • Restoration of flow is usually not indicated in patients with acute, fixed deficits and may in fact worsen symptoms and produce death by causing hemorrhage in the area of infarction. • In patients with an evolving stroke (so-called crescendo TIAs) and fluctuating neurologic deficit, emergent endarterectomy may be of benefit. • Symptomatic stenosis in carotid arteries with ulcerated plaques should undergo endarterectomy because of the propensity of such plaques to activate platelets and form emboli.

ANSWER:
A, B, C, E

4. Which of the following are characteristic of a TIS?

   A. Symptoms lasting longer than 24 hr

   B. Weakness, paralysis, or dysarthria in one side of the face or extremity

   C. Unilateral eye pain lasting 1 second

   D. Unilateral paresthesias, numbness, or aphasia

   E. Incontinence of bowel and bladder

   Ref.: 1–3

COMMENTS: TIAs typically last 2–15 minutes and resolve completely afterward. • Attacks lasting longer than 24 hr but less than 3 weeks are referred to as reversible ischemic neurologic deficits. • After 3 weeks, the attack is completed and referred to as a completed stroke. • TIAs typically involve unilateral motor or sensory deficits of the extremities or face. • Pain is not an associated feature, and episodes lasting only a few seconds are unlikely to be TIAs. • Isolated symptoms of unconsciousness without other symptoms, dizziness alone, dysarthria alone, diplopia alone, incontinence of bowel or bladder, focal symptoms associated with migraines, confusion alone, and amnesia alone are also unlikely to be TIAs.

ANSWER:
B, D

---

5. Which of the following is the best screening test for significant carotid stenosis in a patient with an asymptomatic bruit?

   A. Magnetic resonance angiography

   B. Four-vessel cerebral angiography

   C. Digital subtraction angiography

   D. CT brain scan with infusion

   E. Duplex ultrasound scanning

Ref.: 1, 2

COMMENTS: Because of their sensitivity, safety, and repeatability, noninvasive cerebrovascular studies provide the best means of screening patients with asymptomatic bruits to detect significant stenotic lesions. • **Duplex scanning** (real-time B-mode ultrasound imaging), which combines ultrasound and frequency spectrum analysis, provides a noninvasive method of quantifying the degree of stenosis and assessing morphologic characteristics. • As such, it is the single best screening test for evaluating carotid disease. • **Angiography** is the definitive method of evaluating carotid anatomy in most centers, but it is not advocated as a screening procedure because it carries a 0.5–1.0% combined risk of mortality and major neurologic injury. • **Digital subtraction angiography** has been evaluated as a screening tool in asymptomatic patients but has been found to have limited usefulness. • **CT scanning** of the brain and **electroencephalography** rarely are indicated for screening.

ANSWER:
E

---

6. With regard to the Asymptomatic Carotid Atherosclerosis Study (ACAS), which of the following patients could be recommended for carotid endarterectomy?

   A. A 65-year-old woman with 30% stenosis and complaints of lower-extremity claudication

   B. A 70-year-old man with a carotid bruit and a 60% stenosis revealed on angiogram

   C. An 80-year-old woman with atrial fibrillation, complete left hemiplegia, and a 50% stenosis on duplex ultrasound imaging

   D. A 17-year-old boy with hyperlipidemia, a recent myocardial infarction, and a 50% carotid stenosis

Ref.: 1–3

COMMENTS: The value of prophylactic carotid endarterectomy for patients with asymptomatic stenosis is predicated on a progressive natural history of the disease process and the ability to perform endarterectomy with morbidity and mortality rates of less than 2%. • Several studies have shown that, among *asymptomatic* patients with hemodynamically significant carotid stenosis (exceeding 60%), the percentage of cerebral ischemic events is higher than among patients without stenosis and that carotid endarterectomy in a prophylactic setting probably decreases the expected risk of cerebral ischemic events. • No data to date, however, support the use of endarterectomy for patients with a less than 60% asymptomatic stenosis. • Duplex ultrasound imaging as a diagnostic modality may also under- or overestimate the degree of stenosis, leading to an erroneous conclusion from the study data. • The ACAS and North American Symptomatic Carotid Endarterectomy Trial (NASCET) studies were predicated on angiographic stenosis or diameter reduction, which underestimates area reduction. • Carotid endarterectomy can only be recommended for asymptomatic patients with otherwise low operative risk and few comorbid conditions.

ANSWER:
B

---

7. Of the following changing factors that contribute to flow through a stenotic artery, which is the most important?

   A. Diameter of stenosis

   B. Length of stenosis

   C. Blood viscosity

   D. Blood pressure

Ref.: 1

COMMENTS: Stenosis is usually considered hemodynamically significant if the diameter of the lumen is reduced by 50% or more, which corresponds to a 75% decrease in cross-sectional area. • Blood flow is best described by Poiseuille's law, written as $Q = \pi(P_1 - P_2)r^4/8L\eta$, where Q is flow, P is pressure, r is radius, L is length, and η is viscosity. • Flow is proportional to pressure and inversely proportional to the length of the stenosis and to the blood viscosity, but flow is directly related to the fourth power of the radius. • The radius is the most important factor when determining total blood flow.

ANSWER:
A

---

8. A patient with symptomatic (85%) carotid stenosis is found to have 50% stenosis of the contralateral carotid artery that is asymptomatic. Appropriate initial treatment includes which of the following?

   A. Simultaneous bilateral carotid endarterectomy

   B. Staged bilateral carotid endarterectomy with a 1-week interval between stages

   C. Carotid endarterectomy on the symptomatic side only

   D. Carotid endarterectomy on the side with the greatest stenosis, regardless of symptoms

Ref.: 3

COMMENTS: The long-term risk of asymptomatic carotid stenosis is not fully defined. • The Toronto Asymptomatic Bruit Trial observed an 18% annual incidence of neurologic events in patients with 75% stenosis. • Evaluation of patients with symptomatic disease who are found to have asymptomatic stenosis on the contralateral side suggests that, in 10–15% of patients, TIAs related to the asymptomatic lesion may develop, and approximately 1% of patients suffer stroke. • The latter rate occurs among patients whose lesions have 50–75% stenosis. • The risk for patients with more significant narrowing is not known and may be higher. • It therefore appears that patients with asymptomatic contralateral disease can be managed expectantly and that cerebral ischemic symptoms, when they do develop, are predominantly in the form of TIAs, which can be treated when they are manifested.

ANSWER:
C

9. After elective carotid endarterectomy, a patient is noted to exhibit a new neurologic deficit while in the recovery room. Appropriate management of this perioperative neurologic deficit includes which of the following?

   A. Immediate return of the patient to the operating room for neck exploration

   B. Noninvasive studies in the operating room to determine flow within the operated carotid artery

   C. Cerebral angiography

   D. Observation overnight

Ref.: 3

COMMENTS: The overriding concern for this patient is to be certain that no technical error has been made during surgery. • (The most common technical error is creation of an intimal flap.) • This possibility can be determined most effectively by immediately returning the patient to the operating room for a neck exploration. • The patient should be heparinized once the neck is opened and the artery checked for a pulse, a thrill, or intracarotid thrombosis. • If the pulse is diminished or there is evidence of thrombosis, the artery is reopened to examine it for thrombosis or flap elevation. • If there are no signs of a carotid problem when the neck is opened, an intraoperative duplex scan should be considered to identify intraluminal debris. • Intraoperative angiography also may be a useful maneuver in this desperate situation.

ANSWER:
A, B

10. With regard to long-term results of carotid endarterectomy, which of the following statements is/are true?

    A. The rate of restenosis is 10–15%.

    B. Restenosis is most commonly manifested as stroke.

    C. Ischemic cerebral events are the main cause of late death.

    D. Restenosis rates are higher when endarterectomy is performed for symptomatic disease than for asymptomatic disease.

Ref.: 2

COMMENTS: The combined operative morbidity and mortality rate for carotid endarterectomy should be less than 5%. • Coronary artery disease is the main cause of both immediate and late postoperative death. • There is a significant rate of restenosis (10–15%) after carotid endarterectomy, although most of these lesions are asymptomatic and not hemodynamically significant.

• It is therefore recommended that patients undergo annual B-mode duplex scanning to look for restenosis after having scans two or three times the first year.

ANSWER:
A

11. With regard to symptoms of vertebral basilar insufficiency (VBI) ischemia, which of the following statements is/are correct?

    A. They include diplopia, ataxia, vertigo, and tinnitus.

    B. They are usually indistinguishable from those of carotid insufficiency.

    C. They usually reflect unilateral vertebral disease.

    D. They are most commonly caused by emboli.

Ref.: 2

COMMENTS: Stenosis of the vertebral artery usually involves a localized segment near the origin from the subclavian artery. • Unlike carotid plaques, the stenotic lesions are usually smooth and nonulcerated, and ischemia is generally attributed to decreased flow rather than to an embolic phenomenon. • Although one vertebral artery is usually dominant, unilateral vertebral stenosis rarely produces symptoms. • Symptoms generally reflect bilateral disease. • Associated atherosclerotic involvement of the basilar artery is also common. • Symptoms of VBI ischemia are the same as those of brain stem ischemia and produce a characteristic clinical syndrome (diplopia, dysarthria, vertigo, and tinnitus) quite distinct from the cerebral hemispheric ischemia produced by carotid disease.

ANSWER:
A

12. Most patients with "subclavian steal" syndrome have which of the following conditions?

    A. Reversal of flow in the involved vertebral artery

    B. Disabling neurologic symptoms

    C. Upper-extremity claudication

    D. Decreased systolic blood pressure in the ipsilateral arm

Ref.: 1, 2

COMMENTS: "Subclavian steal" syndrome results from occlusion of a subclavian artery, rarely the innominate, with decreased systolic pressure distal to the obstruction. • This causes blood to flow up the contralateral vertebral area and across the basilar artery (from which more blood is "stolen") as it courses down (in a retrograde manner) the ipsilateral vertebral artery to help supply that subclavian artery. • Most patients with this phenomenon are asymptomatic and do not require intervention, although limb weakness and paresthesias or symptoms of VBI may occur, in which case intervention is appropriate.

ANSWER:
A, D

13. Amaurosis fugax is brought about by occlusion of which of the following arteries?

    A. Facial artery

    B. Occipital artery

C. Retinal artery

D. Posterior auricular artery

D. Horner's syndrome

E. Cerebral ischemia

Ref.: 1, 2

Ref.: 1, 2

COMMENTS: About 75% of patients who suffer a stroke have had a previous TIA. • Amaurosis fugax, one type of TIA (lasting minutes to hours), is manifested as ipsilateral blindness, described by the patient as being like a window shade being pulled across the eye. • It is caused by emboli traveling via the ophthalmic artery—the first intracerebral branch of the internal carotid artery—and lodging in the retinal artery. • These emboli may be seen on funduscopic examination and are called Hollenhorst plaques. • The other arteries listed are branches of the external carotid artery. • There are eight branches of the external carotid artery: superior thyroid, lingual, facial, ascending pharyngeal, occipital, posterior auricular, superficial temporal, and maxillary.

ANSWER:
C

14. Carotid body tumors are most commonly manifested by which of the following?

A. Hypertension

B. Painless neck mass

C. Cranial nerve deficit

COMMENTS: The carotid body is 3–4 mm in size and located within the adventitial tissue of the carotid bifurcation. • It arises from paraganglionic cells of neural crest origin. • Carotid-body tumors (chemodectomas) are uncommon, slow-growing (they may even remain stationary for long periods), and usually manifested as a painless mass. • There are two types of carotid body tumors: *sporadic* (5% of which are bilateral) and *autosomal dominant familial* (32% of which are bilateral). • The criteria for malignancy are controversial, influenced by the tumor's location, its biologic behavior, or evidence of local invasion or distal spread. • Most are benign. • The definitive treatment is excision.

ANSWER:
B

REFERENCES

1. Townsend CM Jr, Beauchamp RD, Evers BM, et al (eds): *Sabiston Textbook of Surgery: The Biological Basis of Modern Surgical Practice,* 17th ed. Saunders, Philadelphia, 2004.
2. Brunicardi FC, Andersen DK, Billiar TR, et al (eds): *Schwartz's Principles of Surgery,* 8th ed. McGraw-Hill, New York, 2004.
3. Ernst CB, Stanley JC: *Current Therapy in Vascular Surgery,* 3rd ed. CV Mosby, St. Louis, 2001.

C. Thoracic Aorta

Apostolos Tassiopolous, M.D., and Walter J. McCarthy, M.D.

1. With regard to ascending aortic aneurysms, which of the following statements is/are true?

   A. They are most often caused by connective tissue abnormalities.

   B. They may be related to earlier venereal disease.

   C. Most dissecting aneurysms begin in the ascending aorta.

   D. They are usually associated with aortic insufficiency.

   E. Death usually is caused by rupture, with resulting pneumothorax.

   Ref.: 1, 2

COMMENTS: Etiologic factors involved in aortic aneurysms vary according to the location of the aneurysm. • In the ascending aorta, a connective tissue abnormality recognized histologically as cystic medial necrosis is the most common underlying abnormality and is the defect seen in aneurysms associated with Marfan's syndrome. • Other known causes, such as syphilitic aneurysms, are steadily decreasing in frequency, and atherosclerotic aneurysms of the ascending aorta are relatively uncommon. • Most dissecting aneurysms do originate in the ascending aorta. • Aortic insufficiency occurs only when there is associated annular dilatation or when one or more aortic cusps are sheared off by an acute dissection. • Death from an ascending aortic aneurysm is usually caused by cardiac failure secondary to chronic untreated aortic insufficiency or to rupture into the pericardium with pericardial tamponade.

ANSWER:
A, B, C

2. With regard to the clinical characteristics and management of ascending aortic aneurysms, which of the following statements is/are true?

   A. Most ascending aortic aneurysms are asymptomatic and are detected primarily by routine chest radiographs.

   B. Valvar murmurs are rare.

   C. Aortography is contraindicated because of the risk of causing dissection of the aneurysm with the catheter.

   D. Operative management with placement of a composite graft of aortic conduit and aortic valve is the treatment of choice for all ascending aortic aneurysms.

   E. CT scanning with contrast is a good noninvasive modality with which to delineate the size and extent of an aortic aneurysm.

   Ref.: 1, 2

COMMENTS: Although relatively uncommon, an ascending aortic aneurysm may be manifested as a mass in the anterior chest wall.

• Patients are usually asymptomatic, in which case the aneurysm is likely to be detected on routine chest radiographs. • Aneurysms can be localized (saccular) or more generalized (fusiform). • When symptoms are present, they are commonly related to congestive heart failure caused by dilatation of the aortic annulus, resulting in aortic insufficiency and its characteristic murmur (an early diastolic murmur at the second interspace along the right sternal border). • This murmur often is present even in asymptomatic patients. • Rupture and cardiac failure are the most common causes of death in patients with thoracic artery aneurysms.

Aortography confirms the diagnosis and is important for defining the dimensional extent of the aneurysm and its relationship to the rest of the aorta, its major branches, and the coronary ostia.

Although surgical correction is clearly the treatment of choice, debate persists over the routine use of a composite valve–conduit graft. • The composite is widely used for aneurysms associated with massive dilatation of the aortic root, aortic annulus, and aortic leaflets (Bentall operation).

CT scanning with intravenous contrast and MRI are excellent noninvasive modalities that delineate the extent and size of an aneurysmal aorta, but they cannot take the place of aortography during the preoperative evaluation.

ANSWER:
A, E

3. Superior vena cava (SVC) syndrome is characterized by which of the following?

   A. Bronchogenic carcinoma with invasion into the mediastinum is the leading cause of SVC syndrome.

   B. Venous pressures in the SVC rarely exceed 15 mmHg.

   C. Acute obstruction of the SVC is rarely clinically significant because of the large number of collateral vessels available.

   D. Occlusion of the SVC between the azygos vein and the right atrium is better tolerated than is occlusion above the azygos vein.

   E. Surgical correction is rarely indicated.

   Ref.: 1, 2

COMMENTS: More than 90% of SVC obstructions are caused by malignant tumors, most often mediastinal invasion by bronchogenic carcinoma. • When obstruction occurs, venous pressures rise to 20–50 mmHg.

Acute complete obstruction allows little time for the formation of collateral vessels and therefore can produce significant edematous laryngeal obstruction and even fatal cerebral edema. • A more *gradual* onset of obstruction results in the characteristic clinical picture of facial swelling and dilatation of the collateral veins of the head and neck, arm, and upper thoracic areas. • Obstruction between the azygos vein and the right atrium is less disabling because the azygos vein provides a large collateral venous channel for drainage of the SVC system into the inferior vena caval system. • Obstruction above the azygos vein eliminates this collateral channel and is not as well tolerated.

The treatment of choice for obstruction caused by associated malignancy is prompt *radiation* therapy, often in association with diuretics and chemotherapy. • Surgery rarely is indicated for management of SVC obstruction because of the technical difficulties associated with vena caval grafts, the underlying poor prognosis in patients with malignant conditions, and the usual adequacy of collateral venous circulation in the rare instances of slowly developing obstruction caused by benign conditions. • The only indication for operation is the unusual instance of a benign problem in which collateral circulation does not relieve the symptoms. • Surgical management consists of either a replacement graft or a bypass. • In general, autologous grafts have performed better than prosthetic grafts. • Balloon angioplasty and stenting can be useful.

ANSWER:
A, D, E

4. Regarding thoracic aortic aneurysms in patients with Marfan's syndrome, which of the following statements is/are true?

A. Less than 50% of patients with Marfan's syndrome survive past the age of 45 years.

B. Ascending aortic aneurysms start at the aortic annulus and involve the coronary sinuses and the aortic valve.

C. All aneurismal dilatations greater than 4 cm should be treated with prophylactic replacement of the aortic root.

D. Surgical repair of an ascending aortic aneurysm usually requires replacement of the entire aortic root with a composite valve-graft.

E. The perioperative mortality rate exceeds 15%.

Ref.: 5

COMMENTS: The severely diminished longevity of patients with Marfan's syndrome has been well documented. • Fewer than 50% of all male and female patients with the syndrome survive past the age of 45 years. • Cardiac deaths account for more than 90% of early deaths of known cause, and 75% of these deaths are secondary to aortic root dilatation or aortic dissections and their complications. • Prophylactic aortic root replacement is recommended for all aneurysms larger than 6 cm in diameter. • In contrast to atherosclerotic aneurismal disease, aneurismal dilatations in patients with Marfan's syndrome involve not only the entire aorta, including the coronary sinuses, but also the cardiac valvular tissues. • Therefore, replacement of the entire aortic root, including the aortic valve, with a composite valve-graft is required in the majority of patients. • Improved techniques in myocardial protection have resulted in perioperative mortality rates of less than 5% in most recent series.

ANSWER:
A, B, D

5. With regard to thoracic trauma, match each statement in the left-hand column with the appropriate item in the right-hand column.

A. Aortography should be performed in most stable patients if injury is suspected.
  a. Penetrating chest injury

B. Cardiac tamponade is a major cause of death.
  b. Deceleration chest injury

C. Fatal hemorrhage is sometimes prevented by the aortic adventitia.
  c. Both

D. Thoracotomy may be indicated.
  d. Neither

Ref.: 1, 2

COMMENTS: Both penetrating and deceleration injuries of the thoracic aorta are commonly fatal. • When the patient is in extremis from exsanguination, thoracotomy in the emergency room to control hemorrhage may be indicated, even though success is unlikely. • In clinically stable patients, aortography is indicated for both types of injury to define the anatomy of the injury because it may influence the choice of surgical approach. • With penetrating injuries, pericardial tamponade, in addition to exsanguination, is a major cause of death. • With deceleration injuries, complete disruption of the aorta is nearly always fatal. • In some instances, however, the adventitia remains intact, confining the hemorrhage and allowing time for surgical correction. • With severe blunt trauma to the chest, the possibility of aortic injury must be suspected, and aortography should be used liberally. • Mediastinal widening (>8.0 cm) with loss of the aortic window contour remains the key to diagnosis. • CT scans and MRI are currently being evaluated as noninvasive screening tests, but they have not been shown to be as valuable as aortography for establishing the diagnosis.

ANSWER:
A-c; B-a; C-b; D-c

6. With regard to aortic dissection, match each item in the left-hand column with the appropriate item or items in the right-hand column.

A. Related to Marfan's syndrome.
  a. Type I

B. Readily accessible to surgical excision
  b. Type II

C. Early causes of death due to cardiac tamponade and acute aortic insufficiency.
  c. Type III-A

D. Can have multiple points of entry and reentry
  d. Type III-B

E. Primarily treated surgically

Ref.: 1, 2

COMMENTS: Aortic dissections have been classified by Michael DeBakey according to their site of origin and extent of aortic involvement. • **Type I** originates in the ascending aorta and dissects throughout the entire thoracic and abdominal aorta. • **Type II** originates in the ascending aorta but is confined to that segment of the aorta and is the type commonly seen in Marfan's syndrome. • **Type III-A** originates distal to the left subclavian artery but remains confined to the descending thoracic aorta. • It is readily accessible to surgical excision. • **Type III-B** originates distal to the left subclavian artery but dissects down into the abdominal aorta, which complicates its surgical repair. • Definition of the origin and extent of aortic dissection is of paramount importance because these considerations dictate therapy. • Most dissections occur in the inner third or half of the aortic wall. • The underlying defect is the destruction of the media from an unknown cause. • Hypertension is present in 80–90% of patients and in well over 95% of those with dissection of the descending aorta. • Dissections originating in the ascending aorta most commonly occur through the entire length, whereas those originating distal to the subclavian artery occur distal to that point. • Multiple entry and reentry points are seen in type I dissections.

After initial presentation and diagnosis, antihypertensive therapy (nitroprusside) should be instituted. • Nearly all patients with ascending aortic dissection (types I and II) should be operated on immediately. • Early causes of death in patients with type I and II dissections are rupture, cardiac tamponade, and acute aortic insufficiency. • The goal of operation is to correct aortic insufficiency and to graft the ascending aorta, with obliteration of the false lumen. • Dissections of the descending aorta require prompt operation if signs of visceral ischemia are present or if rupture has occurred. • In the absence of the aforementioned indications, operation can be postponed. • Thirty percent of such patients ultimately require an operation because of an enlarging aneurysm. • The Stanford classification includes dissections starting in the ascending aorta as type A and those starting in the descending aorta as type B. • Management principles are the same as those for the DeBakey classification.

A N S W E R :
A-b; B-c; C-a, b; D-a; E-a, b

7. Regarding treatment of acute Stanford type B aortic dissections, which of the following statements are/is true?

   A. The most important initial treatment is control of hypertension to prevent proximal extension of the dissection.

   B. Surgical treatment is required for all patients presenting with limb, renal, or mesenteric ischemia.

   C. Surgical treatment always requires a left thoracotomy.

   D. Cardiopulmonary bypass can reduce complications during replacement of the descending thoracic aorta.

   E. Endovascular techniques have no role in these patients.

Ref.: 1, 2

COMMENTS: For patients with acute Stanford type B dissections, hemodynamic stabilization with control of hypertension to levels adequate for maintenance of cerebral, myocardial, and renal perfusion is the immediate goal of medical therapy. • Although sodium nitroprusside is the traditional pharmacologic therapy of choice, intravenous esmolol more effectively reduces the aortic and left ventricular hyperdynamic state and helps prevent proximal extension of the dissection. • Patients presenting with renal, mesenteric, or limb ischemia can be treated nonoperatively with stents, stent grafts, or balloon septostomy. • Placement of a thoracic aortic stent-graft in the proximal descending thoracic aorta results in obliteration of the false lumen and redirection of flow into the true lumen and has been associated with significantly lower perioperative mortality. • If endovascular techniques fail or are not available, patients with ischemic symptoms require surgical revascularization. • This can be accomplished through a left posterolateral thoracotomy, with placement of an interposition graft in the proximal descending aorta and obliteration of the false lumen. • Distal aortic perfusion with the use of left atriofemoral or femorofemoral cardiopulmonary bypass reduces renal, visceral, and spinal cord ischemia time during this procedure and thereby the

incidence of perioperative complications. • An alternative approach is infrarenal aortic graft placement with surgical septostomy and obliteration of the distal false lumen in order to restore lower extremity blood flow. • If only the leg(s) is/are ischemic, femorofemoral or axillobifemoral bypass is a less invasive procedure if leg ischemia cannot be treated with endovascular techniques.

A N S W E R :
A, D

8. With regard to blunt traumatic rupture of the aorta, which of the following statements is/are correct?

   A. The most common site of rupture is distal to the left subclavian artery at the point of insertion of the ligamentum arteriosum.

   B. Nearly 90% of patients die at the scene of the accident.

   C. The intima provides nearly 60% of the strength of the thoracic aorta and must remain intact for the patient to survive.

   D. There is still a high risk of free aortic rupture, even in patients who survive the first 6 weeks after injury.

   E. Bypass support is mandatory for its correction.

Ref.: 1, 2

COMMENTS: About 85–90% of patients who sustain an aortic rupture die at the scene of the accident. • Patients who sustain rupture of the ascending aorta rarely reach the hospital alive. • In most patients who survive, the rupture is located at the aortic isthmus (immediately distal to the origin of the left subclavian artery). • The aortic adventitia provides 60% of the tensile strength of the thoracic aorta. • For someone to survive blunt trauma to the aorta, this layer must remain intact to prevent a free rupture and exsanguinating hemorrhage. • Of the patients who initially survive and are merely observed because the pathologic process is not recognized or for some other reason, 20% die within 6 hr, and 72% die within 1 week. • If a patient survives 6–8 weeks after injury, the risk of free aortic rupture is low. • There is evidence that, if an operation is performed expeditiously with appropriate monitoring of somatosensory potentials to prevent paraplegia, with adequate physiologic support, and with control of blood pressure with nitroprusside, simple aortic clamping without bypass is equally safe, and the operative time and blood loss are significantly less. • Cardiopulmonary bypass is, however, commonly used for these operations.

A N S W E R :
A, B

9. With regard to thoracoabdominal aneurysms, which of the following statements is/are true?

   A. They may present with symptoms of compression of adjacent structures.

   B. Paraplegia and renal failure are the most common complications of elective repair.

   C. Type IV aneurysms are associated with the highest incidence of paraplegia.

   D. Endovascular repair is usually feasible for these aneurysms.

Ref.: 1, 2

COMMENTS: Thoracoabdominal aneurysms occur primarily in older patients with extensive atherosclerosis and are infrequent in comparison with infrarenal aortic aneurysms. • The cephalad location of the abdominal component frequently precludes palpation because of the overlying pancreas and the stomach. • Thirty percent of patients in a large series were asymptomatic, and the condition was first diagnosed on routine chest radiographs, which revealed dilatation of the aorta at the diaphragm. • A major advance in the treatment of these aneurysms was made by E. Stanley Crawford, who developed the intraluminal graft technique. • This procedure has significantly reduced rates of morbidity and mortality associated with surgical repair. • Technical difficulties during surgical repair, including the need to reimplant the celiac, superior mesenteric, and renal arteries, increase the risk of this operation sufficiently that repair is usually warranted only for symptomatic or significantly enlarging aneurysms. • Paraplegia, resulting from temporary or permanent loss of spinal cord blood flow, can occur in 20–40% of cases. • The frequency can be reduced by draining spinal fluid with a lumbar drain. • Distal aortic pressure above 60 mmHg, rather than flow rate, is the key to perfusion of the spinal cord. • Reattachment of large lumbar vessels has helped lower the incidence of paraplegia to 15%.

Thoracoabdominal aneurysms can compress the main stem bronchus, pulmonary tissue, and/or esophagus. • Type IV aneurysms are from the diaphragm distally and have the lowest risk of paraplegia with repair. • Endovascular repair of thoracoabdominal aneurysms is in its infancy, but the use of grafts with side branches and fenestrations is sometimes possible.

ANSWER:
A, B, D

---

10. With regard to transverse aortic arch aneurysms, which of the following statements is/are true?

A. Cystic medial necrosis is a major cause.

B. Repair is associated with the highest operative mortality rate of any of the aortic aneurysms.

C. Differentiation from mediastinal tumors is usually possible on standard chest radiograms.

D. Deep hypothermia with circulatory arrest and cardiopulmonary bypass are associated with a significantly reduced the mortality rate due to repair of these aneurysms.

Ref.: 1, 2

COMMENTS: Transverse aortic arch aneurysms are almost always the result of atherosclerosis. • In asymptomatic individuals, they are most often detected on routine chest radiograms. • Aortography and CT scanning, however, are required to differentiate them from mediastinal tumors and to define the vascular anatomy before repair. • Concomitant association with coronary and cerebrovascular disease, together with the need to disrupt flow to the brain temporarily during repair, has resulted in an operative mortality rate that exceeds that for repair of other aortic aneurysms. • The introduction of cardiopulmonary bypass and hypothermic circulatory arrest has significantly reduced this operative mortality rate. • Spiral CT scanning is used rather than aortography in some centers.

ANSWER:
B, D

---

11. Radiographic signs of aortic injury secondary to blunt chest trauma include which of the following?

A. Widening of the mediastinum

B. Blunting of the aortic knob

C. Left apical capping

D. Depression of the left main bronchus

Ref.: 1, 2

COMMENTS: Blunt injury to the thoracic aorta may occur without clinical signs or symptoms that such an injury is present. • Often, the mechanism of injury (sudden deceleration from vehicular accidents or falls) and a high index of suspicion obligate the examining physician to rule out aortic trauma by aortography. • Radiographic signs of aortic injury, when present, include blunting of the aortic knob, widening of the mediastinum (to 8.0 cm), deviation of the trachea to the right, left apical blunting, and depression of the left main bronchus. • Even when these radiographic signs are present, aortography is required to define precisely the anatomy and the extent of the vascular injury. • Spiral CT scanning is used rather than aortography in some centers.

ANSWER:
A, B, C, D

---

12. With regard to aortic dissections, which of the following statements is/are correct?

A. DeBakey type I aortic dissection begins in the proximal aorta.

B. Stanford type B aortic dissection is limited to the descending thoracic aorta.

C. Hypertension is found in up to 30% of patients with aortic dissection.

D. Atherosclerosis is the most common cause of aortic dissection.

E. Aortic regurgitation is present in 50–75% of patients with acute proximal aortic dissection.

Ref.: 1–3

COMMENTS: *Dissection* is the most common catastrophic event affecting the aorta and is approximately two to three times more frequent than *rupture* of an abdominal aortic aneurysm (AAA). • The most commonly accepted classifications are those of DeBakey and Stanford. • With the Stanford classification, a type A dissection is one involving the ascending aorta, regardless of the site of origin or the distal extent of the process. • Dissection of the descending thoracic aortic is designated type B.

With the DeBakey classification, type I begins in the proximal aorta and involves most of the entire vessel. • Type II involves only the ascending aorta. • Dissection of the descending thoracic aorta is termed type III.

Most authors believe atherosclerosis is coincidental rather than causative of aortic *dissection*. • This is different from thoracic aortic *aneurysms*, in which atherosclerosis is considered a causative factor. • *Hypertension* is found in 60–90% of patients presenting with aortic dissection and is more commonly seen with type B (90%) than with type A (60%) dissection. • *Aortic valve cusps* prolapse in aortic dissection involving the proximal aorta. • The aortic valve can usually be repaired by resuspension of the cusps of the valve. • Preservation of the native valve is possible in 70–90% of patients with acute type A dissections. • Postoperative freedom from the need of valve replacement at 10 years is 90%. • In contrast, patients with dilated aortic roots or with Marfan's syndrome require composite root replacement rather than resuspension or repair of the aortic valve.

ANSWER:
A, B, E

13. With regard to diagnosis and treatment of aortic dissection, which of the following statements is/are true?

A. Aortography and coronary angiography are essential before surgery for type A acute aortic dissection.

B. Transesophageal echocardiography is highly accurate for diagnosing acute aortic dissection.

C. Type B acute aortic dissection is treated primarily medically.

D. Surgical treatment of acute type A dissection is similar in patients with or without Marfan's syndrome.

E. With chronic type B dissection, the indications for surgery are related to the size of the aneurysm, symptoms of pain, and development of visceral, renal, and neurologic ischemia.

Ref.: 1–4

COMMENTS: Coronary angiography before emergency repair of acute proximal aortic dissection is not recommended. • Even in the presence of moderate coronary artery disease, early repair of the dissection has precedence over other procedures. • Since its introduction in 1984, the use of transesophageal echocardiography to diagnose aortic dissection has gained acceptance by many surgeons. • It has a sensitivity and specificity of 99 and 98%, respectively. • Since it can be performed in the emergency room or the operating room, it does not require transferring the patient to a separate area, as does angiography. • It can also assess the function of the left ventricle, the aortic valve, and the mitral valve.

Type B aortic dissection is treated primarily medically by instituting strict control of hypertension. • Indications for surgery for acute type B dissection are limited to prevention or relief of life-threatening complications (i.e., aortic rupture, ischemia of limbs and organ systems, persistent pain, or uncontrolled hypertension).

Patients with Marfan's syndrome have more extensive pathologic involvement of the tissue, which necessitates a more extensive dissection process. • There is general agreement that a composite root replacement with aortic valve and aortic graft, rather than an interposition graft alone, is the surgical treatment of choice for patients with Marfan's syndrome.

ANSWER:
B, C, E

14. A 50-year-old man involved in a deceleration-type motor vehicle accident is brought to the emergency room. He has a systolic blood pressure of 90 mmHg. Chest radiograms reveal a widened mediastinum. He has a bilateral pelvic fracture and a tender abdomen. Which of the following statements is/are true about this patient?

A. Management should begin with aortography to evaluate the widened mediastinum.

B. The most common site of traumatic aortic rupture is distal to the left subclavian artery.

C. Repair of this type of injury virtually always requires cardiopulmonary bypass.

D. Rarely, this type of injury presents 10 years after the accident.

E. The risk of paraplegia following repair of the thoracic aorta can be avoided if certain precautions are taken.

Ref.: 1, 2, 4

COMMENTS: Patients with multiple injuries and suspected aortic tear should have certain associated injuries addressed first (e.g., extensive pelvic fractures or intra-abdominal injuries). • In this patient, diagnostic peritoneal lavage or immediate abdominal CT scanning should be done before evaluating the widened mediastinum. • The most common site of an aortic tear is just distal to the left subclavian artery. • Although cardiopulmonary bypass may be required in certain patients with an extensive aortic tear, tears can be treated by a partial shunt between the left atrium or ascending aorta and the descending aorta. • Although patients with a thoracic aorta tear can have a successful repair, many patients with this injury die at the accident scene. • Some arrive at the hospital and die during initial resuscitation. • Rarely, such patients present with chronic dissection up to 15 years after the accident.

Paraplegia following repair of the thoracic aorta remains one of the most distressing complications associated with the operation. • Aortic cross-clamp time, distal aortic pressure monitoring, and cerebrospinal fluid drainage by spinal tap have been utilized. • However, none of these steps has proved reliable for eliminating the risk of postoperative paraplegia, which is 3–10%.

ANSWER:
B, D

R E F E R E N C E S

1. Townsend CM Jr, Beauchamp RD, Evers BM, et al (eds): *Sabiston Textbook of Surgery: The Biological Basis of Modern Surgical Practice,* 17th ed. Saunders, Philadelphia, 2004.
2. Brunicardi FC, Andersen DK, Billiar TR, et al (eds): *Schwartz's Principles of Surgery*: 8th ed. McGraw-Hill, New York, 2004.
3. Edmunds LH (ed): *Cardiac Surgery in the Adult.* McGraw-Hill, New York, 1997.
4. Crawford ES, Crawford JL, Safi HJ, Coselli JS, et al: Thoracoabdominal aortic aneurysms: preoperative and intraoperative factors determining immediate and long-term results of operations in 605 patients. *J Vasc Surg* 3:389–404, 1986.
5. Mullholland MW, Lillemoe KD, Doherty GM, et al (eds): *Greenfield's Surgery: Scientific Principles and Practice*, 4th ed. Lippincott, Williams & Wilkins, Philadelphia, 2006.

D. Abdominal Aorta

Apostolos Tassiopolous, M.D., and Walter J. McCarthy, M.D.

1. Which of the following may be acceptable treatment for occlusive aortoiliac disease?

   A. Thromboendarterectomy

   B. Aortofemoral bypass

   C. Axillofemoral bypass

   D. Percutaneous balloon angioplasty

Ref.: 1–3

COMMENTS: The basic goal of arterial revascularization for occlusive arterial disease is to reestablish adequate blood flow to the tissue being supplied. • In patients with occlusive aortoiliac disease who require surgery, a variety of techniques are applicable, depending on the site and extent of obstruction, the presence or absence of aneurysmal disease, and the patient's underlying medical condition (Table 1). • **Thromboendarterectomy** (TEA) is appropriate for some patients with disease confined to the distal aorta and common iliac arteries. • Results of TEA are similar to those with aortofemoral bypass grafting. • TEA is contraindicated in the presence of aneurysmal disease and disease that extends to the external iliac arteries and is gradually being abandoned with the development of percutaneous endovascular techniques. • **Aortofemoral bypass grafting** produces excellent results in terms of immediate and long-term patency and relief of claudication. • The long-term patency rates are reported to be as high as 90%. • **Axillofemoral** and **thoracofemoral** bypass grafts have been successful in patients in whom an abdominal operation may pose excessive risk, including those with infected aortic prosthetic grafts, those with previously occluded aortofemoral grafts, and those with a "hostile" abdomen. • **Femorofemoral** and **ileofemoral** bypass grafts are used when only one iliac artery is diseased. • **Percutaneous balloon angioplasty** is successful for isolated short-segment lesions of the iliac arteries in patients with good distal runoff. • This may yield 5-year patency rates as high as 80%. • Angioplasty can also be used to dilate an iliac stenosis before a more distal bypass. • The addition of intraluminal stents has broadened the number and location of lesions amenable to balloon angioplasty and has increased the technical success rates of these procedures. • Disadvantages of percutaneous angioplasty include a lower rate of overall success in patients with poor distal runoff or limb-threatening ischemia and the potential complications of intimal dissection, vascular occlusion or rupture, and distal embolization.

ANSWER:
A, B, C, D

2. Which of the following is the most common graft-related late complication of aortic bypass grafts?

   A. Graft occlusion caused by progressive atherosclerosis

   B. Suture line pseudoaneurysm

   C. Aortoenteric fistula

   D. Distal embolization

   E. Infection caused by transient bacteremia

Ref.: 2

COMMENTS: The long-term patency rates of aortofemoral bypass grafts are reported to range from approximately 65–90%. • The most common graft-related late complication is **graft occlusion**, which develops in 10–35% of cases. • The most common cause of graft occlusion is progressive atherosclerosis, usually occurring at or just beyond the distal anastomosis. • Other late complications include **anastomotic pseudoaneurysm** (1–5%) and **graft infection** (1%), both of which occur more often when a femoral anastomosis is involved. • **Aortoenteric fistula** is rare but carries a high mortality rate (50%). • Therefore, it should be a primary consideration in any patient with a previous abdominal aortic graft who has gastrointestinal bleeding. • Most often, there is bleeding into the third portion of the duodenum from the proximal aortic suture line.

ANSWER:
A

3. What is the most common cause of death after recovery from successful aortic bypass graft?

   A. Rupture of pseudoaneurysm

   B. Acute graft thrombosis

   C. Cerebrovascular accident

   D. Coronary artery disease

   E. Complications of peripheral vascular disease

   F. Renal failure

Ref.: 1, 3

COMMENTS: Associated **coronary artery disease** is the leading cause of death after aortic reconstruction. • Predictive risk factors for postoperative cardiac events include age over 70 years, previous myocardial infarction, history of ventricular arrhythmias, diabetes mellitus, and angina pectoris. • The dipyridamole thallium stress test has an excellent negative predictive value for postoperative cardiac complications. • Combining clinical markers with dipyridamole thallium stress testing increases the specificity of dipyridamole thallium alone. • Aggressive preoperative cardiac evaluation is justified to define a patient's operative risk and to identify patients who would benefit from further invasive cardiac evaluation and therapy.

ANSWER:
D

4. Which of the following is the most common manifestation of an AAA?

 A. Incidental finding on physical examination or by CT scan done for unrelated disease.

 B. Back or abdominal pain

 C. Acute rupture

 D. Spontaneous thrombosis with peripheral ischemia

 E. Peripheral embolization

Ref.: 1, 2, 4

COMMENTS: Approximately three fourths of all AAAs are discovered incidentally and are asymptomatic. • The most common complaint in patients with symptoms is vague abdominal pain. • Patients may also note back or flank pain. • AAAs may expand without symptoms, erode into the adjacent vertebral bodies, partially obstruct the duodenum or ureters (inflammatory aneurysms), embolize, thrombose, or rupture. • Rare manifestations include aortoenteric fistula and aortocaval fistula. • The latter present with an abdominal bruit, venous hypertension, and high-output cardiac failure. • Rupture may mimic other acute intra-abdominal emergencies, such as diverticulitis and renal colic, and may be manifested by acute abdominal pain followed by transient hypotension and eventual vascular collapse. • Signs and symptoms of acute ischemia in the lower extremities may follow thrombosis or embolization from an abdominal aneurysm.

ANSWER:
A

5. With regards to preoperative imaging of AAAs, which of the following statements is/are true?

 A. High-quality CT scanning with and without intravenous contrast provides adequate information for surgical planning in the majority of AAAs.

 B. Arteriography provides more accurate measurements of the size of the aneurysm than does CT scanning.

 C. Arteriography is helpful when there is clinical suspicion of occlusive disease of the renal, mesenteric, or iliofemoral arteries.

 D. Arteriography is the test of choice for identifying candidates for endovascular repair.

 E. The presence of a horseshoe kidney or an ectopic kidney on CT scanning is an indication for arteriography before elective AAA repair.

Ref.: 1, 3, 4

COMMENTS: CT scanning with intravenous contrast is the most commonly used preoperative study to obtain the anatomic information necessary to plan surgical repair of AAAs. • CT scans provide the most accurate measurement of aneurysm size and important anatomic information regarding the proximal and distal extent of the aneurysm, the degree of calcification of the aortic wall, and certain anatomic variants that could complicate surgery. • The new-generation CT scanners offer three-dimensional reconstructions that are particularly helpful in identifying candidates for endovascular repair. • Therefore, CT scanning has largely replaced arteriography in the evaluation of patients with AAAs. • Arteriography is still helpful for patients with occlusive disease of the renal, mesenteric, or iliofemoral arteries who might benefit

from a simultaneous repair. • It is also indicated in the presence of an ectopic or horseshoe kidney for accurate delineation of aberrant renal arteries.

ANSWER:
A, C, E

6. Which of the following are acceptable indications for operation on an AAA?

 A. Any AAA

 B. Symptomatic aneurysm of any size

 C. Symptomatic aneurysm larger than 5 cm in diameter

 D. Asymptomatic aneurysm larger than 5 cm in diameter

 E. Asymptomatic 4.5-cm aneurysm involving the renal arteries

Ref.: 2, 4

COMMENTS: The natural history of most AAAs is progressive enlargement. • The risk of rupture is directly related to the size of the aneurysm. • This relates to the law of Laplace, according to which the mean tension (T) in the wall of a vessel is directly proportional to the product of the radius (R) and the intraluminal pressure (P). • Therefore, an increase in radius (expansion) or pressure (hypertension) results in an increase in wall tension: $T = P \times R$. • Approximately one half of deaths in patients with untreated AAAs are caused by rupture. • The risk of rupture of an aneurysm 5–5.9 cm in diameter is approximately 3.4% per year. • Two recent independent studies in the United States and the United Kingdom have shown no survival benefit for elective repair of asymptomatic aneurysms measuring up to 5.5 cm in diameter. • Since the risk of rupture increases dramatically with diameters larger the 5.5 cm, elective repair is indicated for all aneurysms above that size. • Ruptured aneurysms carry a 50% mortality rate among patients who reach the hospital alive. • Any patients with symptoms suggestive of impending rupture or with a proven contained rupture should be operated on immediately. • Ultrasound imaging provides a reliable noninvasive method for observing patients with small asymptomatic aneurysms. • The anticipated growth rate is 0.4 cm/year. • When growth rate exceeds 0.6 cm/year, the risk of rupture is high, and elective repair is a reasonable approach for aneurysms measuring at least 4.5 cm in diameter, provided the patient is a good surgical candidate. • Diastolic hypertension and severe chronic obstructive pulmonary disease are thought to be predictors of expansion and rupture, especially for large aneurysms. • The decision to operate must therefore be based on considerations of size, shape (saccular is more ominous than fusiform), presence of symptoms, cardiac risk, and presence of cerebrovascular or chronic obstructive pulmonary disease. • The mortality rate of elective repair is approximately 3–5%.

ANSWER:
B, C, E

7. With regard to the operative approach for open repair of AAAs, which of the following statements is/are true?

 A. There is no true indication for a retroperitoneal approach.

 B. Extent of the aneurysm to the right common iliac artery is an absolute contraindication to a retroperitoneal approach.

 C. The retroperitoneal approach is associated with a lower incidence of paralytic ileus.

D. The midline transperitoneal approach is associated with a higher incidence of pulmonary complications.

E. The retroperitoneal approach can be used for ruptured AAA repair.

Ref.: 3

COMMENTS: There are many reported indications for the retroperitoneal approach to the infrarenal aorta. • A "hostile abdomen," usually resulting from multiple transabdominal procedures, irradiation, or the presence of enteric or urinary stomas, is the most common. • The retroperitoneal approach is also useful for patients with ascites, peritoneal dialysis catheters, morbid obesity, inflammatory aneurysms, and a horseshoe kidney. • Relative contraindications to the use of the retroperitoneal approach include the presence of right renal artery stenosis, ruptured AAA, and AAA with a left-sided inferior vena cava (IVC). • The presence of a right common iliac artery aneurysm is not an absolute contraindication to the retroperitoneal approach. • In these cases, the right iliac aneurysm is excluded by oversewing the ostium of the right common iliac artery through the open aorta, making a right lower quadrant transplant incision, ligating the distal neck of the iliac aneurysm, and extending the right limb of the bifurcated aortic graft to the right external iliac or right common femoral artery. • Alternatively, the distal neck of the aneurysm is not ligated, but the distal right external iliac or the proximal right common femoral artery is ligated, followed by extension of the right limb of the graft to the right common femoral artery. • The latter approach has the disadvantage of allowing backflow to the iliac aneurysm via the right internal iliac artery, which may result (on rare occasions) in iliac aneurysm enlargement and rupture. • Although most surgeons avoid the retroperitoneal approach for ruptured AAAs, several centers with extensive experience have reported successful use of this approach in selected cases of ruptured AAAs.

At least four prospective randomized studies have confirmed that the retroperitoneal approach is associated with decreased incidence of postoperative ileus and shorter hospital stay. • There was no significant difference in the incidence of pulmonary complications, perhaps due to the increasing use of epidural analgesia in the postoperative period for patients undergoing AAA repair.

A N S W E R :
C, E

8. With regard to the operative technique of AAA repair, which of the following statements is/are true?

A. Bifurcation grafts are preferred to straight grafts, even if the iliac vessels are not involved.

B. An endoaneurysmal approach is most commonly used today.

C. Bleeding lumbar vessels are routinely ligated from within the aneurysm sac.

D. The inferior mesenteric artery is routinely reimplanted in elderly patients to prevent ischemia of the left colon.

E. Flow should first be restored to the external iliac vessels when the cross-clamps are removed.

F. To avoid tissue necrosis and risk of infection, most of the aneurysm wall is resected before closure.

Ref.: 1, 2, 4

COMMENTS: Details of the operative technique for repair of AAAs vary somewhat, depending on individual circumstances, but several general principles should be emphasized. • Proximal control is established distal to the renal vessels after identifying the left renal vein. • Manipulation of the aorta is kept to a minimum to prevent embolization of aneurysm contents. • After the proximal and distal clamps are applied, the aneurysm is opened and the thrombus evacuated. • The lumbar vessels are ligated from within the aneurysm sac. • The inferior mesenteric artery (IMA) can usually be safely ligated precisely at its origin, thereby avoiding any collateral vessels within the mesentery of the left colon. • If backflow from the inferior mesenteric artery is poor, consideration should be given to reimplanting the artery to the side of the prosthesis. • Some surgeons evaluate backflow by viewing the IMA orifice from inside the opened aneurysm. • Others measure the IMA stump pressure and find that a pressure of less than 40 mmHg is a reason to reimplant.

Flow to at least one hypogastric artery should be preserved to maintain collateral flow to the colon via the middle hemorrhoidal arteries. • If ischemic injury to the left colon is suspected, a second-look laparotomy should be performed 24 hr later.

Because most of the aneurysm sac is preserved, the posterior suture lines consist of a double thickness of aorta. • This provides more suture line strength and hemostasis because the graft is sutured to the aorta from within the aneurysm sac in an end-to-end manner.

A tube graft is preferable to a bifurcation graft when the common iliac arteries are uninvolved. • Tube grafts avoid the need for an additional anastomosis, avoid an increased risk of dissection, and avoid the increased incidence of infection associated with anastomosis performed in the groin.

In some instances in which the aneurysm is extensive, the celiac, superior mesenteric, and renal arteries are involved. • These aneurysms require more complex revascularization procedures, including reimplantation of the vessels previously mentioned.

After graft placement, proper techniques of aortic flushing and sequential unclamping are important to minimize the risk of hypotension, declamping shock, and distal embolization. • The latter is accomplished by adequate flushing before completing the distal anastomosis and opening the circulation first into the internal iliacs and then into the external iliacs.

The surgeon should control the systemic arterial pressure with finger pressure on the graft until appropriate volume replacement has been accomplished.

Hypotension after removal of the aortic cross-clamp is believed to occur on the basis of washout of acidic metabolites and vasoactive substances from the ischemic lower extremities, third-space loss into permeable distal tissues, and sudden flow into vasodilated beds, as well as vascular steal secondary to reactive hyperemia in the lower extremities.

The aneurysm sac is not extensively resected and is closed over the prosthetic graft to isolate the graft from the duodenum and to minimize the risk of erosion and fistulization.

A N S W E R :
B, C

9. Two days after an uncomplicated repair of an AAA, bloody diarrhea develops in the patient, who is still receiving antibiotics. The differential diagnosis includes which of the following?

A. Coagulopathy

B. Pseudomembranous colitis

C. Ischemic colitis

D. Aortoenteric fistula

E. Acute hepatic failure

Ref.: 1–3

COMMENTS: The main concern in this situation is that **ischemic colitis** may have developed as a result of interruption of flow to the inferior mesenteric artery without adequate collateral blood supply from the superior mesenteric or hypogastric artery (or both) to the sigmoid colon. • It is important to realize that diarrhea, whether Hemoccult positive or negative, is one of the first signs of ischemic colitis. • Less commonly, ischemic colitis can also develop as a result of embolization of atheromatous debris into the mesenteric circulation during aneurysm repair. • The reported incidence of clinically significant ischemia is 1–2%. • Additional risk factors related to ischemia include duration and placement of cross-clamping, hypotension, and cardiac arrhythmias. • Ischemia occurs more commonly in patients with previous colon resection and those undergoing total redo aortic graft reoperation. • Immediate proctosigmoidoscopy is important during the initial evaluation of such a patient to assess colonic viability. • The rectum is usually spared, and ischemic changes, seen through the sigmoidoscope as pale, patchy areas with membranes, can be visualized 10–20 cm from the anal verge. • Ischemic colitis may be limited to the mucosa or may be transmural. • Management must be individualized. • The presence of associated increasing abdominal tenderness, peritoneal signs, fever, and elevated white blood cell count point to a transmural process that necessitates operation. • Resection of the descending and sigmoid colon with Hartmann's pouch and end-colostomy is required for transmural necrosis, to prevent gross spillage and graft contamination. • **Pseudomembranous enterocolitis** associated with antibiotic use is also a consideration, although it occurs somewhat later during the postoperative course. • Evaluation of the possibility of pseudomembranous colitis includes proctosigmoidoscopy with biopsy and examination of stool for *Clostridium difficile* toxin. • Treatment involves supportive measures and the administration of vancomycin or metronidazole enterally. • **Aortoenteric fistula** is a late complication of aortic aneurysm repair, resulting from erosion of a false aneurysm at the proximal aortic suture line into the duodenum or, on occasion, the sigmoid colon. • It is not a likely diagnosis in this clinical scenario. • **Coagulopathy** usually is not manifested by bloody diarrhea, but hepatic function and the coagulation profile should be promptly assessed if a bleeding diathesis is suspected.

ANSWER:
B, C

10. With regard to rupture of an AAA, which of the following statements is/are true?

    A. It is the most common cause of death in patients with an untreated AAA.

    B. The rate of associated operative mortality is 30–50%.

    C. Control of the proximal aorta can be accomplished endoluminally.

    D. The highest mortality rates occur in patients with preexisting coronary artery disease.

    E. Female patients with ruptured AAAs have a better chance of survival than do males.

Ref.: 1–4

COMMENTS: Rupture of an AAA is a catastrophic complication that may be heralded by abdominal, back, or flank pain followed by vascular collapse. • It is the most common cause of death among patients with *untreated* abdominal aneurysm, with a mortality rate of 30–50%, although nearly that many patients die of associated atherosclerotic problems, including cardiac, cerebral, or renal disease. • The mortality rate associated with elective resection is 5% or less.

Immediate operation and control of the proximal aorta is mandatory if the patients are to survive. • These procedures are accomplished best transabdominally at a level just below the diaphragm. • Although there are proponents of the retroperitoneal exposure for surgical management of a ruptured AAA, most surgeons believe that a midline incision allows better exposure and control of the ruptured abdominal aorta. • With free abdominal rupture or retroperitoneal rupture above the renal vein, manual compression of the aorta can be used at the level of the crus of the diaphragm for control. • Infrarenal control can then be obtained in the same manner as during an elective aneurysm repair. • A large Foley or Fogarty catheter can be placed in the aneurysm and inflated to achieve immediate control.

The most significant predictors of mortality are the presence of preoperative hypotension and a low hematocrit. • Other factors include age, intraperitoneal rupture, transfusion requirements, and gender (females have a higher mortality rate). • The presence of preexisting coronary disease is not the most significant preoperative factor in the mortality due to a ruptured AAA.

ANSWER:
A, B, D

11. Which one of the following complications occurs most commonly after successful repair of an AAA in a 58-year-old man?

    A. Sexual dysfunction

    B. Ischemic colitis

    C. Renal failure

    D. Peripheral embolization

    E. Leg paralysis

Ref.: 1, 2, 4

COMMENTS: All of these complications may occur after repair of an AAA, but, with appropriate operative technique, most of them are uncommon, except for changes in sexual function. • Retrograde ejaculation has been reported in as many as two thirds and loss of potency in as many as one third of such patients. • These changes may result from injury to the autonomic nerve fibers overlying the anterior aorta near the origin of the inferior mesenteric artery or injury to those fibers overlying the proximal left common iliac artery and aortic bifurcation. • Avoiding excessive aortic dissection in this region can help minimize this complication. • Documentation that sexual dysfunction existed preoperatively is of obvious importance in aortoiliac surgery, inasmuch as the incidence of impotence in men of this age with no aortoiliac occlusive disease is considerable. • Unilateral, isolated iliac artery obstruction in men is often best treated with femorofemoral bypass to avoid the potential for postoperative impotence. • Revascularization of the internal iliacs at the time of aortoiliac reconstruction for occlusive disease can reverse vasculogenic impotence in patients with distal obstructive disease.

ANSWER:
A

12. With regard to inflammatory AAA, which of the following statements is/are true?

    A. Fewer than 1% of AAAs are considered inflammatory.

    B. There is a characteristic gross appearance, consisting of a thick, white fibrotic retroperitoneal process with adherence of the aneurysm to the duodenum and IVC.

C. An infectious cause is responsible for the inflammatory process.

D. The operative approach is the same as for the usual atherosclerotic aneurysm.

E. Most inflammatory AAAs occur in a suprarenal location.

Ref.: 2–4

COMMENTS: Inflammatory AAAs represent 2.5–15.0% of all AAAs. • There is a male predominance. • This type of aneurysm is infrarenal and characterized by an intense adventitial fibroplastic reaction, with adherence of the aneurysm to the third and fourth portions of the duodenum and IVC. • Ureteral entrapment is present in 25% of patients. • No infectious cause has been found, and the inflammatory process is thought to be autoimmune. • Abdominal and back pain, weight loss, and an elevated erythrocyte sedimentation rate (ESR) in a patient with AAA suggest this diagnosis. • Abdominal CT scanning with contrast medium is the most definitive examination for securing a preoperative diagnosis. • This scan demonstrates aortic wall thickening outside the rim of aortic calcification. • In contrast to a leaking AAA, the inflammatory process is enhanced with contrast material and demonstrates less attenuation than does blood. • The operative strategy includes proximal aortic control above the left renal vein and the use of ureteral catheters if the inflammatory process extends to the iliac vessels. • Dissecting off adherent structures (e.g., duodenum) should be avoided. • Ureterolysis is rarely necessary. • The risk of rupture is lower than with the usual atherosclerotic aneurysm. • After aneurysmorrhaphy with graft placement, the inflammatory process gradually resolves, and the ESR returns to normal.

ANSWER:
B

13. A patient who had an AAA repaired 5 years ago presents with fever and positive blood cultures. Which of the following statements are true?

A. CT scanning is the preferred initial imaging technique for suspected graft infection.

B. Published mortality rates following surgery for infected aortic grafts range between 5 and 10%.

C. Graft infections identified within 4 months of AAA repair are associated with a more virulent course than are later infections.

D. *Staphylococcus epidermidis* is the most common infecting pathogen.

E. Upper gastrointestinal bleeding is the most common initial presentation of an infected abdominal aortic graft.

Ref.: 4

COMMENTS: Diagnosis of an infected aortic graft is often a difficult task. • Clinical symptoms can be as subtle as a prolonged ileus, abdominal pain or tenderness, or unexplained sepsis. • The patient should be examined closely for anastomotic pseudoaneurysms or signs of septic embolization. • CT scanning with intravenous contrast material is the preferred initial imaging technique for patients with suspected aortic graft infection. • Fluid or gas around the graft, obliteration of the normal retroperitoneal tissue planes, and pseudoaneurysm formation suggest a graft infection. • Published mortality rates range between 10 and 50%, with subsequent amputation rates ranging from 15 to 60%. • The reasons for the high mortality rates are stump blowout and persistent sepsis.

• Graft infections diagnosed within 4 months are more virulent than those diagnosed later. • *Staphylococcus aureus* and gram-negative bacteria are the pathogens mainly implicated in early graft infection. • Gram-negative bacteria are particularly virulent because the endotoxins (elastase and alkaline protease) they produce can lead to compromise of the structural integrity of the anastomosis. • *S. aureus* was the most prevalent pathogen in infected aortic grafts, although the incidence of *S. epidermidis* infections is on the rise. • *S. epidermidis* infection is more chronic and insidious in nature and is usually diagnosed more than 4 months postoperatively.

ANSWER:
A, C, D

14. Which of the following statements is/are correct regarding endovascular repair of infrarenal AAA?

A. The most common complication with this technique is endoleak.

B. Tube grafts are preferable to bifurcated grafts for endovascular repair of infrarenal AAAs.

C. Anatomic limitations prohibiting endovascular repair include a short neck and large angulation of the aneurysm.

D. Iliac stenosis is an absolute contraindication to endoluminal repair.

E. Use of this technique is more likely to be feasible for large aneurysms.

Ref.: 4, 5

COMMENTS: Complications following endovascular repair of AAAs include endoleaks, microembolization, improper or incomplete placement of the stent, graft migration, graft thrombosis, and delayed aneurysm rupture. • An endoleak is defined as persistent arterial supply of the aneurysmal sac following deployment of the endograft. • The incidence of this complication has been reported to be as high as 40%. • Treatment of endoleaks varies. • Some leaks can be managed conservatively, but others require treatment with further endovascular stenting or conversion to the open technique. • Placement of tube endografts in the infrarenal aorta has been associated with a very high degree of complications (distal endoleaks) and has been abandoned. • Favorable anatomic characteristics for endovascular repair include a proximal neck at least 15 mm in length and a distal neck at least 10 mm in length. • The aneurismal aorta tends to have a significant degree of angulation. • When angulation exceeds 60 degrees, the incidence of graft migration and stent fracture increases significantly. • Therefore, endovascular repair is contraindicated. • Patients with iliac stenosis can have iliac artery angioplasty with or without stent placement that precedes endovascular repair of the aneurysm, thus not making it an absolute contraindication to repair. • The smaller the aneurysm, the more likely it is to have a proximal and distal neck, and the less likely it is to have mural thrombus formation. • About 60% of aneurysms less than 60 mm in diameter fulfill the anatomic criteria for endovascular repair, a number that drops to 50% if all aneurysms are considered.

ANSWER:
A, C

15. With regard to AAA-IVC fistula, which of the following statements is/are true?

A. The preferred exposure is via the retroperitoneal technique.

B. For an unstable patient, the best diagnostic test is abdominal ultrasound studies.

C. Control of the proximal aorta can be accomplished endoluminally.

D. The highest mortality rates occur in patients with preexisting coronary disease.

E. In a stable patient, CT scanning with intravenous contrast material is the gold standard for confirming the diagnosis.

Ref.: 3

COMMENTS: The incidence of an aortocaval fistula caused by AAAs is approximately 1% or less but increases to 2–4% in the presence of rupture. • It is usually the result of an inflammatory response and is more common with larger rather than smaller aneurysms. • The average diameter of AAAs complicated by aortocaval fistula is approximately 11 cm. • The most common presenting symptoms include tachycardia, congestive heart failure, a machinery-like abdominal bruit, abdominal or back pain, a pulsatile abdominal mass, and leg edema with dilated superficial abdominal veins. • Nematuria may also be present, but it is more likely when the fistula involves the aorta and a retroaortic left renal vein. • Proximal and distal control of the aorta is the first step in surgical repair. • Proximal and distal control of the IVC is not necessary and should be avoided because the IVC is very friable in these circumstances. • Venous hemorrhage from the fistula is best controlled by direct finger application over the fistula from within the aortic aneurysm. • Endovascular repair should be considered in patients with appropriate anatomic features for such a graft.

A N S W E R :
A, B, C, E

16. Regarding endovascular repair of AAAs, which of the following statements is/are true?

A. Aneurysm rupture may occur in patients with successful repair in the absence of endoleaks.

B. Type II endoleaks are due to patient lumbar, IMA, or hypogastric arteries.

C. Type I and type III endoleaks must be repaired as soon as they are identified.

D. Endoleaks may develop at any time after endograft placement.

E. Endotension is defined as aneurysm expansion from pressure in the absence of an endoleak.

Ref.: 5

COMMENTS: Continued perfusion and pressurization of the aortic aneurismal sac is called endoleak and is the most common complication of endovascular AAA repair. • Endoleaks have been classified into five different types. • **Type I** results from inadequate seal at the proximal or distal ends of the endograft. • **Type II** is due to branch flow through a patent IMA, lumbar artery, or hypogastric artery. • **Type III** is a mid-graft endoleak originating from fabric holes or an inadequate seal between endograft components. • **Type IV** is due to endograft porosity. • **Type V**, or endotension, is aneurysm pressure and enlargement in the absence of identifiable perigraft flow. • Endoleaks may develop at any time. • Therefore, following a successful endograft deployment, patients are followed with various imaging modalities (commonly spiral CT scans) at 6-month intervals for possible development of a new endoleak. • Although aneurysm rupture in the absence of endoleak has been reported following endovascular repair, several studies have shown that the presence of an endoleak increases the risk of rupture. • This risk is higher with type I and type III endoleaks. • Therefore, once they are identified, these endoleaks require prompt repair. • The risk of rupture from a type II endoleak is significantly smaller, and the need for secondary interventions to address such an endoleak is still a subject of debate. • Usually, if the endoleak is associated with aneurysm growth or it persists for over 6 months, most experts recommend repair.

A N S W E R :
A, B, C, D, E

17. With regard to infected (mycotic) AAAs, which of the following statements is/are true?

A. Infected aneurysms account for 5% of all AAAs.

B. Most infected aneurysms develop when septic emboli infect an artery.

C. *Salmonella* is the most commonly isolated bacterial pathogen.

D. Negative results of intraoperative Gram's staining exclude the diagnosis of an infected AAA.

E. Most patients are treated with aneurysm excision and in-situ aortic reconstruction.

Ref.: 1, 3, 4

COMMENTS: Infected (mycotic) aneurysms are a rare subset of AAAs, constituting only 0.1–1.5%. • Most infected aneurysms are caused by the spread of hematogenous bacteria that infect non-aneurysmal but atherosclerotic arteries, leading to aneurysmal degeneration. • Other causes include arterial trauma, leading to false aneurysm formation with concomitant bacterial contamination; septic emboli of cardiac origin; or infection of a preexisting aneurysm. • *Salmonella* has been identified in almost 40% of patients with infected AAAs. • Infections with gram-negative organisms are less common but are associated with a higher incidence of aneurysm rupture. • The most common symptoms of patients with infected aneurysms are fever and abdominal or back pain. • Laboratory data lack sensitivity and specificity when considered alone. • Blood culture results are positive in approximately 35–50% of patients. • CT scanning is the preferred diagnostic study and may reveal an enhancing and eccentric periaortic mass, an aneurysm at an atypical location, periaortic fluid or gas, retroperitoneal soft-tissue edema, prominent periaortic lymphadenopathy, and evidence of aneurysm rupture. • When the diagnosis of infected AAA is entertained, broad-spectrum antibiotics and prompt surgical intervention are mandatory. • Aneurysm excision with débridement of all involved tissues, secure aortic stump closure, and extra-anatomic reconstruction, such as axillofemoral bypass, is recommended in most cases. • Following surgery, patients are placed on parenteral antibiotics for 4–6 weeks, depending on the virulence of the organism, the extent of infection, and the method of arterial reconstruction. • Aneurysm excision with in-situ aortic reconstruction may be performed in cases with minimal infection and low-virulence organisms, such as *S. epidermidis*. • After in-situ aortic graft reconstruction, lifelong oral antibiotics are advised.

A N S W E R :
B, C

18. With regard to prosthetic aortic graft infections, which of the following statements is/are true?

A. Infected prosthetic aortic grafts occur more commonly after aortofemoral bypass than after aortoiliac bypass.

B. *S. aureus* is the pathogen most commonly isolated from infected prosthetic aortic grafts.

C. Ultrasound imaging is the preferred diagnostic modality for confirming prosthetic aortic graft infection.

D. Most prosthetic aortic graft infections are diagnosed more than 1 year after implantation.

E. Graft excision, secure aortic stump closure, and extra-anatomic reconstruction are required for all infected prosthetic aortic grafts.

Ref.: 1, 3, 4

COMMENTS: Infected prosthetic aortic bypass grafts have an incidence of approximately 1% following aortoiliac bypass and 1.5–2.0% following aortofemoral bypass. • Mortality from infected grafts is as high as 50% in reported series. • The most common pathogen isolated from infected prosthetic aortic grafts is *S. epidermidis.* • Factors that contribute to graft infection include contact between the graft and skin during insertion, break in sterile technique, extension of contaminated wounds, contaminated lymphatics, arterial wall infection, and early transient bacteremia. • CT scanning has proved to be the most sensitive tool for diagnosing infected prosthetic grafts. • Changes on the CT scan suggestive of infected grafts include perigraft fluid or gas, soft-tissue swelling, focal bowel wall thickening, increased soft tissue between the graft and the wrap, and false aneurysm formation. • Radionuclide techniques have similar sensitivity but high false-positive rates due to labeling techniques, especially after graft implantation. • Ultrasound imaging provides limited information. • MRI is limited by its inability to differentiate between infected and sterile fluid, especially during the early postoperative period. • Most prosthetic graft infections are diagnosed more than 1 year after implantation. • Early infection (<4 months) is associated with emergent operation for ruptured AAA, states of impaired immunocompetence, concomitant remote infection, and postoperative colon ischemia. • Most infected prosthetic aortic grafts are treated with graft excision, wide débridement of infected tissues, secure aortic stump closure, and extra-anatomic reconstruction. • Patients with late graft infections of low virulence (*S. epidermidis*) without gross contamination may be treated with segmental graft excision and in-situ graft replacement. • Regardless of the technique of reconstruction, patients are placed on long-term antibiotics and are subjected to close follow-up.

ANSWER:
A, D

19. Which of the following is/are acceptable treatment options for a patient with late aortic graft limb occlusion?

A. Nonoperative therapy

B. Thrombolytic therapy

C. Graft limb thrombectomy

D. Femorofemoral bypass

E. Aortofemoral bypass reoperation

F. Thoracofemoral bypass

Ref.: 1, 3

COMMENTS: The most common graft-related complication following aortofemoral bypass is thrombosis of one limb. • Graft limb occlusion occurs in 10–20% of patients, depending on the duration of follow-up. • Late graft limb occlusion is most commonly due to progressive atherosclerotic disease at or just beyond the distal anastomosis. • Other causes include worsening disease of the outflow vessels, commonly the proximal profunda femoris artery; thrombosis of an anastomotic aneurysm; arterial embolus from a cardiac source; low-output states; hypercoagulable states; and iatrogenic injury to the graft or native vessels following cardiac catheterization or diagnostic angiography. • Except in cases of profound limb ischemia, preoperative angiography should be performed in all patients. • In high-risk or inactive patients without evidence of limb-threatening ischemia, a **nonoperative** approach may be the most prudent course. • **Thrombolytic therapy** has been used in patients with acute graft thrombosis. • Its use is limited in patients with severe limb-threatening ischemia. • Significant complications such as bleeding, distal embolization, and worsening ischemia may occur. • Furthermore, surgical revision of the graft is usually required in most patients. • Therefore, its use is limited to patients with acute occlusion and non–limb-threatening ischemia, particularly high-risk patients. • Most patients with graft limb occlusion are treated with an operative approach. • In patients with graft limb occlusion of short duration, absence of proximal aortic disease, and unilateral occlusion, **graft limb thrombectomy** has been shown to be 90% successful. • To prevent further thrombosis, repair of the distal anastomosis may be required if a defect is present. • Advantages of this approach include the use of a unilateral groin incision and the fact that the procedure may be done under local or regional anesthesia. • A common procedure for those with unilateral limb occlusion is a **femorofemoral bypass**. • This procedure is usually not excessively time consuming, may be done under local or regional anesthesia, and is technically easier than aortic reoperation. • In patients with proximal aortic disease, anastomotic complications, or significant degeneration or dilation of the original prosthesis, **aortofemoral bypass graft reoperation** is the preferred approach. • In patients with multiple occluded grafts or "hostile" abdomens in whom the other, less formidable options are contraindicated, extra-anatomic reconstructions, such as **axillofemoral** or **descending thoracic aortofemoral** bypass, may be utilized. • Regardless of the technique used, revision of the outflow tract must be accomplished if necessary. • It may require profundaplasty, graft limb extension, and bypass to the popliteal or tibial level. • Distal grafts are required in 25–50% of all procedures for graft limb occlusion.

ANSWER:
A, B, C, D, E, F

REFERENCES

1. Mullholland MW, Lillemoe KD, Doherty GM, et al (eds): *Greenfield's Surgery: Scientific Principles and Practice,* 4th ed. Lippincott, Williams & Wilkins, Philadelphia, 2006.
2. Brunicardi FC, Andersen DK, Billiar TR, et al (eds): *Schwartz's Principles of Surgery,* 8th ed. McGraw-Hill, New York, 2004.
3. Ernst CB, Stanley JC: *Current Therapy in Vascular Surgery,* 4th ed. CV Mosby, St. Louis, 2001.
4. Rutherford RB: *Vascular Surgery,* 6th ed. Saunders, Philadelphia, 2005.
5. Ouriel K: Endovascular aneurysm repair: an update. *Semin Vasc Surg* 16(2):87–175, 2003.

E. Peripheral: Lower Extremity

Chad Jacobs, M.D., and Walter J. McCarthy, M.D.

1. Which of the following statements is/are true regarding arterial occlusive disease of the lower extremities?

    A. Intermittent claudication is a symptom of chronic arterial occlusion.

    B. Resting pain usually occurs in the same muscle groups affected by claudication and is often relieved by dependent positioning of the affected extremity.

    C. Changes such as hair loss, brittle nails, and muscle atrophy generally precede symptoms of claudication.

    D. Tissue necrosis is more likely in the presence of multilevel distal arterial disease.

    E. Arterial ulcerations, like those of venous insufficiency, characteristically begin near the malleoli.

Ref.: 1, 2

COMMENTS: Chronic arterial occlusion of the lower extremities is the result of atherosclerotic disease of the aorta and its branches and can be diagnosed from characteristic signs and symptoms. • The classic symptom, intermittent claudication, is cramping pain in specific muscle groups that occurs when blood flow is inadequate for meeting the demands of exercise. • The pain usually occurs below the level of occlusion. • Hence, claudication of the buttock and thigh muscles is suggestive of aortoiliac obstruction, and calf claudication is suggestive of femoral artery obstruction. • As chronic ischemia progresses, trophic changes such as hair loss, nail brittleness, and muscular atrophy occur. • Ischemic pain during rest is a manifestation of end stage disease and characteristically involves the more distal aspects of the arterial circulation, such as the toes and feet. • Pain is typically felt across the metatarsal heads. • Associated physical findings include exacerbation of pain with extremity elevation, relief of pain by dependent positioning of the extremity, and dependent rubor caused by reactive hyperemia. • Tissue necrosis usually signifies multilevel disease of the distal arterial tree, inasmuch as chronic proximal occlusion alone is associated with the development of collateral circulation, which normally is adequate for preventing necrosis and gangrene. • Most ulcers resulting from arterial insufficiency involve the toes or plantar surface of the foot and are painful, whereas venous ulcers are less painful and typically occur near the malleoli.

ANSWER:
A, D

2. Which of the following is the most common site for atherosclerotic occlusion in the lower extremities?

    A. Aortic bifurcation

    B. Common femoral artery

    C. Profunda femoris artery

    D. Proximal superficial femoral artery

    E. Distal superficial femoral artery

Ref.: 2

COMMENTS: Although atherosclerotic disease frequently involves the area of arterial bifurcations, such as the aortic, iliac, and common femoral bifurcations, the most common site of occlusion in the lower extremities is the distal superficial femoral artery. • The occlusion occurs in the adductor canal proximal to the popliteal fossa and may be related to the anatomic relationship of the artery to the adductor magnus tendon at this site. • Affected patients frequently have disease at several levels, however, which emphasizes the need for accurate angiographic assessment before revascularization procedures. • Involvement of the superficial femoral artery alone is usually associated with intermittent claudication but not generally with tissue loss or pain during rest. • The profunda femoris artery is usually not occluded in this situation and serves as an important source of collateral blood flow

ANSWER:
E

3. With regard to aortoiliac atherosclerotic occlusive disease, which of the following statements is/are correct?

    A. Impotence is a common finding that results from decreased blood flow through the external iliac vessels.

    B. Thigh or buttock claudication (or both) is typical, and toe ulceration or gangrene secondary to atherosclerotic emboli is occasionally present.

    C. Lower-extremity hair loss and nail brittleness occur in 60% of patients.

    D. Concomitant coronary artery disease is the principal cause of death after aortoiliac reconstruction.

    E. Percutaneous angioplasty and stenting of iliac lesions only occasionally relieves symptoms.

Ref.: 1–3

COMMENTS: An accurate history and physical examination can help establish the diagnosis of aortoiliac atherosclerotic occlusive disease. • Three common clinical manifestations, often referred to as the Leriche syndrome, include intermittent claudication of the thigh or buttock, impotence, and diminished or absent femoral pulses. • Impotence is caused by hypogastric (internal iliac) arterial occlusion, which reduces blood flow through the internal pudendal artery and the corpora cavernosa. • With aortoiliac involvement alone, however, trophic changes are rarely present because collateral flow originating from the lumbar and epigastric arteries is preserved. • Nutritional changes, such as hair loss and nail brittleness, when present, signify additional distal disease. • Although distal tissue necrosis is often suggestive of more distal occlusive disease, the possibility of emboli from atherosclerotic plaques in the aortoiliac vessels must always be considered. • This has been referred to as the "blue-toe syndrome" and can occur even in the absence of occluding lesions. • The principal cause of death in this group of patients is coronary artery disease. • Iliac angioplasty and stenting are particularly successful in treating short-segment iliac disease. • When multilevel disease necessitates conventional distal bypass techniques, adequate inflow may be established with balloon angioplasty of the iliac arteries.

A N S W E R :
B, D

4. Any patient with intermittent calf claudication should be advised of which of the following?

   A. Angiography should be performed early to determine the extent of arterial disease.

   B. Surgical reconstruction should be performed to prevent progression of disease and the development of pain at rest with gangrene.

   C. Nonoperative treatment is sufficient for 75% of patients.

   D. Patients with claudication benefit from taking aspirin daily.

   E. Claudication progresses to gangrene at a rate of 2–3% of patients per year.

Ref.: 1–3

COMMENTS: The goals of therapy for occlusive arterial disease of the lower extremities are to relieve pain, prevent limb loss, and maintain bipedal gait. • Most patients with intermittent claudication alone remain stable or even improve with appropriate conservative management. • This includes a formal exercise program, smoking cessation, and risk reduction and may include medications such as Pletal. • Daily aspirin administration has been shown to be beneficial for such patients by reducing risk of morbidity from concomitant atherosclerotic disease, such as stroke and myocardial infarction. • Prophylactic surgical intervention is not indicated. • Patients with claudication have a low rate of progression to gangrene. • In fact, more than 75% of these patients remain stable, and the amputation rate is less than 7% in patients treated nonoperatively and observed for up to 8 years. • In patients with severe claudication and marked involvement of the tibial vessels, the disease progresses to gangrene in 2–3% of patients annually. • This is in contrast to patients with pain at rest, ulceration, or gangrene, who are at risk for limb loss and should be evaluated for revascularization. • Surgical intervention may be indicated in the presence of claudication for patients whose lifestyle or livelihood is impaired by their symptoms and who do not otherwise have limiting cardiac disease. • Arteriography is indicated for patients who are considered candidates for operation or angioplasty, but it should be preceded by less invasive testing, such as arterial blood flow studies.

A N S W E R :
C, D, E

5. With regard to nonoperative treatment of occlusive atherosclerotic disease of the lower extremities, which of the following statements is/are true?

   A. Exercising to the point of claudication leads to improved muscle performance due to adaptive changes made in muscle enzymes, leading to more efficient oxygen extraction.

   B. Cessation of cigarette smoking reduces claudication and decreases the risk of gangrene.

   C. Foot protection is important because even minor trauma may lead to gangrene.

   D. Anticoagulant therapy with warfarin (Coumadin) or heparin promotes healing of arterial ulcers.

Ref.: 1, 2

COMMENTS: Most patients in whom intermittent claudication is the only manifestation of peripheral vascular disease respond to conservative measures consisting of abstinence from tobacco and a graduated exercise program. • Continued tobacco use has been associated with an increased risk of gangrene and a higher rate of premature graft failure after reconstructive procedures. • For patients with more advanced ischemia, protection of the lower extremity is critical. • Patients should avoid temperature extremes, improper footwear, or overly aggressive trimming of nails and calluses. • It is not uncommon for relatively minor trauma to result in gangrene and eventual amputation of an already compromised foot. • There is evidence that regular low-dose therapy with acetylsalicylic acid may be of benefit in preventing thrombosis in patients with atherosclerotic disease, but therapy with heparin or warfarin sodium has not proved beneficial.

A N S W E R :
A, B, C

6. Occlusive tibioperoneal disease occurs commonly in patients with which of the following entities?

   A. Buerger's disease

   B. Raynaud's phenomenon

   C. Diabetes mellitus

   D. Arterial emboli

   E. Hyperlipidemia

Ref.: 2, 3

COMMENTS: Whereas the common pattern of atherosclerotic occlusive disease involves the femoral artery or the more proximal aortoiliac system, diabetic patients characteristically acquire a pattern of distal occlusive disease involving the distal popliteal artery and the tibial and metatarsal vessels. • Buerger's disease, or thromboangiitis obliterans, is associated with tobacco use and results in an inflammatory thrombosis of the small and medium-sized vessels of the upper and lower extremity. • This type of distal involvement may also be seen in patients with arterial embolism. • Patients with tibioperoneal involvement often present with advanced ischemia rather than simple claudication, and arterial reconstruction may necessitate bypass grafting to target vessels at the ankle or proximal foot. • Raynaud's syndrome is characterized by vasospasm of the small arteries and arterioles of the most distal portions of the extremities (i.e., the hands, fingers, feet, and toes).

A N S W E R :
A, C, D

7. With regard to the diabetic foot, which of the following statements is/are true?

   A. Foot pain resulting from diabetic neuropathy usually is relieved by dependent positioning.

B. Trophic ulcers rarely occur if pedal pulses are palpable.

C. Débridement of infected tissue should be avoided until revascularization is accomplished because of the risk of nonhealing.

D. Surgical revascularization distal to the popliteal artery may be required to control infection and allow healing if there is arterial occlusion.

E. The ankle brachial index in a diabetic with an ischemic foot is often higher than 1.0 because of calcified vessels.

Ref.: 1, 2

COMMENTS: Diabetic patients are at risk for foot disorders caused by diabetic neuropathy, occlusive arterial disease, and infection. • Diabetic neuropathy has generally adverse consequences. • **Sensory** neuropathy renders the foot susceptible to trauma because of analgesia; **motor** neuropathy causes imbalances in the intrinsic musculature of the foot, leading to ventral subluxation of the metatarsal heads and pressure necrosis of the plantar tissue; and **autonomic** neuropathy may alter the microcirculation, further exacerbating tissue ischemia. • Ischemic pain during rest, unlike pain secondary to neuropathy, may be relieved by dependent positioning. • Trophic ulcers, which are painless, often occur on the plantar surface over the metatarsal heads as the result of pressure necrosis and often occur in the presence of palpable pedal pulses. • Such lesions provide sites of entry for infection, to which the diabetic foot is markedly susceptible. • Control of infection requires aggressive initial débridement of all necrotic tissue, systemic antibiotics, and subsequent arterial revascularization if there is associated occlusive disease. • Arterial reconstruction in diabetic patients usually involves the tibioperoneal vessels and plays an important role in limb salvage. • The ankle brachial index in diabetic patients is typically higher than 1.0 because of lower-extremity arterial calcification and does not accurately reflect the degree of occlusive disease. • Doppler waveforms obtained from noninvasive blood flow studies are a better guide to the degree of ischemia in this setting and are often markedly attenuated in diabetics with peripheral ischemia.

ANSWER:
D, E

8. With regard to femoropopliteal bypass, which of the following statements is/are true?

A. The patency of prosthetic grafts is nearly equal to that of autologous vein grafts in both above- and below-knee bypasses.

B. Patency rates are higher when bypass is performed for claudication than when done for limb salvage.

C. Continued cigarette smoking adversely affects graft patency.

D. Diabetes adversely affects graft patency.

E. Patency rates are unaffected by vein size.

Ref.: 1, 2

COMMENTS: The reversed saphenous vein autograft has been the most successful arterial bypass graft below the inguinal ligament and is the standard against which the success of prosthetic grafts is measured. • Some controversy exists with regard to the primary use of polytetrafluoroethylene or Dacron for above-knee popliteal bypasses, but recent literature supports the preferential use of autologous vein graft even in the above-knee position. • Therefore, autologous vein should be the first choice for all infrainguinal revascularizations. • Patency rates for above-knee saphenous vein grafts are approximately 80–90% at 1 year and approximately 75% at 5 years.

Patency rates generally are higher when bypass is performed for claudication than for salvage of the limb, because of the extent of the underlying pathologic process.

Patency is adversely affected by grafts performed below the knee, continued tobacco use, poor distal runoff, and small vein size (<4 mm). • Small vein size and size mismatch can be corrected through the in-situ technique.

Associated risk factors, such as diabetes, hypertension, and coronary artery disease, have not been shown to exert a detrimental effect on long-term graft patency. • Limb salvage rates generally exceed graft patency rates. • If healing is *complete* after distal bypasses and the bypass subsequently becomes occluded, limb salvage can be maintained in more than 50% of patients.

ANSWER:
B, C

9. Which of the following statements are true regarding endovascular management of lower extremity ischemia?

A. Iliac stenoses may be treated with endovascular techniques, but occlusions must be addressed surgically.

B. Superficial femoral artery stenoses greater than 10 cm in length have much reduced patency when subjected to endovascular treatment.

C. Long-term patency rates for occlusion and stenosis are similar.

D. Endovascular stents should only be placed secondarily to correct a dissection or residual stenosis after initial balloon angioplasty.

Ref.: 3

COMMENTS: Endovascular approaches play an integral role in the management of atherosclerotic occlusive disease. • Long-term patency following angioplasty depends largely on the site being treated. • Proximal, larger-caliber arteries have the best initial and long-term results, while distal sites have decreasing patency rates. • Better results are obtained when treating short, focal stenoses rather than long, diffusely diseased arteries. • Stenoses less than 2 cm are considered ideal lesions for percutaneous treatment, while those longer than 10 cm have poor patency with endovascular repair. • Iliac stenoses and occlusions may both be treated with percutaneous endovascular technique. • Although initial success rates for treating occlusions are somewhat lower, some series have shown similar long-term patency rates for both stenoses and occlusions of the iliac artery. • This may be partly due to increased use of intravascular stents when treating occlusions. • While stents certainly have a role in treating postangioplasty dissections or residual stenoses, primary stent placement may be considered for treating longer, more complex lesions; recurrent lesions; lesions likely to embolize (ulcerated plaque); and occlusions. • In poor operative candidates with limb-threatening ischemia, infrapopliteal angioplasty may be considered. • While the 2-year limb salvage rate for such procedures has been reported as 50–80%, the patency rates are significantly lower, at 30–40%.

ANSWER:
B, C

10. Which of the following statements are true regarding revascularization in patients with end-stage renal disease (ESRD)?

   A. More than half of patients with ESRD will develop symptomatic lower-extremity arterial occlusive disease.

   B. Patients with ESRD have a higher rate of morbidity and mortality compared to the normal population when undergoing infrainguinal revascularization.

   C. At 3 and 5 years, patency rates for infrainguinal revascularization are similar for patients with ESRD and those with normal renal function.

   D. Factors such as length of time on dialysis, availability of autogenous conduit, and size or location of ulceration may be prognostic indicators of successful revascularization for patients with ESRD.

   E. Bypass to the tibial vessels should not be offered to patients with ESRD.

Ref.: 3, 4

COMMENTS: The frequency of infrainguinal revascularization in patients with ESRD has increased over the past decade. • It is expected that by the year 2010, there will be 600,000 patients with ESRD in the United States. • In addition, approximately 20% of patients with ESRD will develop symptoms due to arterial occlusive disease. • Several studies have examined the efficacy of revascularization in this patient population. • While patients with ESRD do have higher rates of morbidity and mortality than the population with normal renal function, the 3- to 5-year graft patency rates are quite similar. • Many prognostic factors have been proposed to help predict success or failure in this tenuous patient population, including length of time on hemodialysis, location of gangrene (heel or forefoot), size of ulceration (>2–4 cm), availability of autogenous conduit, and presence of suitable target vessels. • A global assessment of such patients must be performed, taking into account comorbid conditions, ambulatory status, and the prognostic factors listed above. • When this is performed, tibial bypass can often be successfully undertaken in the renal failure population.

ANSWER:
B, C, D

11. Long-term patency of bypass grafts to the tibioperoneal vessels is influenced by which of the following?

   A. Diabetes

   B. Previous attempts at revascularization

   C. Antiplatelet therapy

   D. Presence of a patent pedal arch

   E. Level of distal anastomosis

Ref.: 1, 2, 3

COMMENTS: Bypass graft procedures to the tibial vessels are typically performed for limb salvage (i.e., rest pain or ischemic tissue loss/gangrene) and in the face of significant multilevel occlusive arterial disease. • As such, they are less successful than bypasses performed for claudication, in which case the atherosclerotic burden is typically much lower. • Patency is better when the pedal arch is angiographically intact, but absence of a pedal arch is not a contraindication to surgery. • Grafts to the anterior or posterior tibial arteries are therefore preferred, but grafts to the peroneal artery are also useful. • Continuity with a patent pedal arch is of paramount importance for graft survival and limb salvage. • Concomitant endarterectomy of the tibial vessels is more likely to result in dissection and is therefore rarely undertaken. • The presence of diabetes does not significantly adversely affect patency on bypasses to the popliteal or tibial levels. • Diabetes is, however, a significant risk factor in the development of tibioperoneal occlusive disease. • Previously performed operative procedures have not adversely affected early or long-term patency rates or limb salvage. • The role of distal vein patches for prosthetic grafts, the addition of an arteriovenous fistula to a bypass graft, and the use of postoperative antiplatelet drugs or anticoagulants have all been proposed as adjuncts to improve infrageniculate bypass graft patency. • The level of the distal anastomosis does not influence graft patency. • However, the quality of the distal runoff is a primary factor.

ANSWER:
C, D

12. Sudden pain and weakness in the left leg develop in a patient with a history of coronary artery disease and atrial fibrillation. Examination reveals a cool, pale extremity with an absence of pulses below the groin and a normal contralateral leg. Which of the following is the most likely diagnosis?

   A. Cerebrovascular accident

   B. Arterial thrombosis

   C. Arterial embolism

   D. Acute thrombophlebitis

   E. Dissecting aortic aneurysm

Ref.: 1, 2

COMMENTS: See Question 14.

13. For the initial evaluation of the patient described in Question 12, which of the following tests is/are mandatory?

   A. Electrocardiography

   B. Venography

   C. Arteriography

   D. Abdominal ultrasound studies

   E. Chest radiography

Ref.: 1, 2

COMMENTS: See Question 14.

14. If the patient described in Question 12 had a history of intermittent left calf claudication and if examination showed, in addition, diminished pulses on the contralateral leg and trophic skin changes bilaterally, which of the following would be true?

   A. Arteriographic findings are unlikely to help plan the appropriate surgical approach.

   B. Venography is mandatory for ruling out phlegmasia alba dolens.

   C. Indications for surgical intervention are unchanged.

   D. The anticipated surgical procedure is unchanged.

Ref.: 1, 2

COMMENTS: The classic signs of acute arterial occlusion are pain, pallor, absence of pulse, paralysis, and paresthesia (the five P's). • The common causes of acute arterial occlusion are embolism, thrombosis, and trauma. • In the patient described in Question 12, the history of atrial fibrillation, coupled with the classic findings of acute arterial occlusion, make arterial embolism the most likely diagnosis.

Clinical findings that suggest arterial thrombosis, rather than embolism, as the cause include an absence of cardiac disease commonly associated with embolization phenomena, symptoms of underlying occlusive atherosclerotic disease, and physical findings suggestive of chronic ischemia. • It can be difficult, however, to differentiate embolism from thrombosis on clinical grounds alone. • Embolism can certainly occur in patients with underlying peripheral vascular disease.

Prompt operative intervention is indicated, regardless of cause, when there is acute limb-threatening ischemia. • It is important, however, to distinguish arterial embolism from arterial thrombosis superimposed on an atherosclerotic plaque because the extent of operation may vary considerably. • Whereas embolism may be successfully treated by simple embolectomy and extraction of the thrombus that forms distal to the embolism, effective treatment of arterial thrombosis can be much more difficult, sometimes requiring arterial reconstruction. • Arteriography may be helpful for differentiating between embolic and thrombotic occlusions. • A careful history and physical examination permit a diagnosis of embolic occlusions in most cases. • Arteriography is not always necessary and should not be performed if it will delay operative reestablishment of blood flow. • Patients with arterial embolism should undergo electrocardiography and radiography of the chest because of the high association with intrinsic cardiac disease and its potential for myocardial infarction.

Acute arterial occlusion can be differentiated from acute venous thrombosis, because venous thrombosis is usually associated with edema and preservation of peripheral pulses. • Severe venous obstruction produces phlegmasia cerulea dolens. • When this is associated with arterial thrombosis and spasm, phlegmasia alba dolens may occur. • Untreated, this process may progress to venous gangrene.

In rare instances, an aortic dissection mimics acute embolism by producing loss of peripheral pulses, but the diagnosis may be suspected because of the presence of back or chest pain and hypertension.

Acute arterial occlusion that rapidly produces paralysis and paresthesia may be mistaken for a stroke. • However, the physical examination should direct attention toward the compromised extremity and eliminate stroke from the differential diagnosis.

Prompt diagnosis of arterial occlusion is critical because irreversible muscular necrosis necessitating amputation may occur within 4–6 hr.

ANSWERS:
Question 12: C
Question 13: A, E
Question 14: C

15. For an acute arterial embolus to the lower extremity with limb-threatening ischemia, appropriate initial treatment includes which of the following?

   A. Intravenous 5,000- to 10,000-unit heparin bolus followed by continuous-drip administration

   B. Delay heparinization until anesthesia is administered because heparinization precludes spinal anesthesia

   C. Routine preoperative trial of vasodilators

   D. Attempt at thrombolytic therapy with drugs such as tissue plasminogen activator

Ref.: 1, 2

COMMENTS: Treatment of arterial embolism must be initiated promptly to prevent irreversible ischemic damage. • Intravenous heparin should be administered to prevent formation and propagation of thrombus distal to the embolus and is the most important first step. • Heparinization should not be delayed, particularly because most embolectomies can be performed with the use of local anesthesia. • Furthermore, the degree of distal thrombus is an important determinant of surgical success and limb salvage. • Although arterial spasm accompanies acute arterial occlusion, the routine use of vasodilators is not advocated. • Fibrinolytic agents have an important role in the treatment of patients with acute thrombosis superimposed on chronic ischemia. • Their routine use to treat acute arterial embolus with limb-threatening ischemia is not advocated, however, particularly because timely intervention is of utmost importance. • Because patients with arterial embolism often have associated cardiac disease and may be compromised further by the metabolic effects of ischemic tissue, preoperative attention must be given to careful physiologic monitoring and to the fluid balance, electrolyte balance, and arterial blood gas status of the patient.

ANSWER:
A

16. With regard to operative management of lower-extremity arterial embolism, which of the following statements is/ are true?

   A. Embolectomy can be performed in most cases.

   B. Suspected aortoiliac emboli should be removed through an abdominal approach.

   C. Brisk back-bleeding is a reliable indicator of successful complete distal embolectomy.

   D. Wide fasciotomy should be avoided in heparinized patients because of the risk of hemorrhage.

   E. Palpable pulses or audible Doppler signals are reliable indicators of complete embolectomy.

Ref.: 1, 2

COMMENTS: In most cases, embolectomy can be performed with the use of balloon catheters introduced through arteriotomies proximal to the embolic lodging site. • Aortoiliac emboli can be removed successfully via bilateral femoral arteriotomies. • Back-bleeding does not necessarily indicate adequate removal of the embolus distally because it may originate from an arterial branch proximal to the thrombus that remains. • For this reason, restoration of distal pulses or Doppler signals and intraoperative arteriography, when necessary, comprise the gold standard used to assess completeness of thromboembolectomy. • Fasciotomy is an important concomitant procedure if the limb has been subjected to ischemia for 4–6 hr or longer. • Fasciotomy should be performed, even in heparinized patients. • Compartment syndrome can develop after reperfusion of an ischemic limb, and close postoperative attention is thus required.

ANSWER:
A, E

17. While a patient is in the recovery room after femoral embolectomy, a palpable pedal pulse disappears. The patient's leg is pale and swollen. Appropriate treatment includes which of the following?

    A. Venography

    B. Fibrinolytic therapy

    C. Arteriography

    D. Immediate reexploration

    E. Fasciotomy

    Ref.: 1, 2

COMMENTS: During the immediate postoperative period, therapy focuses on maintenance of peripheral perfusion, treatment of the patient's underlying cardiac disease, and treatment of the potential metabolic complications after resumption of perfusion of an ischemic limb. • Frequent evaluation of peripheral pulses by palpation and Doppler ultrasound studies and of limb temperature and color is mandatory. • Any change that indicates ischemia warrants *immediate reexploration*. • If swelling threatens the viability of peripheral musculature, *fasciotomy* is indicated. • *Fibrinolytic* therapy has been used for arterial thrombosis but is contraindicated in patients who have undergone a recent operation, because of the risk of hemorrhage at the operative site.

ANSWER:
D, E

18. After undergoing femoral embolectomy and fasciotomy, a patient becomes oliguric, and the urine is brownish red. Immediate treatment includes which of the following?

    A. Cessation of intravenous administration of heparin

    B. Determination of serum potassium level

    C. Intravenous administration of sodium bicarbonate and mannitol

    D. Renal arteriography

    Ref.: 1

COMMENTS: When an extremity has been subjected to ischemia and muscular necrosis occurs, reperfusion can result in metabolic acidosis and profound hyperkalemia. • Rhabdomyolysis releases myoglobulin, which precipitates in acid urine and produces brownish-red urine that is free of red blood cells. • Treatment of patients in this situation requires prompt reversal of hyperkalemia to prevent cardiac arrest (intravenous insulin and glucose), administration of sodium bicarbonate to alkalinize the urine and to treat the systemic metabolic acidosis, and osmotic diuresis with mannitol to prevent renal tubular obstruction. • Fasciotomy is indicated if it has not already been performed. • Continuation of anticoagulation therapy is critical because the patient remains at significant risk of recurrent embolism from the underlying cardiac disease. • Fewer than 10% of arterial emboli involve the renal vessels, and renal arteriography is not indicated in this case.

ANSWER:
B, C

19. Most arterial emboli originate from which one of the following sites?

    A. Cardiac valves

    B. Left atrium

    C. Left ventricle

    D. Thoracic aorta

    E. Abdominal aorta

    Ref.: 1, 2

COMMENTS: By far, most arterial emboli originate in the heart. • Fewer than 10% arise from ulcerated plaques in the aorta, carotid arteries, or subclavian arteries. • The most common intracardiac site is the left atrium, in which thrombi form as the result of stasis in patients with atrial fibrillation, mitral valvular disease, or both. • A rare source of left atrial emboli is a left atrial myxoma. • Left ventricular thrombi are a potential source of embolism in patients with myocardial infarction, left ventricular aneurysm, congestive heart failure, or cardiomyopathy. • Valvular sources of emboli include vegetative endocarditis and thrombi formed on mechanical prosthetic heart valves. • Paradoxical emboli arising from the venous system may reach the arterial circulation through a patent foramen ovale.

ANSWER:
B

20. Arterial emboli of cardiac origin most frequently produce occlusion of which one of the following?

    A. Cerebral vessels

    B. Distal aorta

    C. Common femoral artery

    D. Superficial femoral artery

    E. Popliteal artery

    Ref.: 1, 2

COMMENTS: Arterial emboli usually lodge proximal to arterial bifurcations and most commonly involve the lower extremities. • One third to one half of arterial emboli occlude the common femoral artery at the bifurcation of the superficial femoral and profunda femoris. • Because the embolus lodges proximal to major bifurcations, there is significant and abrupt interruption of potential collateral flow, which results in severe ischemia.

ANSWER:
C

21. After undergoing brachial artery catheterization for coronary angiography, a patient complains of hand numbness, and the previously present radial pulse is noted to be absent. Which of the following is the appropriate treatment?

    A. Administration of systemic vasodilators

    B. Surgical exploration and topical application of papaverine

    C. Percutaneous balloon dilatation of brachial artery

    D. Brachial artery exposure with direct repair of the injured segment

E. Arteriography to determine the presence of thrombus at the catheterization site

Ref.: 1

COMMENTS: Iatrogenic arterial injuries may result from placement of needles and catheters for radiographic studies or monitoring purposes. • Arterial occlusion usually occurs as the result of thrombus in association with intimal injury. • Treatment consists of prompt exploration with arteriotomy and thrombectomy. • Intimal damage may be treated by segmental excision with direct anastomosis. • Surgery should not be delayed by attributing ischemia associated with arterial injury to arterial "spasm." Arteriography to confirm what is already clinically apparent delays the required surgical exploration and usually is not indicated.

ANSWER:
D

22. Which of the following is the most common symptom of thoracic outlet syndrome?

A. Raynaud's phenomenon

B. Pain or paresthesia in the C8–T1 nerve distribution

C. Pain or paresthesia in the radial nerve distribution area

D. Ischemia or pain caused by arterial compression

E. Arm edema caused by venous obstruction

Ref.: 1, 2

COMMENTS: Anatomic compression of the brachial plexus, subclavian-axillary vessels, or both may occur at the thoracic outlet by a variety of mechanisms at several specific sites. • The primary symptoms depend on which anatomic structures are compressed. • Most patients have pain or paresthesias as a result of brachial plexus compression. • Pain and paresthesias may affect any part of the shoulder or upper extremity but most commonly are noted in the C8–T1, or ulnar nerve distribution, area. • Symptoms of arterial compression, such as ischemic pain, fatigue, and decreased temperature, are less common. • Embolic events may produce digital gangrene. • Symptoms of venous compression occur even less frequently than those of arterial compromise and may include edema, venous distention, and discoloration. • In some instances "effort thrombosis" of the subclavian vein (Paget–von Schroetter syndrome) may occur. • Nerve conduction studies, arteriography, and dynamic CT scans may aid in the diagnosis of thoracic outlet syndrome. • Physicians' maneuvers aimed at detecting a pulse deficit have low specificity. • Resection of a cervical rib or a first rib and anterior scalenectomy are performed to decompress the thoracic outlet. • Associated subclavian-axillary arterial lesions are corrected. • A transaxillary or supraclavicular approach may be used.

ANSWER:
B

23. With regard to Buerger's disease, which of the following statements is/are correct?

A. It is most frequently found in African-American men 20–40 years of age.

B. Recurrent migratory superficial phlebitis often predates arterial involvement.

C. Sympathectomy is effective in 50% of patients, but arterial reconstruction offers better long-term results.

D. Cessation of cigarette smoking is the primary therapy.

E. It can be successfully treated with anticoagulants, vasodilators, and steroids.

Ref.: 1, 2

COMMENTS: Buerger's disease (thromboangiitis obliterans) is an inflammatory process of uncertain etiology that produces thrombosis of medium-sized and small arteries and veins. • The disease typically affects young men who are heavy smokers. • It is rare in African-Americans. • Recurrent migratory superficial thrombophlebitis involving the pedal veins often predates arterial involvement by several years. • Both upper and lower extremities can be affected, and ischemic gangrene frequently results. • Complete cessation of tobacco use is the most important aspect of treatment and may produce remission. • Simply decreasing the frequency of tobacco use is ineffective. • Arterial reconstruction usually is not possible, because distal small vessels are frequently involved. • Cervical or lumbar sympathectomy is useful in 50% of patients. • No pharmacologic treatment has proved widely successful.

ANSWER:
B, D

24. With regard to the appropriate management of popliteal aneurysms, which of the following statements is/are true?

A. Popliteal artery aneurysms should be managed conservatively if less than 3 cm in diameter, asymptomatic, and stable.

B. Popliteal aneurysms are bilateral in up to 50% of patients.

C. Proximal and distal ligation with bypass graft is the procedure of choice for popliteal artery aneurysms.

D. The presence of a popliteal aneurysm should heighten suspicion for arterial aneurysms in the abdomen and thorax.

E. Rupture is the most common complication of a popliteal aneurysm.

Ref.: 2

COMMENTS: Peripheral aneurysms are primarily atherosclerotic in origin, associated with hypertension, and frequently multiple. • Popliteal artery aneurysms are the most common, are bilateral in 50–70% of patients, and approximately 50% are associated with femoral or aortic aneurysm. • Patients with bilateral popliteal artery aneurysm have a 70% chance of having an AAA. • Patients with popliteal aneurysms therefore require thorough assessment to rule out other associated aneurysms. • Popliteal aneurysms present a high risk of limb loss as a result of thrombosis or embolus, and rupture is very rare. • Popliteal aneurysms should be operated on even when small, with diameters of 1.5–2.0 cm as a useful guideline. • Proximal and distal ligation with bypass grafting is the procedure of choice. • On occasion, if the aneurysm is small and the artery is tortuous, excision with end-to-end anastomosis is possible.

ANSWER:
B, C, D

25. With regard to Raynaud's disease or phenomenon, which of the following statements is/are correct?

A. It is characterized by upper extremity sequential phases of pallor, cyanosis, and rubor, which are initiated by exposure to heat or emotional stress.

B. It is most frequently seen in elderly women.

C. It is characterized by a pathologic mechanism that involves vasospasm with a reduction in the dermal circulation.

D. Calcium-channel blockers often yield symptomatic control.

E. Cervical sympathectomy is usually the primary therapy.

Ref.: 2

COMMENTS: Raynaud's disease or phenomenon is the most common vasospastic disorder and most commonly affects young women (90% of patients are <40 years old). • It may exist as a primary disorder (Raynaud's disease), or it may be a secondary manifestation (Raynaud's phenomenon) of disorders such as scleroderma, Buerger's disease, or thoracic outlet syndrome. • The classic pattern of pallor, cyanosis, and rubor occurs after exposure to cold or stress. • Vasospasm with a decrease in dermal circulation results in pallor. • Cyanosis occurs as a result of sluggish flow of blood. • Reactive hyperemia then occurs as the vasospasm subsides. • Avoidance of initiating factors is often adequate. • Calcium-channel blockers are the initial drug of choice.

ANSWER:
C, D

26. Appropriate management of frostbite includes which of the following?

A. Rapid rewarming with dry heat rather than rapid rewarming with warm water

B. Rapid rewarming with warm water

C. Slow rewarming at room temperature if heparin or dextran is administered

D. Thorough débridement of blisters and devitalized tissue

E. Sympathectomy in the presence of tissue necrosis to minimize the extent of necrosis and prevent late vasomotor sequelae

Ref.: 2

COMMENTS: The cold-injured extremity is best treated by rapid rewarming in warm water (40–42°C). • This results in less tissue damage than treatment by slow rewarming (i.e., at room temperature). • Dry heat or water at higher temperature risks additional thermal injury because of decreased sensation of the injured part. • The extremity should be elevated and exposed. • Antibiotics are given if there is an open wound, and tetanus prophylaxis is administered as indicated. • Opening of blisters and débridement of apparently devitalized tissue are contraindicated. • True demarcation of nonviable tissue requires many weeks and should be allowed to develop spontaneously. • The initial use of vasodilating drugs or antithrombotic agents such as heparin and dextran has not been shown to be effective. • Sympathectomy may be useful for treatment of the chronic sequelae of frostbite, such as paresthesia, hyperhidrosis, and coldness, but does not minimize the amount of tissue necrosis.

ANSWER:
B

27. With regard to popliteal entrapment syndrome, which of the following is/are true?

A. The syndrome commonly affects men before the age of 40.

B. Limb-threatening ischemia is the most common presentation.

C. Fibrous bands of the popliteus muscle most commonly cause arterial impingement.

D. MRI is the diagnostic procedure of choice.

E. Symptoms are usually treated with exercise and anti-platelet medications.

Ref.: 3, 4

COMMENTS: The popliteal artery entrapment syndrome most commonly affects men before the age of 40. • The most common presentation is mild, intermittent claudication. • Arterial thrombosis or occlusion is rare. • Other, less common causes of claudication in young adults include premature atherosclerosis caused by malignant hyperlipidemia, adventitial cystic degenerative disease, chronic exertional compartment syndrome, and vasculitis secondary to collagen vascular disorders. • Physical examination typically reveals a loss of tibial pulses with plantar flexion. • Noninvasive blood flow studies and duplex scanning may reveal the abnormality when done in conjunction with plantar flexion. • The most sensitive diagnostic study is MRI, which can delineate the musculotendinous structures of the popliteal fossa and document their dynamic relationship with the popliteal vessels. • The most common abnormality encountered is medial deviation of the popliteal artery around the medial head of the gastrocnemius muscle. • Five other anatomic variants have been described. • Surgical repair is the only effective treatment for symptomatic patients. • Resection or release of the variant musculotendinous structures is performed. • Arterial reconstruction is necessary when stenotic or aneurysmal lesions are present. • Surgical repair is also recommended for asymptomatic patients who are noted to have anatomic variants on the opposite side to prevent the development of secondary vascular complications.

ANSWER:
A, D

28. With regard to atheroembolic disease of the lower extremities, which of the following is/are true?

A. Atheroemboli commonly cause acute occlusion of the common femoral bifurcation.

B. Normal pedal pulses are commonly found in patients with atheroembolic disease.

C. The most common source of atheroemboli is aortoiliac atherosclerotic disease.

D. Medical therapy is associated with a low rate of recurrence.

E. Aortofemoral bypass, femoropopliteal bypass, extra-anatomic bypass with aortic exclusion, and localized endarterectomy may be indicated for management of atheroembolic disease.

Ref.: 1–4

COMMENTS: The term *atheroemboli* describes cholesterol or atherothrombotic microemboli. • Both aneurysms and atherosclerotic plaque may be the source of microemboli. • Aortoiliac atherosclerotic disease is the most common source of lower extremity microemboli. • Whereas macroemboli from cardiac sources tend to lodge at the bifurcations of large vessels, microemboli commonly lodge in distal small vessels, such as the digital arteries of the toes. • Cholesterol debris is often found on pathologic review of patients with atheroemboli. • Patients typically present with the sudden appearance of painful, mottled areas on the toes.

• Microemboli may lodge in the capillaries of the skin, leading to livedo reticularis of the knees, thighs, and buttocks. • Typically, patients have palpable pedal pulses. • If the superficial femoral artery is the source, a bruit or thrill may be present. • Duplex scans may help define atherosclerotic lesions, but biplane angiography is the most sensitive diagnostic method for determining the source of emboli.

　　Medical management with antiplatelet agents, steroids, aspirin, or warfarin is associated with a high rate of recurrence. • Warfarin may lead to exacerbation of the condition due to plaque destabilization. • Surgical intervention is indicated to remove the embolic source and reconstruct the arterial tree if necessary. • Aortofemoral bypass, femoropopliteal bypass, extra-anatomic bypass with aortic exclusion, and localized endarterectomy may all be indicated, depending on the location and extent of disease.

ANSWER:
B, C, E

29. True statements regarding anterior tibial compartmental syndrome include which of the following?

　A. It may be caused by severe exertion.

　B. Pain is the dominant symptom and is elicited on palpation of the calf.

　C. The dorsalis pedis pulse is always absent.

　D. Unlike the treatment for other compartment syndromes, fasciotomy is rarely needed.

Ref.: 2

COMMENTS: The anterior tibial compartmental syndrome is related to pressure from tissue fluid within the closed compartment. • The syndrome may be secondary to arterial trauma or arterial embolism and may be seen as a complication of cardiopulmonary bypass or femoropopliteal bypass. • It may also be caused by severe exertion with no proven anatomic lesion. • Pain is characteristically the first and dominant symptom and is located over the anterior compartment. • As with other compartmental syndromes, the presence of pulses does not negate the diagnosis. • Early fasciotomy before neuromuscular necrosis is the treatment of choice and produces excellent results.

ANSWER:
A

REFERENCES

1. Townsend CM Jr, Beauchamp RD, Evers BM, et al (eds): *Sabiston Textbook of Surgery: The Biological Basis of Modern Surgical Practice*, 17th ed. Saunders, Philadelphia, 2004.
2. Brunicardi FC, Andersen DK, Billiar TR, et al (eds): *Schwartz's Principles of Surgery*, 8th ed. McGraw-Hill, New York, 2004.
3. Rutherford RB: *Vascular Surgery*, 6th ed. Saunders, Philadelphia, 2005.
4. Ernst EB, Stanley JE: *Current Therapy in Vascular Surgery*, 4th ed. CV Mosby, St. Louis, 2001.

F. Renal Disease

Apostolos Tassiopolous, M.D., and Walter J. McCarthy, M.D.

1. With regard to the pathophysiology of renovascular hypertension, which of the following statements is/are true?

A. The relationship between unilateral renal artery stenosis and hypertension was established by Harry Goldblatt.

B. Activation of the renin-angiotensin system depends on intact aortic and carotid arch baroreceptors.

C. In response to reduced renal blood flow and pressure, the juxtaglomerular apparatus produces angiotensin I.

D. Angiotensin II elevates blood pressure by increasing peripheral vascular resistance and aldosterone production.

E. Saralasin competitively inhibits angiotensin II and is routinely used to screen for patients with hypertension caused by renin excess.

Ref.: 1, 2

COMMENTS: Renovascular hypertension is the elevation of diastolic and systolic pressures in association with renal artery occlusive disease. • Goldblatt's classic experiment in 1934 confirmed a renovascular source for hypertension. • Renovascular hypertension caused by renal artery stenosis (specifically decreased mean arterial perfusion pressure) stimulates the release of renin, a proteolytic enzyme, from the juxtaglomerular apparatus. • Renin interacts with renin substrate, an α_2-globulin named angiotensinogen (synthesized in the liver), to produce angiotensin I. • Converting enzymes (located primarily in the lung) convert angiotensin I (an inactive, labile decapeptide) to angiotensin II (an active octapeptide).

Angiotensin II, with a half-life of 4 minutes, increases blood pressure by its direct vasoconstrictor properties and by stimulating the release of aldosterone from the zona glomerulosa of the adrenal cortex. • The latter effect increases sodium and water resorption in the renal tubules, leading to increased plasma volume. • Establishment of normal renal artery blood flow can restore normal levels of renin production. • Parenchymal lesions caused by infarction (secondary to emboli, thrombus, or trauma), disease of the distal renal artery branches, arteriolar nephrosclerosis, renal artery aneurysms, spontaneous dissection, and renal artery occlusion with insufficient collateralization can also produce hypertension via renin-angiotensin stimulation.

Saralasin is a specific inhibitor of angiotensin II at the level of the arteriolar receptor site but has not proved reliable for screening patients with presumed renovascular hypertension.

ANSWER:
A, D

2. With regard to surgically correctable hypertension, which of the following statements is/are true?

A. Surgically correctable hypertension, by definition, represents disease of the renal blood vessels and parenchyma.

B. It should be suspected when there is the sudden onset of severe hypertension before the age of 35 or when severe hypertension develops after age 55 in the absence of a family history of hypertension.

C. It should be suspected when easily controllable hypertension becomes labile.

D. It should be suspected in children, adolescents, and premenopausal women with hypertension.

Ref.: 1, 2

COMMENTS: Approximately 5–15% of cases of hypertension are surgically correctable. • Although lesions of the renal artery are the most common cause of surgically correctable hypertension, a number of other causes amenable to surgical correction exist. • They include pheochromocytoma, various causes of Cushing's syndrome (adrenal hyperplasia, cortical adenoma, and adrenal carcinoma), primary hyperaldosteronism, coarctation of the aorta (upper-extremity hypertension), and unilateral renal parenchymal disease, such as renal cell carcinoma associated with renin production. • The diagnostic screening studies of these surgically correctable causes of hypertension include physical examination; family history of multiple endocrine adenomatosis; measurements of levels of serum potassium (three determinations), urinary 17-hydroxy-ketosteroids and 17-ketosteroids, catecholamines, vanillylmandelic acid, and ketosteroids; renal arteriography; and selective renin sampling.

ANSWER:
B, C, D

3. With regard to atherosclerosis and renovascular hypertension, which of the following statements is/are true?

A. Atherosclerosis accounts for up to 80% of renal artery occlusions that produce hypertension.

B. Renovascular hypertension occurs equally in men and women between the ages of 55 and 75.

C. The lesions are most commonly located near the origin of the renal artery, are segmental, and often are less than 1 cm in length.

D. These lesions are the most common source of emboli to the kidney.

E. Up to one third of affected patients have bilateral disease.

Ref.: 1, 2

COMMENTS: Atherosclerosis is the most common cause of renovascular hypertension, accounting for 95% of reported cases. • Fibromuscular dysplasia is another cause. • Renovascular hypertension affects primarily men between the ages of 55 and 75 and is often a segmental defect of the proximal renal artery. • The stenosis is most commonly on the left. • Up to three fourths of affected patients have bilateral disease. • Renal artery atherosclerosis may be associated with renal artery aneurysms and renal emboli. • Most renal emboli, however, originate from the heart. • Hypertension that appears suddenly or that is difficult to control in patients with other stigmata of atherosclerosis is highly suggestive of the diagnosis. • The more severe the hypertension, the more likely there is a correctable cause. • Bruits over the kidneys are common but may represent transmission of sounds from nonrenal arterial stenosis. • Renal bruits in essential hypertension are unusual. • Arterial fibrodysplasia includes intimal fibroplasia, medial fibroplasia, and perimedial dysplasia. • Medial fibroplasia is the most common and accounts for 85% of dysplastic renal artery disease.

A N S W E R :
A, C, E

---

4. A 14-year-old child who complains of headaches presents with marked diastolic hypertension and a soft to-and-fro bruit heard at the right costovertebral angle. Which of the following is/are the most likely diagnoses?

   A. Coarctation of the aorta

   B. Spontaneous segmental renal infarction

   C. Intimal fibromuscular dysplasia

   D. Medial fibromuscular dysplasia

Ref.: 1, 2

COMMENTS: Most asymptomatic children with mildly elevated blood pressure have essential hypertension. • However, children with symptoms and a diastolic blood pressure above 100–110 mmHg usually have secondary hypertension caused by either a renal parenchymal disorder (e.g., glomerulonephritis) or a neurovascular lesion. • One of the common causes of renovascular hypertension in children is **fibromuscular dysplasia,** which causes approximately 5% of all cases of renovascular hypertension. • It is a disease primarily of children and premenopausal women. • The lesions are classified according to the site (intimal, medial, or adventitial) and type (hyperplastic, fibrosing, or both) of involvement. • The most common lesions in children are *intimal* and *medial* dysplasias of unclear cause. • In women, medial fibrodysplasia is most common and may be caused by repeated renal artery stretching during pregnancy, causing damage to the vasa vasorum and mural ischemia, or by the effect of estrogens, which are known to cause medial degeneration. • The right renal artery is affected in 85% of patients. • In comparison, the left renal artery is involved most commonly with atherosclerotic lesions. • Medial fibroplasia can be a systemic process, with the internal carotid and external iliac arteries most often affected. • The lesions frequently are multiple, creating the angiographic "string-of-beads" appearance. • Medial fibromuscular dysplastic lesions may lend themselves to dilatation, whereas intimal and adventitial lesions do not. • In 15% of patients, the lesions progress or new lesions are formed after treatment.

Coarctation is usually associated with brachial femoral pulse discrepancies and a chest radiograph showing rib notching usually after age 11. • Physical examination also reveals a palpable thrill or a hum heard on auscultation over the upper back from well-developed intercostal collateral vessels. • Unilateral blood pressure elevation suggests anomalous origin or stenosis of a subclavian artery. • Due to distal renal hypoperfusion, there may be a renin-angiotensin component to the hypertension as well.

A N S W E R :
C, D

---

5. With regard to the workup of patients in whom renovascular hypertension is suspected, which of the following statements is/are true?

   A. Split-renal function studies provide the most accurate assessment for the presence of renovascular hypertension.

   B. Renal artery stenosis demonstrated on arteriogram is sufficient indication for surgical correction in hypertensive patients.

   C. Intravenous pyelography (IVP) is considered the diagnostic procedure of choice for evaluating patients in whom renovascular hypertension is suspected.

   D. Systemic renin assays are the screening procedure of choice for patients in whom renovascular hypertension is suspected.

   E. Renal vein renin ratios are currently the best means for determining the site of physiologically significant renal artery stenosis.

Ref.: 1, 2

COMMENTS: The goal of the workup for renovascular hypertension is to establish a relationship between an identifiable renal abnormality and altered renin-angiotensin function. • In other words, the functional significance of an angiographically demonstrated renal artery stenosis must be evaluated as well. • The use of **IVP** to screen these patients has some drawbacks. • There is a 75% rate of false-negative findings in children and a 20% rate of false-negative findings in adults with atherosclerosis. • Delayed opacification, reduced kidney size, and ureteral notching are considered positive findings. • IVP is limited for identifying segmental or arterial branch lesions, bilateral parenchymal disease of unequal severity, and bilateral arterial disease. • **Intravenous digital subtraction angiography** may miss fibromuscular lesions, does not enable examination of branch vessels, and requires a large amount of contrast fluid. • **Intra-arterial digital subtraction angiography** offers better detail with less contrast fluid. • **Arteriography** remains the definitive procedure for localization of significant renal artery lesions in patients suitable for operation or percutaneous intervention. • Because **peripheral venous renin** activity is variable, it is not considered a reliable screening test. • **Bilateral renal vein renin** activity, used alone or in combination with peripheral vein renin activity (the ratio of renal vein renin/ systemic renin), is of central importance to the preoperative evaluation. • A renal vein/peripheral vein renin ratio greater than 1.5 is considered positive. • The patient must be on a low-sodium diet and off β-adrenergic blockade before renin levels are determined. • Captopril may be used to amplify the difference in renin activity between the normal and abnormal kidney. • Before renin assays were available, **split-renal function studies** were used to assess the physiologic significance of renal lesions. • They are no longer in wide use because of the high incidence of technical failure, complications, and unreliability. • The advantages of split-renal function studies compared to plasma renin studies are that the former can assess the viability of the ischemic kidney and determine the worse of the two sides when there is bilateral renal artery stenosis.

A N S W E R :
E

---

6. With regard to the selection and preparation of patients for surgery to correct renovascular hypertension, which of the following statements is/are true?

   A. Most patients with renovascular hypertension are hypovolemic and require careful preoperative hydration.

B. Surgery clearly is superior to medical management of hypertension caused by renal artery occlusive disease.

C. Patients with renin levels that are nonlateralizing should not undergo operation.

D. Surgery provides the best outcome for patients with generalized atherosclerosis and renovascular hypertension because hypertension is tolerated least by these patients.

Ref.: 1, 2

COMMENTS: Many patients with renovascular hypertension are hypovolemic and hypokalemic, usually as a result of diuretic therapy. • These deficits must be carefully corrected before surgery. • The importance of discontinuing antihypertensive therapy before operation is debatable. • A diagnosis of renovascular hypertension can truly be made only in retrospect, when correction of a renal artery stenosis leads to correction of the hypertension.

Most patients with unilateral stenosis and lateralizing renin values are helped by surgery. • (False-negative results may result from problems with the screening technique or from the presence of unsuspected bilateral disease.) Medical therapy may control renovascular hypertension, but patients managed medically require close supervision and must comply with the regimen because renovascular hypertension seems to have a more aggressive course than does any other underlying atherosclerosis. • Also, many patients with renovascular hypertension treated with angiotensin-converting enzyme (ACE) inhibitors exhibit deterioration in the glomerular filtration rate, as evidenced by a rising creatinine level.

It is clearly established that renal artery reconstruction provides long-term correction of hypertension. • The same is true in women with fibromuscular dysplastic disease. • The patients with atherosclerosis in whom disease is confined to the renal artery are the ones who do best with reconstruction.

In patients with generalized atherosclerosis and involvement of other organs, surgery may be best reserved for those who fail medical management or in whom renal failure develops as a result of progressive renal artery occlusion.

ANSWER:
A

7. With regard to the choice of procedure for correction of renovascular hypertension, which of the following statements is/are correct?

A. Endarterectomy is rarely indicated because of the risk that emboli will cause parenchymal ischemia and further renin activation.

B. The internal iliac artery is the most common graft used for aortorenal bypass.

C. Partial nephrectomy rather than revascularization may be curative for hypertension caused by segmental infarction, renal artery branch lesions, intrarenal aneurysms, or isolated arteriovenous malformations.

D. Medial fibromuscular dysplasia and renal artery occlusion by plaques originating in the aortic wall adjacent to the renal artery are the lesions most amenable to transluminal angioplasty.

Ref.: 1, 2

COMMENTS: There are many surgical options for the treatment of renovascular hypertension. • Aortorenal bypass with the use of the saphenous vein is most frequently employed. • Since the venous graft tends to dilate in children, internal iliac artery grafts are used in pediatric patients.

Selected bilateral atherosclerotic lesions are amenable to transaortic endarterectomy with good results.

Experience with the technique of transluminal renal angioplasty suggests a technical success rate of up to 90% with proper selection of patients and preprocedure vascular surgery consultation.
• Fibromuscular dysplasia responds best to dilatation, whereas occlusion by atheromas originating in the aorta is least amenable.
• Restenosis after dilatation occurs more frequently in patients with atherosclerosis.

Small branch disease may be treated by benchwork surgery with the use of cold perfusion and ex-vivo surgical repair, followed by reimplantation.

In general, surgical treatment of carefully selected patients with renovascular hypertension is 80–90% successful.

ANSWER:
C

8. Regarding screening for renovascular hypertension, which of the following is/are true?

A. Duplex ultrasound imaging is the preferred initial test, but its accuracy is operator dependent.

B. Measurement of plasma rennin activity is the simplest test to perform, but its sensitivity and specificity are low.

C. Magnetic resonance imaging/magnetic resonance angiogram (MRI/MRA) provides accurate imaging of the renal artery without subjecting the patient to the risks of radiation and contrast nephrotoxicity.

D. Renal arteriography is reserved as the last test before therapy and after physiologic and noninvasive methods have been completed.

Ref.: 1

COMMENTS: In patient with suspected renovascular hypertension, evaluation of the renal artery stenosis and its functional significance is not straightforward, because none of the available diagnostic tests can provide all the information necessary to establish the diagnosis. • A therapeutic intervention is not necessary for every occlusive lesion but only for those affecting renal function to a degree sufficient to impair blood pressure regulation and renal excretory function. • Measurement of plasma rennin activity is the simplest physiologic test, but its sensitivity ranges between 57 and 66% and its specificity between 70 and 75%.

Duplex ultrasound study provides anatomic and functional assessment of the renal artery blood flow and can be safely used in all patients. • It has become the preferred initial imaging modality and in experienced hands has a sensitivity that ranges from 91 to 95%, with specificity from 90 to 97%. • Criteria for a positive test have been established.

MRI and MRA provide excellent imaging of the kidney and renal arteries without subjecting the patient to the risks of catheterization and contrast nephrotoxicity. • The continuous improvement in image analysis software has increased the sensitivity and specificity of this test, with some authors reporting accuracy up to 100%. • It is rapidly becoming the test of choice in the diagnosis of atherosclerotic renal artery stenosis.

Renal arteriography remains the gold standard for identification and assessment of renal artery stenosis but is usually reserved as the last test before therapy and after the completion of the physiologic and noninvasive studies.

ANSWERS:
A, B, C, D

9. Which of the following lesions are best treated by percutaneous transluminal angioplasty (PTA)?

   A. Renal artery occlusion

   B. Transplant renal artery stenosis

   C. Congenital hypoplasia of the renal arteries

   D. Orificial, atherosclerotic renal artery stenosis

   E. Bilateral renal artery stenosis

Ref.: 4, 5

COMMENTS: PTA of significant renal artery stenosis is a growing trend in the treatment of renovascular hypertension and renal insufficiency. • The introduction of stents has led to a lower incidence of restenosis, especially for the treatment of orificial, atherosclerotic disease. • The cause of the stenosis is an important predictor of success. • PTA has become first-line therapy for renal transplant arterial stenosis. • Acceptable results following PTA have been found with nonorificial atherosclerotic disease, unilateral disease, and fibromuscular disease (intimal and medial dysplastic stenosis). • Less favorable results occur with PTA in patients with branch vessel disease, aneurysmal disease, renal artery occlusion, and congenital renal artery hypoplasia.

The consequences of stent placement should be considered before intervention. • They include myointimal hyperplasia, obstruction of a suitable target site for future bypass, and protrusion of the stent into the aortic lumen, creating the potential for thrombus formation and distal embolization or difficulty with subsequent angiographic interventions. • Complications of PTA occur in a small percentage of cases. • Proximal renal artery dilation can result in intimal disruption, with preservation of the flexible elastic media found in this portion of the vessel. • Distal renal artery dilation results in medial disruption due to greater stiffness of this layer in this portion of the vessel. • Myointimal hyperplasia leads to recurrent stenosis after PTA. • Stenting has improved the patency of percutaneous interventions involving the renal arteries. • An initial trial of flexible stents in the renal arteries to reduce myointimal hyperplasia led to greater in-stent restenosis. • Rigid stents are now the configuration of choice for the renal arteries.

ANSWER:
B

10. Which of the following suggest(s) nephrectomy or partial nephrectomy as the treatment of choice for patients with severe hypertension?

   A. The technical success of the procedure has increased with the use of stents.

   B. Improvement of blood pressure control is more probable in patients with fibromuscular dysplasia than in those with atherosclerotic renal artery stenosis.

   C. Restenosis occurs in over 30% of patients with fibromuscular dysplasia.

   D. Complications requiring surgical correction or that result in loss of renal tissue occur in less than 3% of cases.

   E. The overall success of the procedure is similar in children and adults.

Ref.: 1

COMMENTS: Percutaneous balloon angioplasty has been employed with increasing frequency in the treatment of both atherosclerotic and fibromuscular renal artery stenosis. • The technical success of the procedure has been reported to be close to 90%, but with the use of stents it has increased up to 100%. • Restenosis is more common in patients with atherosclerotic lesions than in those with fibromuscular dysplasia (30 versus 11%). • Improvement in blood pressure control is seen in 64% of patients with atherosclerotic stenosis and 85% of patients with stenosis caused by fibromuscular dysplasia. • With recent advances in percutaneous techniques, complications requiring surgical correction or resulting in loss of renal tissue occur in less than 3% of the procedures. • Percutaneous interventions for renovascular hypertension have failed in children and are used only as a short-term temporizing maneuver.

ANSWER:
A, B, D

REFERENCES

1. Ernst CB, Stanley JC: *Current Therapy in Vascular Surgery*, 4th ed. CV Mosby, St. Louis, 2001.
2. Brunicardi FC, Andersen DK, Billiar TR, et al (eds): *Schwartz's Principles of Surgery*, 8th ed. McGraw-Hill, New York, 2004.
3. Moore WS: *Vascular Surgery: A Comprehensive Review.* Saunders, Philadelphia, 1998.
4. Mullholland MW, Lillemoe KD, Doherty GM, et al (eds): *Greenfield's Surgery: Scientific Principles and Practice*, 4th ed. Lippincott, Williams & Wilkins, Philadelphia, 2006.
5. Kidney DD, Deutsch LS: The indications and results of percutaneous transluminal angioplasty and stenting in renal artery stenosis. *Semin Vasc Surg* 9:188–197, 1996.

G. Mesenteric Disease

Apostolos Tassiopolous, M.D., and Walter J. McCarthy, M.D.

1. With regard to the mesenteric circulation, which of the following statements is/are true?

    A. The splanchnic vascular blood flow receives 25–30% of the cardiac output.

    B. Normal portal venous pressure is approximately 12–15 cmH$_2$O as a result of valves in the portal system.

    C. The ileum has more vascular arcades than does the jejunum.

    D. The presence of several sources of collateral blood supply to the superior mesenteric system minimizes the risk of bowel infarction when there is an acute occlusion of the superior mesenteric artery.

    E. The artery of Drummond, also known as the arch of Riolan or meandering mesenteric artery, provides an important collateral pathway between the celiac and superior mesenteric arteries.

    Ref.: 1

COMMENTS: Under resting conditions, the splanchnic vascular bed receives up to 30% of the cardiac output and contains as much as one third of the total blood volume. • This represents a large potential reservoir of blood from which the patient is "autotransfused" in situations of severe hypovolemia. • Normal portal venous pressure is between 12 and 15 cmH$_2$O. • The portal vein contains no valves, and therefore blood flow within the portal vein depends on the pressure gradient between the portal and systemic venous systems. • Blood from the superior mesenteric artery reaches the small bowel via numerous arterial arcades, and, although they become progressively greater in number and complexity in the more distal portion of the small bowel, they do not enhance the ability of the ileum to withstand acute occlusion of the superior mesenteric artery. • Also, although collateral flow does exist between the superior mesenteric and celiac circulations (via the gastroduodenal and the pancreaticoduodenal arteries) and between the superior mesenteric and inferior mesenteric circulations (via the arch of Riolan and the marginal artery of Drummond), these sources of collateral flow only rarely are sufficient to maintain bowel viability in the event of acute occlusion of the superior mesenteric artery. • Occlusion of the celiac or inferior mesenteric artery is much better tolerated and usually asymptomatic.

ANSWER:
A, C

2. With regard to mesenteric vascular occlusion, which of the following statements is/are true?

    A. Occlusion of the inferior mesenteric artery usually causes severe colonic ischemia.

    B. Occlusion of the superior mesenteric artery occurs most often at its origin or at the origin of the middle colic artery.

    C. Intestinal infarctions are caused more often by arterial occlusion than by venous occlusion.

    D. Venous occlusions most often are embolic rather than thrombotic.

    Ref.: 1, 2

COMMENTS: Although acute occlusion of the inferior mesenteric artery can produce symptoms of colonic ischemia, collateral supply from the superior mesenteric system via the marginal artery of Drummond and the branches of the middle and inferior hemorrhoidal arteries from the internal iliac arteries is usually sufficient to preserve the viability of the left colon. • Acute and chronic occlusion of the superior mesenteric artery occurs most often at its origin or near its second branch, the middle colic artery. • Approximately 50% of clinically significant mesenteric vascular accidents are caused by primary arterial occlusion, and 20% are caused by primary venous thrombosis. • The remaining cases are considered nonocclusive, as in low-flow states, spasm, hemoconcentration, and hypovolemia.

ANSWER:
B, C

3. Which of the following statements accurately characterize(s) acute occlusion of the superior mesenteric artery?

    A. Sudden complete occlusion is more often caused by embolism than by thrombosis.

    B. Emboli most commonly arise from atheromatous plaques within the aorta.

    C. Abdominal pain classically is out of proportion to physical findings (e.g., guarding and tenderness).

    D. Acute occlusion of the superior mesenteric artery usually results in complete foregut infarction.

    E. The right and left colon are generally spared as a result of sparing of the middle colic artery.

    Ref.: 1, 2

COMMENTS: Arterial emboli are the most common cause of sudden complete occlusion of the superior mesenteric artery. • These emboli most often arise from the heart, either as mural thrombi from recent myocardial infarction or as auricular thrombi in patients with atrial fibrillation. • Other cardiac arrhythmias, cardiac tumors such as atrial myxoma, and paradoxical emboli through a patent foramen ovale may also be a source of arterial emboli. • One fourth of the patients report previous embolic events. • The initial abdominal pain is severe, often refractory to narcotics, and often out of proportion to the physical findings. • The physical signs of peritonitis imply transmural ischemia and therefore, when present, represent a late stage in the evolution of this process. • Acute occlusion of the superior mesenteric artery results usually in midgut infarction (ligament of Treitz to splenic flexure of the colon). • The proximal jejunum, however, is often spared during acute superior mesenteric artery obstruction because of the location of the embolus beyond the first branch of the artery and the collateral vessels and because of the dual supply by the celiac axis system and the peripancreatic collateral vascular bed. • The latter is formed by anastomosis between the superior pancreaticoduodenal artery (celiac based) and the inferior pancreaticoduodenal artery (first branch of the superior mesenteric artery).

ANSWER:
A, C

4. With regard to the diagnosis and management of acute occlusion of the superior mesenteric artery, which of the following statements is/are true?

A. Early arteriography can be of both diagnostic and therapeutic value.

B. Most patients can avoid operation if arterial infusion of papaverine is begun early during the clinical course.

C. Arteriography should be performed in all patients who present without advanced peritoneal signs.

D. As much as 70% of the small intestine can be resected without creating incapacitating digestive problems.

E. Clinical assessment, Doppler flowmeter analysis, and fluorescein staining are equally accurate for determining intestinal viability.

Ref.: 1, 2

COMMENTS: Early arteriography not only confirms the diagnosis and assists in determining the cause, but it also provides a route by which intra-arterial papaverine can be administered. • Papaverine, a potent vasodilator, assists in dilating the more peripheral mesenteric bed, which frequently is severely constricted as a reflex response to the more proximal mechanical occlusion. • Despite these beneficial effects, most patients require laparotomy.

Serious gastrointestinal disturbances are uncommon if more than 30% of the small bowel can be preserved. • The likelihood of a good result is enhanced if the terminal ileum and ileocecal valve are preserved as well.

Fluorescein dye may be administered intravenously, and assessment of fluorescein staining of the bowel by a Woods lamp may be used to evaluate viability. • The fluorescence pattern is significantly more reliable than either clinical judgment or the Doppler flowmeter for assessing bowel viability in borderline cases at the time of laparotomy. • Reestablishment of the circulation should be attempted before bowel resection is undertaken. • When long segments of intestine are of questionable viability, they are best left in place and reexamined at a second operation 24 hr later to ensure the maximal length of viable intestine.

ANSWER:
A, C, D

5. Which of the following statements correctly characterize a nonocclusive mesenteric infarction?

A. It occurs more frequently but is associated with a lower mortality rate than occlusive mesenteric infarction.

B. It is usually related to a state of low cardiac output and may be exacerbated by digoxin.

C. It is often accompanied by a markedly elevated hematocrit as a result of polycythemia.

D. Arteriography with intra-arterial infusion of papaverine can be effective in selected cases.

Ref.: 2

COMMENTS: Only 20–30% of cases of small-bowel infarction are caused by nonocclusive phenomena. • It is the most lethal form of acute mesenteric ischemia. • The "final common pathway" of nonocclusive infarction appears to be a low cardiac output state, which may accompany numerous processes, including primary cardiac disease as well as septicemia and hypovolemia. • Digoxin induces mesenteric vasoconstriction and therefore worsens the ischemic process. • Papaverine, isoproterenol, and glucagon are vasodilating agents and may be therapeutically beneficial when accompanied by efforts to correct the low-flow state. • Often, however, laparotomy is necessary because of refractory hypotension, because the diagnosis is in question, or because there are signs of peritonitis. • The elevated hematocrit frequently seen in this disease process is caused by third-space loss of serum, not by polycythemia. • Early use of arteriography to distinguish occlusive from nonocclusive mesenteric ischemia can lead to therapeutic intervention with intra-arterial papaverine. • This approach, however, is contraindicated in patients in shock because the vasodilation of the splanchnic bed due to papaverine aggravates the hypovolemia. • Correction of underlying and associated conditions is paramount to the survival of these patients.

ANSWER:
B, D

6. With regard to mesenteric venous occlusion, which of the following statements is/are true?

A. Inflammatory conditions such as appendicitis or diverticulitis can be predisposing factors.

B. Patients with polycythemia vera, those with antithrombin III deficiency, and those taking oral contraceptives may be at increased risk for mesenteric venous occlusion.

C. Bloody diarrhea occurs less commonly with venous occlusion than with arterial occlusion.

D. Shorter segments of intestine are usually involved in venous occlusion in comparison with arterial occlusion.

E. Because of the frequent need for reoperation, heparin is contraindicated in these patients.

Ref.: 2

COMMENTS: Often subacute in its presentation, mesenteric venous occlusion may be idiopathic or secondary to a number of conditions, including appendicitis, diverticulitis, pelvic abscess, hematologic conditions, the postsplenectomy state in some patients (myeloproliferative disorders), use of oral contraceptives, extrinsic compression by tumor, venous trauma, acute portal vein thrombosis, polycythemia vera, and antithrombin III deficiency. • All of these conditions bring into play various pathophysiologic mechanisms predisposing to clotting, including hypercoagulability, inflammatory or mechanical damage to the endothelium of veins, and low flow resulting from a variety of causes. • Bowel-wall edema may be seen on plain films. • CT scanning may reveal thrombus within the portal vein or the superior mesenteric vein. • Mesenteric vein thrombosis is not often diagnosed intraoperatively.

Bloody diarrhea is seen more commonly with venous occlusion but tends to be a later finding than with arterial occlusion.

• The site of venous occlusion tends to be more peripheral within the mesentery than is the site of arterial occlusion, and therefore shorter segments of intestine are involved. • Resection should encompass involved gangrenous bowel and mesentery until veins that appear normal on gross examination are encountered. • Otherwise, extension of residual clot leads to further gangrene. • Anticoagulation with heparin should be started promptly. • Because of a 30–40% recurrent thrombosis rate in untreated patients, lifelong anticoagulation is generally recommended. • A second-look operation should be performed after 24 hr because of the common recurrence of thrombosis. • Most patients with mesenteric venous thrombosis do not require laparotomy, but those with peritoneal signs do.

ANSWER:
A, B, D

7. Regarding splanchnic artery aneurysms, which of the following statements is/are true?

   A. Celiac and hepatic artery aneurysms are more common in men, in contrast to splenic artery aneurysms, which are more common in women.

   B. A left upper quadrant signet ring calcification is highly suggestive of a hepatic artery aneurysm.

   C. Asymptomatic splenic artery aneurysms should be electively repaired when found in women of childbearing age.

   D. All asymptomatic celiac and hepatic artery aneurysms should be electively repaired except in high-risk patients.

   E. Endovascular procedures have no role in the management of splanchnic artery aneurysms.

Ref.: 2

COMMENTS: Splenic artery aneurysms account for approximately 60% of all splanchnic artery aneurysms. • They are four times more common in women than in men. • This is in contrast to celiac and hepatic artery aneurysms, two thirds of which are seen in men. • Most splenic artery aneurysms are incidental findings in studies performed for other indications. • A left upper quadrant signet ring calcification is a classic finding on plain radiograph suggestive of a splenic artery aneurysm. • Splenic artery aneurysms in pregnant patients have a very poor prognosis. • Nearly 95% of splenic aneurysms reported during pregnancy were ruptured, and rupture during pregnancy leads to death in more than half of the women and more than 90% of the fetuses. • Therefore, any women in their childbearing years who are diagnosed with an asymptomatic splenic artery aneurysm should undergo elective repair. • Aneurysms of the other splanchnic arteries should be repaired in patients with acceptable surgical risks, regardless of the absence of symptoms, because the incidence of rupture among these aneurysms approaches 50%. • Endovascular transcatheter embolization or placement of covered stents has been successfully employed in the management of splanchnic artery aneurysms.

ANSWER:
A, C, D

8. With regard to intestinal angina, which of the following statements is/are true?

   A. This term is a misnomer because it bears no pathophysiologic similarity to cardiac angina or claudication.

   B. It is usually characterized by insidious weight loss, food aversion, and postprandial abdominal pain.

   C. Anteroposterior aortography is invaluable for visualizing the origins of the visceral vessels and for demonstrating the large collateral vessels that develop in response to chronic visceral artery occlusion.

   D. Operative correction is almost always indicated, even if only one vessel is diseased.

   E. The operative approach involves primarily transaortic endarterectomy or aortovisceral grafting (antegrade or retrograde).

Ref.: 1, 2

COMMENTS: As with angina pectoris and claudication, intestinal angina represents an imbalance between the metabolic needs of an organ (the intestines) and the blood supply available to meet those needs. • Postprandial abdominal cramping is characteristic and is often accompanied by weight loss (11 kg on average) from food aversion rather than malabsorption. • Although the diagnosis is suggested clinically, *anteroposterior and lateral aortography* is essential for delineating arterial anatomy before operation. • Only lateral views can demonstrate the origins of the visceral vessels. • A long, meandering artery is often demonstrated on the left side of the abdomen. • It results from the collateral circulation between the inferior mesenteric and superior mesenteric arteries through the artery of Drummond (if lateral) and the arch of Riolan (if medial in location). • Noninvasive ultrasonic imaging of the celiac and mesenteric vessels is developing as an important screening tool for patients presenting with weight loss and postprandial pain. • Symptoms typically are not present unless two or more vessels are involved. • Because of the difficulty of exposing the origins of the superior mesenteric and celiac arteries, most surgeons prefer to use bypass grafting for operative correction of these vascular abnormalities. • Antegrade conduits of either prosthetic material or autogenous saphenous vein are preferred. • Trapdoor aortotomy and endarterectomy may be appropriate in the presence of multiple proximal visceral and renal artery stenoses. • Percutaneous angioplasty has been performed on a selective basis, although large series and long-term follow-up are lacking.

ANSWER:
B, E

9. Compression of the celiac artery by the median arcuate ligament is characterized by which of the following statements?

   A. It is always caused by an embryologic anomaly of the diaphragmatic fibers of the median arcuate ligament.

   B. A bruit is classically present over the epigastrium.

   C. Chronic abdominal pain, diarrhea, weight loss, and occasional nausea are the usual presenting symptoms.

   D. Treatment should include transection of the median arcuate ligament to ensure celiac axis patency.

   E. Direct arterial reconstruction to ensure celiac axis patency should be avoided, since the pathologic process involves the abnormal median arcuate ligament.

Ref.: 1, 2

COMMENTS: Compression of the celiac artery by the median arcuate ligament may be caused by an abnormal proximal origin of the celiac artery or abnormally low positioning of the median arcuate ligament. • Chronic abdominal pain, diarrhea, weight loss, and occasional nausea are characteristic symptoms. • The weight loss may be severe because patients stop eating to avoid the fairly predictable postprandial pain. • Classically, a bruit is heard over the epigastrium, but its absence does not negate the diagnosis. • If initial transection of the median arcuate ligament and surrounding neural tissue does not result in restoration of proper blood flow, direct arterial reconstruction may be necessary to ensure celiac axis patency. • Irritation of neural tissue around the origin of the celiac axis by the arcuate ligament may represent another pathophysiologic mechanism for this pain syndrome.

ANSWER:
B, C, D

10. Regarding percutaneous angioplasty and stenting for chronic mesenteric ischemia, which of the following statements is/are true?

A. Initial technical success is approximately 90%, with symptom improvement in 90% of patients with successful procedures.

B. The rate of serious complications is less than 10%.

C. Approximately 30% of patients will develop severe restenosis within 2 years.

D. It should be reserved only for patients who are poor operative candidates.

E. Patients with compression of a mesenteric vessel by the median arcuate ligament do not benefit from angioplasty and stenting.

Ref.: 5

COMMENTS: Percutaneous transluminal angioplasty (PTA) with or without stenting has emerged in recent years as an alternative to surgical bypass for improving chronic intestinal ischemia. • Review of most recent series indicates that the initial success rate is approximately 85–95%. • It is a safe procedure, with major complications reported in only 6% of patients and a 30-day mortality rate of 3%. • Follow-up in the larger series of patients indicates a restenosis rate of less than 10% in 2 years. • Therefore, most authorities suggest that PTA and stenting, when feasible, should be the initial treatment of choice in patients with chronic mesenteric ischemia. • Compression of a mesenteric vessel by the median arcuate ligament can mimic the symptoms of chronic mesenteric ischemia. • These patients do not benefit from PTA and should not have a stent placed. • Surgical release of the median arcuate ligament is the treatment of choice for this condition.

ANSWER:
A, B, E

11. Regarding the diagnosis and surgical management of acute mesenteric ischemia, which of the following is/are causes?

A. Mesenteric venous thrombosis

B. Acute embolic arterial occlusion

C. Acute thrombotic arterial occlusion

D. Nonocclusive mesenteric ischemia

Ref.: 1–4

COMMENTS: Acute mesenteric ischemia is most often secondary to acute embolic arterial occlusion of the superior mesenteric artery (SMA; its 30-degree take-off from the abdominal aorta creates the most accessible visceral vessel for embolic events). • The embolus usually lodges 3–10 cm from the origin of the SMA, at the take-off of the middle colic artery. • The SMA usually feels soft and normal. • Approximately 50% of cases of acute mesenteric ischemia are secondary to arterial emboli. • Thrombotic arterial occlusion is the next most frequent cause, accounting for 25% of cases. • The occlusion usually involves the origin of the SMA, where a hard plaque can be felt in most patients.

The treatment of thrombotic arterial occlusion superimposed on atherosclerotic disease requires a bypass procedure. • Prosthetic arterial conduits can be used in the absence of bowel gangrene or contamination. • When contamination is present, saphenous vein is the conduit of choice. • Patients with atherosclerotic occlusions usually have at least two mesenteric vessels involved when they become symptomatic. • In cases of acute ischemia, revascularization of the SMA has been reported to give results equivalent to those achieved with multiple vessel revascularization. • The long-term graft patency rate is approximately 90%.

ANSWER:
A, B, C, D

REFERENCES

1. Townsend CM Jr, Beauchamp RD, Evers BM, et al (eds): *Sabiston Textbook of Surgery: The Biological Basis of Modern Surgical Practice*, 17th ed. Saunders, Philadelphia, 2004.
2. Brunicardi FC, Andersen DK, Billiar TR, et al (eds): *Schwartz's Principles of Surgery*, 8th ed. McGraw-Hill, New York, 2004.
3. Mullholland MW, Lillemoe KD, Doherty GM, et al (eds): *Greenfield's Surgery: Scientific Principles and Practice*, 4th ed. Lippincott, Williams & Wilkins, Philadelphia, 2006.
4. Moore WS: *Vascular Surgery: A Comprehensive Review*. Saunders, Philadelphia, 2002.
5. Ernst CB, Stanley JC: *Current Therapy in Vascular Surgery*, 4th ed. CV Mosby, St. Louis, 2001.

CHAPTER 45

Peripheral Venous and Lymphatic Disease

Irina Goncharova, M.D., and Walter J. McCarthy III, M.D.

1. A 28-year-old overweight woman comes to the emergency room with a slightly reddened, painful "knot" 8 cm above the medial malleolus. Examination in the standing position demonstrates a palpable vein above and below a tender 2-cm mass. The patient is afebrile and has no other abnormalities on physical examination. Which of the following is the most likely diagnosis?

A. Early deep vein thrombosis (DVT)

B. Superficial venous thrombosis

C. Suppurative thrombophlebitis

D. Cellulitis

E. Hematoma

F. Insect bite

Ref.: 1–3

COMMENTS: Superficial venous thrombi may be associated with thrombophlebitis, which is an acute, nonbacterial inflammation producing pain, redness, and swelling. • Thrombi, however, may form without producing any signs or symptoms. • **Superficial thrombophlebitis** usually appears as a localized process over the known course of a superficial vein. • It occurs in association with intravenous catheters in the upper extremity and is usually seen at the site of varicose veins in the lower extremity. • The presence of distended varicosities above and below the lesion aids in the diagnosis. • The diagnosis is usually readily made based on the history and physical examination findings. • Lack of blood flow through the vein can be confirmed with Doppler ultrasound imaging, but this test usually is unnecessary unless there is concern about a DVT. • Venography is not indicated and may even exacerbate the condition.

The diagnoses of cellulitis, insect bite, subcutaneous hematoma, and traumatic ecchymosis must be considered when evaluating these lesions. • An **insect bite** frequently is associated with itching. • The presence of a hematoma or ecchymosis may indicate **trauma** as the cause. • **Suppurative thrombophlebitis** also must be considered, especially in the presence of fever and leukocytosis. • Suppurative thrombophlebitis is characterized by purulence within the vein and usually is a complication of intravenous cannulation. • The presence of increased redness, pain, fluctuance, fever, and leukocytosis is more typical of bacterial infection than of superficial thrombophlebitis.

ANSWER:
B

2. In a patient with superficial thrombophlebitis associated with varicose veins, the treatment plan may include which of the following measures?

A. Excision of the entire vein and administration of intravenous antibiotics

B. Iodine 125 ([125I])-labeled fibrinogen scan, hospitalization, and heparinization

C. Ligation of the vein proximal and distal to the mass, bed rest, and intravenous antibiotics

D. Bed rest, elastic support hose, leg elevation, and antibiotics

E. Warm moist packs, elastic support hose, nonsteroidal anti-inflammatory drugs, and ambulation with limited sitting or standing

Ref.: 1, 2

COMMENTS: The usual aim when treating superficial thrombophlebitis is to relieve symptoms. • The inflammation is nonbacterial, and antibiotics are not necessary unless there is evidence of secondary infection. • These thrombi almost never embolize to the lungs unless they have propagated to the deep venous system. • Fortunately, superficial venous thrombosis does not usually progress to DVT. • Anticoagulation therefore is not necessary. • Ligation is reserved for superficial lesions in the greater saphenous system above the knee near its junction with the femoral vein and for lesions of the lesser saphenous system near the popliteal fossa, locations from which a thrombus may more easily extend to the deep venous system.

Superficial phlebitis in these locations is best evaluated with duplex ultrasound scanning. • Unlike the recommendations made for DVT, with superficial thrombosis the risk of propagation of the thrombus is lessened by preventing venous stasis. • This is accomplished by frequent walking, use of elastic-stocking support, and keeping the leg elevated above the level of the heart when in the supine position. • In other words, the patient should either walk or lie down with the leg elevated. • Sitting and standing still for extended periods should be avoided whenever possible. • Superficial thrombophlebitis is an acute problem, and symptoms from it usually resolve in several weeks. • Anti-inflammatory drugs are of variable effectiveness. • Aspirin usually suffices. • Recurrent superficial thrombophlebitis may respond to proximal ligation followed by vein stripping.

ANSWER:
E

3. Match the site of thrombosis in the left-hand column with the appropriate signs and symptoms in the right-hand column.

A. Calf vein

B. Femoral vein

C. Ileofemoral vein

D. Pelvic vein

E. Subclavian vein

a. Left side more frequently involved, severe swelling associated with cyanosis and pain

b. No swelling

c. Ankle and calf swelling, venous pressure two to five times normal

d. Minimal swelling, venous pressure normal

e. Swelling in a patient with a central venous catheter

Ref.: 1, 2

COMMENTS: The signs and symptoms of DVT vary according to the vein involved. • The most frequent site of thrombus is the calf, with the lesion usually arising in the sinuses of the soleus muscle. • **Calf vein thrombi** usually produce pain and localized tenderness. • Little swelling occurs (generally less than 1.5-cm diameter difference between the calves, although it is entirely absent in 30% of patients), and venous pressure is normal. • **Femoral vein thrombi** produce pain in the calf, popliteal region, or adductor canal. • Swelling generally is present up to the midcalf, and venous pressure is elevated. • **Ileofemoral thrombi** often are localized but may extend to the calf. • The left leg is involved twice as often as the right, probably because of the longer course of the left iliac vein and its compression by the right iliac artery. • As the venous pressure becomes elevated, the leg becomes painful, edematous, swollen, and pale (phlegmasia alba dolens). • In this condition, the blanched appearance of the limb is the result of edema and not arterial spasm, as previously thought. • More extensive ileofemoral venous thrombosis, in which clot is propagated distally and into the ileofemoral venous tributaries, can obstruct all venous drainage and impair arterial inflow, producing ischemia and threatened loss of the limb. • This condition, phlegmasia cerulea dolens, is a surgical emergency. • **Pelvic vein thrombus** can occur in women with pelvic inflammatory disease or men with prostatic infections. • The condition is detected by pelvic examination, and there are few leg signs. • Venous thrombosis is less frequent in the upper than lower extremity, and most commonly it is the result of **subclavian vein thrombosis** from an indwelling catheter. • **Upper-extremity DVT** may occur in patients with heart failure or cancer. • In otherwise normal patients, it has been termed the Paget–von Schroetter syndrome or "effort thrombosis" and is a subclavian axillary vein thrombosis resulting from injury of the vein at the thoracic outlet. • It presents as arm swelling and heaviness with discomfort made worse by activity.

ANSWER:
A-d; B-c; C-a; D-b; E-e

4. Increased risk of DVT is associated with which of the following factors?

A. Blood group type O

B. Diabetes mellitus

C. Pregnancy

D. General anesthesia

E. Knee joint replacement

Ref.: 3

COMMENTS: Venostasis of the lower extremities is associated with prolonged bed rest, standing, or sitting. • It is also associated with the immobilization and muscular paralysis associated with trauma and general and spinal anesthesia. • The most significant risk factor is a previous DVT. • Additional risk factors include advanced age, obesity, diabetes mellitus, and the presence of malignancy. • Patients with blood group type O are at low risk for DVT, whereas patients with group A blood are at higher risk. • In both instances, the reason is unknown.

Oral contraceptives and pregnancy are associated with increased levels of fibrinogen and factors VII, VIII, IX, and X, and both are associated with increased risk of DVT.

The incidence of DVT in surgical patients is 20–50%. • The incidence in patients with hip fractures or those undergoing knee or hip replacement may exceed 50%.

ANSWER:
B, C, D, E

5. Regarding the workup of patients with DVT, which of the following statements is/are true?

A. Venography as the initial test largely has been replaced by the use of noninvasive tests.

B. Many prefer duplex scanning with B-mode ultrasound imaging as the initial test.

C. Doppler ultrasound imaging and impedance plethysmographic studies are equally useful for diagnosing femoral, popliteal, and major calf vein thrombosis.

D. Doppler ultrasound imaging and impedance plethysmographic studies are equally sensitive for diagnosing ileofemoral venous occlusion.

E. Isotope scanning cannot differentiate between active thrombosis and inflammatory fibrous exudate.

F. Venographic study is considered the definitive test for the diagnosis of DVT.

Ref.: 1–3

COMMENTS: Isotope scans with ^{125}I-labeled human fibrinogen are used to detect clot formation or thrombus propagation. • Studies of even the sickest patient are possible using portable instrumentation. • Isotope scanning is not useful in patients with superficial thrombophlebitis, overlying recent incisions, traumatic injuries, hematomas, cellulitis, active arthritis, or primary lymphedema because it cannot differentiate between active inflammatory fibrous exudate and thrombus formation. • Upper-thigh and pelvic lesions are often confused by the high background counts of the isotope within the pelvic organs. • An isotope scan can be 90% accurate for detecting the onset of thrombus when performed serially (daily) in high-risk patients. • Isotope scanning is now almost never used for a routine clinical diagnosis and is reserved for serial studies of patients in research studies. • It is 80% accurate when testing for suspected established venous thrombosis and generally is reserved for such patients. • **Doppler ultrasound imaging** is useful for detecting occlusions of major venous channels. • It can also detect incompetence of the deep and perforator veins, but it cannot differentiate between old and new thrombi, nor can it help diagnose small, nonobstructing thrombi. • **Duplex scanning with B-mode ultrasound imaging** is the best of the noninvasive studies for DVT. • This test can reliably differentiate extrinsic venous compression from DVT and new thrombi from old, and it can determine valvular competence. • Superficial and deep veins of the calf and thigh as well as the iliac veins and inferior vena cava (IVC) also can be visualized. • These tests are viewed as the preferred initial tests for DVT. • **Impedance plethysmographic study** is more accurate than Doppler ultrasound imaging for diagnosing femoral, popliteal, and major calf vein thromboses but less accurate than duplex scanning. • **Venographic study** is still

considered the definitive test for the diagnosis of DVT and is used to resolve equivocal results obtained by the noninvasive techniques.
• It is rarely used.

ANSWER:
A, B, E, F

6. Which of the following statements is/are true regarding the prevention of venous thrombosis?

   A. Elastic stockings have not been shown to influence the incidence of thrombus formation.

   B. To be effective, pneumatic calf compression must be used for at least 3 days after an operation.

   C. Injury to the intima of veins is an important cause of venous thrombosis.

   D. Sequential pneumatic calf compression and low-dose heparinization are essentially equally effective in preventing venous thrombosis.

   E. Low–molecular-weight heparin is less effective than low-dose heparin in preventing DVT.

Ref.: 1, 2

COMMENTS: Prophylaxis is critical in averting venous thrombosis, and a variety of techniques have been used to accomplish this.
• Attention to technical detail when handling veins so as not to injure their intima and avoidance of leg veins when infusing hypertonic or irritating solutions are two examples of ways to help minimize the risk of thrombosis. • Leg elevation and leg exercises during the postoperative period decrease venous stasis and its predisposition to thrombus formation. • ^{125}I-labeled fibrinogen scans have demonstrated the usefulness of pneumatic compression stockings in decreasing the incidence of thrombus formation. • Pneumatic stockings work by generating fibrinolysin and antithrombin III and, as such, are effective even when placed on an arm rather than the legs. • Sequential pneumatic devices are more effective than nonsequential devices, and, in at least one study, they have been shown to be as effective as low-dose heparinization. • Low-dose heparinization (i.e., 5000 units subcutaneously) given 2 hr preoperatively and continued twice daily until the seventh postoperative day has been shown to decrease the incidence of DVT. • There is evidence, however, that it may increase the rate of postoperative bleeding and wound complications. • Its impact on the incidence of postoperative pulmonary emboli has not been clearly defined.
• Low–molecular-weight heparin has been shown to be superior to low-dose heparin for preventing DVT for patients undergoing both general and orthopedic surgery. • Although no single method of prophylaxis has been shown to be clearly superior, some form of prophylaxis is important, whether it is aimed at preventing venous stasis physically or includes the use of anticoagulants.

ANSWER:
C, D

7. Regarding the medical treatment of DVT, which of the following statements is/are true?

   A. Bed rest is recommended to decrease venous pressure and thus lessen the risk of embolism.

   B. Heparin is given to prevent thrombus attachment to the venous wall.

   C. Platelet counts lower than 75,000/mm^3 imply active clot formation and inadequate levels of heparin.

   D. Anticoagulation should be continued for 1–6 months after the acute event, depending on the site of involvement.

   E. Tissue plasminogen activator and urokinase are contraindicated within 4 weeks of major operations or trauma.

Ref.: 1, 2

COMMENTS: The prevention of embolization from existing thrombi and the inhibition of new thrombus formation are the goals of medical therapy for DVT. • **Bed rest with leg elevation** decreases venous pressure and prevents fluctuations of pressure in the deep venous system. • This allows the thrombus already present to become firmly attached to the vessel wall, minimizes venous distention, and reduces edema and pain. • Elastic support is not needed if there is adequate elevation, but it should be used when ambulation is started.
   Heparin prevents propagation of the thrombus. • It inhibits thrombin by inactivating the thrombin in the presence of antithrombin III (now called antithrombin). • A partial thromboplastin time (PTT) that is two times normal indicates adequate heparinization.
• Giving heparin by continuous intravenous infusion is the preferred method, but intravenous or subcutaneous administration as a bolus can be used. • Heparinization is continued for at least 7 days.
• Some patients receiving heparin therapy develop platelet clots in the arterial and venous system (heparin-induced thrombocytopenia), which can be a catastrophic complication. • Therefore, a platelet count that falls to less than 75,000/mm^3 is thought by some to be a reason to consider discontinuing heparin. • Antiplatelet antibody levels should be evaluated in these patients. • Alternative anticoagulation medications should be used. • Warfarin (Coumadin) derivatives are begun before stopping the heparin to allow anticoagulant therapy to be continued on an outpatient basis. • Treatment usually is continued for 1–3 months, until the risk of recurrence diminishes.
• In cases of ileofemoral thrombosis, anticoagulation is continued for 6 months to allow time for the development of adequate collateral circulation, which decreases the risk of recurrence.
   Tissue plasminogen activator and **urokinase** are capable of lysing thrombi via activation of plasminogen to plasmin. • Their use in combination with heparin may reduce the incidence of late postphlebitic complications when compared with heparin alone.
• Both agents are most effective when given to patients with DVT of less than 5–7 days' duration, and the best results are obtained in patients who have had symptoms for less than 48 hr. • Pyrogenic, allergic, and bleeding complications occur with both agents, and their use is contraindicated within 4 weeks of major operations or injury. • Bleeding complications occur two to five times more frequently in patients treated with heparin alone, and intracranial bleeding may occur in 1% of patients. • Thus, thrombolytic treatment of lower-extremity DVT is best limited to severe cases. • The value of antiplatelet drugs such as aspirin is still undefined, but inhibition of platelet adherence and aggregation with platelet-inhibiting agents does not stop clotting once it has begun. • Such drugs therefore appear to be more useful for prophylaxis than for treatment.

ANSWER:
A, D, E

8. Which of the following statements is/are true? Which is/are false?

   A. The major indication for deep venous thrombectomy is recurrent pulmonary emboli.

   B. Thrombectomy for ileofemoral DVT uniformly results in less swelling, pain, and venous stasis than does conservative therapy.

   C. Thrombectomy is contraindicated for phlegmasia cerulea dolens.

D. Ileofemoral thrombosis from a pelvic infection is best treated with thrombectomy.

E. Caval interruption should always precede ileofemoral thrombectomy.

Ref.: 1, 2

COMMENTS: The role of surgery in the treatment of acute DVT is limited because of the effectiveness of medical management, the high incidence of residual or recurrent venous obstruction, and valvular incompetence that occurs after operative correction. • Operation usually is reserved for major obstruction of the subclavian, iliac, or femoral vein and when the immediate or long-term function of the limb is in jeopardy. • Clinical studies have not demonstrated that thrombectomy leads to less swelling, pain, and venostasis than does nonoperative therapy. • Progression of ileofemoral thrombosis to the stage of near-total occlusion, with tenderness, massive edema, and cyanosis (phlegmasia cerulea dolens) may lead to venous gangrene. • When it occurs, failure of the patient to respond promptly to treatment with leg elevation and heparinization or thrombolytic therapy (or both) is an indication for thrombectomy.

Although there is a theoretic advantage to caval interruption before thrombectomy, ileofemoral thrombectomy can be safely performed without caval interruption.

Septic ileofemoral thrombi (usually as a result of pelvic infection) are a contraindication to thrombectomy.

Operations for subclavian vein thrombosis should include resection of the first rib, cervical rib, or clavicle because most thrombi originate at the point where the clavicle crosses the first rib. • Failure to resect these structures is associated with a high rate of postoperative recurrence.

Success of venous thrombectomy depends on early operation, good technique, and complete removal of the thrombus. • Surgery is not as useful after 7–10 days, and the best results occur when thrombectomy is performed within 48 hr of the appearance of symptoms.

Pulmonary emboli (PE) that recur despite proper medical therapy are best treated with a caval filter.

ANSWER:
A-False; B-False; C-False; D-False; E-False

9. Which of the following statements regarding the evaluation of patients with suspected PE is/are true?

A. The triad of dyspnea, pain, and hemoptysis is present in more than 60% of patients.

B. Normal serum glutamic-oxaloacetic transaminase (SGOT) levels in the presence of elevated serum bilirubin and lactate dehydrogenase (LDH) levels are seen in more than 50% of patients.

C. Pulmonary arteriography requires cardiac catheterization.

D. The arterial blood gas value is characterized by hypoxemia and normal to decreased PCO_2.

E. Ventilation-perfusion scans must be compared with a recent chest radiograph to be of value.

Ref.: 1, 2

COMMENTS: Surgeons must have a low threshold for suspecting PE in postoperative patients. • About 85% of PEs arise from the lower extremity, 10% from the right atrium, and 5% from the pelvic veins, vena cava, or arms. • Up to 30% of patients with PE are free of symptoms, and only one third of patients with PE have physical evidence of DVT at the time of diagnosis. • Emboli produce symptoms either by the direct effects of arterial obstruction or by secondary bronchospasm and vasoconstriction. • The most common symptoms are dyspnea and pleuritic chest pain, and the most common signs are tachypnea, tachycardia, and rales. • The classic triad of dyspnea, pain, and hemoptysis is present in fewer than 25% of patients. • In fact, hemoptysis is indicative of frank pulmonary infarction and is uncommon. • The classic biochemical triad of a normal SGOT level with elevated LDH and bilirubin levels now is considered unreliable. • Few patients show diagnostic electrocardiographic (ECG) changes other than tachycardia. • Wedge-shaped defects on chest radiographs are seen only if infarction occurs. • Decreased vascularity, pulmonary artery distention, and pleural fluid may be detected. • Pulmonary arteriograms are the most specific tests for diagnosis and are performed by contrast infusion through a right atrial or main pulmonary artery catheter. • On ventilation-perfusion scans, areas of the lungs that are normally ventilated but not perfused and that appear normal on chest radiographs should be considered to have PE. • These scans are safe, convenient, and reliable if the findings are strongly positive or normal. • For most patients, they are generally preferred to arteriograms as an initial study. • The arterial blood gas result typically demonstrates hypoxemia and decreased PCO_2. • This is the opposite of what is expected with "dead space" disease (i.e., normal ventilation with decreased perfusion), wherein PO_2 is normal and PCO_2 usually is elevated. • This paradox is explained by a (presumably) chemically mediated right-to-left shunt induced by PE and tachypnea, leading to a normal or slightly decreased PCO_2. • Spiral computed tomographic (CT) scanning is a rapid and excellent way to diagnose PE and is the test of choice in many medical centers but does require a bolus of contrast material.

ANSWER:
D, E

10. Match each location and blood flow pattern in the left-hand column with the appropriate superficial venous system in the right-hand column.

A. Ultimately joins the common femoral vein in the thigh	a. Greater saphenous
B. Ultimately joins the popliteal vein behind the knee	b. Lesser saphenous
C. Anterior and posterior branch in the calf, lateral and medial branch in the thigh	c. Both
D. Receives blood from the deep system via perforators	d. Neither
E. Blood flowing into the deep system via the perforators	
F. Perforators located posterior and superior to the malleoli	

Ref.: 1, 2

COMMENTS: An understanding of normal venous anatomy and blood flow is essential when considering chronic venous insufficiency and its sequelae. • Normal veins of the lower extremity contain valves that direct the flow of blood centrally toward the heart and from the superficial into the deep venous system. • Competent valves resist the force of gravity, which in the erect position tends to pool blood at the ankle. • Forward flow is provided by the action of the left ventricle and compression of the veins as a result of muscular contraction. • During muscular relaxation, deep venous pressure falls, leading to increased emptying of the superficial veins into the deep veins with a resultant fall in superficial venous pressures to below resting levels. • Incompetence of the valves of the deep veins (usually the result of previous venous thrombosis) allows blood pooling and ineffective muscular pumping. • Incompetence of the perforator valves (as a direct result of venous thrombosis or the result of dilation by back pressure from a valveless deep system) allows transmission of this increased deep venous pressure to the superficial system. • When this occurs, the sequelae of venous stasis develop (brawny, nonpitting edema, brown pigmentation, dermatitis, and venous ulceration). • Venous ulcers usually occur over the perforators, which are located dorsal and cephalad to the medial and lateral malleoli. • Superficial venous incompetence, perforator incompetence, and deep vein abnormalities have the potential of causing these changes, and each may occur alone or in combination with the others.

ANSWER:
A-a; B-b; C-a; D-d; E-c; F-a

11. Which of the following patients is/are a candidates for an IVC filter?

    A. A 33-year-old woman, 6 weeks pregnant, with a documented DVT of the femoral vein and a ventilation-perfusion scan suggestive of a small PE

    B. A 65-year-old man, after bilateral total knee replacement, with bilateral femoral DVT

    C. A 50-year-old woman, after total abdominal hysterectomy, with angiographically confirmed PE that occurred despite adequate anticoagulation

    D. A 26-year-old man with an ileofemoral DVT and massive thigh swelling, on heparin, and with a platelet count remaining stable at 90,000/mm³

    E. A 70-year-old woman with evidence of right ileofemoral DVT and a large, loose thrombus in the infrarenal IVC

Ref.: 3

COMMENTS: The primary therapy for PEs in most patients is anticoagulation. • Precise knowledge of the role of thrombolytic agents is still evolving. • For certain patients, caval interruption may be indicated: patients in whom heparin therapy is contraindicated, those with recurrent emboli despite adequate anticoagulation, and those with free-floating ileofemoral thrombi.

Caval interruption may be used prophylactically in high-risk patients (e.g., before major pelvic surgery in those with a history of previous DVT or PE). • In addition, caval interruption is indicated for some patients with septic pulmonary emboli whose condition is refractory to heparin and antibiotics. • Caval interruption may be complete or partial. • Recurrence of PEs after complete interruption is possible through new collaterals, although rare. • Recurrence also results from thrombi arising from the ovarian veins, the IVC between the ligature and the renal veins, the right atrium, the right ventricle, and the veins of the head and neck. • Chronic leg swelling, recurring phlebitis, and the sequelae of deep venous obstruction (edema, discoloration, and ulceration) are more common after complete caval interruption and have been reported to occur with a frequency as high as 35%. • Experience with transvenously placed devices that totally occlude the cava has shown the incidence of these complications to be low (5%) in patients who can be maintained on anticoagulants after caval interruption. • Also, the presence of preexisting deep venous obstruction and chronic venous insufficiency strongly influences late results after caval interruption. • Devices that partially interrupt the IVC produce a lower incidence of postphlebitic sequelae, a higher incidence of nonfatal emboli (7 versus 4%), and a similar incidence of fatal emboli (about 1%). • Caval filters can migrate and have also been associated with injury to adjacent retroperitoneal structures.

Patients with massive PEs producing hypotension who survive the acute event are candidates for pulmonary embolectomy, which is performed using a median sternotomy, cardiopulmonary bypass, and open clot extraction. • An alternative to median sternotomy may be percutaneous catheter embolectomy.

Warfarin is contraindicated during pregnancy because of its teratogenic potential. • Although a pregnant patient with a PE may be treated with long-term therapy with low–molecular-weight heparin, an alternative is a caval filter, especially if the patient is unable to administer subcutaneous heparin.

ANSWER:
C, E

12. A 56-year-old man presents with a history of heaviness, tiredness, and aching of the left lower leg for the past several months. The symptoms are relieved by leg elevation. He mentions that he is awakened from sleep because of calf and foot cramping, but it is relieved by walking or massage. On physical examination, he has thick, darkly pigmented skin, nonpitting edema bilaterally, and a superficial ulcer 2 cm in diameter, 5 cm above and behind the medial malleolus, that is slightly painful. The differential diagnosis includes which of the following?

    A. Arterial insufficiency with ulceration

    B. Isolated symptomatic varicose veins

    C. Varicose veins associated with incompetent perforator veins

    D. Deep venous insufficiency with incompetent perforator veins

    E. Diabetic ulcer

Ref.: 1, 2

COMMENTS: The most common symptoms associated with venous insufficiency are aching, swelling, and night cramps of the involved leg. • The symptoms often occur after periods of sitting or inactive standing. • Leg elevation frequently provides relief. • Although the **edema** of venous insufficiency can occur with varicose veins alone, usually it is associated with deep venous abnormalities and incompetent perforating veins. • **Night cramps** are the result of sustained contractions of the calf and foot muscles and are relieved by massage, ambulation, and proper management of the underlying venous insufficiency. • **Brawny, nonpitting edema** is the result of increased connective tissue in the subcutaneous tissue. • **Brown discoloration** is the result of hemosiderin deposition. • **Ulceration** is most common in patients with deep venous abnormalities and incompetent perforators. • In such cases, the ulcers usually are located above and posterior to the malleoli (medial more than lateral), reinforcing their relationship with perforator abnormalities. • When patients with a history of DVT are followed beyond 10 years, up to 20% ultimately develop ulcers.

In contrast to arterial ulcers, venous ulcers are superficial and rarely penetrate the fascia. • The pain of arterial insufficiency often is increased with leg elevation. • Ulcers associated with arterial insufficiency may occur anywhere on the lower leg but usually occur distally, often involving the toe first. • Arterial ulcers have an associated blue erythematous border and are more painful than venous ulcers. • Patients with diabetes mellitus may develop shallow ulcers of the ankle that closely resemble venous stasis ulcers. • Treating them as venous stasis ulcers (i.e., with leg elevation, an Unna boot, and other measures) may be disastrous because of the associated arterial insufficiency. • The diabetic ulcer often occurs on the calf or ankle but is *not* associated with the edema and other skin changes seen with venous stasis ulcers. • These ulcers result from arterial insufficiency and often begin with minor trauma to the affected area.

ANSWER:
C, D

13. A surgeon has performed a Trendelenburg test on the patient described in Question 12 and has determined that he has

incompetent varicose veins associated with incompetent perforating veins. How should this be interpreted?

A. Negative/negative Trendelenburg test

B. Negative/positive Trendelenburg test

C. Positive/negative Trendelenburg test

D. Positive/positive Trendelenburg test

Ref.: 1, 2

COMMENTS: There are several tests for diagnosing venous insufficiency. • The **Trendelenburg test** is a two-part test used to delineate the competence of the superficial and perforating veins. • While in the supine position, the patient elevates the legs until the superficial veins empty.

In **part I**, the saphenofemoral junction is occluded digitally, and the patient is asked to stand. • The superficial veins are observed for 30 seconds. • This action allows assessment of the competence of the perforator veins. • Slow, ascending, incomplete filling of the superficial veins during compression is a negative (normal) result, whereas rapid filling is a positive result, indicating incompetence of the deep and perforating veins.

In **part II**, the saphenofemoral occlusion is released while the veins are kept under observation. • This action allows assessment of the competence of the superficial veins. • Continued slow ascending filling after saphenofemoral release is a negative (normal) result. • Rapid retrograde filling is a positive result, indicating incompetence of the valves of the superficial system.

The **percussion test** is performed by tapping the superficial veins near the saphenofemoral junction while palpating over the knee for transmitted pulses. • It can also be used to examine the lesser saphenous system. • Transmission of a pulse suggests incompetent valves. • **Venous pressure studies** help delineate abnormalities in the normal venous pressure relationships during exercise. • **Functional phlebography** is performed in patients before and after a standard active exercise and can demonstrate important pathologic and physiologic abnormalities. • The **Perthes' test** involves application of elastic wraps to a leg with varicosities (to occlude the superficial venous system) before the patient is asked to exercise. • Pain during exercise suggests obstruction of the deep venous system.

ANSWER:
D

14. The therapeutic plan for the patient in Question 12 should include which of the following measures?

A. Varicose vein ligation and stripping as soon as possible

B. Ligation of the medial perforating veins as soon as possible

C. Initial treatment with appropriate leg wraps, leg elevation, and ambulation, with avoidance of prolonged sitting or standing still

D. Ulcer débridement, vein stripping, and skin graft

Ref.: 1, 2

COMMENTS: Operative treatment of venous insufficiency in most instances is an adjunct to aggressive conservative management. • Leg elevation, active exercise, and elastic compression form the cornerstones of nonoperative management. • The goals of compression are to relieve symptoms and reduce swelling. • When ulcers are present, local medications should be avoided unless evidence of infection exists. • Ulcers smaller than 3 cm in diameter often heal with the treatment described above.

The indications for superficial vein ligation and stripping are moderate-to-severe symptoms without other signs of venous

insufficiency, venous insufficiency with recurrent ulceration despite aggressive medical management, and occasionally severe varicosities without symptoms. • Ligation of incompetent perforating veins can be an important addition to the treatment of venous insufficiency, particularly if done before ulceration develops. • Ligation is most often performed through a longitudinal incision placed posterior and superior to the malleoli, as first described by Robert Linton. • Subfascial endoscopic techniques have recently reduced the morbidity of this technique. • When present, incompetent superficial veins should be stripped as part of the procedure. • Postoperatively, conservative measures must be continued aggressively. • Obstructions of ileofemoral or femoropopliteal veins have been bypassed using the ipsilateral (femoropopliteal occlusions) or contralateral (ileofemoral occlusions) saphenous veins.

ANSWER:
C

15. Which of the following statements is/are true regarding lymphatic anatomy?

A. The limb lymphatic vessels are valveless.

B. The lymphatic system begins just below the dermis as a network of fine capillaries.

C. Red blood cells, bacteria, and proteins readily enter lymphatic capillaries.

D. Extrinsic factors (e.g., muscle contraction, arterial pulsations, respiratory movement, and massage) aid in the movement of lymph flow.

Ref.: 1, 2

COMMENTS: The lymphatic system begins as a network of valveless capillaries in the superficial dermis. • There is a second valved plexus in the deep or subdermal layer that joins with the first to form the lymphatic vessels, and their course parallels that of the major blood vessels. • The lymphatic vessels also are valved, and lymph flow toward the heart is aided by massage, arterial pulsations, respiratory movement, and muscle contraction. • Intradermal lymphatics can be evaluated by the intradermal injection of patent blue dye. • The capillaries normally become visible as a fine network 30–60 seconds after injection. • Lymphangiography is rarely used to visualize the lymphatic vessels, since it may make lymphedema worse. • Unlike veins, these vessels appear to be of uniform caliber throughout their course.

Lymphatic vessels are entered readily by proteins present in the extracellular fluid. • Red blood cells and lymphocytes enter lymphatic vessels by separating the endothelial cells at their junctions.

Lymphedema occurs when the lymphatics are obstructed, too few in number, or nonfunctional, which results in the retention of interstitial fluid with a high protein concentration. • Tissue oncotic pressure increases, and fluid is drawn into the interstitium. • Measurement of the protein content of edema fluid (normally <1.5 mg/dl) can be used to assess the status of lymphatic function in the edematous extremity.

ANSWER:
C, D

16. Which of the following statements is/are true regarding the cause and complications of lymphedema?

A. Primary lymphedema appears at birth, is more common in females, and occurs in the right leg more often than in the left.

B. Milroy's disease is a form of primary lymphedema that is sex linked.

C. A lymphangiogram usually demonstrates a point of obstruction of the lymphatics in primary lymphedema.

D. Primary lymphedema almost always progresses to involve both lower extremities.

E. The major complication of lymphedema is the later development of lymphangiosarcoma.

Ref.: 1, 2

COMMENTS: Primary lymphedema is caused by abnormal development resulting in aplasia, hypoplasia, or varicosities of the lymphatic vessels. • **Congenital lymphedema** (Milroy's disease) is present at birth and has a familial, sex-linked incidence, but the family history is present in fewer than 5% of patients. • Primary lymphedema usually appears in individuals during their teens, more commonly in females, and it often develops insidiously. • The left limb is more frequently involved than is the right (3:1), and often only one limb is involved.

Secondary lymphedema is the result of obstruction or destruction of normal lymphatic channels and can be caused by tumor, repeated infection, or parasitic infection (particularly filariasis), or it can occur following lymph node dissection. • Lymphangiography often demonstrates a discrete obstruction. • Recurrent infections of venous stasis ulcers can destroy lymphatic vessels and lead to lymphedema.

The inability to clear proteins leads to edema formation that gradually increases over time and becomes woody because of fibrous tissue in the subcutaneous tissue. • Repeated infection hastens formation of this fibrous tissue accumulation. • Some patients develop blisters containing edema fluid, or chyle. • The major complication of lymphedema is recurrent attacks of cellulitis or lymphangitis, often following minor injury. • β-Hemolytic streptococci are the responsible organisms, and the infection spreads rapidly because the protein-containing edema fluid is an excellent culture medium.

Lymphangiosarcoma is a rare complication of long-standing lymphedema most frequently described in patients following radical mastectomy (Stewart-Treves syndrome). • It presents as a blue or purple nodule with a satellite lesion. • Metastases develop early, primarily to the lung.

Rarely, patients with lymphedema develop a protein-losing enteropathy that has been attributed to lymphatic obstruction of the small bowel.

ANSWER:
B

17. Regarding the treatment of lymphedema, which of the following statements is/are true?

A. More than 50% of patients ultimately require an operation.

B. Diuretics have a crucial role in the conservative management of early lymphedema.

C. Pneumatic compression devices can damage the remaining lymphatics and should not be used.

D. Microsurgically constructed lymphovenous shunts are far more effective than are excisional procedures.

E. All surgical procedures have significant failure rates.

Ref.: 1, 2

COMMENTS: The mainstay of management of lymphedema is conservative and nonoperative. • Fewer than 5% of patients require an operation. • The goals of therapy are the prevention of infection and the reduction of subcutaneous fluid volume. • Fluid volume is reduced by elevating the extremity during sleep, the use of pneumatic compression devices, and carefully fitted elastic support stockings. • Diuretics are not used routinely but may be useful in women who retain fluid during the premenstrual period. • Patients prone to recurrent lymphangitis require intermittent long-term antibiotic therapy at the first sign of infection. • The drug of choice is penicillin because streptococci are the usual infecting organisms. • Secondary lymphedema requires treatment of the underlying cause, such as giving diethylcarbamazine for filariasis and appropriate antibiotics for tuberculosis or lymphogranuloma venereum.

Edema that is excessive and interferes with normal activity and the presence of severe recurrent cellulitis are indications for operation. • Patients with minimal edema, gross obesity, and progressing disease are not candidates for surgery. • Excisional procedures include removal of skin, subcutaneous tissue, and fascia followed by split-thickness skin graft reconstruction (the Charles operation); excision of strips of skin and subcutaneous tissue followed by primary closure; and creation of buried dermal flaps. • Physiologic procedures to restore or enhance lymphatic drainage include insertion of silk, Teflon, or polystyrene threads into the subcutaneous tissue; construction of pedicle grafts from the involved limb to the trunk; and microsurgical lymphovenous shunts using dilated lymphatics or the capsule and efferent channels of isolated lymph nodes anastomosed to neighboring veins. • All procedures are associated with significant failure rates.

ANSWER:
E

18. Manifestations of acquired peripheral arteriovenous fistula (AVF) include which of the following?

A. Bacterial endarteritis

B. Distal embolization

C. Peripheral arterial insufficiency

D. Congestive heart failure

E. Venous aneurysm formation

Ref.: 2–4

COMMENTS: Acquired AVF is most commonly the result of penetrating trauma, which causes injury to an adjacent artery and vein. • The upper and lower extremities are the most common sites. • Other causes include suture-ligation of adjacent vessels, vessel catheterization for diagnostic or therapeutic study, erosion of an adjacent vein by an atherosclerotic aneurysm, periarterial abscess, or neoplasm. • Another cause is a remnant fistula following an in-situ peripheral artery bypass. • Small fistulas may close spontaneously. • Fistulas that persist lead to dilation and ectasia of the proximal artery, and the adjacent vein becomes thick walled, dilated, and aneurysmal. • The intimal damage that occurs leads to an increased risk of infection and bacterial endarteritis. • Depending on the size and location of the fistula, significant flow may lead to arterial insufficiency distal to the fistula ("steal phenomenon"). • Venous congestion, chronic venous stasis changes, edema, and venous varicosities may also occur. • In young children, a peripheral fistula may lead to limb length inequality if it is present before closure of the epiphyseal plate. • If the fistula is large, patients may develop signs and symptoms of high-output congestive heart failure. • Temporary compression of the fistula may elicit a Branham-Nicoladoni sign with a rise in diastolic blood pressure and decreased heart rate. • Peripheral AVFs do not cause thrombosis or distal embolization.

ANSWER:
A, C, D, E

19. With regard to the diagnosis and treatment of peripheral acquired AVF, which of the following is/ are true?

A. Acquired AVFs are rarely diagnosed by physical examination.

B. Angiography is the initial preferred diagnostic study.

C. Most AVFs can be observed without surgical intervention.

D. Proximal arterial ligation is the surgical procedure required for repair of most AVFs.

E. Percutaneous techniques, such as detachable balloons and embolization, are used to treat AVFs.

Ref.: 1, 3, 4

COMMENTS: Most AVFs are easily detected with a careful history and physical examination. • A history of penetrating trauma is usually elicited. • Physical findings may include a continuous ("machinery") murmur heard over the site; a palpable thrill; distended, tortuous, or varicose veins; chronic venous stasis changes; elevated skin temperature; and the changes seen with congestive heart failure. • Duplex scanning is useful for establishing a diagnosis. • Arteriography is the preferred diagnostic study to document an AVF. • The fistula is identified by the presence of a dilated afferent artery with early venous filling and simultaneous visualization of both arteries and veins. • There is also diminished contrast distally. • Duplex scanning is useful for diagnosing AVF formation in the groin after catheterization injury. • In this instance, it may be the only test required before surgical repair.

Most acquired AVFs should be repaired soon after diagnosis because of the low rate of spontaneous closure and the long-term sequelae. • The goals of surgical repair include complete closure of the arteriovenous connection and restoration of normal arterial and venous flow. • It may require placement of an interposition arterial graft. • Autogenous vein is preferred when the repair is in the extremity. • Most often, the venous defect is repaired with a lateral suture. • Repair with proximal arterial ligation leads to early distal ischemia and long-term persistence of the fistula due to collateral circulation. • In certain instances, surgical repair is not possible, owing to the location or technical difficulties. • Percutaneous embolization with emboligenic materials or detachable balloons is useful in these situations. • Both surgical repair and percutaneous embolization can lead to distal ischemia, infarction, and closure of an undesired artery. • After repair of a long-standing AVF, long-term surveillance is required because of the risk of arterial aneurysmal degeneration.

ANSWER:
E

20. With regard to axillary-subclavian vein thrombosis (Paget–von Schroetter syndrome), which of the following is/are true?

A. It is commonly associated with thoracic outlet compression syndrome.

B. Severe pain in the affected extremity is usually the presenting symptom.

C. Venography is the gold standard for making the diagnosis.

D. Surgical thrombectomy is highly successful for treating acute disease.

E. Patients treated with thrombolytic and anticoagulation therapy alone have a high rate of recurrence.

Ref.: 3, 4

COMMENTS: Spontaneous thrombosis of the axillary-subclavian vein is termed *effort thrombosis* or Paget–von Schroetter syndrome. • There is a strong male predominance. • Thrombosis typically follows upper-extremity exertion. • Patients invariably develop swelling and complain of heaviness and discomfort in the arm that is exacerbated with activity and relieved with rest. • Severe pain is a rare complaint. • As many as 80% of patients who present with effort thrombosis have an associated thoracic outlet compression syndrome. • As many as 25–75% of patients develop symptoms of disabling venous hypertension if not treated appropriately. • Venography remains the gold standard for diagnosis. • CT scanning, magnetic resonance imaging, and arteriography are often required when planning surgical decompression of the thoracic outlet. • Treatment with thrombolytic therapy and anticoagulation is highly successful for short-term treatment of this disease. • Diagnosis and staged treatment of thoracic outlet compression is mandatory because of the high rate of rethrombosis in those treated with thrombolytic and anticoagulation therapy alone. • This involves removing the first rib.

ANSWER:
A, C, E

21. A 53-year-old female who underwent brain tumor resection 4 days ago developed left lower-extremity pain and swelling. A venous duplex scan was performed, and she was diagnosed with DVT of the femoral and popliteal vein on the left. Which treatment is most appropriate?

A. Begin ambulation and discontinue bed rest.

B. Order emergency venography, and, if results are abnormal, begin intravenous heparin administration.

C. Order spiral CT scanning to rule out PE.

D. Use intermittent leg compression and graduated-compression stockings.

E. Place an IVC filter.

Ref.: 3

COMMENTS: Well-known indications for an IVC filter placement are DVT or PE with contraindications to anticoagulation, recurrent PE or DVT despite proper management, or complications of anticoagulation. • They are also used after pulmonary embolectomy and failure of a previously placed filter. • Among relative indications are the presence of large or free-floating thrombus in the iliofemoral system or vena cava, septic PE, chronic PE in a patient who has significant cardiac or respiratory impairment, trauma patients at high risk, spinal cord injury with paraplegia or quadriplegia, complex pelvic fracture with associated long bone fractures, pregnancy with DVT, patients with cancer, and patients with seizures or gait difficulties who have high risk for Coumadin therapy. • IVC filters are also used for patients with contraindications for anticoagulation. • The list of absolute contraindication to anticoagulation therapy includes recent spinal or brain surgery, eye surgery, major trauma, hemorrhagic stroke, malignant hypertension, and active gastrointestinal hemorrhage. • Relative contraindications to anticoagulation therapy consist of hemorrhagic diathesis, malignant hypertension, and severe renal or hepatic insufficiency.

ANSWER:
E

22. A 17-year-old male comes to the emergency department 1 hr after a strenuous workout involving weight lifting, complaining of left arm swelling and cyanosis. Venography demonstrates subclavian-axillary vein thrombosis. Which treatment is most appropriate?

A. All patients can expect asymptomatic recovery if treated promptly with anticoagulants only.

B. The patient may be effectively treated with acetylsalicylic acid only.

C. The patient will need life-term anticoagulation with Coumadin.

D. The patient requires catheter-directed thrombolysis and first-rib resection if patency is restored and venous narrowing is demonstrated.

E. The patient requires first rib resection only.

Ref.: 3

COMMENTS: Primary DVT of the upper extremity is a rare entity, accounting for 2–3% of all patients with thoracic outlet syndrome. • A young healthy athlete is a typical patient. • Males are affected twice as often as females. • Almost all have a history of strenuous or repetitive physical activity 24–48 hr before presentation. • During hyperabduction of the arm, the subclavian vein is compressed at the costoclavicular space, which is the most medial aspect of the thoracic outlet. • Trauma at this location causes intimal injury, followed by thrombus formation in the axillary and subclavian vein. • All patients complain of swelling and cyanosis of the affected extremity at the presentation, and the majority develop pain.

Catheter-directed thrombolysis is the first line of treatment. • If, after thrombolysis, the resolution of thrombus is documented and extrinsic compression is identified at the level of the costoclavicular space, first-rib resection is recommended. • It is performed through the axillary or supraclavicular approach during the same hospitalization or at a later date. • If the lesion is inside the vein itself, there are several treatment options. • They include anticoagulation and delayed outlet decompression, outlet decompression with external venolysis, outlet decompression followed by angioplasty, and outlet decompression with venous reconstruction. • The decision as to which option to use is based on the level of the patient's discomfort and the venogram.

A N S W E R :
D

23. A 67-year-old male is in the hospital for the treatment of bilateral PE and DVT. Heparin was continued for the last 2 days. On day three, the patient's platelet count was 75,000/mm³, a decrease from an original level of 250,000/mm³. On physical examination, the patient was noted to have ischemic changes on the right upper extremity and right lower extremity. Which of the following statements is/are true?

A. Low–molecular-weight heparin can be safely used as a substitute for unfractionated heparin.

B. Venous thrombosis is the most common likely cause of this patient's problem.

C. Subcutaneous administration of heparin is not associated with this problem.

D. Direct thrombin inhibitors are used as the first line of treatment.

E. Antiplatelet agents are not necessary as additional treatment.

Ref.: 3

COMMENTS: Heparin-induced thrombocytopenia (HIT) is an immune-mediated adverse drug reaction that can occur in up to 5% of patients undergoing treatment with unfractionated heparin. • The initial diagnosis of this condition is clinical. • The occurrence of HIT is independent of the route of administration. • Two forms of acute HIT have been reported. • Mild (type 1) thrombocytopenia occurs 2–7 days after initiation of full-dose heparin therapy. • It is nonimmune in nature. • Platelet counts usually remain above 100,000/mm³, and treatment can be continued without any risk of complications. • Severe (type 2) thrombocytopenia occurs much less frequently, 5–10 days after initiation of full-dose or low-dose heparin therapy. • It is an immune-mediated syndrome. • Platelet counts drop below 100,000/mm³, or there is a more than 50% drop from the baseline. • Laboratory confirmation of the presence of heparin-induced antibodies is available, but not always in a timely fashion for decision making. • Platelet-associated immunoglobulin G (IgG) levels are almost always elevated, but testing for them is not very specific. • The C-serotonin platelet release assay, heparin-induced platelet aggregation assay, and flow cytometric studies are very sensitive and specific. • Paradoxically, severe HIT is associated with thrombotic complications, including arterial thrombosis with platelet-fibrin clot (so-called white clot), which may cause myocardial infarction or stroke or necessitate amputation of a limb. • Up to 75% of the patients may develop arterial or venous thrombosis, and the mortality rate is 25–30%. • Lepirudin and argotroban are the first line of treatment, with the choice of agent depending on the patient's comorbid conditions (lepirudin depends on renal clearance, and argotroban depends on hepatic functional status). • Each agent has a relatively short half-life. • Antiplatelet medications (e.g., aspirin and Plavix) should be used for all patients with HIT.

A N S W E R :
D

24. A 45-year-old female comes to the emergency department complaining of pain in the left foot and calf. She reports that her left leg has been swollen for the last 5 years. She has a fever of 101.5°F (38.6°C). The left leg is swollen from the inguinal ligament down, and she has erythema of the foot and calf. Besides the obvious cellulites, what is the most likely underlying diagnosis?

A. Chronic venous insufficiency

B. DVT

C. Lymphedema tarda

D. Meige's disease

E. Milroy's disease

Ref.: 3

COMMENTS: Extremity swelling secondary to a pathologic condition of the lymphatic system is classified as primary or secondary. • Primary lymphedema is an uncommon condition and is not related to any extrinsic process. • Primary lymphedema is classified into three subtypes based on age of onset of symptoms. • The first group is congenital lymphedema, with onset before 1 year of age. • The lower extremities are more commonly affected, but an upper extremity may be involved also. • No specific therapy is needed. • If associated with a family history, it is referred to as Milroy's disease. • The second group, and the most common form, is lymphedema praecox, with onset of symptoms before 35 years of age. • If associated with a family history, it is referred to as Meige's disease. • Lymphedema tarda represents a minority of the cases. • Patients present with leg swelling after the age of 35. • Secondary lymphedema can be the result of multiple processes, including infection, trauma, filariasis, lymph node dissection, and radiation, among others.

ANSWER:
C

25. A 55-year-old female comes to the physician's office having had bilateral lower-extremity swelling for the last 3 months. The list of differential diagnoses includes all but which of the following?

A. DVT

B. Congestive heart failure

C. Lymphedema

D. Retroperitoneal sarcoma

E. Arterial occlusive disease

Ref.: 3

COMMENTS: Leg swelling may be secondary to a systemic disorder, acute or chronic obstruction of the venous system, or an abnormality of the lymphatic system. • Physical examination and patient's history are usually sufficient to find the cause of limb swelling. • The systemic disorders should be ruled out first. • The list of differential diagnoses includes renal failure, liver disease, constrictive pericarditis, tricuspid regurgitation, congestive heart failure, malnutrition, and other causes of hypoproteinuria. • Rare systemic causes of edema include endocrine disorders, such as myxedema, type 1 allergic reactions, hereditary angioedema, and idiopathic cyclic edema. • Among medications that can cause generalized swelling are angiotensin-converting enzyme (ACE) inhibitors, which most frequently affect the extremities and the face; corticosteroids; antihypertensive drugs; and anti-inflammatory agents. • Local or regional causes of leg swelling include chronic venous insufficiency, lipedema, congenital vascular malformation, AVF, trauma, snake bite, infection, hematoma, soft-tissue tumor, and dependency.

ANSWER:
E

26. A 45-year-old woman reports a recent onset of bilateral edema of the lower extremities. Which of the following statements is true about the appropriate workup?

A. Aspiration of tissue fluid to measure protein content is appropriate.

B. CT scanning is an unnecessary modality in the presence of bilateral disease.

C. The diagnosis can be confirmed by means of lymphoscintigraphic studies.

D. Physical findings are not reliable.

E. Laboratory tests and urinalysis are not very useful for diagnosis.

Ref.: 3

COMMENTS: Although physical examination and patient's history are usually sufficient to find the cause of limb swelling, several diagnostic modalities are available. • Laboratory examinations should include complete blood count, liver function tests, creatinine clearance testing, and urinalysis. • One of the first diagnostic tests is CT scanning, which is used to differentiate inflammatory or infectious processes, enlargement of regional lymph nodes, and underlying local or abdominal malignancy. • Venous Doppler study or strain-gauge plathysmographic study is sufficient to exclude venous thrombosis. • Duplex scanning is used to detect

venous insufficiency. • Magnetic resonance imaging provides the most accurate information in patients with clinical signs of congenital vascular malformation, soft-tissue tumor, or retroperitoneal fibrosis. • Direct contrast lymphangiographic studies are a classic method for diagnosis of lymphedema. • Because it requires cutdown and has a risk of oil embolism and lymphangitis, this test is not longer used, except in very unusual circumstances. • Normal lymphoscintigraphic examination essentially excludes the diagnosis of lymphedema. • Subcutaneous injection of technetium-labeled colloid and a serial gamma camera are used.

ANSWER:
C

27. A 35-year-old woman with three children has a large, painful varicose vein of her left extremity. Diagnosis and treatment should include all but which of the following?

A. Duplex scanning for venous insufficiency and evaluation of the deep venous system

B. Stripping of the left greater saphenous vein (GSV) from the groin to the ankle

C. Stripping of the left GSV from the groin to the knee and excision of the calf varicose vein

D. Treatment of the left GSV with a radiofrequency or laser catheter and excision of the calf varicose vein

E. Treatment of the left GSV with a radiofrequency or laser catheter alone

F. Fitted elastic stockings to reduce symptoms temporally

Ref.: 3

COMMENTS: Duplex scanning is a combination of gray-scale ultrasound and Doppler examination—hence the name *duplex*. • Preoperative examination with duplex scanning defines where the reflux is in the superficial and deep venous systems and ensures that the deep system is present and patent. • If the deep system is occluded, stripping or excising of the superficial system is contraindicated. • If the GSV reflexes significantly, interruption will help the symptoms. • Treatment of the thigh-level GSV is adequate. • Excision of the GSV below the knee risks damage of the saphenous nerve. • Catheter stripping of the GSV is an established technique, but catheter ablation with radiofrequency or laser energy is very effective and less invasive. • After treatment of the incompetent GSV, the residual calf and thigh varicose veins can be observed, excised with small incisions, or injected using a sclerotherapy technique. • Fitted elastic stockings are useful for reducing symptoms for patients who do not desire intervention.

ANSWER:
B

REFERENCES

1. Townsend CM Jr, Beauchamp RD, Evers BM, et al (eds): *Sabiston Textbook of Surgery: The Biological Basis of Modern Surgical Practice*, 17th ed. Saunders, Philadelphia, 2004.
2. Brunicardi FC, Andersen DK, Billiar TR, et al (eds): *Schwartz's Principles of Surgery*, 8th ed. McGraw-Hill, New York, 2004.
3. Rutherford RB (ed): *Vascular Surgery*, 6th ed. Elsevier-Saunders, Philadelphia, 2005.
4. Ernst EB, Stanley JE (eds): *Current Therapy in Vascular Surgery*, 3rd ed. CV Mosby, St. Louis, 1995.

CHAPTER 46

Chest

José M. Velasco, M.D., and Douglas Norman, M.D.

1. Match each of the lung volume measurements in the left-hand column with the appropriate definition in the right-hand column.

   A. Vital capacity (VC)

   B. Total lung capacity

   C. Functional residual capacity (FRC)

   D. Residual volume (RV)

   E. Tidal volume (TV)

   a. Volume in the lungs after a maximal inspiration

   b. Volume in the lungs after a normal expiration

   c. Volume of a spontaneous breath

   d. Volume remaining in the lungs after maximal expiration

   e. Maximum volume that can be expired after a maximal inspiration

   Ref.: 1, 2

COMMENTS: **VC** can be measured as slow or forced, with the forced maneuver producing a lower volume in a patient with chronic obstructive pulmonary disease (COPD). • **FRC** is determined by inspiration of an inert gas or plethysmography. • **RV** is determined by subtracting the expiratory RV (the volume that can be expired from normal end-expiration) from the FRC. • **TV** is easily determined and is a commonly used measurement for management of patients with mechanical ventilators. • **TLC** is determined by adding the VC and RV.

ANSWER:
A-e; B-a; C-b; D-d; E-c

2. Regarding the surgical anatomy of the lung, which of the following statements are true?

   A. The volumes of the right and left lung are approximately equal.

   B. The left main stem bronchus is longer than the right.

   C. The trachea is approximately 20 cm in length.

   D. The right pulmonary artery has a greater length than the left before giving off its first segmental branch.

   E. The angle of takeoff of the right main stem bronchus is the same as that of the left main-stem bronchus.

   Ref.: 1, 2

COMMENTS: See Question 3.

3. Which of the following indicates that the patient is at high risk for respiratory failure following pulmonary resection?

   A. Preoperative 1-second forced expiratory volume (FEV_1) = 800 ml.

   B. Preoperative $PaCO_2$ = 38 mmHg.

   C. Ventilation/perfusion (V/Q) scan shows 30% perfusion to the operative side with an FEV_1 of 1400 ml.

   D. Predicted postoperative FEV_1 = 1.1 L.

   E. Maximum O_2 consumption (MVO_2) = 10 ml/kg/min.

   Ref.: 1–3

COMMENTS: The volume of the left lung is approximately 45%, and that of the right 55%, of the total pulmonary volume. • The right main-stem bronchus is 1.2 cm in length, and the left main-stem bronchus is 4–6 cm in length. • The trachea is 10–13 cm in length, measured from the cricoid cartilage through the takeoff of the left main-stem bronchus. • The right pulmonary artery passes from the left side of the mediastinum to the right pleural cavity before giving off a segmental branch. • Pulmonary aspiration occurs more frequently on the right lung than the left lung due to a sharper left tracheobronchial angle than on the right lung. • During the evaluation of a patient for pulmonary resection, various aspects of pulmonary physiology must be considered. • If the preoperative FEV_1 is 800 ml, or the predicted postoperative FEV_1 is 800–1000 ml, the patient may have inadequate ventilatory reserve for pulmonary resection. • Elevated arterial carbon dioxide tension ($PaCO_2$) suggests serious abnormalities in alveolar ventilation. • The quantitative ventilation perfusion (V/Q) scan is a useful test for predicting what the postoperative FEV_1 of the remaining lung tissue will be after resection. • Adequate pulmonary reserve is related to a MVO_2 over 20 ml/kg/min. • In marginal patients, a maximal oxygen consumption (MVO_2) of less than 10 ml/kg/min is associated with a 29% mortality and 43% morbidity.

ANSWERS:
Question 2: B, D
Question 3: A, E

4. True or false: Flexible bronchoscopy is the preferred method for the following procedures.

   A. Yttrium-aluminum-garnet (YAG) laser therapy

B. Massive hemoptysis

C. Transcarinal needle biopsy

D. Bedside tracheobronchial aspiration

E. Stent placement

Ref.: 1–3

COMMENTS: YAG laser débridement of endobronchial neoplasms is more efficiently accomplished with the rigid bronchoscope than with the flexible one. • Special open-tube bronchoscopes with channels for aspiration and biopsy facilitate tissue procurement and control of bleeding and even expedite the procedure. • In patients with **massive hemoptysis**, the rigid bronchoscope accommodates the use of larger suction tubing for easier clearing of the airway. • In addition, fresh blood frequently splatters the flexible bronchoscope lens, preventing visualization of the tracheobronchial tree. • **Transcarinal** and **transtracheal biopsy** of mediastinal lymph nodes is best accomplished with the flexible bronchoscope. • A special needle-tip catheter is inserted through the channel of the flexible bronchoscope, and selective positioning of the flexible bronchoscope directs the needle to the previously identified mediastinal lymph node. • The flexible bronchoscope greatly enhances the ease and comfort of **bedside aspiration**. • **Stent placement** frequently requires stricture dilatation or tumor débridement. • On occasion, the stent must be repositioned. • All of these maneuvers are more easily accomplished with the rigid bronchoscope.

ANSWER:
A, False; B, False; C, True; D, True; E, False

5. Select the most common complication following pulmonary lobectomy?

A. Retained secretions and atelectasis

B. Bronchopleural fistula

C. Persistent air leakage from the surface of the operated lung

D. Empyema

E. Persistent symptomatic air space

Ref.: 1, 2

COMMENTS: The most common complication following pulmonary lobectomy is related to retained bronchial secretions and consequent atelectasis. • This occurs in 10–30% of patients and is related to reflex splinting of the chest, shallow breathing, and an impaired cough mechanism. • Air leakages, if not originating from the bronchial stump, usually close early. • A small, persistent air space may occur, but it usually causes no problems. • An asymptomatic air space gradually disappears with reabsorption of the air within the space. • Bronchopleural fistula and empyema are uncommon after a lobectomy.

ANSWER:
A

6. In patients who have sustained blunt trauma to the chest, which of the following would most likely be the cause of acute cardiopulmonary collapse?

A. Hemothorax

B. Pulmonary contusion

C. Acute adult respiratory distress syndrome (ARDS)

D. Pneumothorax

E. Multiple segment rib fractures

Ref.: 1, 2

COMMENTS: Rib fractures are the most common injuries to the chest wall, but unless there is a flail segment, they usually do not cause respiratory insufficiency. • Hemothorax can cause respiratory insufficiency but is less common than pneumothorax. • Pulmonary contusion may cause delayed ARDS, resulting in increased alveolar edema, and possible bacterial infection, but it usually does not cause acute cardiopulmonary collapse. • Pneumothorax with progressive buildup of tension can cause sudden cardiorespiratory collapse if not treated.

ANSWER:
D, E

7. Which of the following is the most common malignant primary tumor of the chest wall?

A. Chondrosarcoma

B. Plasmacytoma

C. Osteogenic sarcoma

D. Ewing's sarcoma

E. Fibrosarcoma

Ref.: 1, 2

COMMENTS: Primary tumors of the chest wall are malignant in 60–90% of reported cases. • **Chondrosarcoma** is the most common primary chest wall tumor, occurring in 35–40% of patients. • It commonly occurs in 10- to 40-year-olds and usually in the sternum or adjacent costocartilages. • It occurs more frequently in males and has a favorable cure rate when wide and complete resection is accomplished. • **Plasmacytoma** or **myeloma** is a less frequent tumor of the chest wall that often presents as a painful rib lesion without a palpable mass. • It is most common in 40- to 60-year-olds and more frequently affects males. • Solitary myeloma of the rib is a harbinger of the development of manifestations of the systemic disease of myeloma. • **Osteogenic sarcoma** accounts for 6% of primary bone tumors and is most frequent in males younger than age 20. • Osteogenic sarcoma presents as an enlarged, painful mass, and the radiologic appearance is that of the typical "sunburst" pattern. • **Ewing's sarcoma** occurs most frequently in males younger than age 20 and accounts for 8% of primary bone tumors. • It is associated with fever, malaise, anemia, and an increased erythrocyte sedimentation rate. • The surface of the bone has a typical "onion-skin" appearance, caused by elevation of the periosteum and multiple layers of new bone formation. • **Fibrosarcomas** commonly occur in adults aged 50–70. • They are frequently slightly painful, slowly enlarging masses, which can arise in previously irradiated fields.

ANSWER:
A

8. Which of the following is the most common primary tumor of the anterior mediastinal compartment in adults?

A. Thyroid goiter

B. Thymoma

C. Teratoma

D. Lymphoma

E. Neurogenic tumor

Ref.: 1, 2

COMMENTS: The mediastinum is divided into three compartments: anterior, middle, and posterior. • **Thyroid goiter** may extend into the anterior mediastinum in about 15% of patients with goiter, and, in fact, it is not considered a true primary mediastinal tumor. • **Thymoma** is the most common primary anterior mediastinal tumor, followed by **lymphoma** and, rarely, **teratoma.** • Posterior mediastinal tumors are most likely to be of neurogenic origin. • They arise from the sympathetic ganglia or intercostal nerves. • Pericardial cysts typically occur in the middle compartment adjacent to the heart. • Lymphomas are found usually in the anterior or middle mediastinum. • An esophageal duplication cyst, while posterior, is a rare congenital lesion. • **Neurogenic tumors** are one of the most common primary tumors of the mediastinum but occur in the posterior mediastinum.

ANSWER:
B

9. Management of a posterior mediastinal neurogenic tumor should include which of the following?

A. Surgical resection

B. Computed tomography/magnetic resonance imaging (CT/MRI)

C. Preoperative irradiation of tumor

D. Chemotherapy

E. All of the above

Ref.: 1, 2

COMMENTS: Neurogenic tumors typically occur in the paravertebral space of the posterior mediastinum. • They arise from the intercostal nerves or the sympathetic trunks. • In adults most tumors are benign, but in children they tend to be malignant. • The classical appearance on a lateral chest x-ray is that of a rounded paravertebral mass. • Because of their neural crest origin, some tumors, mainly ganglioneuroma, neurofibroma, and pheochromocytoma, secrete vasoactive peptides. • Neuroblastomas are highly aggressive tumors, best treated with multimodal therapy. • Surgical resection is the treatment of choice. • Since these tumors may involve the intervertebral foramina and vertebral bodies, a preoperative CT/MRI examination helps to identify intraspinal extension. • In such cases, a combined thoracic surgical and neurosurgical procedure is warranted, since failure to recognize intraspinal extension may lead to disastrous paraplegia if only the thoracic portion is excised.

ANSWER:
E

10. Which of the following is the most common cause of acute mediastinitis?

A. Iatrogenic perforation of the esophagus

B. Postoperative infection following median sternotomy for open heart surgery

C. Traumatic injury to the mediastinum and mediastinal structures

D. Intrathoracic leak of an esophageal anastomotic suture line

E. Erosion of tracheobronchial tree or esophagus from a foreign body

Ref.: 1, 2

COMMENTS: Currently, the most common setting of mediastinitis is cardiac surgery performed through a median sternotomy incision. • Prolonged perfusion time, poor postoperative cardiac output, and postoperative bleeding of sufficient magnitude to require reexploration are common predisposing factors. • Perforation of the esophagus, anastomotic leaks, and traumatic injuries can rapidly lead to a fulminating illness. • The standard treatment is appropriate antibiotic therapy, drainage of the contaminated area, and repair or exclusion of the esophagus.

ANSWER:
B

11. Which of the following are characteristics of intralobar pulmonary sequestration?

A. Occurs in the posterobasal portion of the lower lobe

B. Is most frequently seen on the right side

C. Is usually cystic

D. Receives blood supply from the pulmonary artery

E. Does not communicate with the tracheobronchial tree

Ref.: 1, 2

COMMENTS: Intralobar sequestration is typically cystic and presents in the posterobasal segments of the lower lobe, usually the left. • There is usually communication with the tracheobronchial tube and, thus, cystic features appear. • Its blood supply comes from a large anomalous branch off the lower descending thoracic aorta in 70% of cases and from the abdominal aorta in the remainder. • This is important to know, lest unexpected life-threatening bleeding occur.

ANSWER:
A, C

12. All but which of the following tumors have an increased incidence in asbestos workers?

A. Cancer of the lung

B. Pleural mesothelioma

C. Cancer of the esophagus

D. Cancer of the stomach

E. Thymoma

Ref.: 1, 2

COMMENTS: All of the neoplasms listed above occur more commonly in asbestos workers. • There is usually a long latent period (15–35 years) between exposure to asbestos and the development of tumors. • Among asbestos workers, 6–7% of all deaths are due to mesothelioma, and 20% are due to carcinoma of the lung. • The death rate from carcinoma of the esophagus is 2.5 times higher than expected, and the incidence of deaths from stomach cancer is 1.5 times higher.

ANSWER:
E

13. Regarding malignant pleural effusions, which of the following is/are considered effective therapy?

 A. Thoracentesis

 B. Thoracoscopy with instillation of a sclerosing agent

 C. Tube thoracostomy with instillation of a sclerosing agent

 D. Pleurectomy

 E. Irradiation

Ref.: 1, 2

COMMENTS: For treatment of a malignant effusion, **thoracentesis** alone has a 98–99% failure rate. • **Closed-tube thoracostomy** alone also has a high failure rate. • **Closed-tube thoracostomy and instillation** of a sclerosing agent involve the principle of total removal of the fluid and obliteration of the space between the pleura and the lung. • Obliteration of the pleural space can then be accomplished by injecting a sclerosing agent such as bleomycin, doxycycline, or talc into the pleural space through the chest tube. • Video-assisted thoracoscopy has become increasingly useful in the management of these patients. • Occasionally, **parietal pleurectomy** is necessary to obliterate the space, but complications are frequent and mortality rates significant. • **Pleuroperitoneal shunt** is a recent technique that can be effective for refractory benign and malignant pleural effusions. • **Irradiation** alone is not effective in controlling malignant effusions.

ANSWER:
B, C, D

14. Empyema thoracis can be caused by which one or more of the following?

 A. Pneumonia with subsequent pyogenic infection of the associated effusion

 B. Infections associated with a surgical procedure on the lung

 C. Penetration of the pleural space by a foreign body

 D. Extension from a subphrenic abscess

 E. Secondary to systemic sepsis

Ref.: 1, 2

COMMENTS: Most commonly, empyema is secondary to infection of a parapneumonic effusion. • It occurs less frequently now with the early use of antibiotics for pneumonia. • Any trauma, especially penetration of the chest with a nonsterile foreign body, can lead to an empyema. • In one series, patients with subphrenic abscess after abdominal operations or disease constituted 10% of a group of patients who developed empyema. • Empyema also occasionally results from systemic sepsis in immunocompromised patients, trauma victims, and patients who have had cardiac surgery.

ANSWER:
A, B, C, D, E

15. Which of the following modes of therapy is/are useful for treatment of empyema thoracis?

 A. Antibiotic therapy combined with thoracentesis

 B. Video-assisted thoracoscopy with tube drainage

 C. Dependent open drainage of the empyema cavity

 D. Decortication

 E. Muscle flap transposition

Ref.: 1–3

COMMENTS: Antibiotic therapy without additional management of the empyema cavity is ineffective. • If the effusion is still watery, rather than thick viscous fluid, thoracentesis with aggressive antibiotic therapy may abort the process. • Video-assisted thoracoscopy with drainage may also be used during the early empyema stage with improved success. • Frequently, however, it is not possible to remove all the fluid from the pleural space, and so the empyema progresses. • With a well-established empyema, initial drainage is established by closed-tube thoracostomy, followed by dependent open drainage achieved by a rib resection or possibly an Eloesser flap. • Early decortication may be necessary for the cavity of a chronic empyema in which the lung does not reexpand after 4–6 weeks of the standard treatment. • Decortication is also indicated for acute empyema that has not responded to nonoperative therapy. • Pedicle flaps of chest wall muscles, omentum, or, occasionally, abdominal wall muscles are used to obliterate postpneumonectomy and postlobectomy empyema spaces with or without bronchopleural fistula in patients who otherwise are stable.

ANSWER:
A, B, C, D, E

16. A tracheostomy patient is noted to have bright-red blood coming from within and around the tube. What is the presumed diagnosis?

 A. Pulmonary embolism

 B. Necrotizing pneumonia

 C. Stomal granulation tissue bleeding

 D. Tracheoinnominate artery fistula

 E. Pulmonary artery injury (Swan-Ganz catheter)

Ref.: 1, 2

COMMENTS: See Question 18.

17. What is the appropriate treatment for the patient described in Question 16?

 A. Pack around the tracheostomy tube

 B. Type and crossmatch for red blood cells (RBCs)

 C. Inflate the tracheostomy cuff

 D. Notify operating room of emergency case

 E. Emergency arteriogram

Ref.: 1, 2

COMMENTS: See Question 18.

18. What is the appropriate repair of a tracheoinnominate artery fistula?

 A. Exposure by partial or complete sternotomy

 B. Primary suture repair of artery deficit

 C. Excision of deficit and repair with a 10-mm interposed Dacrongraft

 D. Bypass graft of innominate artery

 E. Suture ligation and division of innominate artery

Ref.: 1, 2, 4

COMMENTS: The onset of bright-red bleeding in a tracheostomy should always be considered to be from a feared tracheoinnominate artery fistula (TIF) until proven otherwise. • Half of patients who will eventually have a TIF will have a prodromal sentinel bleeding. • The rest may present with active peristomal or endotracheal bleeding that can be massive. • In 70% of patients, TIF is manifested within the first 3 weeks after tracheostomy. • Pressure necrosis on the posterior aspect of the innominate artery can be due to overinflation of the cuff, a poorly positioned tube with the cannula tip impinging against the tracheal wall, and placement of the tracheostomy tube too low (below the fourth ring). • Failure to recognize this may lead to exsanguinating bleeding if untreated. • All the conditions listed in Question 16 can cause posttracheostomy bleeding. • TIF accounts for 30% of all posttracheostomy bleeding. • Once a TIF is suspected, preparations for taking the patient to the operating room need to be made. • Overinflation of the cuff or finger pressure may temporarily control massive bleeding. • There is no place for arteriography in these circumstances. • Packing the wound only "covers up" the diagnosis and leads to further delay. • Proper exposure for the repair of a TIF requires sternal splitting. • All T-I fistulae should be considered infected. • The use of synthetic graft material will lead to infection and blowout bleeding. • While grafting to restore cerebral circulation is attractive, neurologic sequelae from ligation and division are rare. • The divided, débrided ends should be sutured and covered with healthy muscle flaps.

ANSWERS:
Question 16: D
Question 17: B, C, D
Question 18: A, E

19. Which of the following is the most common primary tumor involving the trachea?

    A. Adenoid cystic carcinoma

    B. Squamous cell carcinoma

    C. Carcinoid

    D. Mucoepidermoid carcinoma

    E. Thyroid cancer

                                                        Ref.: 2

COMMENTS: Tracheal tumors frequently present with stridor, dypsnea, hemoptysis, and pneumonia. • Squamous cell carcinoma remains the most common *primary* tumor of the trachea, accounting for approximately two thirds of primary tracheal tumors. • Mediastinal or pulmonary metastasis are present in approximately one third of patients. • Adenoid cystic carcinoma (formerly called cylindroma) accounts for one fourth of primary tracheal tumors. • Since they spread within the tracheal wall, frozen section of the margins at the time of resection is mandatory. • Since these tumors are radiosensitive, even if the regional lymph nodes are involved or when the margins are positive, long-term survival can be achieved with postoperative radiation therapy. • *Secondary* involvement of the trachea by carcinoma of the esophagus, lung, thyroid gland, or larynx is far more common than are primary tumors of the trachea.

ANSWER:
B

20. The standard therapy for pulmonary abscess includes which of the following?

    A. Antibiotics

    B. Bronchoscopy

    C. Early surgical resection of the involved area of the lung

    D. Catheter drainage of abscess cavity

    E. Muscle flap transposition

                                                        Ref.: 1, 2

COMMENTS: Treatment of pulmonary abscesses consists of (1) diagnostic bronchoscopy to remove any foreign bodies, evaluate for bronchial stenosis or obstruction, and collect secretions for culture and cytology; and (2) administration of the appropriate antibiotics. • With adequate therapy, complete collapse of the abscess cavity wall and complete healing generally take place in 10–14 weeks. • Failure of an abscess cavity to heal should alert the physician to a possible underlying carcinoma. • Patients who have persistent cavities or cavities that are initially 6 cm or larger are candidates for an operation. • Massive bleeding or empyema also necessitates surgery, which should include resection of the entire lobe. • Tube drainage is done only if the abscess cavity is adherent to the pleura. • Muscle flap transposition procedures are not normally used for treatment unless a large empyema cavity occurs as a postoperative complication of surgical resection of a persistent large abscess cavity.

ANSWER:
A, B

21. A patient has been diagnosed with a typical carcinoid tumor in the right upper lobe that protrudes into the right main bronchus. There is no adenopathy noted. What should the treatment be?

    A. Irradiation

    B. Endobronchial excision

    C. Right pneumonectomy

    D. Sleeve right upper lobectomy

    E. Local excision

                                                        Ref.: 1, 2

COMMENTS: Radiation therapy is of little value for carcinoid tumors. • Typical carcinoids have a low potential for spread. • Lung-conserving procedures are indicated when possible. • Local excision with bronchoplasty or sleeve lobectomy is preferred to larger resection, if feasible. • Endobronchial excision by bronchoscopy risks leaving residual tumor. • The typical carcinoid tumor is a neuroendocrine lesion that contains vasoactive peptides. • These peptides are easily identified by histochemistry techniques, but carcinoid syndrome is rare in these lung tumors.

ANSWER:
D, E

22. All but which of the following disease processes can lead to massive hemoptysis?

    A. Bronchogenic carcinoma

    B. Bronchiectasis

    C. Broncholith

D. Tuberculosis

E. Lung abscess

Ref.: 1, 2

COMMENTS: Lung abscess, tuberculosis, and bronchiectasis can frequently lead to massive hemorrhage, that is, more than 600 ml of blood in 24 hr. • Both active tuberculosis and chronic cavitary tuberculosis can present with massive exsanguinating hemorrhage. • Although bronchogenic carcinoma can present with major hemorrhage if the tumor erodes into a major pulmonary artery or vein, this occurrence is less frequent. • Broncholiths almost never cause massive hemorrhage. • The quantity of blood may vary from 1 to 50 ml.

ANSWER:
C

23. Diaphragmatic rupture secondary to blunt trauma is associated with which of the following?

A. Occurs equally on both sides

B. Is frequently an isolated injury

C. Usually develops acute respiratory distress

D. Demands immediate transthoracic repair

E. None of the above

Ref.: 1, 2

COMMENTS: A diaphragm rupture occurs overwhelmingly on the left side. • It is felt that the liver and heart are protective for the right side. • Injuries to other organs usually dictate symptoms. • For this reason, immediate transthoracic repair is not done, since abdominal viscera and bleeding may need urgent treatment. • Delayed respiratory distress usually develops as the progressive displacement of abdominal contents swell with air and compress the left lung. • Treatment of chronic diaphragmatic hernias is probably best done through a thoracotomy because of the potential for adhesion formation to surrounding tissue.

ANSWER:
E

24. Which of the following is the most common cause of spontaneous pneumothorax?

A. Tuberculosis

B. Rupture of small blebs

C. Emphysema and chronic bronchitis

D. Various pulmonary neoplasms

E. Endometriosis

Ref.: 1, 2

COMMENTS: All of the abovementioned conditions can cause spontaneous pneumothorax, but the most common cause is **rupture of small blebs,** generally located in the apex of the lung in persons without underlying lung disease. • The highest incidence is in tall, thin individuals 20–40 years of age. • Men are affected five to six times more frequently than are women. • **Emphysema** and **chronic bronchitis** account for 10% of cases of spontaneous pneumothorax. • Before there was effective drug therapy for

tuberculosis, it was thought to be the most common cause of spontaneous pneumothorax. • **Metastatic sarcoma** is known to erode through the visceral pleura, causing a spontaneous pneumothorax. • **Endometriosis** may cause pneumothorax with menses (catamenial pneumothorax).

ANSWER:
B

25. Which of the following is/are indications for surgical intervention in a patient with spontaneous pneumothorax?

A. Recurrent spontaneous pneumothorax

B. A persistent air leak at the end of a 3-day trial of closed drainage of a spontaneous pneumothorax

C. Complete collapse of the lung in a patient with an initial spontaneous pneumothorax

D. Initial pneumothorax in a commercial airline pilot

E. Pregnancy

Ref.: 1, 2

COMMENTS: Recurrence of a spontaneous pneumothorax is generally considered an indication for its operative repair. • The incidence of recurrence after an initial pneumothorax is 15–20%, and the incidence of a subsequent spontaneous pneumothorax after recurrence is 70–80%. • Operative repair is suggested for a patient with an initial spontaneous pneumothorax whose occupation entails immediate responsibility for the safety of other persons (e.g., an airplane pilot) or who lives in a remote area. • Operative repair of persistent air leaks from spontaneous pneumothorax is usually not considered until at least 7–10 days of closed therapy. • Other indications for early operation are massive air leakage preventing lung reexpansion, hemopneumothorax, or a large solitary bulla. • Treatment should be conservative in a pregnant woman until after delivery, when the indications are as otherwise noted.

ANSWER:
A, D

26. A 62-year-old female cigarette smoker underwent a mastectomy 6 years earlier for adenocarcinoma of the right breast. Although asymptomatic, she now has a routine chest radiograph that demonstrates a 2-cm soft-tissue nodule in the anterior segment of the right upper lobe. Which of the following is/are more useful for further evaluation?

A. Contrast-infusion CT scanning of the chest

B. Positive emission tomographic (PET) scanning

C. Previous chest radiograms

D. Transthoracic percutaneous lung biopsy

E. Bronchoscopic examination

Ref.: 1, 2

COMMENTS: Not all patients with a previous extrathoracic malignancy who have a soft-tissue nodule in the lung can be presumed to have metastatic disease without further evaluation. • Indeed, in the scenario described, the chance that the lung nodule is metastatic is about 50%. • If the extrathoracic malignancy is controlled, the lung abnormality should be approached as if it were a primary neoplasm. • Comparison with any previous chest radiograph would be the next step in the evaluation. • If the nodule was present on previous radiographs (>2 years old) and it is unchanged in size and appearance, by definition it is benign and no further workup is required. • If the nodule is new or has enlarged or if previous films are not available, the abnormality should be investigated as if it were a primary lung nodule. • **Radiographs of the chest** (posteroanterior and lateral views) are the least expensive but also the least sensitive. • In this case, **CT** scanning of the chest would be the next diagnostic procedure to determine whether calcification is present within the peripheral nodule. • CT scanning has the advantage of also allowing evaluation of the mediastinum, hila, and remaining lung. • **Percutaneous biopsy** is not generally indicated because a negative result does not ensure the absence of malignancy and therefore does not change the need for an operation for diagnosis and treatment if the other tests are not conclusive. • It would be unlikely that a bronchoscopic examination would provide histologic diagnosis of a 2-cm peripheral nodule in the anterior segment of the right upper lobe. • The likelihood of confirming a malignant diagnosis is less than 25% for peripheral lesions of the lung. • Bronchoscopic examination is done at the time of pulmonary resection to make certain that the tracheobronchial tree is free of pathologic conditions. • Positive findings on PET scanning are suggestive but cannot substitute for tissue diagnosis.

A N S W E R :
A, B, C, E

27. Which of the following is/are absolute contraindications to surgical resection of a lung tumor?

   A. Vagus nerve involvement, as evidenced by ipsilateral cord paralysis

   B. Pleural effusion

   C. Chest-wall invasion of the tumor

   D. Liver metastases

   E. Mediastinal node involvement on the ipsilateral side

   F. Superior sulcus tumor

Ref.: 1, 2

COMMENTS: Vagus nerve involvement is usually suspected in cases of left vocal cord paralysis, and it indicates invasion of the left recurrent nerve in the aorticopulmonary window. • Tumor in this area is generally considered nonresectable. • Occasionally, however, the left vagus nerve is involved above the aortic arch by direct invasion of the mediastinum. • Although this is classified as stage III disease, it is not an absolute contraindication to resection. • **Pleural effusion** that contains malignant cells makes the disease noncurable by operation. • Such an effusion, however, must be shown cytologically to be malignant before such a patient is denied an operation. • **Chest-wall invasion** and superior sulcus tumor, while locally invasive, can be resected for cure with reasonable survival rates. • **Mediastinal lymph node involvement** on the ipsilateral side, particularly with squamous cell carcinomas, can likewise be resected for cure and with the expectation of reasonable survival rates. • **Liver metastases** constitute a contraindication to pulmonary resection because under these conditions the lung cancer is categorically noncurable.

A N S W E R :
D

28. Which of the following extrapulmonary manifestations of carcinoma of the lung is/are associated with small-cell (oat cell) carcinoma?

   A. Cushing's syndrome

   B. Excessive production of antidiuretic hormone

   C. Hypertrophic pulmonary osteoarthropathy

   D. Hypercalcemia

   E. Carcinomatous neuromyopathy

Ref.: 1, 2

COMMENTS: Hypercalcemia is most frequently associated with squamous cell carcinoma. • **Hypertrophic pulmonary osteoarthropathy** occurs with equal frequency among non–small-cell cancers but does not occur in small-cell cancer. • **Cushing's syndrome** and **excessive production of antidiuretic hormone** are usually associated with small-cell carcinoma. • **Carcinomatous neuromyopathies** are the most frequent (15% incidence when closely looked for) extrathoracic nonmetastatic manifestations of lung cancer. • The most common are a myasthenia-like syndrome and polymyositis. • About 50% of the patients have small-cell cancer.

A N S W E R :
A, B, E

29. In the general population, what percentage of asymptomatic solitary pulmonary nodules are carcinoma?

   A. 5%

   B. 20%

   C. 35%

   D. 50%

   E. 75%

Ref.: 1, 2

COMMENTS: In the general population, only 5% of "coin" lesions discovered on routine screening chest radiographs are carcinomas, most being granulomas. • In patients older than 50 years of age who have undergone resection of such a "coin" lesion, however, the incidence of cancer is 50%. • In those 80 years of age or older, the rate of malignancy of these lesions increases to almost 100%.

A N S W E R :
A

30. What is the overall 5-year survival rate of patients with carcinoma of the lung?

   A. 10%

   B. 20%

   C. 30%

   D. 40%

   E. 50%

Ref.: 1

COMMENTS: The 5-year survival rate of all patients who develop carcinoma of the lung is approximately 10%. • The 5-year salvage rate after surgical resection is 20–35%. • However, for patients who have T1 lesions without nodal involvement and no distant metastasis, the survival rate can be as high as 80%. • Accurate staging is required in all patients to allow one to arrive at a meaningful prognosis.

ANSWER:
A

31. A patient being followed after apparently successful treatment of a squamous cell cancer of the head and neck is found to have a new solitary pulmonary nodule. Which of the following is the most likely diagnosis of this lesion?

    A. Solitary metastasis

    B. Granuloma

    C. Primary lung carcinoma

    D. Benign lung tumor

    Ref.: 1, 2

COMMENTS: Chest radiographs should be evaluated for new lung lesions in the context of the time frame in which a patient is at risk from a previous malignancy. • In general, a new lung lesion in a patient who had had a known primary head and neck tumor, especially a squamous cell carcinoma, is most likely a new primary cancer rather than a solitary metastasis. • In a patient who previously had a melanoma or sarcoma, however, a solitary lesion in the lung is more likely to be a metastasis. • In patients with known cancers of the gastrointestinal tract, genitourinary tract, or breast, a solitary pulmonary nodule has an equal chance of being a metastasis or a new primary lung cancer.

ANSWER:
C

32. A metastasis to the lung from a known malignant tumor elsewhere should not be resected in which of the following situations?

    A. The primary tumor is not controlled.

    B. There are bilateral metastases.

    C. There is metastatic disease in organs in addition to the lung.

    D. There are multiple unilateral metastases.

    E. The cell type is melanoma.

    Ref.: 1, 2

COMMENTS: Before resection of a metastatic neoplasm to the lung, the primary tumor must be under control, and there must be assurance that no other organ is involved with metastasis. • The planned operation must be able to remove all known tumor, and the patient must be able to tolerate removal of involved lung tissue. • Therefore, whether the lesions are multiple or bilateral, these lesions should be resected only if the unresected lung tissue permits adequate pulmonary function. • Several other factors influence the decision to operate, including histologic type, disease-free interval, tumor doubling time, and the presence of secondary nodal metastasis. • Each of these factors has been shown to influence survival, but none of these unfavorable situations is an absolute contraindication to resection.

ANSWER:
A, C

33. Match each of the organisms causing lung infection in the left-hand column with the appropriate clinical statement in the right-hand column.

    A. Actinomycosis   a. Cutaneous and pulmonary infections often occur together.

    B. Histoplasmosis   b. Drainage from the abscess or sinus looks like sulfur granules.

    C. Blastomycosis   c. It has a propensity to colonize a preexisting pulmonary cavity, forming a fungus ball.

    D. Aspergillosis   d. Endemic to Mississippi River basin, is the most common systemic fungal infection in the United States.

    Ref.: 1, 2

COMMENTS: Actinomycosis, unlike the other three infections listed, is caused by a microaerophilic bacterium. • It is often incorrectly called a fungus. • Abscesses and sinus tracts caused by actinomycosis drain a yellow-brown material resembling sulfur granules. • Histoplasmosis, blastomycosis, and aspergillosis are caused by fungi. • **Histoplasmosis** is the most common systemic fungal infection in the United States and is endemic to the Mississippi River basin. • Calcified lymph nodes in the mediastinum are often the result of a past infection caused by histoplasmosis. • **Blastomycosis** is caused by the organism *Blastomyces dermatitidis*. • As the name implies, the cutaneous and pulmonary infections are often seen together. • The organism can readily be cultured from the margins of the skin ulcers it causes. • **Aspergillosis** is usually caused by colonization of a preexisting pulmonary cavity, leading to what is called a "fungus ball," or aspergilloma.

ANSWER:
A-b; B-d; C-a; D-c

34. A 57-year-old man presents to the emergency department with shortness of breath. Scenario 1: A posteroanterior portable view of the chest demonstrates complete opacification of the right hemithorax. The heart and mediastinum are shifted toward the right side. Which of the following is indicated for further evaluation?

    A. Thoracentesis

    B. Bronchoscopy

    C. CT scanning of the chest with infusion

    D. Ultrasound scanning of the chest

    Ref.: 1–3

COMMENTS: See Question 35.

35. Scenario 2: If the radiograph of the patient in Question 34 had demonstrated complete hemithorax opacification and a *midline* heart and mediastinum, which of the following would be indicated for further evaluation?

    A. Thoracentesis

    B. Bronchoscopy

    C. CT scanning of the chest with infusion

    D. Ultrasound scanning of the chest

    Ref.: 1–3

COMMENTS: Scenario 1: The most important radiographic observation in such a setting is the position of the heart and the mediastinum. • The *shift* of the heart and the mediastinum *toward* the opaque hemithorax, as in this case, indicates lung collapse and volume loss, most likely secondary to a central obstructing process. • If the heart and mediastinum are *shifted away* from the abnormally opaque hemithorax, it indicates a space-occupying process, most likely pleural effusion, although an accompanying neoplasm cannot be excluded. • In this clinical setting, lung collapse is the most likely possibility, and bronchoscopy would yield the greatest amount of diagnostic information quickly.

Scenario 2: The radiographic findings described indicate either a combination of balanced lung collapse and pleural effusion or an abnormal process *fixing* the mediastinum in the *midline*, such as a neoplasm or chronic inflammation. • In this setting, further imaging of the chest is essential to plan appropriate diagnostic and therapeutic maneuvers. • **Ultrasound** scans of the chest are usually not valuable because normally aerated lung is an effective sound barrier. • However, with an opaque hemithorax secondary to fluid or collapsed lung, the ultrasound scan can be valuable for distinguishing the component of pleural effusion from an associated solid component. • It can be done quickly and inexpensively and may serve as a guide for follow-up thoracentesis. • A **CT scan** more accurately delineates most structures, however. • **Thoracentesis** performed without radiographic or fluoroscopic guidance may yield fluid positive for malignancy but may not yield a positive diagnosis and could interfere with further imaging. • **Bronchoscopy** would probably have even lower yield in this setting.

ANSWERS:
Question 34: B
Question 35: C

36. A 53-year-old man presents with Horner's syndrome and left arm pain. A posteroanterior chest radiograph demonstrates a 4-cm soft-tissue mass in the left apex. Which of the following would be useful for evaluating this patient?

   A. CT scanning of the chest with infusion

   B. MRI scanning

   C. Percutaneous transthoracic needle biopsy

   D. Bronchoscopy

   F. Selective arteriogram of the left subclavian artery

Ref.: 1, 2

COMMENTS: A left apical mass on a chest radiograph with this clinical presentation is characteristic of a superior sulcus tumor. • With this neoplasm, **bronchoscopy** is usually of little or no value in the diagnosis because the abnormal tissue is located far peripherally. • MRI is better than CT for showing the fine details of vascular and neural structures but is not superior for detecting and assessing mediastinal adenopathy, which is a key aspect during the evaluation of any lung cancer. • The standard evaluation includes a CT scan. • If there is evidence of neural or vascular involvement, MRI is useful. • **Percutaneous needle aspiration biopsy** is mandatory to establish a diagnosis of cancer with the typical presentation and radiographic findings. • A histologic diagnosis is required, since these neoplasms optimally are treated with preoperative radiation.

ANSWER:
A, B, C

37. With regard to myasthenia gravis, which of the following statements is/are true?

   A. It is characterized clinically by abnormal fatigability of voluntary muscles on repetitive activity with recovery after rest.

   B. It is associated with an increased number of postsynaptic acetylcholinesterase (ACh) receptors of the neuromuscular junction.

   C. It is thought to be related to complement-mediated damage to ACh receptors initiated by circulating antibodies to the receptors.

   D. It has no palliative or curative medical or surgical treatment.

   E. It is probably due to an infectious cause.

Ref.: 1

COMMENTS: Myasthenia gravis is a neuromuscular disorder probably of autoimmune cause clinically characterized by abnormal fatigability of voluntary muscles on repetitive activity and recovery with rest. • The ocular muscles are often the first group in which clinical manifestations are seen. • The thymus has been implicated in the disease by producing antibodies to postsynaptic ACh receptors at the neuromuscular junction. • The number of receptors is decreased, and there is alteration in structures, probably as a result of complement-mediated damage of the receptors. • Treatment includes immunosuppressive drugs, steroids, cholinesterase inhibitors, and, in severe cases, plasmapheresis. • Complete thymectomy can be palliative or even curative.

ANSWER:
A, C

38. With regard to thymoma, which of the following statements is/are true?

   A. Determination of whether a lesion is benign or malignant is usually based on histologic evidence.

   B. Fifty percent of patients with thymoma have myasthenia gravis.

   C. Fifty percent of patients with myasthenia gravis have thymoma.

   D. Ninety percent of patients with thymoma are asymptomatic.

   E. Radiation therapy plays no role in the care of patients with thymoma.

Ref.: 1, 2

COMMENTS: Thymomas are notoriously difficult to define as benign or malignant by histologic examination. • Encapsulation and invasion into adjacent structures, determined at the time of surgery, constitute the major criteria for classifying them as benign or malignant. • Of patients with thymoma, 50% have myasthenia gravis. • In contrast, only 10–15% of patients with myasthenia gravis have thymoma. • About one half of patients with thymoma present with local symptoms, most commonly chest pain, shortness of breath, and cough. • Radiation therapy is commonly used after excision of all but the most benign-appearing thymomas and appears to have a beneficial effect on recurrence and survival.

ANSWER:
B

39. A 69-year-old smoker presents with hemoptysis. The CT scan reveals a tumor in the right upper lobe bronchus with distal pneumonia and enlarged (>1 cm) right hilar and paratracheal lymph nodes. What should the next step in the management of this patient be?

A. Bronchoscopy

B. Mediastinoscopy

C. Thoracotomy and resection

D. Referral to an oncologist for chemotherapy

E. Referral for radiation therapy

Ref.: 1–3

COMMENTS: An accurate diagnosis with proper staging is important in patients with bronchogenic carcinomas. • Bronchoscopy usually produces a diagnosis at this proximal site. • With enlarged mediastinal nodes, it is important to differentiate between metastatic disease and simple hyperplastic inflammatory nodes. • Thus, mediastinoscopy is indicated for diagnostic staging. • If the tumor is a non–small-cell carcinoma and positive ipsilateral nodes are found, it is at stage IIIA and is probably best treated with induction chemotherapy and irradiation followed by surgical resection. • Positive contralateral nodes indicate a stage IIIB tumor, which is surgically unresectable. • The patient with small-cell lung cancer is best referred to an oncologist for chemotherapy.

ANSWER:
A, B

40. A patient who underwent transhiatal esophagectomy developed a chylothorax postoperatively. Which is/are the appropriate method(s) of treatment?

A. Multiple thoracentesis

B. Tube thoracostomy

C. Low-fat diet

D. Parenteral nutrition

E. Thoracic duct ligation

Ref.: 1–3

COMMENTS: A chyle leak is most often the result of operative injury to the thoracic duct. • It is less often associated with malignancy and obstruction of lymphatic channels. • Normal daily chyle flow in the thoracic duct can range from 1.5 to 2.5 L/day and varies considerably with diet. • Chyle characteristically has a high lymphocyte count and thus is quite resistant to infection. • Few erythrocytes are found in chyle. • It has an extremely high triglyceride level, often 10 times that of serum. • Diagnostic thoracentesis is performed initially to identify the effusion as chyle. • Once diagnosed, chest tube drainage is initiated to evacuate all fluid and allow full lung expansion. • A low-fat diet provides long-chain triglycerides, which are absorbed in the intestine and produce more chyle. • Adequate nutrition must be maintained while minimizing chyle production. • This is best done by parenteral nutrition, although a strict medium-chain triglyceride diet is used by some. • Conservative treatment may last up to 2 weeks, with a success rate of 50–70%. • Thoracic duct ligation is performed if the chyle leak persists and has an expected 80% success rate. • A pleuroperitoneal shunt may be useful for refractory or recurrent cases.

ANSWER:
B, D, E

41. A 20-year-old white man presents with chest pain and a large bulky anterior mediastinal mass on chest CT scanning. What should an appropriate initial workup include?

A. Fine-needle biopsy

B. Incisional biopsy

C. Human chorionic gonadotropin-β (hCG-β) assay

D. α-Fetoprotein (AFP) assay

E. Thoracotomy/sternotomy

Ref.: 1–3

COMMENTS: This presentation in a young white man is highly suspicious of a malignant germ-cell tumor. • It is important to distinguish between a seminoma and a nonseminomatous germ-cell tumor (NSGCT). • A fine-needle biopsy often gives an accurate diagnosis. • If that is nondiagnostic, an incisional biopsy can be done. • Fully 90% of NSGCTs produce an elevation in AFP and hCG-β levels. • Seminomas, which rarely produce hGB-β and never produce AFP, are highly radiosensitive. • NSGCTs are rarely radiosensitive and are treated by multiagent chemotherapy. • Open excision is rarely possible and is reserved for small local tumors and posttherapy residual disease.

ANSWER:
A, C, D

42. A 60-year-old male smoker is diagnosed with a left lower lobe non–small-cell lung cancer by bronchoscopic biopsy. His CT scan shows a 4-cm peripheral tumor. The mediastinal lymph nodes are all less than 1 cm in size. No distant metastasis is found. What is his *clinical* staging?

A. T3N1M0 stage IIIA

B. T2N0M0 stage IB

C. T2N1M0 stage IIB

D. T1N0M0 stage IA

Ref.: 1, 2

COMMENTS: See Question 44.

43. At surgical exploration, direct local invasion of the chest wall is discovered. A left lower lobectomy with en-bloc chest-wall resection is performed, along with thoracic lymphadenectomy. Final pathologic evaluation reveals that all margins are clear but that the tumor had indeed invaded the chest wall. All lymph nodes were normal. What is the final *pathological* staging?

A. T3N0M0 stage IIB

B. T2N2M0 stage IIIA

C. T3N1M0 stage IIIA

D. T2N2M1 stage IV

Ref.: 1, 2

COMMENTS: See Question 44.

44. What is the most accurate method of diagnosing paratracheal lymph node metastases from lung cancer?

A. Fine-needle aspiration

B. CT scan showing enlarged (>1cm) lymph nodes

C. PET scanning

D. Mediastinoscopy

E. MRI

Ref.: 1, 2

COMMENTS: With a primary lesion larger than 3 cm and no apparent invasion by the mass, the T stage is T2. • If no nodes are larger than 1 cm, the stage is N0. • Without obvious metastases, M0 is appropriate. • Local chest-wall invasion (T3) should not preclude resection. • If the margins are clear and lymph nodes negative (N0), the 5-year survival rate may be as high as 30–40%. • Once mediastinal lymph nodes (N2) are involved, survival drops dramatically. • Staging is important to assess treatment and to predict survival. • A CT scan with enlarged lymph nodes (>1 cm) is suggestive, but not diagnostic, of metastasis. • Hyperplastic nodes may also be enlarged. • MRI has not been proven to be more helpful. • A positive PET scan is indicative of hypermetabolic cell uptake of fluorine-18 labeled deoxyglucose. • All three imaging studies have a significant margin of error. • Fine-needle biopsy may miss small tumor nests. • Mediastinoscopy allows removal of entire nodes from this location to allow accurate tissue diagnosis for staging.

ANSWERS:

Question 42: B

Question 43: A

Question 44: D

REFERENCES

1. Townsend CM Jr, Beauchamp RD, Evers BM, et al (eds): *Sabiston Textbook of Surgery: The Biological Basis of Modern Surgical Practice,* 16th ed. Saunders, Philadelphia, 2001.
2. Schwartz SI, Shires GT, Spencer FC, et al (eds): *Schwartz's Principles of Surgery*, 7th ed. McGraw-Hill, New York, 1999.
3. Sabiston DC Jr, Spencer FC (eds): *Surgery of the Chest*, 6th ed. Saunders, Philadelphia, 1995.
4. Allan JS, Wright CD: Tracheoinnominate fistula: diagnosis and management. *Chest Surg Clin North Am* 2003; 13:331–341.

C H A P T E R   47

Cardiac Surgery

A. Congenital Defects

Eric J. Okum, M.D., R. Anthony Perez-Tamayo, M.D., Ph.D., and Robert S. D. Higgins, M.D.

1. Which of the following statements is/are true regarding fetal circulation?

   A. Blood flows through the ductus arteriosus from the pulmonary artery to the aorta.

   B. Less than 25% of the cardiac output flows through the lungs.

   C. Unoxygenated blood is in the ductus venosus.

   D. The atrial septum is intact.

   E. The right side of the heart pumps against lower resistance than the left side.

Ref.: 1–3

COMMENTS: The circulation in utero differs markedly from postnatal circulation. • Gas exchange occurs in the placenta, which receives blood from the umbilical arteries. • Oxygenated blood then returns through the ductus venosus, which joins the inferior vena cava at the level of the hepatic veins. • This blood is mixed with the venous return from the superior vena cava in the right atrium. • Blood in the right atrium may be shunted across the foramen ovale to the left atrium, where it goes to the left ventricle and is pumped into the circulation. • Blood in the right atrium may also go to the right ventricle and be pumped into the pulmonary artery. • Pulmonary vascular resistance is very high in utero, and much of the blood pumped into the pulmonary artery goes through the ductus arteriosus and into the descending aorta. • Because the ductus arteriosus is large and communicates with the aorta, the pressure in the pulmonary artery is the same as in the aorta (systemic). • After birth, the umbilical cord is cut, decreasing the ductus venosus return to zero, which causes the ductus venosus to constrict and obliterate. • Pulmonary vascular resistance drops with expansion of the lungs, causing pulmonary blood flow to increase. • Because return to the left atrium is increased, left atrial pressure causes the foramen ovale to close. • Increased oxygen tension causes the ductus arteriosus to constrict and close. • The pulmonary and systemic circulations at this point become separate.

ANSWER:
A, B

2. Match each of the defects in the left-hand column with its pathophysiologic effect in the right-hand column.

   A. Obstructive lesions   a. Decreased pulmonary blood flow

   B. Right-to-left shunt   b. Increased pulmonary blood flow

   C. Left-to right shunt   c. Increased ventricular work

Ref.: 1–3

COMMENTS: Congenital heart defects can be divided into four categories, each associated with distinct physiologic abnormalities. • **Obstructive lesions** (e.g., aortic stenosi or coarctation of the aorta) restrict the flow of blood and increase the workload of the obstructed ventricle. • Without an associated lesion, there is no shunting or mixing of blood between the pulmonary and systemic circulations. • **Left-to-right shunts** occur in the setting of a communication between the pulmonary and systemic circulations at the level of the atria (e.g., atrial septal defect [ASD]), ventricles (e.g., ventricular septal defect [VSD]), or great vessels (e.g., patent ductus arteriosus). • When there is no obstruction to pulmonary blood flow, these communications usually result in flow of blood across the defect from the systemic to the pulmonary circuit. • The amount of pulmonary blood flow per minute may be as much as four or five times as great as the amount that flows in the systemic circulation. • Clinically significant shunts occur when pulmonary blood flow is greater than 1.5–2 times the systemic flow. • **Right-to-left shunts** occur in the setting of a similar communication but where there is obstruction to pulmonary blood flow (e.g., Tetralogy of Fallot or subaortic or doubly committed double-outlet right ventricle). • Obstruction of pulmonary blood flow causes blood to flow from the right to left side without having passed through the lungs. • If a sufficient amount of desaturated blood goes into the systemic circuit without passing through the lungs, the patient becomes cyanotic. • Complex lesions include defects such as transposition of the great arteries or hypoplastic left heart syndrome, in which the pathophysiologic features cannot be so easily described. • A child with a complex lesion may suffer from cyanosis, pulmonary overcirculation, and obstructive lesions simultaneously.

ANSWER:
A-c; B-a; C-b

3. With regard to increased pulmonary blood flow (left-to- right shunts), which of the following statements is/are true?

   A. A shunt becomes physiologically important when pulmonary blood flow is 1.5–2.0 times as great as systemic flow.

B. High pulmonary artery pressures preclude surgical correction of the defect.

C. Delivering 100% oxygen to the patient during cardiac catheterization may provide crucial information for determining if the patient is an operative candidate.

D. The rapidity with which pulmonary vascular disease develops depends on the magnitude of the shunt regardless of the anatomic location of the defect.

E. Increased fixed pulmonary vascular resistance precludes surgical correction of the defect.

Ref.: 1–3

COMMENTS: Large left-to-right shunts have, by definition, an increased amount of pulmonary blood flow. • There are often elevated pulmonary artery pressures and elevated left atrial pressures. • The combination of these factors causes increased extravascular fluid in the pulmonary parenchyma and thus congestive heart failure. • A shunt where the pulmonary blood flow is less than 1.5 times systemic flow is unlikely to produce symptoms and usually does not represent an indication for surgical repair. • If a patient has a large communication at the level of the ventricles or the great vessels, the pulmonary artery pressures are systemic, since there is free communication between the systemic pressures and the pulmonary artery. • This does not necessarily imply that the patient has pulmonary vascular disease. • High pulmonary artery pressure with a large pulmonary flow (Qp)/systemic flow (Qs) (e.g., Qp/Qs = 3) implies low pulmonary vascular resistance, making the child an appropriate candidate for repair. • If a child has high pulmonary artery pressures at cardiac catheterization and a relatively low pulmonary blood flow (Qp/Qs < 2), pulmonary vascular resistance is high and the child may not tolerate surgical correction. • Oxygen 100% is a potent pulmonary vasodilator. • If the shunt significantly increases with the administration of 100% oxygen, it implies that the pulmonary vascular disease is reversible and the child may yet be a candidate for surgical correction. • Because development of pulmonary vascular disease depends on pressure as well as flow, patients with large atrial level shunts uncommonly develop severe pulmonary vascular obstructive disease, whereas patients with large ventricular or arterial level shunts usually do.

ANSWER:
A, C, E

4. True or false: Resolution of congestive heart failure without surgical correction in a patient who has had a large left-to-right shunt is a sign of improving prognosis.

Ref.: 1–3

COMMENTS: The natural history of a large left-to-right shunt (especially at the ventricular or arterial level) is progressive pulmonary vascular obstructive disease. • There are considerable variations in the progression of pulmonary vascular disease. • A child with a large VSD usually develops pulmonary vascular disease at 2–4 years of age. • A child with a large left-to-right shunt may have considerable congestive heart failure during the first year of life. • However, as pulmonary vascular obstructive disease progresses, the left-to-right shunt decreases as the pulmonary vascular resistance approaches systemic vascular resistance. • During this period, the child's symptoms may improve, and chest radiographic findings of cardiomegaly and pulmonary plethora may also improve. • However, this finding is grave because the pulmonary vascular disease is usually progressive

at this point, despite surgical correction or any other currently available therapies. • Pulmonary vascular disease progresses until the pulmonary vascular resistance exceeds the systemic vascular resistance. • Shunting ceases to be left to right and becomes right to left, resulting in the patient's becoming cyanotic. • This condition is referred to as Eisenmenger's syndrome. • This process usually continues until it results in the patient's death. • Most patients who succumb from Eisenmenger's syndrome die during their teens or twenties.

ANSWER:
False

5. With regard to obstructive congenital heart lesions, which of the following statements is/are true?

A. The most common obstructive lesions are pulmonary valve stenosis, aortic valve stenosis, and coarctation of the aorta.

B. Obstructive congenital heart lesions produce "systolic" overloading and concentric hypertrophy.

C. Concentric hypertrophy produces marked cardiac enlargement, detected by physical examination and routine chest radiography.

D. Electrocardiographic (ECG) changes occur only after there is marked enlargement of the cardiac silhouette.

E. Angina pectoris, arrhythmia, a predisposition to sudden death, and end-stage cardiac failure result from progressive obstruction.

Ref.: 1–3

COMMENTS: The concentric hypertrophy of obstructive congenital heart lesions is not easily detected by chest radiography. • Auscultation may give some indication of the severity of aortic or pulmonary stenosis. • Coarctation of the aorta may be indicated by differences in the pulses and blood pressures between the arms and legs. • The ECG and echocardiogram with Doppler examination are additional noninvasive tests useful for assessing chamber size, degree of obstruction, and function. • Although often not necessary, cardiac catheterization is the definitive modality for assessing the gradient across obstructive lesions. • Aortic stenosis causes increased myocardial oxygen demand while reducing supply, especially to the subendocardium. • This may lead to myocardial ischemia with all its sequelae.

ANSWER:
A, B, E

6. True or false: Lesions that produce large left-to-right shunts are often symptomatic during the newborn period.

Ref.: 1–3

COMMENTS: Large left-to-right shunting occurs because of a communication between the pulmonary and systemic circuits, combined with lower resistance in the pulmonary circuit. • Blood is directed toward the lower resistance. • The pulmonary vascular resistance of newborns is at systemic levels and then falls during the first few weeks of life. • Thus, there is no left-to-right shunting in the newborn, despite the presence of typical lesions, such as a large VSD. • There are none of the typical signs of VSD, including no murmur, no tachypnea, and no hepatomegaly. • As the pulmonary vascular resistance falls, the shunt becomes greater in magnitude, and signs and symptoms of left-to-right shunting appear.

ANSWER:
False

7. With regard to right-to-left shunts, which of the following statements is/are true?

   A. The degree of cyanosis depends on both the severity of anoxia and the blood hemoglobin concentration.

   B. Systemic emboli are common because the polycythemia may lead to venous thrombosis, which may get shunted through the VSD.

   C. Cardiac catheterization is mandatory to determine the degree of pulmonary stenosis and the suitability of the patient for surgery.

   D. A pO_2 of 45 mmHg is life-threatening and requires immediate surgical treatment if it cannot be increased.

Ref.: 1–3

COMMENTS: Cyanosis is present when the amount of desaturated hemoglobin present in the systemic circulation exceeds 5 g/dl. • Thus, cyanosis is dependent on both the oxygen saturation and the hemoglobin level. • A patient with severe hypoxia who also has a relatively low hemoglobin level may be minimally cyanotic. • Conversely, patients with a similar oxygen saturation may appear profoundly cyanotic if they are polycythemic. • Polycythemia is a physiologic response to cyanosis and can lead to a hematocrit of more than 60%. • A high hematocrit increases blood viscosity and predisposes individuals to venous thrombosis. • Systemic emboli, particularly cerebral emboli, may be life threatening. • In particular, children with right-to-left shunts are at risk for cerebral abscesses. • Most children who have right-to-left shunts can be well evaluated with echocardiography alone. • Cardiac catheterization is reserved for patients who require better delineation of small branch pulmonary arteries. • Children tolerate saturations down to around 75%, which corresponds to a pO_2 of 40 mmHg. • A child who chronically has a pO_2 around 45 mmHg usually does well while waiting for an elective operation.

ANSWER:
A, B

8. Match each of the congenital defects in the left-hand column with its associated radiographic change in the right-hand column.

   A. Tetralogy of Fallot
   B. Transposition of great vessels
   C. Total anomalous pulmonary venous drainage
   D. ASD
   E. Mitral insufficiency
   F. VSD
   G. Ebstein's malformation

   a. Egg-shaped heart
   b. Boot-shaped heart (cour en sabot)
   c. Figure-of-eight abnormality ("snowman")
   d. Left atrial and ventricular enlargement
   e. Right atrial and ventricular enlargement

Ref.: 1–3

COMMENTS: The chest radiograph plays an important role in the evaluation of congenital heart disease. • The right ventricular hypertrophy of tetralogy of Fallot tends to produce a boot-shaped heart with an upturned apex. • With transposition of the great arteries, the great arteries usually overlie each other, leaving a narrow mediastinum. • The heart looks like an egg on a string. • Supracardiac total anomalous pulmonary venous return (TAPVR) has a large vertical vein and a large innominate vein, which make a wide mediastinum and a figure-of-eight contour, or "snowman." ASDs cause right-sided enlargement because of the atrial-level shunt. • VSDs cause left-sided heart enlargement (blood goes through the VSD to the pulmonary artery, left atrium, left ventricle, and then back through the VSD; hence, the *left* atrial and ventricular enlargement). • Atrioventricular (AV) valve regurgitation also causes enlargement on its respective side (Ebstein's anomaly of the tricuspid valve on the right and the mitral valve on the left) secondary to the volume overload.

ANSWER:
A-b; B-a; C-c; D-e; E-d; F-d; G-e

9. Which of the following statements is/are true regarding systemic to pulmonary artery shunts?

   A. They join one of the great vessels with the pulmonary artery, either directly or by means of a prosthetic graft.

   B. They are used to increase pulmonary blood flow in patients with tetralogy of Fallot.

   C. Because less blood goes to the body, the pulse pressure is narrowed after shunt placement.

   D. A successful shunt may make definitive surgery unnecessary.

   E. A shunt may be used in a cyanotic infant to delay definitive surgery until the patient is older.

Ref.: 1–3

COMMENTS: Blalock-Taussig shunts are part of the broader classification of systemic-pulmonary artery shunts. • Although other kinds of shunt connections were made in the past, most shunts today consist of Gore-Tex grafts between the aorta or one of the great vessels (e.g., innominate artery) and the pulmonary artery. • Pulmonary blood flow may be increased to relieve severe hypoxia. • A shunt may delay the need for definitive surgery in young patients with complex heart disease. • Shunt physiology is inherently inefficient, since the blood going through the lungs via the shunt is already partly oxygenated. • Thus, a shunt is never considered the final repair, except in complex cases where definitive repair is not possible. • Because there is runoff through the shunt into the low-resistance pulmonary circuit during diastole, systemic diastolic pressures tend to be low, making pulse pressures wide.

ANSWER:
A, B, E

10. Match each of the comments or pathologic conditions in the left-hand column with the associated auscultatory finding in the right-hand column.

    A. Most common form of "innocent" murmur
    B. Infrequent but, when present, a significant finding
    C. Pulmonary hypertension

    a. Systolic murmurs
    b. Increased second heart sound (S_2)
    c. Diastolic murmurs

D. Pulmonary stenosis or atresia

E. ASD

F. Appearance at 4 weeks of age consistent with a VSD

G. Patent ductus arteriosus (PDA)

d. Widely split and "fixed" S$_2$

e. Continuous murmur

f. Decreased S$_2$

Ref.: 1–3

COMMENTS: Proper auscultation of the heart often leads to the correct diagnosis of a congenital cardiac abnormality. • The S$_2$ is heard best at the left upper sternal border and should be evaluated in terms of its degree of splitting and relative intensity. • The degree of splitting of S$_2$ normally varies with respirations (increases with inspiration and decreases or becomes single with expiration). • An abnormal S$_2$ may be in the form of (1) wide splitting, (2) narrow splitting, (3) single S$_2$, (4) abnormal increase or decrease in the pulmonary component of the second sound (P$_2$), or (5) paradoxical splitting of S$_2$. • Systolic murmurs occur between S$_1$ and S$_2$ and may be (1) ejection (through stenotic semilunar valves or due to increased flow through normal semilunar valves) or (2) regurgitant (pansystolic or holosystolic). • The latter are associated with a VSD, mitral regurgitation, or tricuspid regurgitation. • Diastolic murmurs may occur because of an incompetent semilunar valve or increased flow through an AV valve. • Diastolic murmurs are virtually always pathologic. • Continuous murmurs begin during systole and continue through S$_2$ into all or part of diastole. • They are caused by aortopulmonary or arteriovenous connection (e.g., PDA, arteriovenous fistula, or after a systemic-pulmonary shunt), flow disturbance in veins (e.g., venous hum), or arteries (e.g., coarctation or peripheral pulmonary artery stenosis).

ANSWER:
A-a; B-c; C-b; D-f; E-d; F-a; G-e

11. With regard to echocardiography for the evaluation of congenital heart disease, which of the following statements is/are true?

A. It is the most accurate method by which to delineate intracardiac anatomy.

B. It may precisely define pulmonary artery anatomy.

C. It may indicate whether the right ventricular pressure is at or well below systemic pressures.

D. It may indicate the gradient across a valve.

Ref.: 1–3

COMMENTS: Echocardiography has become the dominant imaging modality for congenital heart disease. • It is the most accurate method by which to delineate intracardiac anatomy, and nearly all diagnoses are determined by echocardiography. • Doppler echocardiography measures velocities across valves and outflow tracts, and these velocities may be translated into gradients by the formula: $\Delta P = 4\ V^2$ (V is velocity). • The velocity of a small amount of tricuspid regurgitation may be translated into the right ventricular/right atrial (RV-RA) gradient and be a good estimate of RV pressure. • Pulmonary artery distortion may be difficult to assess by echocardiography, and better delineation is often needed by cardiac catheterization. • Coronary arteries may be assessed with a good deal of accuracy, although the images obtained do not always yield definitive information.

ANSWER:
A, C, D

12. With regard to pulmonic stenosis, which of the following statements is/are true?

A. The most common morphologic feature is hypoplasia of the pulmonic valve annulus.

B. The physiologic abnormality is obstruction of flow from the right ventricle, with secondary concentric hypertrophy.

C. The intervention of choice is a surgical commissurotomy.

D. The most common symptom is dyspnea on exertion.

E. Echocardiography accurately delineates the anatomy and severity of obstruction.

Ref.: 1–3

COMMENTS: Pulmonic stenosis accounts for 10% of congenital abnormalities. • It most commonly involves fusion of the cusps of the pulmonary valve, poststenotic dilatation of the main pulmonary artery, and concentric hypertrophy of the right ventricle. • Less common morphologic conditions include hypoplasia of the pulmonary valve annulus, supravalvar stenosis, or subvalvular obstruction from hypertrophied muscle (infundibular stenosis). • The condition is usually asymptomatic, but when symptoms are present, the most common is dyspnea on exertion. • Echocardiography accurately delineates the nature and severity of the obstruction by visualizing the anatomy and measuring the velocity of the jet across the obstruction. • The current treatment of choice is balloon valvotomy, which works in most cases that do not have hypoplasia of the valve annulus. • Surgical therapy is reserved for patients who have annular hypoplasia, infundibular obstruction, or failed balloon valvuloplasty.

ANSWER:
B, D, E

13. With regard to coarctation of the aorta, which of the following statements is/are true?

A. The lesion involves narrowing of the descending aorta just distal to the left subclavian artery.

B. Early left ventricular failure requiring surgical correction is common when coarctation presents in a neonate.

C. Coarctation is one of the causes of surgically correctable hypertenison.

D. Arm hypertension, decreased or absent leg pulses, and a systolic murmur over the left hemithorax are the typical physical findings.

E. Late recoarctation occurs in a certain percentage of cases regardless of the repair technique.

Ref.: 1–3

COMMENTS: Coarctation of the aorta accounts for 10–15% of congenital heart defects and occurs twice as frequently in males. • Associated anomalies include bicuspid aortic valve, VSD, PDA, and mitral valve disorders. • Coarctation of the aorta usually occurs distal to the left subclavian artery in association with the ligamentum arteriosum. • When severe, coarctation presents in neonates with severe left ventricular failure, requiring immediate surgical correction. • Patients who present later in childhood often are without symptoms but have severe arm hypertension. • The presence of differential pulses or blood pressures between the arms and legs strongly suggests the diagnosis. • Because collateral flow via the intercostal arteries is sufficient, ischemic symptoms of the lower body are uncommon when the patient presents after the neonatal period. • The findings on physical examination and an ECG showing left ventricular hypertrophy establish the diagnosis. • Echocardiography is the diagnostic method of choice. • Coarctation is one of the classic causes of surgically correctable hypertension (others include pheochromocytoma, aldosterone-secreting tumor, and renal artery stenosis). • Postoperative hypertension may continue to exist even after adequate surgical repair. • Repair may be accomplished by several means, including resection with end-to-end anastomosis, left subclavian flap, and patch aortoplasty. • All are associated with a small but definite percentage of late recoarctation. • Patch aortoplasty is now seldom used because of a high rate of late pseudoaneurysm formation.

ANSWER:
A, B, C, D, E

14. With regard to valvar aortic stenosis, which of the following statements is/are true?

   A. Aortic stenosis predisposes to sudden death, even in children.

   B. There is no valve replacement that grows as the patient grows.

   C. Gradient alone is an indication for intervention, even without symptoms.

   D. Surgical or balloon valvotomy for aortic stenosis has a high likelihood of causing aortic regurgitation.

   E. A bicuspid aortic valve is virtually always stenotic.

Ref.: 1–3

COMMENTS: Valvar aortic stenosis may develop from a bicuspid or tricuspid aortic valve. • Newborns may be affected with critical aortic stenosis, or the stenosis may progress with time and be manifested at any time in the patient's life. • Newborns with critical aortic stenosis present with severe cardiomegaly and heart failure. • The symptoms and indications for surgery for older children are similar as for adults. • Symptoms of congestive heart failure, angina, and syncope may develop. • A gradient of over 50 mmHg is thought to be a risk for sudden death. • The presence of symptoms or an asymptomatic gradient over 50 mmHg is thought to be an indication for intervention. • Unlike the situation in adults, aortic stenosis in children usually does not involve calcified leaflets. • Therefore, valvuloplasty (surgical or balloon) is an option. • Valvuloplasty has produced good results in terms of relieving stenosis as long as the annulus is adequate, but a high rate of postvalvuloplasty aortic regurgitation (20%) is encountered, which often results in valve replacement at a future date. • Both balloon and surgical valvuloplasty have a 50% reintervention rate at 5 years. • An increasingly common valve replacement option is the pulmonary autograft (Ross procedure). • In addition to not requiring anticoagulation, the pulmonary autograft grows as the child grows. • A bicuspid valve constitutes a common underlying morphologic condition for aortic valve stenosis. • However, most people who have a bicuspid aortic valve do not suffer from clinically significant aortic stenosis.

ANSWER:
A, C, D

15. Which of the following statements is/are true regarding subaortic stenosis?

   A. It is usually caused by diffuse narrowing of the subaortic area.

   B. A turbulent bloodstream may hit the aortic valve, causing inflammation and valvar aortic stenosis.

   C. The indications for operation are the same as for valvular aortic stenosis.

   D. Subvalvular aortic stenosis is not amenable to balloon valvuloplasty.

   E. The area of resection of subaortic stenosis is adjacent to the conduction tissue.

Ref.: 1–3

COMMENTS: Subaortic stenosis can occur as a discrete membrane or as a diffuse tunnel-like narrowing, but it is more commonly discrete. • Surgery involves removal of the membrane with or without septal myotomy to further widen the outflow tract. • Because valve replacement is rarely necessary and because the jet from the subaortic stenosis may precipitate aortic regurgitation, the threshold for surgery on a subaortic stenosis is far less than for valvar aortic stenosis. • Because the membrane requires resection with subaortic stenosis, transcatheter interventions have little role. • Despite the fact that the membrane directly overlies the conduction tissue, careful resection of a subaortic membrane rarely leads to heart block.

ANSWER:
D, E

16. True or false: Hypertrophic cardiomyopathy is a diffuse disease of the myocardium, and so surgery has little role.

Ref.: 1, 2, 3

COMMENTS: Hypertrophic cardiomyopathy (also known as idiopathic hypertrophic subaortic stenosis) is a diffuse, inherited myocardial disease. • Patients generally develop asymmetric hypertrophy of the ventricular septum, which may result in dynamic left ventricular outflow tract obstruction. • There are four surgical options for patients with hypertrophic cardiomyopathy. • The first is dual-chambered pacing. • The mechanism of action of cardiac pacing is unclear, but it is thought to work by changing the pathway of spread of the electrical signal throughout the ventricle. • By doing this, the contraction of various parts of the outflow tract may be less coordinated, and there is less dynamic obstruction. • The second option is septal myotomy. • This technique reduces the obstruction by physically removing some of the hypertrophied muscle to enlarge the outflow tract. • The third option is mitral valve replacement to improve outflow tract obstruction or mitral regurgitation. • The fourth option is cardiac transplantation. • Catheter-based alcohol injection of the first septal perforator artery may be used in selected cases.

ANSWER:
False

17. Which of the following statements is/are true regarding aortic regurgitation?

   A. Discrete subaortic stenosis or VSD may be responsible for producing aortic regurgitation.

   B. Symptoms are those of congestive heart failure.

   C. Echocardiography accurately estimates the degree of regurgitation and the chamber sizes.

D. Because effective cardiac output is reduced, the pulses are weak and the pulse pressure is narrowed.

E. Operation is indicated when symptoms develop.

Ref.: 1–3

COMMENTS: Aortic regurgitation causes volume overload on the left ventricle, which eventually results in left ventricular dilatation and left ventricular failure. • There is increased stroke volume because of the regurgitant fraction, resulting in bounding pulses and wide pulse pressure. • Symptoms are those of congestive heart failure. • Angina may occur as a late finding. • Syncope is generally not associated with aortic regurgitation, as it is with aortic stenosis. • The diagnosis is accurately made and the case followed by echocardiography. • Indications for surgery include the onset of symptoms or increased left ventricular dimensions even before symptoms occur. • Aortic regurgitation may occur as the primary valve pathology, secondary to valvuloplasty for aortic stenosis, or after damage to a normal aortic valve caused by discrete subaortic stenosis or a VSD. • The possibility of creating aortic insufficiency is one of the indications for repair of subaortic stenosis and VSDs.

ANSWER:
A, B, C, E

18. With regard to ASDs, which of the following statements is/are true?

A. The magnitude of the shunt is determined by the difference in compliance between the ventricles.

B. The left ventricle frequently becomes enlarged.

C. Patients may develop increased pulmonary vascular resistance.

D. An ASD should be surgically corrected before the patient is 1 year of age to avoid pulmonary hypertension.

E. Surgical closure with cardiopulmonary bypass is the only option for closure.

Ref.: 1–3

COMMENTS: ASDs may produce large left-to-right shunts without high pulmonary artery pressures. • The magnitude of the shunt is determined by the differences in compliance between the two ventricles. • The shunt occurs during diastole, when blood goes from the atria to the ventricles. • Because of the defect, the atria have equal pressures, so the filling pressures for the two ventricles are similar. • The amount of blood that goes to each side depends on the amount that each ventricle distends given that filling pressure. • Because the right ventricle is more compliant, blood from the left atrium has a tendency to cross the defect and enter the right ventricle, creating the left-to-right shunt. • Pulmonary artery pressures may be normal or near normal, since there is no communication between the two sides during systole. • Congestive heart failure eventually develops in about 25% of individuals with ASDs, usually during the third to fourth decade of life, if the ASD if left untreated. • Pulmonary vascular obstructive disease occurs in about 10% if the ASD is left untreated. • Because symptoms rarely occur during the first decade of life, repair is entirely elective. • Repair is usually done when the child is at a preschool age (3–4 years), when he or she is large enough for easy closure but has few psychological effects from undergoing the surgery. • During the current era, many defects are now closed with transcatheter devices by interventional cardiologists.

ANSWER:
A, C

19. Which of the following statements regarding percutaneous ASD closure is/are true?

A. The majority of ASDs are surgically closed today.

B. Sinus venosus defects are easily amenable to device closure.

C. The largest device approved in the United States is 38 mm.

D. The overall complication rate for percutaneous device closure is approximately 8%.

E. The success rate of the device closure is 95–100%.

Ref.: 1–3

COMMENTS: The majority of ASDs are now closed percutaneously. • The published literature shows a success from 80–95% for percutaneous closure and 95–100% for surgical closure. • The largest device is 38 mm (Amplatzer). • Closure of sinus venosus defects is contraindicated secondary to superior vena cava, inferior vena cava, or pulmonary venous obstruction. • The published complication rate of device closure is 8%. • Complications include the following: device malposition or dislocation, early or late embolization, arrhythmias, thrombus formation, atrial or ventricular perforation, mitral regurgitation, or tricuspid regurgitation secondary to interference of the subvalvular apparatus.

ANSWER:
C, D

20. Which of the following statements is/are true regarding total anomalous pulmonary venous return (TAPVR)?

A. TAPVR is categorized as supracardiac, cardiac, infracardiac, or mixed.

B. The pathologic condition occurs when the pulmonary veins fail to empty into the left atrium and, instead, connect directly to the right atrium or one of the large systemic veins.

C. The connection between the pulmonary veins and the systemic veins may be obstructed with equal frequency, regardless of whether the connection is supracardiac, cardiac, or infracardiac.

D. When a patient has obstructed TAPVR, there is reduced pulmonary blood flow, leaving the lungs relatively dark on a chest radiograph.

E. An ASD must be present for survival.

Ref.: 1–3

COMMENTS: During embryologic development, the four pulmonary veins form a confluence that merges with the back of the left atrium. • TAPVR is an anomaly in which this connection fails to occur. • The pulmonary venous flow then goes through an anomolous vessel that most commonly connects to the innominate vein (supracardiac), the coronary sinus (cardiac), or the portal vein (infracardiac). • Supracardiac TAPVR occurs in approximately 50% of cases, cardiac TAPVR in 25% of cases, infracardiac TAPVR in 20% of cases, and 5% are mixed. • Because both the systemic and pulmonary venous return goes to the right side of the heart, an ASD must be present to allow blood into the left side of the heart and the systemic circulation. • The blood returning to the atrium distributes itself between the right and left ventricles according to their relative compliances, as with any large ASD. • Because the right ventricle has greater compliance than the left ventricle, there is more pulmonary flow than systemic flow. • This is equivalent to a large left-to-right shunt. • A serious complication of TAPVR occurs when the connection between the pulmonary venous confluence and the systemic veins is obstructed. • With infracardiac TAPVR, obstruction is the rule because the pulmonary venous return must go through the hepatic capillary bed. • With supracardiac TAPVR, obstruction occurs in only a few patients, and with cardiac TAPVR, obstruction is rare. • When obstruction occurs, pulmonary venous pressure is high, causing severe pulmonary edema.

A N S W E R :
A, B, E

---

21. Match each of the clinical comments in the left-hand column with the associated heart defect in the right-hand column.

   A. More commonly associated with Down's syndrome
   B. Frequently causes symptoms during infancy
   C. An endocardial cushion defect
   D. Long-term risk for mitral insufficiency
   E. Uncommonly causes increased pulmonary vascular resistance
   F. Left axis division

   a. Secundum ASD
   b. Ostium primum defect
   c. Both secundum ASD and ostium primum defect
   d. Neither secundum ASD nor ostium primum defect

Ref.: 1–3

COMMENTS: Secundum ASDs and primum atrial septal defects have in common left-to-right shunting at the atrial level but are different malformations. • Because of their similar atrial level shunting, they rarely cause symptoms during infancy and generally require elective repair at 1–4 years of age. • Secundum ASDs rarely cause any residual problems after closure. • However, primum ASDs are truly part of the spectrum of AV canal defects (endocardial cushion defects). • Therefore, the AV valves are abnormal, and frequently the left AV valve (mitral valve) becomes insufficient with time. • Long-term insufficiency requiring valve repair or replacement is a well-known complication. • Patients with primum ASDs also may develop left ventricular outflow tract obstruction. • Patients with primum ASDs have left axis deviation on their ECGs, which also distinguishes them from secundum ASDs. • Children with Down's syndrome have a high incidence of endocardial cushion defects, although secundum ASDs and typical ventricular septal defects may be found as well.

A N S W E R :
A-b; B-d; C-b; D-b; E-c; F-b

---

22. With regard to partial anomalous pulmonary venous drainage, which of the following statements is/are true?

   A. All patterns of partial anomalous pulmonary venous drainage require surgical correction.

   B. The pathophysiology is similar to that of an ASD (atrial-level left-to-right shunt).

   C. Fifty percent of partial anomalous pulmonary veins are associated with an ASD.

   D. Partial anomalous pulmonary veins arise more commonly from the right lung.

   E. Balloon septostomy is used to palliate infants with partial anomalous pulmonary venous drainage.

Ref.: 1–3

COMMENTS: Only rarely are partial anomalous pulmonary veins found with an intact atrial septum. • They usually arise from a single lung, most commonly the right. • Right anomalous pulmonary veins entering the superior vena cava are usually associated with a high secundum ASD, known as sinus venosus defect. • Single anomalous pulmonary veins (from one lobe of the lung) may result in a small shunt (Qp/Qs < 1.5) and require no treatment. • Because pulmonary venous blood enters the right atrium instead of the left atrium, the end result is physiology similar to other atrial level left-to-right shunts. • Balloon septostomy is virtually never required for palliation, since the atrial septum is usually open and the left pulmonary veins directly empty into the left atrium. • Surgical repair involves closing the ASD with a patch that also covers the anomalous pulmonary vein, such that the pulmonary venous return is kept on the left side of the patch. • Care needs to be taken not to narrow the SVC, often requiring a patch angioplasty.

A N S W E R :
B, D

---

23. With regard to VSDs, which of the following statements is/are true?

   A. Moderate-to-large defects usually become symptomatic at about 1 year of age.

   B. Defects less than 2 cm in diameter are generally well tolerated.

   C. Irreversible pulmonary vascular obstructive disease is uncommon before 1 year of age.

   D. Banding of the pulmonary artery is the operation of choice in infants younger than 2 years of age.

   E. Many small VSDs will close spontaneously.

Ref.: 1–3

COMMENTS: VSDs account for 20–30% of congenital heart defects. • Associated anomalies are common (e.g., patent ductus arteriosus, coarctation, ASD, and aortic insufficiency). • Defects less than 4–5 mm in diameter are associated with pulmonary blood flow less than two times the systemic flow, with few adverse physiologic consequences. • Larger defects can produce cardiac failure, pulmonary hypertension, and death. • VSDs are usually asymptomatic during the newborn period. • Pulmonary vascular resistance is high, which keeps left-to-right shunting and pulmonary overcirculation minimized. • At 1–2 months of age, the pulmonary vascular resistance decreases, allowing a large left-to-right shunt, which produces symptoms of congestive heart failure. • In symptomatic infants with large lesions, surgical correction is indicated. • If such infants are left untreated, increased pulmonary vascular resistance may become irreversible by the age of 2 years. • It is rare for irreversible pulmonary vascular resistance to occur before 1 year of age. • Up to 40% of VSDs close spontaneously by 2 years of age. • Pulmonary artery banding, once widely used in infants with significant VSDs, is now rarely used with the increasing success of definitive closure in younger patients.

ANSWER:
C, E

---

24. True or false: The preferred approach for repair of most VSDs is the transatrial approach.

Ref.: 1–3

COMMENTS: Repair of a VSD was traditionally performed via ventriculotomy. • Advances in operative technique now allow most defects to be closed through the right atrium, with retraction of the tricuspid valve. • This procedure avoids disruption of the ventricular wall and potential coronary artery damage. • Some defects, particularly muscular defects, may still require ventriculotomy.

ANSWER:
True

---

25. True or false: Eisenmenger's syndrome is a classic conduction defect resulting from inappropriate repair of a VSD.

Ref.: 1–3

COMMENTS: Eisenmenger's syndrome is the end stage that results from a large left-to-right shunt with fixed pulmonary hypertension secondary to irreversible pulmonary vascular resistance. • It can occur with VSD, patent ductus arteriosus, AV canal defects, transposition of the great arteries, truncus arteriosus, and, rarely, in association with a large ASD. • The increased pulmonary vascular resistance from the left-to-right shunt eventually exceeds systemic vascular resistance, causing reversal to a right-to-left shunt and producing cyanosis.

ANSWER:
False

---

26. With regard to patent ductus arteriosus (PDA), which of the following statements is/are true?

A. It produces a left-to-right shunt at the level of the great arteries.

B. Irreversible, increased pulmonary vascular disease generally occurs only in association with another defect.

C. Because of low cardiac output, children with PDA tend to have narrow pulse pressures.

D. Indomethacin can be used to close PDAs in term infants but not in premature babies.

E. The presence of cyanosis is a contraindication to closure.

Ref.: 1–3

COMMENTS: PDA is an abnormal communication between the descending aorta and the pulmonary artery. • The ductus arteriosus ordinarily closes after birth in response to rising oxygen tension and numerous other hormonal factors. • PDA in premature babies usually involves a structurally normal ductus that fails to close because of the low oxygen tension and surrounding mediators (e.g., increased prostaglandins) that maintain ductus patency. • By changing the hormonal environment with indomethacin (which blocks prostaglandin production), a PDA in a premature

infant may be closed. • In a term baby, a PDA is caused by a structurally abnormal ductal wall. • Indomethacin therefore has little effect on term infants. • If a PDA is large, there is a large left-to-right shunt, with the pulmonary artery being exposed to systemic pressures. • These children experience the same course of congestive heart failure followed by increased pulmonary vascular resistance as do children with a large VSD. • Like children with a large VSD, children with a large PDA may develop Eisenmenger's syndrome. • Cyanosis from Eisenmenger's syndrome is a contraindication to closure of a PDA. • Because of runoff from the aorta into the low-resistance pulmonary artery during diastole, the diastolic pressure in children with a PDA tends to be low, with large pulse pressures.

ANSWER:
A, E

---

27. True or false: Prostaglandins may be indicated to maintain ductal patency in right-sided obstructive lesions (e.g., tetralogy of Fallot) but not in left-sided obstructive lesions (e.g., interrupted aortic arch).

Ref.: 1–3

COMMENTS: Prostaglandins (PGE_1) are useful for maintaining ductal patency in the newborn. • The indications may be for either right- or left-sided obstructive lesions. • If a patient has a right-sided obstructive lesion (e.g., pulmonary atresia), pulmonary blood flow may be duct dependent. • Prostaglandins may be used to keep the ductus patent until a surgically created systemic-pulmonary artery shunt or definitive repair can be accomplished. • With left-sided lesions, such as an interrupted aortic arch, blood flow to parts of the systemic circulation may be duct dependent; that is, before repair can be undertaken, the ductus is the only means by which part of the systemic circulation can receive blood flow. • Ductal closure is lethal in the setting of a severe left-sided obstruction, such as an interrupted aortic arch. • In this situation, blood through the ductus flows from the pulmonary artery to the aorta.

ANSWER:
False

---

28. Which of the following statements is/are true regarding complete AV canal defects?

A. They are associated with Down's syndrome.

B. There is one AV orifice instead of separate mitral and tricuspid valves.

C. Because most of the shunting occurs at the ventricular level, the natural history of the disease is similar to that of a VSD.

D. The decompression through the atrial part of the defect protects against pulmonary vascular disease.

E. Recurrent ventricular-level shunting is the most common long-term complication of repair.

Ref.: 1–3

COMMENTS: Common AV canal defects involve abnormal endocardial cushion development. • The central point at which the atrial septum, ventricular septum, and AV valves should join fail to meet. • The patient is usually left with a large defect in the inferior atrial septum and inlet ventricular septum. • Instead of the usual mitral and tricuspid valves, there is one large AV valve that separates both atria from both ventricles. • Most patients with complete AV canal defects also have Down's syndrome. • The pathophysiology is that of a large left-to-right shunt, as with a VSD. • Pulmonary vascular disease develops somewhat faster with an AV canal than with a VSD, partly because the shunt is both atrial and ventricular and partly because Down's syndrome children have a tendency to develop early vascular disease. • Patients may develop significant postoperative AV valve regurgitation, usually of the left-sided AV (mitral) valve. • The incidence of reoperation for left-sided AV valve regurgitation is approximately 10–15% at 10 years.

A N S W E R :
A, B, C

29. With regard to tetralogy of Fallot, which of the following statements is/are true?

    A. Cyanosis occurs because of the septal defect associated with the right ventricular hypertrophy.

    B. A right-to-left shunt occurs because of the septal defect associated with the right ventricular outflow tract obstruction.

    C. Patients often become anemic.

    D. Patients learn to squat because it lowers their pulmonary artery pressures.

    E. The aorta is overriding, which exacerbates the right-to-left shunt.

Ref.: 1–3

COMMENTS: The classic congenital abnormality producing a right-to-left shunt is tetralogy of Fallot, a combination of a VSD, pulmonary stenosis, overriding of the aorta, and right ventricular hypertrophy. • The amount of shunting across the VSD is related to the amount of pulmonary stenosis. • In patients with little pulmonary stenosis, the shunting may be left to right, as with an uncomplicated VSD. • Most patients with tetralogy of Fallot have enough pulmonary stenosis that some of the desaturated blood in the right ventricle goes through the VSD to the systemic circulation. • Because of the chronic cyanosis, patients may develop polycythemia with hemoglobin values that exceed 20 mg/dl. • Patients will learn to squat if the problem remains uncorrected past a few years of age. • Squatting increases systemic vascular resistance, forcing more blood to go to the lungs. • Squatting does nothing directly to the pulmonary vasculature.

A N S W E R :
B

30. True or false: Most patients with tetralogy of Fallot require palliative surgery (systemic to pulmonary artery shunt) before complete repair.

Ref.: 1–3

COMMENTS: About 15–20 years ago, most patients with tetralogy of Fallot underwent palliation with a Blalock-Taussig shunt followed by complete repair at 3–6 years of age. • At that time, complete repair during infancy carried significant morbidity and mortality. • Since then, improvements in surgical, anesthetic, and perfusion techniques have allowed single-stage correction during infancy for most patients with tetralogy of Fallot. • Elective repair is usually performed at approximately 6 months of age. • Earlier repair may be done if a child is too cyanotic to wait until 6 months. • A staged approach may still be performed. • One such circumstance is in a patient with very small pulmonary arteries. • VSD closure may cause the right ventricular pressures to become suprasystemic, trying to pump blood through the small pulmonary arteries. • A staged approach may allow time for pulmonary artery growth and a definitive repair at a later date.

A N S W E R :
False

31. Which of the following statements regarding extracorporeal membrane oxygenation (ECMO) are true?

    A. Survival is greater than 75% when placed for neonatal respiratory support.

    B. Survival is equal for adults and children.

    C. Survival for cardiac ECMO is greater than that for respiratory ECMO.

    D. The overall survival rate is 40%.

    E. The lowest survival is for meconium aspiration syndrome.

Ref.: 1–3

COMMENTS: ECMO can be used in infants, children, or adults for acute cardiac or respiratory support. • Common indications in the pediatric population include meconium aspiration, congenital diaphragmatic hernia, sepsis, and primary pulmonary hypertension and for postrepair of intracardiac defects. • Survival in neonates is higher with respiratory than with cardiac causes (77% versus 38%). • Adults have much lower survival rates than do children. • Overall, survival using extracorporeal life support is approximately 40%. • The highest survival rate is for meconium aspiration syndrome (94%).

A N S W E R :
A, D

32. The repair of tetralogy of Fallot may include which of the following?

    A. Repair of aortic override

    B. Closure of the VSD

    C. Division of muscle bundles in the right ventricular outflow tract (RVOT)

    D. Patch augmentation of the pulmonary annulus

    E. Resection of the endocardium of the right ventricle to alleviate right ventricular hypertrophy

Ref.: 1–3

COMMENTS: Repair of tetralogy of Fallot involves closure of the VSD and relief of the RVOT obstruction. • It is usually necessary to resect or divide the thick muscle bundles in the infundibulum to open the subvalvar area of the outflow tract. • If the pulmonary annulus is hypoplastic, the annulus may require augmentation with a transannular patch. • The aortic override is not repaired, and the VSD patch is tilted anteriorly at its superior end to accommodate the aortic override. • The right ventricular hypertrophy subsides when the right ventricle is no longer subjected to systemic pressures.

A N S W E R :
B, C, D

33. With regard to transposition of the great vessels, which of the following statements is/are true?

    A. The aorta arises from the right ventricle and carries unoxygenated blood to the body.

    B. The pulmonary artery arises from the left ventricle and carries unoxygenated blood to the lung.

    C. PDA, VSD, or ASD is necessary for survival (before definitive correction).

    D. Pulmonary stenosis occurs in approximately 10% of patients.

    E. VSD occurs in approximately 25% of patients.

    Ref.: 1–3

COMMENTS: Transposition of the great arteries is a common form of complex cyanotic heart disease. • The aorta arises from the right ventricle, carrying unoxygenated blood to the body. • The pulmonary artery arises from the left ventricle, carrying oxygenated blood to the lungs. • For any oxygen to be delivered to the body, there must be mixing between the systemic and pulmonary circuits. • This mixing is necessary for survival. • The common points of mixing are an ASD, a VSD, and a PDA. • If the patient has an intact ventricular septum and a small ASD, it may be necessary to use a large balloon-tipped catheter to enlarge the atrial septum to stabilize the child preoperatively. • Transposition of the great arteries has many associated defects, the most common being VSDs and pulmonary stenosis (i.e., left ventricular outflow tract obstruction). • Other associations include interrupted aortic arches, coarctation of the aorta, and hypoplastic ventricles. • The associated lesions may greatly affect prognosis and treatment.

ANSWER:
A, C, D, E

34. Which of the following statements regarding the arterial switch operation for transposition of the great arteries is/ are true?

    A. The arterial switch involves redirecting flow from the inferior or superior vena cava to the left ventricle.

    B. Switching the coronary arteries often provides the greatest source of morbidity.

    C. The presence of a VSD is a contraindication for the arterial switch operation.

    D. The presence of pulmonary stenosis is a contraindication for the arterial switch operation.

    E. The arterial switch operation is generally performed at 6 months of age.

    Ref.: 1–3

COMMENTS: The usual surgical treatment for transposition of the great arteries is the arterial switch operation. • This operation involves transecting the great vessels just above the semilunar valves and "switching" their positions, such that the aorta would come off the left ventricle and the pulmonary artery off the right ventricle. • The difficulty of the arterial switch involves switching the coronary arteries. • The small coronary arteries of a newborn may twist and obstruct when being transferred. • The morbidity associated with this procedure has been greatly reduced, since the combined surgical experience with this operation has taught surgeons how the coronaries need to be transferred. • Approximately one third of patients with transposition have abnormal coronary artery branching patterns. • Some of these branching patterns are difficult to switch and dramatically increase the risk of the procedure. • The presence of a VSD does not change one's plan to do an arterial switch. • The VSD is closed as part of the procedure. • The presence of pulmonary stenosis does preclude an arterial switch because, after a switch, the patient would be left with aortic stenosis, which would be poorly tolerated. • Before arterial switch procedures were developed, most patients were treated with atrial switch operations (Mustard or Senning procedures). • They involved redirecting the systemic and pulmonary venous return with baffles inside the atrium, which left the right ventricle still pumping blood to the body and the left ventricle pumping blood to the lungs. • These procedures have been largely abandoned because of the incidence of atrial arrythmias and long-term failure of the right ventricle. • The arterial switch is performed during the neonatal period. • If one waits longer, the left ventricle becomes unable to pump against systemic pressure.

ANSWER:
B, D

35. Which of the following statements is/are true regarding the Fontan procedure (total cavopulmonary anastomosis)?

    A. It involves a direct connection between both venae cavae and the pulmonary artery.

    B. It is used in patients with a single functioning ventricle.

    C. The Fontan procedure is most successful when central venous pressure (CVP) is elevated (>15 mmHg).

    D. Children with moderately elevated pulmonary vascular resistance may not be candidates for a Fontan operation.

    E. The Fontan procedure is performed as soon as the diagnosis is made.

    Ref.: 1–3

COMMENTS: The issue with patients with single-ventricle physiology is how to provide pulmonary blood flow. • Options include the Fontan procedure and a systemic-pulmonary artery shunt. • The Fontan procedure (total cavopulmonary anastomosis) is an operation used for patients with single-ventricle physiology. • It has been in existence since the mid-1970s. • There are a number of techniques for making the connection, but the Fontan procedure in any of its forms involves a connection between the venae cavae and the pulmonary artery. • Blood flow through the pulmonary capillary bed is driven only by the CVP. • After going through the lungs, blood is returned to the single ventricle and is pumped to the body. • Patients remain fully saturated without an extra volume load on the heart. • Neither of these goals is satisfied by providing pulmonary blood flow with a systemic-pulmonary artery shunt. • The problem with a Fontan operation is that patients rarely tolerate a CVP of more than 15 mmHg. • For the CVP to drive blood through the lungs at an acceptable level, the patient must have excellent "Fontan" hemodynamics: pulmonary arteries without stenosis, low pulmonary vascular resistance, no pulmonary venous obstruction, no AV valve regurgitation, and low ventricular filling pressures. • Because the pulmonary resistance is elevated in infants, a Fontan operation is generally not performed until 18–24 months of age.

ANSWER:
A, B, D

36. Which of the following statements is/are true of vascular rings?

A. They may cause decreased perfusion to the lower extremities.

B. The most common form is a double aortic arch.

C. A vascular ring may manifest as recurrent respiratory infections.

D. Repair of a vascular ring requires a bypass graft.

E. Dysphagia may be a sign of a vascular ring.

Ref.: 1–3

COMMENTS: A vascular ring is an encirclement of the trachea and esophagus by an abnormal formation of the arch and great vessels. • The most common form is a double aortic arch. • During early development all fetuses have two aortic arches: a right (posterior) arch and a left (anterior) arch. • These arches encircle the forming trachea and esophagus. • Ordinarily, the right arch regresses. • If both arches persist, the trachea and esophagus become encircled. • A double aortic arch may be asymptomatic, but it often causes compression symptoms. • The trachea is more often affected, and there may be recurrent respiratory infections. • Esophageal compression may be present with or without tracheal symptoms. • Although they may present at any age, symptoms usually develop during infancy or early childhood. • Repair consists of dividing the smaller of the two arches, as determined by ultrasound imaging, magnetic resonance imaging (MRI), or at the time of surgery. • Repair is generally performed through a left thoracotomy and does not involve cardiopulmonary bypass. • A bypass graft is not necessary for repair. • There are other vascular rings in addition to the double aortic arch, and their clinical manifestations, natural history, and principles of repair are similar.

ANSWER:
B, C, E

37. Which of the following regarding pulmonary artery sling are true?

A. The left pulmonary artery originates anomalously from the right pulmonary artery and courses anterior to the trachea.

B. Tracheal abnormalities are found in greater than one third of patients with pulmonary artery sling.

C. Stridor is the most common presenting symptom.

D. The best surgical approach is via a left thoracotomy.

E. Barium esophagram is essentially diagnostic of pulmonary artery sling.

Ref.: 1–3

COMMENTS: Pulmonary artery sling is a vascular congenital anomaly in which the left pulmonary artery originates from the right pulmonary artery and courses posteriorly to the trachea. • Patients present in infancy with stridor or recurrent pulmonary infections. • One third to one half of patients have associated tracheal stenosis or complete rings, giving rise to the term *ring-sling complex.* • The best approach is via sternotomy, in which the left pulmonary artery is reimplanted to the right pulmonary artery. • Tracheal anomalies can be fixed during the same procedure. • Barium esophagram is essentially diagnostic with anterior indentation of the esophagus. • All other vascular rings have lateral or posterior compression. • Bronchoscopy is mandatory before repair.

ANSWER:
B, C, E

38. Which of the following factors affects blood flow across the pulmonary bed in a patient undergoing a Fontan procedure?

A. Presence or absence of AV valve regurgitation

B. Ventricular compliance

C. Pulmonary vascular resistance

D. Blood viscosity

E. The presence or absence of aortopulmonary collaterals

Ref.: 1–3

COMMENTS: In order to minimize morbidity and mortality after the Fontan operation, it is critical to determine whether the patient is a high-risk or low-risk candidate. • Low-risk patients have a low pulmonary vascular resistance, no AV valve regurgitation, normal ventricular compliance and function, no pulmonary artery distortion or stenoses, and no pulmonary venous obstruction. • Blood viscosity or aortopulmonary collaterals do not affect the transpulmonary gradient.

ANSWER:
A, B, C

39. What are possible consequences of a Blalock-Taussig shunt?

A. Volume overload of the ventricle

B. Pulmonary artery distortion

C. Pressure overload of the ventricle

D. Cyanosis

E. Coronary steal

F. Pulmonary overcirculation with systemic underperfusion

Ref.: 1–3

COMMENTS: Blalock-Taussig shunts always result in volume loading of the ventricle owing to the obligatory left-right shunting that occurs. • Coronary steal can occur mainly in patients with a hypoplastic left ventricle after a Norwood procedure, in which the shunt will steal some of the diastolic coronary flow. • A shunt can also result in pulmonary overcirculation (large shunt and low pulmonary vascular resistance), which in turn may result in systemic underperfusion. • Flow through a Blalock-Taussig shunt can be predicted by Pousille's law, which dictates that flow is related to the fourth power of the radius of a given vessel. • Shunt length, proximal and distal anastomosis location, and technical quality are also important determinants of the amount of blood that will flow through a shunt.

ANSWER:
A, B, E, F

40. Which of the following statements regarding pulmonary artery banding is/are true?

A. May result in pulmonary artery distortion

B. May result in pulmonary valve damage

C. May result in development of outflow tract narrowing by muscle band hypertrophy

D. Results in volume loading of the ventricle

E. Will always result in adequate protection of the pulmonary vascular bed

Ref.: 1–3

COMMENTS: Pulmonary artery banding remains a useful palliative maneuver in selected cases with increased pulmonary blood flow. • It may result in pulmonary artery distortion, pulmonary damage, or outflow tract narrowing via muscle band hypertrophy. • It always results in pressure loading of the ventricle. • A loose pulmonary artery band may not adequately protect the pulmonary vascular bed. • However, some patients may "grow into" a loose pulmonary artery band.

ANSWER:

A, B, C

REFERENCES

1. Baue AE, Geha AS, Hammond GL, et al (eds): *Glenn's Thoracic and Cardiovascular Surgery.* Appleton & Lange, Stamford, CT, 1996.
2. Kirklin JW, Barratt-Boyes BG (eds): *Cardiac Surgery.* Churchill Livingstone, New York, 1993.
3. Sellke FW, del Nido RJ, Swanson SJ (eds): *Sabiston and Spencer: Surgery of the Chest,* 7th ed. Elsevier, Philadelphia, 2005.

B. Acquired Diseases

R. Anthony Perez-Tamayo, M.D., Ph.D., Edward B. Savage, M.D., Eric J. Okum, M.D., and Robert S. D. Higgins, M.D.

1. A 60-year-old man is successfully resuscitated after an episode of sudden cardiac death. Appropriate evaluation and treatment may include which of the following?

   A. Cardiac catheterization and coronary angiography

   B. If significant coronary stenoses or left ventricular aneurysm is identified, surgical intervention directed at these targets to achieve satisfactory control of the arrhythmia

   C. Automatic implantable cardioverter defibrillator (AICD) in patients whose ventricular tachycardia cannot be mapped or medically/surgically controlled

   D. Electrophysiologic studies (EPS) to determine the mechanism, origin, inducibility, and suppressibility of the arrhythmia

   E. EPS-directed resection

   Ref.: 1, 2, 5

COMMENTS: Sudden cardiac death is a major cause of morbidity and mortality in the United States. • Most cases are thought to be of arrhythmogenic origin. • The number of survivors is increasing as a result of the rising number of lay people trained in cardiopulmonary resuscitation as well as improved prehospital and emergency medical care. • Survivors, however, have a 60% chance of recurrence during the first 2 years after hospitalization, resulting in sudden death. • During evaluation of these patients, one must include the following: EPS to determine the mechanism of the arrhythmia (automatic versus reentrant), to identify the origin of the arrhythmia, and to identify the inducibility and assess the suppressibility of induced arrhythmias by various pharmacologic agents. • Cardiac catheterization and coronary angiography should be performed to identify significant coronary stenoses and the presence of a ventricular aneurysm, which may be the arrhythmogenic focus. • However, coronary revascularization alone fails to control the arrhythmia, and blind aneurysmectomy (non-EPS directed) often fails because the endocardial origin of the arrhythmia may be distant from the border of the aneurysm. • EPS-directed endocardial resection and encircling endocardial ventriculotomy with or without adjunctive cryoablation have success rates in the range of 90%.

For inpatients whose arrhythmia cannot be mapped or controlled medically and surgically, the AICD is a last alternative. • The AICD is a device that senses ventricular tachycardia/fibrillation through an epicardial or endocardial lead and delivers a defibrillating pulse between two epicardial patches, or using a transvenous coil in the right ventricle. • The AICD terminates more than 98% of episodes of ventricular fibrillation or ventricular tachycardia and provides the greatest benefit for patients with reduced left ventricular systolic function. • A coronary arteriogram should precede the implantation or testing procedure, which has a mortality rate of about 0.5%.

ANSWER:
A, C, D, E

2. Which of the following is the maximum amount of time extracorporeal circulation can be tolerated before significant risk of physiologic injury and metabolic defects occurs?

   A. 2–4 hr

   B. 6–8 hr

   C. 10–12 hr

   D. 14–16 hr

   E. 18–20 hr

   Ref.: 1, 2

COMMENTS: Tolerance of extracorporeal circulation is variable. • Six to 8 hr is an acceptable range, although physiologic injury may occur earlier. • Occasionally, patients undergo longer perfusion with relatively few consequences. • With proper myocardial preservation, the heart can be safely arrested for up to 4 hr. • Physiologic defects observed with extracorporeal circulation include progressive sludging of blood elements in the capillary microcirculation, red blood cell hemolysis, coagulation defects, denaturation of plasma proteins, fibrinolyis, and activation of inflammatory cascades. • The primary culprit within the cardiopulmonary bypass circuit for these derangements is the oxygenator and its vast surface area for blood–foreign body exposure.

ANSWER:
B

3. Which of the following is/are complications of prolonged extracorporeal circulation?

   A. Postoperative bleeding

   B. Pancreatitis

   C. Respiratory insufficiency

   D. Psychosis

   E. Hepatic insufficiency

   Ref.: 1, 2

COMMENTS: The physiologic and metabolic injuries resulting from prolonged extracorporeal circulation are exhibited in several ways. • Postoperative bleeding may occur owing to dilution of clotting factors, destruction of platelets, impairment of platelet function, and improper titration of protamine to reverse systemic heparinization. • The coagulation defect may be transient and usually resolves within the first 12 hr following perfusion. • The importance of meticulous surgical hemostasis is apparent. • Renal and respiratory insufficiency are usually transient and often require only supportive treatment. • Hepatic injury can occur with prolonged support, partly from low cardiac output but potentially from derangements in splanchnic and portal flow. • A variety of central nervous system changes may occur. • These changes have both metabolic and organic causes and may be manifested by localized or generalized deficits of variable severity and duration. • With prolonged nonpulsatile cardiopulmonary bypass and hypothermia, some patients have an elevation of serum amylase levels, which, fortunately, is less frequently associated with signs and symptoms of pancreatitis.

ANSWER:
A, B, C, D, E

4. Following aortic valve replacement for calcific aortic stenosis, a patient experiences seizures. Which of the following are the most likely causes?

   A. Air embolism

   B. Calcium emboli

   C. Emboli from a left atrial thrombus

   D. Emboli from aortic atherosclerosis

   E. Extracorporeal circulation

Ref.: 1, 2

COMMENTS: Seizures may occur as a manifestation of focal injury to the central nervous system. • Air embolism is a result of incomplete evacuation of air from the cardiac chambers following open heart surgery. • Evacuation may be facilitated by use of a left ventricle vent, an aortic vent, or both. • The vents are left in place until after the heart is beating. • During this time, cardiopulmonary bypass is gradually reduced, the patient is rotated, and the heart is manipulated to assist in removing air from within the cardiac chambers. • Calcium fragments may embolize after removal of calcific debris from a diseased aortic valve. • Cannulation or clamping of a diseased aorta may result in dislodgement of arteriosclerotic debris. • Left atrial thrombi are another potential source of cerebral emboli, usually seen in patients with mitral stenosis. • The usual neurologic deficit observed following prolonged extracorporeal circulation is a transient generalized depression of cerebral function related to sludging of blood elements in the cerebral capillaries, resulting in focal areas of stasis and hypoperfusion of the microcirculation.

ANSWER:
A, B, D

5. Indications for coronary artery bypass (CABG) include which of the following?

   A. Severe triple-vessel occlusive disease

   B. Stenosis of the left main coronary

   C. Severe double-vessel occlusive artery disease

   D. Acute myocardial infarction

   E. Development of complications during percutaneous coronary angioplasty (PTCA)

Ref.: 1, 4

COMMENTS: Surgical revascularization provides relief of angina in more than 90% of patients and improves survival in selected groups. • Patients are referred to as having single-, double-, or triple-vessel disease if there are significant stenoses in one, two, or all three of the major coronary arteries. • Numerous studies have concluded that patients with significant triple-vessel disease, especially impaired left ventricular function, are best treated with surgery. • Left main artery disease is also a well-accepted indication. • Most surgeons and cardiologists agree that double-vessel disease is not always an indication for surgery unless the left anterior descending (LAD) artery is involved with a severe (>50%) proximal stenosis. • Acute myocardial infarction is not an unequivocal indication for surgery. • Less than 1% of patients undergoing PTCA develop complications requiring surgery.

ANSWER:
A, B, E

6. Contraindications to coronary artery bypass include which of the following?

   A. Severely depressed left ventricular ejection fraction (<0.20)

   B. Age greater than 70 years

   C. Angiographic inability to visualize a patent distal vessel

   D. Acute myocardial infarction

   E. Refractory congestive heart failure with pulmonary hypertension

Ref.: 1, 3

COMMENTS: Most authorities consider congestive heart failure with pulmonary hypertension (in the absence of mechanical defects, such as left ventricular aneurysm, mitral regurgitation, or VSD) the only cardiac contraindications to bypass grafting. • With current techniques of myocardial preservation and revascularization, bypass can be successfully performed in patients who, for various reasons, were once considered excessive-risk candidates. • Angiographic visualization depends on technique and the collateral circulation and is not a reliable criterion of operability. • Revascularization may be beneficial in the face of an acute, evolving myocardial infarction if the patient can be operated on within the first 3–6 hr. • The role of surgery in relationship to balloon angioplasty and thrombolytic therapy in this setting has not yet been fully defined.

ANSWER:
E

7. The operative mortality rate of coronary artery bypass is approximately 10% in which of the following situations?

   A. Elective operations

   B. Revision of failed coronary artery bypass surgery

   C. Emergency coronary artery bypass surgery

   D. Severely impaired left ventricular function

   E. None of the above

Ref.: 1, 3

COMMENTS: Improvement in anesthetic and surgical techniques and methods of myocardial protection have reduced the mortality rate of elective coronary artery bypass to approximately 2%. • The risk is somewhat higher in certain groups of patients, but even in higher-risk categories, in situations of emergency coronary artery bypass surgery, or during revision of failed surgery, the risk rarely exceeds 3–5%.

A N S W E R :
E

8. With regard to the surgical treatment of atrial fibrillation with the maze procedure, which of the following is/are true?

   A. Greater than 90% of cases of paroxysmal atrial fibrillation arise from an ectopic focus in the pulmonary veins.

   B. The need for mitral valve repair represents a contraindication.

   C. The maze procedure results in a greater than 90% long-term cure rate of atrial fibrillation without antiarrhythmic medications.

   D. The majority of patients will require permanent pacemaker implantation within 1 year of the procedure.

Ref.: 2

COMMENTS: The Cox maze procedure is designed to cure atrial fibrillation by creating a series of lesions in the left and right atria that insulate against conduction and propagation of fibrillatory impulses. • The lesions, created in the earliest forms of the procedure using incision and anastomosis and currently employing different forms of ablating energy, subdivide the atria into a maze of channels, with no channel large enough to allow the formation of macro-reentrant loops. • The set of lesions isolating the pulmonary veins are especially important in patients with paroxysmal atrial fibrillation, which originates from ectopic foci in these structures in 95% of cases. • The maze procedure can be performed alone or in combination with various other cardiac surgery procedures and is ideally applied in patients with pathologic conditions of the mitral valve, since these disease states are often complicated by atrial fibrillation and the exposure to the left atrium is already necessary. • The greater than 90% long-term cure rate for atrial fibrillation without antiarrhythmic medication resulting from the maze procedure will often unmask a dysfunctional AV node, requiring permanent pacemaker implantation in 20% of patients.

A N S W E R :
A, C

9. Following a documented acute myocardial infarction, surgery is indicated in which of the following situations?

   A. Postinfarction angina with anatomic lesions not amenable to PTCA

   B. VSD

   C. Acute mitral regurgitation

   D. Free-wall rupture

Ref.: 2, 4

COMMENTS: Postinfarction angina occurs in 10–15% of patients, with the incidence increasing to 30% if a thrombolytic agent was used. • It generally indicates residual myocardial tissue at risk for subsequent cell death and infarct extension. • In this setting, cardiac angiography is indicated, with PTCA or surgery, depending on the anatomy. • VSDs occur in about 2% of patients following myocardial infarction, generally 3–5 days after myocardial infarction. • Advocates of delayed repair point to better intraoperative demarcation of necrotic and living tissue, with lower incidence of recurrent VSD because of suture-line dehiscence. • Nevertheless, early surgical intervention is indicated, since natural history studies indicate a 25% mortality rate in the untreated at 24 hr and 80% at 4 weeks. • Acute mitral regurgitation resulting from papillary muscle infarction and rupture occurs in fewer than 2% of patients. • Surgery results in a better survival rate than does medical therapy. • Ventricular free-wall rupture occurs 3–6 days following transmural myocardial infarction. • Although the incidence is not precisely known, medical therapy almost certainly leads to death, leaving surgical repair as the only therapeutic option.

A N S W E R :
A, B, C, D

10. A 70-year-old woman in the coronary care unit develops refractory angina 2 days after being hospitalized for acute myocardial infarction. With regard to coronary artery bypass in this situation, which of the following statements is/are true?

   A. It should be performed only if there is left main coronary disease.

   B. Operative mortality and long-term survival rates are poor compared to those for patients who have unstable angina not precipitated by myocardial infarction.

   C. It should be preceded by thrombolytic therapy if multivessel disease is also present.

   D. The operative mortality rate is less than 5%.

Ref.: 1, 2, 4

COMMENTS: Unstable angina is preceded by myocardial infarction in approximately one half of patients. • The initial treatment of patients with unstable angina involves intensive medical therapy with β-blockers, nitrates, and calcium-channel blockers. • Patients with refractory angina should undergo emergent PTCA with stenting or CABG. • PTCA with stenting may be tried for one- and two-vessel disease, but significant left main artery disease should be approached surgically. • Most trials have demonstrated reduced in-hospital and 1-year mortality rates when thrombolytic therapy has been effective in reestablishing flow to ischemic tissue within 4 hr. • PTCA with stenting has been used alone and in conjunction with thrombolytic therapy with a 90% successful reperfusion rate, 10% in-house mortality rate, and 10–30% reocclusion rate within 6 months. • These modalities have been less effective for multivessel disease and in older patients, those in cardiogenic shock, women, and those with poor left ventricular function. • CABG has a 4% mortality rate in patients with unstable angina, with approximately 80% of patients surviving 10 years and 80% experiencing long-term relief of angina.

A N S W E R :
D

11. A patient develops angina 5 years after CABG. Angiography most likely reveals which of the following?

A. Vein graft thrombosis

B. Progressive atherosclerosis in the vein graft

C. Progressive atherosclerosis in the coronary arteries

D. A dominant right coronary system

Ref.: 1, 2, 4

COMMENTS: The rate of recurrence of angina following CABG is approximately 5–7% per year. • Surgery, unfortunately, does not slow the progression of atherosclerosis, which is the primary cause of recurrent symptoms. • Graft occlusion may also occur as a result of thrombosis, intimal fibrosis, or fibrous endarteritis. • Vein grafts may also be involved with atherosclerosis, which usually occurs later during the postoperative course. • Overall, the rate of vein graft patency is approximately 70–80% after 5 years. • Internal mammary artery grafts have significantly higher long-term patency and improved event-free survival compared to vein grafts.

A N S W E R :
C

12. Ventricular aneurysms usually have which of the following characteristics?

A. They result from myocardial infarction.

B. They may involve the posterior left ventricle.

C. They commonly present with peripheral emboli from a mural thrombosis.

D. They commonly cause death because of rupture.

E. Ventricular arrhythmias are uncommon.

Ref.: 1, 2

COMMENTS: Most ventricular aneurysms result from transmural infarction. • They frequently involve the anterior left ventricle in the distribution of the left anterior descending artery. • The most common complication is congestive heart failure, followed by arrhythmias and angina. • Peripheral emboli may occur but are infrequent. • Death due to rupture of a ventricular aneurysm is an unusual event.

A N S W E R :
A, B

13. Indications for surgical resection of a left ventricular aneurysm include which of the following?

A. Angina

B. Congestive heart failure

C. Systemic arterial emboli

D. Ventricular tachyarrhythmias refractory to drug therapy

Ref.: 2, 4

COMMENTS: See Question 14.

14. With regard to surgical treatment of ventricular aneurysm, which of the following statements is/are true?

A. Preservation of the left anterior descending artery is mandatory.

B. All aneurysms should be excised owing to the progressive nature of this lesion and the poor prognosis if it is untreated.

C. Complete aneurysmectomy is preferred.

D. Concomitant coronary bypass is generally performed.

Ref.: 1–3

COMMENTS: Clinical manifestations of ventricular aneurysm resulting from transmural myocardial infarction include those mentioned in Question 13. • Ventricular aneurysms may also be totally asymptomatic, in which case observation rather than resection is usually indicated. • Preservation of the left anterior descending artery is preferred, if possible, to provide blood flow to the septum, but preservation is not mandatory. • Small aneurysms are generally asymptomatic and can be observed. • During surgical resection, total scar removal is generally not performed, but, rather, a rim of scar tissue is left by the surgeon to facilitate closure of the defect. • Because of the high incidence of concomitant multivessel coronary occlusive disease, approximately 75% of patients considered for aneurysm resection also have coronary bypass. • Actual rupture of a true ventricular aneurysm is rare.

A N S W E R S :
Question 13: A, B, C, D
Question 14: D

15. Treatment of acute pyogenic pericarditis may require which of the following?

A. Parenteral antibiotics active against *Streptococcus* and *Mycobacterium*

B. Serial pericardial aspiration

C. Subxiphoid pericardiotomy

D. Radical pericardiectomy

Ref.: 1, 3

COMMENTS: Pyogenic pericarditis is rare. • Today, it is usually seen in infants or young children, in whom it is associated with a high mortality rate. • *Staphylococcus* and gram-negative species are the most common organisms in adults, whereas *Staphylococcus* and *Hemophilus influenzae* predominate in infants and children. • Parenteral antibiotics combined with serial pericardial aspiration and occasional intrapericardial instillation of antibiotics are usually adequate treatment. • Surgical drainage may be necessary, but radical pericardiectomy is not indicated.

A N S W E R :
B, C

16. With regard to chronic constrictive pericarditis, which of the following statements is/are true?

A. It is usually caused by a previous streptococcal infection.

B. It is characterized by equalization of right- and left-sided pressures.

C. It is best treated with a combination of diuretics and β-blocking agents.

D. Pericardiectomy is successful in 50% of patients.

Ref.: 1–3

COMMENTS: Chronic constrictive pericarditis often occurs secondary to a viral infection, although in most cases the true cause is unknown. • Tuberculosis was once thought to be the most frequent cause. • The disease is marked by progressive edema, ascites, hepatic enlargement, and dyspnea on exertion. • Hemodynamic findings include elevation of the right ventricular end-diastolic, right atrial, and central venous pressures to levels equal to those of the pulmonary artery wedge and left ventricular end-diastolic pressures. • Pericardiectomy is the treatment of choice and is successful in 90% of cases if adequate resection is performed.

ANSWER:
B

17. Following open heart surgery, a patient experiences chest pain, fever, tachycardia, and a pericardial friction rub. Which of the following statements is/are true?

A. The most likely diagnosis is postoperative mediastinitis.

B. Primary treatment should include surgical exploration.

C. The patient most likely responds well to antibiotics.

D. There is usually an associated leukocytosis or lymphocytosis.

E. This syndrome is usually accompanied by pleural effusion and shortness of breath.

Ref.: 1, 3

COMMENTS: Following procedures in which the pericardium is entered, transient pericardial inflammation, known as the postpericardiotomy syndrome (or Dressler's syndrome), may occur. • Clinical manifestations include fever, pericarditis, pleuritis, and, sometimes, a pericardial friction rub. • The syndrome usually appears 2–4 weeks postoperatively, and the erythrocyte sedimentation rate is elevated. • There is also leukocytosis, with an increase in lymphocytic cells. • Patients usually respond well to a short course of an anti-inflammatory agent, although some cases require the use of a corticosteroid.

ANSWER:
D

18. Three hours after aortic valve replacement, a patient suddenly becomes hypotensive. The cardiac index has decreased from 2.5 L/min to 1.6 L/min. Central venous pressure is 19 mmHg, with a pulmonary artery wedge pressure of 20 mmHg. Mediastinal drainage over the last hour has been minimal. Immediate treatment should include which of the following?

A. Echocardiogram to assess prosthetic valve function

B. Volume resuscitation to increase cardiac output

C. Afterload reduction with nitroprusside

D. Preload reduction with nitroglycerin

E. Mediastinal exploration

Ref.: 1, 2, 4

COMMENTS: Hypotension and low cardiac output following open heart surgery necessitate prompt, careful evaluation. • Specific causes include inadequate blood volume, occult bleeding, cardiac tamponade, arrhythmias, myocardial insufficiency, and acidosis. • The finding of elevated filling pressures with equalization of right- and left-sided pressures suggests the diagnosis of cardiac tamponade, in which case immediate reoperation is mandatory. • Substantial elevation of filling pressures in association with low cardiac output may also be indicative of cardiac failure, which may be treated with inotropic agents, digitalis, and intraaortic balloon counterpulsation. • Chest radiography is of variable diagnostic value, occasionally allowing detection of occult accumulation of blood in a pleural space.

ANSWER:
E

19. Aortic stenosis presenting in an adult may result from which of the following?

A. Congenital bicuspid valve

B. Marfan's syndrome

C. Rheumatic fever

D. Syphilis

E. Bacterial endocarditis

Ref.: 1, 3

COMMENTS: Aortic stenosis presenting in an adult may result from rheumatic fever or from a congenital valvular deformity. • A congenital bicuspid valve may remain asymptomatic for many years, but the deformed valve is susceptible to endocarditis and eventually develops calcification and symptomatic stenosis. • Aortic insufficiency commonly follows bacterial endocarditis. • Aortic insufficiency may also result from dilatation of the aortic annulus due to an ascending aortic aneurysm, as seen with Marfan's syndrome or, more rarely, syphilis.

ANSWER:
A, C

20. Clinical manifestations of severe aortic valve stenosis include which of the following?

A. Syncope

B. Angina pectoris

C. Dyspnea on exertion

D. Atrial fibrillation

Ref.: 1, 3

COMMENTS: Characteristically, patients with aortic stenosis remain asymptomatic for many years but deteriorate rapidly once symptoms begin. • About two thirds of patients develop angina pectoris. • Left ventricular hypertrophy, increased left ventricular diastolic volume, and prolongation of the isometric contraction phase and systolic ejection time are compensatory mechanisms to allow a longer period for ventricular emptying. • However, the duration of diastolic coronary perfusion to the hypertrophied ventricle is decreased, which gives rise to angina pectoris, even in the absence of primary coronary artery disease. • Syncope, present in one third of patients, also reflects impaired cardiac output. • Signs of left ventricular failure and atrial fibrillation, resulting in elevated left atrial pressures, are evidence of more advanced disease.

ANSWER:
A, B, C, D

21. With regard to the prognosis of adults with aortic stenosis, which of the following statements is/are true?

   A. Intensity of the murmur is correlated with severity of disease and therefore prognosis.

   B. Sudden death accounts for most fatalities.

   C. Symptomatic patients have a greater risk of sudden death than do asymptomatic patients.

   D. Left ventricular failure signifies a worse prognosis than does syncope or chest pain.

Ref.: 1, 3

COMMENTS: Once patients with aortic stenosis develop symptoms, the prognosis is poor. • With angina or syncope, the average life expectancy of untreated patients is 2–3 years. • Death occurs 1–2 years after left ventricular failure. • Sudden death occurs more frequently with aortic stenosis than with any other valvular lesion. • It accounts for approximately 20% of deaths from aortic stenosis and is always a risk, but it occurs more frequently in symptomatic patients. • The loudness of the classic systolic diamond-shaped ejection murmur heard over the aortic area and the apex does not have prognostic significance.

ANSWER:
C, D

22. Indications for operation in patients with aortic stenosis include which of the following?

   A. All symptomatic patients

   B. Systolic pressure gradient greater than 50 mmHg in asymptomatic patients

   C. Valvular cross-sectional area smaller than 1 cm²

   D. Serial radiographic evidence of rapid cardiac enlargement

Ref.: 1, 3

COMMENTS: All symptomatic patients require prompt valve replacement because of the high risk of sudden death and deterioration. • Peak systolic gradients across the valve of more than 50 mmHg and cross-sectional areas of 0.8–1.0 cm² are generally found with moderate-to-severe aortic stenosis and are indications for valve replacement, even if symptoms are absent. • Serial radiographic evidence of rapid cardiac enlargement is an ominous sign in patients with aortic stenosis and is an urgent indication for operation. • Severe stenosis (based on the cross-sectional area) but a low transvalvular gradient may result from compromised ventricular function, which increases the risk of valve replacement. • The 5-year survival rate following aortic valve replacement is approximately 80%.

ANSWER:
A, B, C, D

23. With regard to the selection of prosthetic heart valves, which of the following statements is/are true?

   A. Free aortic homograft valves have a lower incidence of infective endocarditis than do porcine valves.

   B. Bioprosthetic valves should be avoided in patients with chronic renal failure.

   C. Mechanical valves should be avoided in children.

   D. Mechanical valves have better durability than do bioprosthetic valves.

   E. Reconstructed mitral valves have limited durability and offer no advantage over valve replacement.

Ref.: 1–4

COMMENTS: The ideal prosthetic heart valve has yet to be developed. • Selection is based on the patient's characteristics, the operative findings, and the surgeon's preference. • **Bioprosthetic** valves (glutaraldehyde-fixed porcine heterografts or bovine pericardium) have a low rate of associated thromboembolism, and therefore these patients do not require long-term anticoagulation. • The problem with bioprosthetic valves, however, is long-term durability. • Although the latest-generation valves are more durable, the reoperation rate at 10 years is less than 5% for patients over the age of 65. • These valves are contraindicated in children and in patients younger than 20–30 years of age, since they begin to develop structural deterioration at 8–10 years. • In the past, they were not recommended for renal failure patients because of calcification, but recent series show no survival advantage compared to mechanical valves in this population.

   Mechanical heart valves are more durable, but their usefulness is limited by the need for permanent anticoagulation, which is contraindicated in certain clinical states (e.g., pregnancy, coagulopathy, or ulcer disease). • Thromboembolic complications occur at an annual rate of 1–2%, even in patients who are adequately anticoagulated. • Patients with mechanical valves require permanent anticoagulation therapy, which carries a risk of major hemorrhage of approximately 1% per year. • The risk of prosthetic valve endocarditis is about 1–2% per year for both bioprosthetic and mechanical valves. • Because of the low recurrence rate of endocarditis, free-aortic **homograft valves** are advantageous in the setting of active endocarditis. • Even with small valves, there is virtually no gradient across the homograft valve and a markedly decreased incidence of valve cusp calcification in young patients.

   Mitral valve reconstruction is preferred to replacement whenever possible because of the freedom from prosthetic valve complications. • Chronic anticoagulant therapy is not needed, and endocarditis is rare. • Durability has been satisfactory, with approximately 90% of patients remaining free from the need of late valve replacement at 5 years after operation.

ANSWER:
A, D

24. Cardiac catheterization of a 50-year-old man with a recent history of dyspnea on exertion, hemoptysis, and paroxysmal nocturnal dyspnea demonstrates a left atrial pressure of 28 mmHg. The primary determinants of this pressure include which of the following?

   A. Pulmonary artery pressure

   B. Cross-sectional area of the mitral opening

C. Cardiac output

D. Heart rate

E. Size of the left atrium

Ref.: 1, 2

COMMENTS: The primary physiologic consequences of mitral stenosis are increased left atrial pressure, decreased cardiac output, and increased pulmonary vascular resistance. • The clinical manifestations of these changes include the typical symptoms of congestive heart failure, pulmonary edema, and right-sided heart failure, as well as atrial fibrillation and arterial embolism. • The left atrial pressure is determined by the size of the mitral orifice, cardiac output, and heart rate. • The severity of disease is best classified by calculating the cross-sectional area of the valve, which takes into consideration both pressure gradient and cardiac output. • A mitral valve area of approximately 1 cm^2 or less is indicative of significant stenosis, although low flow rates and the presence of mitral regurgitation may influence calculations. • When left atrial pressures exceed the plasma oncotic pressure (24–30 mmHg), pulmonary edema develops.

ANSWER:
B, C, D

25. Indications for valve replacement in patients with significant mitral stenosis include which of the following?

A. Congestive heart failure

B. Pulmonary hypertension

C. Atrial fibrillation

D. Asymptomatic patients

E. Systemic embolization

Ref.: 1

COMMENTS: See Question 26.

26. With regard to results of surgical treatment for symptomatic mitral stenosis, which of the following statements is/are true?

A. Survival rate is increased compared with that after medical therapy.

B. Commissurotomy decreases the risk of systemic embolization and endocarditis.

C. Pulmonary vascular resistance usually diminishes following valve replacement or commissurotomy.

D. Ten-year survival rate exceeds 90%.

Ref.: 1

COMMENTS: The natural history of mitral stenosis is one of progressive manifestation of symptoms. • Treatment of mitral stenosis is a judicious combination of medical and surgical therapy. • Most asymptomatic patients are treated medically and observed. • Symptomatic patients with only medical treatment eventually die from their cardiac disease. • Indications for operative intervention include congestive heart failure (with New York Heart Association class III or IV symptoms), onset of atrial fibrillation with significant mitral stenosis, pulmonary

hypertension, systemic embolization, and infective endocarditis. • Surgical therapy is also recommended for patients who have mild symptoms and a severe reduction in valvular area. • In this situation, mitral commissurotomy can be employed if the leaflet flexibility and subvalvular apparatus are preserved. • This operation produces physiologic and clinical improvement, but these benefits tend to deteriorate. • Recurrent valvular dysfunction that necessitates treatment is almost always best treated by valve replacement.

ANSWERS:
Question 25: A, B, C, E
Question 26: A, B, C, D

27. Which of the following is the most common cause of mitral insufficiency in Western countries?

A. Bacterial endocarditis

B. Degenerative mitral valve disease

C. Marfan's syndrome

D. Silent myocardial infarction

E. Rupture of the chordae tendineae

Ref.: 1–3

COMMENTS: See Question 28.

28. With regard to patients with mitral regurgitation compared to those with mitral stenosis, which of the following statements is/are true?

A. Left ventricular failure is more common.

B. Atrial fibrillation rarely develops.

C. Systemic emboli are less common.

D. Postoperative prognosis is better with repair than replacement.

E. Pulmonary hypertension usually fails to resolve following valve replacement.

Ref.: 1, 4

COMMENTS: Degenerative mitral valve disease (e.g., Barlow's disease) is the most common cause of mitral regurgitation. • Worldwide, rheumatic heart disease is a major cause, producing both stenosis and regurgitation. • Although mitral stenosis almost exclusively results from rheumatic fever, mitral regurgitation may have other causes, including mitral valve prolapse, idiopathic calcification, bacterial endocarditis, chordae rupture, and ischemic heart disease. • A cause other than rheumatic fever is often suspected on the basis of the history and clinical presentation. • The physical signs of pulmonary hypertension and right heart failure produced by mitral regurgitation are similar to those seen with mitral stenosis. • Unlike the case with patients with mitral stenosis, however, moderate-to-severe mitral regurgitation can be tolerated for many years with minor symptoms until left ventricular failure ultimately develops as a result of chronic overload. • Atrial fibrillation is a common manifestation of mitral regurgitation. • Embolization does occur, but it is less common than with mitral stenosis. • The natural history of mitral regurgitation and the results of operative correction are somewhat more variable than those of mitral stenosis because of the different etiologic factors that may produce mitral incompetence. • Clinical severity depends on the degree of regurgitation, the status of left ventricular function, and the course of the valve disease.

In cases of infective endocarditis, trauma, or chordae rupture, emergency operation therapy is required and can be lifesaving. • Long-term prognosis with surgery is poor in patients with ischemic mitral regurgitation and poor ventricular function and in elderly patients with severe associated conditions. • Pulmonary hypertension usually resolves after successful valve repair replacement. • Repair is associated with better survival than is replacement. • Some measure of this advantage may be due to the preservation of the subvalvular apparatus and its relationship to the ventricular walls.

ANSWERS:
Question 27: B
Question 28: A, C, D

29. A 75-year-old man with a history of dyspnea on exertion, palpitations, and episodes of severe diaphoresis has a high-pitched diastolic murmur along the left sternal border. Expected findings include which of the following?

A. Systolic ejection murmur

B. Enlargement of the left ventricle on chest radiographs

C. Atrial fibrillation

D. History of syphilis

E. Bounding peripheral pulses

Ref.: 1

COMMENTS: Common symptoms of aortic insufficiency include angina, progressive dyspnea, palpitations, and peripheral vasomotor changes. • Signs of pulmonary congestion occur later as left ventricular failure develops. • Findings on physical examination include a normal cardiac rhythm and bounding peripheral pulses due to the widened pulse pressure. • The classic diastolic murmur is present and is accentuated when the patient leans forward. • A systolic ejection murmur may also be heard but usually represents aortic stenosis. • Enlargement of the left ventricle is seen on chest radiographs or echocardiogram and represents the ventricular response to the mixed pressure and volume overload of aortic insufficiency.

ANSWER:
B, E

30. The indications for operative intervention to correct aortic insufficiency include which of the following?

A. Progressive symptoms

B. Loudness and length of diastolic murmur

C. Increasing left ventricular size

D. Magnitude of regurgitation

Ref.: 1, 4

COMMENTS: Patients with aortic insufficiency generally remain asymptomatic for many years, although there is substantial variability. • Progressive symptoms of heart failure or ischemia and increasing left ventricular size on chest radiography or echocardiography are considered indications for operation. • The loudness

of the diastolic murmur is not correlated with the severity of the disease. • The length of the murmur reflects to some extent the patient's physiologic status, in that a longer murmur reflects a greater degree of regurgitation. • Short murmurs may be heard, however, in patients with early disease and minimal regurgitation and those with end-stage disease and elevated left ventricular end-diastolic pressures. • Severe ("wide-open") aortic insufficiency is poorly tolerated and indicates the need for replacement.

ANSWER:
A, C, D

31. Which of the following statements commonly applies to tricuspid valvular disease?

A. Replacement carries a significant risk of heart block.

B. Endocarditis is preferentially treated with excision alone.

C. Permanent epicardial pacing leads may be necessary with mechanical valves.

D. The lower-pressure right-sided valve lends itself well to repair.

Ref.: 1, 3

COMMENTS: The location of the AV node along the base of the septal leaflet (triangle of Koch) exposes this structure to injury. • Since transvenous pacing leads are not practical with a mechanical valve replacement, epicardial leads are often left in place in anticipation of treatment of complete heart block. • Isolated organic disease of the tricuspid valve is most commonly seen as a result of endocarditis secondary to intravenous drug abuse. • Total valve excision without replacement has occasionally been an alternative in this difficult situation but is not well tolerated long term. • The lower pressures of the right ventricle and right atrium and the size of the tricuspid annulus allow the opportunity for a variety of repair techniques, including bicuspidalization, wherein a third of the circumference of the valve can be sewn shut.

ANSWER:
A, C, D

32. A 30-year-old man arrives in the emergency department following a high-impact automobile accident. The initial chest radiograph demonstrates a widened mediastinum. Which of the following statements is/are true?

A. Despite normal blood pressure, the patient should be explored to drain the hemopericardium before impending tamponade occurs.

B. The finding of normally palpable femoral pulses makes aortic rupture unlikely, and the patient should be managed medically with β-blocking agents.

C. Aortography is the gold-standard diagnostic evaluation.

D. The most common site of aortic disruption is the proximal arch, which should be approached through a left thoracotomy.

E. Surgical repair of traumatic aortic rupture carries a 15–20% incidence of paraplegia, but it is the only effective therapy.

Ref.: 1, 4

COMMENTS: Traumatic rupture of the aorta requires urgent diagnosis and therapy. • Most patients with this lesion do not reach the hospital alive. • The history of a sudden deceleration injury along with chest radiographic findings of a widened mediastinum and loss of the aortic knob contour are strongly suggestive of the diagnosis. • Aortography demonstrates the site of injury. • Ninety-five percent of traumatic disruptions occur in the proximal descending aorta, just distal to the left subclavian artery, and are best approached through a left thoracotomy. • Surgical repair is the only effective therapy and is associated with paraplegia in approximately 5% of patients. • In the past, simple cross-clamping during repair was often utilized, but techniques that provide distal perfusion during clamping, such as a left atriofemoral bypass, femorofemoral partial bypass, and the Gott shunt, have become the standard of care.

ANSWER:
C

33. Which cardiac chamber is most frequently injured by penetrating trauma?

A. Left ventricle

B. Right ventricle

C. Left atrium

D. Right atrium

Ref.: 1, 2

COMMENTS: The right ventricle is the most anterior chamber of the heart and consequently is the area most susceptible to penetrating injury. • Cardiac injury may produce exsanguination, cardiac tamponade, and, rarely, cardiac failure secondary to damage to a major coronary artery, a valve, or the conduction system. • The key to saving patients who arrive in the emergency department with cardiac injury is prompt recognition and treatment of tamponade while other resuscitative measures are instituted. • Pericardiocentesis can be lifesaving as well as diagnostic while the operating room is made ready. • Most penetrating injuries can be treated without the need to resort to pump support. • Nonpenetrating cardiac trauma usually produces diffuse contusion, which warrants cardiac monitoring.

ANSWER:
B

34. Which of the following is the most common primary cardiac neoplasm?

A. Myxoma

B. Rhabdomyoma

C. Sarcoma

D. Lymphoma

E. Metastatic sarcoma

Ref.: 1, 2

COMMENTS: The most common cardiac neoplasms are metastatic. • Primary cardiac tumors are rare, with an incidence of 0.33% on postmortem studies. • Most primary cardiac neoplasms are benign, and, of them, myxoma is the most common, followed by rhabdomyoma. • Approximately 20% of primary tumors are malignant. • They are almost always rhabdomyosarcomas and

angiosarcomas, and they generally have systemic metastases at the time of diagnosis. • The clinical manifestations of cardiac tumors are due to local invasion, mass effect, embolization, or systemic constitutional signs, such as fever, malaise, weight loss, and autoimmune phenomena, particularly associated with atrial myxomas. • Echocardiography is the initial diagnostic technique of choice, followed by CT, MRI, and transesophageal echocardiography. • Myxomas constitute 50% of benign primary cardiac tumors. • They are most frequently found in female adults and are usually located in the left atrium.

ANSWER:
A

35. Physiologic effects of the intraaortic balloon pump (IABP) include which of following?

A. Increased cardiac afterload

B. Increased coronary blood flow

C. Decreased left ventricular end-diastolic pressure

D. Decreased left ventricular preload

E. Increased left ventricular preload

Ref.: 1, 2

COMMENTS: An electronically synchronized IABP, which inflates during diastole and deflates at the onset of systole, has physiologic effects that both decrease myocardial oxygen consumption and increase coronary blood flow. • The IABP decreases systolic blood pressure, decreases time during systole, and improves emptying of the heart (decreased radius). • Deflation of the IABP reduces impedance to aortic flow, thereby reducing afterload and improving cardiac output. • Left ventricular end-diastolic volume and pressure are reduced, and diastolic coronary blood flow is enhanced, particularly in failing hearts. • The pulmonary artery diastolic pressure is decreased, thereby reducing left ventricular preload.

ANSWER:
B, C, D

36. Which one or more of the following statements describes the clinical effects of the IABP?

A. IABP in myocardial infarction with cardiogenic shock decreases infarct size.

B. IABP effectively relieves pain in patients with unstable angina.

C. IABP is indicated for support of cardiac failure following cardiopulmonary bypass.

D. IABP is indicated in severe aortic insufficiency to decrease peripheral resistance.

Ref.: 1

COMMENTS: Indications for use of the IABP include the following: cardiac failure after cardiopulmonary bypass, refractory unstable angina, preoperative treatment of septal defects, mitral regurgitation, arrhythmias, ventricular aneurysms, and, occasionally, cardiogenic shock. • The IABP is used to treat cardiogenic shock associated with myocardial infarction, but only 15–20% of patients can be weaned successfully from this device, and there is no conclusive evidence that the IABP decreases infarct size. • The IABP is particularly effective in controlling pain in patients with angina refractory to pharmacologic manipulation. • The device has also been successful in the support of patients with cardiac failure following cardiopulmonary bypass. • Most such patients can be weaned successfully, with excellent long-term survival. • Severe aortic insufficiency is a contraindication to use of the IABP because regurgitation and cardiac failure are exacerbated.

ANSWER:
B, C

37. Which of the following is/are indications for placement of a permanent cardiac pacemaker?

   A. Sick sinus syndrome

   B. Complete AV block

   C. Mobitz type I AV block

   D. Mobitz type II AV block

   E. Stokes-Adams attacks

Ref.: 1, 5

COMMENTS: There is some disagreement regarding the indications for temporary or permanent cardiac pacing. • Most agree that indications for permanent pacing include the following: severe or symptomatic sick sinus syndrome; Mobitz type II AV block (because it frequently leads to complete AV block); complete AV block; symptomatic bilateral bundle-branch block; and bifascicular or incomplete trifascicular block with intermittent complete AV block following myocardial infarction. • Stokes-Adams attacks, which consist of intermittent syncopal episodes and sometimes convulsions, are manifestations of complete heart block. • Mobitz type I AV block (Wenckebach's block) rarely necessitates pacing.

ANSWER:
A, B, D, E

38. Open chest massage may be indicated in patients with which of the following?

   A. Blunt thoracic trauma

   B. Penetrating thoracic trauma

   C. Barrel chest

   D. Spinal deformities

Ref.: 1

COMMENTS: External cardiac massage transmits pressure and flow energy to the cardiovascular system by direct cardiac compression. • The stroke work is generated through forceful displacement of the chest wall, which compresses the ventricles, closes the mitral valve, opens the aortic valve, and produces unidirectional pressure and flow. • Intrathoracic pressure, once considered a more plausible explanation for the beneficial effect of closed-chest massage, accounts for less than 25% of cavitary cardiac pressure. • Stroke volume is optimized by compressions of high velocity, moderate force, and brief duration. • Coronary artery flow occurs during diastole and is optimized at a compression rate of 100–120/min. • Open methods are used when arrest occurs after cardiac surgery and in cases of thoracic injury when there is suspected cardiac tamponade, massive intrathoracic hemorrhage, penetrating cardiac injury, or an open pericardium. • It may be necessary in patients with a

barrel chest, emphysema, or spinal deformities because closed-chest resuscitation is sometimes unsuccessful in such settings. • Most patients who arrest in the field following blunt thoracic trauma cannot be successfully resuscitated even by open-chest massage. • Those who survive the initial episode may have a dismal outcome.

ANSWER:
B, C, D

39. With regard to blood conservation during cardiac surgery, which of the following statements is/are true?

   A. Transfusion of blood components during or after cardiac surgery is largely unavoidable.

   B. The risks associated with transfusions are primarily associated with red blood cells, not plasma.

   C. Cardiotomy suction, while it reclaims blood, increases microembolization.

   D. Antifibrinolytics, such as aprotonin, can reduce bleeding.

Ref.: 3

COMMENTS: Strict blood conservation should be practiced, with meticulous hemostasis during surgery and employment of blood reclamation systems such as the Cellsaver suction. • During routine procedures, transfusions can usually be avoided. • The risks associated with the transfusion of blood components such as platelets and plasma are similar to those associated with the transfusion of red blood cells. • Cardiotomy suction returns shed blood from the mediastinum to the cardiopulmonary bypass circuit but in so doing draws up lipid globules and pericardial debris that can escape the filters. • Aprotonin, an antifibrinolytic agent, has been shown to reduce postoperative blood loss and is a common adjunct to reoperative cardiac surgery.

ANSWER:
C, D

40. Which of the following statements regarding adult cardiac transplantation is/are true?

   A. Despite improved immunosuppression, the 5-year survival rate following cardiac transplantation is approximately 50%.

   B. The number of cardiac transplants performed annually in the United States is limited by the number of donors rather than by the number of suitable recipients.

   C. Although rejection and infection are problematic during the early postoperative period, the development of coronary occlusive disease in the transplanted heart affects long-term survival.

   D. With improved medical therapy available, the number of patients awaiting a heart transplant has remained relatively constant.

Ref.: 1, 2, 4

COMMENTS: Results following cardiac transplantation have continued to improve, owing largely to improved immunosuppression. • Currently, the 1-year survival rate is approximately

80%, and the 5-year survival rate is 65–70%. • The number of transplants performed annually is limited almost solely by the number of available donors. • The development of coronary occlusive disease in the transplanted heart, "graft vasculopathy," remains a major determinant of long-term survival. • Many researchers believe that it is a manifestation of a low-intensity, chronic form of rejection. • The number of cardiac transplants performed annually has remained relatively constant, whereas the number of patients waiting continues to increase.

A N S W E R :

B, C

R E F E R E N C E S

1. Sellke FW, del Nido PJ, Swanson SJ (eds): *Sabiston and Spencer: Surgery of the Chest*, 7th ed. Saunders, Philadelphia, 2005.
2. Cohn LH, Edmunds LH (eds): *Cardiac Surgery in the Adult*, 2nd ed. McGraw-Hill, New York, 2003.
3. Kaiser LF, Kron IL, Spray TL (eds): *Mastery of Cardiothoracic Surgery*, Lippincott-Raven, Philadelphia, 1997.
4. Yang SC, Cameron DE (eds): *Current Therapy in Thoracic and Cardiovascular Surgery*. CV Mosby, Philadelphia, 2004.
5. American Heart Association, American College of Cardiology, North American Society of Pacing and Electrophysiology: *2002 Guidelines*. J Am. Coll Cardiol 31:1175–1209, 1998.

CHAPTER 48

Urology

Christopher L. Coogan, M.D.

1. Regarding the management of renal trauma, which of the following statements is/are true?

A. Contusions are treated by observation until the gross hematuria subsides.

B. Parenchymal lacerations secondary to blunt trauma require routine exploration because of the risk of secondary hemorrhage or infection.

C. Retroperitoneal flank hematomas encountered during laparotomy should be explored.

D. On exploring a perinephric hematoma, Gerota's fascia is opened first and vascular control obtained.

E. Nonvisualization of the kidney on computed tomographic (CT) scanning requires immediate operative exploration.

Ref.: 1–6

COMMENTS: As with any visceral organ, a spectrum of renal injuries may occur following **blunt trauma**. • Renal contusions are the most common renal injury and are managed conservatively with bed rest and observation. • Parenchymal lacerations confined to the renal cortex may also be treated nonoperatively if the patient is stable. • Deeper lacerations extending into the calyceal system may require primary surgical repair. • When an expanding retroperitoneal hematoma is encountered, it should be explored. • However, when a nonexpanding perinephric hematoma is encountered, high-dose intravenous urographic studies should be done if no other imaging study is available to evaluate the potentially injured kidney and to confirm the presence of a contralateral functioning kidney. • Preoperative CT scanning provides accurate staging, allowing one to determine the best treatment modality and to manage the majority of patients with observation.

The key surgical principle in the approach to the injured kidney is to *obtain control of the vascular pedicle first*. • Exposure of the pedicle is via an incision in the small-bowel mesentery medial to the inferior mesenteric vein over the aorta. • If Gerota's fascia is incised first, the tamponade effect may be released and a significant hemorrhage can result. • Initial vascular control allows accurate assessment of the extent of injury and may permit primary repair or partial nephrectomy rather than removal of the entire organ. • Also, if a nephrectomy is necessary, the presence of a functioning contralateral kidney is verified via intravenous pyelogram (IVP) or CT before exploration.

Penetrating renal injury usually requires exploration, but patients with a well-staged injury may be managed nonoperatively if they are not undergoing laparatomy for associated injury.

Traditionally, nonvisualization of the kidney has been further evaluated with renal angiographic studies. • Recently, spiral CT scanning has provided adequate evaluation of the renal vessels. • Nonvisualization of the renal artery may be caused by total avulsion of the renal artery and vein, renal artery thrombosis, absence of the kidney, or severe contusion resulting in major vascular spasm. • If a kidney cannot be visualized on the arteriographic image, exploration and revascularization are indicated if salvage of the kidney is possible.

ANSWER:
A

2. Which of the following statements is/are true regarding renal vascular anatomy?

A. Renal arteries are end arteries.

B. The right renal artery usually crosses ventrally to the vena cava.

C. The left renal vein usually crosses ventrally to the aorta.

D. The right adrenal and gonadal veins typically empty into the right renal vein.

E. Multiple renal arteries are seen in approximately 20–30% of patients.

Ref.: 1, 2

COMMENTS: Approximately two thirds of normal kidneys are supplied by a single renal artery arising from the aorta, near the upper aspect of the second lumbar vertebra. • Each renal artery has approximately five segmental branches that are end arteries. • Occlusion of the segmental vessels therefore causes infarction. • Renal arterial anomalies are more often present in abnormally located kidneys. • Venous drainage of the kidney often involves collateral vessels, particularly on the left side, via the gonadal, adrenal, and lumbar veins. • The renal vein itself is usually singular on the left side but is multiple on the right side approximately 10% of the time. • Because the aorta in normal individuals lies to the left side of the vena cava, the right renal artery crosses behind the vena cava, and the left renal vein crosses ventral to the aorta. • This is consistent with the general anatomic principle that major systemic veins pass ventrally to their associated arteries. • The longer length of the left renal vein is advantageous when the left kidney is used as a donor organ during renal transplantation.

ANSWER:
A, C, E

3. Which of the following occurs in most patients with renal cell carcinoma?

   A. Hypertension

   B. Erythrocytosis

   C. Hematuria

   D. Acute varicocele

   E. Fever

Ref.: 1–4

COMMENTS: Among the many symptoms that have been associated with renal cell carcinoma, hematuria, pain, and abdominal mass are the most common. • Only 10% of patients present with the classic triad of hematuria, pain, and abdominal mass. • Hypertension (25% of cases) may result from renal vascular compression but is more commonly seen with Wilms' tumor. • Fever (17%) is thought to result from tumor necrosis. • A small percentage of patients exhibit erythrocytosis (1–5%), which has been related to the production of erythropoietin-like substances by the tumor. • It is more common, however, for patients with renal cell carcinoma to present with anemia than with erythrocytosis. • A small percentage of patients with renal tumors develop renal vein thrombosis and a subsequent acute varicocele (3%). • Hematuria occurs in about 60% of patients. • Renal cell carcinomas occur in an approximate 2:1 male/female ratio. • Most patients are diagnosed during the sixth and seventh decades of life. • Most renal cell carcinomas are now detected incidentally on ultrasound imaging or CT scanning. • Thus, masses are rarely palpable on physical examination.

The TNM staging system classifies a T1/T2 tumor as confined to the kidney, with tumors larger than 7.0 cm at a higher stage (T2). • T3 tumors involve the renal veins, inferior vena cava, or perinephric tissues that are confined by Gerota's fascia. • T4 tumors extend beyond Gerota's fascia. • Nodal status is stratified by size, number of nodes, and whether metastatic disease is present or absent. • Lesions that involve the inferior vena cava may still be cured with surgical therapy, and such involvement is not considered a contraindication to surgery.

ANSWER:
C

4. Transitional-cell cancers of the renal pelvis are best treated by which of the following?

   A. Nephrectomy

   B. Nephroureterectomy with excision of the ureter to the level of the bladder

   C. Nephroureterectomy with excision of the bladder cuff

   D. Nephroureterectomy and total cystectomy

   E. Radiotherapy

Ref.: 1–4

COMMENTS: Transitional-cell cancers of the renal pelvis and ureter are notable for their multicentricity and their tendency to spread by direct extension to other parts of the urothelium. • Approximately 30% of patients have a recurrence in the ureteral stump. • For this reason, nephroureterectomy with excision of a cuff of bladder at the ureteral orifice is the preferred treatment. • There is no specific role for radiotherapy in the primary treatment of these lesions. • Long-term cystoscopic surveillance is necessary postoperatively, since, in approximately 25% of patients, a subsequent bladder tumor arises. • In selected cases (e.g., solitary kidney or chronic renal disease), local resection of low-grade noninvasive tumors of the renal pelvis or ureters has produced long-term survival. • Meticulous long-term postoperative surveillance, including cystoscopic studies, periodic IVP or CT scans, and urine cytologic examination, are essential in these circumstances.

ANSWER:
C

5. Regarding treatment of renal cell carcinoma, which of the following statements is/are true?

   A. Induction chemotherapy followed by nephrectomy yields the best overall results.

   B. Radical nephrectomy involves removal of the kidney, adrenal gland, perinephric fat, Gerota's fascia, and regional lymph nodes.

   C. Regional lymphadenectomy for lesions extending outside the kidney improves postoperative survival.

   D. CT- or ultrasound-guided biopsy of the renal mass should be performed before nephrectomy.

Ref.: 3–5

COMMENTS: The treatment of renal cell carcinoma and the subsequent prognosis are determined by the anatomic extent of the disease. • Treatment of the local disease focuses on tumor removal by radical nephrectomy. • Solid renal masses are rarely biopsied, and they are diagnosed after pathologic examination of the kidney. • Surgery alone offers an excellent prognosis in patients with early lesions confined within the renal cortex.

A survival advantage for those having regional lymphadenectomy has not been established. • Metastases frequently occur by hematogenous routes as well and may negate any theoretic advantage of even more radical local surgery, although the presence of a limited volume of tumor thrombus in the vena cava with right-sided carcinomas may not adversely affect the long-term outcome if the thrombus is completely removed.

In the presence of distant metastases, nephrectomy may still be appropriate to control bleeding, pain, or infection. • A recent randomized controlled study revealed that survival is increased (from 9 to 12 months) in patients who undergo nephrectomy in the face of metastatic disease compared to chemotherapy with interleukin-2 (IL-2) alone. • Chemotherapy for renal cell carcinoma has met with poor results. • Immunotherapy may result in remission of the cancer in a small percentage of cases. • In selected circumstances, patients with isolated metastases have benefited from resection of their metastatic disease.

ANSWER:
B

6. During ultrasonic examination of the abdomen to look for gallstones in a 64-year-old woman with symptoms typical of cholelithiasis, an asymptomatic left solid renal mass is

incidentally detected. Which of the following should be the next examination?

A. Excretory urographic studies

B. Renal angiographic studies

C. CT scanning of the abdomen

D. Radionuclide scanning of the urinary tract

E. Renal biopsy

Ref.: 7

COMMENTS: See Question 7.

7. Precontrast (A) and postcontrast (B) CT scans of the abdomen of this patient is shown. What is the most likely diagnosis?

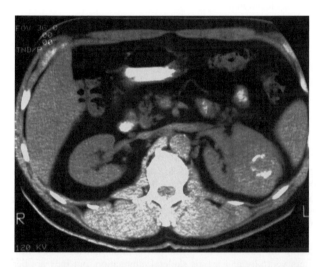

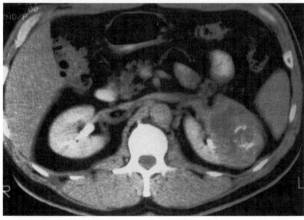

A. Calcified simple cyst

B. Calcified renal artery aneurysm

C. Calcified renal cell carcinoma

D. Calcified metastasis to the kidney

Ref.: 8

COMMENTS: The most likely diagnosis is a calcified **renal cell carcinoma**, since there is a solid intrarenal mass with central calcification. • CT scanning of the abdomen is the single most

useful examination for the workup of patients suspected of having a renal cell carcinoma. • In addition to confirming the solid nature of a renal mass, it can demonstrate local extension, venous and caval involvement, and distant metastases to the liver, adrenal, and visualized skeleton. • Calcification, as seen in this patient, is present in 8–18% of renal cell carcinomas, in contrast to in about 1% of simple renal cysts. • The classic triad of flank pain, gross hematuria, and a palpable renal mass is seen in fewer than 10% of patients at presentation. • Small asymptomatic renal cell carcinomas are frequently discovered during abdominal sonographic and CT examinations done for other reasons. • Renal cell carcinoma, which probably arises from the proximal tubular epithelium, is the most common *primary* renal cancer, accounting for approximately 86% of all primary malignant renal cancers. • Of the remainder, 12% are Wilms' tumor and 2% are renal sarcomas.

The foregoing comments refer to *primary* renal tumors, but the most common *asymptomatic* renal masses are metastatic, with lung as the most frequent primary site. • A **calcified renal artery aneurysm** demonstrates opacification of the lumen on the postinfusion scan. • **Calcified metastases** to the kidney are extremely uncommon, having been reported only in patients with primary osteosarcoma elsewhere. • A **calcified simple cyst** demonstrates a radiolucent center with peripheral ring calcification.

ANSWERS:
Question 6: C
Question 7: C

8. A 45-year-old man presents with severe flank pain and gross hematuria. His urinalysis has 200 red blood cells per high-power field, and his creatinine level is normal. What should the next test be?

A. KUB

B. IVP

C. US imaging

D. CT scanning of the abdomen and pelvis

E. MRI

Ref.: 1–3

COMMENTS: CT scanning of the abdomen and pelvis is currently the best test for diagnosing nephrolithiasis. • It is controversial whether the use of intravenous contrast material is necessary in patients with nephrolithiasis. • The benefits of evaluating renal function and better assessing the degree of obstruction must be weighed against the disadvantages of using contrast material. • Most urologists prefer the use of intravenous contrast media. • The use of oral contrast material is not necessary and may obscure the visibility of stones. • IVP and ultrasound studies are acceptable but are not the preferred choices.

ANSWER:
B, C, D

9. The patient in Question 8 has a 4-mm distal ureteral stone with hydronephrosis. His pain is resolved, and he has no more gross hematuria. What is the best treatment?

A. Extracorporeal shock-wave lithotripsy (ESWL)

B. Ureteroscopy

C. Admission of the patient for intravenous fluids and antibiotics

  D. Open ureterolithotomy

  E. Discharge with a strainer and follow up in the office as an outpatient.

Ref.: 1–3

COMMENTS: Most stones (80%) pass spontaneously without the need for surgical intervention or hospitalization. • Patients are discharged on oral pain medications and instructed to strain their urine. • A repeat KUB may be obtained to assess passage of the stone.

A N S W E R :
E

---

10. For which of the following type(s) of renal calculi is growth not affected by manipulation of urinary pH?

  A. Cystine

  B. Uric acid

  C. Ammonium magnesium phosphate (struvite)

  D. Calcium oxalate

  E. Calcium phosphate

Ref.: 3–5

COMMENTS: Renal calculi result from a variety of metabolic conditions. • Determination of the stone composition is important for both recognition of the underlying abnormality and institution of appropriate therapy aimed at removing the stone and preventing recurrence. • Most urinary calculi (up to 75%) are **calcium oxalate** stones, and approximately one half of these are mixtures of calcium oxalate and phosphate. • Calcium phosphate and calcium oxalate stones are not generally altered by variations of urinary pH within the normal range. • **Ammonium magnesium phosphate (struvite)** stones are next in frequency and are usually associated with infection. • They form in alkaline urine, and their solubility is increased by acidic urine. • Because urea-splitting organisms form ammonias and alkaline urine in the presence of infection, adequate pH manipulation cannot be obtained without control of the infection. • **Uric acid** stones are typically radiolucent, and their solubility is increased by alkalization. • The solubility of cystine is increased in alkaline urine. • However, because **cystine stones** are not crystalline in nature but are composed of amino acids, they are not easily pulverized by extracorporeal shock lithotripsy.

  Stone composition is related to the ability to visualize stones on plain radiographs. • Calcium-containing stones in particular are radiopaque. • Ammonium magnesium phosphate (struvite) and cystine stones may also be visualized.

A N S W E R :
D, E

---

11. Which of the following is/are indications for endoscopic, percutaneous, or open surgical removal of renal calculi?

  A. Progressive renal damage

  B. Intractable pain

  C. Persistent or progressive obstruction

  D. Intractable urinary tract infection

  E. Detection of any calculi

Ref.: 1–4

COMMENTS: The simple presence of a renal or ureteral calculus alone is not an indication for intervention by invasive techniques. • Medical management, including analgesics, antibiotics, and appropriate urinary pH adjustments, often result in the spontaneous passage of stones. • Smaller stones (<4 mm), in particular, can be expected to pass 90% of the time. • There is no evidence that excessive hydration facilitates the passage of renal or ureteral calculi. • Indeed, it may increase pain. • Surgical management is indicated when calculi produce persistent obstruction, intractable pain, or a stone associated with impaired renal function. • Techniques for stone removal include ureteroscopic manipulation, percutaneous nephrolithotomy, open nephrolithotomy, and ESWL.

A N S W E R :
A, B, C, D

---

12. ESWL can fragment stones in which of the following urinary tract locations?

  A. Renal calyx

  B. Upper two thirds of ureter

  C. Ureter overlying sacrum and pelvic bones

  D. Lower ureter

  E. Bladder

Ref.: 3–5

COMMENTS: Initially, only stones in the kidney were considered appropriate for ESWL. • Subsequently, stones located anywhere along the course of the ureter have been successfully treated by this modality. • ESWL is accomplished more readily for calculi at the renal level. • For this reason, some urologists advocate an initial attempt at manipulating a ureteral stone into the kidney. • Ureteral stones located in the bony pelvis can be treated by placing the patient in the prone position, so that the shock wave enters ventrally and avoids skeletal attenuation, but they are best managed with ureteroscopy and intracorporeal lithotripsy.

  Localization of stones for ESWL is usually accomplished fluoroscopically with or without a stent, depending on the size of the stone. • Fifteen percent of stones (mainly uric acid) are not well visualized during fluoroscopy and may require the use of an injectable stent. • Although ESWL has been used to disintegrate bladder stones, most urologists prefer cystoscopic visualization and direct intracorporeal ultrasonic or electrohydraulic lithotripsy. • Lower ureteral stones are most commonly treated with ureteroscopic removal and/or intracorporeal lithotripsy.

A N S W E R :
A, B, C, D, E

---

13. The evaluation of microscopic or gross hematuria consists of which of the following?

  A. Upper tract imaging with IVP, ultrasound imaging, or CT scanning

  B. Cystoscopic studies

  C. Bladder washings

  D. Pelvic examination

  E. Repeat urinalysis

Ref.: 1–3

COMMENTS: All patients with gross hematuria and all patients with microscopic hematuria on two separate urinalyses require evaluation. • Patients should undergo upper tract imaging, cystoscopic studies, bladder washings, and a pelvic examination. • It is important to evaluate the urinalysis for signs of infection or proteinuria. • The differential diagnosis consists of nephrolithiasis, renal or bladder cancer, urinary tract infection, bleeding disorders, trauma, benign essential hematuria (i.e., idiopathic), or prostatic disorders (in men).

ANSWER:
A, B, C, D, E

14. In a male patient with a pelvic fracture due to blunt trauma, retrograde urethrographic examination demonstrates disruption of the membranous urethra. Which one or more of the following constitute(s) appropriate initial treatment?

   A. Passage of a transurethral catheter

   B. Suprapubic cystostomy

   C. Urethrostomy

   D. Retropubic repair

Ref.: 1–5

COMMENTS: Blunt pelvic trauma is the most common cause of urethral injury. • Disruption usually occurs at or above the membranous portion of the urethra, since the anterior prostatic and membranous portions are relatively fixed by the puboprostatic ligaments and the urogenital diaphragm. • Urethral injury should be suspected if blood is noted at the meatus or if the patient is unable to void clear urine. • Passage of a catheter should *not* be attempted under these circumstances. • Rather, a retrograde urethrogram should be obtained. • In selected cases, a urologist may attempt passing a catheter retrograde in patients with minimal disruption. • The risk of inserting the catheter is that partial disruption may convert to complete disruption.

In most cases, if urethral injury is confirmed, treatment initially should be accomplished with suprapubic cystotomy. • A punch cystostomy can be performed if the bladder is palpable and no contraindications exist, such as extreme obesity, suprapubic surgical scars, or the presence of an abdominal hernia. • Perineal urethrostomy does not divert the urine proximal to the site of injury and is of no value in such a situation. • Immediate retropubic surgical realignment has a place in selected clinical situations, such as major bladder-neck laceration, prostatic fragmentation, or severe dislocation of the prostate with severely displaced bony fragments. • In most cases, however, current results suggest that the complications of incontinence, stricture, and impotence are minimized by performance of suprapubic cystostomy and delayed repair. • Penetrating urethral injuries, in contrast, can often be treated by initial repair and urinary diversion.

ANSWER:
B

15. Resection of a sigmoid cancer necessitates excision of a segment of the left pelvic ureter, with the specimen extending 3 cm distal to the bifurcation of the common iliac artery. Possible options for reconstruction include which of the following?

   A. Transureteroureterostomy

   B. Ureteroneocystostomy

   C. Boari bladder flap

   D. Psoas bladder hitch ligatures

   E. Cutaneous ureterostomy

Ref.: 3–5

COMMENTS: In this situation, simple in-situ ureteroneocystostomy is not possible. • An end-to-side anastomosis of the severed ureter to the opposite ureter (transureteroureterostomy) may be successful but may jeopardize the contralateral ureter. • An isolated segment of ileum can be used to bridge the gap between the divided ureter and the bladder. • The ileum can be tapered distally and implanted into the bladder in the fashion of a ureter so as not to reflux (ileal ureter). • A broad U-shaped flap (Boari flap) can be rotated off the bladder, fashioned in the shape of a cylinder, and anastomosed to the severed ureter. • Another solution is to mobilize the bladder extensively and hitch it to the psoas muscle as high as possible, at which point a ureteral implantation is performed (psoas hitch). • With this technique, the bladder can often be brought as high as the common iliac artery. • Mobilization of the kidney may provide 2–3 cm of ureteral length distally. • If time is of the essence or the abdomen is grossly contaminated, the cut end of the ureter can be brought to the skin as an intubated cutaneous ureterostomy, with anticipated later reconstructive repair (rarely performed).

ANSWER:
A, C, D, E

16. Which of the following is/are principles of repair of an intra-operative ureteral injury?

   A. Use of nonabsorbable suture materials

   B. Spatulation of transected ends

   C. Extensive ureteral dissection

   D. Drainage

   E. Intraureteral stent

Ref.: 3–5

COMMENTS: Ureteral injuries are usually iatrogenic and occur during the course of retroperitoneal dissection of various abdominal and pelvic operations. • In cases of transection, repair should be carried out using absorbable suture material and an indwelling intraureteral stent. • Nonabsorbable sutures should be avoided because they may serve as a nidus for calculus formation. • Extensive ureteral dissection should be avoided to preserve the segmental blood supply. • Spatulation reduces the incidence of anastomotic stricture in the severed ureter. • Drains should be placed to accommodate any anastomotic leak. • When injury involves the lowest ureteral segment, ureteroneocystostomy may be preferable. • Percutaneous (or open) nephrostomy serves to divert urine from the repair site, facilitating healing at the anastomotic site.

ANSWER:
B, D, E

17. A properly constructed cutaneous ureteroileostomy (ileal conduit) should do which of the following?

   A. Provide an adequate reservoir for urine storage

   B. Prevent ureteral reflux

C. Require catheterization for emptying

D. Separate the urinary and fecal streams

Ref.: 1–5

COMMENTS: The use of an isolated segment of ileum to serve as a conduit between the ureters and the skin has become the most common form of urinary diversion and is the standard against which all other diversions are measured. • It is used for patients after cystectomy, as well as those with other indications for supravesical diversion. • Large bowel is useful as a conuit because of the ease of creating an antireflux ureterointestinal anastomosis. • Continent urinary reservoirs are fashioned from colon or small bowel (or both) and require periodic catheterization if anastomosed to the skin. • Continent reservoirs offer patients even greater control of urinary function and are well accepted. • In selected cases, complete neobladders, fashioned from bowel, may be attached directly to the urethral remnant, eliminating the need for catheterization. • The purpose of constructing an ileal conduit is to create a route (unidirectionally within the conduit) for transport of urine. • It is not a reservoir for storage. • Stasis in the bowel segment predisposes to infections, stone formation, and ureteral reflux. • Stasis also promotes absorption of electrolytes and may result in hyperchloremic metabolic acidosis. • Some degree of ureteral reflux can be expected normally with an ileal conduit.

ANSWER:
D

18. Regarding bladder cancer, which of the following statements is/are true?

A. Adenocarcinoma is the most common histologic type.

B. Prognosis is related to histologic grade of the tumor.

C. Painless hematuria is the most common presenting symptom.

D. Prognosis is related to the presence or absence of muscular invasion of the bladder wall.

Ref.: 1–4

COMMENTS: Cancer of the urinary bladder has a peak incidence in the 50- to 70-year-old group of patients and is more common in men than in women. • Ninety percent of the tumors are transitional cell in type. • Squamous cell cancer and adenocarcinoma occur infrequently. • Painless hematuria, either gross or microscopic, is the most common initial manifestation. • Approximately 30% of patients present with symptoms of bladder irritability (urgency, frequency, and dysuria). • The prognosis is directly related to both the stage and the histologic grade of the cancer. • It is necessary, therefore, that an attempt be made to obtain adequate tissue during the biopsy to determine the depth of microscopic involvement. • Bladder malignancies metastasize via both lymphatic and hematogenous routes to lung, liver, bone, and other sites.

ANSWER:
B, C, D

19. Appropriate treatment of superficial low-grade transitional-cell bladder tumors may include which of the following?

A. Transurethral resection and electrocoagulation

B. Systemic chemotherapy

C. Intravesical chemotherapy

D. Intravesical bacillus Calmette-GuÈrin (BCG)

Ref.: 3–5

COMMENTS: Only about 10% of patients presenting with superficial low-grade cancers have their lesions progress to invasive cancer. • Generally, endoscopic ablation of superficial cancers is definitive therapy. • Systemic chemotherapy for superficial tumors has not been shown to be of value. • Intravesical chemotherapy, however, with agents such as thiotepa, mitomycin, and doxorubicin, is useful for treatment and prophylaxis of recurrent cancers. • Of all the intravesical agents, immunotherapy with BCG seems most effective against both superficial disease and, in particular, carcinoma in situ.

ANSWER:
A, C, D

20. Preferred treatment for muscle invasive bladder cancer involves which of the following?

A. Radical cystectomy

B. Preoperative irradiation and radical cystectomy

C. Preoperative chemotherapy and radical cystectomy

D. Radiation therapy alone

E. Intravesical chemotherapy

Ref.: 1–5

COMMENTS: In the United States, radical cystectomy is the preferred treatment for muscle-invasive bladder cancer. • Preoperative radiation therapy has not been shown to increase survival after radical cystectomy. • The role of partial cystectomy with muscle invasion is limited secondary to a high local recurrence rate (approximately 50%). • Lesions confined to the mucosa can be treated with transurethral resection, fulguration, or intravesical chemotherapeutic agents. • Then, a careful surveillance program must be maintained. • The treatment of lesions with submucosal invasion has been controversial as to whether intravesical chemotherapy is appropriate and as to the necessary extent of surgical resection. • Certainly, intravesical therapy is of no value for high grade invasive cancer. • In the United States, radical cystectomy is the preferred treatment. • The 5-year survival rate of patients with muscle invasion following cystectomy is only 50%, and the major cause of death is distant metastatic disease. • There is interest in the use of adjuvant chemotherapy before or after cystectomy, but a survival benefit is yet to be proved. • Because combination chemotherapy (with methotrexate, vinblastine, doxorubicin [Adriamycin], and cis-platinum [MVAC]) in patients with advanced disease has yielded response rates of 50–70%, these agents now are being considered before cystectomy when muscle invasion is present. • Complete response rates with MVAC alone have been disappointing (10–15%).

ANSWER:
A

21. Regarding bladder trauma, which of the following statements is/are true?

A. Rupture usually is extraperitoneal when associated with pelvic fracture.

B. A single-view retrograde cystogram in the emergency department demonstrates most significant bladder injuries.

C. Primary closure is generally indicated for extraperitoneal ruptures.

D. Intraoperative injury usually requires repair with a suprapubic cystostomy.

Ref.: 1–5

COMMENTS: Bladder injury may result from blunt or penetrating trauma or may occur during pelvic operations. • When associated with pelvic fracture, the site of injury is usually extraperitoneal, having been caused by the shearing force of the pelvic fracture. • Extraperitoneal rupture without pelvic fracture is an infrequent occurrence. • Isolated extraperitoneal bladder rupture is treated with 7–10 days of Foley catheter drainage. • Blunt injury without pelvic fracture is associated with intraperitoneal rupture, particularly if the bladder is full at the time of injury, and results in perforation, typically at the dome of the bladder. • Bladder injury should be suspected in any patient with lower abdominal trauma if there is any hematuria or if the patient is unable to void. • Single-view cystographic study may miss a significant injury. • Anterior, posterior, lateral, oblique, and, in particular, postvoid films, are necessary.

The usual treatment of intraperitoneal rupture involves a two-layer, watertight closure with absorbable sutures and transurethral or suprapubic bladder drainage. • Iatrogenic injury recognized at the time of an operation generally does not require suprapubic cystotomy but does require repair with absorbable sutures and urethral catheter drainage for 5–7 days. • It is necessary also to be vigilant that the Foley catheter does not become obstructed, such as with blood, causing the bladder to become distended.

ANSWER:
A

22. Which of the following is true regarding management of a patient with benign prostatic hyperplasia (BPH)?

A. All patients with complaints of prostatism should undergo therapy.

B. Patients with BPH have an increased risk of prostate cancer.

C. Initial therapy usually consists of medical therapy with α-blockers (terazosin and doxazosin) or 5α-reductase inhibitors (finasteride).

D. Absolute indications for surgical therapy include recurrent urinary tract infection, recurrent gross hematuria, bladder stones, and renal insufficiency.

Ref.: 1–5

COMMENTS: The indications for treatment of BPH are based on the patient's symptoms. • Most patients are treated initially with medical therapy using 5α-reductase inhibitors or α-blocking agents that act on the prostatic smooth muscle. • 5α-Reductase inhibitors inhibit the conversion of testosterone to dihydrotestosterone, which is the active agent responsible for BPH. • Indications for surgical management include recurrent urinary tract infection, recurrent gross hematuria, worsening renal function, failure of medical management, or the presence of bladder stones. • The presence on rectal examination of a normal-sized prostate does not exclude obstruction by BPH. • BPH occurs in most men with an increased incidence with increasing age. • It is not a risk factor for the development of prostate cancer. • It should be noted, however, that the usual transurethral prostatectomy or open surgery does not remove all the prostate tissue, and prostate cancer can occur following removal of the prostate for benign disease.

ANSWER:
C, D

23. Regarding prostate-specific antigen (PSA), which of the following statements is/are true?

A. It is a better serum marker for prostate cancer than is acid phosphatase.

B. It is produced by both benign and malignant prostate tissue.

C. As an immunohistochemical marker, PSA has been able to establish whether a metastatic adenocarcinoma is of prostatic origin.

D. Elevation of PSA level in a patient with prostatic cancer usually precludes a surgical cure.

E. A normal PSA level is less than 10 ng/ml.

Ref.: 3–5

COMMENTS: PSA is the best marker for prostate cancer and the first organ-specific marker in all of cancer biology. • It is produced by both benign and malignant prostate tissue. • Although age-specific reference ranges have been proposed, most would consider a normal PSA level to be less than 4 ng/ml. • As an immunohistochemical marker, PSA level is much more accurate and specific than is prostatic acid phosphatase level, which can be elevated in association with nonprostatic cancers, bone disorders, and liver abnormalities. • In addition, the acid phosphatase level is not generally elevated with early prostate cancer. • An elevated PSA level does not necessarily imply escape beyond the capsule and surgical incurability, although high values are often associated with bulky lesions. • In contradistinction, an elevated acid phosphatase level in an individual with prostate cancer usually signifies extensive local or metastatic disease.

ANSWER:
A, B, C

24. One hour after a prolonged transurethral prostatectomy (TURP), a 70-year-old man with mild coronary artery disease experiences bradycardia, hypertension, confusion, nausea, and headache. What is the most likely cause?

A. Hyperkalemia

B. Hypokalemia

C. Hypernatremia

D. Hyponatremia

E. Anemia

Ref.: 3–5

COMMENTS: The patient is most likely suffering from transurethral resection (TUR) syndrome, which is caused by excessive absorption of irrigating solution, resulting in hyponatremia. • The usual irrigation fluid is 1.5% glycine, which has an osmolarity of 200 mOsm/L, compared to the normal serum osmolarity of 290 mOsm/L. • Excessive systemic absorption of the irrigating solution can result in a dilutional hyponatremia, hypoproteinemia, and ultimately a decreased serum osmotic pressure. • Extremely low sodium levels (<110 mEq/L) may result in severe cerebral edema, causing seizure. • The treatment of TUR syndrome traditionally consists of terminating the procedure as rapidly as possible, administration of furosemide (Lasix) intra- or postoperatively, and use of 0.9% NaCl (and in severe cases 3% NaCl) solution over 3–6 hr.

ANSWER:
D

25. Which of the following is true regarding BPH?

   A. BPH arises in the periphery of the prostate gland.

   B. The prevalence of BPH increases with age.

   C. All patients with BPH should undergo medical or surgical treatment.

   D. Indications for surgical treatment include recurrent urinary tract infections, bladder stones, renal insufficiency, or persistent hematuria.

   E. Most patients after a TURP experience retrograde ejaculation.

Ref.: 1–5

COMMENTS: Unlike prostate cancer, which arises in the periphery of the gland, BPH arises in the transitional zone of the prostate gland. • The incidence of BPH is approximately 50% at age 50 and increases to approximately 80% with men entering their eighth decade of life. • Patients are traditionally treated with medical therapy first, if symptoms warrant it, and then undergo surgical therapy in the face of medical failure. • Indications for surgical therapy include recurrent urinary tract infections, the presence of bladder stones, worsening renal function, and recurrent hematuria. • Although impotence and incontinence are rare following a TURP, most patients after a TURP experience retrograde ejaculation as a result of resection of the bladder neck. • Patients should be appraised of this preoperatively.

ANSWER:
B, D, E

26. A 60-year-old man in good general health presents with an asymptomatic prostate nodule. The PSA level is 9 ng/ml, and biopsy confirms adenocarcinoma (Gleason III + III) on one side. Bone scanning does not reveal any evidence of metastatic disease. Which of the following therapies is/are appropriate?

   A. Transurethral prostate resection

   B. Radical prostatectomy

   C. Orchiectomy

   D. Diethylstilbestrol

   E. Local radiation therapy

Ref.: 1–7

COMMENTS: When a prostatic nodule is detected, a PSA level should be obtained, followed by transrectal ultrasound imaging and biopsy. • If prostate cancer is found, a bone scan may be obtained to rule out evidence of metastatic disease. • In addition, a chest radiograph and possibly a serum acid phosphatase level are obtained preoperatively.

Treatment of localized prostate cancer is by radical prostatectomy or external beam radiotherapy, depending on the physician's and the patient's preference. • There are many new experimental and investigational modalities utilized for treatment of prostate cancer. • Radical prostatectomy consists of removing the entire prostate and seminal vesicles. • A staging pelvic lymph node dissection is often performed before prostatectomy. • If the lymph nodes are grossly enlarged, they are sent for frozen section, and the operation is usually terminated if cancer has spread to the lymph nodes. • Tables have been established that predict the likelihood of positive margins and lymph node involvement based on the clinical stage, PSA level, and Gleason score.

ANSWER:
B, E

27. An asymptomatic 76-year-old man presents with a hard, irregular prostate, an elevated acid phosphatase level, a PSA level of 53 ng/ml, and multiple osteoblastic lesions in the lumbosacral spine. Biopsy of the prostate reveals a moderately differentiated adenocarcinoma. Which ore of the following therapies is/are indicated?

   A. Transurethral prostate resection

   B. Radical prostatectomy

   C. Hormonal therapy

   D. Radiation therapy

   E. Cytotoxic chemotherapy

Ref.: 1–5

COMMENTS: The treatment of locally advanced or metastatic prostate cancer is palliation. • The primary method of therapy is by hormonal manipulation, consisting of bilateral orchiectomy or the administration of luteinizing hormone-releasing hormone agonists (e.g., leuprolide) and possibly testosterone-blocking agents (e.g., flutamide). • Exogenous estrogens, such as diethylstilbestrol, are not used often because of their associated increased incidence of thromboembolic disease. • Hormonal therapy is the primary means of palliating bone pain, obstructive uropathy, and the general debility of metastatic disease. • Use of early versus delayed hormonal therapy is controversial, and a survival benefit for initiating hormonal therapy before the onset of symptoms has yet to be proven but may benefit select patients with positive nodes. • When hormonal treatment fails to palliate, transurethral resection of the prostate to relieve obstruction or local radiotherapy to palliate painful or bulky metastasis is employed. • Chemotherapy is not particularly useful, although protocols are forthcoming for hormonal-refractory prostate cancer. • Radical prostatectomy is not indicated in the presence of metastatic disease.

ANSWER:
C

28. Regarding prostate cancer, which of the following is/are true?

   A. Prostate cancer causes symptoms early in the course of disease.

   B. Transrectal ultrasound imaging alone (without biopsy) can accurately predict prostate cancer.

   C. Prostate cancer most commonly spreads to the lung and liver.

D. Most lesions are adenocarcinoma.

E. Bony metastases are usually osteolytic.

Ref.: 1–5

COMMENTS: Carcinoma of the prostate is the most common nonskin cancer in men over the age of 65 and is the second most common cause of cancer death in the male population. • Histologically, most of these lesions are adenocarcinomas. • Squamous cell carcinoma and sarcomas of the prostate are rare. • No definite etiologic factors have been established, but age, race, and family history are important predictors. • Most prostate cancers arise in the periphery of the gland and are asymptomatic until urinary obstruction or symptoms of metastases develop. • More than half of the prostate nodules detected on examination are malignant. • PSA determination in conjunction with an annual rectal examination has evolved as the optimal means of early detection of prostate cancer. • Transrectal ultrasound imaging and prostate biopsy are indicated in men with an elevated PSA level or abnormal findings on rectal examination. • After regional lymph nodes, bone metastasis (usually osteoblastic) occur most commonly, but widely metastatic disease can be found at almost any site.

ANSWER:
D

29. Regarding radical prostatectomy, which of the following are true?

A. It may be done via both the retropubic and the perineal routes.

B. Following successful surgical treatment, the PSA level drops to virtually zero within 24 hr.

C. Urinary incontinence develops in most patients after radical prostatectomy.

D. All patients, regardless of age, with localized prostate cancer should undergo this treatment.

Ref.: 3–5

COMMENTS: Radical prostatectomy may be done through the retropubic or the perineal route. • The advantage of a retropubic approach is that a limited staging pelvic lymphadenectomy can be done at the same time. • Fewer than 5% of patients develop total incontinence after radical prostatectomy. • A higher percentage, however, do develop some mild stress incontinence. • Almost all patients develop erectile dysfunction immediately postoperatively, but the use of a nerve-sparing prostatectomy preserves potency in up to 80% of selected patients. • The PSA level drops to zero after successful prostatectomy, but because the half-life of PSA is approximately 2–3 days, the PSA does not reach its nadir for approximately 3 weeks postoperatively. • Patients considered candidates for surgical therapy should have localized disease and a life expectancy of at least 10 years.

ANSWER:
A

30. Match the illustrations with the following pathologic conditions.

A. Testicular tumor

B. Spermatocele

C. Chronic epididymitis

D. Acute or subacute epididymitis

E. Hydrocele

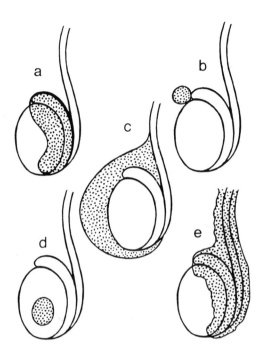

Ref.: 1–5

COMMENTS: Hydrocele can be idiopathic or secondary to a disease process, such as epididymitis, trauma, mumps, or tuberculosis. • Typically, it is a nontender, translucent mass. • It can obscure palpation of the testis, and it is important to be aware of this in young men, because as many as 20% of acute hydroceles are secondary to testicular tumors. • If a mass with all the characteristics of a hydrocele empties when the patient is in the supine position, there is likely a patent processus vaginalis. • Hydroceles in adults require treatment only when symptomatic, but in children they may require treatment if persistent. • **Spermatocele** is a simple or multiloculated cyst at the head of the epididymis and usually requires no treatment unless it is symptomatic. • It transilluminates and can be palpated as being discrete from the testes. • **Epididymitis**, if acute, leaves the patient with an exquisitely tender scrotum whose skin may be red and edematous. • There may be a mass, but often this is difficult to appreciate because the patient does not permit a deliberate examination. • With **chronic epididymitis**, the mass is nontender and firm and can cause beading of the entire vas deferens. • If, in addition, a draining sinus tract is present, the most likely cause is tuberculosis. • **Testicular cancer** is the most serious condition present in the scrotum, and a solid mass arising from the testicle is considered cancer. • The mass is usually firm, cannot be transilluminated, and is not tender. • If it is tender, it may be as a result of bleeding of a tumor into the testicle. • Ultrasonic examination of the testicle, along with tumor markers, have greatly facilitated making a diagnosis in such a clinical setting.

ANSWER:
A-d; B-b; C-e; D-a; E-c

31. A 14-year-old boy presents to the emergency room with a 4-hr history of acute, severe left scrotal pain. Examination reveals a left high-riding testicle with severe pain upon palpation. Urinalysis does not reveal any evidence of red or white blood cells. Which of the following is/are the treatment of choice at this point?

A. Heat, scrotal elevation, and antibiotics

B. Manual attempt at detorsion

C. Analgesics and reexamination

D. Doppler examination to assess testicular blood flow

E. Radioisotope scanning to assess testicular blood flow

F. Surgical exploration

Ref.: 1–5

COMMENTS: When examining the acutely painful scrotum, one should attempt to differentiate epididymitis from testicular torsion, but it may not be possible. • Doubtful cases should be treated as testicular torsion until proved otherwise. • Because irreversible testicular ischemia occurs within 4 hr when there is complete torsion, prompt surgical exploration is indicated even if there is diagnostic uncertainty. • Use of a Doppler examination may be helpful for assessing the testicular blood flow. • Nuclear medicine scans also are reliable and must be used judiciously. • Manual detorsion is not usually successful but can be done when the scrotum is not swollen. • It may relieve pain, but exploration is still necessary because residual torsion may still exist. • At the time of exploration, the involved testis should be anatomically fixated as well as detorsed. • The contralateral testis should undergo a similar procedure prophylactically, since the same anatomic abnormality may be found in both testes.

ANSWER:
F

32. The anatomic abnormality found with torsion of the testicle in adolescents most commonly involves which of the following?

A. Intravaginal torsion of the spermatic cord

B. Extravaginal torsion of the spermatic cord

C. Torsion of the appendix testis

D. Torsion of the appendix epididymis

Ref.: 1–5

COMMENTS: There are two types of torsion of the testicle. • In the neonate, torsion of the spermatic cord occurs before attachment of the gubernaculum, allowing torsion of the entire testicle and tunica vaginalis. • This is called **extravaginal torsion**. • The second type of torsion usually occurs in adolescents and older men and is called **intravaginal torsion** of the spermatic cord. • By this time, the tunica vaginalis is fixed to the dartos fascia and cannot twist. • Intravaginal torsion is most commonly associated with a long mesenteric attachment between the cord and the testes and epididymis, which allows the testicle to rotate (producing the "bell clapper" deformity), and torsion can therefore occur within the tunica vaginalis. • Since this deformity is often bilateral, fixation of the contralateral testis should be performed at the time the testicular torsion is corrected. • Regarding the appendix testis and the appendix epididymis, torsion of these appendages

can produce acute pain and swelling similar to torsion of the spermatic cord, but it does not result in testicular infarction. • Transillumination may reveal the "blue dot" sign representing the infarcted structure. • Exploration is sometimes required to exclude testicular torsion.

ANSWER:
A

33. Which of the following is/are true regarding varicocele?

A. Varicoceles occur more commonly on the left side

B. Varicoceles are associated with infertility

C. Varicoceles occur in about 40% of men

D. Varicoceles are often associated with testicular tumors

E. Varicoceles feel like a "bag of worms" on physical examination

Ref.: 1–5

COMMENTS: Varicoceles are found in approximately 15–20% of the adult male population but are seen even more commonly in infertile men. • Varicoceles have not been found to be associated with testicular tumors. • They have been associated with diminished sperm count, decreased sperm motility, and abnormal sperm morphology. • In infertile patients with an abnormal semen analysis, varicocelectomy often improves the semen analysis. • Physical examination of the scrotum reveals a large group of veins palpable within the scrotum that has been described as a "bag of worms."

ANSWER:
A, B, E

34. A 65-year-old man is unable to void after an abdominoperineal resection. Postvoid residuals have been 600–800 ml. The treatment of choice is which of the following?

A. Chronic Foley catheterization

B. TURP

C. Clean intermittent catheterization

D. Transurethral sphincterotomy

E. α-Blockers alone

Ref.: 1–5

COMMENTS: Bladder dysfunction has been reported in 10–50% of patients following abdominal perineal resection or other major pelvic surgery. • The type of voiding dysfunction that occurs is dependent on the specific nerve involved and the degree of the injury. • Patients are best treated by clean intermittent catheterization. • Most (>80%) resolve over 3–6 months. • The use of a chronic indwelling catheter is a reasonable choice in some patients, but the risk of infection is higher with chronic catheterization than with intermittent catheterization. • The use of α-blockers alone or TURP is unlikely to be successful. • Transurethral sphincterotomy does not treat the underlying problem and may result in incontinence.

ANSWER:
C

35. Match the following regarding testicular tumors in the left-hand column with the appropriate treatment or sign in the right-hand column.

A. Seminoma

B. Nonseminomatous

a. Radiation therapy

b. Retroperitoneal lymph node dissection

c. Elevated α-fetoprotein (AFP)

d. Elevated human chorionic gonadotropin (hCG)

e. Chemotherapy for advanced disease

Ref.: 1–5

COMMENTS: The most common solid tumor in a young male is a seminoma. • About 95% of testicular masses are of a germ-cell origin. • Germ-cell tumors are divided into seminoma and nonseminomatous germ-cell tumors. • Nonseminomatous germ-cell tumors include tumors of the following histologic types: embryonal cell carcinoma, yolk sac tumor, choriocarcinoma, and teratoma. • Clinically, stage I seminomas (confined to the testis) are treated with prophylactic radiotherapy to the retroperitoneal lymph nodes to eliminate any chance of failure in the retroperitoneum. • Selected patients are now treated with surveillance alone. • Higher-stage seminomas (visible adenopathy in the retroperitoneum or lung metastasis) are best treated with chemotherapy. • An elevated hCG level is seen in 5–10% of seminomas, but if an elevated AFP level is found, the tumor is considered nonseminomatous. • The treatment of clinical stage I nonseminomatous germ-cell tumors is controversial but consists of either retroperitoneal lymph node dissection or surveillance. • Elevated AFP and the β-subunit of human gonadotropin (β-hCG) levels may be seen in patients with nonseminomatous germ-cell tumors. • For patients with bulky retroperitoneal disease or visceral metastasis, treatment consists of combination chemotherapy.

ANSWER:
A-a,d,e; B-b,c,d,e

36. Appropriate treatment of a painless solid testicular mass in a 28-year-old man includes which of the following?

A. Preoperative determination of tumor markers

B. Incisional biopsy via a scrotal incision

C. Incisional biopsy via an inguinal incision

D. Orchiectomy via a scrotal incision

E. Orchiectomy via an inguinal incision

Ref.: 1–4

COMMENTS: During the workup of a patient with a testicular tumor, serum should be obtained for determination of the AFP level and β-hCG, since these tumor markers are elevated in many patients with testicular cancer. • The primary diagnostic and therapeutic maneuver is orchiectomy and should be carried out via an inguinal incision with early clamping of the vessels. • If the presence of a testicular mass is confirmed, an orchiectomy should be performed. • Rarely, the testicle suspected of being involved with cancer may be affected by a benign condition. • Yet, even in this situation, the best treatment is often orchiectomy. • A scrotal approach is contraindicated, since it does not permit control of the testicular vessels before manipulation of the testicle, which may dislodge tumor cells into the venous drainage. • Also, with such an approach, cells from the biopsy specimen may spill into the scrotum and subsequently spread tumor via the scrotal lymphatic drainage to the superficial inguinal nodes, or they may seed locally.

ANSWER:
A, E

37. Which of the following is/are true regarding testicular tumors?

A. Solid masses of the testis are usually malignant.

B. Testicular tumors are the most common solid tumor in men aged 18–35.

C. The overall survival for patients with testicular cancer exceeds 90%.

D. The most common testicular tumor is seminoma.

E. They are associated with cryptorchidism (undescended testis) as a cause.

Ref.: 1–3

COMMENTS: The most common non–skin-cell tumors in men ages 18–35 are testicular tumors of germ-cell origin. • These tumors, unlike extratesticular tumors within the scrotum, which are benign, are almost always malignant. • The most common solid testicular mass is a seminoma. • Today, survival of patients with testicular tumor exceeds 90%, owing to the development of aggressive surgical therapy, tumor markers (AFP and hCG), and *cis*-platinum–based combination chemotherapy. • Thirty percent of premature male neonates have an undescended testis, but spontaneous descent occurs in most of these infants by 1 year of age. • The incidence of undescended testes is approximately 0.8% in 1-year-old infants. • Undescended testes must be placed in the scrotum (orchiopexy). • They often have an associated indirect hernia, which should be repaired by ligation of the sac at the time of orchiopexy. • Patients who are found to have cryptorchidism of the testes have a higher chance (1–5%) of developing cancer in both the affected and contralateral testes.

ANSWER:
A, B, C, D, E

38. A 32-year-old man presents in the emergency department with an exquisitely painful and "woody"-feeling penile erection of 18 hours' duration. Effective therapy includes which of the following?

A. Aspiration of blood from the corpora cavernosa

B. Irrigation of the corpora cavernosa with a dilute solution of papaverine

C. Creation of a communication between the glans penis and a corporal body with a biopsy needle or scalpel blade

D. Side-to-side anastomosis between the corpus spongiosum and the corpus cavernosum

E. Exchange transfusions

Ref.: 3–5

COMMENTS: Most cases of prolonged pathologic penile erection in the absence of sexual stimulation (priapism) are idiopathic. • Some known causes are sickle cell disease, leukemic infiltration of veins draining the penis, and certain medications, such as anticoagulants and antidepressants. • Often, simple aspiration of blood from the corpus cavernosum alone can cause lasting detumescence.

• If this fails, irrigation of the corpus with a dilute solution of epinephrine or norepinephrine may work. • This has the dual effect of decompressing the corpus and the venous obstruction that goes with it, as well as diminishing arterial flow. • Papaverine is used to treat impotence. • It increases penile blood flow by directly relaxing vascular smooth muscle. • The glans penis is an extension of the corpus spongiosum and is usually not affected by priapism. • Shunts between it and the corpus cavernosa created with biopsy needles or scalpel blades or removal of a portion of the glandular corporal septum may provide a path of egress for blood trapped in the penis. • If all else fails, formal spongiosum-to-cavernosum shunts may be created. • There is a high incidence of impotence after priapism of 24 hr or more. • When priapism is secondary to sickle cell anemia, exchange transfusions and other medical therapies, including oxygenation, hydration, and alkalinization, may be indicated.

ANSWER:
A, C, D, E

39. Regarding vasectomy, which of the following statements is/are true?

   A. It produces prompt sterility.

   B. Duplication of the vas deferens is a common cause of failure.

   C. It may be performed through a midline scrotal incision.

   D. The pregnancy rate after vasovasotomy performed to reestablish patency approaches 50%.

Ref.: 1–5

COMMENTS: Vasectomy for the purpose of sterilization has become a commonplace procedure safely performed in the outpatient setting. • Careful attention must be given to appropriate screening of patients, preoperative education of patients, and informing patients of the risk and alternative methods of birth control. • Patients must also be instructed that viable spermatozoa remain in the seminal tract distal to the site of vasectomy for several weeks after the operation. • Careful follow-up examination of the semen must be performed at 6–8 weeks to confirm that the patient is in fact sterile. • Vasectomy may be done through a midline scrotal incision or two smaller incisions on either side of the scrotum. • The procedure should be considered a permanent form of sterilization, although, with microsurgical techniques, reanastomosis of the vas deferens can be performed in more than 90% of cases, with an average success rate (as attested to by subsequent pregnancy) approaching 50%. • The presence of high antisperm antibody levels and a prolonged interval between vasectomy and reanastomosis have a negative effect on pregnancy rates after vasovasotomy. • Duplication of the vas deferens is a rare cause of failure after vasectomy.

ANSWER:
C, D

40. Match the conditions in the left-hand column with the symptoms in the right-hand column.

   A. Dysuria   a. Painful urination

   B. Strangury   b. Difficulty or straining with voiding

   C. Hesitancy   c. Delayed voiding in response to attempts at voiding

   D. Prostatism   d. Symptoms associated with benign prostatic hypertrophy

Ref.: 3–5

COMMENTS: Dysuria is defined as painful urination, and strangury is defined as difficulty or straining with voiding. • Pneumaturia refers to the presence of air in the urine and is associated with recent instrumentation or enterovesical fistula. • Prostatism refers to the symptoms of obstruction associated with benign prostatic hyperplasia, and it may be defined as having both obstructive and irritation components. • Nocturia, hesitancy, and intermittency are associated with prostatic obstruction. • Urgency and daytime frequency are considered urge-related prostatism.

ANSWER:
A-a; B-b; C-c; D-d

REFERENCES

1. Sabiston DC Jr: *Textbook of Surgery*, 15th ed. WB Saunders, Philadelphia, 1997.
2. Schwartz SI, Shires GT, Spencer FC: *Principles of Surgery*, 7th ed. McGraw-Hill, New York, 1999.
3. Mulholland M: *Greenfield's Surgery*. Lippincott, Williams & Wilkins, Philadelphia, 2005.
4. Gillenwater JY, Grayhack JT, Howard SJ, et al: *Adult and Pediatric Urology*, 3rd ed. CV Mosby, St. Louis, 1996.
5. Walsh PC, Retik AB, Vaughan ED, et al: *Campbell's Urology*, 7th ed. WB Saunders, Philadelphia, 1998.
6. Wessels H, McAnich JW, Meyer A, et al: Criteria for nonoperative treatment of significant penetrating renal lacerations. *J Urol* 157:24–27, 1997.
7. Partin AW, Yoo J, Carter HB, et al: The use of prostate specific antigen, clinical stage and Gleason score to predict pathological stage in men with localized prostate cancer. *J Urol* 150:110–115, 1993.
8. Pollack HM: *Clinical Urography*. WB Saunders, Philadelphia, 1990.

CHAPTER 49

Gynecology

Eric R. Brown, M.D., Ph.D.

1. Match the congenital abnormality with the appropriate embryologic developmental error.

A. Uterine didelphys	a. Failure of the sinovaginal bulb and mullerian tubercle to canalize
B. Bicornuate uterus	b. Partial fusion of the mullerian ducts
C. Unicornuate uterus	c. Failure of one mullerian duct to develop
D. Transverse vaginal septum	d. Failure of the mullerian ducts to fuse

Ref.: 1–3

COMMENTS: Genitourinary development in the male and female results from appropriate migration and fusion of the *wolffian* (mesonephric) and *mullerian* (paramesonephric) ducts, respectively. • The mullerian ducts, which form in the absence of antimullerian hormone, lead to the development of the fallopian tubes, the uterus, and the upper vagina. • Failure of both mullerian ducts to develop results in an absent uterus, absent cervix, and frequently vaginal agenesis. • Unilateral failure leads to unicornuate uterus. • During normal development, the mullerian ducts fuse at the midline, with subsequent resorption of the midline septum. • Failure of the mullerian ducts to fuse leads to uterine didelphys (double uterus and double cervix), while partial fusion can lead to a bicornuate uterus. • Failure of the midline septum to resorb can result in a septate uterus and/or a longitudinal vaginal septum (double vagina). • The vagina develops from the sinovaginal bulbs. • These bulbs unite with the fused mullerian ducts at the mullerian tubercle, with subsequent canalization. • A transverse vaginal septum develops when the bulbs and mullerian tubercle fail to canalize. • Developmental failure of the sinovaginal bulbs leads to vaginal agenesis. • Mullerian developmental failure is frequently associated with renal system abnormalities. • Therefore, a urological evaluation of patients presenting with these abnormalities should be considered.

ANSWER:
A-d; B-b; C-c; D-a

2. All but which of the following are considered major pelvic spaces?

A. Retroperitoneal space

B. Retrorectal space

C. Retropubic space

D. Paravesical space

Ref.: 4

COMMENTS: In general, there are eight major pelvic spaces: two paravesical, two pararectal, one retropubic, one vesicovaginal, one rectovaginal, and one retrorectal space. • Familiarity with these spaces is essential in order to successfully perform pelvic surgery and manage intraoperative complications. • The retroperitoneal space, although important in abdominal and pelvic surgery, is not considered one of the major pelvic spaces.

ANSWER:
A

3. Regarding endometriosis, which of the following is/are true?

A. Total abdominal hysterectomy with bilateral salpingo-oophorectomy is considered definitive surgical therapy.

B. Adenomyosis is a clinical variant of the disease.

C. Laparoscopy is considered the gold standard for diagnosis.

D. Minimal and mild stages of the disease can be associated with infertility.

Ref.: 3

COMMENTS: Endometriosis is defined as endometrial tissue outside of the uterus. • Symptoms can include pelvic pain, dysmenorrhea, and infertility. • Minimal and mild stages of the diseases have been associated with infertility. • The diagnosis can be empirically made if the patient's symptoms are ameliorated after a short (3-month) trial of a gonadotropin-releasing hormone (GnRH) agonist and after all other causes have been ruled out. • Laparoscopy, however, is considered the gold standard for diagnosis. • Definitive surgery for endometriosis consists of total abdominal hysterectomy with bilateral salpingo-oophorectomy. • Bilateral salpingo-oophorectomy is the key component, since it causes surgical menopause. • Adenomyosis, which refers to endometrial tissue *within* the myometrium, is not considered a variant of the disease. • Symptoms of adenomyosis include abnormal uterine bleeding and dysmenorrhea. • Medical therapy for adenomyosis is usually ineffective, and surgery (hysterectomy) is usually required for persistent symptoms.

ANSWER:
A, C, D

4. Regarding endometriosis, which of the following is/are true?

A. Clinical stage is correlated with the severity of pain.

B. Lesions do not need to be visualized at the time of surgery to make the diagnosis.

C. Multiple medical options exist for suppressing the disease.

D. Histologically, endometrial glands, endometrial stroma, and/or hemosiderin-laden macrophages should be present to make the diagnosis.

Ref.: 3

COMMENTS: Lesions of endometriosis vary in appearance from clear to red, blue, black, or white. • Early lesions are usually red, while later ones are white or clear (peritoneal window). • White and clear lesions are difficult to visualize at laparoscopy. • Ideally, suspicious lesions should be biopsied to allow pathologic evaluation. • Histologically, the presence of endometrial glands, stroma, and/or hemosiderin-laden macrophages supports the diagnosis. • Endometriosis is surgically staged as minimal, mild, moderate, or severe. • Staging is based on fertility potential and is not well correlated with the extent of pain. • Medical options for suppressing the disease include oral contraceptives, progestins, or short courses of GnRH agonists.

A N S W E R :
B, C, D

5. Regarding uterine leiomyomas, which of the following is/are true?

A. GnRH agonists can be used for short-term treatment.

B. Recurrence after myomectomy is less than 5%.

C. Symptoms include abnormal uterine bleeding, pelvic pain, and urinary frequency.

D. Hysterectomy is considered definitive therapy.

Ref.: 1–5

COMMENTS: Uterine leiomyomas (fibroids) are benign tumors that originate from myometrial smooth muscle cells. • They may be single or multiple and asymptomatic or symptomatic. • Symptoms include pelvic pain, abnormal uterine bleeding, or bulk-related symptoms, such as urinary frequency or constipation. • Management of symptomatic disease includes surgical and short-term medical therapy. • GnRH agonists, which induce a hypoestrogenic state, can be used for a 3-month period, usually in anticipation of surgery. • Surgical options include myomectomy, uterine artery embolization, and hysterectomy (definitive therapy). • Uterine leiomyomas do recur after conservative surgical management. • Symptomatic recurrence rates range from 25 to 50%. • Symptomatic recurrences appear to be related to the patient's age at initial treatment and the number of fibroids removed.

A N S W E R :
A, C, D

6. Match the patient presenting with uterine leiomyoma with the appropriate treatment.

A. A 43-year-old asymptomatic woman presents for an annual examination. An 11-week size, irregularly shaped uterus is felt on pelvic examination. Ultrasound study reveals an 11-by-7-by-5 cm uterus with multiple leiomyomas and normal adnexa.

B. A 58-year-old woman, postmenopausal for 6 years, with a history of uterine leiomyomas is noted to have an enlarging uterus.

C. A 28-year-old woman desiring fertility presents with abnormal uterine bleeding. Imaging studies reveal a 2.7-cm submucous fibroid.

D. A 32-year-old woman desiring fertility presents with abnormal uterine bleeding and anemia. Ultrasound study reveals multiple uterine leiomyomas.

a. Hysteroscopic myomectomy

b. Observation

c. Hysterectomy

d. Myomectomy

Ref.: 1–5

COMMENTS: Asymptomatic uterine leiomyomas can generally be observed unless they undergo rapid growth. • If this occurs, one may suspect malignancy (leiomyosarcoma), but the evidence to support this conclusion is sparse. • Patients who desire fertility should undergo uterine-preserving surgery when possible. • Myomectomy is the most common conservative surgical procedure for symptomatic uterine leiomyomas. • Uterine leiomyomas can be submucosal, intramural, subserosal, or pedunculated. • In symptomatic patients, the size, location, and number of uterine leiomyomas, coupled with the patient's surgical history and health, usually guide the surgical approach. • Multiple large leiomyomas are generally removed via laparotomy. • Pedunculated and subserosal leiomyomas can be resected laparoscopically, while submucosal ones are generally managed via hysteroscopic resection.

A N S W E R :
A-b; B-c; C-a; D-d

7. Regarding amenorrhea, which of the following is/are true?

A. It can be classified as primary or secondary.

B. Primary pituitary pathologic states are the most common cause of secondary amenorrhea.

C. Anorexia nervosa is a common cause in adolescent girls.

D. Various abnormalities of the hypothalamic-pituitary-ovarian axis can lead to amenorrhea.

Ref.: 3

COMMENTS: *Primary* amenorrhea is defined as the failure to menstruate by age 14 in the absence of secondary sexual characteristics or the failure to menstruate by age 16 in the presence of secondary sexual characteristics. • Gonadal failure is the most common cause of primary amenorrhea. • Other causes include constitutional delay, congenital absence of the vagina, or imperforate hymen. • *Secondary* amenorrhea is defined as the absence of menses for 6 months in someone who previously menstruated. • Chronic anovulation is the most common cause of secondary amenorrhea. • Other causes include pregnancy, anorexia nervosa, weight loss, hypothyroidism, hyperprolactinemia, primary pituitary or hypothalamic pathologic conditions, and ovarian failure.

A N S W E R :
A, C, D

8. Which of the following is/are common cause(s) of bloody vaginal discharge in a 6-year-old girl presenting for evaluation?

A. Vaginitis

B. Foreign body in the vagina

C. Sexual assault

D. Germ-cell ovarian tumor

Ref.: 3, 6

COMMENTS: Bloody vaginal discharge is a rare problem in preadolescent girls. • However, when it does occur, a detailed investigation is warranted. • Common causes of vaginal bleeding in preadolescent girls include the presence of a foreign body in the vagina, vulvovaginitis, sexual assault, trauma, genital tumors, urethral prolapse, and vulvar lesions. • The presence of a foreign body in the vagina commonly presents as a foul-smelling, bloody discharge. • Toilet paper is the most commonly discovered foreign body. • Vulvovaginitis occurs because of poor hygiene, but infectious organisms, including those responsible for sexually transmitted diseases, should be considered, especially when sexual abuse is suspected. • Although ovarian germ-cell tumors are the most common tumors in preadolescent girls, they infrequently cause bloody vaginal discharge. • These patients usually present with abdominal pain and a palpable abdominal mass. • Estrogen-secreting tumors, such as granulosa-cell ovarian tumors, may lead to precocious puberty and vaginal bleeding in preadolescent girls. • Once discovered, these tumors should be resected.

ANSWER:
A, B, C

9. Physiologic changes in pregnancy include which of the following?

A. Dilutional anemia

B. Mild, compensated respiratory acidosis

C. Increased cardiac output

D. Decreased gastric and intestinal motility

Ref.: 7, 8

COMMENTS: Pregnancy is characterized by numerous physiologic changes that occur as a result of hormonal changes, increased circulatory volume, and the mass affect of the gravid uterus. • The physiologic increase in plasma volume that occurs during pregnancy can lead to dilutional anemia. • The increased plasma volume is also responsible for increased cardiac output in pregnancy, which can reach levels up to 50% above normal. • Increased progesterone levels, coupled with the mass affect of the gravid uterus, are believed to be responsible for the decreased gastric and intestinal motility observed during pregnancy. • Both tidal volume and minute ventilation increase during pregnancy. • The decreased pCO2 that results from these changes commonly leads to a mild, compensated respiratory alkalosis.

ANSWER:
A, C, D

10. A 28-year-old woman at 35 weeks' gestation presents with acute onset of right upper quadrant pain. Which of the following should be considered in the differential diagnosis?

A. Acute cholecystitis or appendicitis

B. Right-sided pyelonephritis

C. Severe preeclampsia

D. Placental abruption

Ref.: 7, 8

COMMENTS: Acute appendicitis and acute cholecystitis are the two most common general surgical conditions encountered during pregnancy. • The gravid uterus causes gradual displacement of the appendix into the upper abdomen. • This anatomic migration accounts for the fact that appendicitis in the third trimester presents as right upper quadrant pain in over 50% of instances. • The enhancing effects of estrogen on gallstone formation coupled with the inhibitory effects of progesterone on gallbladder contractility may predispose the pregnant patient to cholecystitis. • During pregnancy, pyelonephritis occurs preferentially on the right side, presumably because the presence of the sigmoid colon causes dextrorotation of the gravid uterus. • A mild right ureter may predispose to right-sided pyelonephritis. • Preeclampsia, a pregnancy-specific syndrome of hypertension and proteinuria, may involve the liver. • Laboratory and clinical manifestations of hepatic involvement include elevated transaminase levels and right upper quadrant pain. • The pain occurs as a result of a transient hepatitis and/or stretching of the liver capsule by blood. • Placental abruption, or placental separation from the uterus, may result in right upper quadrant or diffuse abdominopelvic pain. • Uterine contractions are believed to be responsible for the pain resulting from placental abruption.

ANSWER:
A, B, C, D

11. Regarding laparoscopy during pregnancy, which of the following is/are true?

A. Pregnancy in general is not considered a contraindication to laparoscopy.

B. Open trocar placement with direct visualization is preferred over blind placement.

C. Increased insufflation pressures of at least 18 mmHg should be used.

D. When possible, the procedure should be deferred until the second trimester.

Ref.: 3, 4

COMMENTS: In general, laparoscopy during pregnancy is not contraindicated. • Maternal and fetal complications may be minimized by delaying surgery until the second trimester when possible, using an open technique for trocar placement, limiting insufflation pressures to no greater than 15 mmHg, and careful intraoperative and postoperative monitoring of maternal ventilation and acid-base status.

ANSWER:
A, B, D

12. Which of the following patients with irregular uterine bleeding should undergo endometrial biopsy?

A. A 54-year-old postmenopausal woman with an endometrial thickness of 7.4 mm

B. A 44-year-old with a strong family history of breast cancer who is on tamoxifen for chemoprevention.

C. A 29-year-old, poorly compliant with her oral contraceptives, who presents with intermenstrual bleeding

D. A 29-year-old diabetic woman with at least a 10-year history of anovulatory cycles

Ref.: 3, 9

COMMENTS: The differential diagnosis of irregular uterine bleeding is extensive. • However, one of the key features of management is ruling out atypical endometrial hyperplasia or endometrial cancer. • Postmenopausal women who present with uterine bleeding and have an endometrial thickness of greater than 4 mm are at increased risk of endometrial cancer and should undergo endometrial sampling. • This can be done in the office setting, when feasible, or in the operating room (dilation and curettage). • The effects of prolonged unopposed endogenous or exogenous estrogen on the endometrium also increase the risk of atypical endometrial hyperplasia and cancer. • A longstanding history of anovulatory cycles may result in prolonged unopposed endogenous estrogen. • Thus, these patients should undergo endometrial assessment. • Tamoxifen is a selective estrogen-receptor modulator that has a stimulatory (estrogenic) effect on the endometrium. • Patients on tamoxifen who present with irregular bleeding should undergo endometrial sampling.

A N S W E R :
A, B, D

13. A 34-year-old with history of infertility who has recently undergone ovulation induction presents to the emergency department with abdominal distention and complaints of shortness of breath. A chest radiograph reveals bilateral pleural effusions. A pelvic ultrasound study shows large amount of ascites and enlarged ovaries with multiple large ovarian cysts, the largest being 28 mm. What is the most likely diagnosis?

A. Meigs' syndrome

B. Ovarian hyperstimulation syndrome

C. Ovarian cancer

D. Ruptured ovarian cyst

Ref.: 1, 2, 6, 10

COMMENTS: Meigs' syndrome, a malignancy mimic, involves the coexistence of hydrothorax, ascites, and an underlying benign ovarian tumor, usually a fibroma. • Multiple large ovarian cysts are not commonly seen in this condition, and the presentation is generally not acute. • A ruptured ovarian cyst may result in acute or subacute pelvic pain and pelvic fluid seen on ultrasound imaging. • However, the other symptoms described in this patient are not seen. • Advanced stages of ovarian cancer usually do not cause acute symptoms. • Ovarian hyperstimulation syndrome is an infrequent complication of ovulation induction that may affect women with elevated estradiol levels and multiple ovarian follicles. • Central to the syndrome is fluid shift from the intravascular compartment. • This can result in hemoconcentration, hypercoagulability, pleural effusions, and abdominopelvic ascites. • Patients usually present with the acute onset of symptoms.

A N S W E R :
B

14. Regarding cervical carcinoma, which of the following statements is/are true?

A. It is the most common malignancy of the female genital tract in the United States.

B. There is a possible viral cause.

C. The death rate from this malignancy has declined in recent years.

D. Most are squamous cell type.

Ref.: 1, 2, 6, 9, 11

COMMENTS: Cervical cancer is the second most common gynecologic malignancy in the United States and the most common worldwide. • Endometrial cancer is the most common gynecological cancer in the United States. • Approximately 95% of cervical cancers are of the squamous cell type. • They usually begin at the squamocolumnar junction of the cervix. • The Papanicolau (Pap) smear is believed to be responsible for the decline in the cervical cancer death rate. • There appears to be an increased incidence of cervical cancer in women with a history of multiple sexual partners, suggesting a possible viral cause. • High-risk subtypes of the human papillomavirus (HPV) have been associated with cervical cancer.

A N S W E R :
B, C, D

15. Regarding treatment of cervical carcinoma, which of the following is/are true?

A. Primary surgical therapy is preferred for patients staged beyond stage IIA.

B. Primary surgical or radiation therapy can be employed for lesions staged below stage IIA.

C. Cervical conization can be used to treat stage IA1 lesions.

D. Chemosensitization can be utilized to augment the efficacy of radiation therapy.

Ref.: 4, 6, 11

COMMENTS: Surgery and radiation are commonly employed in the treatment of cervical cancer. • The stage of the disease determines treatment. • Although either surgical or radiation therapy can be used in patients with disease of stage IIA and below with equal results, surgical therapy is preferred in otherwise healthy patients. • In patients staged above IIA, radiation therapy is generally the preferred treatment. • During radiation treatment, chemotherapy is frequently utilized as a sensitizer and has been shown to augment radiation effects in squamous cell cancer. • In patients with microinvasive disease (stage IA1) desiring conservative treatment, cervical conization can be done.

A N S W E R :
B, C, D

16. Which of the following is/are true of a radical hysterectomy?

A. It can be used as a primary surgical modality in treating stage III cervical cancer.

B. Parametrial tissue is resected.

C. The upper third of the vagina is removed.

D. There is a higher incidence of ureteral and bladder fistula than with extrafascial hysterectomy.

Ref.: 4, 6

COMMENTS: Radical hysterectomy involves removal of the uterus, resection of parametrial tissue lateral to the ureter, ligation of the uterine arteries at their origin on the hypogastric arteries, transection of the uterosacral ligaments near the rectum, and removal of the upper third of vagina. • Pelvic lymphadenectomy is commonly done at the time of radical hysterectomy. • The ovaries are preserved if they appear normal. • Extrafascial hysterectomy involves removal of the uterus, preservation of the parametrium, ligation of the uterine vessels at the level of the cervical os, transection of the uterosacral ligaments at the uterus, and preservation of the vaginal cuff. • Because of the more extensive and lateral dissection done during a radical hysterectomy, there is a higher incidence of ureteral and bladder complications than with extrafascial hysterectomy.

A N S W E R :
B, C, D

17. Regarding the Pap smear, which of the following statements is/are true?

A. It is approximately 95% accurate when screening for cervical cancer.

B. Abnormal-appearing epithelial cells that are not frankly malignant suggest an underlying inflammatory process.

C. A definitive histologic diagnosis cannot be made on the basis of the smear results alone.

D. All patients with atypical squamous cells of undetermined significance (ASC-US) results should under colposcopic evaluation.

Ref.: 1–3, 5

COMMENTS: Wide use of the Pap smear has made it possible to screen large populations of women for cervical cancer. • Results of the Pap smear are accurate in approximately 95%. • Because it is a cytologic examination, it may indicate the presence of malignant cells but cannot give information about the degree of invasion. • Definitive diagnosis requires colposcopic evaluation and a tissue diagnosis. • Patients with ASC-US Pap results can be managed in one of three ways: they can undergo immediate colposcopic evaluation, undergo a repeat Pap smear in 3–6 months, or have reflex DNA testing for high-risk HPV serotypes. • If testing reveals the absence of high-risk HPV serotypes, the Pap smear result is treated as normal. • Patients with positive high-risk HPV serotypes should undergo colposcopic evaluation.

A N S W E R :
A, B, C

18. Match each of the clinical findings for cervical carcinoma with the appropriate clinical stage.

A. Confined to the cervix, with stromal invasion greater than 3 mm

B. Clinical lesion 4 cm in size confined to the cervix

C. Metastases to the upper two thirds of the vagina

D. Involves the bladder mucosa

a. Stage IV

b. Stage II

c. Stage IB

d. Stage IA2

Ref.: 1, 2, 10, 11

COMMENTS: Cervical carcinoma is **clinically** staged. • Clinical staging involves a physical examination and may involve intravenous pyelographic (IVP) studies, cystoscopic studies, proctoscopic examination, or computed tomographic (CT) scanning. • Stage I tumors are confined to the cervix. • Stage IA lesions are microinvasive. • Stage IA1 lesions do not invade the stroma beyond 3 mm and are not wider than 7 mm. • Stage IA2 lesions invade more than 3 mm but not greater than 5 mm. • Stage IB are visible tumors. • Stage 1B1 lesions are less than 4 cm, and stage IB2 lesions are greater than 4 cm. • Stage II tumors may involve the upper two thirds of the vagina (IIA) or the parametrial tissue (IIB). • Stage III tumors extend through the parametrial tissue to the pelvic side wall or to the lower third of the vagina (IIIA) or result in ureteral obstruction (IIIB). • Stage IV tumors may invade the bladder or rectal mucosa (IVA), or they may spread outside the pelvis (IVB).

A N S W E R :
A-d; B-c; C-b; D-a

19. All but which of the following are risk factors for endometrial cancer?

A. Early menopause

B. Tamoxifen use

C. Nulliparity

D. Obesity

Ref.: 1–3

COMMENTS: Prolonged endometrial exposure to unopposed estrogen increases the risk of endometrial cancer. • Additional risk factors include nulliparity, early menarche, late menopause, obesity, and anovulatory cycles. • Tamoxifen, a selective estrogen receptor modulator, has stimulatory effects on the endometrium and increases endometrial cancer risk.

A N S W E R :
A

20. Regarding endometrial cancer, which of the following is/are true?

A. Currently, there is no role for radiation therapy.

B. It is usually clinically staged.

C. It is the most common gynecologicl cancer in the United States.

D. Most patients present with stage III disease.

Ref.: 1, 2, 3, 10

COMMENTS: Endometrial cancer is the most common gynecologic cancer in the United States. • Fortunately, most patients present with early stage, or stage I, disease. • Endometrial cancer, unlike cervical cancer, is **surgically** staged. • Hysterectomy is usually curative for patients with early-stage (stage IA) low-grade (grade 1–2) disease. • However, patients with higher-stage and -grade disease usually receive adjuvant radiation therapy.

ANSWER:
C

21. Match the clinical finding with the appropriate stage for endometrial cancer.

A. Invasion of cervical stroma

B. Tumor confined to the endometrium

C. Metastases to the pelvic lymph nodes

D. Tumor involvement of less than half of the myometrium

a. Stage IIIC

b. Stage IB

c. Stage IIB

d. Stage IA

Ref.: 1, 2, 3, 6

COMMENTS: Endometrial cancer is **surgically staged.** • This process may involve a total abdominal hysterectomy with bilateral salpingo-oophorectomy, peritoneal washings for cytologic study, and pelvic and/or para-aortic lymph node evaluation. • Stage I are tumors confined to the uterus. • They can be confined to the endometrium (IA), invade up to halfway through the myometrium (IB), or invade to a depth greater than halfway through the myometrium (IC). • Stage II tumors have spread to the cervix. • Those involving the endocervical glands only are stage IIA, while those involving the cervical stroma are stage IIB. • Stage III tumors involve the adnexa or the serosa or result in positive peritoneal cytologic findings (IIIA), involve the vagina (IIIB), or involve the pelvic or para-aortic lymph nodes (IIIC). • Stage IV tumors have invaded the bowel or bladder (IVA) or have spread beyond the pelvis (IVB).

ANSWER:
A-c; B-d; C-a; D-b

22. Which of the following is the most common uterine sarcoma?

A. Stromal sarcoma

B. Leiomyosarcoma

C. Mixed mullerian tumor

D. Endolymphatic stromal myosis

Ref.: 1, 2, 6

COMMENTS: Uterine sarcomas comprise up to 5% of all uterine cancers. • They may arise from the myometrium, the endometrial stroma and glands, or both. • These tumors are very malignant and frequently metastasize to the lung. • *Rapid uterine growth is a common presentation.* • Mixed mullerian tumors, which contain both adenocarcinomatous and sarcomatous elements, are the most common. • Leiomyosarcoma, which was once thought to be the most common uterine sarcoma, is the second most common. • Mixed mullerian tumors are generally more aggressive. • Hysterectomy is usually the first-line treatment. • Adjuvant radiation and/or chemotherapy may be used in selected patients and may confer some benefit.

ANSWER:
C

23. Match the clinical finding with the appropriate stage of ovarian cancer.

A. Metastases to the liver parenchyma

B. Retroperitoneal node involvement

C. Tumor involvement of the fallopian tubes

D. Tumor confined to one ovary and positive findings on peritoneal washing

a. Stage IV

b. Stage II

c. Stage III

d. Stage IC

Ref.: 3, 6, 10, 11

COMMENTS: Primary adenocarcinomas of the ovary may be serous, mucinous, or endometroid. • Ovarian cancer is staged **surgically** by total abdominal hysterectomy with bilateral salpingo-oophorectomy, omentectomy, lymph node evaluation, peritoneal washing for cytologic study, and biopsies of suspicious areas. • Stage I lesions are confined to the ovaries, stage IA denotes unilateral involvement, and stage IB is bilateral disease. • Stage IC disease is defined by involvement of the ovarian surface or capsular rupture or by positive peritoneal cytologic findings. • Stage II tumors involve one or both ovaries, with pelvic extension. • The tumor may spread to the fallopian tubes or uterus (IIA) or to other pelvic organs (IIB). • Stage IIC are stage IIA or B tumors with ovarian capsule involvement, rupture, or positive peritoneal cytologic results. • Stage III tumors are peritoneal implants beyond the pelvis and/or positive retroperitoneal or inguinal lymph nodes. • *Most patients present with stage III disease.* • Peritoneal lesions may be microscopic (IIIA), up to 2 cm (IIIB), or greater than 2 cm (IIIC). • Stage IV tumors are those that have spread distantly (liver, lungs).

ANSWER:
A-a; B-c; C-b; D-d

24. Match the ovarian tumor with the appropriate characteristic

A. Masculinizing

B. α-Fetoprotein (AFP)

C. Human chorionic gonadotropin (hCG)

D. Elaborates estrogen

a. Sertoli-Leydig cell tumor

b. Granulosa-Theca cell tumor

c. Endodermal sinus tumor (yolk sac)

d. Choriocarcinoma

Ref.: 10, 11

COMMENTS: Ovarian tumors are frequently characterized by their ability to produce hormones or biologic markers. • **Sertoli-Leydig** cell tumors produce androgens and frequently cause masculinization. • **Granulosa-theca** cell tumors frequently produce estrogen and have been associated with precocious puberty in young patients and endometrial cancer in older patients. • **Endodermal sinus tumor** (yolk sac tumor), which is the second most common germ-cell ovarian tumor, secretes AFP. • **Choriocarcinoma** produces hCG, which can be used as a marker to gauge response to treatment.

ANSWER:
A-a; B-c; C-d; D-b

25. Regarding ovarian adenocarcinoma, which of the following is/are true?

    A. The disease is clinically staged.

    B. Most patients present with stage III disease.

    C. For most patients, adjuvant single-regimen chemotherapy is sufficient.

    D. There are currently no reliable methods for screening.

Ref.: 10, 11

COMMENTS: Ovarian cancer represents approximately one fourth of all gynecologic cancer but is the leading cause of gynecologic cancer deaths. • Lack of a good screening tool and delay in diagnosis largely contribute to this fact. • Moreover, up to 50% of ovarian cancers are inoperable at the time of diagnosis. • *Most patients present with stage III disease.* • Ovarian cancer is **surgically** staged by total abdominal hysterectomy with bilateral salpingo-oophorectomy, omentectomy, lymph node evaluation, peritoneal washing for cytologic study, and biopsy of suspicious areas. • Adjuvant chemotherapy with a platinum-based drug and paclitaxel is often used. • This combination is associated with a response rate of up to 80%.

A N S W E R :
B, D

26. Regarding treatment of ovarian adenocarcinoma, which of the following is/are true?

    A. For most patients, total abdominal hysterectomy with bilateral salpingo-oophorectomy is curative.

    B. If adjuvant chemotherapy is employed, a single-agent regimen is usually sufficient.

    C. Debulking of the tumor (surgical removal of as much tumor as possible) may contribute to improved survival.

    D. At laparotomy, peritoneal fluid or washings should be routinely sent for cytologic evaluation.

Ref.: 3, 6, 10

COMMENTS: Since most patients with ovarian cancer present with advanced-stage disease, total abdominal hysterectomy with bilateral salpingectomy is usually not curative. • Complete surgical staging should include cytologic evaluation of peritoneal fluid to rule out microscopic disease. • Up to 30% of patients who have disease apparently confined to the ovary have microscopic metastatic disease. • In the presence of gross or macroscopic metastatic disease, surgical debulking of as much tumor as possible may contribute to improved survival. • Dual-agent chemotherapy is used as adjuvant treatment.

A N S W E R :
C, D

27. Meigs' syndrome is characterized by all but which of the following?

    A. Hydrothorax

    B. Ascites

    C. Presence of fibroma

    D. Malignant ovarian tumor

Ref.: 1–3

COMMENTS: Findings common in Meigs' syndrome can mimic those found with malignancy. • Meigs' syndrome involves the coexistence of hydrothorax, ascites, and an underlying benign ovarian tumor, usually a fibroma. • The pathophysiologic mechanism of the ascites and pleural effusion is unclear. • It is believed to be the result of lymphatic obstruction of the ovary. • Removal of the ovarian fibroma usually results in resolution of the findings.

A N S W E R :
D

28. Match each vaginal cancer with its appropriate characteristic.

    A. Clear-cell carcinoma

    B. Sarcoma botryoides

    C. Squamous cell carcinoma

    D. Direct spread of cancer from adjacent organs

    a. Most common primary vaginal cancer

    b. Most common vaginal cancer

    c. Diethylstilbestrol (DES) exposure

    d. Seen in young girls

Ref.: 6, 10, 11

COMMENTS: Squamous cell carcinoma is the most common primary vaginal malignancy. • Most vaginal cancers are direct extensions from cancers arising in adjacent organs. • Sarcoma botryoides is a bulky polypoid sarcoma commonly found in infants or young children. • Clear-cell carcinoma can develop in adolescent or adult children of mothers who took diethylstilbestrol during pregnancy.

A N S W E R :
A-c; B-d; C-a; D-b

29. Regarding vaginal cancer, which of the following is/are true?

    A. It is rare.

    B. In general, primary vaginal cancer involving the upper third of the vagina should be treated as is cervical cancer, while that involving the lower third should be treated as is vulvar cancer.

    C. Tumor extending to the pelvic side wall is considered stage II disease.

    D. It is predominantly a disease of older women.

Ref.: 6, 9, 11

COMMENTS: Primary vaginal cancer is predominantly a disease of older women but is rare overall. • Primary vaginal cancers involving the upper third of the vagina generally behave as and are treated as cervical cancer. • Similarly, tumors involving the lower third of the vagina are treated as vulvar cancer. • Management of tumors involving the middle third of the vagina is challenging. • Vaginal carcinoma is **clinically** staged. • The tumor may be limited to the vaginal wall (stage I), extend to the subvaginal tissue (stage II), extend to the pelvic side wall (stage III), spread to adjacent organs or to areas outside of the true pelvis (stage IVA), or spread to distant organs (stage IVB).

A N S W E R :
A, B, D

30. Which of the following vulvar abnormalities is/are considered risk factors for invasive malignancy?

A. Vulvar intraepithelial neoplasm III (VIN-III)

B. Paget's disease

C. Lichen sclerosis

D. Hypertrophic dystrophy without atypia

Ref.: 3, 6

COMMENTS: Suspicious vulvar lesions should be biopsied to rule out malignancy. • There are numerous risk factors for vulvar cancer, including a history of vulvar dysplasia, smoking, hypertension, diabetes, and chronic steroid use. • Lichen sclerosis and hypertrophic dystrophy without atypia are the two types of vulvar, nonneoplastic epithelial disorders that are not considered risk factors for malignancy. • Paget's disease is an intraepithelial lesion of the vulva associated with vulvar adenocarcinoma. • Untreated VIN can progress to vulvar cancer in 5% of cases. • VIN is commonly multifocal, and multiple biopsies are needed to determine the extent of the disease. • Acetic acid can be used to help identify dysplastic vulvar lesions. • Treatment of VIN consists of observation, wide local excision, skinning vulvectomy, laser ablation, or topical 5-fluorouracil (5-FU). • Most lesions that undergo spontaneous regression do so within 6 months. • Wide local excision requires removal of full thickness of skin with a 2–3 cm free margin. • Laser treatment to a depth of 1 mm in non–hair-bearing areas and 3 mm in hair-bearing areas is required for effective treatment. • Topical 5-FU can be very effective but requires good compliance on the part of the patient and is associated with significant skin reactions.

ANSWER:
A, B

31. Regarding vulvar carcinoma, which of the following is/are true?

A. Adenocarcinoma is the most common type.

B. There is an association with HPV infection in young patients.

C. Pruritus is one the most common symptoms.

D. The disease is clinically staged.

Ref.: 3, 6

COMMENTS: Squamous cell cancer is the most common vulvar malignancy. • Pruritus and the presence of an abnormal or ulcerating lesion are common presenting complaints. • High-risk subtypes of HPV have been associated with vulvar cancer in younger patients. • Patients often have a history of cervical or vulvar dysplasias. • Vulvar cancer, unlike cervical cancer, is surgically staged. • The staging assists in guiding treatment and determining prognosis.

ANSWER:
B, C

32. Regarding treatment of vulvar squamous cell carcinoma, which of the following is/are true?

A. Adequate local resection should involve a 2-cm free margin.

B. For central (<1 cm lateral of midline) invasive lesions, unilateral groin node dissection is usually sufficient.

C. Radical local excision of an invasive lesion with bilateral inguinal and pelvic node dissection may produce therapeutic results similar to those of radical vulvar excision and bilateral inguinal and pelvic node dissection in selected patients.

D. The 5-year survival rate of patients with positive inguinal nodes is about 50%.

Ref.: 6, 10, 11

COMMENTS: Primary treatment of vulvar cancer is surgical. • Wide local resection of the lesion with a free margin of at least 2 cm is considered optimal. • Groin lymph node sampling should be undertaken if the lesion has invaded greater than 1 mm. • For centrally invasive lesions less than 1 cm from the midline, bilateral groin lymph node sampling is recommended. • For selected patients with lateral lesions, unilateral groin lymph node sampling may be sufficient. • Patients with positive groin nodes usually have a 5-year survival rate of about 50%. • For selected patients, radical local excision of invasive lesions with bilateral inguinal and pelvic node dissection may produce therapeutic results similar to those of radical vulvar excision and bilateral inguinal and pelvic node dissection, with significantly less morbidity.

ANSWER:
A, C, D

33. Risk factors for pelvic organ prolapse include which of the following?

A. Vaginal delivery

B. Chronic asthma

C. Cesarean delivery

D. Previous total abdominal hysterectomy

Ref.: 3, 4, 12

COMMENTS: Damaged or weakened support structures can lead to vaginal support deficits and/or vaginal prolapse. • The muscles of the pelvic floor and the endopelvic fascia provide support to the pelvic organs. • Events that adversely affect their structure and function increase the likelihood of subsequent pelvic organ prolapse. • Vaginal delivery can directly damage endopelvic fascial support and weaken pelvic floor muscles and is a major risk factor for the development of pelvic organ prolapse. • During total abdominal hysterectomy, endopelvic fascial support, specifically the uterosacral cardinal ligament complex, is frequently transected. • Failure to recognize and appropriately repair these support structures can lead to pelvic organ prolapse. • Chronic coughing, chronic asthma, heavy lifting, and obesity can all lead to increased intra-abdominal pressure, which can weaken pelvic support structures. • For patients who have not labored, cesarean delivery is believed to be protective against the development of pelvic organ prolapse.

ANSWER:
A, B, D

34. Match the clinical pelvic organ prolapse with the appropriate description.

A. Rectocele

B. Cystocele

C. Enterocele

D. Uterovaginal prolapse

a. Defect in pubocervical fascia

b. Defect in rectovaginal septum

c. Uterosacral ligament defect

d. Pouch of Douglas herniation between the uterosacral ligaments

Ref.: 3, 12

COMMENTS: Damage to endopelvic fascial support structures can lead to pelvic organ prolapse. • The **pubocervical fascia** provides major support to the urethra and bladder. • Damage to this support structure can lead to a cystocele, which causes protrusion of the bladder through the anterior vaginal wall. • The **rectovaginal septum** lies between the posterior vagina wall and the anterior rectum. • Damage to this results in a rectocele, which is a herniation of the rectum anteriorly. • In addition to distressing symptoms from the bulge itself, rectoceles can cause a sensation of obstructed defecation from stool trapping. • The **uterosacral ligaments**, along with the cardinal ligaments, provide major support to the cervix and upper vagina. • Weakened or damaged uterosacral ligaments can lead to uterovaginal prolapse. • The uterosacral ligaments also prevent the development of enterocele, or herniation of small bowel into the pouch of Douglas.

ANSWER:
A-b; B-a; C-d; D-c

35. Which of the following provides major support to the upper vagina?

A. Uterosacral-cardinal ligament complex

B. Infundibulopelvic ligament

C. Broad ligament

D. Round ligament

Ref.: 3, 4, 12

COMMENTS: The uterosacral-cardinal ligament complex provides major support to the upper vagina through its attachment at the cervix. • It helps maintain the cervix and upper vagina above the levator plate. • The infundibulopelvic ligament, which is usually transected during oophorectomy, contains the ovarian vessels and nerves. • It also provides some support to the ovary. • The broad ligament provides a route for blood vessels and lymphatics of the pelvis and is not considered a major pelvic support structure. • The round ligament provides accessory support to maintain anteversion of the uterus. • It does not provide any significant support to the vagina.

ANSWER:
A

36. Potential sites for ureteral injury during an abdominal hysterectomy with bilateral salpingo-oophorectomy include which of the following?

A. Transection of the round ligaments

B. Transection of the uterine arteries

C. Transection of the cardinal ligaments

D. Transection of the infundibulopelvic ligaments

Ref.: 3, 4

COMMENTS: Anatomical knowledge of the course of the ureters in the pelvis is essential for preventing ureteral injury. • The ureters travel in the retroperitoneal space in abdominal and pelvic segments. • In the abdomen, they run downward and medially along the anterior surface of the psoas muscle. • The iliopectineal line serves as the marker for the pelvic segment of the ureter. • The ureters cross the iliac vessels as they enter the pelvis and travel in the medial leaf of the parietal peritoneum. • They course near the ovarian and uterine vessels. • Thus, they are susceptible to injury during transection of the infundibulopelvic ligaments and uterine arteries. • The ureters travel through the cardinal ligaments about 1–2 cm lateral to the cervix. • Removal of the cervix during hysterectomy places the ureter at risk for injury. • In general, the ureters do not travel near the round ligaments. • In a pelvis with normal anatomy, this is not regarded as a common site for ureteral injury.

ANSWER:
B, C, D

37. All but which of the following are acceptable therapies for stress urinary incontinence in women?

A. Suburethral sling procedure

B. Retropubic urethropexy

C. Kegel pelvic muscle exercises

D. Oxybutynin

Ref.: 3, 12

COMMENTS: Oxybutynin is an anticholinergic drug used primarily to treat overactive bladder with or without incontinence. • It has not been shown to effectively treat primary stress urinary incontinence. • Suburethral sling procedures are very effective in treating stress urinary incontinence. • Although the complete mechanism as to how they work is unclear, they appear to exert their positive effects through increasing urethral pressures and providing additional support to the bladder neck. • These procedures can be done either abdominally or vaginally. • The retropubic urethropexy procedures, such as the Marshall-Marchetti-Krantz and Burch procedures, are performed abdominally. • They are very effective in treating stress urinary incontinence and appear to do so by supporting the bladder neck. • Kegel exercises, which involve training of the levator ani muscles through intermittent contractions, are very effective in treating mild stress urinary incontinence.

ANSWER:
D

38. Which of the following is the major cause of overactive bladder in women?

A. Detrusor dysnergia or hyperreflexia

B. Hypoestrogenism

C. Interstitial cystitis

D. Idiopathic

Ref.: 3, 12

COMMENTS: The major cause of overactive bladder in women is unknown. • Although interstitial cystitis and hypoestrogenic states can lead to urge symptoms, they are not very common causes of overactive bladder. • *Detrussor dysnergia* is an old term used to describe overactive bladder due to detrusor instability. • *Detrusor hyperreflexia* is used to describe detrusor instability caused by a known central nervous system lesion, such as multiple sclerosis.

ANSWER:
D

39. Which of the following is/are considered risk factors for stress urinary incontinence in women?

A. Previous operative vaginal delivery

B. Multiple sclerosis

C. Previous bladder neck surgery

D. Cystocele

Ref.: 3, 4, 12

COMMENTS: Stress urinary incontinence, or loss of urine with increased intra-abdominal pressure, is caused by either urethral hypermobility or intrinsic urethral sphincter damage. • The result is loss of urine with coughing, sneezing, or heavy activity. • Previous vaginal delivery with forceps, which may damage pubocervical fascial support, is a major risk factor for the development of urethral hypermobility and subsequent stress urinary incontinence. • Patients who have had previous bladder neck surgery may sustain urethral sphincter damage. • A cystocele, or herniation of the bladder through the anterior vaginal wall, is frequently associated with urethral hypermobility. • Patients with multiple sclerosis are at increased risk for overactive bladder.

ANSWER:
A, C, D

40. Regarding menopause, which of the following is/are true?

A. The average age of onset in the United States is 51.4 years.

B. It occurs as result of gradual depletion of functional ovarian follicles.

C. Vaginal atrophy, vasomotor symptoms, and osteoporosis are sequelae.

D. Unopposed estrogen is acceptable therapy for women with a uterus and vasomotor symptoms.

Ref.: 3

COMMENTS: The average age of menopause in the United States is 51.4 years old. • A gradual decrease in the number of ovarian follicles usually precedes its onset. • The result is diminished estrogen production. • This hypoestrogenic state may lead to vasomotor symptoms, vaginal atrophy, and osteoporosis. • Menopausal hormone therapy is usually highly effective in ameliorating all of these symptoms. • For patients who have contraindications to menopausal hormone therapy, alternative therapies exist for each of these symptoms. • If menopausal hormone therapy is prescribed, it should never be given as an unopposed oral estrogen formulation in women with a uterus. • Unopposed estrogen has been associated with an increased incidence of endometrial hyperplasia with atypia, the precursor to endometrial cancer. • Combination oral menopausal hormonal therapy has been reported in a recent randomized controlled trial to be associated with increased risk of breast cancer, coronary heart disease, dementia, and venous thromboembolic events.

ANSWER:
A, B, C

41. Results of the Women's Health Initiative showed an increased risk of which of following in postmenopausal women treated with combination (conjugated equine estrogen and medroxyprogesterone acetate) hormone therapy?

A. Breast cancer

B. Colon cancer

C. Stroke

D. Osteoporosis

Ref.: 3, 13

COMMENTS: The Women's Health Initiative was a randomized, double-masked, placebo-controlled trial designed as a primary prevention trial of menopausal hormone therapy in women with an average age of 63 years. • The primary outcome event was coronary heart disease, while the primary adverse outcome was invasive breast cancer. • Results of the trial indicated a significant increase in invasive breast cancer, coronary heart disease, and stroke in women who took menopausal hormone therapy compared to those on placebo. • There was a significant decrease in colon cancer and osteoporosis in the treatment groups.

ANSWER:
A, C

42. For a postmenopausal patient presenting with hot flashes, alternatives to hormonal therapy include which of the following?

A. Raloxifene

B. Selective serotonin-reuptake inhibitors

C. Clonidine

D. Gabapentin

Ref.: 3, 13

COMMENTS: As a result of the Women's Health Initiative, practitioners and patients are becoming increasingly interested in alternatives to hormonal therapy in treating menopausal symptoms. • Clonidine, selective serotonin-reuptake inhibitors, and gabapentin have all been shown to reduce hot flashes and vasomotor symptoms when compared to placebo. • Raloxifene, which is a selective estrogen-receptor modulator, can be used as an alternative for the treatment of osteoporosis. • However, it can worsen menopausal vasomotor symptoms.

ANSWER:
B, C, D

43. Regarding pelvic inflammatory disease (PID), which of the following is/are true?

A. *Neisseria gonorrhoeae* is the most common causative organism.

B. Physical examination is considered the gold standard for diagnosis.

C. Chronic pelvic pain and ectopic pregnancy are sequelae.

D. It is the most common reason for gynecologic hospital admission.

Ref.: 3

COMMENTS: Treatment PID is the most common reason for gynecologic hospital admissions in the United States. • PID is a spectrum of inflammatory disorders of the upper genital tract in women that include salpingitis, endometritis, and tubo-ovarian abscess. • Bacterial organisms involved include *N. gonorrhoeae, Chlamydia trachomatis,* endogenous aerobic and anaerobic bacteria, and *Mycoplasma.* • *C. trachomatis* is the causative organism more often than is *N. gonorrhoeae.* • Although physical examination is frequently used to diagnose PID, laparoscopy is considered the gold standard for diagnosis. • Patients who meet diagnostic criteria can be treated as outpatients with broad-spectrum antibiotics, but a follow-up evaluation should be scheduled for 48 hr later. • Patients who fail outpatient therapy should be admitted and treated with intravenous broad-spectrum antibiotics. • Imaging studies are required if one suspects a tubo-ovarian abscess. • All patients with PID should be counseled about the common sequelae of the disease, which include chronic pelvic pain, infertility, and increased risk of ectopic pregnancies.

ANSWER:
C, D

44. All but which of the following are true of ectopic pregnancy?

    A. A history of PID is a risk factor.

    B. The rate of ectopic pregnancy has been declining over the past 20 years in the United States.

    C. Medical therapy can be used in selected patients.

    D. Serial serum β-hCG level measurements can aid in diagnosis.

Ref.: 3, 9

COMMENTS: Ectopic pregnancy is any pregnancy that occurs outside of the uterus. • Most occur in the fallopian tubes. • Risk factors for ectopic pregnancy include a history of previous ectopic pregnancy, tubal surgery, PID, and concurrent intrauterine device use. • The rate of ectopic pregnancies has increased over the past 20 years, presumably because of the increased incidence of treated PID. • Up to 7 weeks' gestation, the serum β-hCG level roughly doubles in normal pregnancies. • An abnormal rise in serum β-hCG level and sonographic absence of an intrauterine gestation should raise suspicion of an ectopic pregnancy.

An ectopic pregnancy can be treated medically or surgically. • Medical therapy is generally reserved for compliant, hemodynamically stable patients. • Methotrexate is the current drug of choice, provided patients have no contraindications to its use. • Surgical treatment usually consists of salpingostomy, with removal of the ectopic pregnancy, or salpingectomy. • Laparotomy or laparoscopy may be performed, depending on the surgeon's preference. • Follow-up serum β-hCG level determinations should be obtained to confirm the absence of residual trophoblastic tissue.

ANSWER:
A, C, D

45. Regarding Bartholin's gland cysts, which of the following is/are true?

    A. They are most common in postmenopausal women.

    B. Most are caused by sexually transmitted diseases.

    C. Acute vulvar pain is a common symptom.

    D. Incision and drainage with insertion of a Word catheter can be used for treatment.

Ref.: 3, 4

COMMENTS: Bartholin's gland cysts are fairly common. • Most are not due to infection, but, when infected, they are referred to as abscesses. • Organisms that cause sexually transmitted diseases can be cultured from the abscess, although they are not the usual causative agents. • Bartholin's gland cysts or abscesses are not common in postmenopausal patients. • Therefore, vulvar masses presenting in this age group should raise the suspicion for malignancy. • Acute vulvar pain is one of the most common presenting symptoms for a Bartholin's cyst or abscess. • Incision and drainage of the cyst or abscess is usually required for these patients. • After incision and drainage, a small inflatable catheter, or Word catheter, can be placed in the cyst to allow complete drainage. • Alternatively, the cyst can be sutured open (marsupialized) or excised. • Excision of a Bartholin's cyst is generally reserved for recurrences.

ANSWER:
C, D

46. Ultrasound study is based on the reflection of sound in human tissues. Which of the following conditions affect reflectivity?

    A. Size of the transducer head

    B. Acoustic impedance

    C. Frequency of the transducer

    D. Angle of the incident sound beam

Ref.: 14

COMMENTS: Ultrasound study uses sound waves with frequencies measured in megahertz (millions of cycles per second). • In general, the strength of the echoes returning to the probe (reflectivity) during ultrasound study is related to the angle at which the beam strikes the acoustic interface. • Thus, the more perpendicular the beam, the stronger the returning echoes. • In addition, acoustic impedance, which is determined by multiplying the acoustic density of the tissue by the speed of sound in the tissue, also affects returning echoes. • The greater the difference between adjacent structures, the stronger the returning echoes. • Neither the frequency of the transducer nor the size of the transducer head has any affect on reflectivity.

ANSWER:
B, D

47. Match the clinical symptom with the appropriate diagnosis.

    A. First-trimester bleeding, closed cervical os, no fetal tissue passed, and fetal heartbeat seen on ultrasound imaging

    B. First-trimester bleeding, closed cervical, no fetal tissue passed, irregularly shaped intrauterine gestational sac, and absent fetal heartbeat on ultrasound imaging

    C. First-trimester bleeding and fetal tissue protruding through the cervical os

    D. First-trimester bleeding, passage of fetal tissue, ultrasound imaging showing an empty uterus

    a. Complete abortion

b. Incomplete abortion

c. Missed abortion

d. Threatened abortion

Ref.: 3

COMMENTS: First-trimester bleeding occurs through 13 weeks of gestation. • About one third of women have first-trimester bleeding, and approximately 50% of them will go on to spontaneously abort. • Any woman with first-trimester bleeding should be suspected of having an ectopic pregnancy and should be evaluated accordingly. • Abortion, by definition, is a pregnancy loss that occurs before 20 weeks' gestation. • A **complete** abortion occurs when all fetal tissue passes. • The cervical os is generally closed, and ultrasound study reveals an empty uterus. • With an **incomplete** abortion, there is some passage of fetal tissue. • The cervical os is usually open, and fetal tissue may be seen protruding through it. • A **missed** abortion is defined as a sonographically detectable intrauterine gestation with absent cardiac activity. • Usually no fetal tissue has passed, and the cervical os is closed. • A **threatened** abortion is diagnosed when first-trimester bleeding occurs and ultrasound study reveals cardiac activity. • The cervical os is generally closed. • If the cervical os is opened, the patient is deemed to have an inevitable abortion. • A **septic** abortion is any type of abortion accompanied by uterine infection. • The Rhesus status of all women with first-trimester bleeding should be ascertained. • If the patient is found to be Rhesus negative, Rhesus D immunoglobulin should be given to help prevent Rhesus alloimmunization.

ANSWER:
A-d; B-c; C-b; D-a

48. Match the venereal infection with its appropriate characteristic.

A. Syphilis

B. Herpes

C. Gonorrhea

D. Condyloma acuminatum

a. Painful vesicles and intranuclear inclusion bodies

b. Purulent vaginal discharge and intracellular diplococci

c. Painless ulcer and positive findings on dark-field microscopic examination

d. Associated with cervical dysplasia

Ref.: 3

COMMENTS: Primary **syphilis** usually presents with a painless ulcer (chancre), which may resolve with or without antibiotic treatment. • The diagnosis is made by serologic tests that include a reactive plasma reagent test, a fluorescent treponemal antibody test, or a microhemagglutination assay of antibodies to *Treponema pallidum*. • Genital **herpes** is a viral disease that begins as multiple painful vesicles in the genital area. • Cytologic evaluation of herpes lesions may show intranuclear inclusion bodies and multinucleated giant cells. • There is currently no known cure for genital herpes. • Antiviral therapy, such as acyclovir, may accelerate healing but does not eradicate the infection. • **Gonorrhea** can present as a purulent urethritis or cervicitis, although most women are asymptomatic. • The diagnosis is made by identifying intracellular gram-negative diplococci in the vaginal discharge or

with positive culture results. • Concomittant treatment for chlamydia should be given to patients diagnosed with gonorrhea. • In addition, the sexual partner should be treated. • **Condyloma acuminatum**, or venereal warts, is caused HPV. • There is a strong association between this virus and genital dysplasia. • There is currently no known cure for HPV. • The lesions may be treated by various methods, including application of podophyllum and excision with laser, electrocautery, or cryotherapy.

ANSWER:
A-c; B-a; C-b; D-d

49. Noncontraceptive effects of combination (estrogen-progestin) oral contraceptives include all but which of the following?

A. Decreased incidence of dysmenorrhea

B. Decreased incidence of PID

C. Increased menstrual cycle regularity with decreased blood loss

D. Increased incidence of benign breast disease

Ref.: 3, 9

COMMENTS: When taken correctly, oral contraceptives provide excellent protection against unwanted pregnancies. • Patients are often unaware of the numerous noncontraceptive benefits of oral contraceptives. • It is essential that the clinician include discussion of these potential benefits when counseling patients. • Noncontraceptive benefits of oral contraceptives include reduction in dysmenorrhea, increased cycle regularity, decreased blood loss, decreased incidence of recurrent PID, decreased incidence of benign breast disease, decreased incidence of endometrial and ovarian cancers, and decreased incidence of functional ovarian cysts.

ANSWER:
D

50. Regarding triphasic oral contraceptives, which of the following is/are true?

A. The progestin dose varies throughout the cycle.

B. The estrogen dose varies throughout the cycle.

C. Both progestin and estrogen doses vary throughout the cycle.

D. Neither the progestin nor the estrogen dose varies throughout the cycle.

Ref.: 3, 9

COMMENTS: Triphasic and biphasic oral contraceptives are regarded as multiphasic. • In general, the estrogen dose in multiphasic pills does not vary. • There are three variations of the progestin dose in triphasic pills. • It is theorized that this decrease in total progestin dose would decrease breakthrough bleeding. • To date, there are no published, well-designed clinical trials comparing breakthrough bleeding in triphasic versus monophasic oral contraceptive pills.

ANSWER:
A

51. Match the clinical condition with its appropriate description.

 A. Bacterial vaginosis

 B. Trichomonal vaginitis

 C. Candidal vaginitis

 D. Atrophic vaginitis

 a. "Clue cells" seen on microscopic examination, vaginal discharge with fishy odor, and pH greater than 6.0

 b. Acid environment, cottage cheese–like vaginal discharge, and marked pruritus

 c. "Strawberry" cervix; considered a sexually transmitted disease

 d. Estrogen withdrawal

Ref.: 3

COMMENTS: Vaginitis can be caused by infections, allergic reactions, neoplasms, or foreign bodies. • **Bacterial vaginosis** occurs when there is an overgrowth of anaerobic bacteria. • This generally leads to an increase in vaginal pH. • Epithelial cells lined with bacteria ("clue cells") are commonly seen on microscopic evaluation of the vaginal fluid. • The addition of potassium hydroxide to the vaginal discharge results in an amide reaction and an abnormal fishy odor ("whiff test"). • **Trichomonal vaginitis** is a sexually transmitted disease caused by *Trichomonas vaginalis*. • These ovoid-shaped, flagellated organisms can be seen on microscopic examination. • Patients may have petechial subepithelial redness of the cervix, which gives a strawberry appearance. • **Atrophic vaginitis** occurs when estrogen levels available to the vagina fall below physiologic levels. • Patients with **candidal vaginitis** frequently have a cottage cheese–like discharge and/or pruritus. • Evaluation of the vaginal discharge frequently reveals an acidic environment.

ANSWER:
A-a; B-c; C-b; D-d

52. Regarding hormonal contraception, which of the following is/are currently approved routes of administration?

 A. Intramuscular

 B. Intranasal

 C. Transdermal

 D. Intravaginal

Ref.: 3, 9

COMMENTS: Hormonal contraception provides excellent protection against unwanted pregnancies when taken correctly. • To date, hormonal contraceptives can be administered by intramuscular, transdermal, and intravaginal routes. • Currently, there are no commercially available hormonal contraceptives that can be administered intranasally.

ANSWER:
A, C, D

53. Regarding adnexal masses, ultrasound features suggestive of malignancy include which of the following?

 A. Multiple thick septations

 B. Solid components

 C. Presence of ascites

 D. Increased resistive index of ovarian vessels

Ref.: 4, 14

COMMENTS: In the absence of extensive disease in the pelvis, ultrasonographic diagnosis of ovarian malignancy may be difficult. • Ultrasonographic features of adnexal masses suggestive of malignancy include bilaterality, presence of solid components, irregular borders, multiple thick septations, presence of ascites, persistent size greater than 6–8 cm, and decreased resistive index of ovarian vessels. • The decrease in the resistive index likely occurs as a result of neovascularization.

ANSWER:
A, B, C

54. All but which of the following is/are true of the menstrual cycle?

 A. Estrogen has two separate peaks.

 B. Progesterone peaks during the follicular phase.

 C. The slight decrease in estrogen seen after the luteinizing hormone (LH) surge is a result of a shift in steroid synthesis favoring progesterone.

 D. An estrogen level of at least 200 pg/ml for 2 days is required for the LH surge.

Ref.: 3, 9

COMMENTS: The typical menstrual cycle occurs as a result of fluctuating levels of gonadotropic and steroid hormones. • Estrogen predominates during the proliferative or follicular phase, enabling follicular development and endometrial proliferation. • An estrogen level of at least 200 pg/ml for 2 days is required for the LH surge. • A small decrease in estrogen occurs after the LH surge. • It is believed to occur as a result of a shift in steroid synthesis favoring progesterone. • Estrogen levels rise again and peak in the luteal phase. • Progesterone levels peak during and dominate the luteal phase.

ANSWER:
B

55. All but which of the following is/are true of the two-cell system of steroid hormone synthesis?

 A. LH receptors are present on thecal cells.

 B. Follicle-stimulating hormone (FSH) receptors are present on granulosal cells.

 C. LH induces aromatization of androgen in the thecal cells.

 D. FSH can induce LH receptor presence on granulosal cells.

Ref.: 3, 9

COMMENTS: The two-cell system of steroid synthesis involves the thecal and the granulosal cells. • LH receptors are present on thecal cells. • Binding of LH to these receptors results in androgen synthesis in the thecal cells. • The granulosal cells possess FSH receptors. • Androgens are transported to the granulosal cells, and under the influence of FSH, they undergo aromatization with production of estrogen. • During mid-cycle, an LH surge occurs, and FSH induces the presence of LH receptors on the granulosal cells (luteinization), enabling survival of the dominant follicle.

ANSWER:
C

56. Regarding tuboovarian abscesses (TOAs), which of the following is/are true?

   A. Initial outpatient oral antibiotic therapy is currently considered suboptimal treatment.

   B. Initial therapy should be nonsurgical.

   C. TOAs are present in approximately 50% of patients with PID.

   D. Unilateral removal can be used as conservative therapy for women desiring fertility.

Ref.: 3, 4

COMMENTS: TOAs are present in 10% of women with PID. • They are more common in women with concurrent bacterial vaginosis or human immunodeficiency virus. • TOAs contain a mixture of anaerobic and facultative or aerobic organisms. • Therefore, antibiotic therapy should cover a wide range of organisms, including *N. gonorrhoeae* and *C. trachomatis.* • Initial therapy with oral antibiotics does not appear to provide sufficient serum antibiotic levels necessary to treat TOAs. • In general, broad-spectrum intravenous antibiotics should be used as initial therapy. • If the patient's symptoms do not improve over 24–48 hr, alternative interventions, such as surgery, should be considered. • TOAs can be drained laparoscopically or under radiologic guidance. • There appears to be no difference in outcome between these approaches. • Midline pelvic TOAs may be drained through a posterior colpotomy. • Often, a temporary intraperitoneal catheter for drainage is left in place. • For patients who are not candidates for conservative procedures, resection of TOAs via laparotomy is commonly done. • TOAs involving both ovaries or the uterus are treated with hysterectomy and bilateral salpingo-oophorectomy. • Unilateral TOAs can be treated with unilateral adnexectomy for patients desiring fertility. • The abdominopelvic cavity should be extensively irrigated. • Ideally, the vaginal cuff should be left open or an intraperitoneal catheter placed for postoperative drainage. • Ruptured TOAs are surgical emergencies. • Patients should undergo prompt surgical treatment via laparotomy after they are hemodynamically stabilized. • These patients usually present with acute and progressive pelvic pain, and they may be hemodynamically unstable. • The mortality rate associated with a ruptured TOA is 5–10%. • Delay in diagnosis and treatment results in higher mortality rates. • Most patients undergo hysterectomy with bilateral salpingo-oophorectomy. • Conservative surgeries for ruptured TOAs have not been well studied. • Broad-spectrum intravenous antibiotics are continued until the patient is able to tolerate oral intake, and oral antibiotics are continued until the patient is afebrile.

ANSWER:
A, B, D

57. Regarding cervical intraepithelial neoplasia (CIN), which of the following is/are true?

   A. Dysplasia involving the middle third of the epithelium is considered CIN-III.

   B. The regression rate of CIN-II is about 40%.

   C. Cervical cone biopsy, cryotherapy, and laser ablation are all acceptable therapies for CIN-II.

   D. Compliant patients diagnosed with CIN-I can be observed.

Ref.: 3, 10

COMMENTS: CIN is a histologic diagnosis. • Abnormal cytologic findings on Pap smear usually prompt colposcopic evaluation with cervical biopsies. • Dysplasia involving the lower, middle, and upper third of the cervical epithelium are designated as CIN-I (mild dysplasia), CIN-II (moderate dysplasia), and CIN-III (severe dysplasia), respectively. • Progression of CIN to invasive cervical cancer is well established. • In general, higher-grade lesions are associated with higher rates of progression. • The rates of progression for CIN-I, -II, and -III lesions are 1%, 5%, and 12%, respectively, while the rates of regression for these lesions are 57%, 43%, and 32%, respectively. • Given the high rate of regression of CIN-I lesions, they can be observed over time, provided there is good patient compliance. • CIN-II and -III lesions are generally treated once diagnosed. • Treatment options include cervical conization, cryoablation, laser ablation, electrocautery ablation, and hysterectomy. • Cervical conization has the advantage of providing a pathologic specimen to rule out invasive disease. • Hysterectomy is reserved for patients with high-grade lesions or persistent low-grade lesions who have completed childbearing.

ANSWER:
B, C, D

58. Which of the following statements is/are true regarding trophoblastic disease?

   A. The risk of malignant metastatic trophoblastic disease following partial hydatidiform mole is 3–5%.

   B. Patients at high risk for metastatic trophoblastic disease include women with twins and women who smoke more than two packs of cigarettes per day.

   C. Hysterotomy is preferable to suction curettage when emptying a 16-week gestational-size uterus.

   D. Patients with nonmetastatic or low-risk gestational trophoblastic disease are 100% curable by chemotherapy.

   E. Complete hydatidiform moles are of paternal origin and carry a 20% risk of malignant sequelae.

Ref.: 1, 2, 3, 6

COMMENTS: Gestational trophoblastic disease is categorized as hydatidiform mole (partial or complete) and gestational trophoblastic neoplasia (metastatic and nonmetastatic). • About one half of the cases of gestational trophoblastic neoplasia follow molar pregnancy, one fourth follow normal pregnancy, and one fourth follow ectopic pregnancy or abortion. • Complete moles are of paternal origin are diploid and carry a 20% risk of malignant sequelae. • Partial moles are of maternal and paternal origin are triploid and rarely are followed by gestational trophoblastic neoplasia. • Hydatidiform moles are effectively and safely evacuated using suction curettage. • *Low-risk* gestational trophoblastic neoplasia is one in which the initial serum hCG titer is less than 40,000 mIU/ml, the disease has been present for less than 4 months, and there has been no previous chemotherapy. • It usually is treated with single-agent chemotherapy. • *High-risk* gestational trophoblastic neoplasia is characterized by one or more of the following: an initial serum hCG titer of more than 40,000 mIU/ml, disease present longer than 4 months, brain or liver metastases, and failure of previous chemotherapy. • It is treated with multiple-agent chemotherapy.

Prognostic Classification of Gestational Trophoblastic Neoplasia

1. Nonmetastatic GTN
2. Metastatic GTN: Disease outside the uterus
   A. Good prognosis:
      1. Disease present less than 4 months (short duration)
      2. Pretreatment hGC less than 40,000 mIU/ml
      3. No previous chemotherapy
   B. Poor prognosis:
      1. Disease present more than 4 months (long duration), or
      2. Pretreatment hCG greater than 40,000 mIU/ml, or
      3. Presence of brain or liver metastases, or
      4. Failure of previous chemotherapy

From Herbst AL, Mishell DR Jr, Stenchever MA, et al: *Comprehensive Gynecology*, 2nd ed. Mosby Year Book, St. Louis, 1992, p 934..

ANSWER:
A, D, E

REFERENCES

1. Townsend CM Jr, Beauchamp RD, Evers BM, et al (eds): *Sabiston Textbook of Surgery: The Biological Basis of Modern Surgical Practice*, 17th ed. WB Saunders, Philadelphia, 2004.
2. Brunicardi FC, Andersen DK, Billiar TR, et al (eds): *Schwartz's Principles of Surgery*, 8th ed. McGraw-Hill, New York, 2004.
3. Herbst AL, Mishell DR, Stenchever MA, et al: *Comprehensive Gynecology*, 4th ed. Mosby Year Book, St. Louis 2001.
4. Thompson JD, Rock AR: *Te Linde's Operative Gynecology*, 9th ed. Lippincott, Williams & Wilkins, Philadelphia, 2003.
5. Mullholland MW, Lillemoe KD, Doherty GM, et al (eds): *Greenfield's Surgery: Scientific Principles and Practice*, 4th ed. Lippincott, Williams & Wilkins, Philadelphia, 2006.
6. Hoskins WJ: *Principles and Practice of Gynecologic Oncology*, 3rd ed. Lippincott, Williams & Wilkins, Philadelphia, 2000.
7. Gabbe SG: *Obstetrics*, 4th ed. Churchill-Livingstone, New York, 2001.
8. Cunningham FG: *Williams Obstetrics*, 21st ed. McGraw-Hill, New York, 2001.
9. Speroff L: *A Clinical Guide for Contraception*, 3rd ed. Lippincott, Williams & Wilkins, Philadelphia, 2000.
10. Berek JS: *Practical Gynecologic Oncology*, 3rd ed. Lippincott, Williams & Wilkins, Philadelphia, 2000.
11. DiSaia PJ: *Clinical Gynecologic Oncology*, 6th ed. CV Mosby, St. Louis, 2002.
12. Bent AE: *Ostergard's Urogynecology and Pelvic Floor Dysfunction*, 5th ed. Lippincott, Williams & Wilkins, Philadelphia, 2003.
13. Rossouw JE, Anderson GL, Prentice RL, et al: Writing Group for the Women's Health Initiative Investigators. Risks and benefits of estrogen plus progestin in healthy postmenopausal women: principal results from the Women's Health Initiative randomized controlled trial. *JAMA*. 288:321–333, 2002.
14. Callen PW: *Ultrasound study in Obstetrics and Gynecology*, 4th ed. WB Saunders, Philadelphia, 2000.

C H A P T E R **50**

Neurosurgery

Richard W. Byrne, M.D.

1. Which of the following statements regarding neuronal function is/are true?

    A. The resting membrane potential is dependent on sodium and potassium ion concentrations and the sodium/potassium-dependent ATPase pump. The action potential is dependent on changes in the permeability to ions, specifically sodium and potassium.

    B. Myelin provides the axon with necessary insulation to slow the action potential.

    C. γ-Aminobutyric acid (GABA) is the major neurotransmitter at the neuromuscular junction.

    D. The sections of myelin along the axon are known as nodes of Ranvier.

Ref.: 1

COMMENTS: Neuronal physiology depends on a semipermeable membrane that, along with a membrane-bound ATPase pump, keeps two important ions—sodium and potassium—at markedly different concentrations. • An action potential is a self-propagating ionic current that results from opening voltage gated channels, allowing a drastic change in the permeability of sodium and potassium ions. • Myelin is produced by Schwann cells to cover axons on the peripheral nerves and by oligodendrocytes to cover axons of the brain and spinal cord. • Myelin offers insulation to decrease the diffusion of ionic current needed to propagate the axon potential and therefore increase the velocity of the action potential. • The axon is lined by myelin sheaths, which are interrupted by areas of bare axon called nodes of Ranvier. • This arrangement allows a faster, interrupted style of conduction known as saltatory conduction. • The neuromuscular junction involves the release of acetylcholine from synaptic vesicles as a result of an action potential and the acetylcholine receptor on the muscle cell. • Activation of this receptor causes ionic permeability changes, leading to release of calcium from the sarcoplasmic reticulum with activation of actinomycin and subsequent muscular contraction. • The hallmark neurologic disorder involving the neuromuscular junction is myasthenia gravis, which is an autoimmune disorder involving the blocking of an acetylcholine receptor.

ANSWER:
A

2. Which of the following statements regarding diagnostic procedures used to evaluate the central nervous system (CNS) is/are true?

    A. Magnetic resonance imaging (MRI) is the most useful initial test in the evaluation of spinal cord compression.

    B. Magnetic resonance angiography (MRA) eliminates the risk associated with cerebral angiography.

    C. Water-soluble contrast material has decreased the incidence of arachnoiditis following myelography.

    D. Computed tomographic (CT) scanning is the best available radiographic test for soft tissue evaluation.

Ref.: 2–4, 11

COMMENTS: Angiography is the main method of demonstrating vascular lesions and is useful for preoperative evaluation of neoplasms and certain cases of trauma. • Its major stroke danger—as a result of vessel manipulation—may be eliminated by the use of **MRA**, but the images obtained with MRA are of slightly inferior quality. • **Myelography** is the radiographic study of the spinal cord and spinal canal after subarachnoid injection of contrast material. • The use of water-soluble contrast media has decreased the incidence of postprocedure arachnoiditis. • In most institutions, myelography is used with CT scanning. • This method is most useful for the evaluation of intervertebral disc disease. • The **CT scan** is at present the most useful diagnostic tool for identifying acute hemorrhage or fracture. • Modern units provide resolution in the range of 1 mm. • The major disadvantage of CT scans is the artifact created by the bone coverings of the CNS. • In the evaluation of intracranial processes, **MRI** is superior to CT scanning in many cases because it does not expose the patient to radiation, is associated with minimal bone artifact, yields high-grade differentiation of gray-white matter, and can directly scan in multiple planes. • MRI is the best diagnostic tool for soft-tissue evaluation. • Hence, MRI is the most useful initial test for cord compression.

ANSWER:
A, B, C

3. Which of the following statements regarding scalp injuries is/are true?

    A. The blood supply to the scalp lies between the periosteum and the galea.

B. Most scalp laceration hemorrhages can be controlled by applying direct pressure.

C. Subgaleal hematomas must be drained to avoid abscess formation and extensive scalp elevation.

D. If a scalp laceration extends below the zygoma, the ipsilateral vagus nerve may be injured.

Ref.: 2, 3

COMMENTS: The scalp consists of five layers: skin, subcutaneous, galea aponeurotica, loose areolar tissue, periosteum (SCALP). • The skin and galea are the layers of surgical importance, with the blood supply lying between the skin above and the galea below. • Since the blood supply to the scalp is rich, lacerations can be accompanied by significant blood loss. • When the underlying skull is intact, this blood loss can be controlled by simple pressure. • If the skull is fractured, direct pressure may be hazardous to the underlying brain. • Pulling the retracted galea back over the wound edge with forceps often controls such hemorrhage. • Contusions causing subgaleal hemorrhage can lead to the formation of large subgaleal hematomas that can elevate extensive portions of the scalp off the skull. • For this condition, compression dressings can reduce the extent of hematoma formation. • If the overlying scalp is viable and there is no evidence of infection, subgaleal hematomas should be left alone to resolve naturally, a process that may require several weeks. • If the hematoma is infected, it is necessary to evacuate it. • The occipitalis and frontalis muscles insert on the galea, and their contraction tends to separate areas of galeal disruptions. • Therefore, even small lacerations of the galea should be closed. • As for nonoperative treatment of subgaleal hematomas, large lacerations with significant loss of galeal or subgaleal tissue should be treated with compression dressings after appropriate débridement and closure to minimize the chances of postoperative subgaleal hematoma and infection. • The largest arteries supplying the scalp, the superficial temporal and occipital arteries, originate from the external carotid arteries. • The facial nerve runs below the zygoma, and it may be injured if a laceration extends into the face.

ANSWER:
B

4. Which of the following statements regarding hydrocephalus is the most accurate?

A. It represents a primary process in up to two thirds of patients.

B. It is classified as communicating or noncommunicating, depending on where the obstruction to cerebrospinal fluid (CSF) flow occurs.

C. With proper shunting, patients with hydrocephalus usually have intelligence equal to that of matched control groups without hydrocephalus.

D. Hydrocephalus ex vacuo is more common in the young.

Ref.: 2, 3

COMMENTS: Hydrocephalus is a secondary, not a primary, problem. • Causes of hydrocephalus include aqueductal stenosis, dysfunction of arachnoid granulations, subarachnoid scarring, and CSF blockage by clot or tumor. • Hydrocephalus is classified as communicating or noncommunicating. • With **communicating hydrocephalus**, obstruction to flow is outside the ventricular system. • With **noncommunicating hydrocephalus**, there is obstruction to flow of the CSF inside the ventricular system. • The clinical features of **infantile hydrocephalus** include diastasis of the cranial sutures, weakness of upward gaze (the "setting sun" sign), enlarging head circumference, and a bulging anterior fontanelle. • Clinical features of hydrocephalus past 1 year of age (when the cranial sutures are closed) include headache, nausea, vomiting, visual loss, and lethargy. • In some cases, this progresses to coma and death without proper treatment. • Most cases of hydrocephalus are treated by pressure-activated shunts, the most common being the ventriculoperitoneal (VP) shunt. • Although treated patients usually attain acceptable levels of intelligence (and some, in fact, are very bright), overall, patients with shunts do not do as well intellectually as nonhydrocephalic matched control groups. • The outcome largely depends on the cause of the hydrocephalus. • **Hydrocephalus ex vacuo** refers to enlarged ventricles secondary to cerebral insult or atrophy. • Therefore, it is more common in the elderly.

ANSWER:
B

5. Which of the following statements regarding intracranial pressure (ICP) monitoring is/are true?

A. Although ventricular pressure monitoring is the reference standard for ICP, it has a higher risk of causing hemorrhage and infection.

B. In patients with a Glasgow Coma Scale (GCS) score of 3–8 after resuscitation who have an abnormal head CT scan, intracranial pressure monitoring may be appropriate.

C. Risk factors for elevated ICP after head injury include age less than 40, open basal cisterns on CT scanning, and systolic blood pressure over 90 mmHg.

D. Normal ICP is 0–15 mmHg or 0–20 cmH$_2$O.

Ref.: 5, 6, 11

COMMENTS: Because of the approximately 1% risk of hemorrhage and 5% infection risk with ICP monitoring, this procedure is not appropriate for all patients with head injury. • ICP monitoring is appropriate in patients with a GCS score of 3–8 with an abnormal head CT scan or for select patients with normal CT and risk factors for elevated ICP, such as age over 40 and systolic blood pressure less than 90 mmHg. • Ventricular catheter ICP measurements are accurate but carry a higher risk of complications than do intraparenchymal monitors. • The normal ICP is 0–15 mmHg, but the ICP is usually not treated in most centers until it rises to 20 mmHg or higher.

ANSWERS:
A, B, D

6. Which of the following statements regarding traumatic CSF leaks is/are true?

A. Most are due to basilar skull fractures and close spontaneously.

B. The risk of infection is greater with rhinorrhea than with otorrhea.

C. They require immediate surgical repair to avert infection.

D. They may be observed for up to 14 days if there is no evidence of infection.

Ref.: 2, 3, 5

COMMENTS: Most traumatic CSF fistulas close spontaneously. • They should be managed in the hospital under close supervision. • Placement of a lumbar drain to divert the fistula can be helpful. • The risk of persistent drainage and infection is greater with rhinorrhea than with otorrhea. • Otorrhea or rhinorrhea that persists for more than 10–14 days despite lumbar drainage is an indication for repair of the torn dura if the site of the CSF leak can be found. • Some patients can go on for years with a CSF leak without sequelae. • The overall incidence of CSF leak with head injury is 0.25–0.50%.

ANSWER:
A, B, D

7. Which of the following statements regarding brain injury is/are true?

   A. The extent of brain injury is a function of the mechanism of injury.

   B. Contusions tend to involve the anterior portions of the frontal and temporal lobes.

   C. Diffuse axonal injury is usually an incidental finding.

   D. The effects of secondary edema and hematoma enlargement may be delayed for several days.

Ref.: 2, 3, 5, 11

COMMENTS: **Localized force** can cause damage to the scalp, skull, and underlying brain in the immediate area of injury. • The resulting neurologic deficit is related to the area of the brain directly involved and usually produces brief or no loss of consciousness. • Applications of **generalized force** to the skull, such as that caused by impact of the head against an immovable object, allow diffuse transmission of energy, causing injury to the whole brain. • In such a case, the brain insult is generalized, often producing altered consciousness, and its severity is related to the mechanism of injury. • For example, the injury may be the result of linear or rotational acceleration-deceleration of the brain against the confining cranium, such as when the head hits an immovable object. • When the brain strikes the rigid skull, contusions occur in the area where the force is applied as well as against the opposite inner surface of the skull (contrecoup injury). • Rotation of the brain within the skull may cause tearing of axons, resulting in diffuse axonal injury within the white matter, a so-called shearing injury, which is often severe. • The undersurface of the frontal lobes, the anterior portions of the temporal lobes, the posterior portions of the occipital lobes, and the upper portion of the midbrain are more likely to suffer contusions because they are relatively more confined by bone or dural shelves. • The contusion may be clinically silent initially if the involved area of the brain has no demonstrable clinical function. • These injuries often become apparent days after the injury as edema accumulates, creating the effects of an intracranial mass. • Occasionally, a hematoma accumulates in the area of contusion 24–72 hr after injury, a situation seen more often in elderly persons. • Gunshot brain injuries are often severe because of damage caused by the bullet and the associated shock wave that travels along the path. • The primary injury, bleeding, swelling, and infection result in high mortality rates.

ANSWER:
A, B, D

8. Which of the following statements regarding the evaluation and care of head-injured patients is the most accurate?

   A. Hypotension is often the direct result of intracranial trauma.

   B. Decerebrate posturing is a common response to diffuse cortical injury.

   C. A score of 5 on the GCS is associated with a poor prognosis.

   D. Inappropriate secretion of antidiuretic hormone (ADH) should be suspected when the serum sodium level exceeds 150 mEq/L.

Ref.: 2, 3, 11

COMMENTS: The initial care of the head-injured patient must focus on maintenance of ventilation, control of hemorrhage, and maintenance of the peripheral circulation. • Continued hypotension and tachycardia are rarely the direct result of head trauma and should alert the examiner to the existence of a systemic hemorrhage. • In fact, intracranial hemorrhage with elevated intracranial pressure often manifests as hypertension and bradycardia. • As soon as possible, there should be a careful neurologic examination and documentation of the level of consciousness to obtain a baseline against which the patient's progress is measured. • Decerebrate posturing (extension and internal rotation of the extremities, neck extension, and arching of the back) implies compression of or damage to the brain stem and often requires immediate therapy. • In a patient unconscious for more than 6 hr, the GCS is useful for predicting eventual outcome. • It measures motor (M), verbal (V), and eye (E) responses on scales of 1–6, 1–5, and 1–4, respectively. • It is recorded as a sum of the highest score in each category. • Patients with a score lower than 5 have a mortality rate higher than 50%. • Patients who have lost the reflex capability to protect their airway should be intubated and their stomachs decompressed by a nasogastric tube. • A Foley catheter should be placed and serum and urine electrolytes monitored. • Inappropriate secretion of ADH should be suspected when serum osmolality and sodium levels fall in association with an increase in urinary osmolality. • Restriction of water intake or the use of solute diuretics may be necessary to control this problem. • The body temperature must be closely monitored because head injuries may be accompanied by the loss of capacity for superficial cutaneous vasodilation and sweating, leading to hyperthermia.

ANSWER:
C

9. Which of the following statements regarding cerebral edema caused by head injury is the most accurate?

   A. CT scans should be obtained to exclude the diagnosis of intracranial hemorrhage or a mass lesion before starting therapy.

   B. Cerebral edema caused by head injury is vasogenic and not cytotoxic in origin.

   C. Steroids are useful for treatment of head trauma.

   D. Hypercapnea induces cerebral vasoconstriction and is useful for decreasing intracerebral blood volume.

Ref.: 2, 3, 5

COMMENTS: The brain responds to injury by forming edema. • The bony confines of the skull impose a narrow tolerance for swelling before the intracranial pressure equals the arterial pressure. • When this occurs, perfusion stops and neuronal death follows in 4–5 minutes. • The onset of edema usually is slow and reaches a maximal level within 48–72 hr after injury. • The progress of cerebral edema can be followed by the neurologic exam, CT scanning, and the use of intracranial pressure-monitoring devices. • These devices are commonly used to monitor patients with altered consciousness following head injury or patients with GCS scores lower than 8. • After a baseline CT scan is obtained to rule out intracranial hemorrhage or a mass lesion, treatment is started as soon as possible to counter the progress of edema. • This can be accomplished by (1) elevating the head of the bed 15–30 degrees, (2) intermittent drainage of CSF by a pressure-monitoring catheter placed in the frontal horn of the lateral ventricle, (3) hyperventilation to PCO_2 levels of 30–35 mmHg to induce vasoconstriction, and (4) the use of fluid restriction and solute diuretics to minimize edema. • Steroids are thought to decrease inflammation and swelling, but their effectiveness in the treatment of cytotoxic cerebral edema resulting from head trauma has not been established. • Steroids are useful in tumor cases where vasogenic edema predominates.

ANSWER:
A

10. Which of the following statements regarding subarachnoid hemorrhage (SAH) is the most accurate?

A. A normal CT scan of the brain excludes the possibility of a subarachnoid hemorrhage.

B. Aneurysms occur most frequently on the basilar artery.

C. Surgical or endovascular correction within 48–72 hr is recommended in patients who are neurologically intact and have an uncomplicated aneurysm.

D. The use of hypertension, hypervolemia, and calcium-channel blockers is contraindicated for treatment of vasospasm.

Ref.: 2, 3, 6

COMMENTS: Sudden headache followed by altered consciousness is the usual clinical pattern following SAH. • Focal neurologic deficits may occur, but they are less common than those seen after occlusion of major intracranial arteries. • The sequelae vary, depending on the size of the hemorrhage, and range from headache to death. • Although CT scanning is the diagnostic method of choice to confirm an SAH, approximately 10% of patients with documented hemorrhages have a normal CT scan within 24 hr of SAH. • It is important, therefore, to perform a lumbar puncture when SAH is suspected and the CT scan is negative for SAH. • Angiography is helpful to confirm the presence of an aneurysm. • Most intracranial aneurysms arise from the large intracranial arteries of the circle of Willis and at the origin of the vertebrobasilar arteries. • The most common sites of SAH, in decreasing order of prevalence, are the internal carotid artery, anterior cerebral artery, middle cerebral artery, and vertebrobasilar system. • Multiple aneurysms are present 20% of the time. • When multiple, they tend to be symmetric in distribution or arise from the same parent artery. • Most aneurysms are the result of defects in the muscular and elastic layers of the intracerebral arteries. • They have a saccular or berry-like shape, hence the name *berry aneurysm*. • The incidence of silent aneurysms is the same in patients with and without hypertension, but rupture is more common in patients with hypertension. • The incidence of rupture is highest in patients between the ages of 40 and 60 years.

The goal of treatment is to isolate the aneurysm from the force of systolic blood flow. • This should be attempted as early as possible because the likelihood of secondary rupture is approximately 20% by 2 weeks after SAH. • It is recommended that surgical correction be performed within 48–72 hr in patients who are neurologically intact with an approachable aneurysm. • A relative contraindication to early surgical intervention is the presence of a neurologic deficit resulting from spasm of the circle of Willis

caused by the irritating effect of blood in the CSF. • The rationale for early surgical correction—that the patient then can be treated aggressively for vasospasm—is based on the concept of maximizing cerebral perfusion. • A calcium-channel–blocking agent (nimodipine), relative hypertension, and hypervolemia are recommended for treatment of vasospasm. • Other treatments are advocated, however, and there is no proven effective treatment for symptomatic cerebral vasospasm as a result of subarachnoid hemorrhage. • The incidence of hydrocephalus is 15–20% in patients after a subarachnoid hemorrhage, and many of these patients eventually require a shunt for this complication. • Some aneurysms with a narrow neck can be coiled or stented under fluoroscopy. • Short-term results of this approach are promising, but long-term data are pending.

ANSWER:
C

11. Which of the following statements regarding subdural hematomas is/are true?

A. Acute subdural hematomas are usually unilateral and have a poorer prognosis than do chronic subdural hematomas.

B. Adequate treatment of an acute subdural hematoma generally consists of drainage through burr holes.

C. Chronic subdural hematomas frequently recur.

D. Chronic subdural hematomas should be suspected in elderly patients with progressive changes in mental status, even without a definite history of trauma.

Ref.: 2, 3, 5, 11

COMMENTS: Subdural hematomas are caused by rupture of veins traversing the subdural space or by arterial bleeding from parenchymal laceration. • Their presentation and treatment depend on the rapidity of hematoma formation. • All types of subdural hematomas (acute, subacute, and chronic) have in common the presence of a decreased level of consciousness out of proportion to the observed focal neurologic deficit.

Acute subdural hematomas are those that cause progressive neurologic deficit within 48 hr of injury. • They usually follow severe head trauma, are unilateral, have both arterial and venous sources of bleeding, and can progress rapidly. • The diagnosis should be considered in any patient with a severe head injury who shows deteriorated neurologic status or who is unresponsive with a focal neurologic deficit. • The hematomas are solid and easily visualized by CT scan. • They can be bilateral, and adjacent intracerebral hematomas often are present. • Treatment requires formal craniotomy with removal of solid clot and control of bleeding points.

Subacute subdural hematomas are defined as those more than 48 hr but less than 2 weeks old. • The patients usually are less severely injured than those with acute subdural hematomas, and marked fluctuation of the level of consciousness or headache should alert surgeons to the diagnosis. • With large hematomas, third-nerve paresis with pupil dilatation is a warning that midbrain compression due to temporal lobe herniation is occurring. • CT scans may not identify the mass because the hematoma becomes isodense 10–12 days after its formation, and there may be bilateral hematomas. • If the clot is completely liquefied, burr holes are therapeutic as well.

Chronic subdural hematomas most often occur in elderly people, frequently without a clear history of antecedent trauma. • They can occur months after the initial injury and should be suspected in patients with a decreasing or fluctuating mental status out of proportion to the focal neurologic deficit. • The hematoma is liquid, and drainage via burr holes is usually all that is necessary for treatment. • Chronic subdural hematomas frequently recur when they are associated with multiple subdural membranes. • In some of these cases, craniotomy to strip the membranes is necessary. • Subdural peritoneal shunting may also be necessary.

ANSWER:
A, C, D

12. Which of the following statements regarding surgical treatment of epilepsy is the most accurate?

   A. Surgery for focal epilepsy without an associated lesion is considered only after a significant trial of medical therapy.

   B. Surgery for primary generalized epilepsy is often successful.

   C. The chance for rendering a patient seizure free with temporal lobectomy for temporal epilepsy is about 20%.

   D. With modern medicines now available, epilepsy surgery is becoming less common.

Ref.: 2, 3, 6, 7

COMMENTS: The surgical treatment of epilepsy is a valuable option for well-selected patients. • Patients who are medically intractable, who are proven to have a localizable seizure focus, and who can accept the risks and consequences of surgery are candidates for surgery. • Most seizure foci in adults are in the temporal lobe, where surgical removal is associated with a seizure-free rate of 60–70% in most series. • Primary generalized (idiopathic) epilepsy is rarely aided by surgery, although the vagal nerve stimulator is an option. • Advances in differentiating primary and focal onset seizures and advances in surgery have made epilepsy surgery a progressively more common therapeutic choice. • Other surgical treatments are tailor made for specific problems. • **Corpus callosotomy** for drop attacks and **hemispherectomy** for a patient with a dysfunctional epileptogenic hemisphere are rare but useful procedures in carefully selected patients. • Most recently, **multiple subpial transection**, a procedure that selectively isolates a seizure focus, has been shown to be useful.

ANSWER:
A

13. Current uses of stereotaxis in neurosurgery include which of the following?

   A. Treatment of spinal cord injury

   B. Biopsy of brain tumors

   C. Stimulation of the ventralis intermedius nucleus thalamus for essential tumor

   D. Radiosurgery for treatment of arteriovenous malformation (AVM)

Ref.: 3, 6

COMMENTS: Stereotaxis has been a useful aid in localizing, biopsying, or ablating lesions in the brain. • A stereotactic frame is placed on the patient's head, and a CT or MRI scan is obtained. • This image shows the lesion or target in relationship to posts on the head frame. • With these points as a reference, X, Y, and Z coordinates with possible trajectories to the target are chosen.

• This allows the surgeon to pass a probe through a small hole in the skull to the target with millimeter accuracy. • This approach is being used in some patients with Parkinson's disease and patients with essential tremor. • The basic idea of stereotaxis with a frame is being used for **stereotactic irradiation** targeted at AVMs and some tumors.

ANSWER
B, C, D

14. Which of the following statements regarding subarachnoid hemorrhage following trauma is/are true?

   A. It is one of the most common intracranial hemorrhages following head trauma.

   B. It usually produces meningismus (stiff neck and headache).

   C. Mass effect from the subarachnoid blood is a major concern.

   D. It may produce communicating hydrocephalus as a late complication.

Ref.: 2, 3, 11

COMMENTS: One of the most common intracranial hemorrhages following head injury is subarachnoid hemorrhage. • It usually causes signs of meningismus (stiff neck and headache) and changes in the patient's mental status. • Because the hemorrhage is small and rapidly diluted by the CSF, no localized mass effect occurs. • Therefore, this type of hemorrhage after trauma has little surgical significance. • Rarely, it leads to progressive communicating hydrocephalus requiring shunting.

ANSWER:
A, B, D

15. Which of the following statements regarding intracranial vascular malformations is the most accurate?

   A. AVMs are the most common vascular malformations in the brain.

   B. Venous angiomas commonly bleed, and surgical removal is usually required.

   C. To plan surgical excision of a cavernous angioma properly, angiography should be performed.

   D. AVMs have a 2–4% incidence of hemorrhage per year.

Ref.: 2, 6

COMMENTS: Vascular malformations in the brain include venous angiomas, cavernous angiomas, capillary telangiectasias, and **AVMs**. • AVMs receive more attention than do the other, more common lesions because of their propensity to cause seizure or life-threatening hemorrhage. • Most AVMs are symptomatic when found. • During the era of MRI, the other lesions are commonly incidental findings. • In fact, CT scanning or MRI is necessary to find a **cavernous angioma**, which is not visible on the angiogram. • AVMs have irregular vessel walls, and 10% have aneurysms. • These irregularities lead to a 2–3% incidence of hemorrhage per year. • This risk must be balanced against surgical risks as measured by lesion size, location, and drainage pattern.

ANSWER:
D

16. Which of the following statements regarding peripheral nerve injuries is/are true?

   A. Neuraproxia requires surgical resection of the nerve root involved if pain is to be eliminated.

   B. Axonal regeneration progresses at a rate of 1 mm per day after a 10- to 20-day lag period.

   C. Denervation atrophy of muscles becomes irreversible after 12–15 months.

   D. Restoration of sensory loss is not possible after the muscle atrophy following denervation is complete.

Ref.: 2, 3, 11

COMMENTS: There are several classifications of nerve injuries. • The Seddon classification uses three terms to classify nerve injuries: neuropraxia, axonotmesis, and neurotmesis. • With **neurapraxia**, anatomic continuity of the nerve is preserved, and often there is incomplete motor paralysis with little muscle atrophy and considerable sparing of sensory and autonomic function. • Operative repair is not indicated, and the quality of recovery is excellent. • **Axonotmesis** is the loss of axonal continuity without interruption of the investing myelin tissue. • There is complete motor, sensory, and autonomic paralysis and progressive muscle atrophy. • Operative repair is not indicated, and recovery occurs at the rate of about 1 mm/day. • **Neurotmesis** is a more severe injury, with significant disorganization within the nerve or actual disruption of continuity of the nerve and its investing tissues.

Recovery is impossible without operative repair. • After disruption, axonal sprouting begins within 10–20 days. • If the injury is not repaired, scar tissue blocks the entrance of axonal sprouts into the distal nerve, and the axons coil into a disorganized neuroma that can be quite painful. • After operative repair, distal growth occurs at the rate of 1 mm/day after the initial 10- to 20-day lag period. • The degree of recovery is a function of the patient's age (with greater recovery in younger patients), type of nerve involved (pure motor or sensory nerves recover better than do mixed nerves), level of nerve injury (distal is better), and duration of denervation (shorter is better). • If more than 12–15 months are required for regenerating axons to reach a denervated muscle, a significant degree of denervation atrophy will have occurred, which is irreversible. • In contrast, sensory loss may be recovered after prolonged periods of denervation, and thus a nerve repair can provide protective sensory function in the atrophied distal extremity.

ANSWER:
B, C

17. Match the brain tumor type in the left-hand column with the most appropriate statement in the right-hand column.

   A. Glioma   a. Most common type of brain tumor

   B. Meningioma   b. Most common type of primary brain tumor

   C. Cerebral metastasis   c. Arises from the eighth cranial nerve

   D. Acoustic neuroma d. More common in women, is extra-axial, and is commonly found parasagittally

Ref.: 2, 3, 6, 7, 11

COMMENTS: No uniformly accepted system of classification for brain tumors has been developed. • One system, developed by

J.W. Kernohan and G.P. Sayre, is based on naming the tumor for the cells present in the adult nervous system, vascular tissue, and developmental defects (e.g., astrocytoma, medulloblastoma, and oligodendrocytoma) combined with grading the malignancy (where appropriate) from grade I (least malignant) to grade IV (most malignant). • Another method classifies tumors according to location: intra-axial neuroectodermal (gliomas), intra-axial nonneuroectodermal (e.g., metastases and blood vessel tumors), and extra-axial (meningiomas). • Most primary brain tumors are **gliomas**, the most common of which, in adults, is the highly malignant glioblastoma multiforme (astrocytoma grade IV). • The most commonly used grading system for astrocytomas is that of the World Health Organization, which includes low-grade astrocytomas, anaplastic astrocytomas (intermediate malignant potential), and glioblastoma multiforme (malignant). • Other gliomas include medulloblastomas, oligodendrogliomas, and ependymomas. • **Nonglial tumors** include meningiomas, pituitary tumors, neurilemmomas, blood vessel tumors, and metastatic tumors. • Approximately 25% of patients who die of cancer have **brain metastases** on autopsy. • The most common brain metastases are from lung, breast, melanoma, and kidney cancers. • Half of all patients with brain metastases will have a single metastasis. • If these patients do not have widespread disease, they are considered for surgery. • Meningiomas arise from the arachnoid layer over the surface of the brain and are therefore extra-axial. • Acoustic neuromas arise from the vestibulochoclear nerve (eighth), causing hearing loss and deficits related to local mass effect on the brain stem or other cranial nerves.

ANSWER:
A-b; B-d; C-a; D-c

18. A 53-year-old banker with a history of lung cancer presents to the physician's office with difficulty ambulating. On examination, he has nystagmus, dysmetria, and an ataxic gait. What statement is the single best answer concerning this patient?

   A. There is likely to be an abnormality in the corpus callosum.

   B. The most common tumor in the adult posterior fossa is an acoustic neuroma.

   C. A posterior fossa mass is likely. Additional symptoms in this patient, including confusion, nuchal rigidity, and cranial nerve palsies, are highly suggestive of meningeal carcinomatosis.

   D. Radiation therapy is better than surgical treatment when dealing with solitary metastatic brain lesions.

Ref.: 2, 3, 7

COMMENTS: Metastatic brain tumors constitute at least 25% of adult brain tumors. • This patient's symptoms are suggestive of cerebellar dysfunction. • In the adult population, the most common tumors found in the posterior fossa are metastatic lesions. • Another common presentation of metastatic disease of the CNS is **meningeal carcinomatosis**. • Symptoms suggestive of this disease include confusion, nuchal rigidity, pain, and multiple cranial nerve palsies. • Diagnosis is usually obtained by performing a lumbar puncture with isolation of malignant cells and CSF cytologic studies. • When dealing with patients with a metastatic brain lesion, the first question to address is whether it is a solitary lesion or multiple lesions. • If it is a solitary lesion, the patient has at least a 6-month expected longevity from the systemic cancer, and the lesion is in a surgically accessible region, surgical resection followed by limited brain radiation therapy is strongly recommended.

• If the lesions are multiple, biopsy may be done (to confirm the diagnosis only), and whole-brain radiation therapy is strongly recommended.

ANSWER

C

19. Which of the following statements regarding peripheral nerve injury is the most accurate?

A. Recovery is influenced by the cause of the injury, the patient's age, the type of nerve injured, and the severity of injury to nearby vessels and bone.

B. Injuries of peripheral nerves during surgical positioning are usually neurotmesis and have a good prognosis for recovery.

C. Electromyography (EMG) is useful during the first week of peripheral nerve injury.

D. *Causalgia* refers to the cause of nerve injury.

Ref.: 1–3, 7, 11

COMMENTS: Traumatic peripheral nerve injury requires surgical repair in cases of neurotmesis, where a nerve and its connective tissues are disrupted. • This is common with penetrating trauma and less common with compression injury, such as that seen with surgical positioning. • Early repair of the severed nerve has the advantage of clearer anatomy and a longer period for regeneration, but late repair also has advantages. • The timing of surgical repair is controversial and depends on many factors, which are weighed in each case. • When the repair is done, a primary repair in a pure nerve (pure motor or pure sensory) near the target muscle gives the best results. • With peripheral nerve injury, the site of injury and nerve activity can be detected by EMG only after 2–3 weeks. • A rare late consequence of peripheral nerve injury is **causalgia**, a painful condition causing burning sensations in the distribution of a partially injured mixed peripheral nerve. • Treatment is with phenoxybenzamine or sympathectomy in intractable cases.

ANSWER:

A

20. Match the spinal tumor in the left-hand column with the most appropriate characterization in the right-hand column.

A. Schwannoma   a. Associated with a sinus tract, congenital

B. Metastasis   b. Intradural, extramedullary

C. Ependymoma   c. Epidural, causes bone erosion

D. Dermoid   d. Intramedullary

Ref.: 2, 3, 7

COMMENTS: Spinal cord tumors are one sixth as common as intracranial tumors. • Although most intracranial adult tumors are malignant, 60% of spinal cord tumors are benign. • Many malignant spinal cord tumors seem to have a better prognosis than do their intracranial counterparts. • **Metastatic** tumors occur as frequently as primary tumors. • Spinal metastases and primary spinal neoplasms (malignant and benign) are classified according to their relationship to the dura and spinal cord. • They are divided into extradural and intradural groups, the intradural group being divided into the extramedullary and intramedullary locations.

• Most extradural spinal tumors are metastatic. • Common intradural, extramedullary tumors in the spine are **schwannomas**, meningiomas, and neurofibromas. • Common intramedullary tumors are astrocytomas and **ependymomas**. • Dermoid tumors of the lumbar spine are usually associated with a sinus tract, which reaches the skin. • Dermoid sinus tracts can be mistaken for pilonidal cysts. • **Dermoid** sinus tracts extend intradurally, and therefore surgery is more complicated.

ANSWER:

A-b; B-c; C-d; D-a

21. Match the nerve root in the left-hand column with the dermatome and myotome it innervates in the right-hand column.

A. C7   a. Dermatome: posterior thigh, large toe; myotome: extensor hallucis longus and anterior tibialis

B. T4   b. Dermatome: inguinal area; myotome: iliopsoas

C. L1   c. Dermatome: finger tips of middle fingers; myotome: triceps

D. L5   d. Dermatome: anterior and posterior chest; myotome: intercostal muscles

Ref.: 6, 7

COMMENTS: Thirty-one paired spinal nerves provide afferent and efferent innervation to the body. • Compression of a spinal nerve can lead to pain, numbness, or weakness in the distribution of that spinal nerve. • This is known as **radiculopathy**. • When the radiculopathy presents with pain only, certain ones mimic common medical conditions. • A left-sided midthoracic radiculopathy can be mistaken for cardiac disease, a right-sided lower thoracic radiculopathy can mimic gallbladder disease, and an L1 or L2 radiculopathy can be mistaken for hernia symptoms. • Disc herniations at these levels are uncommon. • Common levels for disc herniation are C5-6, C6-7, L4-5, and L5-S1. • The disc herniation usually causes a radiculopathy in the nerve root paired with the lower vertebra (e.g., C5-6 causes C6 radiculopathy).

ANSWER:

A-c; B-d; C-b; D-a

22. Which of the following statements regarding cervical spine fractures is the most accurate?

A. Cervical spine fractures are usually not visible on plain x-rays but require CT scanning or MRI for diagnosis.

B. Tachycardia is a common response to cervical spinal cord injury.

C. In a patient with a complete cervical spinal cord injury, early surgery has been shown to make a significant impact on neurologic recovery.

D. Subluxation with locked facets usually can be reduced with traction but often requires open surgery to maintain stability.

Ref.: 2, 4,11

COMMENTS: Plain x-rays are an excellent diagnostic study for evaluating cervical spine fractures. • Most fractures can be diagnosed with a lateral spine film. • Additional views can be obtained when a specific case warrants them. • CT scanning and MRI can add complementary information in some cases. • In cases of complete neurologic injury in the cervical spine, bradycardia is often seen as a result of the loss of sympathetic cardiac tone. • This may be treated if significant hypotension results. • Unfortunately, in the great majority of cases of complete traumatic cervical spinal cord injury, early intervention does not improve the prognosis for neurologic recovery. • Surgery may still be necessary to stabilize the spine and to reduce pain, for example, in cases of subluxation with locked facets. • Although cervical traction may reduce the subluxation, surgery is usually necessary to maintain stability.

ANSWER:
D

23. Which of the following statements regarding blood supply to the brain is the most accurate?

    A. The cervical portion of the internal carotid artery gives off the internal and external maxillary arteries.

    B. The circle of Willis is fully developed in only 18% of the population.

    C. Because of collateral flow, occlusion of the middle cerebral artery is usually well tolerated.

    D. Occlusion of the cervical carotid artery invariably leads to a stroke.

Ref.: 2, 3

COMMENTS: The major blood supply to the brain is conveyed by the paired internal carotid and vertebral arteries. • The internal carotid artery is divided proximally to distally into the cervical portion (which has no branches) and the **petrous**, **cavernous**, and **intradural** portions. • The **petrous portion** has branches that anastomose with the internal maxillary artery, a branch of the external carotid artery. • Branches of the **cavernous portion** include arteries to the cavernous sinus, semilunar arteries, and meningeal arteries (which anastomose with meningeal branches of the internal maxillary artery). • These communications create important extracranial-intracranial anastomoses that become significant with certain occlusive lesions. • The **intradural branches** of the internal carotid artery include the ophthalmic artery (which has anastomoses with terminal branches of the external maxillary artery) and the anterior cerebral, middle cerebral, posterior communicating, and anterior choroidal arteries. • The vertebral arteries have anastomotic branches to the thyrocervical trunk of the subclavian artery and to the posterior branches of the external carotid artery. • After crossing the dura, the vertebral arteries join to form the basilar artery, which supplies the brain stem. • The basilar artery ultimately divides into the posterior cerebral arteries. • The circle of Willis, fully developed in 18% of the population, is therefore formed by branches of the internal carotid and vertebral arteries. • The anterior cerebral arteries (joined by the anterior communicating artery) and the posterior communicating arteries of the internal carotid artery join the posterior cerebral arteries of the basilar artery to create the circle of Willis. • Because of these anastamoses, occlusion of a carotid artery may be tolerated in an individual with good collateral flow. • End arteries, such as the middle cerebral artery, cannot be occluded without some area of infarction and subsequent deficit.

ANSWER:
B

24. Regarding spinal cord injury, match the syndrome in the left-hand column with its definition in the right-hand column.

    A. Anterior spinal   a. Unilateral or bilateral loss of motor and sensory in the distribution of multiple nerve roots

    B. Posterior spinal   b. Bilateral motor and pain sensation loss in the arms more than in the legs

    C. Central cord   c. Ipsilateral motor and position sense loss, contralateral pain, and temperature loss

    D. Brown-Sequard   d. Bilateral loss of position and vibration sense with preservation of motor and pain sensation

    E. Cauda equina   e. Bilateral loss of motor and pain below the lesion, with position and vibratory sense spared

Ref.: 2, 7, 8

COMMENTS: The syndromes of spinal cord injury are named according to the area of injury and have deficits related to the tracts running in that area of the spinal cord. • The **anterior** two thirds of the spinal cord holds the corticospinal tracts and the spinothalamic tract. • Injury to this area via compression or infarct leads to paralysis and loss of pain and temperature sense below the level of the lesion. • The **posterior** spinal cord holds the dorsal columns, which are involved in position and vibratory sense. • Lesions in this area result in loss of these modalities below the level of the lesion. • The **cervical central** spinal cord consists of gray matter, crossing fibers of the spinothalamic tract, and motor fibers to the upper extremities. • Injury here is often caused by neck hyperextension and leads to weakness and pain loss in the arms more than in the legs, along with loss of bowel and bladder control. • An axial hemisection of the spinal cord leads to the **Brown-Sequard** syndrome. • Deficits associated with this syndrome are ipsilateral motor loss, position and vibratory sense loss, contralateral pain, and temperature loss due to the crossing fibers of the spinothalamic tracts. • The nerve roots of the **cauda equina** arise from the distal spinal cord at L1–L2. • Compression of nerve roots of the cauda equina leads to variable loss of all functions in the nerve roots involved, along with radicular pain.

ANSWER:
A-d; B-e; C-b; D-c; E-a

25. Which of the following is/are common early complications of acute cervical spinal cord injury?

    A. Ileus

    B. Hydronephrosis

    C. Hypertension

    D. Spasticity

    E. Bradycardia

    F. Deep vein thrombosis

Ref.: 2, 8, 11

COMMENTS: With cervical spinal cord injury, there is a loss of **sympathetic tone**, since the outflow of the sympathetic fibers is mainly through the thoracic spinal cord. • This loss of tone leads to an imbalance in autonomic control favoring the parasympathetic system. • The result is a slowing of gastrointestinal motility, weakening of bladder contracture leading to distention and hydronephrosis, and loss of peripheral vascular tone with secondary venous pooling, hypotension, and thrombosis. • Bradycardia results from unopposed vagal tone. • Reflexes are usually hypoactive initially with a spinal cord injury, with spasticity a late complication.

ANSWER:
A, B, E, F

26. Which of the following statements regarding brain abscesses is/are true?

    A. The brain is highly susceptible to infection as a result of its high glucose content.

    B. The brain is extremely effective in walling off infections.

    C. Brain abscesses are classified as acute, chronic, and subacute.

    D. Prompt drainage is indicated for all types of brain abscess.

    E. Corticosteroids may inhibit abscess wall formation.

Ref.: 2, 3, 6

COMMENTS: The brain is generally resistant to infection unless previously damaged by trauma, hemorrhage, or anoxia. • Once infected, the brain is effective in walling off the infection and is capable of isolating the abscess from the uninvolved brain and systemic circulation, making sterilization by systemic antibiotics difficult. • The three major sources of brain abscesses include (1) direct extension from middle ear, mastoid, and nasal sinus infections (commonly affecting the temporal lobe and cerebellar hemispheres); (2) hematogenous spread (as occurs in cyanotic heart defects with right-to-left shunts); and (3) direct trauma. • The most common organisms are *Streptococcus* and *Staphylococcus* and *Pneumococci*. • Brain abscesses are classified as **acute**, following a course similar to and difficult to differentiate from subdural empyema; **chronic**, often presenting with progressive neurologic deficit and an expanding mass with a longer history (2 weeks to 2 months); and **subacute**, presenting with a picture somewhere between acute and chronic. • MRI is the most accurate indirect means of making the diagnosis and is helpful before performing surgical drainage.

The treatment consists of medical measures (antibiotics) or surgical drainage or excision. • Medical therapy requires 6–8 weeks of intravenous antibiotics and the use of corticosteroids if severe edema and mass effect are present. • On follow-up films, if an increase in the size occurs, surgical drainage must be considered. • Medical therapy is best used in patients with multiple lesions and those with relatively small lesions. • Abscesses also can be treated with surgical drainage or excision. • Again, antibiotics for 6–8 weeks are required, and, as with medical treatment, it may take longer than 10 weeks for significant resolution of the capsule and its enhancement to be seen on CT scan. • Seizures are common sequelae of brain abscess. • Brain abscess recurs in 8–10% of patients who initially present with a brain abscess.

ANSWER:
B, C, E

27. Match each clinical description with the appropriate unenhanced CT brain film shown here (a–d).

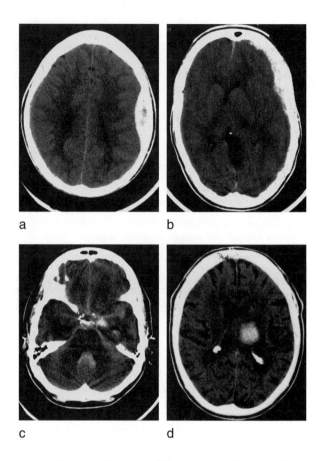

a   b

c   d

    A. A 61-year-old woman fell at home and presented to the emergency department with lethargy and confusion.

    B. A 75-year-old man with a long history of hypertension became acutely unresponsive.

    C. A 24-year-old man was involved in a motor vehicle accident. Plain skull films in the emergency department revealed a fracture.

    D. A 52-year-old woman had an acute onset of severe headache and shortly thereafter became unresponsive.

Ref.: 5, 9, 11

COMMENTS: All of the CT images shown demonstrate intracranial hemorrhage appearing as high-density collections that can be either intra-axial (within the brain parenchyma) or extra-axial (outside the brain parenchyma). • Extra-axial hemorrhage is further subdivided into epidural hematoma (EDH), subdural hematoma (SDH), and subarachnoid hemorrhage (SAH).

EDH, which is often associated with skull fracture, occurs following significant head trauma and is usually the result of arterial bleeding between the dura and inner table of the calvarium. • The dura does not strip easily from the inner table, even under arterial pressure. • As a consequence, an EDH acquires a biconvex configuration, as seen in image *a*.

SDH also occurs following head trauma, but the injury may be mild, particularly in the elderly. • Bridging veins between the dura and arachnoid are torn, because the arachnoid strips easily from the dura, and the SDH assumes a crescentic configuration around the hemisphere, as seen in image *b*.

SAH may be posttraumatic or spontaneous, as a result of a ruptured aneurysm. • Spontaneous SAH typically presents with acute, severe headache. • The subarachnoid space—the space between the arachnoid and pia mater—is filled with CSF. • Blood in this compartment can flow relatively freely among the basal cisterns, sylvian fissure, and cortical sulci and may rupture into the ventricular system. • In image *c*, which shows a spontaneous SAH secondary to a ruptured aneurysm, blood is noted in the basal cisterns as well as in the fourth ventricle. • Posttraumatic SAH tends to remain localized in association with the region of contusion.

Individuals with hypertension are predisposed to spontaneous **intraparenchymal hemorrhage** (IPH). • Hypertensive hemorrhage occurs most frequently in the basal ganglia, followed in frequency by the brain stem, cerebellum, and occasionally the cortex. • In image *d*, a spontaneous thalamic hemorrhage is shown. • IPH also may be the result of underlying lesions, including infarction, tumor, and vascular malformation, or it may occur following a trauma (e.g., contusion).

ANSWER:
A-b; B-d; C-a; D-c

28. Match each clinical description with the appropriate gadolinium-enhanced MRI images shown here (a–d).

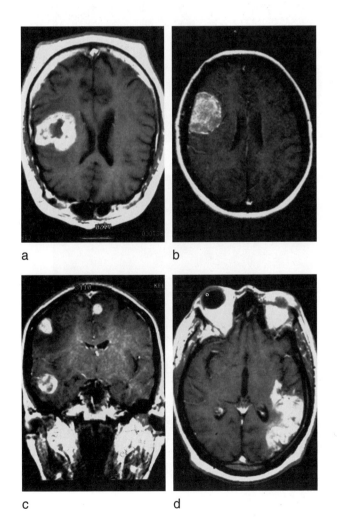

a   b

c   d

   A. A 43-year-old woman with a history of breast carcinoma presented with confusion.

   B. A 61-year-old man with no significant past medical history developed seizures and the gradual onset of hemiparesis.

   C. A 52-year-old woman had mild head trauma, and plain films of the skull demonstrated sclerosis of the calvarium.

   D. An 81-year-old man had an acute onset of aphasia 2 weeks before the scan.

Ref.: 6, 9

COMMENTS: Gadolinium-DTPA is an MRI contrast medium that increases the intensity ("brightness") of tissues in which it is distributed. • Thus, it changes the appearance of MRI scans in the same way that radiopaque contrast medium changes the appearance of CT scans. • Gadolinium-enhanced MRI is highly sensitive for detecting a wide variety of CNS lesions. • Although not always specific, there are features that help distinguish various lesions.

Image *a* is that of a **glioblastoma multiforme** (high-grade astrocytoma) and demonstrates a single peripherally enhancing lesion with central necrosis and surrounding edema. • The tumor margins are somewhat ill-defined and irregular, and the thickness of the enhancing wall varies. • Pathologically, viable tumor cells are almost invariably found outside of the enhancing portion of the tumor.

Meningioma, demonstrated in image *b*, is a (usually) benign nonglial neoplasm thought to arise from meningothelial cells of arachnoid villi. • Therefore, it typically occurs along dural surfaces. • Because of their slow growth, meningiomas may produce few or no symptoms. • Radiographically, meningiomas usually are smooth, rounded, sharply defined extra-axial masses that enhance homogeneously following administration of contrast media. • Hemorrhage and necrosis are uncommon. • Often, sclerosis of the overlying calvarium can be seen on plain radiographs or a CT scan.

Most **cerebral metastases**, as seen in image *c*, are multiple and supratentorial and tend to occur at the junction of gray and white matter. • Lung, breast, melanoma, kidney, and colon are the most common sites of origin. • Radiographically, metastases typically are enhanced, and hemorrhage and necrosis within them are common. • Even small lesions may have significant surrounding edema and mass effect. • Not all enhancing intracranial lesions, however, are neoplastic.

Image *d* demonstrates gyriform enhancement in a **subacute cortical infarction**. • This enhancement occurs approximately 1–3 weeks following the acute event. • Cortical enhancement also may be seen in cases of encephalitis. • Intracranial abscesses and granulomas may be indistinguishable from primary tumors or metastatic disease, although they tend to have thinner, more uniform walls.

ANSWER:
A-c; B-a; C-b; D-d

29. Which of the following statements regarding cerebral perfusion pressure (CPP) is/are true?

   A. CPP is defined as the mean arterial pressure (MAP) minus the intracranial pressure (ICP).

   B. CPP should be kept above a minimum of 30 mmHg.

   C. With head trauma, low CPP may aggravate cerebral ischemia caused by mass lesions, vasospasm, and altered vascular autoregulation.

   D. ICP increases dramatically with blood pressure changes up to 30 mmHg in head-injured patients.

Ref.: 5, 11

COMMENTS: CPP is defined as the MAP minus ICP. • Studies have shown that the management of critically ill head-injured patients should take into account the CPP. • This was a logical extension of evidence indicating that cerebral ischemia (global and local) was a major factor in the poor outcome of those with severe head injury. • Because CPP is a direct factor in cerebral blood flow, increasing the CPP in a patient at risk for cerebral ischemia may improve the outcome. • Experimental evidence shows that modest increases in MAP increase CPP without significant changes in ICP.

ANSWER:
A, C

30. Match the following clinical history and physical examination findings with the MRI scan most likely causing the scenario.

A. Severe thoracolumbar pain, numbness, and weakness in proximal legs bilaterally after a fall; lumbar spine tenderness

B. Severe neck pain, especially with flexion after a motor vehicle accident; no neurologic deficit

C. Sudden onset of low back pain with radiating pain and numbness to the left foot; positive straight leg raise on physical examination

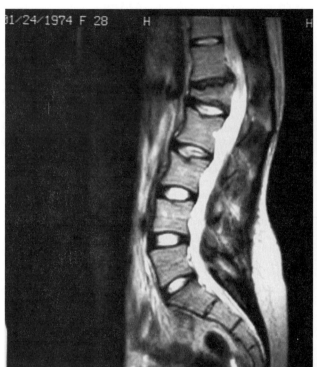

a

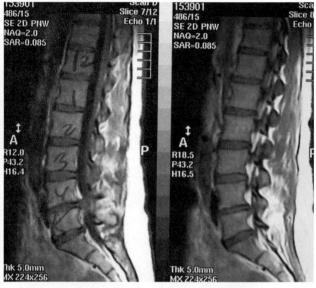

b

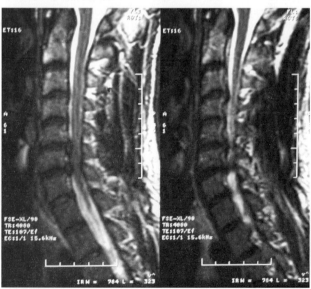

c

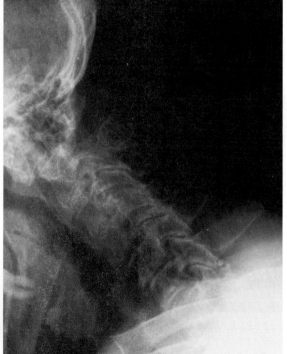

d

D. Gradual onset of numbness and weakness in hands and legs; hyperreflexia on physical examination

Ref.: 2, 3, 11

COMMENTS: Lumbar compression fractures cause severe low back pain, and, if there is compression of the cauda equina, radiating leg pain, numbness, weakness, or incontinence may result. • Some of these cases are managed with bracing and some with surgery. • Odontoid fractures often cause severe pain at the craniovertebral junction. • Normal findings on neurologic examination are not uncommon if the neck is stabilized soon after the accident. • Lumbar herniated discs commonly occur without an identifiable traumatic cause. • If the herniated disc compresses the nerve root passing posteriorly, a **radiculopathy** with radiating pain, numbness, and weakness often results. • Many of these cases can be managed without surgery. • Herniated discs in the cervical spine may or may not cause neck pain. • If they compress the spinal cord significantly, an insidious progressive **myelopathy**, with numbness, weakness, gait or bowel or bladder problems, may result. • These patients usually are found to be hyperreflexive on physical examination and may have clonus or Babinski's sign.

A N S W E R :
A-a; B-d; C-b; D-c

R E F E R E N C E S

1. Kandel ER, Schwartz JH (eds): *Principles of Neural Sciences*, Part II. Edward Arnold, London, 1981.
2. Schwartz SI, Shires GT, Spencer FC: *Principles of Surgery*, 7th ed. McGraw-Hill, New York, 1999.
3. Sabiston DC Jr: *Textbook of Surgery*, 15th ed. WB Saunders, Philadelphia, 1997.
4. Ross JS, Masaryk TJ, Modic MT, et al: Intracranial aneurysms: evaluation of MR angiography. *AJR* 155:159–165, 1990.
5. Narayan RK, Rosner MJ, Pitts LH, et al: *Guidelines for the Management of Severe Head Injury*. Brain Trauma Foundation, Chicago, 1995.
6. Schmidek HH, Sweet WH: *Operative Neurosurgical Techniques*, 3rd ed. WB Saunders, Philadelphia, 1995.
7. Way LW: *Current Surgical Diagnosis and Treatment*, 10th ed. Appleton & Lange, Norwalk, CT, 1994.
8. Menezes AH, Sonntag VK, Benzel EC, et al: *Principles of Spinal Surgery*. McGraw-Hill, New York, 1996.
9. Atlas SW: *Magnetic Resonance Imaging of the Brain and Spine*. Raven Press, New York, 1991.
10. Aston S, Seasley R, Thorne C (eds): *Grabb and Smith's Plastic Surgery*, 5th ed. Lippincott-Raven, Philadelphia, 1997.
11. Greenfield LJ: *Surgery*, 3rd edition. Lippincott, Williams & Wilkins, Philadelphia, 2001.

C H A P T E R 51

Orthopedics

A. Clinicopathologic Principles

Edward H. Kolb, M.D., and Eric M. Berkson, M.D.

1. With regard to normal articular cartilage, which of the following statements is/are true?

   A. It contains predominantly type II collagen.

   B. It is relatively hypercellular.

   C. It receives its nutrition via capillaries in the subchondral bone.

   D. Its mechanical behavior can be described as viscoelastic.

   Ref.: 1

COMMENTS: Articular cartilage is composed of relatively few cells within an extracellular matrix consisting predominantly of type II collagen and proteoglycans. • The large, highly negatively charged proteoglycans hold positively charged ions and water in the tissue by electrostatic and osmotic forces. • Under compressive loading, these smaller molecules are expressed from the tissue, which results in a greater negative charge density in the tissue. • When the load is removed, the positive ions and water are reabsorbed. • This is the molecular basis for the viscoelastic property of the tissue, which is vital to its role of smoothly transmitting forces across bony articulations. • The cartilage receives its nutrition from the synovial fluid. • Movement of nutrients into and out of the tissue is dependent on the cyclic loading of the tissue, which occurs during use of the joint. • When musculoskeletal injuries are treated, the advantages of immobilization (e.g., fracture healing) must be weighed against the potential metabolic injury to the cartilage of associated joints.

ANSWER:
A, D

2. Osteoclasts have receptors for which one of the following substances?

   A. Parathyroid hormone

   B. Calcitonin

   C. 1-25 Vitamin D_3

   D. Estrogen

   E. Thyroxine

   Ref.: 6

COMMENTS: Osteoblasts are responsible for bone formation, whereas osteoclasts are responsible for bone resorption. • Osteocytes represent former osteoblasts, comprising 90% of cells in the mature skeleton. • Parathyroid hormone, 1-25 Vitamin D_3, and thyroxine all cause bone resorption via indirect means with receptors on osteoblastic cells. • Estrogen is responsible for bone production via its receptor on osteoblasts. • Calcitonin works to inhibit bone resorption by binding to its receptor on the osteoclast.

ANSWER:
B

3. With regard to bone growth and repair, match each term in the left-hand column with one or more appropriate characteristics in the right-hand column.

   A. Endochondral ossification   a. Longitudinal growth (physis)

   B. Intramembranous ossification   b. Fracture callus

   C. Heterotopic ossification   c. Flat bone growth (clavicle, pelvis, and scapula)

      d. Soft tissue injury

      e. Elbow dislocation with concomitant head injury

   Ref.: 1, 2

COMMENTS: Bone growth occurs primarily by endochondral ossification or intramembranous ossification. • The truncal bones and spine are formed principally by **endochondral ossification**. • The process consists of formation of a cartilage model and subsequent replacement of the cartilage by bone. • This process occurs at the growth plate. • The skull, mandible, and clavicles are formed primarily by **intramembranous ossification**, a process that consists of the development of bone directly from mesenchymal cells of the periosteum without a cartilage anlage. • Fracture healing is a complex process in which a composite tissue of bone, cartilage, and fibrous tissue is formed and subsequently is remodeled to form mature bone. • The reparative tissue is bone callus. • **Heterotopic ossification** is the formation of bone within the soft tissue. • It is associated with certain fractures (especially elbow fractures or dislocations with concomitant head injury), and surgical procedures and may be a significant source of morbidity.

ANSWER:
A-a, b; B-c; C-d,e

---

4. Lateral herniation of the sixth cervical intervertebral disc usually produces which of the following?

A. Compression of the fifth cervical nerve root

B. Compression of the sixth cervical nerve root

C. Compression of the seventh cervical nerve root

D. Spinal cord compression alone

E. Concurrent nerve root and spinal cord compression

Ref.: 1, 2

COMMENTS: Most patients with cervical disc degeneration have only symptoms of local and referred pain. • **Lateral herniation** of a cervical disc may produce nerve root compression with radicular symptoms. • **Central (posterior) herniation** occurs less commonly and may result in spinal cord compression. • There are eight cervical nerve roots. • The first exits from the spinal canal between the occiput and the atlas. • Nerve root compression produced by herniation of a cervical disc affects the nerve root immediately below it.

ANSWER:
C

---

5. Which of the following diagnostic studies may be useful in the evaluation of de Quervain's disease?

A. Adson test

B. Finkelstein test

C. Two-point discrimination test

D. Cervical spine radiograph

E. Allen test

Ref.: 1, 2

COMMENTS: Pain in the hand or forearm (or both) may result from various musculoskeletal or neurologic disorders. • Neurogenic pain may reflect involvement at any level from the spinal cord to peripheral nerves. • The cause can be determined from the history, physical examination, and appropriate laboratory tests. • Radiologic studies are important for evaluation of cervical vertebral abnormalities and lung tumors. • Nerve conduction studies confirm the clinical diagnosis of median nerve compression. • The Adson test involves elevation of the first rib (a deep breath), contraction of the scalene muscle (turn head to examined side), and stretching it (extending the neck). • The test results may be positive with thoracic outlet syndrome (as may other such test results), but they are not diagnostic. • The Finkelstein test (patient grasps own thumb within clenched fist and then makes an ulnar deviation of the wrist) produces pain in patients with tenosynovitis of the abductor pollicis longus and extensor pollicis brevis (de Quervain's disease). • Two-point discrimination is used to assess integrity of the digital nerves. • Normal two-point discrimination is checked at the tip of the finger and should be less than or equal to 5 mm on both the ulnar and the radial side of the digit. • The Allen test is used to individually assess the radial and ulnar arterial supply to the hand.

• Pressure is applied to the radial and ulnar arteries at the level of the wrist while the patient is making a clenched fist. • The fist is then opened, revealing a bloodless hand. • Pressure on the radial artery is released, and blood flow to the hand is assessed. • The test is repeated, with pressure on the ulnar artery being released. • The Allen test is useful in assessing the contribution of both arteries to blood flow in the hand.

ANSWER:
B

---

6. Match each spinal condition in the left-hand column with the appropriate phrase in the right-hand column.

A. Spondylolisthesis   a. Defined as forward slippage of one vertebra on another

B. Spondylolysis   b. One hundred percent anterior translation of one vertebral body over another

C. Spinal stenosis   c. Defined as a defect in the pars interarticularis caused by repetitive hyperextension

D. Spondyloptosis   d. Common cause of back pain in children and adolescents

   e. Narrowing of the spinal canal or neural foramina

Ref.: 1, 2

COMMENTS: Spondylolisthesis is anterior subluxation of a vertebral body on another. • Its cause may be congenital, isthmic, degenerative, traumatic, pathologic, or postsurgical. • When associated with a pars interarticularis defect (isthmic type), the spondylolisthesis typically occurs at the L5–S1 level. • **Spondylolysis** is a defect in the pars interarticularis (part of the neural arch) that may lead to subsequent spondylolisthesis. • Spondylolysis is most common in gymnasts and football lineman, who perform repetitive hyperextension movements. • **Spinal stenosis** is defined as a narrowing of the spinal canal or neural foramina. • Spinal stenosis may cause nerve root compression, root ischemia, and variable degrees of back and leg pain. • **Spondyloptosis** is severe spondylolisthesis in which one vertebral body translates completely over the vertebral body below it.

ANSWER:
A-a; B-c, d; C-e; D-b

---

7. Which of the following tumors is seen most frequently in the spine in women?

A. Primary central nervous system (CNS) tumor

B. Primary bone tumor

C. Metastatic breast cancer

D. Metastatic colon cancer

E. Metastatic prostate cancer

Ref.: 1, 2

COMMENTS: Spinal tumors are classified as intradural or extradural. • **Extradural** tumors are usually metastatic cancers or primary bone tumors (the metastatic lesions are more common). • Prostate, thyroid, breast, lung, and kidney are frequent primary sites (remember: **P.T. Barnum Loves Kids**). • Other malignant extradural tumors include myeloma, lymphoma, plasmacytoma, chordoma, and osteogenic sarcoma. • **Intradural** tumors are usually primary CNS tumors. • They may be benign or malignant. • Primary bone tumors and CNS tumors are rare compared to metastatic tumors.

ANSWER:
C

8. What disorders make up the female athlete triad?

   A. Eating disorder, amenorrhea, and osteoporosis

   B. Hypothyroidism, tendinitis, and recurrent fractures

   C. Hypothyroidism, eating disorder, and tendinitis

   D. Malnutrition, hyperthyroidism, and obsessive compulsive disorder

   E. Osteomalacia, eating disorder, and hyperthyroidism

Ref.: 8

COMMENTS: The female athlete triad consists of three interrelated components identifiable in the female athlete succumbing to the pressure of achieving or maintaining an unrealistically low body weight. • The eating disorder may be anorexia nervosa, bulimia, or other eating disorders. • Amenorrhea is also present, resulting in diminished estrogen levels. • The diminished estrogen levels secondary to amenorrhea, in combination with the typical diminished body weight, leads to osteoporosis and increased fracture risk. • Thyroid dysfunction, tendinitis, and obsessive compulsive disorder are not part of the female athlete triad.

ANSWER:
A

9. A previously healthy 20-year-old college football player sustains a direct blow to the head while being tackled during a football game. After the play, he complains of an intense, sharp, burning pain radiating from the neck down into the right arm. When questioned, he is oriented to time, person, and place. He does not appear to be confused. Physical examination reveals 4/5 strength with elbow flexion on the right, with no other positive physical findings. He is the star running back of his football team and would like to return to play. What is the most appropriate next step of action?

   A. Have the patient rushed to the hospital for evaluation of transient quadriplegia.

   B. Reassure the patient that his concussion has not affected his consciousness and he may immediately return to play.

   C. Explain to the patient that he has suffered a "stinger," or "burner," and send him back on the football field.

   D. Explain to the patient that he has suffered a "stinger" and may not return to play until all symptoms are completely resolved.

   E. Transport the patient to nearest hospital for cervical spine x-rays and evaluation.

Ref.: 8

COMMENTS: The football player is suffering from a "stinger," or "burner," which occurs in 50–70% of college football players during their 4-year career. • The physical findings of intense, sharp, burning pain radiating down the arm are classic. • Stingers occur as a result of nerve root compression or a traction injury to the upper part of the brachial plexus typically in the C5 and C6 distribution. • Often, associated weakness or numbness occurs concomitantly. • The player should not return to play until all symptoms have resolved and the neurologic examination findings are normal.

Transient quadriplegia is a temporary neuropraxia of the spinal cord that occurs without fracture or bilateral involvement and is often accompanied by complete paralysis. • The symptoms completely resolve in most patients within 10 minutes, and full recovery is expected. • A concussion occurs when a patient with a head injury experiences postconcussvie symptoms consisting of headache, dizziness, nausea, confusion, or blurred vision. • The patient should be prohibited to return to play if loss of consciousness has occurred or symptoms last more than 15 minutes. • X-rays of the cervical spine are not warranted in this case.

ANSWER:
D

10. With regard to coccydynia, which of the following statements is/are true?

    A. It is often associated with radicular symptoms.

    B. It may be of traumatic origin.

    C. It is best treated by excision of the coccyx.

    D. It is often associated with anal sphincter incompetence.

    E. It is secondary to lumbar spondylosis.

Ref.: 1, 2

COMMENTS: Pain in the coccyx or lower sacrum can be caused by trauma, arthritis, or disc protrusion. • The pain must be clinically differentiated from other forms of perineal pain, including proctalgia fugax, intergluteal fold inflammation, low pilonidal cyst infection, and dorsal perirectal abscess. • The symptoms of coccydynia may be aggravating and progressive, but there is no radicular component or impairment of sphincter function. • Treatment is usually nonoperative, consisting of heat, cushioned seating, and anti-inflammatory medications. • Only rarely is operative intervention required. • Lumbar spondylosis is degenerative arthritis of the lumbar spine.

ANSWER:
B

11. All but which of the following may be common initial symptoms of lumbar intervertebral disc herniation?

    A. Low backache

    B. Sciatic pain

    C. Positive contralateral straight leg-raise test

    D. Pain at the tip of the tailbone

Ref.: 6, 8

COMMENTS: Most lumbar disc herniations occur in the posterolateral direction where the posterior longitudinal ligament of the spine is weakest. • Symptoms of disc protrusion include back pain and sciatica involving the lower nerve root at the involved level (e.g., L4–5 posterolateral disc herniation would involve the L5 nerve root). • The contralateral straight leg-raise examination is the most specific test for herniated nucleus pulposus. • Pain at the tip of the tailbone is not suggestive of a herniated disc.

ANSWER:
D

12. Which of the following physical findings is/are not consistent with an L5–S1 disc herniation?

    A. Positive straight leg-raise test results on the side of the herniation

    B. Positive Lasègue's sign on the side of the herniation

    C. Sensory deficit

    D. Absent knee jerk

    E. Absent ankle jerk.

Ref.: 1, 2

COMMENTS: Examination of a patient with low back pain includes careful observation of movement, spinal curvature, and range of motion. • **Straight leg-raising** with the patient in the supine position produces ipsilateral pain when there is nerve root compression. • Aggravation of the pain may be produced by subsequent dorsiflexion of the foot. • **Lasègue's sign** is elicited with the patient in the supine position and the hip and knee flexed to 90 degrees. • The knee is then extended. • Pain in the back and leg with less than 180 degrees of knee extension constitutes a positive result. • Neurologic examination may reveal **hypesthesia** and **weakness** according to the nerve root involved. • Herniation at the L5–S1 level may be accompanied by a diminished **ankle jerk**. • If the **knee jerk** is absent, compression is occurring at a higher level (L3–L4). • Results of the **femoral stretch test** (extension of the hip with flexion of the knee) may be positive in this instance.

ANSWER:
D

13. With regard to treatment of a herniated intervertebral disc, which of the following statements is/are true?

    A. Rest, analgesics, and use of heat and cold modalities provide relief in most cases.

    B. Laminectomy is performed in all cases to prevent paraplegia.

    C. Epidural steroid injections are contraindicated.

    D. Injection of chymopapain is indicated in patients with extruded disc fragments.

Ref.: 1, 2

COMMENTS: An initial trial of **conservative treatment** is indicated in patients without progressive neurologic deficits. • Most patients (>85%) have substantial improvement within 6 weeks. • Epidural steroids have been found effective in patients with spinal stenosis and may have some beneficial effect in patients with sciatica. • **Operative management** is indicated for substantial or progressive neurologic deficit, in refractory cases, or for those with severe sciatica. • Paraplegia rarely occurs with isolated disc injury. • **Chymopapain (proteolytic enzyme) injection** into the disc was historically used in selected patients with small central disc

herniations but was not effective when frank extrusion of the disc was present. • Chymopapain is no longer used because of the risk of complications.

ANSWER:
A

14. With regard to pyogenic osteomyelitis of the vertebral column, which of the following statements is/are true?

    A. It is most commonly caused by tuberculosis.

    B. It is usually associated with paravertebral abscess.

    C. It is most common in the thoracic region.

    D. It is most common in young, healthy adults.

    E. The organism is typically hematogenous in origin.

Ref.: 1, 2

COMMENTS: Pyogenic osteomyelitis of the vertebral column is most commonly caused by hematogenous spread of *Staphylococcus aureus* from other sites. • These infections most commonly occur in older debilitated patients and intravenous drug users and most commonly involve the lumbar region. • Paravertebral abscess formation, although rare, is seen with increasing frequency in immunocompromised patients. • Tuberculosis of the spine, the most common extrapulmonary site of tuberculosis, may occur in patients with active human immunodeficiency virus (HIV) syndrome. • The organism is usually hematogenous in origin. • Treatment of pyogenic osteomyelitis includes immobilization, antibiotics, and surgical débridement or drainage. • An anterior operative approach is usually advised.

ANSWER:
E

15. All but which of the following principles of tendon transfer are true?

    A. The muscle used should retain its full strength after transfer.

    B. Joint contractures should be corrected before operation.

    C. The transfer of synergistic muscles provide better results.

    D. The selected muscle must have adequate excursion.

Ref.: 1, 2

COMMENTS: Tendon transfer is used to restore function, muscle balance, and strength to joint motions in patients with various paralytic conditions. • There are four main requirements for tendon transfer. • (1) A muscle with adequate strength must be available, because one grade of strength is lost after transfer as a result of loss of the direct line of action between the muscle origin and insertion. • (2) The muscle must have adequate excursion to allow sufficient range of motion of the joint. • (3) The joint must have passive range of motion before transfer. • (4) Synergistic muscles generally provide better results, although tendon transfers of nonsynergistic muscles can be successful with proper rehabilitation.

ANSWER:
A

16. With regard to Dupuytren's contracture, which of the following statements is/are true?

    A. It may be treated with steroid injection and close observation.

    B. It is most common among manual laborers.

    C. It results from severe tenosynovitis.

    D. Successful surgical treatment always requires complete excision of the palmar fascia.

    Ref.: **1, 6**

COMMENTS: Contracture of the palmar aponeurosis is believed to be inherited, although other factors affect the extent of its expression. • It is associated with diabetes, epilepsy, tuberculosis, and alcoholism. • Contrary to common notions, its incidence is not higher in manual laborers. • There are several clinical types of involvement, and they vary in severity. • In most cases, Duputren's contracture can be treated with steroid injection and close observation. • Surgical intervention, usually partial fasciectomy, is useful for severe joint contractures.

A N S W E R :
A

17. Volkmann's ischemic contracture involves which of the following?

    A. Ischemic injury to the deep flexor muscles of the thigh

    B. Ischemic injury to the extensor muscles of the forearm

    C. Compromised blood flow in the anterior interosseous artery

    D. Compromised blood flow in the posterior interosseous artery

    Ref.: **1, 2**

COMMENTS: Volkmann's contracture is the result of ischemic damage to the muscles of the deep flexor compartment of the forearm (flexor digitorum profundus and flexor pollicis longus) secondary to compromise of flow in the anterior interosseous artery. • This contracture can be a complication of supracondylar fracture, forearm fracture, brachial artery puncture, hemophilia, and various forms of trauma. • The median nerve, which lies close to the anterior interosseous artery, may be involved in this process. • In severe cases, the ulnar nerve can be involved as well. • Because the damage occurs within a few hours of the insult, initial treatment must be prompt and definitive.

A N S W E R :
C

18. A 17-year-old, thin female cross-country runner has recently taken a 2-week vacation in Cancun, Mexico, where she refrained from running. She has had irregular menses for the past 2 years. Upon returning home, she begins a rigorous running schedule to get in shape for the upcoming cross-country season. After her third day of returning to the track, she notices progressively increasing pain in the right groin. She states that the pain is present only with activity and completely resolves with rest. She is seen by her local primary care doctor. She is found to have groin pain with internal and external rotation of the right hip. Her doctor decides to order x-rays of her pelvis and right hip. The x-rays are normal. What is the next step in treatment?

    A. Encourage the patient to supplement her diet with calcium, perform adequate pre-exercise stretching, and continue her current running regimen.

    B. Reassure the patient that she is fine and that her iliopsoas tendinitis will resolve with time.

    C. Order a computed tomographic (CT) scan of the right hip.

    D. Obtain a bone scan.

    E. Refer the patient to her obstetrician-gynecologist for hormone replacement therapy.

    Ref.: **8**

COMMENTS: Repetitive exercise can cause strain within bone that exceeds its local strength and causes microdamage. • Bone subjected to repetitive strain attempts to strengthen itself by remodeling, involving reabsorbtion followed by new bone formation. • If high strains continue during the reabsorption phase, the microdamage in the bone may progress to a stress fracture. • Hip fractures typically present with groin pain, which occasionally radiates to the thigh and/or knee. • Risk factors for stress fracture include rapid increase in exercise time or intensity, decreased lower-extremity strength, and a history of menstrual disturbance. • Plain radiographs are often initially negative. • This patient's history and clinical examination findings are very suspicious for a stress fracture of the femoral neck. • Displacement of a femoral neck fracture in a 17-year-old girl could have devastating sequelae. • It is therefore necessary to proceed with a bone scan to evaluate for a femoral neck fracture, which may require operative intervention. • Magnetic resonance imaging (MRI) is also an excellent test for diagnosing a stress fracture and the surrounding soft tissue. • A CT scan is not effective at detecting stress fractures, since it can easily miss fracture lines.

A N S W E R :
D

19. Which of the following statements is/are true?

    A. Osgood Schlatter disease involves inflammation of the calcaneal aphophysis.

    B. Toxic synovitis may be confused with septic arthritis of the hip.

    C. Slipped capital femoral epiphysis (SCFE) most commonly occurs in thin adolescent girls.

    D. Legg-Calvé-Perthes disease and toxic synovitis of the hip typically occur at a later age than does SCFE.

    Ref.: **3, 7**

COMMENTS: Traction apophysitis may occur in rapidly growing children as an overuse type of injury. • **Osgood's** (tibial tubercle) and **Sever's** (calcaneus) disease are the most common. • Numerous factors have been implicated, including vascular disturbance, repetitive overuse, and genetic factors. • Symptomatic improvement is generally the rule with rest, analgesics, and occasional immobilization. • **Legg-Calvé-Perthes** is the pediatric equivalent of avascular necrosis of the proximal femur. • It is most common in the 6- to 11-year age group. • Symptoms include acute or subacute onset of hip pain, limp, and loss of motion, which may be confused with septic arthritis. • Bone scans or MRI may be helpful, although hip aspiration may be necessary to rule out joint infection. • **SCFE** presents with similar symptoms but is usually seen in endomorphic boys between the ages of 11 and 15 years of age. • Treatment of SCFE is surgical stabilization with screw fixation or open epiphyseodesis. • **Toxic synovitis** is commonly confused with septic arthritis of the hip. • One must have a high clinical suspicion for arthritis, given the associated potential morbidity. • Four factors used to help identify a potential infection include erythrocyte sedimentation rate (ESR) greater than 40 mm/hr, history of a fever greater than 100.4°F (38°C), a white blood cell (WBC) count greater 12,000/mm³, and inability to walk. • Patients with three or more of these factors have a greater than 90% chance of having a septic hip, according to a recent study.

ANSWER:
B

20. Match the following neurovascular structures with their anatomic locations.

A. Posterior humeral circumflex artery and axillary nerve	a. Guyon's canal
B. Circumflex scapular artery	b. Quadrangular space
C. Radial nerve and deep brachial artery	c. Triangular space
D. Lateral thoracic artery	d. Triangular interval
E. Ulnar nerve	e. Second part of the axillary artery

Ref.: 6

COMMENTS: The subclavian artery becomes the axillary artery at the lateral border of the first rib. • The axillary artery is divided into three parts based on their relationship to the pectoralis minor muscle (medial to, under, and lateral to the pectoralis minor). • One artery comes off the first branch (supreme thoracic), two arteries come off the second branch (throracoacromial and lateral thoracic), and three arteries come off the third branch (subscapular artery and anterior and posterior humeral circumflex). • The triangular space is bordered by the teres minor superiorly, teres major inferiorly, and the long head of the triceps laterally, which contains the circumflex scapular artery. • The quadrangular space—bordered by the teres minor superiorly, teres major inferiorly, long head of triceps medially, and lateral head of triceps laterally—contains the posterior humeral circumflex artery and the axillary nerve. • The deep brachial artery and radial nerve may be found in the triangular interval bordered by the teres major superiorly, the long head of the triceps medially, and the lateral head of triceps or humerus laterally.

ANSWER:
A-b; B-c; C-d; D-e; E-a

21. While obtaining a posterior iliac crest bone graft, the surgeon encounters major arterial bleeding at the base of the wound. Which artery is most likely to be damaged?

 A. Inferior gluteal

 B. Iliohypogastric

 C. Lateral femoral circumflex

 D. Superior gluteal

Ref.: 4

COMMENTS: The superior gluteal artery exits the pelvis via the sciatic notch just above the piriformis muscle. • Lying deep to the gluteus medius muscle, the artery may be lacerated during bone graft harvesting. • The lacerated artery may retract back into the pelvis, making hemostasis difficult to obtain. • Arterial embolization or retroperitoneal exploration may be necessary for control.

ANSWER:
D

22. Which of the following is a consistent feature of osteoporosis?

 A. Increased serum alkaline phosphatase levels

 B. Decreased serum phosphorus levels

 C. Impaired mineralization of osteoid

 D. Increased susceptibility to fracture

 E. Hyperparathyroidism

Ref.: 5

COMMENTS: Osteoporosis, defined as decreased bone mass, most commonly occurs in postmenopausal women. • A relative lifelong calcium deficiency, early menopause, and genetic factors contribute to the cause. • Serum laboratory values are normal and are used to exclude other conditions. • Bone density is best measured using radiographic techniques (DEXA scanning) of the spine, radius, or calcaneus. • To minimize the increased risk of fracture, treatment strategies include calcium supplementation and hormonal replacement. • Some medications (alendronate) may increase bone mass.

ANSWER:
D

23. After lifting a heavy box, a 33-year-old patient has numbness of the lateral and plantar aspect of the foot, no Achilles tendon reflex, and weakness with plantar flexion of the ankle. Which nerve root is involved?

 A. First sacral

 B. Second lumbar

 C. Third lumbar

 D. Fourth lumbar

 E. Fifth lumbar

Ref.: 5

COMMENTS: See Question 24.

24. What is the most appropriate diagnostic test for the patient in Question 23?

 A. Electromyography

 B. Bone scanning

 C. MRI

 D. CT scanning

Ref.: 5

COMMENTS: The patient presents with complaints typical of sciatica due to a herniated disc between the fifth lumbar and first sacral vertebrae affecting the S1 nerve root. • Electromyography is commonly used in cases of suspected peripheral neuropathy or cervical radiculopathy but rarely for isolated herniated disc of the lumbar or sacral spine. • Bone scanning or CT imaging may be helpful in suspected cases of spondylolysis or spondylolithesis. • MRI provides the best examination of soft tissues, including the intervertebral discs and nerve roots.

ANSWERS:
Question 23: A
Question 24: C

25. The parents of an 11-month-old child indicate that she has been crying and has refused to walk since she fell last night. She had recently begun to walk. Radiographs reveal a displaced spiral midshaft fracture of the femur. In addition to stabilization of the fracture, what should the physician order?

   A. Serum calcium, phosphorus, and alkaline phosphastase assays

   B. Skeletal survey

   C. MRI of the femur

   D. Bone biopsy

   E. Urine mucopolysaccharide screening

Ref.: 3

COMMENTS: Spiral fractures are due to a twist or torsional injury and are rare in children less than 1 year of age. • A skeletal survey is indicated to rule out injuries in various stages of healing in cases of suspected child abuse. • Fractures due to metabolic bone disease (e.g., nutritional rickets) occur more commonly as transverse metaphyseal fractures and are associated with chronic radiographic changes.

ANSWER:
B

REFERENCES

1. Brunicardi FC, Andersen DK, Billiar TR, et al (eds): *Schwartz's Principles of Surgery*, 8th ed. McGraw-Hill, New York, 2004.
2. Townsend CM Jr, Beauchamp RD, Evers BM, et al: *Sabiston Textbook of Surgery: The Biological Basis of Modern Surgical Practice,* 17th ed. Saunders, Philadelphia, 2004.
3. Morrissey RT, Weinstien SL: *Lovell and Winters Pediatric Orthopaedics*, 4th ed. Lippincott, Philadelphia, 1996.
4. Browner BD, Jupiter JB, Levine AM, et al: *Skeletal Trauma.* Saunders, Philadelphia, 1992.
5. Deg R: *Principles of Orthopaedic Practice.* McGraw-Hill, New York, 1992.
6. Miller MD: *Review of Orthopaedics*, 3rd ed. Saunders, Philadelphia, 2000.
7. Sponseller PD: *Orthopaedic Knowledge Update: Pediatrics, vol. 2.* American Academy of Orthopaedic Surgeons, Rosemont, IL, 2002.
8. Koval KJ: *Orthopaedic Knowledge Update: Pediatrics, vol. 7.* American Academy of Orthopaedic Surgeons, Rosemont, IL, 2002.

B. Trauma

Edward H. Kolb, M.D., and Eric M. Berkson, M.D.

1. Proper emergency room management of an open fracture generally includes all but which of the following?

   A. Culture of the wound

   B. Antibiotic prophylaxis

   C. Tetanus prophylaxis

   D. X-rays one joint above and below the region of injury

   E. Provisional reduction and splinting

   Ref.: 1, 2

   COMMENTS: Open fractures are associated with a high rate of infection. • They constitute a surgical emergency because irrigation and débridement of the wound less than 8 hr after injury have been shown to dramatically lower the incidence of wound infection and osteomyelitis. • In the emergency department, a careful clinical and radiographic examination is performed. • Antibiotic and tetanus prophylaxis is initiated. • A saline-solution–soaked sterile dressing is applied to the wound without significant irrigation or débridement. • Irrigation of the wound and foreign-body removal in the emergency department setting may force debris further into the wound and should be performed in the operating room. • The extremity should be provisionally reduced and splinted. • Culture specimens are not obtained from wounds associated with open fractures because they have been found not to be correlated with future infective sources.

   ANSWER:
   A

2. Low–molecular-weight heparin has a primary inhibitory effect on which of the following?

   A. Antithrombin III

   B. Factor VII and factor IX

   C. Cyclooxygenase

   D. Factor Xa

   E. Protein C

   Ref.: 1

   COMMENTS: The importance of adequate prophylaxis for thromboembolism in orthopedics cannot be understated. • Depending on the study and prophylaxis, approximately 7–50% of patients following major orthopedic procedures will develop deep venous thrombosis (DVT). • Low–molecular-weight heparin inhibits primarily factor Xa. • To some extent, it promotes antithrombin III activity. • Because it has a minimal effect on thrombin, there is minimal elevation of the partial thromboplastin time (PTT). • Factors II, VII, IX, and X are the vitamin K–dependent clotting factors that are inhibited by warfarin. • Cyclo-oxygenase is inhibited by aspirin.

   ANSWER:
   D

3. Torus fractures and greenstick fractures have which of the following characteristics in common?

   A. At least partial continuity of the cortex

   B. Higher rate of nonunion than with other fractures

   C. Best treated by internal fixation

   D. Caused by repeated stress

   E. Occur only in adults

   Ref.: 1, 2

   COMMENTS: A torus fracture is a buckle of the metaphyseal cortex of bones, such as the distal radius, which occurs in pediatric populations. • The fracture results from failure of the cortex under compression. • There may be angulation of alignment, but displacement does not occur. • Greenstick fractures, in contrast, are pediatric fractures that involve disruption of the cortex under tension. • Partial continuity of the cortex is present with both fractures. • These fractures occur in children and heal readily. • They rarely necessitate internal fixation. • Whereas repeated stress results in a fatigue or stress fracture, it plays no role in the mechanism of injury for torus or greenstick fractures.

   ANSWER:
   A

4. Which of the following types of peripheral nerve injury associated with extremity trauma is/are usually best treated by delayed surgical repair?

   A. Neurapraxia

   B. Neurotmesis

   C. Axonotmesis

   D. Digital nerve injury

   Ref.: 2

   COMMENTS: Fractures of the extremities may be associated with peripheral nerve injuries, of which there are three major types. • Neurapraxia implies a physiologic interruption of nerve conduction caused by the inability of the neurons to reestablish their membrane potentials. • With severe stretch injuries, the motor deficit is typically more prominent than the sensory loss. • The abnormality usually resolves within 6 weeks after injury. • Axonotmesis occurs when there is both axonal and myelin loss (wallerian degeneration) even though the Schwann sheath is intact. • In this circumstance, there may be complete motor and sensory loss, although axonal regeneration usually ensues in a proximal-to-distal manner. • Most fractures cause nerve injuries in continuity (neurapraxia or axonotmesis). • These deficits require follow-up observation and electrodiagnostic studies and should be allowed to heal spontaneously. • The most severe lesion is neurotmesis, or complete division of the nerve. • Neurotmesis necessitates precise apposition of the nerve ends. • Primary repair is most appropriate in the presence of sharp lacerations without adjacent stretch and for digital nerve injuries. • Most cases are best treated by delayed repair once the soft-tissue injury has resolved.

A N S W E R :
B

5. Match each fracture or dislocation in the left-hand column with one or more appropriate associated injuries in the right-hand column (each of which may be selected once, more than once, or not at all).

A. Anterior dislocation of the shoulder	a. Median nerve
B. Fracture of the distal radius	b. Axillary nerve
C. Posterior dislocation of the knee	c. Peroneal nerve
D. Fracture of the neck of the fibula	d. Popliteal artery

Ref.: 8

COMMENTS: Blunt trauma can produce a variety of limb-threatening injuries. • Anterior dislocation of the shoulder results from axial loading of the externally rotated, extended arm. • The humeral head is driven forward out of the glenoid cavity. • The axillary nerve is injured in 5–30% of cases. • Most supracondylar fractures of the humerus are of the extension type. • The end of the proximal fragment is driven through the overlying brachialis muscle into the brachial artery and the median nerve. • Posterior dislocations of the knee often compromise the popliteal artery. • Fractures of the distal radius and the fibular neck can produce compression of the median nerve and common peroneal nerve, respectively.

A N S W E R :
A-b; B-a; C-d; D-c

6. Pathologic fractures may result from which of the following?

A. Primary bone tumors

B. Metastatic bone tumors

C. Benign bone cysts

D. Osteogenesis imperfecta

E. All of the above

Ref.: 1, 2

COMMENTS: Pathologic fractures include any fracture in bone weakened by a preexisting pathologic condition. • Although any primary or metastatic malignant process may be responsible, benign conditions frequently are the cause. • In adults, osteoporosis may result in pathologic fractures. • In children, developmental and metabolic diseases, such as osteogenesis imperfecta, osteopetrosis,

and nutritional deficiencies, may lead to fractures. • Benign bone cysts and tumors also may be associated with fractures.

A N S W E R :
E

7. With regard to stress fractures, which of the following statements is/are false?

A. They are typically associated with an underlying congenital disorder of bone formation.

B. They commonly affect the femoral neck.

C. They are best detected as a result of strong clinical suspicion.

D. Risk factors include repetitive excessive exercise and osteoporosis.

Ref.: 1, 2

COMMENTS: Stress, or fatigue, fractures are the result of repeated forces that cause accelerated osteoclastic activity with a loss of normal structural mass and subsequent new periosteal bone formation. • Patients complain of local pain during the early phase. • Radiographic findings at this time reveal only subtle osteoporosis and further diagnostic tests, including a bone scan or an MRI, may be necessary to establish the diagnosis. • Should the repetitive stress continue, a fracture results. • Stress fractures may occur in the femoral neck, the distal second and third metatarsal shafts, the proximal tibia, the distal fibula, the calcaneus, and other bones. • The treatment of stress fracture is immobilization and cessation of the responsible activity, but internal fixation may be necessary, depending on the location of the fracture.

A N S W E R :
A

8. Match each Salter and Harris classification with the corresponding physeal injury in children illustrated below.

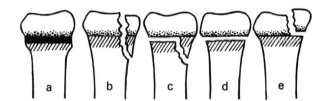

A. Salter I

B. Salter II

C. Salter III

D. Salter IV

E. Salter V

Ref.: 2

COMMENTS: The Salter and Harris classification applies to fractures through and around the growth plate in patients in whom the physeal plate has not yet fused. • Salter I injury is a transphyseal fracture that may appear as widening of the physis on plain radiographs. • Salter II injury is a transphyseal fracture that exits through the metaphysis. • This extra-articular fracture commonly occurs at the distal radial or tibial physis. • Salter III injury is a transphyseal fracture that exits through the epiphysis. • It represents an intra-articular fracture. • A Salter IV injury is a fracture that extends from the metaphysis to the bony epiphysis, crossing the physeal plate. • The most common injury is fracture of the lateral condyle of the humerus. • A Salter V injury is a crush injury to the physeal plate. • It is important to recognize the presence and type of epiphyseal plate injury because the physeal plate is the center of longitudinal bone growth, and injuries may result in abnormalities of length or in angular deformities. • Type I and type II fractures are treated by closed reduction and usually carry an excellent prognosis. • Accurate reduction is necessary for type III injuries because of an intra-articular component. • Nevertheless, the prognosis is good if the blood supply to the fractured portion is not impaired. • Type IV and type V injuries are more likely to cause growth disturbances. • Whenever a physeal fracture exists, the patient and the parents should be cautioned that growth abnormalities may result.

ANSWER:
A-d; B-c; C-e; D-b; E-a

9. When pain persists after closed reduction and casting, what should the immediate concern be?

    A. Inadequate immobilization

    B. Pressure point necrosis

    C. Neural injury

    D. Muscle spasm

    E. Ischemia

Ref.: 2

COMMENTS: Although several factors may be responsible for limb pain after casting, ischemia is the most serious. • After plaster casting, the extremity should be elevated and the digits exposed. • Adequate immobilization should substantially relieve pain. • Unrelenting pain is always suggestive of ischemia and is an indication for splitting the cast with parallel cuts through the padding on both sides of the extremities. • Other causes of pain include nerve injury, muscle spasm, and pressure-point necrosis. • Persistent pain suggests a compartment syndrome or ischemia and must be ruled out in all cases. • Localized burning pain may occur as a result of pressure-point necrosis from the cast over a bony prominence and is treated by cutting a cast window.

ANSWER:
E

10. With regard to dislocation of the acromioclavicular joint, which of the following statements is true?

    A. It is most common in elderly patients with lax ligaments.

    B. Radiologic diagnosis is usually made by CT scan.

    C. It is best detected with the patient examined in the supine position.

    D. Operative treatment is usually not necessary.

Ref.: 2

COMMENTS: In young patients, a sudden strong, downward force on the shoulder produces acromioclavicular dislocation as a result of disruption of the acromioclavicular and coracoclavicular ligaments. • The stability of the distal clavicle is dependent primarily on the coracoclavicular ligaments. • In elderly patients, whose bones are more osteoporotic, a similar mechanism of injury results in fracture of the distal clavicle. • Patients are best examined in the seated position, since the dislocation may reduce spontaneously in the supine patient. • Radiologic confirmation is made with plain films of both acromioclavicular joints for comparison. • Treatment, which is focused primarily on relieving symptoms, consists of wearing a sling to support the weight of the arm. • Operative treatment is seldom indicated.

ANSWER:
D

11. Which of the following are indications for immediate operative treatment of humeral shaft fractures?

    A. Radial nerve injury

    B. Median nerve injury

    C. Brachial artery injury

    D. Fractures in adults

    E. Unsuccessful closed reduction

Ref.: 1, 2

COMMENTS: Neurovascular injuries are not uncommon with humeral shaft fractures, the most common being traction injury to the radial nerve. • As with other nerve injuries secondary to fractures, function is usually recovered spontaneously. • The median nerve is not in sufficient proximity to be at serious risk. • Surgical exploration is indicated if nerve function has not recovered in 4–6 months. • When repair of the brachial artery is required, open reduction with internal fixation of the humeral shaft is necessary to protect the vascular repair. • Although most fractures can be treated by closed reduction through some form of casting or traction, open reduction for closed shaft fractures is necessary for fractures extending into the elbow or shoulder joint, bilateral fractures, impending pathologic fractures, or associated spinal cord or brachial plexus injuries. • Age is not a criterion for open versus closed reduction of fractures of the humeral shaft.

ANSWER:
C

12. A 7-year-old is brought to the emergency department complaining of pain and deformity in his right elbow. His mother states that he fell from a tree on an extended, outstretched arm. The radial pulse is absent, and findings on neurologic examination are normal. Prompt radiographs demonstrate a displaced extension-type supracondylar humerus fracture. Appropriate management at this time should consist of which one of the following?

    A. Immediate arteriography

    B. Closed reduction, reexamination of vascular status, and percutaneous pinning

    C. Closed reduction, reexamination of vascular status, and immobilization in maximal flexion at the elbow

    D. Immediate open exploration of the brachial artery

Ref.: 4

COMMENTS: Supracondylar fractures of the humerus in children most often occur from a fall on an extended, outstretched arm.

• Because of the high incidence of neurovascular injury associated with this fracture, accurate assessment of the median, radial, and ulnar nerves and the brachial artery is imperative. • Immediate reduction under general anesthesia using fluoroscopy in most cases restores the radial pulse and peripheral circulation. • Reduction is achieved by traction on the extended arm followed by pronation and maximal flexion at the elbow to restore alignment. • The elbow is reextended to ensure adequacy of the radial pulse, but fractures with significant displacement and brachial artery compression are often unstable, precluding cast immobilization. • These fractures are stabilized with percutaneous pinning to maintain bone stability while allowing more extension at the elbow. • Forearm compartment fasciotomy is indicated with any extended ischemia.

ANSWER:
B

13. Which one of the following humeral fractures in children usually necessitates open reduction internal fixation?

A. Anatomic neck

B. Surgical neck

C. Shaft

D. Supracondylar

E. Lateral epicondyle

Ref.: 1, 2

COMMENTS: Humeral fractures of the surgical neck, anatomic neck, and shaft are best treated by closed reduction. • Supracondylar fractures are common fractures about the elbow in children and usually are treated satisfactorily by closed reduction and percutaneous pinning. • Fractures of the lateral epicondyle in children are Salter type IV injuries and are therefore intra-articular. • Malunion or nonunion may result in limb deformity, limitation of motion, or both. • Operative correction is therefore indicated. • All of the other fractures listed above are best treated by closed reduction.

ANSWER:
E

14. Monteggia's fracture is best described as which of the following?

A. Radial head fracture and proximal ulnar subluxation

B. Distal radius fracture and proximal ulnar subluxation

C. Ulnar styloid fracture and radial head subluxation

D. Proximal ulnar fracture and radial head subluxation

Ref.: 1, 2

COMMENTS: Monteggia's fracture, usually sustained by a fall on the extended, outstretched arm, is characterized by a fracture of the proximal ulna with subluxation of the radial head. • The radial head dislocates anteriorly in 60% of cases. • Treatment consists of closed reduction for children. • Adults, however, require rigid internal fixation of the ulna with the forearm placed in supination to maintain reduction of the radial head.

ANSWER:
D

15. Complications of distal radius fractures include which of the following?

A. Osteoarthritis

B. Wrist stiffness

C. Carpal tunnel syndrome

D. Loss of grip strength

E. All of the above

Ref.: 1, 2, 4

COMMENTS: Fractures of the distal radius, which may involve the articular surface, are common in adults over the age of 50 years. • More common in women than in men, the injury occurs from a fall on the outstretched hand. • Examination typically reveals a dorsal deformity of the wrist and hand and occasionally median nerve injury. • An anatomic reduction must be performed to retain radial length and dorsal tilt. • Unstable fractures require use of external fixation and plate or pin fixation. • Posttraumatic osteoarthritis of the radiocarpal joint can result from articular injury. • Prolonged cast immobilization or positioning of the wrist in excessive palmar flexion can result in joint stiffness and median nerve compression.

ANSWER:
E

16. A 25-year-old skater complains of wrist pain after slipping on the ice and falling on an outstretched hand. There is specific point tenderness over the anatomic snuffbox. There is no deformity. Which of the following is the most likely diagnosis?

A. Colles' fracture

B. Scaphoid fracture

C. Scaphoid-lunate subluxation

D. Lunate subluxation

Ref.: 1, 2

COMMENTS: See Question 18.

17. Which of the following radiographs should be obtained on the patient described in Question 16?

A. Posteroanterior (PA) view of the wrist

B. Lateral view of the wrist

C. Oblique view of the wrist

D. Ulnar deviated view of the wrist

E. All of the above

Ref.: 1. 2

COMMENTS: See Question 18.

18. Radiographs of the patient described in Question 16 reveal no fracture or dislocation. Appropriate treatment at this time should be which of the following?

A. Ice packs, elastic wrap, and rest

B. Dorsal wrist splint

C. A short arm plaster splint, including the thumb, but excluding the elbow

D. A long arm plaster splint, including the thumb and elbow

Ref.: 1, 2

COMMENTS: Schaphoid fractures can be an isolated finding or associated with other fractures of the upper extremity. • It is not uncommon for this fracture to go undetected on initial radiographs. • Less commonly, hyperextension injuries of the wrist may cause lunate dislocation or disruption of the normal scaphoid-lunate relationship. • The ulnar-deviated PA view of the wrist brings the scaphoid into full profile. • PA and lateral views demonstrate displacement of the lunate. • Oblique radiographs may demonstrate a nondisplaced scaphoid fracture. • If the patient has tenderness over the scaphoid, a fracture should be suspected despite negative radiographs. • The patient should be treated with a thumb spica splint including the thumb and elbow. • After 3 weeks, radiographs with the arm out of plaster should be repeated. • If the tenderness is gone and the radiographs still are negative, no further cast immobilization is necessary. • A bone scan or CT scan can be performed to exclude a scaphoid fracture if uncertainty continues. • Adequate treatment is important because of the risk of avascular necrosis of the proximal fragment of the scaphoid (the arterial supply enters the distal third of the scaphoid bone). • Most scaphoid fractures require at least 6 weeks of immobilization, and up to 3 months may be needed.

ANSWERS:
Question 16: B
Question 17: E
Question 18: D

19. A 25-year-old man sustains a laceration to his wrist from a knife injury during a fight. Upon presentation to the emergency department, the patient appears intoxicated and is unable to provide accurate information regarding sensation to the fingertips. An Allen test is performed, revealing no blood flow to the hand during compression of the radial artery. Which of the following functions is likely impaired in this patient?

A. Extension of the wrist

B. Flexion of the distal interphalangeal joint of the index finger

C. Abduction and adduction of all fingers

D. Flexion of the interphalangeal joint of the thumb

E. Extension of the metacarpophalageal joint of the middle finger

Ref.: 6

COMMENTS: The Allen test is performed by having the patient make a tight fist while the examiner compresses the radial artery and ulnar artery at the wrist. • The hand is opened and pressure released from the radial artery, revealing collateral flow to the hand via the ulnar artery. • This is performed a second time, releasing pressure from the ulnar artery and noting collateral flow from the radial artery. • This patient has an obvious ulnar arterial insufficiency. • Accompanying the ulnar artery in Guyon's canal at the wrist is the ulnar nerve, which is just ulnar to the ulnar artery. • Extension of the wrist is controlled by the radial nerve. • Flexion of the distal interphalageal joint of the index finger is median nerve. • Flexion of the interphalangeal joint of the thumb is controlled by the anterior interosseous branch of the median nerve.

• Extension of the metacarpophalangeal joint of the middle finger is controlled by the posterior interosseous branch of the radial nerve. • In this patient, the ulnar nerve, which allows abduction and adduction of the fingers via the interossei muscles, is severed, given its ulnar relationship to the ulnar artery.

ANSWER:
C

20. Which of the following physical findings is most indicative of a posterior shoulder dislocation?

A. Limited forward elevation of the shoulder

B. Loss of sensation over the deltoid region of the shoulder

C. Pain over the acromioclavicular joint of the shoulder

D. Limited external rotation of the shoulder

E. Loss of abduction and adduction of the fingers

Ref.: 6, 7

COMMENTS: Anterior shoulder dislocations are far more common than are posterior shoulder dislocations, making up approximately 95% of all shoulder dislocations. • Posterior shoulder dislocations are associated with the three E's: ethanol, epilepsy, and electrocution. • Posterior shoulder dislocations are missed up to 50 percent of time upon initial presentation. • It is essential to obtain adequate x-rays of the involved shoulder consisting of AP, scapular-Y, and axillary lateral views to avoid this mistake. • The hallmark clinical finding seen in patients with a posterior shoulder dislocation is lack of external rotation of the shoulder.

ANSWER:
D

21. With regard to fractures of the bones of the hand, which of the following statements is/are true?

A. Moderate rotational deformity is acceptable with boxer's fractures.

B. A mallet finger is an avulsion of the flexor digitorum profundus.

C. Crush injuries of the distal phalanx can be treated by finger splinting.

D. Bennett's fracture involves an intra-articular fracture of the carpometacarpal joint of the index finger.

Ref.: 1, 2

COMMENTS: Fractures of the bones of the hand are among the most common problems encountered in the emergency department, and they must be treated properly to avoid or minimize any subsequent disability. • Boxer's fractures are metacarpal neck fractures, typically of the fifth metacarpal. • Correction of rotational deformities with these and other metacarpal fractures is important and is determined clinically: each finger should point toward the scaphoid. • Correction of angulation in the ulnar and radial planes is also important. • Intra-articular fractures generally necessitate anatomic reduction. • A mallet finger results from avulsion of the extensor tendon, with or without a bone fragment, from its insertion on the distal phalanx. • This causes dropping of the finger and loss of the last 20 degrees of active extension. • When avulsion occurs with a fragment of bone involving one third or more of the articular surface, open reduction and wire fixation are required.

• If the bone chip is small or does not involve the joint, treatment is the same as with pure tendon avulsion, that is, finger splint with the distal phalanx in hyperextension. • A crushed finger requires meticulous débridement and repair of the soft tissues, including the nail bed. • The often associated comminuted fracture of the distal phalanx requires only finger splinting for relief of pain. • Bennett's fracture involves the carpometacarpal joint of the thumb and usually is sustained by a blow against the tip of the outstretched thumb.

ANSWER:
C

---

22. A 52-year-old complains of elbow pain after falling off a bicycle. During the fall, the patient landed on a right flexed elbow. Examination is significant for focal tenderness over the olecranon, with an obvious joint effusion. The elbow is stable to varus and valgus stresses. The patient is neurovascularly intact. Radiographs show a comminuted intra-articular olecranon fracture. Which of the following is true?

    A. Operative treatment is the standard of care for all olecranon fractures.

    B. An elbow effusion is uncommon with an olecranon fracture.

    C. It is permissible to remove up to 50% of the olecranon in severely comminuted fractures.

    D. Casting is the treatment of choice for a patient unable to actively extend the elbow against gravity.

Ref.: 8

COMMENTS: Olecranon fractures predictably result from direct falls on the point of the elbow or indirectly from sudden contracture of the triceps and brachialis during a fall on the upper extremity. • Standard anteroposterior and lateral radiographs should be obtained, and other fractures and dislocations about the elbow should be excluded. • Clinically, a thorough neurovascular examination should be performed. • Most olecranon fractures are intra-articular, and a hemorrhagic effusion of the elbow joint is common. • The patient's ability to actively extend the elbow against gravity must be assessed to determine the continuity of the triceps mechanism. • Operative intervention must be performed if there is greater than 2 mm of displacement, an increase in degree of separation with 90-degree flexion of the elbow, or an inability to extend the elbow actively against gravity. • Fractures that do not meet these criteria can be treated with immobilization and gradual return to full range of motion. • Operative treatments include both tension band wiring and plate fixation. • Excision of fracture fragments is a reasonable alternative for severely comminuted fractures or for fractures in elderly patients with osteopenia. • Recent research suggests that up to 50% of the olecranon can be excised as long as the triceps is repaired.

ANSWER:
C

---

23. A 40-year-old patient presents to a trauma center after falling vertically from a 15-foot ladder. He has no motor or sensory function below the T10 level and has no perirectal sensation. He has no detectable bulbocavernosus reflex. Which of the following is correct?

    A. The lack of a bulbocavernosus reflex is a poor prognostic sign.

    B. The patient is in spinal shock.

    C. Hypotension from neurogenic shock can be differentiated from cardiac shock by the presence of tachycardia.

    D. Spinal shock usually resolves within several months.

    E. The bulbocavernosus reflex is the contraction of the glans penis in response to digital rectal examination.

Ref.: 8

COMMENTS: The bulbocavernosus reflex is the contraction of the anal sphincter in response to stimulation of the trigone of the bladder. • This can be accomplished with a squeeze of the glans penis or a pull on a urethral catheter. • The absence of a bulbocavernosus reflex signals that the patient is in spinal shock and a physiologic disruption of reflex arcs within the spinal cord exists in addition to any structural disruption. • The bulbocavernosis reflex (S2–3) usually returns within 24–48 hr after injury and signals the end of spinal shock. • The presence of a complete spinal cord lesion after spinal shock has ended indicates a poor prognosis for neurologic recovery. • Neurogenic shock is a disruption of the sympathetic chain at the T1–L2 level and results in unopposed parasympathetic tone. • Hypotension from neurogenic shock, while initially resulting in tachycardia and hypertension, results in bradycardia and hypotension.

ANSWER:
B

---

24. Appropriate treatment of pediatric femoral shaft fractures includes which of the following?

    A. Internal fixation at the fracture site

    B. Closed intramedullary nailing

    C. Skeletal traction followed by spica casting

    D. Spica casting

    E. All of the above

Ref.: 1, 2

COMMENTS: Whereas closed antegrade intramedullary nailing has become the standard of care in adult femoral shaft fractures, pediatric femur fractures can be treated using multiple modalities. • Pediatric fractures are complicated by the potential for growth abnormalities surrounding the proximal and distal physes. • Intramedullary nails can lead to aseptic necrosis of the pediatric femoral head if placed too medially on the greater trochanter. • Nonetheless, closed nailing remains a viable option in children more than 7 years old if the distal physis is avoided. • Other options include spica casting, skeletal traction, or internal fixation.

ANSWER:
E

---

25. With regard to the technique of inserting a Steinmann pin for skeletal traction and femoral shaft fractures, which of the following statements is/are true?

    A. The pin should be placed as anteriorly as possible in the distal femur.

    B. The pin is placed in the proximal tibia when there is an associated knee injury.

C. The pin is inserted laterally to medially at the level of the tibial tubercle.

D. The pin is inserted laterally to medially in the supracondylar femur.

Ref.: 2

COMMENTS: Steinmann pins for skeletal traction are easily inserted after administration of a local anesthetic and may be placed proximally to the femoral condyles or across the proximal tibia. • The position of the pin can be controlled with greater precision at the point of entry than at its exit. • Hence, the side involving more hazard is penetrated first. • In the supracondylar position, the pin is placed as far posteriorly as possible to avoid the suprapatellar pouch and is advanced medially to laterally to avoid injury to the femoral vessels. • At the tibial tubercle, the pin is inserted laterally to medially to avoid injury to the common peroneal nerve. • When there is associated knee injury, the pin is inserted above the knee so that traction is not applied across the injured joint.

ANSWER:
C

26. A 19-year-old man jumps over a fence. Upon landing, his knee suddenly gives out. Although he is able to stand and ambulate, he complains that his knee is unstable. Examination reveals moderate swelling and tenderness. Results of the Lachman test are positive. Plain radiographs of the knee are normal. Aspiration of the knee reveals hemarthrosis without fat droplets. What is the likelihood that the patient suffered a tear of the anterior cruciate ligament (ACL)?

A. 10%

B. 30%

C. 50%

D. 75%

E. 100%

Ref.: 4

COMMENTS: Traumatic hemarthrosis of the knee due to ACL tears most commonly occurs with twisting, noncontact injuries. • The most sensitive clinical method for identifying tears of the ACL is the Lachman test. • It is performed by applying an anterior force on the tibia with the knee held at 30 degrees of flexion. • Tears of the ACL are noted with increased anterior movement of the tibia relative to the femur compared to that of the uninjured extremity. • This finding must not be confused with periarticular fractures around the knee, which may permit the same anterior translation. • Immediate swelling of a joint or extremity is usually due to fracture. • Ligament injuries typically produce joint swelling within 2–4 hr after the injury, whereas meniscal injuries typically swell within 12–24 hr. • The presence of a traumatic hemarthrosis without evidence of fracture may represent tears of the ACL in as many as 75% of cases. • Associated meniscal tears may be present in up to 65% of cases. • Although a careful history, physical examination, and plain radiographs allow diagnosis in most cases, the accuracy of MRI is 85–100%.

ANSWER:
D

27. A 17-year-old football player sustains a direct blow to the lateral aspect of the knee. Clinical examination reveals a grade III tear of the medial collateral ligament (MCL). He has no other demonstrable injury. What should the physician recommend?

A. A hinged knee brace for 8 weeks

B. A brace locked at 5 degrees of flexion for 6 weeks, then unlocked for 6 weeks

C. A cylinder cast for 6 weeks

D. Arthroscopic repair of the deep MCL

E. Open repair of the superficial MCL

Ref.: 4

COMMENTS: The MCL is the primary restraint to valgus loads of the knee and is injured with direct blows to the lateral aspect of the knee. • Unlike the cruciate ligaments, the MCL is an extra-articular structure with an excellent ability to heal with functional treatment. • Diagnosis of MCL injuries is confirmed by the presence of abnormal valgus laxity of the knee when held at 25 degrees of flexion. • Patients with excessive valgus laxity with the knee in full extension have a more complex injury involving the capsule and cruciate ligaments. • Patients treated with immediate protected motion obtain a stronger, more rapid healing response than those treated operatively or those immobilized in a cast.

ANSWER:
A

28. Which of the following is best treated without surgery?

A. An injury to the Lisfranc ligament and a dislocation of the tarsometatarsal joint

B. An open clavicle fracture

C. A 27-year-old with a femoral neck fracture

D. A displaced talus fracture

E. A nondisplaced patella fracture

Ref.: 4, 5, 8

COMMENTS: The Lisfranc ligament attaches the medial cuneiform to the base of the second metatarsal and maintains stability across the tarsometatarsal joint (the Lisfranc joint). • Patients present with deformity and pain. • Operative treatment should be considered for displacement of the tarsometatarsal joint greater than 2 mm to avoid significant posttraumatic arthritis. • Clavicle fractures are primarily treated conservatively because the rate of fracture union is high and nonunions of this bone are generally well tolerated. • Operative indications for clavicle fractures include all open fractures, fractures with neurovascular injury, and fractures with severe associated injuries, such as a floating shoulder. • Talar fractures result from high-energy injuries and have a high rate of osteonecrosis. • Displaced talar fractures should be reduced emergently. • Patellar fractures can be treated nonoperatively if there is less than 2 mm of displacement and if the patient's extensor mechanism remains intact.

ANSWER:
E

29. With regard to meniscal injuries, which of the following statements is/are true?

A. Mechanism involves rotational forces.

B. The lateral meniscus is injured more commonly than is the medial meniscus.

C. Diagnosis requires arthroscopy.

D. Operative correction always requires meniscectomy.

Ref.: 2

COMMENTS: The tibia rotates slightly as the knee flexes and extends. • Forceful rotation causes the cartilage to straighten and become taut. • If the force is excessive or continuous, a tear results. • The medial meniscus is injured three times more frequently than is the lateral meniscus. • Diagnosis is usually made clinically and occasionally verified with MRI, which can provide accurate information regarding ligamentous and meniscal injuries and associated fractures. • When the tear is within the peripheral third of the meniscus, consideration may be given to direct repair of the meniscus.

ANSWER:
A

30. With regard to tibial fractures, match each characteristic in the left-hand column with the appropriate location of the fracture in the right-hand column.

A. Associated ligamentous injury	a. Shaft
B. Inramedullary nailing is gold standard operative treatment	b. Plateau
C. Open fracture	c. Both
D. More common in the elderly	d. Neither

Ref.: 1, 2

COMMENTS: Tibial shaft fractures are usually the result of direct trauma, whereas plateau fractures usually result from indirect forces. • Plateau fractures are more common among middle-aged and elderly persons. • Tibial plateau fractures may necessitate surgical repair if the medial collateral ligament is disrupted or there is displacement or compression of the tibial plateau. • Tibial shaft fractures are caused by substantial trauma and are often associated with severe soft-tissue injury, and 30% are open fractures. • Intramedullary nailing is the gold standard for operative intervention. • Careful observation is mandatory for all tibial shaft fractures, and prompt measurement of compartmental pressures, fasciotomy, or both should be performed whenever signs of the compartmental syndrome are present.

ANSWER:
A-b; B-a; C-a; D-b

31. A 7-year-old child is brought to the emergency department following a fall off of the monkey bars during recess. There is significant swelling of her right elbow. On examination, the patient has no radial pulse and is neurologically intact. She is significantly tender over the supracondylar humerus. Radiographic examination demonstrates a large anterior and posterior fat pad with an extension-type supracondylar humerus fracture. Which one of the following is true is regarding this fracture?

A. Immediate arteriography is indicated.

B. Closed reduction, reexamination of vascular status, and immediate percutaneous pinning should be performed.

C. A posterior fat pad sign is usually a normal finding on plain radiographs.

D. Pediatric elbow fractures are simple to diagnose and treat.

Ref.: 3, 9

COMMENTS: Pediatric elbow fractures are difficult to diagnose and treat because of variable ossification of the elements of the elbow. • Displaced fractures through cartilogenous portions of the elbow may not be visualized on plain radiographs. • Significant morbidity, including angular deformities and neurovascular injuries, is associated with supracondylar humerus fractures. • Immediate reduction under general anesthesia using fluoroscopy in most cases restores the radial pulse and peripheral circulation. • Neurologic injury may result directly from the injury or as a result of subsequent swelling. • Volkmann ischemic contractures, which are compartment syndromes of the forearm secondary to brachial artery injury, may result in contractures of the hand. • For these reasons, displaced supracondylar humerus fractures are usually treated with surgical stabilization. • The reduction is held with flexion of the elbow, but extreme flexion of a swollen elbow may cause neurovascular compromise. • An anterior fat pad may be a normal finding on plain radiographs of the elbow, but the presence of a posterior fat pad sign (fluid filling the olecranon fossa) suggests a large elbow effusion.

ANSWER:
B

32. A 25-year-old man is brought into the emergency department after sustaining a closed displaced right tibia fracture after falling 10 feet off a ladder. Pain is limited to the right leg. Physical examination reveals severe tenderness of the right tibia with moderate swelling of the calf. The patient has severe tenderness over the leg with passive dorsiflexion and plantar flexion of the foot. The patient also complains of mild parasthesias diffusely about the foot. His blood pressure upon presentation is 140/80. Which of the following is indicative of a compartment syndrome?

A. Deep posterior compartment pressure within 30 mmHg of the diastolic blood pressure

B. Superficial compartment pressure of 25 mmHg

C. Anterior compartment pressure within 70 mmHg of the mean arterial pressure

D. Diastolic blood pressure of 50 mmHg

E. An open fracture

Ref.: 4, 8

COMMENTS: Compartment syndrome occurs when end-capillary perfusion pressure is less than intracompartmental pressure. • Compartment syndromes typically occur in the setting of trauma. • Typical presenting symptoms include pain disproportionate to the injury, pain on passive stretching of the tendons traversing the compartment, and parasthesias. • The deep posterior and anterior compartments in the leg are most commonly involved, although any muscular compartment in the body may be at risk. • A pulse may be present even with a compartment syndrome. • Recent investigations have reported that perfusion gradients (diastolic blood pressure minus compartment pressure) of 30 mmHg or less are indicative of a compartment syndrome. • An open fracture does not preclude a compartment syndrome. • Compartment syndromes are treated by immediate fasciotomy.

ANSWER:
A

33. With regard to the assessment of ankle injury, which of the following statements is/are true?

    A. Ability to walk immediately after injury excludes fracture.

    B. Medial tenderness in the presence of an ankle fracture is suggestive of injury to the deltoid ligament or its bony attachment.

    C. Lateral tenderness after adduction injury is suggestive of osteonecrosis.

    D. Stress radiographs should be avoided because they are painful and do not help with the diagnosis.

Ref.: 4, 6

COMMENTS: Ligamentous and bony injuries of the ankle frequently result from rotational or abduction-adduction forces. • An anatomic reduction and a symmetric ankle mortise is necessary to maintain ankle stability and prevent premature ankle arthritis. • Initial evaluation should include a history of the mechanism of injury and examination for the site of tenderness, swelling, or deformity. • If the patient was able to walk after the injury, the ankle may be stable, but fracture cannot be excluded. • Adequate radiologic evaluation requires standard anteroposterior and lateral views as well as a mortise view obtained in a 10- to 15-degree medial oblique position. • The most common ankle injury is lateral collateral ligament strain. • Tenderness distal to the medial malleolus is suggestive of deltoid ligament injury. • This injury is seen with abduction and external rotation injuries. • Integrity of the lateral collateral ligament and deltoid ligament can be assessed with stress films, which may require the help of local or general anesthesia.

ANSWER:
B

34. Complications of hip dislocation include all but which of the following?

    A. Sciatic nerve injury

    B. Avascular necrosis

    C. Degenerative arthritis

    D. Compartmental syndromes

Ref.: 2

COMMENTS: Avascular necrosis of the femoral head and the later development of degenerative arthritis are the most common complications of hip dislocations. • Avascular necrosis occurs in about 20% of patients, and the incidence is directly related to delay in reduction. • Approximately half of patients who have a hip dislocation later acquire posttraumatic arthritis. • Chondral and osteochondral fractures of the femoral head are more common with posterior dislocations, increasing the risk for arthritic deterioration. • CT scanning is the most effective diagnostic imaging test used to evaluate bone injury. • Sciatic nerve injury is a potential complication when the hip dislocates posteriorly. • A compartmental syndrome is not a complication of hip dislocation.

ANSWER:
D

35. Match each mechanism of injury in the left-hand column with a fracture of the spine in the right-hand column.

    A. Hyperflexion   a. Hangman's fracture

    B. Axial load on the head   b. Teardrop fracture

    C. Extension   c. Jefferson fracture

    D. Flexion-rotation   d. Dislocation

    E. Avulsion   e. Clay shoveler's fracture

Ref.: 1, 2

COMMENTS: Although spinal fractures are common, fewer than 10% are associated with neurologic deficit. • In patients with a history of trauma who complain of pain or tenderness in the neck, a fracture must be suspected. • The neck should be immobilized. • A complete neurologic examination, followed by adequate radiographic evaluation with full view of levels C1–T1, is mandatory. • Fractures of the posterior arch of the atlas (Jefferson's fracture) are caused by an axial load. • A fracture through the pedicles of C2 (hangman's fracture) is caused by a severe extension injury. • Compression fracture of the cervical spine (teardrop fracture) is frequently caused by hyperflexion of the neck, as in diving accidents, and is associated with a high incidence of neurologic injury. • Dislocation of the cervical spine occurs most commonly between C5 and C6. • The injury results from a flexion-rotation force, with dislocation of the facets and concomitant capsular ligament rupture. • Severe muscular contraction can avulse the spinous processes, as in the clay shoveler's fracture.

ANSWER:
A-b; B-c; C-a; D-d; E-e

36. Indications for operation in patients with acute fractures or dislocations of the cervical spine include all but which of the following?

    A. Unstable fractures or dislocations

    B. Progressive neurologic deficits

    C. Established neurologic deficit

    D. Persistent bone fragments in the spinal canal

Ref.: 1, 2

COMMENTS: Patients with unstable fractures or dislocations may be treated by stabilization procedures. • Reduction and stabilization are indicated in patients who present with minimal neurologic findings that subsequently progress. • In patients with fragments in the spinal canal, operative intervention is mandatory in the presence of a neurologic deficit. • The role of surgery for patients with acute fractures and dislocations and established neurologic deficits is controversial.

ANSWER:
C

37. Which of the following statements regarding spinal cord trauma is false?

A. Immediate intravenous infusion of methylprednisolone following spinal cord injury may improve motor recovery.

B. Progressive neurologic deficit warrants surgical intervention.

C. Most (85%) cervical spinal injuries are detected on plain lateral radiographs.

D. A soft cervical collar provides adequate stability for most bone cervical injuries.

Ref.: 4

COMMENTS: Multicenter studies have verified the efficacy of intravenous steroid infusion for decreasing spinal cord injury with trauma. • The best results occur if treatment begins within the first 8 hr after the accident (30 mg/kg within 8 hr and then 5.4 mg/kg/hr for the next 24 hr). • Controversy persists as to the timing and method of surgery following spinal cord injury associated with malalignment or canal compromise. • However, progressive neurologic deficit requires immediate decompression and stabilization. • Radiographs of the cervical spine, including open-mouth views, are essential for diagnosing the fracture, with lateral radiographs being the most sensitive. • CT scanning remains the standard for evaluating spinal fractures and canal compromise. • Soft cervical collars are ineffective in providing stability. • Rigid collars can restrict flexion-extension, but a halo vest is necessary to control rotation and is indicated for unstable cervical spine injuries.

ANSWER:
D

38. A 42-year-old man feels a sudden sharp pain in the lower calf after jumping for a basketball. Examination reveals weak plantar flexion and dorsiflexion of the ankle with diffuse ecchymosis. Examining the patient prone with his legs over the edge of the examining table shows that he has no palpable defect, but squeezing the calf muscle fails to produce ankle plantar flexion. What is the diagnosis?

A. Subfascial hematoma

B. Torn Achilles tendon

C. Torn plantaris tendon

D. Torn gastrocnemius muscle

E. Torn posterior tibial tendon

Ref.: 4, 5

COMMENTS: Eccentric contraction of the calf muscles in middle-aged men can result in lower leg muscle and tendon injuries. • Those with occasional participation in recreational sports are at greatest risk. • The Thompson test, performed by squeezing the calf muscles to assess ankle plantar flexion with the patient in the prone position, is pathognomic for tears of the Achilles tendon. • Gastrocnemius muscle tears occur under similar circumstances, but patients typically have more proximal swelling and a negative Thompson test.

ANSWER:
B

39. A 31-year-old man is involved in an altercation and is forced to jump out of a second-story window. He presents to the emergency department with pain localized to the distal right tibia. The patient is alert and oriented, with no other systemic complaints. Physical examination reveals a 2-cm opening over the anterior aspect of the distal tibia. The patient is neurovascularly intact. The right distal tibia is found to have moderate swelling. X-rays reveal the patient to have a severely displaced and comminuted fracture of the distal tibia involving the metaphysis and extending into the articular surface. The fracture is found to have 30 degrees of angulation in the sagittal plane. X-rays of the chest, pelvis, and cervical spine are normal. What is the best option for management of the patient's fracture?

A. Irrigation and débridement in the operating room followed by application of a short leg cast

B. Irrigation and débridement in the emergency room followed by application of a sugar-tong splint

C. Irrigation and débridement followed by open reduction and internal fixation via an extensile approach of the tibia fracture

D. Irrigation and débridement of the wound followed by application of an external fixator with limited internal fixation

E. Administration of antibiotics in the emergency department followed by application of a long leg cast

Ref.: 8

COMMENTS: Distal tibial fractures involving the articular surface are referred to as tibial pilon or tibial plafond fractures. • These fractures may be classified as low-energy and high-energy injuries. • Low-energy injuries may be amenable to immediate open reduction and internal fixation. • However, this patient's injury is an example of a high-energy injury. • The most devastating complication associated with this type of injury is extensive wound dehiscence, which may be avoided by respecting the soft tissues. • Initial management of any open fracture should consist of irrigation, débridement, and administration of intravenous antibiotics. • Soft-tissue stripping should be minimized to avoid the complication of wound dehiscence. • The immediate goals of pilon fracture treatment are to avoid complications and restore overall limb alignment. • Definitive reconstruction may be performed 1–2 weeks after injury, once the soft-tissue envelope has had a chance to recover.

ANSWER:
D

40. Which of the following is most closely associated with the development of heterotopic ossification (HO)?

A. Tibia fracture with concomitant ankle dislocation

B. Acetabular fracture with a ruptured spleen

C. Dislocated shoulder with associated glenoid rim fracture

D. Elbow fracture dislocation with concomitant head injury

E. Acute ACL tear with associated medial meniscal tear

Ref.: 6

COMMENTS: HO is the formation of extraosseous bone. • The development of HO is most clearly associated with elbow fracture dislocations with associated head or spinal cord injury. • This typically leads to pain around the elbow and eventual ankylosis of the elbow. • The cause is unclear at this time, although reports state that up to 80% of patients with concomitant elbow fracture dislocation and head injury will develop HO. • The key to treatment is prevention. • Patients at risk should be treated with a course of indomethacin or postoperative radiation therapy to the elbow. • HO may be excised once complete maturation has occurred, typically requiring 12–18 months.

ANSWER:
D

41. A 16-year-old boy is seen in the emergency department with a gunshot wound to the thigh. Examination reveals one bullet wound in the posterior lateral aspect of the mid-thigh. There is obvious deformity of the femur and a peroneal nerve palsy. Anteroposterior and lateral radiographs of the femur are shown. What should the physician recommend?

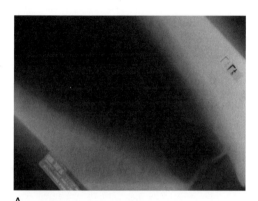

A

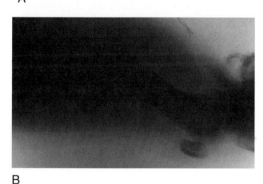

B

A. Skeletal traction followed by long leg casting

B. Closed intramedullary (IM) nailing of the femur with a locked nail

C. Exploration of the peroneal nerve and plating of the femur

D. Bullet extraction, peroneal nerve exploration, and IM nailing of the femur

Ref.: 4

COMMENTS: Gunshot injuries to the femur are generally treated in the same manner as is a closed femoral shaft fracture. • With low-velocity gunshot wounds, the track is débrided locally at the skin, but a formal, extensive débridement is not necessary. • Most nerve injuries in such cases are neurapraxias due to the concussive effect of the bullet and do not require exploration. • A small percentage of gunshot fractures are due to a close-range shotgun blast or military-style high-velocity bullets. • These fractures are similar to type III open fractures and require extensive débridement, delayed fixation, and possibly external fixation.

ANSWER:
B

42. A 25-year-old man is seen in the emergency department with a gunshot wound to the shoulder. The radiograph reveals the bullet near the glenoid with a fracture of the inferior glenoid rim. The CT scan reveals that the bullet remains intra-articularly. What should the physician recommend?

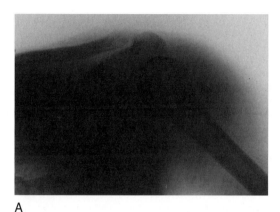

A

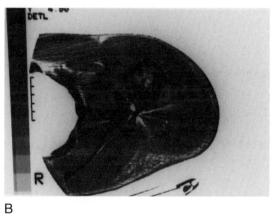

B

A. Sling immobilization with oral antibiotics

B. Sling immobilization with intravenous antibiotics

C. Open or arthroscopic débridement of the bullet fragments and intravenous antibiotics

D. Delayed exploration if infection develops

Ref.: 4, 5

COMMENTS: Whereas the bullet in bullet wounds in the soft tissues of extremities rarely requires removal, retained intra-articular foreign bodies should be débrided while the joint is inspected. Damage to the articular surfaces should be treated. • Arthroscopic débridement is the method of choice unless fracture care necessitates wide exposure.

ANSWER:
C

R E F E R E N C E S

1. Brunicardi FC, Andersen DK, Billiar TR, et al (eds): *Schwartz's Principles of Surgery*, 8th ed. McGraw-Hill, New York, 2004.
2. Townsend CM Jr, Beauchamp RD, Evers BM, et al: *Sabiston Textbook of Surgery: The Biological Basis of Modern Surgical Practice,* 17th ed. Saunders, Philadelphia, 2004.
3. Morrissey RT, Weinstien SL: *Lovell and Winters Pediatric Orthopaedics*, 4th ed. Lippincott, Philadelphia, 1996.
4. Browner BD, Jupiter JB, Levine AM, et al: *Skeletal Trauma.* Saunders, Philadelphia, 1992.
5. Deg R: *Principles of Orthopaedic Practice.* McGraw-Hill, New York, 1992.
6. Miller MD: *Review of Orthopaedics*, 3rd ed. Saunders, Philadelphia, 2000.
7. Norris TR: *Orthopaedic Knowledge Update: Shoulder and Elbow, vol. 2,* 2nd ed. American Academy of Orthopaedic Surgeons, Rosemont, IL, 2002.
8. Koval KJ: *Orthopaedic Knowledge Update, vol. 7.* American Academy of Orthopaedic Surgeons, Rosemont, IL, 2002.
9. Sponseller PD: *Orthopaedic Knowledge Update: Pediatrics, vol. 2.* American Academy of Orthopaedic Surgeons, Rosemont, IL, 2002.

C. Acquired Diseases

Edward H. Kolb, M.D., and Eric M. Berkson, M.D.

1. Match each type of joint in the left-hand column with the appropriate example in the right-hand column.

   A. Fibrous joint   a. Hip

   B. Fibrocartilaginous joint   b. Skull sutures

   C. Synovial joint   c. Intervertebral disc

   Ref.: 1

COMMENTS: Joints may be categorized according to the tissue type by which they are joined. • A **fibrous** joint (synarthrosis) represents two bones joined by fibrous tissue, as exemplified by the suture lines in the skull. • **Fibrocartilaginous** joints (symphyses) are those in which the bones are joined by hyaline cartilage or fibrocartilage, such as the pubic symphysis and the intervertebral discs. • **Synovial** (diarthrodial) joints are movable joints in which cartilage-covered bone ends articulate within a synovium-lined capsule, permitting more motion to occur. • Most joints of the extremities are synovial joints. • The type of motion a synovial joint permits is determined by the contour of the articular surfaces, the anatomy of the supporting connective tissues (capsule and ligaments), and the external forces applied to it.

ANSWER:
A-b; B-c; C-a

2. Which of the following organisms is most commonly found in pyogenic arthritis?

   A. *Escherichia coli*

   B. *Staphylococcus aureus*

   C. *Hemophilus influenzae*

   D. *Pseudomonas* spp.

   Ref.: 6, 8

COMMENTS: Pyogenic, or septic, arthritis is a severe joint condition that, if not diagnosed and managed early in the clinical course, will likely result in permanent joint disability. • This orthopedic emergency is most often caused by hematogenous spread of organisms from other infected sites. • Direct infection by way of traumatic wounds and extension of adjacent osteomyelitis are also seen. • The most common causative organism is *S. aureus*. • Other common organisms include *Streptococcus pyogenes, Streptococcus pneumoniae, Staphylococcus epidermidis, Neisseria gonorrhoeae*. • *H. influenzae* is less common since the advent of the childhood vaccine.

The clinical manifestation is that of local tenderness, swelling, and extreme pain on motion. • The specific diagnosis is made by joint aspiration with immediate Gram's staining and culture.

• Crystal analysis should be performed on the joint fluid to rule out crystalline arthropathy, specifically, gout and pseudogout. • Administration of systemic antibiotics should be started promptly and the joint surgically drained on an urgent basis. • Drainage can be performed using arthroscopic or open surgical techniques. • Adequate débridement of all devitalized tissue is necessary to prevent recurrent abcess formation.

ANSWER:
B

3. Which metabolic bone disease is described as a quantitative decrease in bone mass and microarchitectural deterioration of bone tissue?

   A. Osteomalacia

   B. Rickets

   C. Osteoporosis

   D. Osteopetrosis

   E. Paget's disease

   Ref.: 6, 8

COMMENTS: Osteomalacia is a metabolic disorder in which the total amount (quantitative) of bone is normal but there is inadequate mineralization (qualitative) of newly formed bone. • Osteomalacia occurs in adults, whereas rickets occurs in children. • Rickets is characterized by an inadequate mineralization of the growth plate. • Both osteomalacia and rickets may be caused by various disorders affecting calcium and phosphate metabolism. • Osteopetrosis (Albers-Schönberg disease, or marble bone disease) is a rare disorder characterized by a decrease in bone resorption by osteoclasts with normal bone formation. • This results in increased bone density and obliteration of the marrow space. • Paget's disease is second to osteoporosis as the most common metabolic bone disease, with some evidence supporting a viral (paramyxovirus) cause. • Paget's disease, usually asymptomatic, is characterized by abnormal bone remodeling manifested by coarsened bone trabeculae and remodeled cortices, resulting in a "mosaic" bone pattern. • Osteoporosis is a quantitative decrease in bone mass that increases a patient's overall risk of fracture. • Risk factors for osteoporosis include a sedentary life style, low body weight, smoking, and poor nutrition. • Dual-energy x-ray absorptiometry (DEXA) is the gold standard for diagnosis when bone mass is less than 2.5 standard deviations below the mean peak bone mass measurements defined as osteoporosis.

ANSWER:
C

4. The most common site of skeletal tuberculosis is which of the following?

   A. Knee

   B. Hip

   C. Spine

   D. Humerus

Ref.: 6, 7, 8

COMMENTS: Skeletal tuberculosis remains a significant problem in most of the Asian and African countries. • Tuberculosis is now more commonly seen in immunocompromised patients (e.g., HIV infection and chemotherapy), typically in large urban areas. • Although skeletal tuberculosis is rare in the United States (1% of all cases of tuberculosis), its incidence has increased since 1980. • The most common site of involvement is the spine. • Peripheral joint tuberculosis also occurs and usually involves synovium, bone, and cartilage. • If untreated, joint tuberculosis usually results in complete joint destruction, deformity, and pain. • In contrast to septic arthritis, the clinical course of skeletal tuberculosis is insidious. • Symptoms may last weeks to months before the patient seeks medical advice. • Worsening of the pain at night is a characteristic feature. • The diagnosis requires recovery of organisms from the involved joint or bone. • Treatment involves antituberculous drug therapy, rest (bracing), and general supportive and nutritional measures. • Surgical management is indicated for patients with advanced lesions, including those with caseation or severe joint destruction.

A N S W E R :
C

5. An 8-year-old African American boy with sickle cell anemia has a 1-week history of progressive right tibia pain, swelling, and erythema and a limp after a superficial skin abrasion. He is seen in the emergency department, at which time thorough clinical and radiographic evaluations are performed. His WBC count is 18,000/mm^3 with greater than 90% neutrophils, his ESR is 105, and his CRP is 78. Blood culture results are negative, and x-ray evaluation reveals signs of periosteal elevation with soft-tissue extension. The patient is felt to have osteomyelitis. What is the most common causative organism?

   A. Group B streptococcus

   B. *Salmonella multilocida*

   C. *N. gonorrhoeae*

   D. *S. aureus*

   E. *H. influenzae*

Ref.: 9

COMMENTS: The patient presents with a typical history of osteomyelitis. • Although patients with sickle cell anemia are at increased risk for infection with *Salmonella* spp., *S. aureus* is the most common organism. • *H. influenzae* has been relatively uncommon since routine vaccinations have been initiated. • Group B streptococcus is a common cause of infection in newborn infants. • *N. gonorrhoeae* is a common infecting organism in adult septic arthritis, developing in 1–3% of patients with gonococcal infection.

A N S W E R :
D

6. Which one of the following is true regarding an autosomal dominant disorder of collagen synthesis caused by a mutation in the *FBN1* gene exhibiting musculoskeletal, ocular, and cardiovascular abnormalities.

   A. The disorder is referred to as Ehlers-Danlos syndrome.

   B. Cardiovascular factors are the primary factors contributing to increased morbidity and mortality.

   C. The diagnosis may be made by demonstrating homocysteine in the urine.

   D. It is not usually associated with arachnodactyly, scoliosis, or lens dislocations.

   E. It is often referred to as brittle bone disease.

Ref.: 6, 8

COMMENTS: Ehlers-Danlos syndrome is an autosomal dominant connective tissue disorder caused by a mutation in the COL5A, COL5A2, or COL3A1 genes. • Patients typically exhibit skin extensibility, articular hypermobility, and tissue fragility. • Ocular abnormalities are not typically present. • Homocystinuria, an autosomal recessive inborn error of methionine metabolism, demonstrates increased homocysteine in the urine. • These patients exhibit marfanoid-like habitus. • Brittle bone disease is another name for osteogenesis imperfecta (OI), caused by an abnormality in quantity or quality of type I collagen production. • OI results in osteopenia, variable degrees of short stature, and progressive skeletal deformity, with an increased incidence of fractures. • This question is describing Marfan's syndrome, a disorder of collagen synthesis in which patients exhibit arachnodactyly (long, slender fingers), pectus deformities, scoliosis, cardiac abnormalities, and ocular pathologic conditions (e.g., superior lens dislocations).

A N S W E R :
B

7. Which one of the following statements regarding HIV syndrome is true?

   A. Musculoskeletal involvement is rare.

   B. HIV arthropathy is best treated with methotrexate and azathioprine (AZT).

   C. Pyogenic arthritis may occur despite low synovial WBC counts (<10,000/mm^3).

   D. HIV septic arthopathy is a benign disorder managed with conservative antimicrobial therapy.

Ref.: 1

COMMENTS: Infection with HIV can lead to a variety of musculoskeletal manifestations. • The most common is a sterile polyarthritis, which presents in a manner similar to that of psoriatic arthropathy, with atypical skin lesions, joint swelling, and arthralgias. • Treatment typically involves nonsteroidal antiinflammatory drugs (NSAIDs), although some patients respond to a combination of AZT and etidronate. • Immunosuppressive medications, including methotrexate, are not recommended. • Pyogenic joint infections, although uncommon, can be difficult to diagnose. • HIV patients may be unable to mount the appropriate response, leading to false-negative synovial analysis results. • The synovial WBC count may remain within normal limits, making diagnosis difficult. • Treatment, however, is similar to that for non-HIV patients: aggressive surgical drainage and intravenous antibiotics.

A N S W E R :
C

8. With regard to the clinical features of gonococcal arthritis, which of the following statements is/are true?

A. It occurs predominantly in elderly males.

B. It usually begins as a migratory polyarthralgia.

C. The hip, knee, and shoulder are the most common sites of infection.

D. Even with proper treatment, mild residual loss of joint motion usually results.

Ref.: 6, 8

COMMENTS: Gonococcal urethritis in males usually is symptomatic and causes the patient to seek early medical treatment. • In contrast, gonococcal cervicitis or vaginitis in females frequently is asymptomatic, and the sequelae of septicemia and arthritis are therefore more common among females (4:1). • Initial symptoms usually include migratory polyarthralgia, with a variable febrile course. • The infection usually localizes in the knee, elbow, or wrist. • Diagnosis requires recovery of gonococcal organisms from the septic joint. • Treatment includes a 2-week course of penicillin and appropriate joint immobilization. • With proper treatment, there is usually full recovery of joint function.

ANSWER:
B

9. Radiographic findings of rheumatoid arthritis include which of the following?

A. Subluxation

B. Osteoporosis

C. Bone erosions

D. Joint deformity

E. All of the above

Ref.: 6, 8

COMMENTS: There are many radiographic abnormalities in patients with rheumatoid arthritis, depending on the stage of the disease process and the specific joints involved. • The earliest findings are those related to the destructive effects of the hyperplastic synovium and are best seen on radiographs of the hands. • Fusiform swelling, particularly in the area of the proximal interphalangeal or metacarpophalangeal joints, is common. • As the disease progresses, periarticular bone erosions produced by osteoclastic resorption occur. • This cortical irregularity is made apparent by the development of periosteal new bone formation in response to the synovial inflammation. • Osteoporosis occurs as a result of disuse as well as inflammation in the surrounding tissues. • Further progression results in subluxation of the involved joints and joint deformity (particularly ulnar deviation at the metacarpophalangeal joints).

ANSWER:
E

10. With regard to joint fluid assessment, which one of the following statements is correct?

A. Joints should be aspirated with a 22-gauge or smaller needle to prevent hemarthrosis.

B. The mucin clot test helps differentiate inflammatory from degenerative joint abnormalities.

C. The normal gradient of glucose concentration between plasma and joint fluid is approximately 50 mg/dl.

D. Most joint fluid crystals can be adequately assessed with standard microscopic illumination techniques.

Ref.: 4, 6

COMMENTS: Aspiration of a joint to obtain fluid for testing is commonly required for evaluation of joint abnormalities. • It should be accomplished through scrupulously sterile technique. • In general, the use of an 18-gauge or larger needle is recommended in order to be able to aspirate the more viscous fluid associated with certain pathologic processes. • The fluid obtained should be routinely examined for color, appearance, and viscosity and should undergo Gram's stain examination, bacterial culture, mucin clot test, WBC count, crystal examination, and measurement of glucose concentration. • The mucin clot test is a good qualitative assessment of the character of the protein-polysaccharide complex of synovial fluid. • A firm, rope-like clot that does not easily fragment suggests normal polymerization and is seen in normal joints and those with degenerative arthritis. • Poor mucin clots suggest the presence of one of the inflammatory arthritides. • Similarly, the gradient between joint fluid and plasma glucose concentration may suggest the presence of infection or rheumatoid arthritis. • Under such conditions, this gradient may be 50 mg/dl or greater. • Normally, the gradient is less than 10 mg/dl. • Assessment of joint fluid crystals also is important, particularly if gout and pseudogout are possible diagnoses. • Such assessment requires examination of the joint fluid under polarized light. • Rod-shaped urate crystals, which manifest a strongly negative birefringence, are seen with gout, while rhomboid crystals with weakly positive birefringence are seen with pseudogout.

ANSWER:
B

11. With regard to rheumatoid arthritis, which of the following statements is/are true?

A. Its incidence peaks during the fourth and fifth decades of life.

B. It occurs more commonly in men.

C. It is easily distinguished from other autoimmune disorders.

D. A negative rheumatoid factor assay result rules out the disease.

E. The clinical manifestations of rheumatoid arthritis are limited to joint disorders.

Ref.: 6, 8

COMMENTS: Rheumatoid arthritis is a systemic disease that may involve the musculoskeletal, cardiovascular, respiratory, and nervous systems. • Its incidence peaks during the fourth and fifth decades of life, and it has a marked predominance in females. • Because multiple systems may be involved, it is sometimes difficult to differentiate rheumatoid arthritis from other autoimmune disorders. • A positive rheumatoid factor is seen in 90% of adult patients and in only 20% of juvenile patients with rheumatoid arthritis. • Thus, a negative assay result does not rule out the disease.

From a surgical standpoint, the most significant changes in rheumatoid arthritis are those affecting the synovial joints and the adjacent tendons, tendon sheaths, and bursae. • Surgeons treating these disorders must be aware of the cardiopulmonary and other systemic effects of rheumatoid arthritis as well as the side effects of drugs (e.g., steroids, NSAIDs, and methotrexate) used to treat this disease.

ANSWER:
A

12. With regard to the management of rheumatoid arthritis, which one of the following statements is true?

A. Medical management is the mainstay of treatment of early rheumatoid arthritis.

B. As opposed to osteoarthritis, physical therapy does not reduce the pain of rheumatoid arthritis or affect the progressive joint destruction and disability from the underlying disease.

C. Synovectomy of involved joints should be performed along with initial medical therapy in newly diagnosed cases to prevent progression of the disease.

D. Synovectomy is contraindicated in rheumatoid arthritis.

Ref.: 6, 8

COMMENTS: Patients with rheumatoid arthritis are best managed in a multidisciplinary way, with input from a rheumatologist, an orthopedist, and physical and occupational therapists. • Although management of early or less severe cases involves appropriate medical intervention (i.e., analgesics and anti-inflammatory medications), physical therapy and counseling with regard to physical activities may be of great benefit early in the course of the disease process. • Such therapy not only relieves the associated pain but also plays a major role in maintaining strength and joint mobility and delaying joint deformity.

Synovectomy has been beneficial in relieving pain and preventing or delaying joint destruction in selected patients. • However, it should be performed only when there is evidence of disease progression despite adequate anti-inflammatory treatment and modification of activity. • Synovectomy appears to have the greatest benefit in the management of rheumatoid arthritis of the knee and does not appear to modify the disease process when it involves the metacarpophalangeal or metatarsophalangeal joints.

A N S W E R :
A

13. Which one of the following statements characterizes osteoarthritis?

A. The earliest recognizable changes occur in the subchondral bone.

B. Radiographic changes include joint-space narrowing, osteophyte formation, sclerosis, and cyst formation.

C. There is a strong correlation between clinical symptoms and radiographic changes.

D. The amount of chondroitin sulfate is increased in the articular cartilage.

E. The articular cartilage is involved late in the disease process.

Ref.: 6, 8

COMMENTS: Osteoarthritis is a term that refers to degenerative changes in synovial joints. • The earliest changes seen are those in the articular cartilage. • On gross examination, the cartilage may appear softer and yellower than usual, while on biochemical examination, a decrease in the normal amount of chondroitin sulfate is seen. • Because cartilage is not normally seen on radiographs, these early changes, which may be symptomatic, are not seen radiographically. • Thus, at times there is a poor correlation between the clinical and radiographic findings. • This process is more one of degeneration than of inflammation. • Accordingly, some authors believe that the terms **degenerative joint disease** and

osteoarthrosis more accurately describe the process. • Joint-space narrowing, osteophyte formation, bony sclerosis, and subchondral cysts are common radiographic findings in osteoarthritis.

A N S W E R :
B

14. The classic clinical manifestation of osteoarthritis includes which of the following?

A. Joint pain occurring on motion and relieved by rest

B. Frequent involvement of the metacarpophalangeal joints

C. An elevated serum–synovial fluid glucose gradient

D. Fairly abrupt onset of symptoms

Ref.: 6, 8

COMMENTS: Osteoarthritis may be considered a primary disease in which there is no antecedent joint disorder or a secondary entity that is related to previous joint trauma, rheumatoid disease, gout, or other forms of inflammatory arthritis. • The onset is usually insidious, and the primary symptom is joint pain brought on by motion and weight bearing and relieved by rest. • Primary osteoarthritis is a disease of the elderly, usually manifesting in persons 60 years and older. • It is most common in the large weight-bearing joints, especially the hips, knees, and spine. • Secondary osteoarthritis may be found in any joint that has been previously altered by trauma, rheumatoid arthritis, or other inflammatory conditions. • The elbows, wrists, and metacarpophalangeal joints are rarely involved. • Laboratory examinations are usually unrevealing, and in the absence of an underlying inflammatory process, the synovial fluid reveals few abnormalities.

A N S W E R :
A

15. Match each surgical procedure used for osteoarthritis of the hip in the left-hand column with the appropriate descriptive statement in the right-hand column.

A. Arthrodesis	a. An 80-year-old woman with a displaced femoral neck fracture without arthritic changes on the acetabulum
B. Proximal femoral osteotomy	b. A 24-year-old male heavy laborer with a destroyed hip joint secondary to recurrent infections
C. Hemiarthroplasty (replacement of the femoral head and neck)	c. A 10-year-old boy with hip dysplasia and a valgus deformity of the femoral neck
D. Total hip arthroplasty	d. A 60-year-old man with severe osteoarthritis of the hip

Ref.: 6, 8

COMMENTS: A number of operative procedures are available to treat disorders of the hip. • **Arthrodesis** (fusion of the hip joint) is most frequently indicated when the presence of pyogenic or tuberculous sepsis precludes prosthetic arthroplasty. • It also represents an alternative for young patients with severe degenerative joint changes.

• **Osteotomy** of the proximal femur involves transection of the femoral shaft and displacement or angulation of the femoral head and neck. • It allows articulation of less severely involved cartilage of the femoral head with the acetabulum. • It results in excellent pain relief and improved joint motion in carefully selected young patients with early osteoarthritis or hip dysplasia. • **Hemiarthroplasty** (replacement of the femoral head and neck) is used mainly for femoral head and neck fractures. • It requires a normal acetabulum. • **Total hip replacement** is indicated when both the femoral head and acetabulum are involved. • It has the best overall results of all of the procedures available. • However, complications from infection or loosening of the prostheses may be severe and debilitating. • The tendency to avoid its use in the young population has been based on unanswered questions about the long-term performance of the prostheses, particularly the risk of loosening. • Research in the fields of bioengineering and bioprosthetics is extremely active in this regard.

ANSWER:
A-b; B-c; C-a; D-d

16. With regard to chondromalacia of the patella, which one of the following statements is true?

   A. The initial changes usually occur on the lateral aspect of the patella.

   B. Patellectomy is the only form of surgical therapy that has proved successful.

   C. Radiographs show characteristic changes early in the course of the disease process.

   D. The progressive nature of the disease warrants early surgical intervention.

   E. The pain is aggravated by knee flexion, kneeling, and descending stairs.

Ref.: 6, 8

COMMENTS: Chondromalacia of the patella, as its name implies, is a disease process of the cartilage of the patella. • The hallmarks are softening and discoloration of the cartilage. • The initial changes are usually seen on the medial aspect of the patella. • The characteristic clinical manifestation is an insidious onset of anterior knee or peripatellar pain aggravated by knee flexion, direct pressure (as when kneeling), and descending stairs. • As with other forms of cartilage injury, radiographs are frequently negative and not diagnostic, especially during the early stages of the disease. • Most patients with this problem are adequately managed by conservative treatment, which involves strengthening the quadriceps muscle. • For advanced cases, surgical intervention may be warranted. • The spectrum of surgical management includes local shaving or resection of the involved cartilage (chondroplasty), realignment of the quadriceps mechanism, and total knee replacement (for degeneration involving the trochlea of the femur). • Patellectomy is rarely performed.

ANSWER:
E

17. With regard to hallux valgus, which of the following statements is/are true?

   A. Exostosis removal is usually effective.

   B. Surgical intervention should be considered before the patient experiences any type of pain.

   C. It is much more common in populations in which shoes are not worn.

   D. Silastic arthroplasty is the surgical procedure of choice in most instances.

   E. Most patients with hallux valgus are asymptomatic and do not require surgical intervention.

Ref.: 6, 8

COMMENTS: Hallux valgus refers to the lateral deviation of the great toe and medial deviation of the first metatarsal. • It is popularly considered synonymous with **bunion**, which refers more specifically to the large exostosis and overlying soft-tissue bursa that frequently occur in association with hallux valgus. • This is primarily a disease of the shoe-wearing population (improper shoe fitting). • Whereas the anatomic abnormality is fairly common, the associated symptoms of intermittent pain over the involved metatarsophalangeal joint occur relatively infrequently. • Conservative treatment with the use of molded insoles and metatarsal arches to redistribute the body weight is usually successful. • When symptoms persist despite conservative measures, surgical intervention may be warranted. • Surgical management may include simple exostectomy, soft-tissue repair, osteotomy of the metatarsal, or fusion, depending on the pathophysiologic mechanism and other factors. • Prosthetic arthroplasty generally is not employed for this condition.

ANSWER:
E

18. A 62-year-old man with a past medical history significant only for hypertension is admitted to the hospital with a 3-day history of progressive right knee pain and low-grade fever. The patient does not recall a history of trauma to the knee. On physical examination, the right knee is found to be erythematous, with a moderate effusion. There is diffuse tenderness with palpation about the knee, and the patient refuses to place the knee through range-of-motion movements because of severe pain. The WBC count is 13,500/mm^3, the ESR is 80, and the CRP is 110. The knee is aspirated, revealing a WBC of 98,000/mm^3, with 98% neutrophils, no uric acid crystals, no calcium pyrophosphate crystals, and gram-positive cocci in clusters revealed on Gram's staining. X-rays are normal. What should the definitive treatment at this point be?

   A. Treat with Ancef 1 g intravenously every 8 hr for 6 weeks.

   B. Perform serial aspirations of the right knee, and administer a 1-week course of intravenous Ancef.

   C. Treat initially with intravenous colchicine, followed by a course of indomethacin for the acute pain.

   D. Treat the patient with observation only, and reassess in 12 hr.

   E. Immediately irrigate and débride the right knee in the operating room, followed by a course of intravenous antibiotics.

Ref.: 5, 6, 8

COMMENTS: This patient has a typical presentation of septic arthritis. • Severe pain with active or passive range of motion of the knee in the absence of preceding trauma should lead one to be suspicious of a septic joint. • Other processes to consider include gout, chondrocalcinosis, inflammatory arthritis, hemorrhagic arthritis, and noninflammatory arthritis. • Septic joints typically present with intra-articular WBC counts greater than 75,000/mm^3, except in immunocompromised patients (e.g., patients with HIV or chronic steroid users), when a lower threshold for infection should be maintained. • The positive Gram's stain result in this case is indicative of infection. • Antibiotics should not be started until fluid is attained from the joint and subjected to Gram's staining and culture. • Operative irrigation and débridement constitute the treatment of choice. • Broad-spectrum antibiotics should be started until definitive antibiotic sensitivities are known.

ANSWER:
E

19. A 2-year-old child is brought to the emergency department by his mother for an apparent limp. The patient's mother states that her son was fine until 2 days before, when he began limping on his right leg. She cannot recall a history of trauma. The patient has no history of fever or chills, although he did have an upper respiratory infection about 1 week ago. His temperature is 99.4°F (37.4°C). Physical examination reveals a healthy-appearing 2-year-old boy who walks with a pronounced limp. The patient resists passive range-of-motion movements of the right hip, although knee and ankle range-of-motion movements do not appear to bother him. His WBC count is 10,000/mm³, with an ESR of 14 and a CRP of 5. X-rays include an anteroposterior view of the pelvis as well as right hip, knee, and ankle films, all of which are negative. What is the most likely diagnosis?

   A. Legg-Calvé-Perthes disease

   B. Septic arthritis of the right hip

   C. Avascular necrosis of the right hip

   D. Transient synovitis

   E. Slipped capital femoral epiphysis (SCFE)

Ref.: 9

COMMENTS: Legg-Calvé-Perthes disease is a poorly understood disorder, usually affecting children 3–8 years old, associated with a disturbance of the blood supply to the femoral head. • X-rays typically reveal sclerosis, fragmentation, and collapse of the femoral head, which is typically treated conservatively with maintenance of hip range of motion being the mainstay of treatment. • Slipped capital femoral epiphysis typically occurs in adolescents, and patients are typically obese. • The femoral head is displaced posteriorly and medially, leaving the patient with an out-toeing gait. • Avascular necrosis of the hip usually occurs in adults typically after trauma, although causes such as steroid use, sickle cell disease, caisson disease, and hypercoagulable disorders may be responsible.

Septic arthritis is often difficult to differentiate from the benign disorder of transient synovitis. • Symptoms including fever greater than 100.4°F (38°C), WBC count greater than 12,000/mm³, inability to ambulate, and ESR greater than 40 are suggestive of septic arthritis. • If three or more of these signs are present, the likelihood of septic arthritis is greater than 90%, and hip aspiration is necessary, followed by immediate irrigation and débridement if indeed infected. • Transient synovitis typically occurs preceding a viral infection and is self limited in nature. • If clinical suspicion for transient synovitis is high, close observation with serial examinations is warranted.

ANSWER:
D

20. With regard to gout, which of the following statements is/are true?

   A. It commonly manifests as a monoarticular arthritis of the metatarsophalangeal joint of the great toe.

   B. Diagnosis requires demonstration of calcium pyrophosphate crystals in synovial fluid.

   C. There is a direct correlation between clinical evidence of gout and the serum uric acid level.

   D. Because of the inability of medical management to control chronic disease, surgical intervention is usually required at some point in the clinical course.

Ref.: 6, 8

COMMENTS: Gout is a metabolic disease that may manifest in a primary form (inborn error of metabolism) or a secondary form (e.g., myeloproliferative disorders, leukemia, or hemolytic anemia). • The clinical manifestations of gouty arthritis are caused by the effects of inflammation on the surrounding cartilage, subchondral bone, and periarticular soft tissues as a result of urate crystal deposition in the synovial fluid. • Calcium pyrophosphate deposition is seen with pseudogout. • Although the likelihood of clinical symptoms increases with higher serum uric acid levels, it is not uncommon for significant hyperuricemia to be present without clinical symptoms and for clinical symptoms to be present without hyperuricemia. • The classic clinical manifestation is that of an acute attack of monoarticular arthritis, most often involving the metatarsophalangeal joint of the great toe and occurring in men over age 30.

Management of the acute attack involves rest and anti-inflammatory medication (e.g., colchicine or NSAIDs). • Upon resolution of the acute symptoms, long-term management with allopurinol to reduce serum uric acid levels may be needed. • Surgery is rarely indicated for management of acute or chronic gouty arthritis, but excision of large tophaceous deposits may provide symptomatic relief, and joints that are severely involved may require arthrodesis or arthroplasty.

ANSWER:
A

21. With regard to slipped capital femoral epiphysis, which of the following statements is/are true?

   A. It is more prevalent in females.

   B. It is rarely bilateral.

   C. It commonly resolves spontaneously and typically warrants conservative treatment.

   D. It is often associated with loss of normal internal rotation and knee pain.

   E. It is rarely managed surgically because of the risk of permanent epiphyseal damage.

Ref.: 9

COMMENTS: Slipped capital femoral epiphysis is a relatively rare entity that occurs predominantly in adolescent boys. • It represents a separation of the capital femoral epiphysis through the growth plate region above the zone of calcified cartilage. • The cause of the physeal disruption is unknown, but the muscular forces across the hip result in the characteristic medial and posterior displacement of the capital epiphysis. • The clinical findings include pain in the area of the hip aggravated by motion, pain referred to the knee, and loss of normal internal rotation. • The process is bilateral in 25% of cases. • Treatment is based on the principles of preventing further slippage and minimizing existing deformity by early fusion of the growth plate. • This is achieved most often by surgically pinning the femoral head and neck to engage the epiphysis.

ANSWER:
D

22. Which of the following statements accurately characterize Charcot's joint?

 A. It occurs as a consequence of long term osteoporosis or osteomalacia.

 B. Its onset is usually acute.

 C. Characteristic radiographic findings are those of dense sclerosis of the subchondral bone.

 D. Treatment may involve arthrodesis.

Ref.: 6, 8

COMMENTS: Charcot's joint, or neuropathic joint, is caused by significant articular and periarticular destruction secondary to repeated trauma to structures rendered insensitive by underlying neurologic disorders (e.g., tabes dorsalis, diabetes, or syringomyelia). • The clinical course usually begins with insidious onset, and the patient is often unaware of the joint disability until it becomes severe with gross instability and significant effusion. • Radiographs usually reveal marked bone destruction and abnormality of the joint space, which may contain loose bone fragments. • The foot is most commonly involved in diabetic patients, but the hip and knee are frequently involved. • When conservative management with a properly fitted weight-bearing brace fails, arthrodesis is frequently indicated.

ANSWER:
D

23. Shoulder pain may be caused by all but which of the following?

 A. Spinal arthritis

 B. Lung cancer

 C. Umbilical hernia

 D. Diaphragmatic irritation

 E. Angina

Ref.: 2, 6

COMMENTS: See Question 24.

24. Match each primary shoulder disorder in the left-hand column with the appropriate clinical characteristic in the right-hand column.

 A. Subacromial bursitis

 B. Bicipital tendinitis

 C. Subscapularis tendon tear

 a. A 38-year-old man with positive Speed and Yergason test results and pain extending along the proximal humeral groove

 b. A 60-year-old man with pain over the superior aspect of the shoulder and three fifths strength with external rotation of the shoulder

 c. A 56-year-old man with pain over the anterior aspect of the shoulder and associated weakness with internal rotation of the shoulder

 D. Supraspinatus or infraspinatus rotator cuff tear

 d. A 40-year-old man with pain over the anterolateral aspect of the shoulder reproduced with flexion and internal rotation of the shoulder, and five-fifths strength with all shoulder activity

 e. Pain relieved with injection given from the lateral shoulder just inferior to the acromion

Ref.: 2

COMMENTS: When evaluating shoulder pain, clinicians must be alert to the numerous clinical entities that, although anatomically unrelated, may cause pain referred to the shoulder. • These entities include cervical arthritis with nerve root irritation, Pancoast's tumor, cardiac angina, and abdominal conditions associated with diaphragmatic irritation. • Of the primary shoulder disorders that characteristically produce pain, lesions of the rotator cuff, bicipital tendinitis, and subacromial bursitis are the most common.

The **rotator cuff** consists of the common tendinous insertion of the supraspinatus, infraspinatus, teres minor, and subscapularis muscles. • In positions of full elevation or abduction, the rotator cuff may contact the acromion or coracoacromial ligament and cause irritation of the intervening bursa.

Repeated injury may cause degeneration and lead to **subacromial bursitis**. • This entity is usually characterized by fairly severe and unrelenting pain that is not improved by position and may even necessitate the use of narcotics for relief.

A **rotator cuff tear** is a physical disruption of the tendinous structure, with varying degrees of associated inflammation. • Most rotator cuff tears are partial, and initial conservative management with shoulder immobilization is usually successful. • With total rupture, open surgical repair of the tear is often preferred, but conservative management can be successful.

With **supraspinatus tendinitis**, the pain is more insidious in onset and of lesser degree. • It frequently limits the motions of internal rotation and full abduction, which are painful. • **Bicipital tendinitis** produces symptoms similar to those of supraspinatus tendinitis. • However, the distribution of pain and tenderness is more distal over the proximal humeral or bicipital groove.

With these four inflammatory entities, treatment with rest, analgesics, NSAIDs, and occasionally steroid injection is usually successful.

ANSWERS:
Question 23: C
Question 24: A-d; B-a; C-c; D-b

25. All but which of the following statements about osteomyelitis in adults are true?

 A. MRI is most effective for evaluating medullary involvement.

 B. Surgery is rarely if ever indicated.

 C. Treatment includes appropriate antibiotics, excision of all necrotic tissue augmented by the use of antibiotic-impregnated beads, and dead-space management.

 D. Chronic osteomyelitis can lead to the development of squamous cell carcinoma.

Ref.: 3

COMMENTS: The diagnosis of osteomyelitis is based on clinical judgment coupled with laboratory studies and imaging techniques. • Plain radiographs are helpful but may fail to identify early infection. • Indium-labeled leukocyte scintigraphy is more accurate than is technetium- or gallium-labeled scintigraphy for the diagnosis, but MRI is the most effective technique for evaluating medullary involvement. • MRI is unable to identify cortical osteomyelitis if there is no cortical disruption or medullary involvement. • Appropriate antibiotics and aggressive surgical management are the mainstays of treatment, but late reconstruction of bone loss can be difficult. • A complication of long-standing chronic osteomyelitis is the development of squamous cell carcinoma, which occurs in 0.2–1.7% of patients. • Treatment in these cases often requires amputation.

A N S W E R :

B

R E F E R E N C E S

1. Brunicardi FC, Andersen DK, Billiar TR, et al (eds): *Schwartz's Principles of Surgery*, 8th ed. McGraw-Hill, New York, 2004.
2. *Orthopaedic Knowledge Update: Shoulder and Elbow, vol. 2*, 2nd ed. American Academy of Orthopaedic Surgeons, Rosemont, IL, 2002.
3. Morrissey RT, Weinstien SL: *Lovell and Winters Pediatric Orthopaedics*, 4th ed. Lippincott, Philadelphia, 1996.
4. Browner BD, Jupiter JB, Levine AM, et al: *Skeletal Trauma*. Saunders, Philadelphia, 1992.
5. Deg R: *Principles of Orthopaedic Practice*. McGraw-Hill, New York, 1992.
6. Miller MD: *Review of Orthopaedics*, 3rd ed. Saunders, Philadelphia, 2000.
7. Menendez LR: *Orthopaedic Knowledge Update: Musculoskeletal Tumors*. American Academy of Orthopaedic Surgeons, Rosemont, IL, 2002.
8. Koval KJ: *Orthopaedic Knowledge Update, vol. 7*, American Academy of Orthopaedic Surgeons, Rosemont, IL, 2002.
9. Sponseller PD: *Orthopaedic Knowledge Update: Pediatrics, vol. 2*. American Academy of Orthopaedic Surgeons, Rosemont, IL, 2002.

D. Neoplasms

Edward H. Kolb, M.D., and Eric M. Berkson, M.D.

1. With regard to suspected soft-tissue tumors of the musculoskeletal system, which is the imaging modality of choice?

   A. Plain tomographic scanning

   B. CT scanning

   C. MRI

   D. Thermographic studies

   E. Ultrasound imaging

   Ref.: 1

COMMENTS: For the workup of suspected soft-tissue tumors, plain films are always obtained first, but their contrast resolution is not always sufficient for differentiating between soft-tissue tumors and adjacent normal tissue. • They may, however, demonstrate phleboliths in hemangiomas, bone destruction secondary to adjacent malignant tumors, and dystrophic calcification within tumors. • Plain films are excellent for ruling out bone lesions and detecting myositis ossificans.

   It is generally agreed that MRI is the next step in imaging evaluation. • MRI has superb soft-tissue contrast, enabling immediate delineation of tumors and adjacent normal tissue, such as fat and muscle. • In addition, MRI demonstrates the anatomy with great clarity, enabling anatomic localization of the tumor.

   Plain tomographic scanning shows little that is not obvious on plain films. • CT scanning often does not demonstrate the margins of lesions, particularly intramuscular lesions, as well as does MRI. • Thermographic studies, which are basically maps of regions of increased temperature, have no role in the evaluation of soft-tissue masses. • Ultrasound imaging is helpful for distinguishing cystic from solid lesions but does not depict the anatomy as well as does MRI.

ANSWER:
C

2. A 13-year-old girl comes to the emergency department with severe right knee pain that has been present for 3 months and that has become progressively more severe. There is no history of trauma. The pain has been characteristically worse in the evening, inhibiting the patient from sleeping. Her past medical history is otherwise unremarkable. On physical examination, there is a large, extremely tender soft-tissue mass fixed to the distal femur posteromedially. There is knee flexion contracture measuring 10 degrees and severe pain on range-of-motion movements of the knee beyond 90 degrees of flexion. Results of all the laboratory examinations are within normal limits except for an alkaline phosphatase level of 340 IU/L. A technetium-99 disphosphonate bone scan reveals a monostotic lesion with intense update in the right distal femur. A CT scan of this area shows a destructive lesion of the distal femur with a large posteromedially based soft-tissue mass. A chest radiograph and a CT scan of the chest are normal. The figure shows anteroposterior and lateral radiographs of the right distal femur. An incisional biopsy of this lesion confirms the pathologic diagnosis. Which of the following is the most appropriate treatment for this patient?

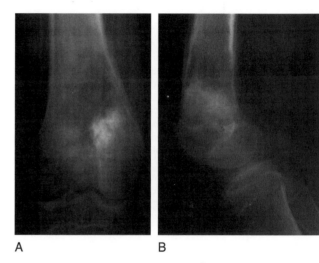

A   B

   A. Excision of the lesion followed by grafting with autogenous iliac crest

   B. Systemic chemotherapy followed by radiation

   C. Neoadjuvant systemic chemotherapy followed by wide resection of the distal femur with reconstruction

   D. Above-knee amputation or hip disarticulation

   Ref.: 1, 3

COMMENTS: There is a destructive lesion of the metaphysis of the distal femur with matrix ossification within the lesion. • In addition, there is evidence of cortical destruction with soft-tissue extension. • These radiographic findings are consistent with an osteosarcoma. • The current treatment of osteosarcoma consists of neoadjuvant chemotherapy for approximately 3 months, followed by reconstruction and limb salvage. • Limb salvage has largely replaced amputation, even in growing children, largely due to advances in reconstruction techniques. • Excision with autogenous iliac crest bone graft is not indicated for this sarcoma of the distal femur. • This procedure is reserved exclusively for benign tumors of bone. • Chemotherapy plus irradiation would be a reasonable choice for Ewing's sarcoma, but Ewing's sarcoma has a different radiographic manifestation and location.

ANSWER:
C

3. A 7-year-old child comes to the emergency department with a complaint of pain in the upper aspect of his right arm following a fall off the monkey bars. Examination reveals focal tenderness at the upper metaphyseal area of his right humerus. Radiographs at the time of presentation demonstrate a pathologic fracture through a centrally located lytic lesion in the metaphysis of his humerus. The lesion is well marginated, and a fallen-leaf sign is present. Which of the following statements is not correct?

A. This condition is more commonly found in the humerus than in the distal femur.

B. Aspiration of the lesion before the fall would have produced yellow fluid.

C. This condition, if left alone, will most likely regress spontaneously.

D. The lesion is not malignant.

E. This is a Codman's tumor.

Ref.: 3, 4

COMMENTS: The young patient presents with a pathologic fracture through a lytic lesion. • While the differential diagnosis includes a unicameral bone cyst, an aneurysmal bone cyst, or a nonossifying fibroma, the central location of the lesion and the fallen-leaf sign identify the lesion as a unicameral bone cyst (simple bone cyst). • The most common presentation in this young age group for a unicameral bone cyst is a pathologic fracture. • Lesions are more often found in the metaphyseal region of the humerus, proximal femur, and calcaneus but are rare around the knees. • These lesions are thought to regress spontaneously but may be treated with methylprednisolone or curettage and bone grafting to prevent recurrent fracture. • A Codman's tumor is an eponym for a chondroblastoma.

ANSWER:
E

4. Features of osteogenic sarcoma include all but which of the following?

A. The most common site of involvement is the metaphysis of the femur.

B. It occurs in 10% of male patients with Paget's disease.

C. Metastases occur mainly via the lymphatic system.

D. The first symptom usually is pain not relieved by rest.

E. Spicules of bone within the tumor produce a typical appearance on radiograms.

Ref.: 1–3

COMMENTS: Osteogenic sarcoma is uncommon, occurring in about 1 in 775,000 population. • It is, however, the most common primary malignant tumor of bone. • As a primary tumor, it is seen most commonly during the second decade of life. • The most common site of involvement is the metaphysis of the distal femur. • In 90% of cases, it presents as a high-grade tumor with soft-tissue extension. • Osteogenic sarcoma can arise from preexisting Paget's disease. • Such sarcomatous degeneration occurs in 10% of male patients with Paget's disease, and it carries a poorer prognosis than does primary osteogenic sarcoma. • Metastatic spread is primarily hematogenous and most commonly to the lungs. • When the tumor extends to or originates underneath the periosteum, the periosteum is raised off the bone, producing a soft-tissue swelling. • Spicules of bone within the tumor produce a sunburst

appearance on the radiograph. • Usually, the first symptom is pain unrelieved by rest, secondary to periosteal irritation. • This pain often precludes ambulation. • Pathologic fractures are thus an uncommon occurrence.

In the past, standard treatment was local radiation therapy with delayed amputation, and the 5-year survival rate was 20%. • Current treatment combines surgery with multiple cytotoxic drugs, including methotrexate, cisplatin, ifosfamide, and doxorubicin. • The 5-year survival rate is now greater than 70%. • Considerable success is being reported with limb salvage surgery in combination with pre- and postoperative chemotherapy.

ANSWER:
C

5. With regard to Ewing's tumor and lymphoma of bone, all but which of the following statements is/are true?

A. Both tumors mostly affect patients under 20 years of age.

B. Ewing's tumor is frequently associated with intermittent fevers and an increased ESR.

C. Ewing's tumor begins in the diaphyseal marrow, and as it extends to the periosteum, new bone formation occurs, creating so-called onion skinning.

D. Lymphoma of bone responds well to irradiation and chemotherapy

Ref.: 1–3

COMMENTS: Ewing's tumor is a small, round-cell malignancy typically arising from the diaphyseal marrow of long bones in patients under 20 years of age. • The tumor extends from the medullary canal to the periosteum, and as new bone is formed, "onion skinning" parallel to the shaft is visible on radiographs. • A history of trauma is not uncommon, and there are frequently associated febrile attacks and leukocytosis. • The tumor is capable of lymphatic and hematogenous spread, and death usually results from pulmonary metastases. • The tumors are radiosensitive but tend to recur.

Newer treatments involving the use of various chemotherapeutic agents have improved survival. • In carefully selected patients, the limb can be salvaged. • Lymphoma of bone occurs in patients between ages 20 and 40 and commonly affects the femur, tibia, ilium, and humerus. • Pain, which precedes formation of a visible tumor, is often the first complaint. • On radiographs, the lesions appear osteolytic at the end of the diaphysis, later extending throughout the length of the bone. • Radiation therapy combined with surgery and chemotherapy has given the best survival rates.

ANSWER:
A

6. Which of the following is not an indication for bone scintigraphy?

A. Evaluation of the nature and physical limits of a primary bone tumor

B. Elevation of alkaline phosphatase levels that is not explained by obvious liver disease

C. Bone pain unexplained by pertinent radiographs

D. Abnormal evaluation of serum calcium phosphate levels

E. Workup of potentially metastasizing tumors

Ref.: 5

COMMENTS: Bone scintigraphy often provides the most direct answer to whether the skeleton is responsible for aberrations in serum alkaline phosphatase and calcium phosphate levels, pinpointing offending bones and frequently defining the pathologic process involved. • Bone pain, which cannot be adequately explained by radiographs of the offending site, remains one of the more important and frequently employed indications for skeletal scintigraphy. • Bone scintigraphy does not define the nature or the extent of the primary lesion. • CT scanning, plain and tomographic roentgenography, and MRI are more productive in this regard. • However, the bone scan remains the most efficient and effective tool for differentiating monostotic from polyostotic disease.

A N S W E R :
A

7. A 24-year-old right-hand–dominant college student presents to a community surgeon for evaluation of a soft-tissue mass on her right upper arm that has been present for the past year. The mass is approximately 5 cm and has become somewhat painful at night. The patient believes it to have grown in size over the past 2 months. After a full physical examination, plain radiographs, and an MRI, the decision is made to perform an incisional biopsy of the lesion. Which one of the following statements is true?

A. The biopsy should be performed in the community setting before referral to a specialist.

B. The biopsy should be performed through intermuscular planes

C. The radial nerve should be exposed and protected during the procedure.

D. The incision should be longitudinal.

E. It is permissible to approach the lesion through more than one compartment.

Ref.: 3

COMMENTS: Biopsies of musculoskeletal tumors must be carefully planned to avoid complications and to facilitate care. • Biopsies should be performed by experienced individuals to avoid unnecessary contamination of tissues and to increase diagnostic accuracy. • For this reason, the Musculoskeletal Tumor Society recommends referral to a tumor specialist for biopsy and definitive care of a suspected malignant mass.

An incisional biopsy is a procedure in which a sample of tumor is removed from within the lesion without removing the entire lesion. • During this procedure, all tissue that has been exposed is considered potentially contaminated with tumor. • At the time of definitive resection of a malignant lesion, the entire incisional biopsy tract (including skin) is excised. • To minimize risk to adjacent structures, no neurovascular structures should be unnecessarily exposed, and uninvolved compartments should be avoided. • Intermuscular planes should not be contaminated. • Meticulous hemostatis should be maintained to prevent hematoma formation. • The incision should be longitudinal to facilitate extensile exposure and excision and coverage of the biopsy tract at time of definitive procedure.

A N S W E R :
D

8. A 31-year-old woman has an enlarging and painful mass of the right thigh. Since its first appearance approximately 6 weeks ago, it has progressively enlarged. The patient has otherwise been healthy, and there is no history of trauma. On examination, there is a mass involving the medial aspect of her right thigh. The mass is extremely tender but mobile with no obvious fixation to the underlying bone. Results of the neurovascular examination of the right lower extremity are within normal limits. Results of all laboratory studies, including complete blood cell count, serum chemistry studies, and chest radiograph, are within normal limits. The accompanying figure shows a CT scan of the right thigh and T1- and T2-weighted MRI studies of the same area of the thigh. Which of the following is the most likely diagnosis?

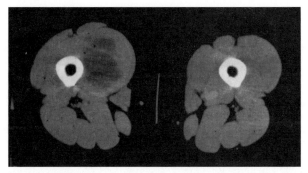

A

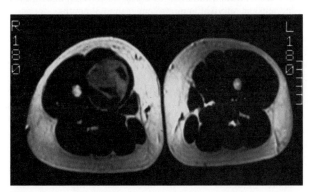

B

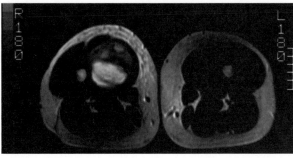

C

A. Aneurysm of the femoral artery

B. Hematoma

C. Lipoma

D. Liposarcoma

Ref.: 1, 3

COMMENTS: Imaging of the extremity shows a heterogeneous mass of the medial thigh composed of several tissue densities. • This is evident on both the CT scan (Figure A) and MRI (Figure B). • The T2-weighted MRI scan (Figure C) reveals areas of significant tumor enhancement surrounded by areas that are less enhanced, confirming the heterogeneity of the tumor. • This is a typical appearance of a soft-tissue sarcoma (liposarcoma). • The other choices are not consistent with the clinical and radiographic scenario. • Aneurysm of the femoral artery is unlikely because the artery is well visualized on the CT scan and MRI studies without evidence of abnormality. • A hematoma is also unlikely because of the lack of history of trauma and the heterogeneity on the imaging studies. • Lipoma may be excluded, since the tumor shown is not a fat-density tumor and has a heterogeneous signal on MRI.

ANSWER:
D

9. With regard to metastatic tumors of bone, all but which of the following statements is true?

   A. Skeletal metastases can arise from virtually all types of malignant tumors but most frequently are from tumors of the breasts, prostate, thyroid, kidneys, and lungs.

   B. Metastatic bone tumors are the result of hematogenous spread ending in bony capillary beds.

   C. Most patients with bone metastases complain of pain.

   D. Bone metastases are a grave prognostic sign, once they are present, survival is rarely longer than 3 months.

Ref.: 2

COMMENTS: Although the most common cancers metastasizing to bone are those of the breasts, prostate, thyroid, kidneys, and lungs, nearly all types of malignant tumors can metastasize to bone. • The usual route is via the bloodstream, originating in veins leaving the primary tumor and then passing through the pulmonary circulation and on to the bony capillary beds. • The high incidence of metastasis to the axial skeleton probably is attributable to hematogenous dissemination through the vertebral venous plexus (of Batson). • Sixty-five percent of patients with radiographic evidence of bone metastases complain of pain. • Tenderness to palpation is present in fewer than 20%. • Many patients with bone metastases live many months or years, particularly those with breast and prostate cancer responsive to hormonal manipulation.

ANSWER:
D

10. Which method of diagnosis is most sensitive for the detection of bone metastases?

    A. History and physical examination

    B. Plain radiographs

    C. Technetium bone scanning

    D. Measurement of serum alkaline phosphatase levels

    E. Measurement of serum calcium levels

Ref.: 1, 3

COMMENTS: About 65% of patients with bone metastases complain of pain, and about 15% have palpable tenderness. • The alkaline phosphatase level is normal in up to 40% of patients. • Radiographs are not reliable, since 50% bone loss occurs before a lesion is seen on a plain film. • Technetium bone scanning is by far the most sensitive screening test for bone metastases. • Hypercalcemia may be the result of bone destruction secondary to metastases. • With properly functioning kidneys, hypercalcuria is usually found in the presence of normal serum calcium levels.

ANSWER:
C

11. A 37-year-old male office worker presents with a 2-month history of right distal thigh mass, which the patient believes has been growing in size. Physical examination reveals a nontender mass approximately 7cm in diameter located in the anteromedial portion of the distal thigh. There are no skin changes. Plain radiographs, followed by MRI, demonstrate a deep-seated heterogeneous mass adjacent to the deep tissues of the vastus lateralis with some bone erosion around the distal femur. Biopsy is performed demonstrating spindle-shaped cells in a storiform (cartwheel) pattern. What is the most likely diagnosis?

    A. Malignant fibrous histiocytoma

    B. Extra-abdominal desmoid tumor

    C. Giant-cell tumor

    D. Liposarcoma

Ref.: 3

COMMENTS: The patient has a malignant fibrous soft-tissue tumor, as evidenced by the spindle-shaped cells in the biopsy specimen and the aggressive nature of the lesion within the soft tissues. • There are two types of malignant fibrous soft-tissue tumors: malignant fibrous histiocytoma and fibrosarcoma. • These tumors have similar clinical and radiographic presentations and are treated similarly. • The most common presentation is that of an enlarging, painless mass. • Symptoms are not common until the mass reaches a large enough size. • Treatment is wide local excision, with consideration of radiation therapy if the lesion exceeds 5 cm. • Malignant fibrous histiocytoma is the most common soft-tissue sarcoma in adults.

An extra-abdominal desmoid tumor is a poorly circumscribed, usually locally invasive, tumor with "rock-hard" character. • Desmoid tumors do not metastasize but have high local recurrence rates. • While giant-cell tumors are commonly located in the distal femur, they are not a primary soft-tissue tumor. • A liposarcoma is a tumor of fatty tissue.

ANSWER:
A

12. With regard to treatment of skeletal metastases, which one of the following statements is true?

    A. The pain that arises from skeletal metastases may be diminished if the hypercalcemia is treated.

    B. Large lytic lesions, particularly of the femur, should be treated initially with radiation, followed by internal fixation to avoid a pathologic fracture.

C. There is an 80–90% chance of pain relief after hormonal therapy.

D. Radiotherapy to the localized area of pain is never indicated for the treatment of metastatic lesions.

Ref.: 5

COMMENTS: In most instances, treatment of skeletal metastases is palliative in nature. • Pain occurs in association with hypercalcemia. • Once the latter is treated, the pain may be relieved. • Patients with hormonally dependent tumors often experience significant relief from pain after hormonal manipulation, but not all skeletal metastases are hormonally sensitive. • If hormonal therapy fails or for tumors that are not hormonally dependent, radiotherapy to a localized area of pain often produces relief. • Large lytic lesions with impending fracture should undergo prompt internal fixation followed by irradiation. • Radiotherapy given preoperatively may predispose the patient to pathologic fracture, lessening the effectiveness of the fixation. • Vertebral metastases with subsequent compression fracture involving the spinal cord may be treated by decompression laminectomy. • Radiotherapy alone in this setting can control pain but does not improve an established paraplegia.

ANSWER:
A

13. A 32-year-old woman has a 3-month history of left knee pain that began after a 2-hr aerobic exercise class. Since that time, the pain has become progressively worse and is now present with activity and at rest. On examination, there are an antalgic component to her gait and marked tenderness over the medial femoral condyle. The range of motion of the knee is normal, and no effusion is present. Results of all laboratory tests are within normal limits, including a complete blood cell count and determinations of calcium, phosphorus, and alkaline phosphatase levels. The figures shown below are anteroposterior and lateral radiographs of the left distal femur and knee joint. A technetium-99 diphosphonate bone scan shows intense uptake in the medial femoral condyle. No other osseous lesions are noted. Which of the following is the most likely diagnosis in this patient?

A. Metastatic carcinoma to bone

B. Hyperparathyroidism

C. Giant-cell tumor

D. Osteosarcoma

Ref.: 1, 3

COMMENTS: Giant-cell tumor of bone occurs in skeletally mature individuals. • It usually manifests as an eccentric lytic lesion of bone located in the epiphysis and metaphysis. • The knee is the most common location. • Metastatic carcinoma is unlikely because of the age of the patient and because the bone scan shows it be a monostotic lesion. • Metastatic carcinoma rarely involves the epiphysis and metaphysis of the bone. • Hyperparathyroidism can radiographically resemble a giant-cell tumor, but normal serum calcium, phosphorus, and alkaline phosphatase levels make this diagnosis unlikely. • Osteosarcoma is a bone-forming tumor occurring in the metaphysis around the knee joint. • There is no evidence of bone formation on these radiographs.

ANSWER:
C

14. Which one of the following statements regarding fibrous dysplasia is true?

A. It may be linked to phenytoin toxicity.

B. The polyostotic form is malignant.

C. Deformity of bone may be a significant feature.

D. Fibrous dysplasia can be associated with café-au-lait spots with regular borders.

E. Lesions are typically bilaterally symmetric.

Ref.: 3

COMMENTS: Fibrous dysplasia is a benign, nonhereditary dysplastic condition of bone in which fibro-osseous tissue replaces the normal bony architecture. • There is no known link to phenytoin toxicity. • Deformity of bone may be a significant feature, especially around the hip, with the classic "shepherd's crook" deformity. • It may be monostotic or polyostotic. • The monostotic form commonly affects the ribs and diaphyseal-metaphyseal regions of long bones. • The polyostotic form tends to affect only one side of the body. • McCune-Albright syndrome is a condition in which polyostotic fibrous dysplasia is accompanied by endocrine abnormalities, including precocious puberty. • Typically, irregularly bordered café-au-lait spots are associated with this condition. • Café-au-lait spots with regular borders are typically associated with neurofibromatosis.

ANSWER:
C

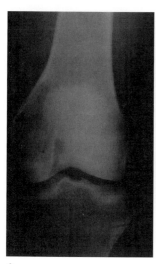
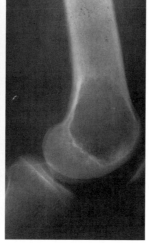

A   B

REFERENCES

1. Brunicardi FC, Andersen DK, Billiar TR, et al (eds): *Schwartz's Principles of Surgery*, 8th ed. McGraw-Hill, New York, 2004.
2. Townsend CM Jr, Beauchamp RD, Evers BM, et al: *Sabiston Textbook of Surgery: The Biological Basis of Modern Surgical Practice,* 17th ed. Saunders, Philadelphia, 2004.
3. Menendez LR: *Orthopaedic Knowledge Update: Musculoskeletal Tumors*. American Academy of Orthopaedic Surgeons, Rosemont, IL, 2002.
4. Sponseller PD: *Orthopaedic Knowledge Update: Pediatrics, vol. 2.* American Academy of Orthopaedic Surgeons, Rosemont, IL, 2002.
5. Schajowicz F: *Tumors and Tumor-Like Lesions of Bone and Joints.* Springer-Verlag, New York, 1981.

CHAPTER 52

Amputations

Chad Jacobs, M.D., and Walter J. McCarthy, M.D.

1. Match the amputation in the left-hand column with the appropriate characteristic in the right-hand column.

A. Conventional

B. Osteomyoplastic

C. Myodesis

D. Open "guillotine"

   a. Tissues are cut circularly and allowed to retract initially, and the wound may be closed secondarily or placed with skin traction.

   b. Antagonist muscles are sutured across the bone end.

   c. Transected muscles are attached to bone by suturing through drill holes placed at the distal bone.

   d. Skin, fascia, and muscle are transected based at the level of amputation and then closed over the bone.

   e. It is used when the extremity is grossly infected and the patient is septic.

   f. It usually requires revision.

Ref.: 1

COMMENTS: The **conventional** amputation uses curved skin and fascial flaps based at the level of amputation. • When care is taken to ensure proper approximation of soft tissue over the bony stump, it lends itself to the potential of good rehabilitation. • Fitting for a prosthesis is delayed until healing has occurred. • The **osteomyoplastic** amputation (suturing antagonistic muscles across the bone end) and the **myodesis** amputation (attaching muscles directly to the bone) typically are used for special situations (e.g., young patients with trauma). • They provide improved function and allow the application of immediate postsurgical prosthetic devices. • The **open**, or **"guillotine,"** amputation is reserved for emergency situations, unstable patients, or the presence of severe sepsis. • The wound is left completely open, and the bone usually protrudes after soft-tissue contraction occurs, thus requiring revision. • This situation can be obviated by employing appropriately elongated skin flaps or even by countering this tendency with postoperative skin traction. • The stump usually is not amenable to easy rehabilitation.

ANSWER:
A-d; B-b; C-c; D-a,e,f

2. Principles of postoperative management after amputation include which of the following?

A. Splinting of the stump dressing to avoid shifting in position

B. Compression dressing over the stump to avoid postoperative edema and hematoma formation

C. Exercise and positioning to avoid contracture

D. Early evaluation and care by a qualified physical therapist and prosthetist

E. Use of a stump stocking to mold the stump for eventual prosthesis fitting

Ref.: 1, 2

COMMENTS: Conventional postoperative care begins with application of a light compression dressing in the operating room, followed by repeated application of elastic dressings to avoid stump edema. • Damage to the skin can result from excessively compressive dressings applied over bony prominences (e.g., the anterior tibial area in a below-knee stump). • Stump exercises and stretching prevent contracture after primary wound healing has taken place. • Progressive training after suture removal allows the eventual application of a permanent prosthesis. • Alternatively, application of a rigid dressing in the operating room allows the immediate use of a prosthetic device, but a rigid dressing may also be used without immediate prosthetic fitting. • Rigid dressings offer the advantage of immediate use of the extremity. • Wound healing may be enhanced by maximum control of edema and hematoma and by better tissue immobilization. • When treatment is successful, resumption of full activity can be expected to occur within 4–6 weeks. • All of the listed choices are important for proper amputation management.

ANSWER:
A, B, C, D, E.

3. True or false: The absence of a pulse is a contraindication for amputation beyond that point.

COMMENTS: See Question 4.

Ref.: 1–3

4. Useful preoperative methods of evaluating adequacy of blood flow in patients with peripheral vascular disease undergoing amputation include which of the following?

A. Clinical assessment of cutaneous blood flow

B. Determinations of transcutaneous PO_2 and PCO_2

C. Assessment of the status of peripheral pulses

D. Segmental Doppler systolic blood pressure determinations

E. Laser Doppler velocimetric studies

Ref.: 1–3

COMMENTS: The healing ability of an amputation stump is determined by the adequacy of the nutritional blood flow to the skin. • Clinical assessment is successful in determining the level of amputation in approximately 80% of below-knee amputations and 90% of above-knee amputations. • For amputations below the ankle, clinical judgment alone has been shown to be less effective, achieving a healing rate of only 40%. • Physical examination findings such as the extent of tissue necrosis, skin temperature, capillary refill, and pulse assessment help determine the clinical assessment. • The presence of pulses immediately above the proposed amputation site is a good prognostic indicator, but the absence of such a pulse does not necessarily preclude adequate wound healing.

Several other methods have been employed to preoperatively select amputation levels, including Doppler segmental blood pressure measurements, transcutaneous oxygen and carbon dioxide measurements, fluorescein dye measurements, laser Doppler velocimetric studies, isotope measurement of skin perfusion, conventional or magnetic resonance angiography, and others. • Segmental Doppler blood pressure measurement is probably the most commonly used first test to assist in determining the level of amputation. • An absolute pressure of at least 50–70 mmHg at the calf and 80 mmHg at the thigh is highly predictive of successful healing of a below-knee amputation. • However, a major caveat of this test modality is the falsely elevated pressures that result from calcification of the arterial wall, particularly in the tibial vessels of diabetic patients. • Transcutaneous PO_2 levels can also be measured and may help to determine whether a particular level of amputation will heal. • A transcutaneous PO_2 greater than 40 mmHg is associated with successful healing and a value below 20 mmHg is associated with failure.

ANSWER:
A, B, C, D, E

5. Which of the following statements regarding proper selection of the level of amputation is/are true?

A. The extent of resection for malignant tumors must not be compromised for functional considerations.

B. The use of skin grafts and flaps to conserve bony length is appropriate in healthy, stable trauma patients.

C. Unless 4 inches or more of tibia can be preserved, the knee joint should be sacrificed.

D. The presence of contracture should not influence the level of amputation.

Ref.: 1–3

COMMENTS: As a general principle, the longer the amputation stump, the more functional the limb. • However, when performing amputations for malignancy, adequate tumor excision, not preservation of stump length, is the primary concern. • The irregular

damage to skin caused by trauma can be treated by skin grafts and flaps to preserve bony length. • Full-thickness skin should be maintained for weight-bearing surfaces. • Amputations in patients with peripheral vascular disease succeed best when performed at levels that have adequate nutritional blood flow to the skin. • Below-knee stumps as short as 2 inches can be successfully fitted with prostheses, but function is much better if at least 4 inches of stump is maintained. • Preservation of the knee joint allows a bent-knee, end–weight-bearing prosthesis to be used and is usually preferable to a long above-knee stump. • Amputations above the knee should remove at least 4 inches of femur to facilitate fitting a prosthetic knee joint. • Relative contraindications to below-knee amputation include the presence of hip or knee contracture, which negates its functional advantage.

ANSWERS:
Question 3: False
Question 4: A, B

6. Which of the following statements regarding toe amputation is/are true?

A. Empirical selection and clinical judgment provide a 95% healing rate regardless of the presence of pedal pulses.

B. When the entire toe must be removed, disarticulation is preferred over transmetatarsal amputation.

C. Toe amputations should not be attempted in patients who do not have pedal pulses.

D. Rehabilitation after a transmetatarsal amputation of all five toes is improved by a shoe-filler prosthesis.

Ref.: 1–3

COMMENTS: Empirical selection for toe amputation provides a 75% healing rate in the absence of palpable pedal pulses and a 98% healing rate in the presence of palpable pulses. • Patients with palpable popliteal and pedal pulses who have toe or transmetatarsal amputations do better than those without, but their absence is not considered an absolute contraindication. • Therefore, if pedal pulses are not palpable, other measures, such as Doppler toe and ankle pressure measurements, should be used. • Toe and ankle pressures greater than 35 mmHg are associated with a higher rate of successful healing. • When the entire toe is to be amputated, a transmetatarsal procedure, rather than a simple joint disarticulation, is performed. • The former prevents exposure of the avascular cartilage of the proximal joint capsule. • Ambulation may be started after the incision is healed. • No special shoe is required, but a shoe filler improves gait. • A shoe modification incorporating a steel shank in the sole allows normal toe pushoff and prevents excessive dorsiflexion.

ANSWER:
D

7. A Syme amputation is best suited for which of the following?

A. Preservation of leg length

B. Gangrene involving the heel pad

C. A distal foot destroyed by trauma

D. A patient with a patent anterior tibial artery but a chronically occluded posterior tibial artery

E. Distal forefoot necrosis involving the plantar skin

Ref.: 1–3

COMMENTS: The Syme amputation is created at a bone level just distal to the tibial flare, with preservation of the heel pad. • Therefore, any gangrene, infection, or open lesions of the heel create a contraindication to this amputation. • It maintains the length of the lower extremity and allows creation of an end–weight-bearing stump. • It is usually performed when most of the forefoot has been destroyed by trauma or tissue necrosis. • Since the heel flap for this amputation derives its entire blood supply from the posterior tibial artery, the patency of this vessel must be certain. • A patient with a well-healed Syme amputation and a properly constructed prosthesis has only a 10% increase in ambulatory energy consumption compared to nonamputees.

ANSWER:
A, C, E

8. Knee disarticulation has which of the following advantages?

   A. For children, it is useful for maintaining the epiphysis for bony growth.

   B. For adults, it is used to preserve bony length when severe ischemia contraindicates a below-knee amputation.

   C. It provides maximal length with good end–weight-bearing characteristics.

   D. It is easily fitted with a simple prosthesis.

   Ref.: 1, 2

COMMENTS: Knee disarticulation is most often used for children because it allows maintenance of the epiphysis for bony growth. • It is rarely used in situations in which there is impaired circulation and is rarely performed on adults. • The procedure preserves maximum length, provides a good end–weight-bearing stump, and lends itself to a good fit between stump and socket. • However, because the femoral condyles are preserved, the stump is bulky, which can make prosthesis fitting difficult. • The anterior flap is left longer than the posterior flap, and the patella is preserved if it is not involved by disease.

ANSWER:
A, C

9. Which of the following statements regarding below-knee amputation is/are true?

   A. It may be performed on patients with significant knee contracture.

   B. Compared to above-knee amputation, below-knee amputation provides higher potential for prosthetic ambulation.

   C. A below-knee prosthesis does not significantly increase the energy expenditure required for ambulation.

   D. The commonly used posterior myocutaneous flap involves the soleus and gastrocnemius muscles.

   E. The level of tibial transection should be 10–12 cm (one handbreadth) below the tibial tuberosity.

   Ref.: 3

COMMENTS: Below-knee amputation is performed on patients who have gangrene, infection, or ischemic ulcers that preclude a more distal amputation and are not amenable to vascular reconstruction. • A patient with a fixed contracture of the knee is not a candidate for a below-knee amputation. • In such cases, fitting a prosthesis is not possible, use of the joint for ambulation is unlikely, and the stump is vulnerable to decubitus ulceration. • However, in patients with a normal knee joint and distal disease, a below-knee amputation provides far superior rehabilitation potential than does an above-knee amputation. • Nonetheless, ambulation with a below-knee prosthesis increases the energy expenditure of ambulation by 10–40%.

Although several skin-flap techniques have been utilized for below-knee amputation, the most commonly used is the posterior flap technique. • The posterior myocutaneous flap is based on the underlying soleus and gastrocnemius muscles. • The level of transection of the tibia should be approximately 10-12 cm below the tibial tuberosity. • However, the absolute minimal length for a functional result is just below the tibial tuberosity. • This preserves the insertion of the patellar tendon, which is critical for knee extension and successful ambulation.

ANSWER:
B, D, E

10. Indications for an above-knee amputation include which of the following?

    A. Absent popliteal pulses

    B. Diabetes mellitus

    C. Gangrene at the tibial tuberosity

    D. Calf muscle rigor

    E. Knee or hip contractures

    F. Patient with minimal potential for rehabilitation and ambulation

    Ref.: 1, 2

COMMENTS: Assessment of the vascular status at the level of amputation is important, but the absence of popliteal pulses or the presence of diabetes is not in itself an absolute indication for an above-knee amputation. • The rigor of the calf muscles and the presence of gangrene of the skin at the level where the flaps would be constructed for the below-knee amputation are sufficient indications for an above-knee amputation. • Because knee and hip contractures make rehabilitation after below-knee amputation unlikely and because the above-knee amputation has the highest healing rate and the lowest reamputation rate in patients with severe peripheral vascular disease, patients so afflicted do best with an above-knee amputation.

ANSWER:
C, D, E, F

11. Which of the following statements regarding hip disarticulation and hemipelvectomy is/are true?

    A. Prostheses are unavailable for ambulation.

    B. The usual indications are bone tumors, soft-tissue tumors, and, occasionally, extensive trauma.

    C. Flaps are brought together posteriorly after hip disarticulation.

    D. The entire ilium must be removed during hemipelvectomy.

    Ref.: 1, 2

COMMENTS: The most common indications for hip disarticulation include tumors of bone or soft tissue and, in some cases, extensive trauma. • Hemipelvectomy is indicated when an upper thigh tumor cannot be excised by disarticulation alone. • The posterior flap after hip disarticulation is closed anteriorly so that the patient can sit comfortably on the socket of the prosthesis. • Whenever possible, leaves of ilium and the pelvic rami are preserved during the hemipelvectomy to act as support points for the prosthesis. • Both amputations can be fitted with a prosthesis that allows ambulation.

ANSWER:
B.

12. Which of the following statements regarding lower limb prostheses is/are true?

   A. They require less energy to use than does crutch walking.

   B. The shorter the stump, the greater the stump tip pressure.

   C. The main pressure point in the below-knee prosthesis is the stump end.

   D. A suspension belt is used for all above-knee prostheses.

Ref.: 1, 2

COMMENTS: Prostheses are designed to restore function, mobility, and appearance. • Properly fitted prostheses have lower energy requirements than does crutch walking. • Socket design has as its goals patient comfort and an even distribution of forces on the stump. • The longer the stump, the greater the surface area over which these forces can be distributed. • Above-knee sockets are usually of the quadrilateral total contact design and are suspended by stump suction or pelvic belts. • The below-knee prostheses most commonly used are the patellar tendon-bearing type and the patellar tendon supracondylar type.

ANSWER:
A, B

13. Which of the following statements regarding amputations distal to the elbow is/are true?

   A. Digital tourniquets should be avoided when possible.

   B. The length of forearm preserved has little bearing on functional status.

   C. After suprametacarpal amputation, opposing tendons should be fixed to preserve muscle tone and strength.

   D. The precise nature of the operation requires a general anesthetic.

Ref.: 1–3

COMMENTS: Most patients undergoing lower-extremity amputations have peripheral vascular disease, and the use of tourniquets is not necessary. • For the upper extremity, however, tourniquets are frequently used to provide a blood-free field so that critical nerve and tendon structures can be identified. • Because of the risk of thrombosis, digital tourniquets such as rubber bands should be avoided. • To best preserve muscle strength, tone, and hence function, opposing tendons should be fixed anatomically. • The goal of amputation of the proximal arm is preservation of as much viable tissue as possible. • For distal arm amputations, the goal is to preserve the grasping function of the hand. • Leaving as much forearm length as possible results in higher functionality of the residual limb and easier prosthesis fitting. • Adequate anesthesia

can often be accomplished by regional block. • This is preferred in trauma patients, who may have a full stomach, because it avoids the risk of aspiration.

ANSWER:
A, C

14. Which of the following statements regarding amputation of digits is/are true?

   A. A shorter volar flap and a longer dorsal flap are desired.

   B. The root of the nail should always be preserved.

   C. During removal of the distal phalanx, the distal middle phalangeal cartilage should be preserved.

   D. Amputation at the metacarpophalangeal joint is preferable to amputation through the proximal phalanx.

   E. Even the smallest stump of the thumb is preferable to complete amputation with prosthesis.

Ref.: 1, 2

COMMENTS: A longer volar flap is desired so that the scar can be positioned away from pressure-bearing surfaces. • However, bone and viable tissue should never be sacrificed to obtain ideal scar placement. • Unless more than half of the nail bed can be preserved, the nail root should be removed. • If the distal phalanx must be removed, the exposed middle phalangeal cartilage should be resected. • Given a choice, resection through the proximal phalanx is preferred over a metacarpophalangeal amputation. • As is the case with the thumb, any stump, no matter how short, has function. • When a digit must be removed in its entirety, preservation of function of the hand as a unit is the goal and may require a variety of secondary procedures.

ANSWER:
E

15. Which of the following statements regarding wrist disarticulation is/are true?

   A. It provides better prosthesis control than does a long forearm amputation.

   B. The stump is stronger than that left when the amputation is through the carpal bones.

   C. The severed tendons and ligaments of the hand must be fixed to prevent their retraction and atrophy.

   D. Preservation of the styloid processes is necessary for prosthetic fitting.

Ref.: 1, 2

COMMENTS: Wrist disarticulation has several advantages over more proximal amputations. • It preserves length and provides better control of the prosthesis. • Although it is weaker than when the carpal bones remain, it accommodates a less conspicuous prosthesis. • The styloid processes are removed to permit a smoother fit. • The tendons of the hand are transected with the muscles at rest and fixed to periosteum to prevent retraction and atrophy.

ANSWER:
A, C

16. Which of the following statements is/are true regarding forearm amputations?

A. Unless significant forearm muscle mass and length can be preserved, an above-elbow amputation is preferred to enhance prosthetic function.

B. Skin mobility is preserved by avoiding excessive dissection between skin and fascia.

C. A short stump of the ulna or radius can be lengthened secondarily.

D. Cineplastic operations using biceps or pectoralis muscles can provide function to artificial limbs when the amputation stump is extremely short.

Ref.: 1, 2

COMMENTS: Dissection is kept to a minimum to avoid immobilization of skin by subsequent scar formation. • Pronation and supination are preserved by striving for a longer stump. • Also, the procedure is conducted as atraumatically as possible to avoid fibrosis. • Even an extremely short forearm stump is preferable to an above-elbow amputation. • Functional control of a prosthesis fitted over a short stump can be provided by a cineplastic operation using the ipsilateral biceps or pectoralis muscle after the initial stump has healed. • Other secondary procedures include the use of bone flaps or grafts to lengthen short stumps of the ulna or radius.

ANSWER:
B, C, D

17. Which of the following statements regarding infection of a diabetic patient's foot is/are true?

A. The infection within the foot usually is less severe than it appears on clinical evaluation.

B. The pain expressed by the patient usually is less than one would expect in relationship to the degree of infection.

C. The infection rarely has a bony or tendinous element at its base.

D. The factors contributing to the ulceration and infection in the foot of a diabetic patient are neuropathy, peripheral arterial occlusive disease, and perhaps impaired leukocyte phagocytic function.

E. Conservative measures rarely succeed, often necessitating amputation.

Ref.: 1, 2

COMMENTS: The foot ulcer in a diabetic patient may be due to pressure on a dysesthetic extremity that may or may not be associated with peripheral vascular arterial insufficiency. • There often is a bony or tendinous element at the base of the ulcer. • The infection usually is more extensive in the foot than appears clinically. • After adequate débridement, many extremities are salvageable. • Aggressive open débridement is essential. • Unless the need for amputation is urgent, an evaluation for arterial reconstruction should be made first.

ANSWER:
B, D

REFERENCES

1. Frymoyer JW (ed): *Orthopaedic Basic Science*. American Academy of Orthopaedic Surgeons, Rosemont, IL, 1993.
2. Kasser JR (ed): *Orthopaedic Knowledge Update 5*. American Academy of Orthopaedic Surgeons, Rosemont, IL, 1996.
3. Rutherford RB: *Vascular Surgery*, 6th ed. Saunders, Philadelphia, 2005.

CHAPTER 53

Hand Surgery

Srdjan A. Ostric, M.D., and Gordon H. Derman, M.D.

1. Match each of the following nerves with the correct labeled structure on the diagram.

   A. Median nerve

   B. Radial nerve

   C. Ulnar nerve

Ref.: 1–4

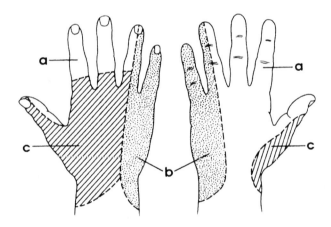

COMMENTS: There is considerable overlap in the sensory innervation of the hand. • The usual innervation is as depicted in the illustration. • Despite the overlap, there are certain autonomous zones useful for evaluating individual nerve function: the **median** nerve, on the flexor aspect of the index finger beyond the distal interphalangeal (DIP) joint; the **ulnar** nerve, on the flexor aspect of the little finger beyond the DIP joint; and the **radial** nerve, on the dorsal web space of the thumb. • Two-point discrimination and light touch with a piece of cotton are the most valuable sensory tests, particularly on an emergency basis. • Soaking a digit in water and looking for wrinkling ("pruning") of the skin or checking for sweating or moisture of the skin can also be helpful when examining uncooperative patients or children.

ANSWER:
A-a; B-c; C-b

2. Which of the following statements regarding the intrinsic muscles of the hand is/are true?

   A. The intrinsic muscles originate in the forearm and insert on the metacarpals.

   B. The palmar interossei pull the fingers to the midline and flex the metacarpophalangeal (MCP) joints of the index, ring, and little fingers.

   C. Their innervation is derived from the radial, median, and ulnar nerves.

   D. The dorsal interosseous muscles spread the fingers, flex the MCP joints, and extend the proximal interphalangeal (PIP) and DIP joints.

   E. The intrinsic muscles of the index, long, and ring fingers consist of the palmar and dorsal interossei and the lumbrical muscles.

Ref.: 1–3

COMMENTS: The intrinsic muscles have their entire course confined to the hand and include the thenar and hypothenar muscles, the lumbrical muscles, and the interosseous muscles. • Together they flex the MCP joints, extend the interphalangeal (IP) joints, and spread and close the fingers. • When functioning normally, they provide the hand with a transverse and longitudinal arch. • The thumb thenar muscles provide radial abduction, palmar abduction, and opposition of the thumb. • Their innervation is derived from the median and ulnar nerves, the distribution of which is variable. • The classic pattern is **median innervation** of the first two lumbrical muscles and the muscles of the thenar eminence, excluding the ulnar head of the flexor pollicis brevis. • The **ulnar nerve** innervates the hypothenar muscles, the interosseous muscles, the ulnar head of the flexor pollicis brevis, and two ulnar lumbrical muscles. • The median nerve is tested by **palmar** abduction of the thumb and opposition. • The ulnar-innervated intrinsic muscles are responsible for finger abduction and adduction, providing the physiologic basis for the classic test for ulnar nerve motor function, which is abduction and adduction of the long finger. • The lumbrical muscles have their origins on the flexor tendons and insert on the extensor hood mechanism, providing additional balance and smooth motion of the digits. • They also flex the MCP joint and extend the PIP joints.

ANSWER:
B, D, E

3. Which of the following statements regarding examination of the acutely injured hand is/are true?

A. All fingers (except the thumb) when flexed at the MCP and PIP joints point to the scaphoid tubercle.

B. Normal two-point discrimination in the hand is 4 mm or less.

C. A laceration over the proximal phalanx of a finger raises suspicion for a zone II flexor tendon injury.

D. A severed finger should be soaked in a cool, dilute antiseptic solution (e.g., 1:100,000 Betadine/normal saline solution) until replantation is possible.

E. Pain on palpation in the area of the anatomic "snuffbox" should raise suspicion of a fracture of the scaphoid bone.

Ref.: 1–4

COMMENTS: Examination of the acutely injured hand should be a systematic process that includes thorough evaluation of both bony and soft-tissue structures. • A complete history and physical examination are mandatory. • The time, place, and method of injury, as well as the hand dominance of the patient, are essential components of any hand examination. • Neurovascular status is then checked. • The Allen test is used to assess the vascular supply to the hand, while the neurologic examination can be assessed accurately via light touch and two-point discrimination. • These tests should always be performed in any hand examination. • Two-point discrimination can be easily assessed by unfolding a paper clip and placing the points 4 mm apart (sharp needles should not be used). • If the patient can discriminate between one point and two, this is normal. • However, two-point discrimination greater than 8 mm should raise suspicion of a nerve injury.

The bony architecture of the hand is evaluated through both x-ray examination and physical examination. • If they are not open, many types of fractures (e.g., boxer's fractures) can be reduced and splinted in an emergency-department situation with the aid of a hematoma block or a wrist block. • Metacarpal fractures need special attention because, even though radiographic evidence may suggest a stable, nondisplaced fracture, a rotational deformity may exist, which, if not treated, will cause functional disability. • The best way of assessing a rotational deformity is by observing the hand as it is flexed at the MCP and PIP joints. • Normal fingers point to the scaphoid tubercle.

Flexor tendon injuries are categorized according to five anatomic zones. • Zone II begins proximally at the distal palmar creases and ends distally over the middle portion of the middle phalanx. • Anatomically, this area includes Camper's chiasm, the insertion of the flexor digitorum sublimis and the point where the flexor digitorum profundus becomes superficial to the sublimis tendon before its insertion at the base of the distal phalanx. • Bunnell called this area "no-man's land" because—even though injuries may be relatively easy to repair—both flexor tendons run through the area inside the sheath, and subsequently there can be significant scarring, with difficulty in restoring long-term function.

An amputated finger part should be wrapped in sterile, saline solution–soaked gauze only and placed in a plastic bag or sterile urine cup, if available, which is then placed in ice water until replantation is possible. • Although the finger or hand may appear to be badly mutilated, its salvage (even of certain parts only) may be possible and should ultimately be decided by a hand surgeon. • Soaking the finger in antiseptics may injure tissue and adversely affect the ability to replant.

The scaphoid is the most commonly injured wrist bone (accounting for almost two thirds of all carpal bone fractures), and a history of a fall onto outstretched hands should prompt an examiner to look for a scaphoid fracture. • Tenderness in the anatomic snuffbox, formed by the abductor pollicis longus and the extensor pollicis longus on the dorsum of the hand, should raise suspicion of a scaphoid fracture, which can be seen on x-ray. • However, sometimes standard X-ray is not diagnostic, and further studies are necessary (i.e., magnetic resonance imaging [MRI], computed tomographic [CT] scanning, or a bone scan) to rule out the diagnosis. • A missed scaphoid fracture can lead to serious complications of avascular necrosis of the bone, chronic arthritis, and chronic wrist pain.

ANSWER:
A, B, C, E

4. Which of the following statements regarding the placement of hand incisions is/are true?

A. Palm incisions should parallel the skin creases or cross them obliquely.

B. It is better to err on the volar aspect than the dorsal aspect when placing incisions on the side of the digit.

C. Incisions on the volar side of the digit must cross the IP flexion creases transversely.

D. Dorsal skin incisions should cross skin creases transversely or obliquely.

Ref.: 1–3

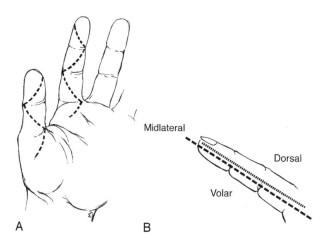

COMMENTS: There are several key principles of planning hand incisions. • Whenever possible, the incision should be designed along lines that undergo no change of length with motion. • Those on the palm should run parallel to the skin creases or across them obliquely, since the blood supply in this region comes straight upward into the skin. • Digital incisions should be placed dorsally to the midlateral line through the midaxial line, which is exactly neutral between flexion and extension. • This line is determined by connecting the most dorsal points of the IP joint creases when the finger is in a flexed position. • Oblique incisions connecting these points, (Bruner's) volar zigzag incisions, are also an excellent approach, giving full exposure to the entire palmar side of the digit. • A line marking the change in character between the dorsal and volar skin of the digit is also a useful landmark. • Given a choice, it is far better to err in placing an incision dorsally rather than on the volar aspect of the side of the digit, because the volar incisions may form a bridging scar. • Skin incisions on the dorsum of the hand and digits should cross skin creases transversely, obliquely, or over the mid-dorsum when between joints. • In the rheumatoid hand, incisions that cross the skin of the dorsal wrist should be longitudinal or minimally curved to avoid slough of a distally based flap.

ANSWER:
A, D

5. Which of the following statements regarding evaluation of the extrinsic flexors and extensors of the hand is/are true?

   A. The flexor digitorum profundus flexes the PIP joint.

   B. The flexor digitorum profundus flexes the DIP joint.

   C. The flexor digitorum superficialis inserts on the proximal end of the distal phalanx.

   D. The flexor pollicis longus flexes the MCP joint.

   E. There are two extensor tendons to the little finger.

Ref.: 1–3

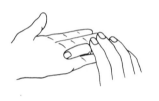 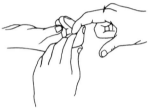

Superficialis testing   Profundus testing

COMMENTS: The extrinsic muscles, or long flexors and extensors, of the hand originate in the forearm, and their tendons insert on the phalanges (flexor digitorum profundus, flexor digitorum superficialis, and extensor digitorum communis) and thumb (flexor pollicis longus, abductor pollicis longus, and extensor pollicis brevis). • The flexor digitorum profundus inserts on the base of the distal phalanx and flexes the DIP and PIP joints. • Isolated function of the flexor digitorum profundus to the index finger is present in 85% of patients. • The tendons to the ulnar three digits often act as a single unit and should be tested both simultaneously and individually. • Profundus function is evaluated by fixing and holding the PIP and MCP joints of the finger being examined in extension. • The **flexor digitorum superficialis** inserts on the volar surface of the middle phalanx and flexes the PIP joint. • It is evaluated by holding the adjacent fingers in extension and asking the patient to flex the PIP joint of the involved finger. • When examining superficialis injuries to the little finger, simultaneous flexion of both the ring and little fingers at the PIP joint should be tested because their superficialis tendons may share a common muscle belly. • The flexor pollicis longus is responsible for flexion of the distal phalanx of the thumb but also flexes the **MCP** joint. • The main extensors of the MCP joints are the extensor digitorum communis passing to each of the four fingers. • In addition, there is the extensor digiti minimi to the little finger and the extensor indicis proprius to the index finger. • These are independent extensors and must be taken into account when assessing the extent of injury. • Transection of an extensor tendon results in extensor lag of that digit at the MCP joint. • The presence of double tendons to the index and little fingers may confuse the diagnosis. • The extensor pollicis brevis extends the proximal phalanx of the thumb, and the abductor pollicis longus extends the first MCP joint. • Injury to either of these tendons results in loss of their corresponding function.

ANSWER:
A, B, D, E

6. Match the muscle tendon unit in the left-hand column with its appropriate innervation in the right-hand column.

   A. Flexor digitorum superficialis

   B. Extensor digitorum communis, extensor indicis proprius, extensor digiti minimi, extensor pollicis brevis, and abductor pollicis longus

   C. Flexor digitorum profundus to index and middle fingers

   D. Flexor digitorum profundus to ring and little fingers

   a. Median nerve

   b. Radial nerve

   c. Ulnar nerve

Ref.: 1–3

COMMENTS: Innervation of the extrinsic muscles is derived from the radial, median, and ulnar nerves. • Although variations may occur, the usual patterns of innervation to the extrinsic muscles of the hands are as follows. • The innervation of the flexor digitorum superficialis is entirely median, and that of the extensor group is entirely radial. • The ulnar nerve innervates the flexor digitorum profundus tendons to the fingers on the ulnar half of the hand, and the median nerve innervates the profundus tendons to the index and middle fingers. • Injury to the forearm can potentially lead to abnormalities of digit and thumb flexion and extension due to nerve or muscle injury. • Flexion and extension of the digits and thumb should always be evaluated in patients presenting with forearm injuries.

ANSWER:
A-a; B-b; C-a; D-c

7. A surgeon is called to examine a 30-year-old painter who cut the palm of his right hand with a fresh razor blade. Examination reveals a 2-cm, clean laceration at the base of the long finger. MCP joint flexion is intact, but the patient cannot flex either IP joint in that finger. The injury is 1 hr old. What is the diagnosis?

   A. Lacerated flexor digitorum superficialis tendon

   B. Lacerated flexor digitorum profundus tendon

   C. Combined flexor digitorum superficialis and profundus laceration

   D. Laceration of the intrinsic muscles to the long finger

   E. Median nerve transection

Ref.: 1–3

COMMENTS: See Question 8.

8. The immediate treatment plan for the patient described in Question 7 should include which of the following?

   A. Plans for immediate tendon repair (within 6 hr) to avoid the hazards of delayed tendon anastomosis

   B. Wrist block anesthesia, extension of the skin wound along proper incision lines, and exploration to confirm the diagnosis

   C. Careful cleansing and irrigation of the wound, placement of an appropriate dressing or simple sutures, and hand immobilization before definitive primary surgical repair some time within 2 weeks

   D. Cleansing of the wound, primary skin closure, hand immobilization, and outpatient follow-up visits, because this injury will require free-tendon graft reconstruction 6 weeks after injury

Ref.: 1–3

COMMENTS: Flexion of the MCP joint is a function of the intrinsic muscles and can persist in the face of extrinsic flexor muscle and tendon injury. • The goal of flexor tendon repair is restoration of IP joint flexion. • Flexor tendon repair demands meticulous attention to detail and, whenever possible, should be performed by a hand surgeon. • The character of the wound, the nature of the injury, the degree of contamination, and the time between injury and definitive treatment determine whether primary or delayed repair is performed. • Proper wound cleansing, dressing, immobilization, and prophylactic antibiotics allow delay of primary repair if a hand surgeon is not immediately available. • If there is a question about the degree of contamination or if the initial wound treatment has been delayed beyond several hours, making primary closure hazardous, delayed repair after 2–14 days may be performed. • This allows the presence or absence of infection to be clearly established. • Many experts believe this type of delay does not significantly alter the ultimate outcome of the repair. • Tendon injuries with grossly contaminated wounds, those with significant tendon loss, or wounds with significant associated injuries to the soft tissue, bone, nerve, or blood vessels should be treated by secondary repair in 3–6 weeks, after the wounds have been stabilized, the infection has cleared, and edema formation has subsided.

ANSWERS:
Question 7: C
Question 8: C

9. Which of the following statements regarding the most common metacarpal fractures is/are true?

   A. They are commonly known as Bennett's fractures.

   B. They are commonly known as boxer's fractures.

   C. They most often involve the distal metacarpal of the little and ring fingers.

   D. Physical examination is the most effective means of assessing the degree of angulation.

Ref.: 1–3

COMMENTS: Metacarpal fractures commonly result from hitting an object with a clenched fist. • They usually involve the distal metacarpal of the fifth and occasionally fourth fingers and are known as "boxer's fractures." The metacarpal head is displaced palmward, and pain, swelling, and some loss of knuckle prominence are the usual physical findings. • Associated lacerations should be treated as human bites until proven otherwise, and early exploration, with administration of intravenous antibiotics, is recommended. • Swelling usually masks the degree of angulation, and a lateral radiograph is needed for accurate evaluation. • Each finger should be individually flexed to the palm to assess the degree of rotational deformity. • During flexion, the fingers normally point to the scaphoid tubercle. • Deviation from this alignment allows estimation of the rotational deformity. • The usual treatment is closed reduction followed by immobilization of the involved and adjacent digits, placing the MCP joint in 65–90 degrees of flexion and the IP joints in full extension. • Unstable or multiple metacarpal fractures often require open reduction and internal fixation. • Metacarpal shaft fractures require reduction and immobilization. • Percutaneous K wires or plate and screws for internal fixation often are required if the fracture is unstable, particularly if the fracture is oblique or comminuted.

ANSWER:
B, C

10. Which of the following statements regarding injuries of the thumb is/are true?

    A. Bennett's fracture is an intra-articular avulsion fracture of the base of the metacarpal.

    B. Abduction force applied to the thumb most often injures the IP joint.

    C. The valgus stress test is used to diagnose disruption of the ulnar collateral ligament system at the first MCP joint.

    D. The term *gamekeeper's thumb* refers to injuries of the MCP joint of the thumb.

    E. The valgus stress test should not be performed when a fracture is suspected or in children suspected of having epiphyseal injury.

Ref.: 1–4

COMMENTS: Bennett's fracture is an intra-articular avulsion fracture at the base of the thumb metacarpal. • The ligaments remain attached to the distal bone fragment, the abductor pollicis longus subluxes the metacarpal laterally, and the fracture becomes unstable. • The usual treatment is traction reduction with percutaneous wire fixation of the metacarpal to the trapezium and adjacent carpus, although open reduction and internal fixation may be required. • Abduction force applied to the thumb may result in disruption of the ulnar collateral ligament system at the first MCP joint. • This injury commonly occurs while skiing, ball handling, or supporting a fall with the thumbs. • It also may result from repetitive low-grade abduction force, as is encountered when using the thumb to dislocate rabbit's necks, hence the name *gamekeeper's thumb*. • The diagnosis is based on the finding of valgus instability of the MCP joint. • An angle of more than 30 degrees of laxity is usually considered a complete rupture. • When the diagnosis is made, open repair of the ligament is indicated because the ulnar collateral ligament has retracted proximally to the adductor aponeurosis to the thumb. • This interposed aponeurosis now prevents the ligament from healing back to its insertion, even with casting and immobilization. • The valgus stress test should be performed judiciously on children with an epiphyseal fracture or adults with avulsion fractures at this level so as to avoid distraction of the fracture, thus requiring open reduction.

ANSWER:
A, C, D, E

11. Which of the following statements regarding phalangeal fractures is/are true?

    A. Volar angulation of proximal phalangeal fractures causes a flexion deformity of the PIP joint.

    B. Collateral ligament tears of the IP joints require open repair.

    C. Fractures of the base of the middle phalanx tend to have apical dorsal angulation.

    D. Fractures of the neck of the middle phalanx tend to have apical volar angulation.

    E. In the presence of distal phalange fracture, an associated subungual hematoma must not be opened, to avoid osteomyelitis.

Ref.: 1–3

COMMENTS: Closed **distal phalangeal fractures** are often the result of crush injury and involve nail bed damage as well. • If the nail bed and plate are intact, subungual hematomas are drained, and the nail bed underneath is meticulously repaired after careful antiseptic preparation of the digit. • Displaced fractures involving injury to the nail matrix require exploration to ensure that no matrix is interposed in the fracture, and repair of the nail bed tends to better reduce the fragments of bone. • It is most important with open fractures of the distal phalanx to repair the skin and soft-tissue injury rather than the fracture itself. • Failure to do so predisposes to malalignment, nail deformity, and osteomyelitis.

Fractures of the middle phalanx may or may not involve injury to the collateral ligaments at the IP joints. • Tears of these ligaments with or without small chip fractures usually respond to closed realignment, splinting, and appropriate rehabilitative motion. • Dorsal and volar fracture dislocations at the IP joints require precise reduction, and open procedures with internal fixation are frequently necessary. • Distal fractures of the middle phalanx usually have apex volar angulation because the proximal segment is flexed by the flexor digitorum superficialis. • Fractures at the base of the middle phalanx usually have apical dorsal angulation because of distal segment flexion by the flexor digitorum superficialis and proximal segment extension by the central slip of the extensor mechanism. • Most middle phalangeal fractures respond to closed reduction and external immobilization.

Proximal phalangeal fractures have a relatively long fulcrum, and even minimal displacement or rotational abnormalities exhibit significant rotation and deviation of the digit distally. • For that reason, meticulous reduction is required, and postreduction examinations should assess extension and flexion for rotation or orientation in both positions.

ANSWER:
A, C, D

12. Which of the following statements regarding extensor tendon injuries is/are true?

　A. Extensor tendon lacerations have a good prognosis because of their subcutaneous location.

　B. The extensor retinaculum must be closed over extensor tendon repairs to prevent bow stringing.

　C. Avulsion of the extensor tendon at the base of the distal phalanx results in the boutonniére deformity.

　D. Disruption of the central extensor tendon at the base of the middle phalanx results in the mallet deformity.

Ref.: 1–3

COMMENTS: The extensor tendons occupy a subcutaneous position, except at the wrist. • The overlying skin is nearly as mobile as the excursion of the extensor tendons and, after repair, rarely restricts their function. • An exception to this is at the wrist, where the extensor retinaculum overlies the tendons. • Injuries at this level are repaired by transposition of the tendons into the subcutaneous tissue, with closure of the retinaculum deep to the repair or complete release of the retinaculum if tendon gliding is impeded.

The **boutonniére deformity** results from disruption of the central extensor tendon at its insertion into the dorsum of the base of the middle phalanx. • Eventually, the lateral bands are displaced toward the palm and, with this repositioning, lose their extensor function and become PIP joint flexors. • The patient is unable to initiate extension from the flexed position but sometimes can maintain extension if the digit is passively placed in that position. • Without treatment, the PIP joint develops a flexion contracture, and the

DIP joint assumes a position of hyperextension. • Immobilization of the PIP joint at zero degrees of extension with dynamic extension splinting for 6–8 weeks is recommended whenever possible. • Because this immobilization allows DIP joint motion and tendon gliding, the lateral bands will dynamically "snap back" up into their proper position.

Injuries to the extensor insertion into the dorsum of the distal phalanx result in the **mallet deformity**. • Often, no fracture can be seen. • If such an injury is associated with a fracture and the fragment is small, dorsal splinting with the joint in 0–10 degrees of hyperextension for 6–8 weeks provides good results. • If more than one third of the articular surface is displaced with the avulsed tendon and volar subluxation of the distal phalanx occurs, open reduction and internal fixation are advised.

ANSWER:
A

13. Which of the following statements regarding hand infections is/are true?

　A. The relatively avascular environment of the synovial sheaths makes them resistant to infection.

　B. One third of hand infections have a mixed flora.

　C. Treatment of human bite wounds includes aggressive cleansing and antibiotic therapy before suturing.

　D. A common organism isolated in a human bite injury to the hand is *Eikenella corrodens*.

　E. The organisms most commonly isolated from hand infections are penicillinase-producing staphylococci.

Ref.: 1–4

COMMENTS: Hand infections are potentially serious because of the superficial location of the hand's bones and joints; the high density of relatively avascular tendons, fat, and synovium; and the ease of spread through the synovial sheaths due to constant flexion and extension. • Staphylococci are present in nearly 80% of hand infections and are frequently penicillin resistant. • One third of hand infections contain mixed flora and frequently include β-hemolytic streptococci, *Escherichia coli*, *Proteus* spp., and *Pseudomonas* spp. • In human bites, a high percentage of anaerobic organisms may also be present, with *E. corrodens* known to be a significant contributor. • Drainage procedures are reserved to decompress loculations of pus. • Cellulitis without fluctuance is treated with immobilization, elevation, antibiotics, and frequent reexamination. • The empiric use of antibiotics is indicated for severe infections, with appropriate changes in therapy being made when culture and sensitivity results are available. • All complex infections should be drained in the operating room with proximal tourniquet control. • Distal-to-proximal wrapping to obtain a bloodless field, as used during elective hand surgery, **is contraindicated** in order not to spread infection. • Human bites should be vigorously cleansed, treated with antibiotics (including anaerobic coverage), and left open to close secondarily. • Because of the superficial location of the tendons and MCP joints, human bites (usually from a punch) should be vigorously treated. • The motion of the skin, tendon, and joints in various planes helps spread infection and cover drainage paths, trapping bacteria. • Extension of the wound, with formal joint exploration in an operating room, is often required.

ANSWER:
B, D, E

14. Which of the following statements is/are true?

A. Paronychia occurs in the digital pulp of the finger.

B. A felon is an infection around the margin of the nail bed.

C. Finger felon, or paronychia, has the potential to cause tenosynovitis.

D. The deep structures of the hand are protected from subcutaneous abscesses of the palm by the superficial palmar fascia.

E. The versatile "fish-mouth" incision is used for draining both pulp and paronychial infections.

Ref.: 1, 2, 4

COMMENTS: Subcutaneous abscesses of the volar surface of the hand often follow small puncture wounds or infection of superficial blisters. • Pain and swelling are confined to the area of inflammation and are not increased with minor tendon motion. • Loculations should be drained, since they have the potential of tracking to the dorsum of the hand. • A **felon** is an infection of the pulp of the fingertip that can lead to deep ischemic necrosis, osteomyelitis, or both because of the presence of compartmentalizing septa that prevent expansion as pressure increases. • Sharp pain and tenderness out of proportion to the amount of swelling are characteristic. • The pulp space must be drained by dividing the septa before tissue necrosis occurs. • As a result of the proximity of the pulp and paronychial space to the tendon sheath, extension of this infection can lead to tenosynovitis. • The once popular fish-mouth incision is now discouraged because of the potential for painful scarring and neuroma formation. • **Paronychial** infections are around the margins of the nail plate, often caused by hangnails, manicure trauma, or small foreign bodies. • *Staphylococcus* is the usual offending organism. • Early cases can be treated with warm soaks and antibiotics, but abscesses must be drained, often requiring resection of a portion of the overlying proximal nail plate. • Unattended superficial infections may spread to deeper compartments, such as the tendon sheaths. • Likewise, deep compartment infections frequently spread to neighboring bursa and web spaces.

ANSWER:
C

15. Which of the following statements regarding tenosynovitis is/are true?

A. Infections of the flexor sheath of the little finger more often extend to the thumb than to the adjacent ring finger.

B. A flexor tendon sheath infection causes the involved finger to assume a position of mild extension at all joints.

C. The involved digit becomes uniformly swollen, and active or passive extension elicits pain.

D. By definition, deep palmar space infections involve the flexor tendons.

Ref.: 1–4

COMMENTS: Infection of the synovial sheaths of the flexor tendons is a serious problem that requires prompt appropriate treatment. • The tendons are relatively avascular and are characterized by poor natural resistance to infection. • Although anatomy varies, the sheath of the little finger is often continuous with the ulnar bursa, which in turn is directly adjacent to the radial bursa, which extends to the flexor sheath of the thumb. • A. Kanavel (from Cook County Hospital, in Illinois) described three cardinal findings of pyogenic tenosynovitis: (1) the infected digit becomes uniformly swollen along the length of the flexor tendon sheath, (2) the involved digit assumes a slightly flexed position, and (3) passive flexion elicits exquisite local pain. • If there is no frank purulence, conservative measures may be successful, and surgery may be avoided. • These measures include elevating the extremity, splint immobilization, intravenous antibiotics, and close observation. • If there is no response within 24–48 hr, surgical drainage with copious irrigation is indicated. • Immediate surgical drainage should be considered at any time if there is progression of the disease process in spite of treatment. • Surgical drainage is accomplished by a longitudinal incision on the side of the digit along the axis of joint motion. • The incision is placed on the ulnar side of the digit if palmar spread is suspected. • Placement of irrigating catheters within the sheath and systemic antibiotics may be used as adjuncts to surgical therapy, but they are not always needed if thorough irrigation is performed. • The deep palmar space is located between the flexor tendons and the metacarpals in the palm. • It is divided into the thenar space and the midpalmar space at the level of the third metacarpal, where a vertical septum extends between the metacarpal and sheath of the long finger flexor tendons. • Infection here is manifested by localized, tender swelling and must be drained using an appropriate incision.

ANSWER:
A, C

16. Which of the following statements regarding the forearm compartment syndrome is/are true?

A. The four P's—pain, pallor, paralysis, and pulselessness (radial or ulnar arteries)—accurately describe the syndrome.

B. The underlying cause is increased tissue pressure in the deep flexor compartment of the forearm.

C. The deep flexor compartment obtains its blood supply only by the anterior interosseous artery, which becomes occluded as tissue pressure rises.

D. The median, radial, and ulnar nerves become strangulated by deep flexor compartment fibrosis.

E. The hand loses intrinsic muscle function and becomes numb in the median and ulnar distributions.

Ref.: 1–4

COMMENTS: The elevation of tissue pressure in the deep flexor compartment of the forearm leads ultimately to occlusion of flow through the anterior interosseous artery. • **Volkmans' ischemic contracture** is the long-term result of this occlusion if left untreated. • A supracondylar fracture in a child should always raise the suspicion of a compartment syndrome, since it can commonly be missed, resulting in Volkmans' ischemic contracture. • Dense fibrotic degeneration of the muscular contents of the deep flexor compartment occurs, which causes a fixed flexion contracture of the wrist and fingers and a "strangulation neuropathy" of the median and ulnar nerves. • The nerve involvement causes loss of intrinsic muscle function and numbness in the respective sensory distributions of the ulnar and median nerves.

Compartment syndrome is an acute syndrome that can be caused by a number of insults, including a wringer injury, extravasation of blood or drugs into the forearm, snake and insect bites, and a tight cast or dressing. • These mechanisms are characterized by elevation of tissue pressure as their common denominator. • Needle testing of compartment pressures can be of great assistance in establishing an early diagnosis so that treatment with complete fasciotomy may be performed.

The radial artery does not pass through the deep flexor compartment and maintains its patency until late in the course of the process. • The early clinical signs of increasing tissue pressure are tenderness over the forearm muscles, pain with passive finger extension, and paresthesias in the distribution of the median and ulnar nerves. • Once the diagnosis is made, complete fasciotomy from elbow to wrist is indicated. • Treatment of late cases that develop Volkman's ischemic contracture involves major reconstructive surgery.

ANSWER:
B, C, E

17. Which of the following statements regarding replantation of the hand is/are true?

   A. Single digits (other than the thumb) are uncommonly replanted except in children.

   B. The amputated part may tolerate cool ischemia for up to 24 hr if there is no significant avascular muscle mass.

   C. Bleeding from the proximal part is ideally treated with pressure rather than clamping.

   D. A history of heavy smoking, diabetes mellitus, hypertension, and Raynaud's phenomenon are relative contraindications to replantation.

   E. Replantation above the elbow is contraindicated.

Ref.: 1–4

COMMENTS: Replantation is a highly specialized procedure best performed by a team of replantation surgeons. • The procedure is long and requires that the patient be carefully evaluated for associated injuries before committing to a replantation attempt. • Distal amputations properly cooled immediately after injury may be viable for up to 24 hr. • The part should be wrapped in sterile saline solution–soaked dressings and placed in a plastic container (a sterile urine cup if one is readily available), which is then submerged in ice water. • The part should never be frozen or "salted" or come in contact with the surrounding liquid. • Single digits are less frequently replanted, except in children or if there is a sharp noncrushing cut at the level of the middle phalanx distal to the splitting of the superficialis tendon. • The hand and thumb are always considered for replantation unless definite contraindications exist or the extremity was not properly preserved. • Amputations above the elbow are considered for replantation (particularly in children), since even partial success can convert an above-elbow to a below-elbow stump for future rehabilitation. • Guillotine amputations are the injuries that present most favorably for replantation.

ANSWER:
A, B, C, D

18. Which of the following statements regarding digit amputations is/are false?

   A. Any length of thumb that can be saved should be preserved.

   B. The middle finger can assume the role of primary pinch if the index finger is lost.

   C. Any length of index finger that can be saved should be preserved to maintain its pinching function.

   D. MCP joint amputations of the middle and ring fingers leave a space open in the clenched fist through which objects held in the palm may fall.

   E. Traumatic loss of the thumb can be treated by digital transposition or by toe transfer.

Ref.: 1–3

COMMENTS: Planned or traumatic amputations within the hand must take into consideration a number of factors, including the patient's handedness, age, and occupation and concern for aesthetics. • The thumb is the most important digit, and as much of its length as possible should be preserved. • The index finger amputated proximally to the PIP joint loses its ability to pinch, and the brain naturally switches the pinching to the long finger. • Attempts to preserve length distal to the PIP joint should be made, but if the digit is painful, insensate, or "gets in the way," the patient may be best served by transection through the metacarpal (ray amputation), since the long finger can assume the role of primary pinch. • Loss of little finger length proximal to the PIP joint may also be best treated by ray amputation. • Central finger amputations (long and ring fingers) near the MCP joint can cause bothersome spaces in the clenched fist that can be treated by transfer of the adjacent peripheral finger with its metacarpal to fill the space. • Using this basic principle, when multiple digits are amputated at once, combinations of digits, or "on-top-plasties," should be considered at the time of original surgery so that parts can be utilized and not discarded.

ANSWER:
C

19. Which of the following statements regarding carpal tunnel syndrome is/are true?

   A. The carpal tunnel syndrome is entrapment of the ulnar nerve in the carpal canal.

   B. It is most commonly traumatic in origin.

   C. The associated pain and numbness is often nocturnal, with referral of the pain to the shoulder and neck.

   D. Injection of steroids into the carpal canal is contraindicated.

   E. Electromyography and nerve conduction studies help confirm the diagnosis and exclude more proximal nerve entrapment.

Ref.: 1–4

COMMENTS: Carpal tunnel syndrome is entrapment of the median nerve in the carpal canal, with resultant nerve injury. • Most commonly, it is idiopathic in origin, but it can be seen following trauma, such as Colles' and Smith's fractures or lunate and perilunate dislocations, or it can be part of the presenting symptoms of systemic diseases, such as rheumatoid arthritis, gout, diabetes mellitus, hypothyroidism, or amyloidosis. • Carpal tunnel syndrome may also be related to the patient's occupation, caused by repetitive strain, such as working on an assembly line or on a computer keyboard for prolonged periods. • Proximal entrapment due to Pancoast tumors, brachial plexus abnormalities, cervical spine disease, and compression in the forearm (pronator teres syndrome) must be excluded as a diagnosis.

Presenting symptoms include pain and numbness along the median nerve distribution that are often nocturnal because of peripheral vasodilation that increases venous congestion or fluid shifts owing to a recumbent position, which causes pressure on the nerve. • Sleeping in the fetal position with the wrists flexed can also increase pressure inside the carpal canal at night. • The pain may be referred to the shoulder and neck, making the diagnosis more difficult. • Classic physical findings include reproduction of the symptoms with forced wrist flexion (Phalen's test) and a positive Tinel's sign (tingling felt after percussion over the nerve at the wrist). • Altered sensibility and thenar atrophy may also be present in advanced cases. • Initial treatment consists of splinting, non-steroidal anti-inflammatory agents, and possibly a steroid injection into the carpal canal. • Thenar atrophy, pain, weakness, and persistence of symptoms despite conservative therapy are indications for surgery, which involves release of the portion of the flexor retinaculum that is entrapping the nerve. • This release can be performed with an open procedure with small incisions or in some cases endoscopically with excellent success.

A N S W E R :
C, E

20. True statements regarding stenosing tenovaginitis include which of the following?

    A. One form is also known as trigger finger.

    B. It is also known as the swan-neck deformity.

    C. It can cause locking of the digit in flexion or extension.

    D. Surgical correction should be performed with wrist-block anesthesia.

    E. When seen at the wrist level, it is called Dupuytren's contracture.

Ref.: 1–4

COMMENTS: Stenosing tenovaginitis of the fingers and thumb is a common cause of hand pain and loss of function. • Limitation of free gliding of the tendon within its fibroosseous tunnel is due to a disproportion in size between the flexor tendons and the fibroosseous sheath. • It is associated with a popping or snapping sensation that, in extreme situations, can even cause locking of the digit in extension or flexion. • Treatment is with nonsteroidal anti-inflammatory agents and steroid injections.

Failure to respond to medical treatment is an indication for surgical decompression, with release of the A-1 pulley. • Local infiltration or wrist-block anesthesia is used with tourniquet control for the operation so that free active excursion of the tendon can be demonstrated following release of the constricting area.

DeQuervain's syndrome is tenovaginitis of the first dorsal compartment, leading to pain and tenderness on the radial dorsal aspect of the wrist. • If conservative measures fail, release of this compartment surgically is recommended. • Multiple tendon slips and intracompartmental bands may be identified and require full release.

A N S W E R :
A, C, D

21. Which of the following statements regarding Dupuytren's contracture is/are true?

    A. Dupuytren's contracture involves the palmar aponeurosis.

    B. Males are affected more often than females, and the contracture is primarily caused by excessive alcohol consumption.

    C. It begins as a nodule formation, ultimately leading to contracture at the MCP and PIP joints.

    D. Four clinical types have been described.

    E. Aggressive nonsurgical treatment can influence the course of the disease.

Ref.: 1–4

COMMENTS: Dupuytren's contracture occurs 10 times more frequently in males and primarily affects people of northern European origin. • It appears to be transmitted as an autosomal gene influenced by multiple exogenous factors, such as injury, liver disease, alcoholism, pulmonary disease, seizure disorders, and chronic bowel disease. • It begins as nodule formation within the palmar fascia in line with the pretendinous bands. • Gradually, the skin becomes dimpled, and contractures form at the level of the MCP and PIP joints. • Four clinical types—senile, middle-aged, young fulminant, and feminine—have been identified. • There is no known effective medical therapy.

Surgical options include open fasciotomy (performed in high-risk patients), radical excision of the palmar fascia and skin, and partial palmar fasciectomy (which is most often performed). • Postoperative splinting and hand therapy are critically important to the success of such therapy. • Care must be taken to avoid injury to skin flaps and the digital nerves, which can be pushed to the surface and out of anatomic position, especially when associated with spiral bands.

A N S W E R :
A, C, D

22. Which of the following statements regarding peripheral nerve injury is/are true?

    A. Nerve repair is progressively less effective if delayed beyond 2 months after surgery.

    B. Nerve repair is best performed using 4–15 times magnification.

    C. Nerve repair is best performed in a fashion that minimizes tension across the repair.

    D. Regeneration may be followed clinically by observing the distal progression of Tinel's sign.

Ref.: 1–3

COMMENTS: Nerve injuries result from stretching or compression (neurapraxia) or transection. • Neurapractic injuries carry a better prognosis than do transection injuries. • Nerve injuries do not need to be repaired at the time of injury, but it is thought that the results are progressively worse if repair is delayed beyond 6 months when the distal nerve tubules have contracted and the new axons can no longer grow distally. • Occasionally, repair delayed for up to 2 years has been successful, particularly in children. • Most surgeons perform a careful epineural repair, but repair of the individual fascicular bundle is also required in large, mixed peripheral nerves.

Recovery after repair begins with return of function starting proximally. • Regenerating axons grow down the distal nerve sheath at a rate of approximately 1 mm/day. • Distal progression of Tinel's sign (tingling felt after percussion over the growing nerve) usually follows the start of regeneration. • Recently, successful nerve regeneration with improved healing has been achieved with vein grafts, which act as conduits for nerve growth across the repair.

A N S W E R :
B, C, D

23. Match each item in the left-hand column with the appropriate item in the right-hand column.

A. Median nerve palsy   a. Claw deformity of ring and little fingers

B. Ulnar nerve palsy   b. Loss of wrist extension

C. Radial nerve palsy   c. Loss of thumb palmar abduction and opposition

               d. Ring finger superficialis transfer used to restore function when injured in the forearm

Ref.: 1–3

COMMENTS: Median nerve palsy at the wrist results in an inability to perform proper thumb opposition or palmar abduction. • Transfer of the flexor digitorum superficialis of the ring finger (median nerve innervation proximal to the wrist) to the insertion of the abductor pollicis brevis is frequently the treatment of choice (superficialis opponens plasty). • Median nerve injuries at the elbow result in denervation of the flexor digitorum superficialis, and in this case transfer of the abductor digiti minimi (ulnar innervation) or extensor indicis proprius (radial innervation) is used.

    Ulnar nerve palsy at the wrist results in a claw deformity of the third and fourth fingers. • It results from MCP joint hyperextension with secondary flexion of the IP and distal phalangeal joints. • The flexor digitorum superficialis to the little finger can be moved to the base of the proximal phalanx of the ring and little fingers to restore MCP joint flexion. • The profundus tendons to the small and ring finger are innervated by the ulnar nerve.

    Radial nerve disruption over the mid- or distal humerus causes loss of wrist extension, MCP joint finger extension, and thumb abduction and extension. • The common transfer used to repair this deformity is the pronator teres to the extensor carpi radialis brevis, the flexor carpi ulnaris (ulnar innervation) to the extensor digitorum communis, and the palmaris longus (median innervation) to the extensor pollicis longus.

A N S W E R :
A-c; B-a; C-b

24. Which of the following statements regarding syndactyly is/are true?

A. Syndactyly is often associated with polydactyly.

B. Release should be accomplished by the age of 1 year if digits of differing growth rates are involved.

C. It may be related to an autosomal dominant genetic pattern.

D. Males are more frequently affected than females.

Ref.: 1–3

COMMENTS: Syndactyly is a common congenital deformity that varies in severity from a thin skin web between normal digits to complete fusion of bony elements with a common nail. • It may be inherited in an autosomal dominant pattern and is associated with several syndromes, including Poland's and Apert's syndromes. • Often, both hands and feet are involved, and males are affected more frequently than females.

    The timing of operation is debatable. • Syndactyly involving distal bony structures in digits of differing growth rates is often treated by surgical division of the distal portion of the syndactyly before 1 year of age to allow for normal unrestrained growth. • Because of reports of recurrences when performed earlier, complete release of syndactyly before age 1 frequently results in an unacceptable degree of scarring. • When there is no concern about the differential growth rate, surgery is delayed 2–3 years. • When more than two digits are involved, the releases are staged with 6 months between operations to avoid compromise of the middle digits' blood supply. • Most frequently (unless the syndactyly is small), full-thickness skin grafts are harvested from the groin as needed to close a portion of the surgical defect. • Geometric calculations reveal that separating two digits always requires addition of tissue.

A N S W E R :
B, C, D

25. Match the hand lesions in the left column with the descriptive common features in the right column.

A. Ganglion cyst   a. Arises from the short vinculum near the IP joints

B. Giant-cell tumor of tendon   b. Called a mucous cyst when arising from the DIP joint

C. Inclusion cyst   c. Fibrous capsule lined with squamous epithelium found on the flexor aspect of the palm and fingers

D. Lipoma   d. Most commonly found around the thenar eminence and possibly in the carpal canal

E. Glomus tumor   e. Painful tumor found underneath the nail

Ref.: 1–4

COMMENTS: Ganglion cysts are often seen in any of four locations: the dorsum of the hand or wrist, the flexor side of the wrist adjacent to the radial artery, arising from the flexor sheaths (often at the base of the digit), or arising from the DIP joints (where they are known as mucous cysts). • **Giant-cell tumors** of the tendons are benign and arise from the short vinculum near the IP joints or from the joint synovium itself. • Both tendons in the flexor sheath are usually involved by the tumor, which lies deep to the neurovascular bundle. • **Inclusion cysts** result from implantation of the epithelium with or without a foreign body and occur on the flexor aspect of the palm or finger. • **Lipomas** often appear over the thenar eminence but can even be found within the carpal canal and have been associated with carpal tunnel syndrome. • The **glomus tumor** originates from the vasculomusculoneuroglomus of the nail bed, which regulates blood flow. • Growth of this tissue within the closed space of the fingertip may cause nerve pressure and exquisite pain beyond the degree expected. • MRI is highly successful for confirming the diagnosis, and surgical treatment involves removal of the nail plate with complete excision.

A N S W E R :
A-b; B-a; C-c; D-d; E-e

26. Match the common anatomic defect in the left column with the associated type of arthritis in the right column.

A. MCP joint anterior subluxation-dislocation with extensor lag and ulnar drift   a. Rheumatoid arthritis

B. Can be diagnosed with
   a blood test
C. Related to repetitive strain
   at high-stress joints
D. IP joints of fingers and
   thumb and the MCP joint
   of the thumb often affected
E. Heberden's nodes
F. Bouchard's nodes

b. Osteoarthritis

Ref.: 1–3

COMMENTS: Rheumatoid arthritis is a systemic disease that can involve any or all of the tendon systems and joints of the hand. • Often, there is significant involvement at the wrist and in the MCP and IP areas. • The management of rheumatoid arthritis is complex and involves hand surgeons, rheumatologists, hand therapists, and social workers. • **Osteoarthritis** commonly involves multiple hand joints and most frequently occurs in postmenopausal women. • The joints most commonly involved are the IP joints of the fingers and thumb and the metacarpocarpal (i.e., trapeziometacarpal) joint of the thumb. • Heberden's nodes are osteophytes at the DIP joint, and Bouchard's nodes are found at the PIP joint. • Disabling involvement of the DIP joint is often treated with arthrodesis. • Severe involvement of the first MCP joint of the thumb often requires autologous or implant arthroplasty or fusion.

ANSWER:
A-a; B-a; C-b; D-b; E-b; F-b

27. A 35-year-old mechanic presents 1 hr after a high-pressure oil solvent injection injury to his right index finger sustained while cleaning his spray apparatus. The finger is slightly swollen and erythematous. Sensation is intact. He is able to flex and extend all joints with mild discomfort. What is the most appropriate treatment at this point?

A. Ice, elevation, and reexamination in 24 hr

B. Ice, elevation, oral antibiotics, and reexamination in 24 hr

C. Elevation, intravenous antibiotics, and hospital admission for close observation with frequent assessment of vital signs, sensibility, and circulation

D. Urgent wide surgical drainage and débridement of the digit and palm to remove all tissue containing the solvent

Ref.: 1, 2

COMMENTS: High-pressure solvent injection injuries often initially appear deceptively benign. • The entrance site is small, the digit is not necessarily painful, and the patient tends to minimize the degree of injury. • Despite this appearance, urgent wide surgical drainage, irrigation, and débridement of the digit and hand are required to prevent rapid progression of a severe inflammatory response, compartment syndrome, and digital loss. • Similar problems can be seen with paint, paint thinners, and grease injected under pressure. • Extensive cases have been known to have fluid forced all the way up to the wrist. • Application of ice, elevation, and antibiotics are all important aspects of management to reduce the inflammatory response and prevent digital compartment syndrome and infection, but they are only temporizing measures. • The intense inflammatory response to the solvent will lead to digital compartment syndrome and tissue necrosis unless wide surgical drainage of the digit and hand is performed

urgently (even before the inflammatory response is obvious). • As with tendon sheath infections, the solvent quickly tracks proximally along the flexor tendon sheath into the palm, and aggressive, wide opening and débridement into the palm are required. • Subcutaneous tissue containing the solvent should be débrided while vital structures are preserved whenever possible. • Repeated débridement is often required. • Standard x-rays often reveal radiopaque material and help define the extent of extravasation. • Stiffness is a common long-term complication, if the digit can be salvaged at all. • Even with appropriate management, results are often not optimal.

ANSWER:
D

28. Match the organism with the most likely method of transfer.

A. *Eikenella corrodens*
B. *Pasteurella multocida*
C. *Sporothrix schenckii*
D. *Staphylococcus epidermis*

a. Human bite
b. Cat bite, dog bite
c. Gardening
d. Human bite, cat bite, dog bite, and intravenous drug use

E. *Aeromonas hydrophila*
F. *Mycobacterium marinum*

e. Leeches
f. Cleaning fish tanks

Ref.: 1–3

COMMENTS: The putative agent in many types of hand infections can be ascertained by a detailed history. • Human bites are notoriously infective, since human saliva contains a variety of pathogens, including *Staphylococcus aureus*, *S. epidermis*, *Streptococcus* spp., and *E. corrodens*.

Dog and cat saliva both contain the agent *P. multicoda*. • With aggressive cleaning and débridement, direct repair at the time of emergency department evaluation is feasible in these types of bites, while human bites are never closed initially. • Instead, they are left to drain after incision, treated with antibiotics, and often allowed to close via secondary intention.

Gardeners, especially those who works with roses, should be suspected to have sporotrichosis. • This organism spreads through the lymphatics of the arm, causing red, hard nodules and local ulceration. • Treatment with oral potassium iodide and, in severe cases, amphotericin B is indicated.

The first known use of leeches dates back 3500 years, as evidenced in Egyptian tomb painting, and medical leeches are used with frequency in free tissue transfer and replantation surgery to relieve venous congestion. • However, the use of leeches is not without risk. • *A. hydrophila* is a gram-negative rod that lives within the gut of the leech and can cause infection at a rate of up to 20% after their use. • This organism is sensitive to ciprofloxacin. • Infection can be extensive owing to compromise of the blood supply to the tissues being treated.

M. marinum must be suspected in those handling fish or cleaning fish tanks. • It is known as the swimming-pool granuloma. • This atypical mycobacterium causes a cutaneous infection, which results in a chronic, indolent tenosynovitis. • In non-immunosuppressed patients, it responds well to antibiotics, and no surgical intervention is required beyond biopsy and culture acquisition. • Special cultures must be taken on Löwenstein-Jensen culture medium at 30–32°C, as opposed to 37°C.

ANSWER:
A-a; B-b; C-c; D-a; E-e; F-f

29. A 36-year-old man is involved in a common industrial mishap in which he sustains a phenol burn. Which of the following antidotes can most effectively minimize skin destruction?

A. Alcohol

B. Sodium bicarbonate

C. Propylethylene glycol

D. Calcium gluconate

E. Balanced salt solution

Ref.: 4, 5

COMMENTS: Propylethylene glycol applied directly to the burn areas is the treatment of choice. • If it is not available, glycerol is the best second choice. • Phenol burns not only affect the skin locally but also, if absorbed systemically, can cause toxic effects. • For this reason, using soap and water is not recommended, since it would dilute the concentration in the phenol burns and prevent formation of a thick eschar, which acts as a barrier preventing further absorption of phenol.

Calcium gluconate is used for the immediate treatment of hydrofluoric acid exposure. • Patients exposed to hydrofluoric acid usually present several hours after exposure (most commonly when etching glass or cleaning aluminum) with pain about the nails and fingertips. • Injection of a 10% solution of calcium gluconate is required without delay to prevent further symptoms and tissue destruction.

ANSWER:
C

30. A 70-year-old mechanic sustains "pinching" amputation when his dominant long finger is caught between a garage door pulley and the belt. There is loss of the volar two thirds of the pulp skin, with exposed subcutaneous tissue. What is the most appropriate reconstruction?

A. Sterile dressing changes with topical antibiotics and closure by contracture and epithelialization

B. Full-thickness hypothenar skin graft

C. Split-thickness skin graft

D. V-Y advancement flap

E. Replantation

Ref.: 1–3

COMMENTS: Fingertip amputation is one of the most common hand injuries. • The mechanism of injury, the orientation and location of the amputation, and the age, gender, general condition, and hand dominance of the patient are integral to decision making and planning of the reconstruction. • Reconstructions that require prolonged immobilization in "unsafe" positions, such as a thenar flap or a cross-finger flap, are not recommended in older individuals. • If properly cared for and free of crush avulsion injury, the amputated part can be defatted, meticulously sutured back, and used for a salvage procedure. • Microvascular replantations have been successful even as far distal as the midnail but generally are not performed for fingertip injuries, except in certain countries where complete digits are of cultural significance.

In this particular case, a hypothenar skin graft is best. • It provides glabrous skin (the unique non–hair-bearing skin found on the volar aspect of the digits and palms as well as the soles), which matches the other digits and resists contracture and hypersensitivity. • The donor site for a hypothenar graft can also be closed primarily. • Sensibility, which is an important factor with all of hand grafts, is similar to those achieved with the flaps.

The V-Y advancement flap would have been a good option, except that the orientation of this amputation does not lend itself to its use. • It is best used with straight transverse amputations. • A split-thickness skin graft would be too thin and entails texture- and color-match problems as well as difficulties with wound breakdown and hypersensitivity. • Allowing the wound to heal by contracture and epithelialization is a good option when there is only soft-tissue loss, but the orientation should be such that the tissues can contract to cover the defect. • The broad surface area described here would not be satisfactory for this method of healing.

ANSWER:
B

31. Which of the following statements regarding the brachial plexus is/are true?

A. An axillary block will frequently miss the musculocutaneous nerve.

B. The origin of the thoracodorsal nerve is the brachial plexus.

C. The fourth intercostobrachial nerve has an origin at the root of the brachial plexus.

D. The radial nerve originates from the posterior cord.

Ref.: 1–3

COMMENTS: The brachial plexus originates at C5–T1. • An axillary block, which is performed by injecting local anesthetic into the brachial plexus at the level of the axilla, often misses the musculocutaneous nerve because the nerve originates at a higher level than that at which the block is given. • Therefore, the patient will have sensation in the area of the lateral antebrachium, and a supplemental injection is required.

The thoracodorsal nerve originates from the posterior cord of the brachial plexus. • General surgeons often encounter the thoracodorsal neurovascular bundle during axillary node dissection. • Of particular significance to plastic surgeons, this bundle supplies the latissimus dorsi, which is often used in breast reconstruction. • Every attempt should be made to save the neurovascular bundle, particularly when breast reconstruction is anticipated.

The fourth intercostobrachial nerve does not originate from the brachial plexus. • It provides sensation to the medial arm and should not be sacrificed for an easier dissection because transection can result in pain, neuroma formation, and numbness of the medial arm.

The mnemonic *STAR* can be used to remember the posterior cord nerves: subscapular, thoracodorsal, axillary, and radial nerves all derive their origin from the posterior cord of the brachial plexus.

ANSWER:
A, B, D

32. True or false: Do the following eponyms match their definitions?

A. Jersey finger: intra-articular fracture of the DIP joint

B. Mallet finger: traumatic avulsion of the extensor tendon insertion into the distal phalanx

C. Gamekeeper's thumb: laxity of the radial collateral ligament at the thumb MP joint

D. Skier's (ski-pole injury) thumb: disruption of the ulnar collateral ligament at the thumb MP

E. Preiser's disease: avascular necrosis of the hamate

F. Kienböck's disease: idiopathic lunatomalacia

G. Rolando's fracture: comminuted, intra-articular fracture of the thumb IP joint

H. Bennett's fracture: comminuted trapezium fracture

Ref.: 1–3

COMMENTS: There are numerous common names for disorders of the hand. • Understanding the cause of the disorder sheds light on the common name. • For instance, jersey finger is traumatic avulsion of the flexor digitorum profundus at the DIP level. • It is an injury sustained most commonly by rugby and/or football players as the tendon avulses from the bone with forceful gripping, such as when grabbing a jersey. • Mallet finger is the extensor counterpart of jersey finger and is a traumatic disruption of the extensor mechanism at its insertion into the distal phalanx, usually caused by forced flexion at the joint, such as occurs when "jamming" one's thumb while catching a softball.

The name *gamekeeper's thumb* is derived from the Scottish gamekeeper's practice of breaking the neck of rabbits by twisting their necks. • Repetitive trauma of this type tended to weaken the ulnar collateral ligament of the thumb, causing both pain and laxity of the thumb at the MP joint in this area. • Skier's (ski-pole injury) thumb is specifically an acute traumatic avulsion of the ulnar collateral ligament, although *gamekeeper's thumb* is sometimes used incorrectly to describe this situation.

Robert Kienböck, an Austrian professor of radiology, was the first to describe a syndrome of idiopathic lunatomalacia in 1910. • Although Keinbock's disease may be related to antecedent trauma, its cause is obscure. • It is most commonly manifested as a stiff, painful, and weak wrist in a young adult male. • Preiser's disease is idiopathic avascular necrosis of the scaphoid. • Debate still exists about its cause, since some scaphoid fractures may be hard to detect and tend to lead to avascular necrosis in many cases.

A Bennett's fracture is a fracture at the base of the thumb metacarpal. • It is inherently unstable owing to divergent pull forces of the adductor pollicis longissimus at the fracture site. • Its management tends to be less complicated and its prognosis much better than those for a Rolando's fracture. • The latter is a comminuted, intra-articular fracture at the base of the thumb metacarpal that exhibits a T or Y fracture pattern splitting the articular surface at the base of the first metacarpal.

ANSWER:
A-false; B-true; C-false; D-true; E-false; F-true; G-false; H-false

33. Which of the following statements regarding burns of the hands is/are true?

A. Full-thickness dorsal burns cause scarring, which prevents flexion contractures.

B. Loss of the extensor tendons is often treated by joint fusion to prevent contractures due to unopposed flexion forces.

C. An important part of treatment includes splinting in the "safe" position.

D. Partial-thickness burns are best treated with whirlpool débridement and splinting.

E. Deep partial-thickness burns require meticulous application of topical antibiotics and débridement after "declaration" of full-thickness losses over 2–3 weeks.

Ref.: 1–3

COMMENTS: Treatment of hand burns must begin as soon as possible. • Although the injury to the hand may be complex, certain principles must be followed. • Proper dressing should be applied and the hand splinted in a "safe" position whenever possible. • Destruction of extensor tendons results in flexion contractures unless the tendons and skin are reconstructed or the joints are fused in the appropriate position. • Superficial partial-thickness burns should be débrided of superficial necrotic tissue using whirlpool baths. • Deep partial-thickness and full-thickness burns are best treated by early full-thickness or tangential excision and skin grafting. • This allows early initiation of occupational hand therapy to prevent stiffness and contractures.

ANSWER:
B, C, D

34. A surgeon is called to the emergency department to evaluate a 42-year-old man who, after 14 hr in subfreezing temperatures, has frostbite of his left index, middle, and ring fingers down to the level of the PIP joint. What treatment should be undertaken?

A. Plan to amputate the involved areas within the next 6 hr.

B. Begin gradual rewarming of the involved area by immersion in a water bath (35–39°C).

C. Splint the hand and administer tetanus immunoglobulin, provide elevation, begin oral antibiotics, and discharge for follow-up in 48 hr.

D. Begin rapid rewarming of the involved area by immersion in a water bath at 40–44°C.

Ref.: 1–3

COMMENTS: Tissue destruction secondary to frostbite is the result of direct cellular injury through the formation of extracellular ice crystals and through vascular impairment as the result of intense invasive constriction, shunting, stasis, and endothelial damage. • The frozen extremity should be rewarmed rapidly in a warm bath carefully maintained at 40–44°C until flushing of the digital pads is observed (usually about 30 minutes). • Gradual warming allows continued tissue injury and is not indicated. • Parenteral analgesics may be required during the rewarming period. • Loose dressings and topical aloe vera or bacitracin should be applied to intact blebs and Silvadene dressings to ruptured blebs and exposed skin. • Because it takes at least 2 weeks for demarcation to occur, amputation should be delayed until after this acute period. • Splinting and elevation do not address the issue of tissue damage. • The intense care listed above requires hospitalization, especially for observation during the first 48 hr. • The patient should not be discharged until the wounds are under control, although the patient need not remain in the hospital until demarcation and surgery, if the latter should become necessary. • The tetanus immunization status must always be checked and supplemented as necessary for frostbite and burn injuries.

ANSWER:
D

REFERENCES

1. Townsend CM Jr, Beauchamp RD, Evers BM, et al (eds): *Sabiston Textbook of Surgery: The Biological Basis of Modern Surgical Practice,* 17th ed. Saunders, Philadelphia, 2004.
2. Brunicardi FC, Andersen DK, Billiar TR, et al (eds): *Schwartz's Principles of Surgery*, 8th ed. McGraw-Hill, New York, 2004.
3. Canale ST (ed): *Campbell's Operative Orthopaedics*, 10th ed. CV Mosby, St. Louis, 2002.
4. Green DP, Hotchkiss RN, Pederson WC, Wolfe SW (eds): *Green's Operative Hand Surgery,* 5th ed. Churchill-Livingstone, Philadelphia, 2005.
5. Bentivegna PE, Deane LM: Chemical burns of the upper extremity. *Hand Clin* 6:253–259, 1990.

CHAPTER 54

Plastic and Reconstructive Surgery

Alberto J. Aviles, M.D.

1. Which of the following statements regarding the skin is/are true?

A. The skin is composed of dermis, epidermis, and an underlying subcutaneous padding, all derived from mesoderm.

B. The amount of pigmentation of the skin is determined by the absolute number of melanocytes present.

C. Skin thickness varies widely according to anatomic location, and this difference is due almost entirely to the varying thickness of the epidermis.

D. The epidermis minimizes skin tension during wound closure.

Ref.: 1, 2

COMMENTS: The **epidermis** is composed of four cell types: keratinocytes (the most common); Merkel cells, which originate from neural crest cells (ectodermal in origin); Langerhans cells, which are mesenchymal; and melanocytes. • The **dermis** is mesodermal except for its neural supply. • The melanocyte secretes melanin from melanosomes and is absorbed by adjacent keratinocytes. • Melanosome activity influences the amount of pigmentation and is stimulated by sunlight and various hormones (melanocyte-stimulating hormone, adrenocorticotropic hormone, estrogen, and progesterone). • The **dermis** provides variable thickness and is made up of 80% type I collagen and 15% type III collagen. The collagen content provides strength in the wound when dermal sutures are placed and minimizes tension. • The thickness of the epidermis varies little, and epidermal sutures are used to align the skin edges.

ANSWER:
B

2. Which of the following statements regarding skin incisions and excisions is/are correct?

A. Skin incisions should usually be oriented parallel to the long axis of the underlying muscle.

B. Lines of minimal tension parallel skin lines.

C. The long axis of underlying muscles is usually perpendicular to skin lines.

D. During an excisional biopsy, the long axis should be two times the length of the short axis.

Ref.: 1–4

COMMENTS: In most anatomic areas, skin lines represent lines of minimal tension (Langer's lines), or relaxed skin tension lines (RSTLs). • Incisions in these areas should be made parallel to these lines to result in the narrowest possible scar. • These lines of minimal tension generally run perpendicular to the long axis of underlying muscles. • When excising lesions of the skin, the long axis should be four times the length of the short axis along an RSTL. • This approach will minimize skin tension and scarring.

ANSWER:
B, C

3. Which of the following statements regarding the blood supply of a skin graft is/are true?

A. The active uptake of nutrients and serum by the skin graft is a process called imbibition.

B. Before imbibition, inosculation, or capillary alignment, is essential for graft survival.

C. The process of capillary ingrowth begins approximately 48 hr after grafting, with generalized blood flow established by the fifth or sixth postgraft day.

D. Capillary buds from recipient bed vessels have been shown to form anastomoses with graft vessels and to invade the graft directly.

Ref.: 1–4, 5

COMMENTS: A skin graft survives initially by plasmatic circulation, a *passive* imbibition of serum by the graft. • This phase lasts 24–48 hr, depending on the degree of proliferation of the grafted wound. • During this phase, the graft is ischemic and undergoes significant weight gain, since the plasmatic circulation occurs essentially from bed to graft only. • At the end of 48 hr, a process of inosculation, or graft revascularization, occurs. • Capillary buds grow from the recipient bed, probably in response to a vasoactive agent released by the anaerobic metabolism of the graft. • These buds grow across the fibrin meshwork between the graft and the recipient bed. • Evidence suggests that circulation is ultimately restored by a combination of actions. • Anastomoses are formed between invading vessels and graft arteries and veins. • Capillary ingrowth may occur directly into the graft, or neovascularization may occur along preexisting degenerated graft vessels. • By the end of the first postgraft week, some of the final remodeling of the microvasculature has begun, with differentiation into afferent and efferent vessels. • It is at this point that true circulation is restored. • Return of the venous circulation occurs later in the process, and its delayed return is one of the reasons for the required elevation of the extremity after grafting. • This explains the initial pink appearance of the early graft, which changes to blue or purple because of venous insufficiency later.

ANSWER:
C, D

4. Which of the following statements regarding the techniques of wound closure is/are true?

A. Forceps with fine teeth are less traumatic to skin than are forceps without teeth.

B. Absorbable braided sutures are used to approximate skin edges and minimize inflammation.

C. Sutures on the face should be kept in for approximately 10–14 days to reduce tension on the wound during that time.

D. Even modest undermining of skin edges should be avoided, because it devascularizes the overlying skin and impedes wound healing.

Ref.: 1, 2, 4

COMMENTS: Successful closure of a surgically created or traumatic wound requires proper coaptation of well-vascularized tissues without tension. • Gentle handling of tissues is always recommended and is facilitated by the use of small "piercing" forceps rather than "crushing" forceps (i.e., those without teeth). • Skin hooks may even be used to tug gently on the edges. • Devitalized or questionably viable tissue should be removed before closure when the tissue is not deemed critical. • Tension on a wound impedes healing and leads to widening of the scar. • At times tension can be avoided by undermining the wound edges. • A rich network of subdermal vessels provides adequate vascular supply to the skin edges as long as the undermining has not been excessive. • For best cosmetic results, sutures are removed at varying times, depending on the vascularity and tension of the tissues coapted. • On the abdomen, sutures may be removed at 5–7 days, with the edges then reinforced with adhesive strips. • On the face, sutures are removed sooner. • The sutures themselves do not add to the cosmetic appearance but are a "necessary evil" to coapt the tissues properly. • Preferably, smooth monofilament sutures that are nonabsorbable should be used in skin closure to minimize inflammation and scarring. • Early removal of sutures or staples with the addition of adhesive strips allows support of the wound without leading to the crosshatch marks created by permanent epithelialization of the sutures or staple holes themselves. • Cyanoacrylates are now being used as "surgical glue" in an effort to reduce inflammation and provide adhesion at the coapted edges, thereby avoiding the use of sutures, with their associated complications.

ANSWER:
A

5. Which of the following statements regarding open wounds and débridement is/are true?

A. When assessing an open wound, the local causes should determine the treatment.

B. A traumatic wound should be closed as soon as possible.

C. Wet-to-dry dressings are not traumatic to wounds and therefore promote wound healing.

D. Delayed débridement of a wound can often lead to necrosis of borderline viable tissue.

Ref.: 1, 5

COMMENTS: Wound assessment involves evaluation of systemic and regional, in addition to local, causes. • **Systemic** impairments to wound healing include diabetes, malnutrition, congestive heart failure, hepatic and renal insufficiency, and immunosuppression and steroid usage. • **Regional** effects include peripheral neuropathy and arterial and venous insufficiency. • The **local** causes, such as pressure, trauma, radiation, and infection, should include both regional and systemic influences to optimize wound healing and treatment. • A nonsurgical treatment option for open wounds that harbor devitalized and contaminated tissue is the use of wet-to-dry dressings. • This form of débridement is mechanical and does not discriminate between viable and nonviable tissue, which can hinder the wound healing process. • Viable tissue can be difficult to assess in a traumatic wound. • Therefore, delayed débridement can be employed, leading to dessication and necrosis of marginal tissue. • Traumatic wounds are typically closed within 6 hr to minimize dessication and contamination. • One and a half liters of lactated Ringer's solution should be used to irrigate the wound in a pulsatile manner before primary closure.

ANSWER:
B, D

6. Which of the following recipient beds is/are unlikely to support a split-thickness skin graft?

A. Muscle with overlying fascia intact

B. Muscle without overlying fascia

C. Tendon with paratenon intact

D. Tendon without paratenon

E. Nerve with perineurium intact

F. Bone without periosteum

Ref.: 1–4

COMMENTS: Proper "take" of a split-thickness skin graft applied to a recipient bed depends on adequate vascularization of the bed. • Avoidance of shear forces and tenting of the graft over the bed can be prevented using a tie-over compression dressing to allow for fibrous adherence and revascularization. • Furthermore, prevention of seroma or hematoma formation (the most common reason for graft failure), minimization of dead space, and absence of infection within the wound (defined as <10⁵ bacteria per gram of tissue) will aid in graft survival. • Often, the skin graft may be meshed, or "pie-crusted," to provide more surface area and facilitate fluid drainage at the expense of cosmesis. • Muscle with or without its fascia intact is an excellent recipient site for split-thickness skin grafts. • Although less well vascularized, tendon with its paratenon intact, nerve with its perineurium intact, and bone with its periosteum intact can also support a split-thickness skin graft.

ANSWER:
D, F

7. Which of the following statements regarding the use of split-thickness and full-thickness skin grafts is/are true?

A. A split-thickness skin graft undergoes approximately 10% shrinkage of its surface area immediately after harvesting.

B. A full-thickness skin graft undergoes approximately 40% shrinkage of its surface area immediately after harvesting.

C. Secondary contraction is more likely to occur after adequate healing of a full-thickness skin graft than of a split-thickness skin graft.

D. Sensation does not return to areas that have undergone skin grafting.

E. Skin grafts may be exposed to moderate amounts of sunlight without changing pigmentation.

Ref.: 1–4

COMMENTS: Skin grafts are considered to be *full-thickness* when they are harvested at the dermal-subcutaneous junction. • *Split-thickness* skin grafts are those that contain epidermis and variable partial thicknesses of underlying dermis. • They may be thin, medium, or thick split-thickness skin grafts and usually are in the range of 0.018–0.060 inch in thickness. • Cells from epidermal appendages deep to the plane of graft harvest resurface the donor site of a split-thickness skin graft in approximately 1–3 weeks, depending on the depth. • The donor site requires a moist environment to promote epithelialization, and such an environment is maintained using polyurethane or hydrocolloid dressings. • Because a full-thickness graft does not leave epidermal appendages behind, defects must be closed primarily.

When a skin graft is harvested, there is immediate shrinkage of the surface area of the graft. • This process is known as primary contraction and is due to recoil of the elastic fibers of the dermis. • The thicker the skin graft, the greater this immediate shrinkage, with full-thickness grafts shrinking by approximately 40% of their initial surface area and split-thickness grafts shrinking by approximately 10% of their initial surface area. • This must be considered when planning the amount of skin to harvest for coverage of a defect of a given size.

Contractile myofibroblasts in the bed of a granulating wound interact with collagen fibers to cause a decrease in the wound's surface area, a process known as *secondary contraction.* • Secondary contraction is greater in wounds covered with split-thickness grafts than in those covered with full-thickness grafts. • The amount of secondary contracture is inversely proportional to the amount of dermis included in the graft, not to the absolute thickness of the graft. • Dermal elements hasten the displacement of myofibroblasts from the wound bed.

Sensation may return to areas that have been grafted as long as the bed is proper and not significantly scarred. • Although sensation is not completely normal, it is usually adequate for protection. • This process begins at about 10 weeks and is maximal at 2 years.

Skin grafts appear to be more sensitive to melanocyte stimulation during ultraviolet sunlight exposure than is the normal surrounding skin. • Early exposure to sunlight after grafting may lead to permanently increased pigmentation of the graft and should be avoided. • Dermabrasion or application of hydroquinones may be of benefit for reducing this pigmentation.

ANSWER:
A, B

8. Situations in which a full-thickness skin graft is preferred to a split-thickness skin graft include which of the following?

A. Contaminated wounds

B. Small facial wounds

C. Wounds in an irradiated field

D. Burn wounds

E. Wounds in hair-bearing regions

Ref.: 1, 2, 4

COMMENTS: Thicker grafts have a higher rate of failure when a wound is more likely to be compromised by vascular insufficiency, hematoma, or infection. • For this reason, thinner split-thickness skin grafts generally are preferred when the recipient site for a graft is suboptimal. • With extensive burn injury, multiple grafts are often required from limited donor sites. • Therefore, the technique of harvesting thin split-thickness grafts—and earlier skin regrowth—may increase the availability of donor tissue. • For wounds in which the most normal final appearance and the least contraction is desired, as on the face or hands, full-thickness skin grafts are preferred. • Donor sites are typically from the upper eyelid or the postauricular region. • Full-thickness grafts are also used when hair production is required. • Accessory skin structures (i.e., hair follicles, sweat glands, and sebaceous glands) transplanted with a graft survive but must be included in the graft. • Partial-thickness or full-thickness grafts are the only ones deep enough to include the pilosebaceous apparatus.

ANSWER:
B, E

9. Match the type of flap in the left column with the appropriate nature of its blood supply in the right column.

A. Z-plasty	a. Random pattern
B. Forehead flap	b. Axial pattern
C. Deltopectoral flap	
D. Omental flap	
E. Rhomboid flap	

Ref.: 1–4

COMMENTS: See Question 10.

10. Match the type of flap in the left column with the appropriate description or example from the right column.

A. Transposition flap	a. Moved directly forward without rotation
B. Interpolation flap	b. Microvascular anastomosis required
C. Advancement flap	c. Rotation about a point to an adjacent defect
D. Island flap	d. Rotation about a point to a defect near but not directly adjacent to the donor site
E. Myocutaneous flap	e. Attached pedicle of vessels
F. Free flap	f. Transverse rectus abdominis myocutaneous (TRAM) flap

Ref.: 1–4, 5

COMMENTS: Flaps are defined according to the nature of their blood supply. • A **random flap** derives its blood supply from the dermal-subdermal plexus, in contrast to an **axial flap**, which derives its blood supply by a direct, usually named, cutaneous artery. • The vessel that supplies a specific region is described as an angiosome.

Random flaps usually are those used to reorient a wound in a different direction or to close small defects. • Examples of random flaps include the Z-plasty, simple rotation flap, advancement flap, and transposition flap. • A *simple rotation flap* is usually semicircular and is "slid" over the recipient site for closure. • An *advancement flap* is moved directly forward to cover a defect without rotation around a pivot point. • A *V-Y flap*, a commonly employed *advancement flap*, frequently is used to close small defects in the finger or eyelid areas. • *Transposition flaps* involve rotation around a pivot point to a defect that is adjacent to the donor site. • A *rhomboid flap* is a type of transposition flap in which a rhomboid-shaped flap is transposed to cover an adjacent defect with primary closure of the donor site. • An *interpolation flap* is another type of transposition flap. • It involves rotation around a pivot point but is used to cover a defect that is nearby but not directly adjacent to the donor site.

Axial flaps generally are used to cover larger defects more distant from the donor site. • Historically, the primary determinant for the design of skin flaps has been the length/width ratio, and axial flaps can be designed with a much greater length/width ratio than can random flaps. • The knowledge of angiosomes can determine the length of flap needed without compromising the periphery. • A flap that crosses two angiosomes will undergo necrosis of the "watershed" area. • Examples are the midline forehead flap (supratrochlear artery), deltopectoral flap (perforating branches of the internal mammary artery), and omental flap (gastroepiploic arteries). • An *island flap* is a type of axial flap in which a segment of tissue is carried on a vascular pedicle that has been skeletonized and is without overlying skin at the base to allow greater flap mobility. • A *myocutaneous flap* provides blood supply through the overlying skin or subcutaneous tissue (or both) via muscular perforators. • Examples are the perforators emanating from the rectus muscles about the umbilical region supplying the *TRAM flap* or the latissimus dorsi myocutaneous flap. • *Free flaps* involve complete severing of the nutrient vessels with reanastomosis to vessels in the vicinity of the recipient site. • This nearly always requires microvascular surgical technique.

ANSWERS:
Question 9: A-a; B-b; C-b; D-b; E-a
Question 10: A-c; B-d; C-a; D-e; E-f; F-b

11. Necrosis of a pedicle flap is usually due to which of the following?

   A. Arterial thrombosis

   B. Venous thrombosis

   C. Arterial spasm

   D. Venous spasm

   E. Trauma from manipulation of a compromised flap

Ref.: 2

COMMENTS: All flaps must be observed closely during the immediate postoperative period following transfer because of possible compromise of their circulation. • An initial dusky coloration may be due to venous spasm or excess tension on the flap, each resulting in compromised venous return. • Development of a sharp line of color demarcation portends venous thrombosis, which is the most common cause of flap necrosis. • Arterial insufficiency is not usually responsible for flap failure. • Complications such as

excessive tension, infection, or hematoma can eventually lead to venous thrombosis. • A seriously compromised flap requires immediate attention, and treatment may involve taking down a dressing; removing tight sutures; changing the position of an extremity or the head and neck; returning a flap to its donor site; using heparin, aspirin, or low–molecular-weight dextran; and (experimentally) using hyperbaric oxygen. • The patient must also be examined for systemic causes such as hypovolemia, hypotension, or hypoxia.

ANSWER:
B

12. Which of the following statements regarding myocutaneous flaps is/are true?

   A. A myocutaneous flap is a free graft of full-thickness skin with a small shaving of underlying muscle.

   B. A myocutaneous flap is predicated on the fact that the skin receives its blood supply from perforating vessels from the underlying musculature.

   C. A myocutaneous flap fails if it is transferred to a poorly vascularized wound.

   D. Only myocutaneous flaps supplied by arteries larger than 0.8 mm in diameter can be transferred as free flaps.

   E. Rib, with its overlying pectoralis muscle and skin used for mandibular reconstruction, is an example of an osseomyocutaneous flap.

Ref.: 2, 4, 5

COMMENTS: The development of myocutaneous flaps for reconstruction of soft-tissue defects is based on the fact that skin frequently receives blood supply from vessels perforating the underlying somatic musculature. • More specifically, the vascular supply to the skeletal muscle can be found in five discernable patterns: types I–V. • Only the type IV pattern relies on small multiple perforators, as seen in the sartorius muscle flap. • When the blood supply to the underlying muscle is by way of a discrete vessel(s), the muscle and its overlying skin may be transferred to a distant site on a pedicle containing only the nutrient vessels. • It is critical that both the artery and the vein within the pedicle remain patent for successful transfer of the flap.

In some circumstances, bone closely associated with the muscle and skin may be transferred en bloc, providing an osseomyocutaneous flap (e.g., rib and its overlying pectoralis muscle and skin used for mandible reconstruction or latissimus dorsi muscle with a portion of scapula). • Transfer of these flaps to distant sites requires the use of microvascular surgery. • The vessels that supply the flap are isolated, transected, and anastomosed to vessels near the recipient site. • Refinements in technique and instrumentation allow the routine transfer of flaps on vessels as small as 0.5 mm in diameter. • Myocutaneous flaps are widely used in head and neck, breast, upper and lower extremities, and other areas of reconstructive surgery where well-vascularized soft-tissue covering of bone, tendon, nerve, or vascular structures is required. • Myocutaneous or muscle flaps can be used to introduce additional blood supply to an area of impaired vascularity. • Clinical examples include transfer of a latissimus dorsi myocutaneous flap to the anterior chest wall to correct an area of necrosis after radiation therapy and transfer of vascularized muscle to the lower extremity after débridement of chronic osteomyelitis. • In both of these examples, tissue with an excellent blood supply is imported to bring about the healing of a wound or infection not responding to more conservative measures.

ANSWER:
B, E

13. Which of the following statements is/are true?

 A. Reduction mammoplasty only rarely relieves the back pain that accompanies macromastia.

 B. A suprasternal notch–to–nipple distance of less than 40 cm requires nipple grafting during reduction mammoplasty.

 C. Gynecomastia in the adolescent should be treated surgically if the condition does not resolve in 6 months.

 D. Ptosis of the breast is said to exist when the nipple lies below the level of the inframammary fold.

Ref.: 1–3

COMMENTS: Macromastia is an abnormal enlargement of the breast, which may be a result of hormonal imbalance or obesity or may be idiopathic. • For some women, the breasts become so large that they cause chronic back, shoulder, or neck pain. • Women may also develop numbness of the ulnar side of the hand due to brachial plexus compression about the chest and shoulder region, skin changes on the shoulders from pressure of brassiere straps, and skin maceration or infection in inframammary areas from constant moisture. • These conditions usually are markedly improved by reduction mammoplasty, which involves resecting portions of the breast parenchyma and overlying skin and repositioning the nipple and areola. • The inferior pyramid (or pedicle) technique is used when the suprasternal notch–to–nipple distance is less than 40 cm. • This method preserves the pedicle to the nipple, but scarring cannot be avoided. • When the distance is less than 40 cm, free-nipple grafting is necessary, resulting in excellent cosmesis, but sensation and lactation are lost when the pedicle is not included in the tissue transfer. • Extremely large breasts may require partial mastectomy with recontouring of the breast and free-nipple grafting.

    Gynecomastia is enlargement of the male breast due to an increase in glandular tissue. • In adolescents, it is frequently a physiologic response to the hormonal changes of puberty. • In such cases, it may be unilateral or bilateral, and it usually reverses itself. • For this reason, surgery should be postponed until gynecomastia has been present for 2 years. • In adults, gynecomastia may result from underlying liver disease; pituitary, testicular, or adrenal tumors; or the use of certain drugs (e.g., digitalis, estrogens, some antihypertensives, and even marijuana). • It must be differentiated from male breast carcinoma, especially when it is unilateral and presents with pain, drainage, or rapid enlargement. • Resection of the breast tissue confirms the diagnosis and corrects the cosmetic abnormality.

    Ptosis of the breast exists when the nipple is present at a level below that of the inframammary crease. • This may occur in breasts of any size and may lead to chronic skin changes in the inframammary crease. • Reduction of the skin envelope (mastopexy) can alleviate the ptosis. • This is a common procedure also performed in breast reconstruction after mastectomy to obtain symmetry.

ANSWER:
D

14. Which of the following statements regarding techniques of breast reconstruction is/are true?

 A. When a silicone implant is used for a single-stage breast reconstruction, frequent problems include an inadequate

skin envelope, leading to excess tension, with possible skin necrosis or wound dehiscence.

 B. Breast reconstruction with a tissue expander involves placement of the expander in a submuscular pocket, closure of the wound, and immediate introduction of sufficient saline solution to match the size of the opposite breast.

 C. When a latissimus dorsi myocutaneous flap is used for breast reconstruction, a silicone implant is usually placed underneath the flap.

 D. A trapezius myocutaneous flap may be used to reconstruct a breast even if the vascular pedicle to the latissimus dorsi muscle has been interrupted.

 E. A TRAM flap survives on vessels that run longitudinally in a plane superficial to the anterior rectus sheath.

Ref.: 1–4, 5

COMMENTS: Breast reconstruction following mastectomy is an important aspect of breast cancer therapy for cosmetic and psychological reasons. • There are two main avenues available for breast reconstruction: (1) the use of tissue expanders and silicone implants and (2) transfer of vascularized tissue by means of a myocutaneous flap. • **Tissue expander** breast reconstruction has several advantages: the avoidance of scars other than the mastectomy incision, creation of natural native breast skin that has the best textural and color match, less operative morbidity, and a shorter operative time. • The simplest method of breast reconstruction is placement of a **silicone implant** in a submuscular pocket. • This method has three potential disadvantages: (1) inability to reach a symmetric volume, (2) poor projection due to an inadequate skin envelope, and (3) the lack of a naturally ptotic breast shape with a well-defined inframammary fold. • The surgeon may avoid these disadvantages by placing a **tissue expander** (*not* a simple silicone implant) in a subpectoral, subserratus pocket. • Saline solution is added to the expander intermittently over a several-month period. • It leads to stretching of the overlying muscle and skin and the creation of some additional skin as well, due to increased mitosis at the epidermal level. • At a second-stage operation, the surgeon replaces the expander with a permanent implant. • An alternative is the use of a single-stage expander, which has a removable valve. • Although the morbidity is minimized with the implant approach, 4–6 months is typically required for complete reconstruction. • **Myocutaneous flap** reconstruction is particularly well suited to patients who have an *inadequate amount* of local skin remaining after the mastectomy, a poor-quality skin envelope, skin that has been damaged from previous radiation therapy, or loss of the pectoralis major muscle, such as with the defect following radical mastectomy. • In addition, flap reconstruction provides more immediate results as well as dynamic tissue. • Modifications in the patient's appearance may occur with weight gain or loss.

    The **latissimus dorsi** myocutaneous flap is considered a hybrid procedure, in which autogenous tissue is used but an implant is also required. • The flap pedicled on the thoracodorsal vessels can transfer sufficient skin to the chest wall and is particularly useful for replacing the pectoralis major muscle in a radical mastectomy defect. • Usually an implant must be placed underneath this flap to achieve adequate volume and projection of the breast mound. • The **TRAM** flap obtains its blood supply from the superior epigastric vessels that run *within* the rectus abdominis sheath, with perforating branches supplying the overlying skin and fat of the abdominal wall. • When there is sufficient volume of skin and fat, a natural breast mound can be created without the need for an implant. • The TRAM flap, or a free gluteal flap,

with the patient's own fatty tissue and skin, offers one of the best methods for matching the shape of a broadly based ptotic breast.
• The short pedicle and improper arc of rotation of the **trapezius** myocutaneous flap precludes its use for breast reconstruction.

ANSWER:
A, C

15. Which of the following statements regarding postmastectomy breast reconstruction is/are true?

   A. The presence of cancer-positive axillary nodes is a contraindication to reconstruction.

   B. Delayed reconstruction (i.e., 3 months or longer after mastectomy) is generally preferred over immediate reconstruction.

   C. The status of the skin flaps (vascular supply and degree of tension) is the key consideration when deciding on immediate versus delayed reconstruction.

   D. Nipple reconstruction is usually delayed for several months following reconstruction of the breast mound.

   E. In most cases, excellent symmetry can be achieved without the need for surgery on the uninvolved breast.

Ref.: 1–3

COMMENTS: The presence of cancer-positive axillary lymph nodes, anticipated adjuvant chemotherapy, and postoperative chest wall irradiation are not in themselves absolute contraindications to reconstruction. • However, one must weigh the possible increased risk of infection (related to chemotherapy-induced leukopenia) and the possibility of a suboptimal cosmetic result due to postreconstruction irradiation against the psychological advantage to the patient of the reconstruction itself. • Postmastectomy reconstruction may be carried out immediately or in a delayed fashion (at least 3 months after mastectomy), depending on the desires of the patient, the anticipated need for adjuvant treatment, and, most important, the status of the skin flaps in terms of vascular supply and degree of tension on closure. • Excess tension or poor vascular supply to the mastectomy flaps necessitates delayed reconstruction. • Comparing immediate with delayed reconstruction, there does not appear to be any significant difference in the final cosmetic outcome. • In either case, **nipple reconstruction** is usually deferred for several months following completion of the breast mound reconstruction to allow the breast to settle into its final position. • The prominent papule of the nipple can be created from a flap of skin and subcutaneous tissue on the breast mound. • A skin graft can then be used for the surrounding areolar part of the nipple, or it can be done after the flap has healed. • Some advocate that the nipple and areola be tattooed to the appropriate color. • This approach avoids the need to harvest skin from remote sites and minimizes patient discomfort. • The ultimate goal of breast reconstruction is to achieve **symmetry** of the two breasts. • In many patients, this necessitates a reduction mammoplasty, mastopexy, or submuscular augmentation on the uninvolved side.

ANSWER:
C, D

16. Which of the following statements is/are true?

   A. Women with breast augmentation implants have a significantly increased risk of developing breast carcinoma compared to those with nonaugmented breasts.

   B. When breast cancer is diagnosed in a patient with silicone breast augmentation implants, it is more likely to be at an advanced stage than when diagnosed in nonaugmented breasts.

   C. Patients with silicone breast implants require a modification of conventional mammographic techniques to obtain optimal visualization of the breast parenchyma.

   D. Silicone deposits have been noted in the lymph nodes of patients with silicone breast augmentation implants but not in the lymph nodes of patients with other implanted silicone medical devices.

   E. Epidemiologic studies have clearly demonstrated a cause-and-effect relationship between breast implants and the development of collagen vascular diseases.

Ref.: 6

COMMENTS: Recent media coverage of the possible hazards of breast implants has produced a great deal of confusion among patients with these medical devices. • It is important to base recommendations to patients on scientifically valid data. • Well-designed studies have demonstrated that patients with breast implants *do not have* an increased risk of developing breast carcinoma. • In addition, when breast carcinoma is diagnosed in a patient with breast implants, it is not at a more advanced stage than when it develops in a patient without breast implants.

It is important to be aware of the need to modify conventional mammographic techniques when performing imaging studies on patients with breast implants. • The Eklund modification involves compression of the implant and displacement of the breast parenchyma away from the implant, with a modification of the conventional mammographic views. • If this modified technique is not employed, significant portions of the breast parenchyma are obscured by the radiopaque silicone. • Although reports have occasionally surfaced documenting the presence of minute deposits of silicone in the lymph nodes of patients with breast implants, such deposits have also been found in the lymph nodes of patients with other implanted silicone medical devices (e.g., joint implants) as well. • The significance of this finding is unclear and its association with other disease states unproved. • At present, there is no clear-cut documentation of an increased incidence of collagen vascular disease in patients with silicone breast implants, nor is there any proven cause-effect relationship between the two.

ANSWER:
C

17. Which of the following statements regarding maxillomandibular disproportion is/are true?

   A. Retrognathia is defined as an abnormally small mandible positioned abnormally posteriorly.

   B. Prognathism is not satisfactorily correctable without the use of synthetic prostheses.

   C. Most operative corrections of developmental mandibular problems with wire fixation allow normal use of the mandible within 3 weeks of the surgery.

   D. Hypoplasia is the most common developmental deformity of the maxilla.

   E. Maxillary osteotomies are used for correction of both hypoplasia and hyperplasia of the maxilla.

Ref.: 1–3

COMMENTS: Developmental mandibular deformities may result from the mandible's being malpositioned or abnormally large or small. • With **retrognathia**, the mandible is of normal size but is malpositioned posteriorly. • Correction involves osteotomies through the mandibular rami. • With **micrognathia**, the mandible is properly positioned but is abnormally small in its anterior portion. • It can be corrected by a horizontal osteotomy, which brings the chin prominence forward. • With **prognathism**, the mandible is overdeveloped and prominent. • Surgical treatment involves osteotomy with posterior repositioning. • For all of these surgical corrections, if the bone segments are held in position by wires, intermaxillary fixation of the mandible is required for 10–12 weeks for proper healing of the osteotomies. • An increasing number of surgeons make use of rigid fixation techniques involving plates and screws. • With rigid immobilization of the fragments, the time in intermaxillary fixation is reduced or even eliminated. • Of the maxillary anomalies, **hypoplasia** is the most common and is often seen in association with cleft palate. • It may be treated by a maxillary osteotomy with repositioning of the isolated lower maxillary segment. • Maxillary **hyperplasia** is evidenced clinically by a long face with exposure of the gingiva when smiling. • This may be corrected with maxillary osteotomy and a resection of a vertical segment of maxilla with an upward repositioning of the lower segment of the maxilla.

ANSWER:
D, E

18. Match each vascular abnormality in the left column with one or more appropriate descriptive statements in the right column.

A. Capillary hemangioma (port-wine stain)	a. It is flat and dark red, does not involute, and is best treated with a tunable dye laser.
B. Immature hemangioma (strawberry mark)	b. It is associated with gigantism of the affected part.
C. Cavernous hemangioma	c. It may enlarge during periods of infection, but there are no documented cases of the development of carcinoma.
D. Cystic hygroma	d. Most spontaneously involute.
	e. Microembolization may be required.

Ref.: 1–4

COMMENTS: The surgeon must be aware of the differential characteristics of the above-listed vascular lesions, since their natural history, size, and location may affect the appropriateness and difficulty of surgical intervention. • The **capillary hemangioma** (port-wine stain) is a vascular malformation that results in a flat, uniformly dark-red cutaneous lesion that is present at birth and does not involute. • The tunable dye laser, which can select the appropriate wavelength for destroying the lesion, has markedly improved treatment of this lesion. • **Immature hemangioma** (strawberry mark) is a form of capillary hemangioma and is raised and brighter red in color than a port-wine stain. • Usually, it is not present at birth but may become apparent within several weeks and then grow rapidly during the early months of life. • Observation is appropriate, since most of these lesions involute spontaneously by age 7 years. • Often, anxious parents wishing for prompt erasure of such a blemish need repeated reassurance. • Corticosteroids, radiation therapy, and even emergency surgery may be required for large lesions obstructing the rapidly maturing eyes, airways, or small lumens. • These cases must be treated immediately, as must lesions that bleed or are large enough to consume platelets,

leading to coagulopathy (Kasabach-Merritt syndrome). • The **cavernous hemangioma** (venous malformation, in recent terminology) is situated in deeper subcutaneous tissues and appears as a swollen blue mass. • It may be associated with gigantism of the involved part of the body. • It is present at birth and seldom involutes. • Excision may be hazardous because of the risk of hemorrhage and should be reserved for patients with significant associated functional or cosmetic disability. • In certain situations, microembolization treatment may be required to thrombose vessels and reduce lesion size. • The **cystic hygroma** is a lymphatic malformation that most often presents in the head and lateral neck region. • These lesions may enlarge and become tender during periods of upper respiratory infection. • Some cystic hygromas involute, but those with a venous component do not. • Complete excision of both venous and lymphatic malformations is frequently impossible because of the diffuse insinuation of these lesions into local tissues without regard to tissue planes.

ANSWER:
A-a; B-d; C-b,e; D-c

19. Which of the following statements regarding the embryologic development and anatomy of the craniofacial region is/are true?

A. The first embryonic structures that form the face are not evident until late during the first trimester (week 10).

B. The maxillary and mandibular processes differentiate from the first branchial arch.

C. The external ear develops from a single mesenchymal projection, the absence of which causes microtia.

D. Ossification of the craniofacial skeleton occurs by endochondral and intramembranous bone formation.

E. Normal development of the soft tissues of the face depends on normal bone growth, an independent process inherent in the bone itself.

Ref.: 2

COMMENTS: By the *fourth week* of embryonic life, primitive facial structures are evident. • Migration of *mesenchyme* forms the frontonasal prominence; the nasal, otic, and optic placodes; and the maxillary and mandibular processes. • By the eighth week, rapid morphologic change creates a nearly completely developed face. • The external ear develops from six small hillocks surrounding the first and second branchial arches. • Bony development is thought to occur in response to soft-tissue forces. • A distinction of the craniofacial skeleton is that ossification occurs by two separate processes: **endochondral** (replacement of preformed cartilage by bone) at the cranial base and **intramembranous** (mesenchymal differentiation to osteoblasts, which lay down bone without a cartilaginous framework) throughout the rest of the craniofacial skeleton. • This distinction has clinical significance with regard to craniofacial bone grafting and the improved results seen with bone grafts using a cranial donor site.

ANSWER:
B, D

20. Which of the following statements regarding cosmetic and reconstructive procedures of the nose is/are true?

A. A composite graft of cartilage and skin from the ear should not be employed for reconstruction of the nasal alar rim because of the high risk of graft necrosis.

B. A full-thickness skin graft is an appropriate form of reconstruction for soft-tissue loss at the tip of the nose.

C. A forehead rotation flap is useful for reconstruction of major nasal defects.

D. An intranasal approach allows for direct vision of the nasal skeleton.

E. Osteotomies along the nasal bones and maxilla allow the surgeon to narrow the width of the upper two thirds of the nose.

Ref.: 1, 5

COMMENTS: Reconstruction of soft-tissue defects in the upper two thirds of the nose (e.g., following excision of a superficial basal cell carcinoma) may be achieved by a full-thickness skin graft if the defect is 1.5–2 mm. • A rotation flap can be constructed adjacent to a defect 0.5–1 mm in size. • Defects smaller than 0.5 mm are often closed primarily. • When there is loss of cartilage, as may occur at the nasal ala, a composite graft of skin and cartilage taken from the ear results in an excellent reconstruction when the defect is less than 1 cm. • This helical rim tissue is similar to the alar rim and can be found nowhere else in the body. • *Major* nasal losses require a bone graft or cartilage grafts for the framework and provision of internal and external soft-tissue lining. • *Total* nasal reconstruction is accomplished by anterior mobilization of the septal cartilage to provide midline support and reconstruction of lateral support with cartilage grafts. • Lining is provided from adjacent mucosa, and skin coverage is provided with a two-staged midline forehead flap based on the supratrochlear vessels. • A tissue expander in the forehead allows for linear closure.

In aesthetic rhinoplasty, either an intranasal or an external approach can be used to access the dorsum. • The intranasal approach typically involves incisions in the inferior borders of the lateral cartilage in order to gain access to the nasal tip and dorsum, but exposure is limited. • Direct visualization of the nasal skeleton is achieved through the external, or open, approach, in which an incision is made through the columnella and carried along the border of the lower lateral cartilages. • The skin is elevated from the dorsum, and modifications performed on the nasal cartilages and bones are made with more precision. • Narrowing of the upper portions of the nose is accomplished by osteotomies along the nasal bones and maxilla. • The tip is improved by altering the anatomy of the alar cartilages through a combination of scoring, partial resection, internal sutures, and cartilage grafts. • Most rhinoplasties, with the exception of nostril reduction, can be accomplished without external incisions.

ANSWER:
B, C, E

---

21. True or false: The proper alignment of the vermilion border is the most important cosmetic aspect of primary closure of lip defects.

Ref.: 1–3

COMMENTS: Defects of the **lip** usually can be closed primarily unless they involve more than one third the length of the upper lip or are in close approximation to the commissure. • The most important cosmetic aspects of primary closure of a lip defect are *proper apposition* of the vermilion border and multilayered closure. • Even a slight "step-off" of vermilion apposition is noticeable. • *Large* lip defects or those near the commissure require rotation flaps from the opposite lip (Estlander flaps) or cheeks and

advancement of buccal mucosa. • The Abbe, or lip-switch, flap uses a full-thickness wedge of up to one third of either the upper or lower lip. • Based on the marginal artery, this flap is rotated to cover the defect, with the pedicle divided 10 days later. • This technique is best for reconstruction of the central philtral area of the upper lip. • The lower lip is longer, and up to one half of this lip can be resected while retaining good function and cosmesis.

ANSWER:
True

---

22. Which of the following statements regarding ear surgery is/are true?

A. The optimal time for the performance of ear surgery is 1 year of age.

B. Prosthetic ears are preferable to autogenous grafts in children.

C. Cartilage may be used from the opposite ear for reconstruction.

D. Loss of the antihelix and hypertrophy of the concha result in prominent ears.

Ref.: 1, 5

COMMENTS: The optimal time for the performance of ear surgery is after age 6, since 85–90% of full size is achieved. • In children, ear reconstruction is best done with autogenous tissue. • Specifically, the postauricular skin is expanded while costal cartilage is harvested to provide the framework for the ear. • In adults, a prosthetic ear is often used, with placement of a 3-mm implant in the mastoid bone for 3 months and attachment of a silicone prosthesis to clips or magnets held in place by the implants. • The lost tissue is replaced by various flaps from within the ear (intrinsic) or locally with flaps from the retroauricular region. • Sometimes cartilagenous grafts are taken from the opposite ear for more extensive defects.

Otoplasty is the surgical procedure used to correct prominent ears. • Protruding ears are a result of hypertrophy of the concha, absence of the antihelical fold, or both. • Correction requires resection of the cartilage at the base of the concha through a posterior incision. • The antihelical fold is addressed through a similar approach, but small incisions are made in the anterior cartilage and weakened with a dermabrader. • In general, the helix should be 17–23 mm from the temporal scalp.

ANSWER:
C, D

---

23. Which of the following statements regarding eyelid reconstruction and blepharoplasty is/are true?

A. Resection of the tarsal plate should follow a wedge shape.

B. Small defects (>6 mm) can often be closed primarily, while larger defects (<12 mm) require a regional flap.

C. Lower eyelid blepharoplasty may consist of preorbital fat repositioning rather than fat resection.

D. Access to the preorbital fat can be achieved only through external incisions.

Ref.: 1, 5

COMMENTS: In eyelid reconstruction, often the levator muscle, tarsal plate, medial and lateral canthal ligaments, and conjuctiva require surgery. • The tarsal plate, when resected for trauma or a neoplasm, should follow a rectangular shape. • This will facilitate eversion of the eyelid margin. • In general, 6–8 mm of tissue loss can be closed primarily. • For up to 12 mm of tissue loss, an advancement of the eyelid with a lateral flap is required, and a defect larger than 12 mm requires a tarsoconjuctival flap with a full-thickness skin graft from the upper opposite eyelid. • Any injury to the lacrimal system should be repaired with stenting of the duct.

In blepharoplasty, removal of eyelid skin and excision or repositioning of fat from both upper and lower eyelids is performed. • Incisions are made in the supratarsal crease in the upper eyelid and 1–2 mm below the lowest lashes on the lower eyelid. • Access to the preorbital fat is gained through the orbital septum, where two compartments are located in the upper eyelid and three in the lower eyelid. • Conservative resection of fat is performed in the upper eyelid, while repositioning of the lower preorbital fat over the inferior orbital rim typically occurs with excision of any redundant skin. • A transconjuctival approach can be used for the lower eyelid so that no external scars are visible.

ANSWER:
B, C

24. Which of the following statements regarding cleft lip and cleft palate is/are true?

  A. Cleft lip is an uncommon abnormality, occurring in approximately 1 of every 50,000 live births.

  B. Repair of the cleft lip generally is delayed until the patient is at least 6 months old.

  C. Structures anterior to the incisive foramen are part of the primary palate.

  D. With a soft palate cleft, the palatal musculature is abnormally inserted onto the posterior margin of the hard palate.

  E. Speech development is optimized if the palate is closed before age 12 months.

Ref.: 1, 2, 4

COMMENTS: Cleft lip is one of the more common anomalies treated by the plastic surgeon, with an incidence of approximately 1 in 1000 live births. • Cleft lip may occur as an isolated abnormality or may be associated with clefts of the alveolar ridge, hard palate, and soft palate. • Typically, the "rule of 10's" determines the timing of lip repair: when the hemoglobin is more than 10 g/100 ml, the patient is more than 10 weeks old, and the patient weighs more than 10 pounds. • At some centers, clefts of the lip are repaired at even earlier ages.

The primary palate (the lip and hard palate anterior to the incisive foramen) and the secondary palate (the hard palate posterior to the incisive foramen) develop from different embryologic structures, resulting in different degrees of susceptibility to genetic and environmental influences. • Hence, it is possible to have isolated clefts of either the primary or secondary palate as well as complete clefts of the entire palate. • When the soft palate is cleft, the levator palatini muscle, which normally forms a muscular sling across the palate, is abnormally inserted on the posterior border of the hard palate.

Restoration of the normal muscular anatomy is thought to play an important role in normal speech development. • Contraction of normal palatal musculature propels the posterior margin of the soft palate against the posterior pharyngeal wall to produce velopharyngeal closure. • This closing off of the nasopharynx is critical to the normal production of most sounds in the English language. • Patients who lack this closure mechanism have hypernasal speech. • Most consonants require the buildup of nasal pressure.

• Patients with cleft palate have velopharyngeal incompetence and are therefore unable to produce sufficient nasal pressure to produce most consonant sounds. • This situation results in characteristic speech marked by hypernasality; nasal air emissions; weak pressure consonants, or plosives (*p*, *t*, and *d*); and compensatory articulation consisting of consonant omissions ("og" for "dog"), substitutions, or distortions. • It is well known that patients with cleft palate have an increased incidence of middle ear infections and resultant hearing loss, probably related to abnormal muscular dynamics of the eustachian tubes. • The development of normal speech in patients with cleft palate appears to be optimized if the palate is closed before the age of 12 months, before abnormal compensatory habits are formed.

ANSWER:
C, D, E

25. Match the stage of pressure sore development in the left column with its appropriate characteristics in the right column, according to the National Pressure Ulcer Advisory Panel staging system.

  A. Stage I   a. Requires sharp débridement but underlying bone usually not exposed

  B. Stage II   b. Partial skin loss

  C. Stage III c. Nonblanchable erythema and no skin loss

  D. Stage IV   d. Complete necrosis of tissue superficial to bony prominence, often with infection of the bony cortex

Ref.: 2, 4

COMMENTS: Continuous pressure on tissues, if severe enough for a long enough time, results in venous, then capillary, and then arterial compression, with subsequent ischemic necrosis of the tissue, leading to a pressure ulcer. • A pressure of 40–80 mmHg applied continuously to tissue over 4 hr results in temporary microvascular changes and edema. • If the pressure continues for an 8-hr period, it may lead to permanent microvascular changes and the development of a pressure ulcer. • This process is most commonly seen in the sacral, trochanteric, and ischial regions.

Stage I pressure sores appear as nonblanching erythema with some edema and tenderness while the skin is intact. • Treatment is removal of pressure from these areas with frequent turning or the use of specially designed beds to distribute pressure evenly (Clinitron). • Meticulous skin care to avoid maceration, friction, and shear forces is also necessary. • **Stage II** ulcers have areas of partial skin loss with a yellow debris often seen as a shallow crater. • They can be treated with the conservative means listed above plus topical antibiotics (e.g., Silvadene). • Superficial ulcers usually heal spontaneously as long as there is no devitalized tissue and subsequent pressure is avoided. • **Stage III** ulcers have areas of full-thickness skin loss and subcutaneous tissue exposure. • Sharp débridement of devitalized, infected tissue and conservative treatment may allow closure by secondary contracture and scarring with epithelialization. • **Stage IV** pressure sores represent full-thickness loss of skin and underlying soft tissue, usually with involvement of the bony cortex of the underlying bony prominence. • These sores require débridement, control of the septic cellulitic process, and usually excision of the bony prominence and flap closure. • Myocutaneous flaps are generally preferable to random rotational flaps because they provide more durable coverage and a better blood supply to deal with infection.

ANSWER:
A-c; B-b; C-a; D-d

26. Which of the following statements regarding myocutaneous flap repair of pressure ulcers is/are true?

   A. Before planning a flap closure of a pressure ulcer, devitalized tissue needs to be débrided.

   B. A pressure ulcer has to be rendered sterile before flap repair.

   C. Incisions are planned solely with regard to achieving wound closure.

   D. The bursa is excised, but the bony prominence usually does not require removal.

   E. Wound-approximating sutures or staples are not removed until 3–5 weeks.

   Ref.: 2

COMMENTS: Superficial ulcers usually heal spontaneously if devitalized tissue is débrided and subsequent pressure is avoided. • Deeper ulcers, especially those involving exposed bone in the base of the ulcer, also require débridement, followed by the transfer of well-vascularized tissue into the defect. • Reduction of the underlying bony prominence is critical to preventing recurrence of the pressure sore. • Local skin flaps often fail because of tension and poor vascularity. • The most successful closure of deep pressure ulcers involves the placement of myocutaneous flaps into the defect. • Before operative repair of a pressure ulcer with a myocutaneous flap, it is necessary to excise devitalized tissue, assess the extent of the wound, and allow resolution of the cellulitic reaction or infection at the viable margins. • The open base of the wound, often with exposed bone, is not sterile. • The cellulitic process must be controlled with débridement, wound care, and frequently antibiotics. • The entire ulcer bursa and usually the exposed bony prominence are excised to remove devitalized tissue and provide a more even surface for pressure distribution. • The incisions are not placed over potential pressure areas, and previous trauma and surgeries, with their associated incisions or alterations in skin blood supply, must be taken into account. • These wounds are large and slow in healing, with varied tension forces. • It is best to have approximated tissues supported by sutures or staples for 3–5 weeks while the healing proceeds. • Inherent in all surgical treatment modalities is proper nutrition and the correction of systemic problems such as hypoxia, anemia, hypovolemia, or hypotension. • It is important to choose the appropriate antibiotics for treatment of infection and to prevent direct pressure with turning or alternating pressure. • The use of pressure-distribution beds or mats is usually required. • It should be noted that, although these beds can reduce pressures to a safe level of 30 mmHg over most bony prominences, the heel must still be protected. • Pressure sores along the heels and other unusual areas can develop even on a pressure-distribution bed.

ANSWER:
A, E

27. Which of the following statements regarding wound healing is/are true?

   A. Granulation tissue is seen only during the inflammatory phase.

   B. Platelet-derived growth factor (PDGF) stimulates fibroblasts and the production of transforming growth factor β (TGF-β).

   C. The mediators interleukin-1 (IL-1) and TFN-α dominate the proliferative phase.

   D. A keloid grows beyond the boundaries of the initial scar or injury.

   E. Hypertrophic scars and keloids both exhibit increased lysis of collagen at the cellular level.

   Ref.: 1, 7

COMMENTS: The process of wound healing undergoes three phases: inflammatory, proliferative, and maturation. • Chronic wounds often become "stalled" in the inflammatory phase owing to necrotic or heavily contaminated tissue, even though evidence of all three phases is present. • This stimulates platelets, lymphocytes, and neutrophils to secrete IL-1 and TFN-β, which are proinflammatory mediators. • The rationale for administering recombinant PDGF (Regranex) is to "push" the wound into the proliferative phase. • PDGF stimulates fibroblasts to proliferate and to secrete fibronectin and collagen. • In addition, it indirectly stimulates T cells to secrete TGF-β. • Once the levels of TGF-β rise, the wound moves into the proliferative phase of angiogenesis, fibroplasia, and epithelialization. • A granulating wound is considered to be in the proliferative phase.

Increased collagen deposition results in a keloid or hypertrophic scar if it exceeds collagen degradation. • Again, elevated levels of TGF-β stimulate fibroblasts and collagen deposition. • Current studies are exploring how to block such activity with antibodies to the cytokine. • The differentiation between hypertrophic scarring and a keloid is based mainly on clinical examination. • A keloid scar overgrows the boundaries of the initial injury, whereas a hypertrophic scar is a raised, indurated, erythematous scar.

ANSWER:
B, D

28. Which of the following statements regarding differentiation of keloid from hypertrophic scar is/are true?

   A. A keloid grows beyond the boundaries of the initial scar or injury.

   B. Differentiation between the two is by histologic diagnosis and cannot be determined clinically.

   C. Keloids are most often seen in dark-skinned individuals.

   D. If left chronically neglected, a keloid can degenerate into a malignancy.

   E. They both have increased lysis of collagen at the cellular level.

   Ref.: 7

COMMENTS: The differentiation between hypertrophic scarring and keloid is based mainly on clinical examination. • A keloid scar overgrows the boundaries of the initial injury, whereas a hypertrophic scar is a raised, indurated, erythematous scar. • There may be wound breakdown, pain, itching, or decreased function across joints. • Light microscopic examination alone shows the same basic architecture for both lesions: increased collagen production and decreased lysis of the collagen with perivascular sclerosis. • Keloid and hypertrophic scars occur more commonly in persons with dark skin, but this fact in itself does not help differentiate between the two, and certainly they are seen in all groups. • Malignant degeneration to squamous cell carcinoma (Marjolin's ulcer) is seen with chronic open wounds, burns, or ulcers but not with keloid formation.

ANSWER:
A, C

29. Which of the following wounds would most likely require free-flap reconstruction?

A. Open wound of the knee with an exposed total knee prosthesis

B. Open wound with exposed sternum following coronary artery bypass surgery

C. Full-thickness resection of the chest wall for tumor with exposed lung

D. Fracture of the distal one third of the tibia with an open wound and exposed bone without hardware in the wound

Ref.: 8

COMMENTS: Open tibial fractures have a high incidence of infection and nonunion, and they necessitate extended hospital stays. • The zone of injury is always larger than is clinically apparent. • Replacement of the tissue deficit is a critical part of the treatment, and myocutaneous flaps have led to a significant decrease in the incidence of infection and nonunion. • Local muscle flaps are not dependable in this region, since they are usually involved in the zone of injury and may not be available that far distally. • For this reason, free-flap transfer of muscle or skin (or both) from a distant site is the treatment of choice, especially for lower-extremity defects. • When considering free-flap coverage for traumatic wounds, it should be noted that the recipient vessels are often traumatized within the zone of injury and require extensive débridement. • These defects are often repaired in less than 1 week, or repair is delayed after 3 months for successful reconstruction. • The other wounds mentioned above require muscle coverage but can be treated with a local muscle flap, unless the flap has been previously used and failed. • In such instances, a free flap can be used in a salvage procedure.

ANSWER:
D

30. Match the composite tissue transfer on the left with its predominant blood supply on the right.

A. Rectus abdominis myocutaneous free flap
B. Latissimus dorsi myocutaneous free flap
C. Fibula osteocutaneous free flap
D. Dorsalis pedis fasciocutaneous flap

a. Thoracodorsal artery
b. Superior epigastric artery
c. Inferior epigastric artery
d. Anterior tibular artery
e. Peroneal artery

Ref.: 4

COMMENTS: The above-mentioned free flaps are widely used for free tissue transfer. • Their use should follow three principles: (1) the flap should be of adequate size, with a constant pedicle, (2) use of the flap should result in a mild secondary defect, and (3) the flap should provide functionality as well as adequate cosmesis. • The pedicle of the **latissimus dorsi flap** comes from the thoracodorsal artery, which gives one branch to the latissimus dorsi and another to the serratus anterior muscles. • The latissimus dorsi can be transferred on the thoracodorsal artery itself, or it can be harvested at the level of the subscapular artery to provide a longer, larger pedicle. • The **rectus abdominis free flap** is classically based on the inferior epigastric artery. • When it is used as a pedicle flap (e.g., TRAM flap for breast reconstruction), it is usually based on the superior epigastric artery. • The inferior epigastric artery is a branch of the external iliac artery. • The **fibular osteocutaneous flap** is based on the peroneal artery. • The **dorsalis**

pedis flap (dorsum of the foot) is based on the anterior tibial artery. • Documenting the blood flow present in the three leg vessels is critical before harvesting these flaps, and it is also extremely helpful when the leg is the recipient site as well. • Arteriograms are usually necessary to assist in planning and in helping to avoid tissue necrosis or loss of the foot.

ANSWER:
A-c; B-a; C-e; D-d

31. Which of the following statements regarding microvascular free tissue transfers and technique is/are true?

A. End-to-side anastomoses are preferred when recipient vessels are limited.

B. 10-0 suture on a cutting needle is used for vessels up to 3 mm in diameter.

C. The arterial anastomosis should be performed before the venous repair.

D. Thrombosis typically occurs in the initial postoperative period (48 hr).

Ref.: 9, 10

COMMENTS: Microvascular anastomoses can be performed in an end-to-end or end-to-side fashion, with similar patency rates (>95%) for vessels smaller than 1 mm in diameter. • However end-to-side repairs should be reserved for recipient sites with few vessels. • Often, the extremity has end arteries, and an end-to-side technique is needed to preserve flow distally. • For vessels between 0.5 and 3 mm in diameter, 10-0 suture is commonly used, while 8-0 suture is acceptable for vessels larger than 3 mm in diameter. • All sutures should be on tapered needles to minimize trauma to the vessel. • Débridement of the vessel edges is paramount for proper coaptation and to lessen intimal flap formation. • The venous anastomosis should be performed first to avoid flap engorgement and prevent clamping of the arterial anastomosis during the repair.

Ischemia time is crucial for a successful transfer, whether at the time of initial surgery or following thrombotic events postoperatively. • For this reason, prompt recognition of postoperative thrombosis is essential, and immediate intervention is mandatory for a successful outcome. • Thrombosis typically occurs within the first 24 hr but can be seen up to 10 days postoperatively. • The flap should be frequently monitored in the initial postoperative period for arterial or venous obstruction. • A flap that is cool, pale, and with sluggish capillary refill may need further assessment by rubbing gauze on the surface to check arterial perfusion. • Brisk refill, dark oozing from the flap edges, and engorgement may signify venous obstruction.

ANSWER:
A, D

32. Which of the following statements regarding face-lifts and Botox is/are true?

A. Wrinkles are caused by the repeated contraction of the muscles of expression.

B. Performing a deep face-lift often minimizes risk of bleeding and nerve injury.

C. Botulinum toxin A causes an increase in muscular contraction, tightening wrinkled skin.

D. The effects of botulinum toxin A are reversible.

Ref.: 4, 5

COMMENTS: Wrinkles are caused by aging and repeated contraction of the underlying muscles. • They are generally corrected surgically by stretching skin and fascia, resecting redundant skin, and repositioning fat. • The deep face-lift requires dissection in the subperiosteal plane, allowing easier repositioning of fat at the expense of increased risk of bleeding and nerve injury. • Hyperkinetic wrinkles can be treated temporarily with botulinum toxin A (Botox). • The toxin is produced by *Clostridium botulinum* and functions by preventing the release of acetylcholine at the neuromuscular junction and thus preventing muscle contraction. • Since acetylcholine production is not inhibited, the effect is reversible in months. • After injection, the results are typically seen in 3–10 days and last approximately 3–6 months. • The procerus and corrugator muscles are targeted to remove wrinkles of the upper one third of the face. • Botulinum toxin A can be used around the mouth and neck, but the risks of causing asymmetry and functional paralysis (Bell's palsy) are increased. • In addition to local complications such as pain, bruising, infection, and edema, the toxin may cause loss of sensation, eyelid ptosis, and dysplopia.

ANSWER:
A, D

33. A 12-year-old girl is brought to a surgeon's office because she has hypoplasia of the breasts. On closer examination, she is also found to have asymmetry of the chest wall itself. Which of the following is most likely associated with this syndrome?

    A. Absence of the nipple and areola

    B. Deformity of the thoracoacromial joint

    C. Absence of the sternum

    D. Absence of the sternal head of the pectoralis muscle

Ref.: 4, 7, 11

COMMENTS: Poland's syndrome is a congenital defect with an incidence of about 1 in every 30,000 births. • The chest wall anomaly is a hallmark of the syndrome, which includes partial absence of the sternal head of the pectoralis major muscle and possibly complete absence of the pectoralis minor muscle. • Other muscles around the chest wall may be affected, including the serratus anterior, supraspinatus, external oblique, and latissimus dorsi muscles. • Although the sternum may be normal, the ribs may be hypoplastic or absent. • Absence of the nipple is rare and not associated with this syndrome. • The upper extremities and the hand may be affected in the form of hypoplasia, possibly with syndactyly. • Reconstruction can be started early with a temporary expandable prosthesis that is inflated periodically to match the growing opposite side. • Ultimately, during adulthood the chest wall asymmetry must be addressed by reconstruction to obtain maximum aesthetic results.

ANSWER:
D

34. Which of the following are indications for repair of orbital blowout fractures?

    A. Cosmetically unacceptable enophthalmos

    B. Disabling diplopia

    C. Associated facial fractures

    D. Accompanying severe permanent visual loss

Ref.: 4

COMMENTS: The indications for surgery for orbital blowout fractures are not always clear-cut. • A fracture in the absence of significant physical signs or symptoms does not invariably require operative intervention. • Significant, cosmetically unacceptable enophthalmos and disabling diplopia are the most obvious indications for exploration. • If these indications are not present, the need for surgical repair is not established. • Likewise, if a patient has permanent visual loss accompanying an orbital blowout fracture, repair of the floor fracture is probably not justified unless there is marked enophthalmos. • Exploration of the orbital floor is not considered an emergency measure, and surgery can safely be delayed for up to 14 days without risking irreversible scarring and fibrosis. • Patients who initially have no diplopia or lose the diplopia within 14 days of injury should not undergo surgery unless radiographic films show extensive defects in the orbital floor that could cause delayed, marked enophthalmos if not repaired. • Surgery under emergency conditions is not justified unless the patient is undergoing a necessary operation for other, simultaneously sustained facial trauma. • In summary, the basic indications for repairing an orbital floor fracture are prevention of subsequent subjective diplopia and cosmetically significant enophthalmos.

ANSWER:
A, B

35. Which of the following statements regarding midface trauma is/are true?

    A. If the nose is swollen, it is best to delay treatment of a nasal fracture until the swelling subsides so that the fragments may be reduced more precisely.

    B. If a hematoma of the nasal septum is detected during physical examination, it should not be drained, since drainage would increase the likelihood of infection.

    C. Complex nasoorbital fractures are best approached through a coronal incision.

    D. A depressed fracture of the zygomatic arch may cause difficulty in opening the jaw by impinging on the motor nerve to the muscles of mastication.

Ref.: 1, 4

COMMENTS: Fractures of the nasal bones are best evaluated by physical examination, since radiographs are notoriously misleading. • Frequently, the patient with a nasal injury presents with a marked degree of swelling. • Reduction is best delayed for several days to allow the swelling to subside so that the fragments can be reduced more precisely. • Even then, many patients require later surgical revision after the fracture fragments have healed. • Examination of patients with midface trauma should always include inspection of the nasal septum for a hematoma. • An undrained septal hematoma can lead to necrosis of the septal cartilage, with loss of midline nasal support and resultant saddle-nose deformity.

Application of craniofacial techniques has improved the treatment of midfacial trauma. • Complex midfacial injuries, including nasoorbital fractures, are best approached through a coronal incision. • Incisions at the upper gingivobuccal sulcus and lower eyelid complete the exposure of a multiply injured midface. • A depressed fracture of the zygomatic arch may interfere with jaw motion by directly impinging on the coronoid process or muscles of mastication.

ANSWER:
A, C

36. A 65-year-old woman with insulin-dependent diabetes mellitus underwent coronary artery bypass grafting using the left inferior mammary artery (IMA). She developed a sternal wound infection. Which of the following flaps is/are appropriate for repair?

A. Bilateral pectoralis flaps

B. Omental flap

C. Bilateral rectus abdominis flaps

D. Latissimus flap

Ref.: 3, 7, 11

COMMENTS: Sternal wound infections are a potential complication of heart surgery. • When the IMA is used in diabetic patients, there is an increased risk of a sternal wound infection. • The use of the IMA interrupts the blood flow to the superior epigastric artery (SEA). • The SEA provides the blood supply to the pedicled rectus abdominis flap. • In this patient, the bilateral rectus abdominis flap is a poor choice because the left rectus muscle's superior vascular pedicle (i.e., the SEA) has been interrupted. • Bilateral pectoralis muscle flaps are an excellent choice for sternal wound repair. • Each pectoralis muscle is fully dissected and advanced to the midline. • Each muscle can be dismissed for additional mobility. • The thoracoacromial artery supplies the pectoralis muscle. • The omental flap is also a viable choice. • It may be based on the right or the left gastroepiploic vessels. • The latissimus flap, although not ideal, can be mobilized to repair a sternal wound. • It is based on the thoracodorsal vessels.

ANSWER:
A, B, D

REFERENCES

1. Townsend CM Jr, Beauchamp RD, Evers BM, et al (eds): *Sabiston Textbook of Surgery: The Biological Basis of Modern Surgical Practice*, 16th ed. WB Saunders, Philadelphia, 2001.
2. Schwartz SI, Shires GT, Spencer FC, et al (eds): *Schwartz's Principles of Surgery*, 7th ed. McGraw-Hill, New York, 1999.
3. Jurkiewicz MJ (ed): *Plastic Surgery: Principles and Practice.* CV Mosby, St. Louis, 1990.
4. Aston S, Seasley R, Thorne C (eds): *Grabb and Smith's Plastic Surgery*, 5th ed. Lippincott-Raven, Philadelphia, 1997.
5. Greenfield LG, Mulholland MW, Oldham KT, et al (eds): *Surgery: Scientific Principles and Practice*, 3rd ed. Lippincott, Williams & Wilkins, Philadelphia, 2001.
6. Habal MB (ed): *Advances in Plastic and Reconstructive Surgery*, vol 15. CV Mosby, St. Louis, 1999, Ch 1.
7. McCarthy JG (ed): *Plastic Surgery.* WB Saunders, Philadelphia, 1990.
8. Shaw WW, Hidalgo DA (eds): *Microsurgery in Trauma.* Futura Publishing, Mount Kisco, NY, 1987.
9. Serafin D (ed): *Atlas of Microsurgical Composite Tissue Transplantation.* Saunders, Philadelphia, 1996.
10. Strauch B (ed): *Atlas of Microvascular Surgery: Anatomy and Operative Approaches.* Theime, New York, 1993.
11. Cohen M: *Mastery of Plastic and Reconstructive Surgery.* Little, Brown, Boston, 1999, p 1252.

C H A P T E R 55

Genetics

Michael J. Gaffud, M.D., and Steven D. Bines, M.D.

1. What risk do female *BRCA 1* mutation carriers have of developing breast cancer?

   A. 100%

   B. 60–80%

   C. 40–60%

   D. 20–40%

   Ref.: 1, 2

COMMENTS: The frequency of *BRCA1* or *BRCA2* mutations in North America ranges from 1 in 150 to 1 in 800. • *BRCA1* and *BRCA2* function as tumor suppressor genes. • *BRCA1* is located on chromosome 17, and *BRCA2* is located on chromosome 13. • For carriers of either *BRCA1* or *BRCA2*, the lifetime risk of developing breast cancer is between 60 and 80%. • Guidelines regarding screening for carriers include annual mammograms beginning at around 25–30 years of age, monthly breast self-examinations, and clinical breast examination once or twice a year.

ANSWER:
B

2. What risk do female *BRCA 1* mutation carriers have of developing ovarian cancer?

   A. 100%

   B. 60–80%

   C. 40–60%

   D. 20–40%

   Ref.: 2

COMMENTS: Female carriers of *BRCA1* are also at risk of developing ovarian cancer. • There is currently no established screening method for ovarian cancer. • Ultrasound imaging and determination of serum CA-125 levels are not sensitive methods of detecting stage I or stage II ovarian cancer.

ANSWER:
D

3. What risk do male *BRCA 2* mutation carriers have of developing breast cancer?

   A. 3%

   B. 6%

   C. 12%

   D. 25%

   Ref.: 3

COMMENTS: The *BRCA2* mutation is associated with the majority on hereditary male breast cancer. • Due to wide variance in population, the estimate of male breast cancer associated with *BRCA2* is not precisely established. • The 6% risk is 150-fold greater than the risk for the general population. • *BRCA1* mutations are rare in hereditary male breast cancer.

ANSWER:
B

4. After the initial diagnosis of breast cancer in a *BRCA1* or *BRCA2* carrier, what is the approximate annual risk of developing cancer in the contralateral breast?

   A. 3%

   B. 6%

   C. 9%

   D. 12%

   Ref.: 2

COMMENTS: Following the initial diagnosis of breast cancer in a *BRCA1* or *BRCA2* carrier, the annual risk of developing cancer in the contralateral breast is 3%. • A prophylactic mastectomy on the contralateral side is an option in patients with established genotyping. • Tamoxifen or prophylactic oophorectomy is an option for reducing the risk of contralateral breast cancer. • Each therapy reduces the risk of contralateral breast cancer by 50%.

ANSWER:
A

5. Which of the following is/are associated with an increased risk of breast cancer?

   A. Turner's syndrome

   B. Down's syndrome

   C. Klinefelter's syndrome

   D. Patau's syndrome

Ref.: 4

COMMENTS: Klinefelter's syndrome is a 47 XXY karyotype abnormality that occurs in 1 in 1000 men. • This hereditary disorder is associated with microtestes, gynecomastia, infertility, and an increased risk of breast cancer, which is 20 times more common in males with the syndrome than in males without it. • Three to 4% of male breast cancer cases are associated with Klinefelter's syndrome, and patients typically develop breast cancer at a younger age (55–65 years) than do patients without the syndrome.

   Turner's syndrome is an XO karyotype abnormality associated with infertility and amenorrhea. • Down's syndrome is a trisomy 21 karyotype abnormality associated with low-set ears, slanted eyes, cardiac defects, and early Alzheimer's disease. • Patau's syndrome is a trisomy 13 karyotype abnormality associated with rocker-bottom feet, severe mitral regurgitation, and deafness. • Turner's and Down's syndromes are not associated with an increased risk of breast cancer. • Patau's syndrome is associated with an 85% mortality rate within the first year of life.

ANSWER:
C

6. Familial pheochromocytomas are associated with all but which of the following?

   A. Multiple endocrine neoplasia (MEN) type 2 *RET* proto-oncogene, located on chromosome 10q11

   B. Von Hippel-Lindau tumor-suppressor gene, located on chromosome 3p25

   C. Neurofibromatosis type 1 gene, located on chromosome 17q11

   D. *MEN1* gene, located on chromosome 11q13

Ref.: 5

COMMENTS: Thirty percent of pheochromocytomas are associated with a hereditary syndrome. • The *RET* proto-oncongene is associated with MEN type 2 syndromes and causes abnormal cellular proliferation, resulting in medullary hyperplasia and pheochromocytoma. • Thirty to 50% of patients with MEN type 2 are at risk of developing pheochromocytoma. • Von Hippel-Lindau tumor-suppressor gene is also associated with pheochromocytoma, which will develop in 15–20% of patients with von Hippel-Lindau syndrome. • Five percent of patients with neurofibromatosis will develop pheochromocytomas. • The *MEN1* gene is not associated with pheochromocytomas.

ANSWER:
D

7. The *RET* proto-oncogene is associated with all but which of the following?

   A. Medullary thyroid carcinoma

   B. Pheochromocytoma

   C. Zollinger-Ellison syndrome

   D. Hyperparathyroidism

Ref.: 6

COMMENTS: The *RET* proto-oncogene, located on chromosome 10, is associated with MEN type 2 syndromes, resulting in medullary thyroid cancer, pheochromocytoma, and hyperparathyroidism. • Medullary thyroid cancer and pheochromocytoma are associated with both MEN type 2A and MEN type 2B. • Hyperparathyroidism is associated with MEN 2A only. • Zollinger-Ellison syndrome is associated with MEN 1. • Gastrinoma is a very common functional neuroendocrine tumor in MEN 1 patients. • The hypergastrinemia associated with MEN 1 presents as epigastric pain, reflux esophagitis, secretory diarrhea, and weight loss.

ANSWER:
C

8. What percentage of carriers of the *RET* proto-oncogene mutation will develop medullary thyroid carcinoma?

   A. 25%

   B. 40%

   C. 65%

   D. 100%

Ref.: 6

COMMENTS: One hundred percent of patients with mutation of the *RET* proto-oncogene will develop medullary thyroid cancer associated with the MEN 2 syndromes and familial medullary thyroid cancer. • Twenty-five percent of cases of medullary thyroid cancer are familial and present multifocally and bilaterally. • Prophylactic screening and surgery are recommended for patients with a family history of medullary thyroid cancer.

ANSWER:
D

9. Screening recommendations for hereditary nonpolyposis colorectal cancer (HNPCC) include all but which of the following?

   A. Colonoscopy every 2 years, beginning at age 20, and annually after age 40 or the youngest age at which a family member was diagnosed minus 10 years

   B. Transvaginal ultrasound imaging every 1–2 years, beginning at age 25–35

   C. Urinalysis every 1–2 years

   D. Thyroid examination every 1–2 years

Ref.: 6

COMMENTS: HNPCC is the most common hereditary colorectal cancer in the United States. • It is estimated to be associated with 3% of all colorectal cancer cases and 15% of colorectal cancer cases associated with an established family history. • Close surveillance of patients carrying the mutation is necessary. • Colonoscopy is recommended at an early age. • Transvaginal ultrasound imaging is recommended for endometrial cancer. • Urinalysis and ultrasound imaging are recommended for upper urinary tract cancer. • Thyroid examination is not recommended for HNPCC. • Thyroid examination is recommended annually for patients with an established family history of familial adenomatous polyposis (FAP). • There is a 2% lifetime risk of thyroid cancer with FAP.

ANSWER:
D

10. What is the most common trait expressed in MEN 1?

    A. Parathyroid adenoma

    B. Gastrinoma

    C. Pituitary adenoma

    D. Thymic carcinoid

Ref.: 6

COMMENTS: Parathyroid adenomas occur in more than 95% of patients with MEN 1. • Typically, all four glands are involved. • Hypercalcemia is the first biochemical abnormality, and symptoms are similar to those of primary hyperparathyroidism. • Neuroendocrine tumors of the duodenum or pancreas (gastrinomas) occur with a frequency between 30 and 80%. • Pituitary tumors occur in 15–50% of patients with MEN 1. • Thymic carcinoids occur in less than 8% of patients with MEN 1.

ANSWER:
A

11. Peutz-Jeghers syndrome is associated with a defect in which of the following genes?

    A. *STK 11*

    B. *PTEN*

    C. *MSH2*

    D. *APC*

Ref.: 6

COMMENTS: *STK 11*, serine/threonine kinase 11, causes Peutz-Jeghers syndrome. • It is an autosomal dominant syndrome consisting of hamartomatous polyps of the intestinal tract and pigmented lesions of the buccal mucosa, lips, and digits. • The *PTEN* mutation is associated with Cowden's syndrome. • The *MSH2* mutation is associated with HNPCC. • The *APC* mutation is associated with familial adenomatous polyposis, or Gardner's syndrome.

ANSWER:
A

12. Patients with Cowden's syndrome are at increased risk for which of the following?

    A. Adenocarcinoma of the pancreas

    B. Adenocarcinoma of the breast

    C. Renal clear-cell carcinoma

    D. Cerebellar medulloblastoma

Ref.: 6

COMMENTS: Cowden's syndrome is a hereditary hamartomatous polyposis syndrome. • In addition to the risk of hamartomatous polyps of the colon, there is a 50% risk of developing adenocarcinoma of the breast. • Increased risk of pancreatic cancer is associated with

familial juvenile polyposis. • Increased risk of renal cell carcinoma is associated with HNPCC. • Increased risk of medulloblastoma is associated with Turcot's syndrome.

ANSWER:
B

13. Complications of skin wound healing is reported in all but which of the following heritable connective tissue diseases?

    A. Ehler-Danlos syndrome

    B. Marfan's syndrome

    C. Acrodermatitis enteropathica

    D. Epidemolysis bullosa

Ref.: 7

COMMENTS: Marfan's syndrome is characterized by tall stature, lax ligaments, myopia, aneurysm of the ascending aorta, and hernias. • The genetic defect is associated with the elastic fibers. • Although a dissecting aneurysm may be difficult to repair owing to the soft connective tissue, the skin is only hyperextensible and there is no wound healing delay.

Ehlers-Danlos syndrome consists of 10 disorders of collagen formation characterized by poor wound healing, easy bruising, and abnormal scar formation. • This syndrome should be considered in children with recurrent hernias and coagulation disorders.

Acrodermatitis enteropathica is an autosomal recessive disease causing an inability to absorb zinc by the intestine. • Zinc is a necessary cofactor for DNA polymerase and reverse transcriptase. • The deficiency causes impaired wound healing and erythematous pustular dermatitis.

Epidermolysis bullosa causes impairment of tissue adhesion within the epidermis, basement membrane, or dermis with minimal trauma. • In addition to poor wound healing, patients can easily blister and ulcerate.

ANSWER:
B

14. The majority of Li-Fraumeni syndrome germ-line mutations are caused by which of the following?

    A. *WT*

    B. *rb1*

    C. *p53*

    D. *TSC*

Ref.: 7

COMMENTS: Approximately 70% of patients diagnosed with Li-Fraumeni syndrome have mutations in the tumor suppressor gene *p53*. • Criteria for diagnosis of Li-Fraumeni syndrome include a bone or soft-tissue sarcoma before 45 years of age, a first-degree relative with any type of cancer before 45 years of age, and another first- or second-degree relative with a sarcoma at any age or any cancer diagnosed before 45 years of age. • *WT* is associated with Wilms' tumor. • It consists of embryonal tumor of renal origin, aniridia, and genitourinary abnormalities. • *Rb1* is a tumor suppressor gene associated with retinoblastoma. • In addition to the retinal tumor, patients are found to have a higher incidence of sarcoma, brain neoplasms, and malignant melanoma. • *TSC* is associated with tuberous sclerosis and the syndrome of multiple hamartomas, renal cell carcinoma, and astrocytoma.

ANSWER:
C

15. All but which of the following are manifestations of cystic fibrosis?

A. Esophageal dysmotility

B. Gastroesophageal reflux

C. Distal intestinal obstruction syndrome

D. Intussusception

Ref.: 8

COMMENTS: Although cystic fibrosis is considered predominantly a lung disease, improved life expectancy has necessitated management of gastrointestinal complications. • Gastroesophageal reflux in children with cystic fibrosis presents with the typical symptoms of heartburn and regurgitation, and the pathophysiologic features are the same as in other populations. • However, it occurs more frequently in children with cystic fibrosis than in other pediatric patients.

Distal intestinal obstruction syndrome is the pediatric or adult equivalent of meconium ileus due to pancreatic insufficiency. • It is a complication of cystic fibrosis most common after 20 years of age. • Although surgery has been the classic treatment for distal intestinal obstruction syndrome, attempts to remove the inspissated plug with enemas and laxatives should be made.

Intussusception is also a complication of cystic fibrosis. • It may also be due to pancreatic insufficiency, with inspissated bowel contents as first symptom. • Surgery is necessary for failed medical management or the development of peritonitis.

Esophageal dysmotility is not a complication of cystic fibrosis.

ANSWER:
A

16. Extracolonic manifestations of familial adenomatous polyposis (FAP) may include all but which of the following?

A. Congenital hypertrophy of the retinal pigmented epithelium

B. Adenocarcinoma of the breast

C. Osteomas of the skull

D. Desmoid tumors

Ref.: 6

COMMENTS: FAP is associated with the *APC* gene, located on chromosome 5q21. • Congenital hypertrophy of the retinal pigmented epithelium is an ophthalmologic finding associated with 75% of patients with FAP. • Osteomas of the skull and desmoid tumors are also associated with FAP. • Adenocarcinoma of the breast is associated with Cowden's syndrome.

ANSWER:
B

17. For carriers of DNA-mismatch repair gene mutations, what is the lifetime risk of developing colorectal cancer?

A. 70%

B. 80%

C. 90%

D. 100%

Ref.: 9

COMMENTS: Mutations of the DNA-mismatch repair genes are associated with HNPCC or Lynch's syndrome. • People with an established family history of HNPCC or Lynch's syndrome should undergo routine screening at an earlier age for colon, endometrial, and upper urinary tract cancer.

ANSWER:
B

18. Hereditary diffuse gastric cancer is most commonly associated with mutations in which of the following genes?

A. *CDH1*

B. *NOD2*

C. *IBD2*

D. *SDHD*

Ref.: 10

COMMENTS: Gastric cancer is associated with Li-Fraumeni syndrome, HNPCC, and FAP, but not as a diffuse lesion. • Diffuse gastric cancer is associated with mutations in *CDH1*, the e-cadherin gene on chromosome 16. • Mutations are found in up to 48% of diffuse gastric cancer patients. • The tumor spreads through the submucosa, and biopsies detect less than 50% of cases. • This difficulty in detection has prompted the recommendation of prophylactic gastrectomy for patients with the syndrome. • Mutations in the *NOD2* and *IBD2* genes are associated with Crohn's disease. • Mutations in the *SDHD* gene are associated with paragangliomas.

ANSWER:
A

19. Hereditary pancreatic cancer syndromes are associated with mutations in all but which of the following genes?

A. *PRSS1*

B. *MLH1*

C. *SKT11*

D. *RET*

Ref.: 10

COMMENTS: *RET* is associated with the MEN syndromes, which most frequently involve medullary thyroid cancer and not pancreatic cancer. • *PRSS1* is associated with hereditary pancreatitis as well as pancreatic cancer. • *MLH1* is a DNA-mismatch repair gene associated with HNPCC and pancreatic cancer. • *SKT11* is associated with pancreatic cancer and Peutz-Jeghers syndrome.

ANSWER:
D

20. Familial melanoma syndromes are most frequently associated with which of the following genes?

A. *CDKN2A*

B. *PTH*

C. *LKB1*

D. *PMS1*

Ref.: 10

COMMENTS: Familial melanoma syndromes are associated with *CDKN2A*, with a 65% penetrance by age 80 years. • *PTH* is thought to be associated with nevoid basal cell carcinoma. • *LKB1* is another mutation associated with Peutz-Jeghers syndrome. • It causes hyperpigmentation but not melanoma. • *PMS1* is one of the mutations associated with HNPCC. • It can be associated with sebaceous gland adenomas and keratacanthomas in its Muir-Torre variant.

A N S W E R :
A

21. Soft-tissue sarcomas are associated with all but which of the following?

A. Werner's syndrome

B. Neurofibromatosis type 1

C. Neurofibromatosis type 2

D. Li-Fraumeni syndrome

Ref.: 11

COMMENTS: Neurofibromatosis type 2 is associated with neural tumors, including acoustic neuromas, meningiomas, gliomas, and ependymomas. • Werner's syndrome, or adult progeria, is an autosomal recessive disorder associated with a decreased life expectancy due to atherosclerosis and various cancers, most commonly sarcoma.

• Neurofibromatosis type 1 is an autosomal dominant trait causing neurogenic sarcomas and, in children, rhabdomyosarcoma, fibrosarcoma, and liposarcoma. • Li-Fraumeni syndrome is an autosomal dominant disorder associated with a spectrum of disease, including possible soft-tissue sarcomas, osteosarcomas, breast cancer, and brain tumors.

A N S W E R :
C

R E F E R E N C E S

1. Martin AM, Weber BL: Genetic and hormonal risk factors in breast cancer. *J Natl Cancer Inst* 92:1126–1134, 2002.
2. Narod SA, Offit K: Prevention and management of hereditary breast cancer. *J Clin Oncol* 23:1656–1663, 2005.
3. Giordano SH, Cohen DS, Buzdar AU, et al: Breast carcinoma in men: a population-based study. *Cancer* 101:51–57, 2004.
4. Weiss JR, Moysich KB, Swede H: Epidemiology of male breast cancer. *Cancer Epidemiol Biomarkers Prev* 14(1):20–26, 2005.
5. Pacak K, Linehan WM, Eisenhofer G, et al: Recent advances in genetics, diagnosis, localization, and treatment of pheochromocytoma. *Ann Intern Med* 134(4):315–326, 2001.
6. Townsend CM Jr, Beauchamp RD, Evers BM, et al (eds): *Sabiston Textbook of Surgery: The Biological Basis of Modern Surgical Practice,* 17th ed. Saunders, Philadelphia, 2004.
7. Brunicardi FC, Andersen DK, Billiar TR, et al (eds): *Schwartz's Principles of Surgery*, 8th ed. McGraw-Hill, New York, 2004.
8. Riedel BD: Gastrointestinal manifestations of cystic fibrosis. *Pediatr Ann* 26(4):235–241, 1997.
9. Aarnio M, Sankila R, Pukkala E, et al: Cancer risk in mutation carriers of DNA-mismatch repair genes. *Int J Cancer* 81:214–218, 1999.
10. Garber JE, Offit K: Hereditary cancer predisposition syndromes. *J Clin Oncol* 23:276–292, 2005.
11. Hoar Zahm S, Fraumeni JF: The epidemiology of soft tissue sarcoma. *Semin Oncol* 24:504–514, 1997.

CHAPTER 56

Biostatistics and Data Management

Linnea S. Hauge, Ph.D., and Steven D. Bines, M.D.

1. Which of the following describes this data set: 2, 3, 3, 4, 5, 8, 10?

    A. Mean = 5, median = 4, mode = 3.

    B. Mean = 4, median = 4, mode = 5.

    C. Mean = 4, median = 3, mode = 5.

    D. Mean = 5, median = 3, mode = 4.

Ref.: 1

COMMENTS: The mean, median, and mode are all measures of central tendency of a data set. • The arithmetic **mean** is the measure of central tendency for interval and ratio data. It is calculated as summing all of the observations (?*x*) and dividing by the number of observations (*N*). • The **median** is the measure of central tendency for ordinal data. The median is that value such that half of the data points fall above it and half below it. To calculate the median, rank the data in the sample. The median is the middle point of the ranked data. For odd sample sizes, half of the remaining observations fall to the left of this value, and the other half fall to the right of this value. For even sample sizes, the median is the mean of the two middle values. • The measure of central tendency for nominal data is the **mode**. The mode is the most frequently occurring value in the data set. • For a normal distribution, the mean, median, and mode are approximately the same value.

ANSWER:
A

2. Match each statistical measure of dispersion with its unique characteristic.

    A. Variance

    a. Sum of the squares of the deviation of each sample point about the mean

    B. Standard deviation

    b. Variability of sample means drawn from the same population

    C. Standard error

    c. Variability of sample data points about the mean in natural units

Ref.: 1

COMMENTS: The ability to test hypotheses of a sample mean is critically dependent on the degree to which the data points deviate from the mean. • The **variance** is the sum of the squares of the difference between each sample point and the mean. • The **standard deviation** is the square root of the variance. The standard

deviation is a more familiar and frequently reported quantity because it is in the same units as the mean and is not dependent on sample size. • The **standard error** of the mean is the standard deviation divided by the square root of the sample size. The standard error decreases as the sample size increases. The accuracy of a sample estimate of a population mean is dependent on the standard error. If the standard error is large, the mean is an unreliable measure. • If the standard deviation is small and the sample size is large (yielding a small standard error), the sample mean is an accurate estimate of the population mean.

ANSWER:
A-a; B-c; C-b

3. The notation P (A or B) is read as "the probability that A or B or both occur." The conditional probability notation P (A/B) is read as "the probability that A occurs given that B occurs." Match the left side of each probability definition equation in the left column with that in the right column.

    A. P (A or B)

    a. P (A) + P (B)

    B. P (A and B)

    b. P (A) × P (B)

    C. For mutually exclusive events A, B: P (A or B)

    c. P (B) × P (A/B)

    D. For independent events A, B: P (A and B)

    d. P (A) + P (B) - P (A and B)

    E. P (A/B)

    e. P (A and B)/P (B)

Ref.: 1

COMMENTS: A basic understanding of the probability theory is required for the proper use of statistics. All probabilities fall between zero and one ($0 \leq P (x) \leq 1$). The probability of A occurring or A not occurring is always equal to 1 (a specific example of mutually exclusive events). For two events, A and B, that cannot happen at the same time (mutually exclusive events), the probability that A or B occurs is the probability that A occurs plus the probability that B occurs: P (A or B) = P (A) + P (B). However, if both can happen at the same time, the probability that they do would be counted twice, and we must therefore subtract the probability that both occur: P (A or B) = P (A) + P (B) − P (A and B). Similarly, the joint probability of two independent events both occurring is the simple product of the probabilities: P (A and B) = P (A) × P (B). However, if the events are not independent (e.g., the probability of having a high glucose level, given that one has diabetes), one must multiply one event by the conditional probability of the other event: P (A and B) = P (A) × P (B/A), also P (A and B) = P (B) × P (A/B).

A N S W E R :
A-d; B-c; C-a; D-b; E-e

4. Which of the following is/are true about descriptive statistics?

A. Histograms and frequency polygons are graphic depictions of group means.

B. A percentile indicates the rank of a data point within a distribution.

C. A normal distribution of data points is bell-shaped.

D. Kurtosis is the symmetry of a graphic depiction of a frequency distribution.

Ref.: 1, 3

COMMENTS: A **frequency distribution** lists each value in the sample data set and the frequency of each data point's occurrence. These data can be depicted graphically in bar charts, histograms, and frequency polygons. • **Percentile ranks** are used to describe the location of a data point within a data set. A percentile is a value on a scale of 0 to 100 that specifies the percentage of a distribution that is equal to or below it. For example, an individual who scores in the 80th percentile on an examination has performed as well as or better than 80% of all examinees. The 50th percentile of any data set is equivalent to the median. • Data are considered normally distributed if the frequency polygon is continuous from positive to negative and has a characteristic bell-shaped curve. For a **normal** (or **Gaussian**) **distribution**, the mean, median, and mode all have approximately the same value. For a normal distribution, approximately 68% of the data points fall within 1 standard deviation of the mean, and approximately 95% of the data points fall within 2 standard deviations of the mean. • The symmetry of a distribution is known as its **skewness**, and the flat or peaked shape of a distribution curve is known as its **kurtosis**.

A N S W E R :
B, C

5. Which of the following is/are true about statistical testing?

A. Researchers aim to generalize their results to a specific sample.

B. A normal distribution is required for most statistical tests.

C. In hypothesis testing, the null hypothesis is rejected if $p = 0.50$.

D. Confidence intervals can be used for hypothesis testing.

Ref.: 1, 3

COMMENTS: The term **sample** refers to the individuals, subjects, or participants in a specific study. The term **population** describes the hypothetical group of people from which a sample is derived. Researchers aim to draw conclusions about a specific population based on their study of a sample of that population. • The **central limit theorem** states that, as sample size increases, the sample mean approaches normality. This theorem allows us to perform statistical testing on the sample mean of nonnormal data *if* the sample is large enough. • **Hypothesis testing** is the process by which conclusions are drawn in an objective, probabilistic way. **Statistical significance**, confirmed by a test's *p* value, is the likelihood that there is a

difference that is not due to chance. Generally, conclusive studies are those in which the probability is less than 5% that the sample data were obtained by chance ($p < 0.05$). In this circumstance, we reject the null hypothesis (i.e., the experimental group data are different from the control group data). However, when the probability of a chance finding is greater than 5% ($p > 0.05$), we draw no conclusions and retain the null hypothesis. • The **confidence interval (CI)** is a calculated range that encompasses a specified percentage of the sample data. • Calculation of the 95% CI is analogous to hypothesis testing. Generally, if the expected value (null hypothesis) does not fall within the 95% CI, the null hypothesis can be rejected.

A N S W E R :
D

6. Which of the following is/are true about hypothesis testing?

A. Type I error is the probability of concluding that no difference exists when in fact it does.

B. Type II error is the probability of concluding that a difference exists when it does not.

C. The Bonferroni adjustment ensures that significant differences are detected during multiple comparisons.

D. Power is influenced by alpha, sample size, and effect size.

Ref.: 1, 3

COMMENTS: Type I error (alpha) is the probability of falsely rejecting the null hypothesis, or saying there is a difference between groups when there actually is not. The alpha level is set a priori, or before a study is conducted. Alpha is typically set at 0.01 or 0.05 for clinical, behavioral, and basic science research. Type I error increases in proportion to the number of tests performed on the same data set. When performing multiple group comparisons, the **Bonferroni adjustment** can be used to ensure that alpha is maintained at the a priori, fixed level.

Type II error (beta) is the probability of failing to reject the null hypothesis when it is in fact false or, in other words, concluding that a difference exists when it does not. Power is the probability of detecting a significant difference when it exists. The **power** of a test is equal to one minus beta. Power is the confidence that one's results are accurate.

Statistical tests are chosen to minimize type I error and type II errors and to maximize power. However, any action to minimize one tends to increase the other. In practice, alpha is set at a specified level and power is maximized by increasing the sample size or the effect size (the relative strength of a treatment). Optimally, power calculations are performed before initiating a study to determine the sample size required to achieve an acceptable level of power (0.80) or to determine the power for a specific sample size.

A N S W E R :
C, D

7. Match each data type with the variable it best describes.

A. Ordinal	a. Systemic blood pressure
B. Ratio	b. Gender
C. Nominal	c. USMLE Step I score
D. Interval	d. A 7-point pain scale

Ref.: 1, 3

COMMENTS: Variables in a study can yield four types of data: nominal, ordinal, interval, and ratio. **Nominal data** are classified into groups or named categories without any specific order (e.g. medicine, surgery, and pediatrics). **Ordinal data** are ordered (small, medium, and large), but the distance between values cannot be considered equal. Calculating arithmetic means for ordinal data is not meaningful. **Interval data** are on an ordered scale with equal distance between values but an arbitrary zero point (e.g., an IQ test). Calculations of arithmetic means and standard deviations can be performed on interval data. **Ratio data** have an ordered scale with equal intervals between values and a meaningful zero point (e.g., the Celsius temperature scale).

Specific methods of statistical inference are chosen based on the nature of the data to be compared. Flowcharts can be constructed to outline the decision process for choosing the appropriate statistical test. **Parametric methods** are used for interval and ratio data. Parametric methods are based on the parameters of the normal distribution, such as means and variances. The independent sample t test and the Analysis of Variance test (ANOVA) are parametric methods commonly used to compare group means.
• **Nonparametric methods** are used when there is no underlying distribution to describe the data, which is typical of nominal and ordinal data types. Chi-square, Wilcoxon rank sum, and Kruskall-Wallis test statistics are nonparametric methods typically used with ordinal data.

ANSWER:
A-d; B-a; C-b; D-c

8. Which of the following is/are true about regression and correlation?

A. The dependent variable is used to predict the independent variable.

B. Multiple regression generally refers to more than one outcome variable.

C. In logistic regression, the outcome variable is categorical.

D. Two variables are uncorrelated if they have a negative correlation coefficient.

Ref.: 1

COMMENTS: Regression methods are statistical models used to predict the value of a dependent variable from one or more independent variables. • **Multiple regression** generally refers to models with more than one independent variable. • In **linear regression** the outcome variable is normally distributed, whereas in **logistic regression** the outcome variable is dichotomous. • Often, instead of predicting one variable or another, we wish to determine if there is a relationship between two variables. A **correlation coefficient** quantifies the relationship between two variables. • A positive **correlation coefficient** means that, as one variable increases, the other variable increases. A negative correlation means that, as one variable increases, the other variable decreases.

ANSWER:
C

For Questions 9 through 11, please use the table on this page. The table represents the results of performing the same diagnostic test for the same diagnosis in two different patient populations.

Diagnostic Test	Disease +	Disease −	Total
Population 1	(True +) = 90	(False +) = 90	180
Test +	(False −) = 10	(True −) = 810	820
Test −	100	900	1000
Total			
Population 2	(True +) = 9	(False +) = 99	108
Test +	(False −) = 1	(True −) = 891	892
Test −	10	990	1000
Total			

9. For each population, calculate the prevalence of disease in percentages and the relative risk of disease in those who test positive (versus those who test negative).

A. Prevalence of disease in population 1   a. 81
B. Prevalence of disease in population 2   b. 1
C. Odds ratio in population 1   c. 89.1
D. Odds ratio in population 2   d. 10

Ref.: 2

COMMENTS: **Prevalence** is the number of patients in a sample who currently have disease divided by the total number of patients sampled. The prevalence is calculated from the column totals only. • It is important to distinguish **incidence** from prevalence. Often, in epidemiologic studies, we wish to determine the number of new cases of a disease that occur during a specified time period (incidence). When we do this, we must be certain not to count all diagnosed cases but only those newly diagnosed during the study period. We can then calculate the relative risk of disease: the incidence in one population divided by the incidence in another population. • If incidence cannot be determined, we can still compare risk of disease in two populations using the **odds ratio** (the odds of disease in the exposed divided by the odds of disease in the nonexposed). • In the table, the incidence of disease cannot be directly calculated, but the relative risk of disease (in those who test positive versus those who test negative) is approximated using the odds ratio TP × TN/FP × FN.

ANSWER:
A-d; B-b; C-a; D-a

10. What are the sensitivity and specificity of the test in the table?

A. Sensitivity   a. 82%
B. Specificity   b. 18%
                          c. 90%
                          d. 10.8%
                          e. 89.2%

Ref.: 2

COMMENTS: Sensitivity and specificity are characteristics of tests that are independent of the population tested. **Sensitivity** is defined as the number of patients with disease who also test positive divided by the total number with disease in the sample TP/(TP + FN). **Specificity** is defined as the number of patients without disease who also test negative divided by the total number without disease in the sample TN/(TN + FP). Sensitivity is a measure of the test's ability to detect the disease, whereas specificity is a measure of the test's ability to detect the absence of disease. Recall that the prevalence of disease in these two populations is different, but the sensitivity and specificity of the test do not change across the populations tested. For this test, the sensitivity happens to be equal to the specificity (90%). In general, as one improves either the sensitivity or the specificity of a test, the other is degraded.

ANSWER:
A-c; B-c

---

11. What are the positive predictive value (PPV) and negative predictive value (NPV) of the test for each population?

A. PPV for population 1   a. 99.9%
B. NPV for population 1   b. 50%
C. PPV for population 2   c. 99%
D. NPV for population 2   d. 8%

Ref.: 2

COMMENTS: PPV and NPV are characteristics of tests that are dependent on the prevalence of disease in the population tested. **PPV** is defined as the number of patients who test positive who also have the disease divided by the total number who test positive in the sample: TP/(TP + FP). **NPV** is defined as the number of patients who test negative who also do not have the disease divided by the total number who test negative in the sample: TN/(TN + FN). PPV is a measure of the test's ability to predict the presence of disease, whereas NPV is a measure of the test's ability to predict the absence of disease. Note that the PPV and NPV can change dramatically as the prevalence of disease in a population changes. In this example, as the prevalence changes from 10 to 1%, the PPV falls from 50 to 8%. Thus, this may be a good screening test for the first population but a poor screening test for the second. In fact, in the second population, most positive tests are falsely positive. This is often the case when testing low-prevalence populations (even with a highly sensitive and specific test). It is therefore important to use tests selectively for a specific purpose. For example, the above-mentioned test may be extremely useful for the second population to be confident that a patient is not a rare individual with the disease (high NPV).

ANSWER:
A-b; B-c; C-d; D-a

---

12. Which of the following is/are true of the characteristics of screening tests?

A. The population to be screened should have a high prevalence of preclinical disease.

B. Treatment before the development of clinical disease must reduce cause-specific morbidity and mortality more than treatment does after clinical manifestations of disease.

C. Increasing the specificity of the test often increases the PPV.

D. Determining feasibility is as important as efficacy when determining the effectiveness of a screening program.

Ref.: 2

COMMENTS: The PPV of a screening test improves if the test is applied to a population with a high prevalence of disease. In addition, measures taken to improve the specificity in a given population tend to increase the PPV because, as the number of negative test results increase, a positive test result is more likely in a disease-positive patient. Since the measures taken to improve specificity tend to decrease sensitivity, there is always a trade-off. Obviously, treatment is useful only when it diminishes morbidity and mortality rates. Furthermore, successful screening requires

that early treatment based on screening test results improves morbidity and mortality rates more than does treatment initiated later, when disease is clinically detected. Bias in measurement of survival based on earlier detection of disease (lead-time bias) must also be accounted for. Screening tests are of no value if they are not feasible. Considerations of feasibility include acceptability to the population screened, cost-effectiveness, and case yield.

ANSWER:
A, B, C, D

---

13. Which type of validity is threatened in each of the following scenarios?

A. Internal validity   a. Study findings were due to chance.
B. External validity   b. A high percentage of patients do not complete a study.
    c. A study yields findings that are implausible.
    d. Unbeknownst to the investigators, a group of patients enrolled in their postoperative quality-of-life study begin an exercise program.
    e. A sample of urban, East Coast medical students is selected for a study of national medical student debt.

Ref.: 2

COMMENTS: Good **internal validity** is defined by a statistical association that is not due to chance, confounding by other causal factors, or bias introduced in the study design. In other words, a planned intervention is the actual cause of a study's outcome. A **confounding factor** is defined as an effect that independently causes the outcome and that is unevenly distributed among patients with and without the exposure risk. **Bias** enters when there is a methodologic difference in the handling of exposed and unexposed populations and, as such, poses a threat to internal validity. For example, bias occurs when participants are enrolled by different criteria (selection bias), when there is participant attrition, when noncomparable information is collected from the various groups (observational bias), or when inaccuracies are introduced during data collection (classification bias).

The **external validity** of a clinical study is the degree to which its findings can be generalized to other patients in other settings. Good external validity is also required to postulate a cause-and-effect relationship. A study is considered to have good external validity if the association demonstrated is **biologically credible** (i.e., consistent with other observations and theories) and is **generalizable** to clinically relevant populations beyond the narrow group selected for study. Selecting the appropriate population for study can be challenging and often requires balancing internal validity against external validity.

ANSWER:
A-a,b,d; B-c,e

---

14. Match the observational study designs with their relevant advantages.

A. Case-control   a. Quick and inexpensive
B. Cohort   b. Valuable when the exposure is rare
    c. Useful when the disease has a long latent period
    d. Optimal for evaluating rare diseases

e. Can demonstrate temporal relationships and multiple effects of an exposure
f. Minimizes bias
g. Allows direct measurement of incidence

Ref.: 2

COMMENTS: When conducted properly, observational studies can provide conclusions as compelling as those drawn from interventional studies (randomized, controlled trials). In **case-control studies**, patients with the disease of interest are selected from a population and compared with representative nondiseased individuals selected from the same population. There are several advantages of case-control design. They are generally quick and inexpensive. Case-control studies are useful when there is a long latent period between exposure and disease or the disease is rare. Multiple causes of a single disease can be studied with a case-control design. There are also several disadvantages of case-control studies. They are inefficient when the exposure is rare. In addition, the incidence of disease or the relative risk cannot be directly calculated (the odds ratio must be used instead). Temporal relationships can be difficult to measure in case-control studies, and case-control design is prone to bias.

In **cohort studies**, a population is selected and followed for the development of exposures and disease over time. Advantages of using a cohort study design include that (1) it is valuable when exposure is rare, (2) it can examine multiple effects of an exposure, (3) it can demonstrate temporal relationships, (4) when performed prospectively, bias is minimized, and (5) it allows for direct measure of incidence and relative risk. Disadvantages include greater expense, inefficiency for studying rare diseases, and the need for complete follow-up and detailed record keeping.

ANSWER:
A-a,c,d; B-b,e,f,g

15. Which of the following is/are true with regard to interventional studies (randomized, controlled trials)?

A. Randomization and large sample size generally eliminate the effects of confounding variables.

B. Randomization serves to eliminate observational bias.

C. The effects of poor compliance with therapy can be eliminated with an "intention-to-treat" design.

D. High costs can make interventional studies impractical.

Ref.: 2

COMMENTS: Interventional studies that are designed well and conducted properly can generate a level of validity greater than that of observational studies. Interventional studies include an adequate sample of a study population, and subjects are randomly assigned to treatment or control conditions. Proper randomization not only equalizes the prevalence of known confounding factors in each group, it also makes the prevalence of unknown factors equal. In a double-blind study, both the investigator and the patient are unaware of the assignment to the intervention or control conditions. Double-blind designs serve to eliminate observation bias. The "intention-to-treat" research design requires that a patient be assigned to the treatment group for the duration of a study, whether or not treatment can be completed. This method can enhance the generalizability of a study.

There are, however, unique problems when performing controlled trials. Subjects' poor compliance with therapy can bias study results toward the null hypothesis. This problem can be avoided by selecting a population that is known to be compliant. The ethical considerations of randomizing a potentially effective therapy to a treatment group are significant for researchers considering an interventional study design. Feasibility issues, such as high cost and time-intensive data collection, can make interventional studies impractical. In addition, the placebo effect—the phenomenon by which the perception of receiving a therapy tends to improve an individual's assessment of well-being—can dramatically alter results.

ANSWER:
A, D

16. Which of the following is/are true with regard to meta-analysis?

A. Meta-analysis techniques can be used to answer a research question about treatment efficacy.

B. Meta-analysis methods can eliminate observational or selection bias.

C. Many of the statistical techniques used in meta-analysis are unique to meta-analysis.

D. The choice to use a fixed-effect or a random-effect model is moderated by the nature of the research question.

Ref.: 2

COMMENTS: Meta-analysis is a statistical technique used to synthesize the literature on a particular topic. A meta-analysis is essentially a study of a group of studies and is conducted to increase the power of an investigation or to resolve inconsistencies among study results. Meta-analysis methods can not control for bias in the original studies. The steps of a meta-analysis are to (1) formulate a research question, (2) perform a literature search, (3) establish selection criteria for including studies in the meta-analysis, (4) extract and organize data, and (5) perform statistical analysis on extracted data according to a selected model. Statistical analyses conducted as part of a meta-analysis typically include calculations of effect size and confidence intervals, as well as homogeneity tests.

Two models of meta-analysis include the fixed-effects model and the random-effects model. The fixed-effects model can be used to answer questions about whether a treatment, on average, produces a particular effect. A fixed-effects model considers only within-study variation. Random-effects models are used to answer questions about whether a treatment produces a certain result. A random-effects model is computationally more intense because it considers both between- and within-study variation.

ANSWER:
A, D

17. Which of the following statements regarding research on human subjects is/are true?

A. Informed consent procedures are designed to protect human subjects who are considering study participation.

B. Surgical procedures, blood draws, and quality-of-life surveys are examples of research interventions.

C. Vulnerable populations include prisoners, children, pregnant women, fetuses, and persons with disabilities.

D. Research utilizing existing data is not subject to review by an institutional review board (IRB).

Ref.: 4

COMMENTS: The conduct of responsible and ethical research on human subjects begins with an appreciation of federal regulations and definitions relevant to research. **Research** is defined as a systematic investigation, including research development, testing, and evaluation designed to develop or contribute to generalizable knowledge. • Research **intervention** includes both physical procedures by which data are gathered (e.g., venipuncture) and manipulations of the subject or the subject's environment that are performed for research purposes. • **Informed consent** procedures are designed to enable persons to voluntarily decide whether to participate as a research subject. • **Minimal risk** means that the probability and magnitude of harm or discomfort anticipated in the research are not greater in and of themselves than those ordinarily encountered in daily life or during the performance of routine physical or psychological examinations or tests. • **Vulnerable populations** have been defined by federal regulation as pregnant women, fetuses, prisoners, children, and persons with disabilities.

Federal regulations on research on human subjects require review of research protocols by a recognized IRB. Research may qualify for exemption from *continuing* review if it involves the collection or study of existing data, documents, records, pathologic specimens, or diagnostic specimens if these sources are publicly available or if the information is recorded by the investigator in such a manner that subjects cannot be identified directly or through identifiers linked to the subjects. An IRB must designate a study to be exempt from continuing review. Therefore, all research studies of human subjects, including studies of existing data, must be submitted to an IRB for review.

ANSWER:
A, B, C

REFERENCES

1. Rosner B: *Fundamentals of Biostatistics*, 5th ed. Wadsworth Publishing, Belmont, CA, 2000.
2. Hennekens CH, Buring JE: *Epidemiology in Medicine*. Little, Brown, Boston, 1987.
3. Norman G, Streiner D: *Biostatistics: The Bare Essentials*. BC Decker, Hamilton, Ontario, Canada, 1998.
4. Retrieved May 30, 2006 from U.S. Department of Health and Human Services, Office for Human Research Protections, <http://www.hhs.gov/ohrp/>